Veterinary Computed Tomography

VETERINARY COMPUTED TOMOGRAPHY

Edited by

Tobias Schwarz
MA Dr. med. vet. DVR DipECVDI DACVR MRCVS
Royal (Dick) School of Veterinary Studies
The University of Edinburgh
Roslin, Scotland
UK

Jimmy Saunders
Dr. med. vet. PhD CertVR DipECVDI
Faculty of Veterinary Medicine
Ghent University
Merelbeke
Belgium

WILEY-BLACKWELL
A John Wiley & Sons, Ltd., Publication

This edition first published 2011 by John Wiley & Sons Ltd

Wiley-Blackwell is an imprint of John Wiley & Sons, formed by the merger of Wiley's global Scientific, Technical and Medical business with Blackwell Publishing.

Registered office: John Wiley & Sons Ltd, The Atrium, Southern Gate, Chichester, West Sussex, PO19 8SQ, UK

Editorial offices: 9600 Garsington Road, Oxford, OX4 2DQ, UK
The Atrium, Southern Gate, Chichester, West Sussex, PO19 8SQ, UK
2121 State Avenue, Ames, Iowa 50014-8300, USA

For details of our global editorial offices, for customer services and for information about how to apply for permission to reuse the copyright material in this book please see our website at www.wiley.com/wiley-blackwell.

Library of Congress Cataloging-in-Publication Data

Veterinary computed tomography / edited by Tobias Schwarz, Jimmy Saunders.
p. ; cm.
Includes bibliographical references and index.
ISBN 978-0-8138-1747-7 (hardcover : alk. paper) 1. Veterinary tomography.
2. Radiography, Medical—Digital techniques. I. Schwarz, Tobias. II. Saunders, Jimmy, 1965-
[DNLM: 1. Tomography, X-Ray Computed—veterinary—Practice Guideline. SF 757.8]
SF757.8.V48 2011
636.089'60757–dc22

2010051093

A catalogue record for this book is available from the British Library.

This book is published in the following electronic formats: ePDF 9780470960127; ePub 9780470960134; Mobi 9780470960141

Set in 10/12.5 pt Palatino by Toppan Best-set Premedia Limited

1 2011

Contents

Contributors

William H. Chess Adams, BS DVM DACVR DACVR-RO
School of Veterinary Medicine
University of Wisconsin-Madison
Madison
Wisconsin
USA

Hendrik-Jan Bergman, DVM DipECAR certISELP
Lingehoeve Diergeneeskunde Equine Referral Hospital
Lienden
The Netherlands

Susanne Boroffka, MA Dr. med. vet. PhD DipECVDI
University Clinic for Companion Animals
Utrecht University
The Netherlands

Ana V. Cáceres, BS DVM DACVR
University of Pennsylvania
School of Veterinary Medicine
Philadelphia
Pennsylvania
USA

Laurent Couturier, Dr Med Vet DipECVDI, AZURVET
Referral Center in Diagnostic Imaging and Neurology
Cagnes sur Mer
France

Marc-André d'Anjou, DMV DACVR
Université de Montréal
Saint-Hyacinthe
Québec
Canada

Sophie Dennison, BVM&S DACVR MRCVS
San Francisco
California
USA

Randi Drees, Dr. med. vet. DipECVDI DACVR
School of Veterinary Medicine
University of Wisconsin-Madison
Madison
Wisconsin
USA

Lisa J. Forrest, VMD DACVR DACVR-RO
School of Veterinary Medicine
University of Wisconsin-Madison
Madison
Wisconsin
USA

Ingrid Gielen, MSc Dr Med Vet PhD
Faculty of Veterinary Medicine
Ghent University
Merelbeke
Belgium

Michaela Gumpenberger, Dr. med. vet.
Clinic of Diagnostic Imaging
University of Veterinary Medicine
Vienna
Austria

Silke Hecht, Dr. med. vet. DipECVDI DACVR
University of Tennessee
College of Veterinary Medicine
Knoxville
Tennessee
USA

Victoria Johnson, BVSc DVR DipECVDI MRCVS
Vet CT Specialists Ltd
Cambridge
UK

Ingmar Kiefer, Dr. med. vet.
Department of Small Animal Medicine
Veterinary Faculty
University of Leipzig
Germany

Jennifer Kinns, BSc VetMB DipECVDI DACVR MRCVS
VDIC-Idexx
Stirling
UK

Robert Kirberger, BVSc MMedVet(Rad) DipECVDI
Faculty of Veterinary Science
University of Pretoria
Onderstepoort
South Africa

Marcel Kovalik, Dr. Med. Vet. PhD MRCVS
Royal (Dick) School of Veterinary Studies
The University of Edinburgh
Roslin
UK

Eberhard Ludewig, Dr. med. vet. DipECVDI
Department of Small Animal Medicine
Veterinary Faculty
University of Leipzig
Germany

Wilfried Mai, MS Dr. Med. Vet. PhD DipECVDI DACVR
University of Pennsylvania
School of Veterinary Medicine
Philadelphia
Pennsylvania
USA

Robert Malinowski, MA DVM
College of Veterinary Medicine
Michigan State University
East Lansing
Michigan
USA

Fintan McEvoy, MVB PhD DVR DipECVDI
Faculty of Life Sciences
University of Copenhagen
Copenhagen
Denmark

Federica Morandi, MS Dr. Med. Vet. DipECVDI, DACVR
College of Veterinary Medicine
The University of Tennessee
Knoxville
Tennessee
USA

Alastair Nelson, MA VetMB CertVR CertESM MRCVS†
Rainbow Equine Clinic
Old Malton
North Yorkshire
UK

Robert O'Brien, MS DVM DACVR
Department of Veterinary Clinical Medicine
University of Illinois
Urbana
Illinois
USA

Stefanie Ohlerth, Dr. med. vet. habil. DipECVDI
Division of Diagnostic Imaging
Vetsuisse Faculty
University of Zürich
Zürich
Switzerland

Michail Patsikas, MD DVM PhD DipECVDI
School of Veterinary Medicine
Aristotle University of Thessaloniki
Thessaloniki
Makedonia
Greece

Audrey Petite, Dr. med. vet. DVDI DipECVDI MRCVS
Pixelvet
Kent
UK

Rachel Pollard, DVM PhD DACVR
University of California Davis
School of Veterinary Medicine
Davis
California
USA

Sarah Puchalski, BSc DVM DACVR
School of Veterinary Medicine
University of California Davis
Davis
California
USA

Victor Rendano Jr., MSc VMD DACVR DACVR-RO
Veterinary Multi-Imaging Pllc
Lansing
New York
USA

Federica Rossi, Dr. med. vet. SRV DipECVDI
Clinica Veterinaria dell'Orologio
Sasso Marconi
Bologna
Italy

Valerie Samii, DVM DACVR
College of Veterinary Medicine
The Ohio State University
Columbus
Ohio
USA

Jimmy Saunders, Dr. med. vet. PhD CertVR DipECVDI
Faculty of Veterinary Medicine
Ghent University
Merelbeke
Belgium

Ryan M. Schultz, DVM DACVR
Seattle Veterinary Specialists
Kirkland
Washington
USA

Tobias Schwarz, MA Dr. med. vet. DVR DipECVDI DACVR MRCVS
Royal (Dick) School of Veterinary Studies
The University of Edinburgh
Roslin
UK

Gabriela Seiler, Dr. med. vet. DipECVDI DACVR
College of Veterinary Medicine
North Carolina State University
Raleigh
North Carolina
USA

Olivier Taeymans, DVM PhD DipECVDI
Cummings School of Veterinary Medicine
Tufts University
North Grafton
Massachusetts
USA

Russ Tucker, DVM DACVR
Veterinary Clinical Sciences
College of Veterinary Medicine
Washington State University
Pullman
Washington
USA

Henri van Bree, DVM PhD DipECVS DipECVDI
Faculty of Veterinary Medicine
Ghent University
Merelbeke
Belgium

Katrien Vanderperren, DVM PhD
Faculty of Veterinary Medicine
Ghent University
Merelbeke
Belgium

Massimo Vignoli, Dr. med. vet. PhD SRV DipECVDI
Clinica Veterinaria dell'Orologio
Sasso Marconi
Bologna
Italy

Zoe Windley, BVetMed Hons MRCVS
Royal Veterinary College
North Mymms
UK

Erik R. Wisner, DVM DACVR
School of Veterinary Medicine
University of California Davis
Davis
California
USA

Allison Zwingenberger, DVM MAS DipECVDI DACVR
School of Veterinary Medicine
University of California Davis
Davis
California
USA

Preface

Since its development in the 1970s computed tomography (CT) has undergone continuous technological improvement and refinement, contributing greatly to the advancements in clinical medicine. As radiography in the 1890s, CT was initially developed by physicists and engineers but was very quickly adapted to the needs of clinical medicine. The first scanners offered an amazing new way to indirectly visualize the brain and other organs, something that had previously been impossible. Veterinary CT was introduced in the late 1980s, initially by scanning animal patients in human medical institutions. The installation of a CT scanner at the Centre Radiothérapie-Scanner on the campus of the École Nationale Vétérinaire d'Alfort in Paris in 1989 perhaps marks the beginning of dedicated *veterinary* CT. At first it was primarily used for imaging of the head in dogs and cats with neurological or nasal diseases. The development of slip ring technology, which allowed helical scanning, and the design of better and smaller detectors, opened up new avenues for veterinary use, including thoracic imaging and high-definition scanning of lungs and bone. With the advancement of multi-detector-row technology a new chapter begins for veterinary CT. Long body parts can be scanned within a couple of seconds in amazing detail and with minimal image artifacts. For large domestic animals, small mammals, birds, reptiles, and even wildlife and zoo animals, CT enables us to obtain a quick and accurate diagnosis of many disorders. Computed tomography is now widely used in veterinary practice, it is comparable with or superior to other imaging modalities for many disorders, and has immense potential as a rapid and efficient diagnostic tool for a wide range of indications.

Several atlases (Assheuer and Sager, 1997; Davies *et al.*, 1987; Mihaljević *et al.*, 2009) and articles have been published depicting the computed tomographic anatomy of the dog and selected other species. The reader is referred to these for detailed anatomic information. A large body of scientific publications describing the computed tomographic features of diseases in animals has also been published to date. This book closes a gap as the first comprehensive textbook of CT, including technological concepts, imaging protocols and computed tomographic disease features for most species treated in veterinary practice. We have been fortunate enough to attract more than forty veterinary specialists from 13 different countries to provide state-of-the-art expertise on the wide spectrum of veterinary computed tomography.

We wish you pleasant reading and hope that we can provide some answers for you and stimulate your curiosity for veterinary CT.

Tobias Schwarz & Jimmy Saunders
Edinburgh & Ghent, January 2011

References

Assheuer J and Sager M (1997) *MRI and CT atlas of the dog*. Berlin: Blackwell Science.

Davies AS, Garden KL, Young MJ and Reid CSW (1987) *An atlas of X-ray tomographic anatomy of the sheep*. DSIR Bulletin No 243. Wellington, New Zealand: Department of Scientific and Industrial Research.

Mihaljević M, Kramer M and Gomerčić H (2009) *CT und MRT atlas. Transversalanatomie des Hundes*. Stuttgart: Parey.

Acknowledgements

This book represents the collaborative effort of more than 40 authors to whom we are extremely grateful. The high quality of their contributions and their timely manuscript submissions deserve a special thank you. We are also indebted to Marcel Kovalik for providing the wonderful illustrations, often at very short notice. We would like to thank Edouard Cauvin for help in translation of Chapter 21 and all other individuals who kindly contributed images to this textbook as acknowledged in the figure legends.

This textbook would not have been possible without the hard work and endless patience of the publishing team at Wiley-Blackwell, in particular Justinia Wood and Nancy Turner whose effort and dedication are greatly appreciated.

Our colleagues have assisted us a great deal in the clinics while we were working on this textbook and we would like to express our gratitude in this regard to Maya Esmans, Carolina Urraca, Tiziana Liuti, Mairi Frame, Elizabeth Munro, Pascaline Pey, Elke Van der Vekens, Anais Combes, Els Raes, Yseult Baeumlin, Hendrik Haers, Stijn Hauspie and others, such as Simon Kidd and David Williamson, who helped us with difficult technical issues.

We are particularly appreciative of the support we received from our families throughout this project and would like to thank our wives Aaike and Deborah for their patience and understanding. Also Aurélie, Deborah, Virginie, Alice, Ingrid and Misha receive our thanks for understanding why we could spend so little time with them. We are all happy that this project has now come to a conclusion.

This book is a tribute to our friend, colleague and co-author Alastair Nelson, a true pioneer in equine computed tomography, whose untimely death meant a great loss to all of us.

A final mention goes to all animals who patiently sat, stood or laid down for their CT examinations and whose images provide the core of this book.

Tobias Schwarz & Jimmy Saunders
Edinburgh & Ghent, January 2011

CHAPTER ONE

CT Physics and Instrumentation – Mechanical Design

Jimmy Saunders and Stefanie Ohlerth

Basic CT Unit Anatomy

A computed tomography (CT) unit consists of a gantry, a patient table, hardware equipment, an operator console and optionally additional workstations.

The gantry is a doughnut-shaped ring containing the X-ray tube, the detector array and associated equipment. The central hole in the gantry accommodates the patient on a sliding table. The X-ray tube rotates around a slice of patient anatomy. This slice represents the X-Y plane, with the X-axis being horizontal and the Y-axis vertical. The isocenter of the gantry is the central point of this plane. The third dimension is represented by the Z-axis, which is along the orientation of the patient table. The patient bed is a sliding tray on a fixed table with an adjustable height and a defined capacity of forward motion. The operator console is located in another room or behind radioprotective screening, and allows operation of the CT units. Additional workstations can be used to review processed image data, but usually not raw data processing.

X-Ray Tube

Basic anatomy of the X-ray tube

An X-ray tube is a vacuum tube that produces X-rays. It is composed of a cathode (filament) and an anode (target). The cathode cup is negatively charged and incorporates a wound tungsten filament that emits electrons when heated. The anode consists of a disk of tungsten or a tungsten alloy with an annular target, called the focal track, close to the edge. The anode disk is supported on a long stem that is supported by ball bearings within the tube. The anode can be rotated by electromagnetic induction from a series of stator windings outside the evacuated tube.

The X-ray tube is enclosed in a housing unit filled with insulating oil. This oil provides electric shielding from the tube voltage, X-ray protection and transmits heat generated in the housing unit to the unit's surface. The exterior of the housing unit is cooled with a fan, and insulating oil is cooled by passing it through a heat exchanger.

Low-power applications use stationary anode tubes, while for most mid-range and high-performance applications there is a need to utilize rotating anode tubes.

Basic physiology of the X-ray tube

A current of a few amperes (4–8 A) heats the tungsten filament that releases electrons (thermoionic emission) in the vacuum. A high-voltage power source ('tube voltage') ranging from 30 to 150 kilovolts (kV) is connected across cathode and anode to accelerate the electrons producing an electron flow ('tube current'). These electrons collide with the anode material and about 1% of their kinetic energy is converted into X-rays, usually perpendicular to the path of the electron beam. The remainder of energy is converted into heat, causing the

Veterinary Computed Tomography, First Edition. Edited by Tobias Schwarz, Jimmy Saunders.

X-ray tube to warm up during operation. The temperature of the focal track can increase quickly to 1000–1500°C. Heat diffuses by conduction throughout the anode body and by thermal radiation (infrared radiation) to the tube housing (80%). Heat is removed from the tube housing by convection to the surrounding atmosphere.

Many X-ray systems, including CT, have built-in safety features that will not allow the equipment to be operated in 'overheated' conditions. The temperature cannot be measured directly in the focal track. It has to be evaluated based on indirect values that characterize the ability of the anode to store the heat generated during the X-ray emission, such as the anode heat capacity, the anode dissipation/cooling rate or the tube dissipation.

Specificities for CT

Since the invention of CT, its demands regarding the X-ray source never ceased to increase and are largely superior to those of radiography. These specific requirements can be summarized with higher scan power, shorter rotation times (maximum rotation speed), shorter cool-down times and smaller focal spots without compromise on resolution and image quality. In older CTs, the generator capacities and anode disk's heat storage capacities were insufficient and long time interruptions were needed.

Scan power: typical values for the maximum power are 20/40–100 kW with the high voltage range ranging from 80 to 150 kV.

Focal spots: X-ray tubes use typical focal spot sizes of 0.5–1.2 mm. Specific innovations for CT are the 'flying focus' allowing for control of the focus position on the anode during the scan or the electromagnetic control of the electron beam, which allows switching of the focal spot position both in the fan and in the Z-direction, providing overlapping sampling.

Rotation speed: the traditional glass tube technology is not adequate in terms of required precision and stability to sustain the very high rotation speed, up to 10 500 rotation/min, of high-performance tubes. Despite its higher thermic dissipation and lower cost, glass has been replaced by the metal ceramic technology, which is more precise and better able to sustain the constraints related to the rotation speed.

Cool-down time: different approaches can be used on their own or in combination to shorten the cool-down times and improve the heat storage capacities of CT.

- The '***brute force approach***' was the main way used for three decades. This approach consists of an increase in the thermal capacity of the anode by increasing its diameter and mass. This system has obvious limitations, as it still uses radiative cooling.
- The '***material approach***' is based on a slow evolution in the materials used for the anode.

  Direct:
  - Use of circular grooves in the anode support to increase the contact and improve cooling.
  - Use of special liquid metal vacuum bearings that allow faster anode rotation.
  - Focal track made of a mixture of rhenium and tungsten. Rhenium has a higher linear expansibility than tungsten and slows the rate at which anode crazing occurs.
  - Anode 'compound'/increased thermal capacities: use of molybdenum or graphite with tungsten in the anode disk. Molybdenum has twice the specific heat capacity and half the density of tungsten. Graphite has an even higher specific heat capacity and a quarter of the density of molybdenum. It increases thermal capacity.
  - Replacement of the ball bearings by a liquid metal (gallium) that allows the evacuation of heat by conduction.

  Indirect:
  - Multiple detectors allow reduction of the heat produced via reduced scan duration by a factor approximately equivalent to the number of rows. Manufacturers developed systems with up to 1000 rows.
- The '***paradigm shift***' corresponds to innovations in X-ray tubes.

In 2000, Siemens developed the Straton tube, also called the rotating envelope tube, for its high-tech scanner. This tube uses direct convective cooling, exclusively of the anode, with a cooling oil stream at the anode's back surface. As a result, the cooling rate is vastly increased to 4.8 MHU/min, eliminating the need for large heat storage capacities of the anode disk and reducing waiting times due to anode cooling in the clinical workflow.

This lighter tube also presents a solution for the acceleration/pressure centrifuge high G (above 20 G).

Another innovation on the X-ray tube in relation to CT is the dual-source CT (two tubes, two detector fans); the main advantage of this architecture is its improved temporal resolution. In today's CT scanners, the gantry rotation time is reduced to about 0.35 s and it is mechanically challenging to reduce that time even further, which justifies the renewed interest in multi-source architectures.

Collimators and Filtration

CT systems feature various collimators, filters and shielding designs, which provide filtration of the X-ray spectra, definition of the measured slices, guarding detectors against scattered radiation and general radiation protection. These vary from scan to scan but always offer the same functions.

Collimation

Collimation in CT serves to ensure good image quality and to reduce unnecessary radiation doses for the patient.

Collimators are present between the X-ray source and the patient (tube or pre-patient collimators) and between the patient and the detectors (detector or post-patient collimators).

The tube collimator is used to shape the X-ray fan beam before it penetrates the patient (restrict the X-ray flux applied to a narrow region defines the shape of the X-ray beam). It consists of a set of collimator blades made of highly absorbing materials such as tungsten or molybdenum. The opening of these blades is adjusted according to the selected slice width and the size and position of the focal spot. It defines slice thickness for single-slice CT. Tube collimators define the dose profile according to the required slice thickness. Post-patient collimators improve the slice sensitivity profile by giving a more rectangular shape. Table 1.1 shows the features of CT collimators.

Filtration

The X-ray photons emitted by the X-ray tube exhibit a wide spectrum. The soft, low-energy X-rays, which contribute strongly to the patient dose and scatter radiation but less to the detected signal, should be removed. To achieve this goal, most CT manufacturers use X-ray filters.

The inherent filtration of the X-ray-tube, typically 3 mm aluminium equivalent thickness, is the first filter. In addition, flat or shaped filters can be used. Flat filters, made of copper or aluminium, are placed between the X-ray source and the patient. They modify the X-ray spectrum uniformly across the entire field of view. Because the cross-section of a patient is mostly oval-shaped, some manufacturers use shaped (or bow-tie) filters. These filters have an increased thickness from center to periphery, allowing them to attenuate radiation hardly at all in the center but strongly in the periphery. They are made from a material with a low atomic number and high density, such as Teflon.

In some machines comb-shaped collimators close to the detector array are used to decrease the effective detector element width and thus increase the achievable geometrical resolution.

Detector Systems

The detector is the system for quantitative recoring of the incident ionizing radiation. It acts in two steps.

Table 1.1
CT collimator features.

Collimator type	Tube side – detector side	Location	Fixed/ adjustable	Aim
Pre patient	Tube	Very close to the focus (tube housing)	Fixed	– To reduce the generated radiation roughly to the maximally anticipated beam for the given detector and geometry – Blocks 99% of the photons emitted by the tube
Pre patient	Tube		Fixed	– To exactly define the maximum permitted beam
Pre patient	Tube	As far as possible from the focus (close to gantry housing)	Adjustable	– Variable collimation to the desired slice width or multiple slice widths – To minimize penumbra caused by finite focus size
Post patient	Detector		Fixed	– To minimize signal contributions from scattered radiation – Width = maximal collimation
Post patient	Detector* (optional)	Between the single detector elements	Adjustable	– To minimize signal contributions from scattered radiation

*Can only be implemented in scanners with a rotating detector.

1. The reception of the incident X-ray photon via X-ray-sensitive detector elements with a specific geometrical configuration.
2. The transformation of the X-ray photon into a corresponding electrical signal, that is then amplified and converted from an analog to a digital form (via analog-to-digital converters). This step is relatively easily specified and submitted to few fluctuations.

There are two detector types.

- Ionization chambers, mostly filled with the noble gas xenon under high pressure. Gas detectors have become obsolete due to their limited detection efficiency and the difficulty in manufacturing them for multi-row design.
- Scintillation detectors, in the form of crystals such as cesium iodide or cadmium tungstate, and ceramic materials such as gadolinium oxysulfide. These detectors are now predominantly used mainly because of their short decay time, which is an essential factor in subsecond scanning times since. Ultra-fast ceramic (gadolinium oxysulfide based) have superior characteristics in this area, making them the best choice for spatial resolution and image quality.

The alternative detector concept is the flat-panel technology. Potential advantages are the possibility to scan with wider cone angles without the need to develop detectors with 1024 rows or more and the high spatial resolution, particularly in medium to large field of view scans. Flat-panel detectors were developed for digital radiography and their use for CT is currently being explored by manufacturers.

Gantry Anatomy

Third generation

With third-generation CT, simultaneous rotation of the X-ray tube and detector array became possible (rotate/rotate geometry, rotating gantry). Moreover, the number of detectors and the angle of the fan beam were increased considerably so that the X-ray beam could scan the entire patient. The translational motion of first- and second-generation CT scanners could therefore be eliminated, which reduced the scan times substantially.

In the beginning, third-generation scanners suffered from the problem of ring artifacts. Each detector in third-generation scanners is responsible for the data corresponding to a ring in the image. Detectors close to the center of the detector array are responsible for a ring with a smaller diameter than those detectors towards the periphery of the detector array. Because there is always a certain amount of electronic drift associated with each detector, this causes gain changes between detectors, finally leading to ring artifacts. Today, modern technology has overcome this problem so that third-generation CT scanners are free of ring artifacts.

Multislice CT systems always use a third-generation technology and they provide scan times as short as 0.5 s.

Fourth generation

Because of the problem of ring artifacts with third-generation scanners, fourth-generation CT scanners were designed. The detectors are placed separately in a stationary 360° ring around the patient and only the X-ray tube rotates (rotate/stationary geometry). Whereas in third-generation scanners, data are acquired by the detector array simultaneously, a single detector collects the data in fourth-generation CT over the period of time that is needed for the X-ray tube to rotate through the arc angle of the fan beam. Each detector also represents its own reference detector. In this way, ring artifacts were avoided in fourth-generation scanners.

This technology requires many detectors because the detector array covers a 360° angle. It is not used nowadays to design multislice CT units because of the high costs for such an immense number of detectors.

Slip-ring technology

In third- and fourth-generation scanners, the X-ray tube rotates around the object. This also applies to the detectors in third-generation scanners. In combination, this is also referred to as a 'rotating gantry', although not all parts of the gantry rotate. These components require a number of electrical connections for high-voltage power, data transmission and control. In most early CT systems, the connections between the components on the rotating side of the gantry bearing and the power sources, computers, etc., on the stationary side of the bearing were made using cables. They were of finite length and allowed a rotation of perhaps 700°. As a result, these systems had to stop and reverse rotation directions between images.

The alternative to this cable system is the slip-ring technology. It allows the continuous circular rotation of the X-ray tube and other components of a CT system. In a slip ring, electrical brushes allow connections between continuously rotating and stationary components. The slip-ring design made it possible to achieve greater rotational velocities allowing shorter scan times. It finally enabled the design of the modern helical CT scanner.

Multislice CT

Helical CT represents a CT system using slip-ring technology in which continuous X-ray tube rotation is used along with simultaneous and continuous table translation through the gantry. The X-ray tube describes a helical path around the object. The term 'helical CT' is equivalent to spiral CT, which is actually an inaccurate term (a spiral decreases in diameter). Helical CT scanners are named single section (single slice, single detector row), dual section (dual slice, dual detector row) or multisection (multislice, multidetector, multirow) according to the maximum number of slice images generated per gantry rotation.

Helical CT technology makes it possible to image a given volume much more quickly (e.g. 30 s for the entire abdomen). More importantly, though, it allows a volume to be imaged during a more consistent phase of contrast enhancement. It is of significant benefit for CT angiography and multiphase abdominal imaging. The extent of sequential coverage, or the total time of scanning, is generally limited by X-ray tube heating.

The relationship between the incremental table movement and the selected slice width during one rotation of the gantry is described as 'pitch'. In single-slice CT the pitch describes the ratio of the table movement per 360° gantry rotation to the collimator width (*collimator pitch*). In multislice CT, the *detector pitch* describes the ratio of the table movement per 360° gantry rotation to the detector width. The *collimator pitch*, then, defines the ratio of the detector pitch to the number of detector rows in multislice technology. The pitch influences patient dose, scan time and image quality. Increasing the pitch decreases scan time and reduces motion artifacts. However, the effective section thickness as well as image noise increases, too. For clinical studies, a pitch of 1–1.5 is commonly used.

Since the helical data set does not correspond to sequential plane data, it needs to be reconstructed via interpolation into planar image data sets before the actual CT reconstruction.

With single-slice CT, detectors are rather wide in the Z-axis, e.g. 1 × 20 mm. Almost the entire detector element is actively detecting radiation, and slice thickness is determined by the collimator width. Per default, the collimator width is always smaller than the detector width. Therefore, for single-slice CT, slice thickness can be decreased via smaller collimator width; however, utilization of the X-ray beam is lower, therefore signal-to-noise-ratio decreases as well. This may be partially compensated by increasing the mAs. As an advantage, partial volume averaging decreases and spatial resolution is improved with thinner slice thickness.

With multislice CT, detectors are much smaller (e.g. <1 × 1 mm). The detector size determines the smallest possible slice thickness and the collimators determine the number of detectors used. If only the central two detectors are used, the slice width can be reduced below the detector width. To allow for variation in slice width and to decrease scan time, the signals from multiple rows of detector elements can be combined, so-called binning. Binning can be performed during the requisition or from raw data after scanning.

There are two detector array designs in multislice systems: those with detector elements of equal width (equal-width design) in each detector row and those with detector elements of unequal width in the different detector rows (unequal-width design).

With multislice CT, a much higher anatomic coverage can be achieved with the same pitch and slice thickness than in single-slice CT. For the same anatomic coverage and scan time, with single-slice CT one has to either increase the pitch or the slice thickness. But image quality is then degraded considerably.

There are many advantages with multislice CT. Scanning is faster, providing better temporal and contrast resolution and fewer motion artifacts. Consequently, multiphase studies (e.g. arterial, venous, portal phase studies) became possible. Thinner slice thicknesses are possible, which improves spatial resolution and reduces partial volume averaging. Due to more patient length scanning per rotation, higher X-ray tube current settings may be used, which in turn reduces image noise.

Table 1.2 shows typical performance characteristics for a CT scanner in 2010.

Moving gantry

Most CT units include a moving table and a fixed gantry housing. However, for certain purposes, moving or sliding gantries have been developed. Instead of the table moving into the gantry, as in conventional CT, in

Table 1.2
Performance characteristics for a CT scanner in 2010.

Power	60–100 kW
Rotating time per 360°	0.33–0.4 s
Slice width	0.5–0.6 mm
Simultaneously scanned slices	64
Data per helical scan	200–4000 MB
Image matrix	512 × 512
z-coverage per rotation	20–40 mm
Scan times 'whole body'	10–30 s
Scan range	>1000 mm
Isotropic spatial resolution	0.4–0.6 mm
Contrast resolution	3 HU
Effective dose	1–20 mSv

this case the table is fixed and scanning is accomplished by moving the gantry over the patient. In human oncology, for example, it may be an advantage during the course of irradiation if a CT scan can be performed for treatment planning adjustments immediately prior to irradiation. For this, patients are positioned on a common and fixed treatment table, which is integrated in a combined CT and linear accelarator irradiation system. The irradiation system and the CT gantry are positioned on opposite ends of the table so that, by rotating the treatment table, linac radiotherapy or CT scanning can be performed. Moving gantry systems are also designed for usage during surgery or angiography.

Scanning Modes

A routine scan requires a scout radiograph for anatomical orientation and scan region (slice) selection and scan performed in sequential or helical mode.

Scout radiograph (survey radiograph, localizer radiograph, scanogram, topogram, scout view)

A survey radiograph, similar to a conventional radiograph, is very useful for selection of single slices or complete scan regions. This radiograph is taken with a low dose and low spatial resolution by transporting the patient slowly through the field of measurement with the X-ray tube in a fixed position with radiation emitted continuously or in pulsed mode. Lateral scanograms are particularly useful to select the gantry tilt according to anatomy.

Sequential scanning (axial scanning, single-slice scanning)

For a long time, CT examinations consisted of scanning single slices sequentially. A single slice is scanned, then the patient is transported for a scan increment, mostly equal to the chosen slice thickness. Then, a second scan is taken and the procedure is repeated. This examination mode is relatively time-consuming and has been largely replaced by the faster helical CT. One fundamental disadvantage is that overlapping images for 3D image reconstruction are generally not available.

Modern scanners offer automated and therefore fast modes for scanning single slices sequentially. Cardiac scanning may be a future indication.

Dynamic scanning (serial scanning)

Dynamic CT is used to record temporal changes in the density characteristics of an object. Typically, dynamic scanning is used to assess contrast medium dynamics. A representative selected slice is scanned repeatedly or multiphase examination of a complete organ is performed before, during and/or after administration of contrast medium. The observed changes may represent physiological processes, such as heart motion or breathing, or pathological processes such as portosystemic shunts. Dual-phase CT angiography is a minimally invasive technique, which provides an excellent 3D representation of portal and hepatic vascular anatomy.

Material-selective scanning (dual-energy CT)

Dual-energy methods serve to obtain information about the material composition in the tissues examined. To achieve this, a selected slice is scanned with two different spectra, i.e. with different high-voltage values and possibly with different filtration. This can be done in two successive scans or by switching the high voltage rapidly from projection to projection.

Table Design

Many CT tables are made of a carbon fiber material because it will not cause artifacts when scanned. The movement of the table is referred to as incrementation (incrementation indexing). All table designs have weight limits that if exceeded may compromise increment accuracy. The maximum table load on actual CT machines is between 200 kg and 330 kg. Various table attachments and positional aids are available for specific body parts. For large animal CT these are usually custom made (for details, *see* Chapter 39).

Proprietary CT Terminology (Table 1.3)

Table 1.3
Proprietary CT terminology.

	GE Medical	Siemens	Philips	Toshiba
X-ray tube preparation				
Warm up and calibration	Tube warm-up	Check-up calibration	Tube conditioning	Warm-up
Scanning modes				
Planning radiograph	Scout	Topogram	Pilot or surview	Scano
Planning single CT scan	N/A	N/A	N/A	S&V (scan & view)
Sequential scan mode	Axial	Sequential	Axial	S&S (scan &scan)
Thick slice reformatting of sequential thin slices	Addition	Average	N/A	StackScan
Helical scan mode	Spiral	Helical	Spiral	Helical
Dynamic CT	Dynamic cine (continuous scanning)	Cine (dynamic, serio)	Dynamic	Dynamic
Scan planning				
Table	Couch	Couch	Patient table	Couch
Tube heat	Heat units	Heat	Tube heat (load)	Tube (OLP)
Scan range, length	Range	Range	1500	Range
Scan FOV	Scan FOV	Scan FOV	Scan FOV	C FOV
Reconstruction FOV	D FOV	Recon FOV (ZOOM)	FOV	D FOV
Bolus tracking	Smart prep	Care bolus	Bolus Pro	SureStart
Collimator pitch	Pitch	Pitch	Pitch	(Thickness)
Dose management software	Smart mA & Auto mA	Care dose 4D	Dose Wise	Sure Exposure
Image reconstruction interval	Interval	Increment	Continuous, Overlapping	Interval
Image reconstruction algorithm	Algorithms	Kernels	Recon algorithm	Recon FC
Additional image filtration	E1-4	Filters	Custom Image Filters	Filter (QDS)
Matrix, reconstruction	Center X,Y (0,0)	Center X,Y (0,0)	Center X,Y (0,0)	Center X,Y (256,256)
Cone beam reconstruction algorithm	Cross beam	AMPR/ASSR	COBRA	TCOT

(*Continued*)

Table 1.3
(Continued)

	GE Medical	Siemens	Philips	Toshiba
Post-processing				
Archive	Image works	Browser	Patient catalogue	Directory
Visualization software	Image display	Sub-tree	Viewer	I-selector
Multiplanar reconstruction (MPR)	Direct MPR	Real-time MPR	Real-time MPR	Multiview (auto MPR)
DICOM protocols transfer	Network	Export	Copy series	Transfer
Subtraction software	Innova 3D	Subtraction Syngo neuro DSA	Subtraction	Sure Subtraction
Cardio software	CT Cardiac Imaging	Syngo circulation	Cardiac tools/Best to beat	Sure Cardio
Plaque analysis software	Color mapping	Syngo plaque MAP	Plaque Analysis	SurePlaque
Gating software application	SnapShot Pulse	Syngo circulation	Step & shoot cardiac	SureCardio Prospective
Fluoro CT software	CT fluoro	Care vision	CCT (continuous CT)	CT Fluoro SureFluoro
CT endoscopy/endo 3D	Navigator	Fly	Endoview	3D

Further Reading

Bushberg JT, Seibert JA, Leidholdt EM and Boone JM (2002) Computed tomography. In: Bushberg JT, Seibert JA, Leidholdt EM and Boone JM (eds) *The essential physics of medical imaging* (2e), pp 327–72. Philadelphia, PA: Lippincott Williams & Wilkins.

CHAPTER TWO

CT Acquisition Principles

Tobias Schwarz and Robert O'Brien

Image Parameter Selection

Introduction

When running a CT scan the operator of a CT unit is faced with a large number of selectable settings, which can be intimidating. The following guidelines are designed to help in the selection process and can be used to set up individual CT protocols.

Body part selection

In all modern CT units, the operator needs to preselect a body part folder, which contains different protocol options. The body part selection includes hardware choices such as selection of specifically shaped bow-tie filters for beam hardening compensation. These are not adapted to veterinary patients and therefore it is worth testing other body parts protocol groups as well. There are often restrictions on protocol uses and topogram selections and it is not always possible to reuse topograms when changing protocol groups.

Tube rotation time

The tube rotation time selected should be as short as possible (usually between 0.5 and 1 s) for all body parts with anticipated movement, such as thorax, abdomen and spine, to avoid motion blur. For non-moving body parts in anesthetized patients, such as head, neck and extremities, it can be advantageous to increase the tube rotation time to 2 s to reduce view aliasing artifact (*see* Chapter 4). However, this might not be necessary in modern CT units, where the software is designed to ensure a sufficient number of views even with shorter rotation times. It is worth running some tests and comparing 1 and 2 s rotation time images for artifact magnitude. When selecting the tube rotation time, the effect on the mAs needs to be considered. In some units, changing the tube rotation time will automatically adapt the mA to result in the same mAs and vice versa, whereas in other units the mAs will change according to the selected product of mA and time.

Current and mAs product (Figure 2.1)

The current ranges usually from about 50 mA to 400 mA in modern CT units and there are either a large number of selectable settings or it can be selected freely within that range. The deciding factor is the applied current during the entire rotation of the tube, or mAs product. In some units, it is the mAs that is selected, whereas in others the mA is selected.

There is an inverse proportional relationship between mAs and image noise. Thus higher mAs settings will reduce noise. Small slice thickness increases image noise. Therefore if a small slice thickness is selected (2 mm or less) the mAs should be increased to keep the noise at an acceptable level.

The mAs and the kilovoltage both contribute to the heat load of the X-ray tube. Depending on the heat capacity of the tube, the combination of very high mAs and kilovoltage settings is usually limited.

All CT units have special protocols with low mAs setting (usually 80 mAs or lower) for infants to minimize radiation exposure levels. Despite the fact that most small animals usually are close in size to an infant, these low mAs settings do not always generate high-quality images for the head, spine and abdomen in dogs and cats. In small animals, mAs settings between 100 mAs (thorax) and 250 mAs (head and spine) are usually adequate.

Veterinary Computed Tomography, First Edition. Edited by Tobias Schwarz, Jimmy Saunders.

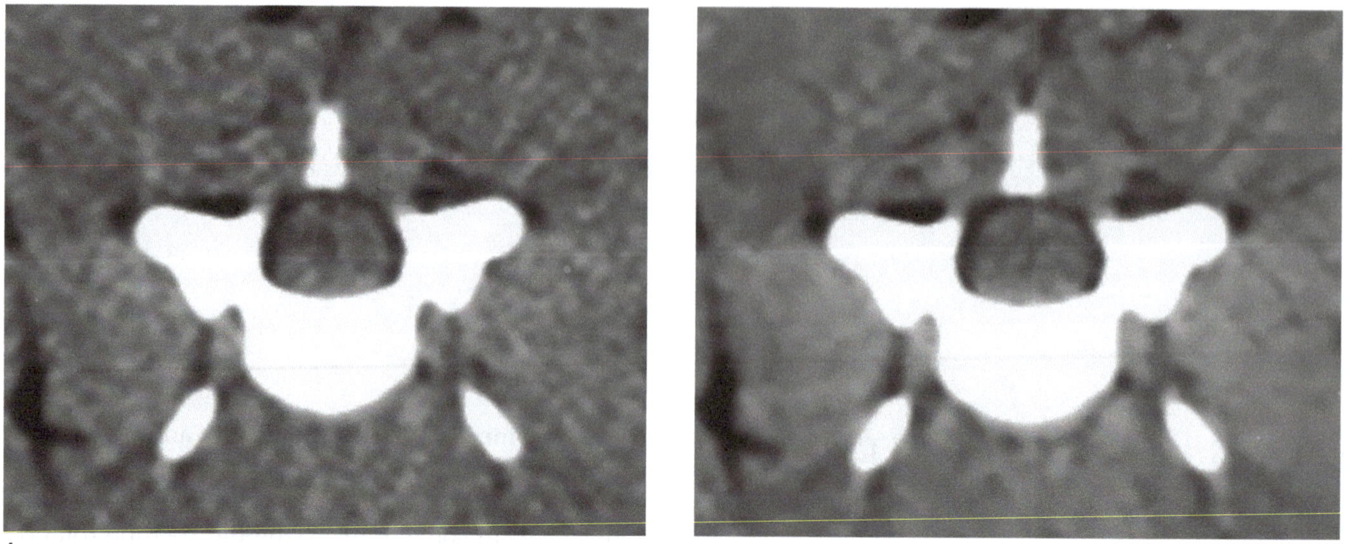

Figure 2.1 CT images of a canine cervical spine acquired with (A) 100 mAs and (B) 200 mAs, and otherwise identical settings. The image noise is represented by the general graininess of the image, which is reduced in (B).

All modern CT units have one or two adaptive mAs output options that can modulate the current along the Z plane and/ or the X–Y plane. The shoulder region is a good example where both can be applied. As the patient's neck travels through the gantry, the increase in body thickness at the shoulder region (Z plane current adaptation) requires an increase in mAs settings to minimize noise. But since the shoulder area is also wider than high, different mAs settings are optimal at different positions of the gantry circle (X–Y plane current adaptation). Adaptive mAs settings are designed to minimize radiation exposure and tube load and therefore do not always improve image quality in veterinary patients. This should be tested before using it.

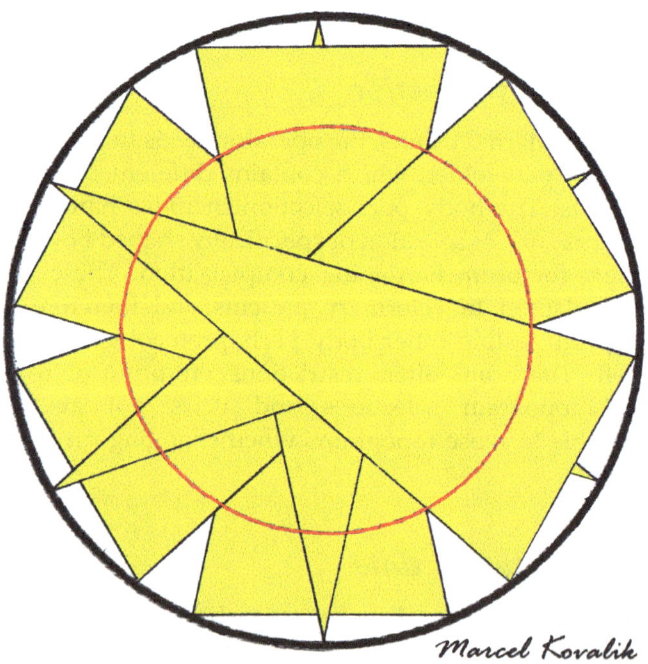

Figure 2.2 Illustration of the gantry with the trace of the rotating X-ray tube (black ring) and wedge-shaped projections obtained along its course (yellow wedges). The SFOV (within the red ring) is the area that is included in all projections. Only for this area is a full set of data acquired and images can only be reconstructed from within the SFOV.

Kilovoltage

In CT, the kilovoltage settings are usually high and there is a limited number of choices, usually 80, 120 and 140 kV. The 120 kV setting is adequate for almost all small animal patients, and can be applied universally. In large patients, the 140 kV setting would be preferential to ensure adequate penetration; however, the maximum kV settings usually only work in combination with relatively low mAs settings. Maximizing the mAs at the expense of the kilovoltage settings is usually the better option in this case.

Scan field of view (Figure 2.2)

During a CT image acquisition, the X-ray tube emits radiation that is collimated on all sides to match a fan-shaped array of detectors on the opposite side of the gantry, resulting in a wedge-shaped area of the gantry being exposed to radiation. The X-ray tube and the detectors circle around the gantry center during the exposure, resulting in an area of circularly overlapping

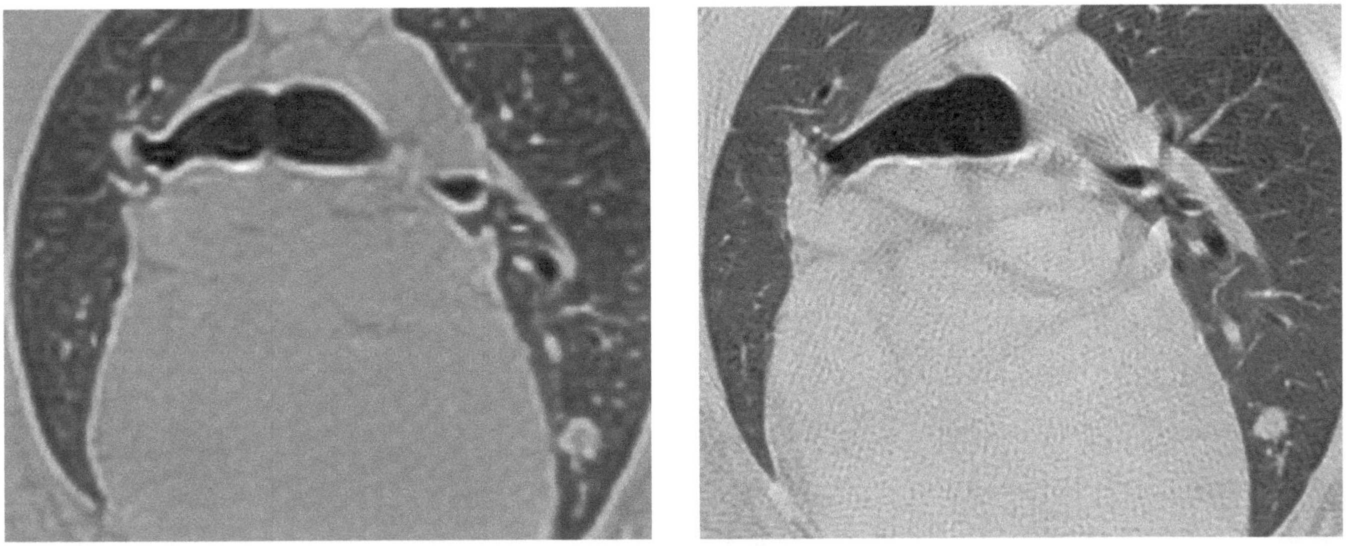

A B

Figure 2.3 Thoracic CT image of a dog obtained with (A) a 42 cm DFOV and (B) a 14 cm DFOV and otherwise identical settings. There is a dramatic increase in image resolution in (B) compared with (A), best visible in the small lung vessels, bronchi and the lung nodule. Coning down the DFOV improves image resolution.

wedges of exposed areas within the gantry. The scan field of view (SFOV) is the area of the gantry where there is complete overlap of these wedges. Image reconstruction in a matrix requires all data from all projections. As a result, a CT image can only be selected from within the SFOV. In most modern CT units, the SFOV is no longer selectable, because the maximum SFOV is always preselected. However, in General Electrics scanners, the SFOV is selected by the operator, and it is important to select the SFOV larger than the maximal patient diameter to avoid out-of-field artifacts (*see* Chapter 4). Keeping the SFOV only as big as necessary improves spatial resolution marginally.

Display field of view (Figure 2.3)

The display field of view (DFOV, synonym *FOV*) is the area of the SFOV from which an image is reconstructed. The DFOV cannot exceed the SFOV and should be kept as small as possible. During the reconstruction of a digital image, the matrix size defines the number of pixels used to form the image. For instance, in a 512^2 matrix, each image will be composed of 262 144 pixels. Displayed over a 40 cm DFOV, the pixel length will be 0.78 mm; displayed over a 15 cm DFOV, the pixel length will be 0.29 mm. Thus sizing of the DFOV has a significant impact on image resolution.

It is often essential to include the whole body cross-sectional area to assess the entire patient, so that coning down too far may not be practical. However, all newer CT scanners allow a targeted retrospective reconstruction from the raw data so that images with a smaller DFOV of specific areas can be obtained after the procedure. Due to the size and geometry of the detectors, decreasing the DFOV below 10 cm usually does not further increase the image resolution.

Gantry tilt (Figures 2.4 and 2.5)

In most CT units the gantry can be tilted to up to 30° in both directions. The topographic radiographs usually cannot be obtained with tilt, but all CT studies can be done tilted. Some older CT unit such as Elscint scanners even had a table swivel to align in the lateral orientation. Gantry tilt is useful for optimal alignment of the image plane with anatomic planes of interest to achieve optimally aligned sequentially reconstructed images. The most common use of gantry tilt is to align the scanning plane with the lumbar and particular cervical spine. Gantry tilt can be essential to achieve artifact-free images of patients with metallic foreign material or to avoid inclusion of artifact-inducing patient structures such as the head in elbow CT.

There are several caveats when using gantry tilt. It is preferable to adjust tilt at the gantry itself for patient safety reasons. Since the gantry tilts only in one plane, it is essential to position the patient in the appropriate recumbency. For instance, aligning with intervertebral disk spaces via gantry tilt is not possible in lateral recumbency. When the gantry is tilted, the scan direction remains along the Z plane, not the tilted plane. This requires for instance for longer spine sequences

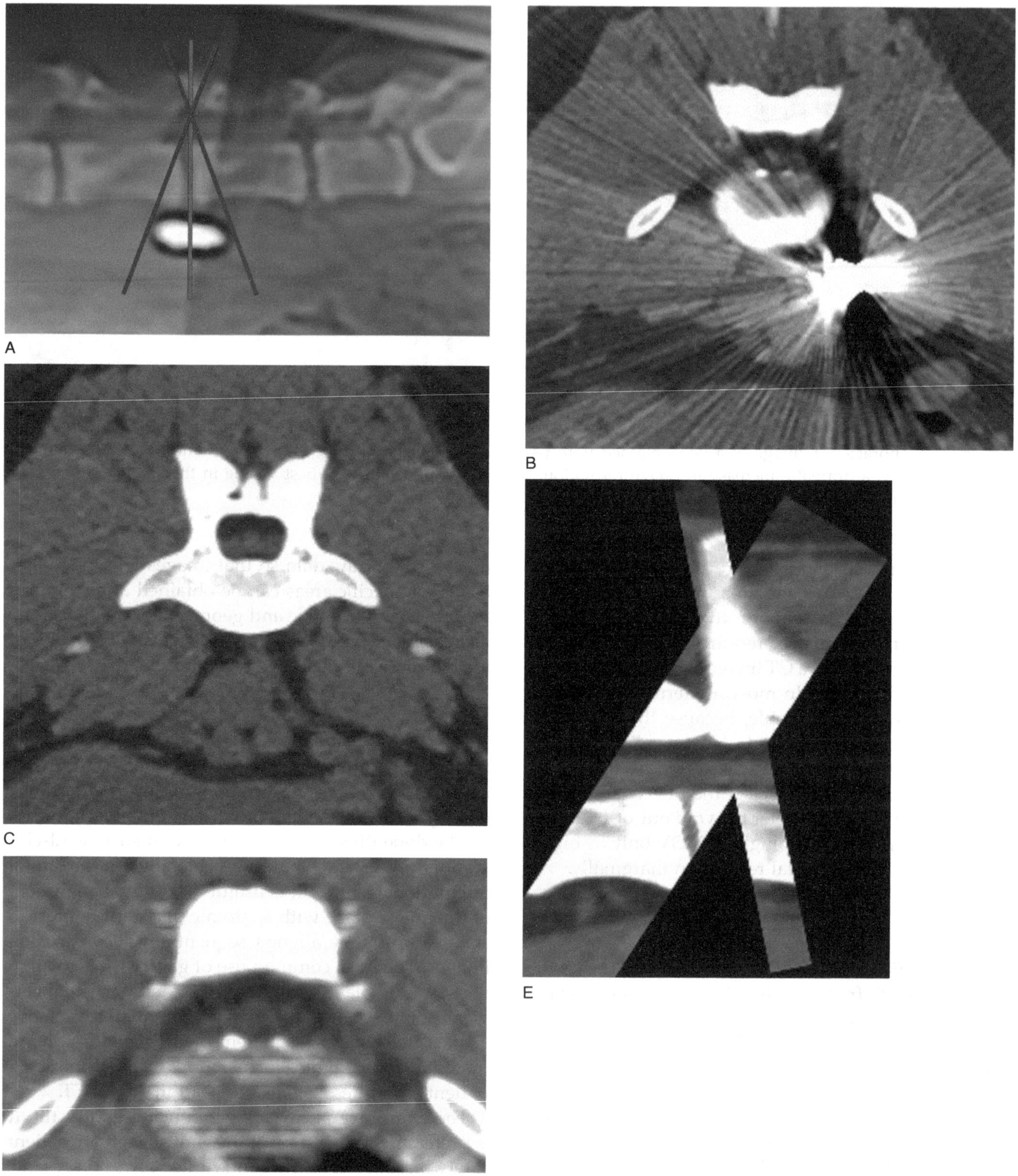
A
B
C
D
E

Figure 2.4 The creative use of gantry tilt can facilitate diagnostic images in challenging patients, such as in this dog with a paraspinal bullet seen on the topogram in (A). The transverse scan plane (red line) results in a non-diagnostic transverse CT image (B) for the area of interest due to the strong metallic artifact. The tilted (blue line in A) CT image (C) eliminates the artifact. These images can be retrospectively reconstructed into a transverse aligned CT image (D). A combination of the sagittal reconstructions from both tilted acquisitions (E) displays the diagnostic information from almost all areas obtained with this strategy.

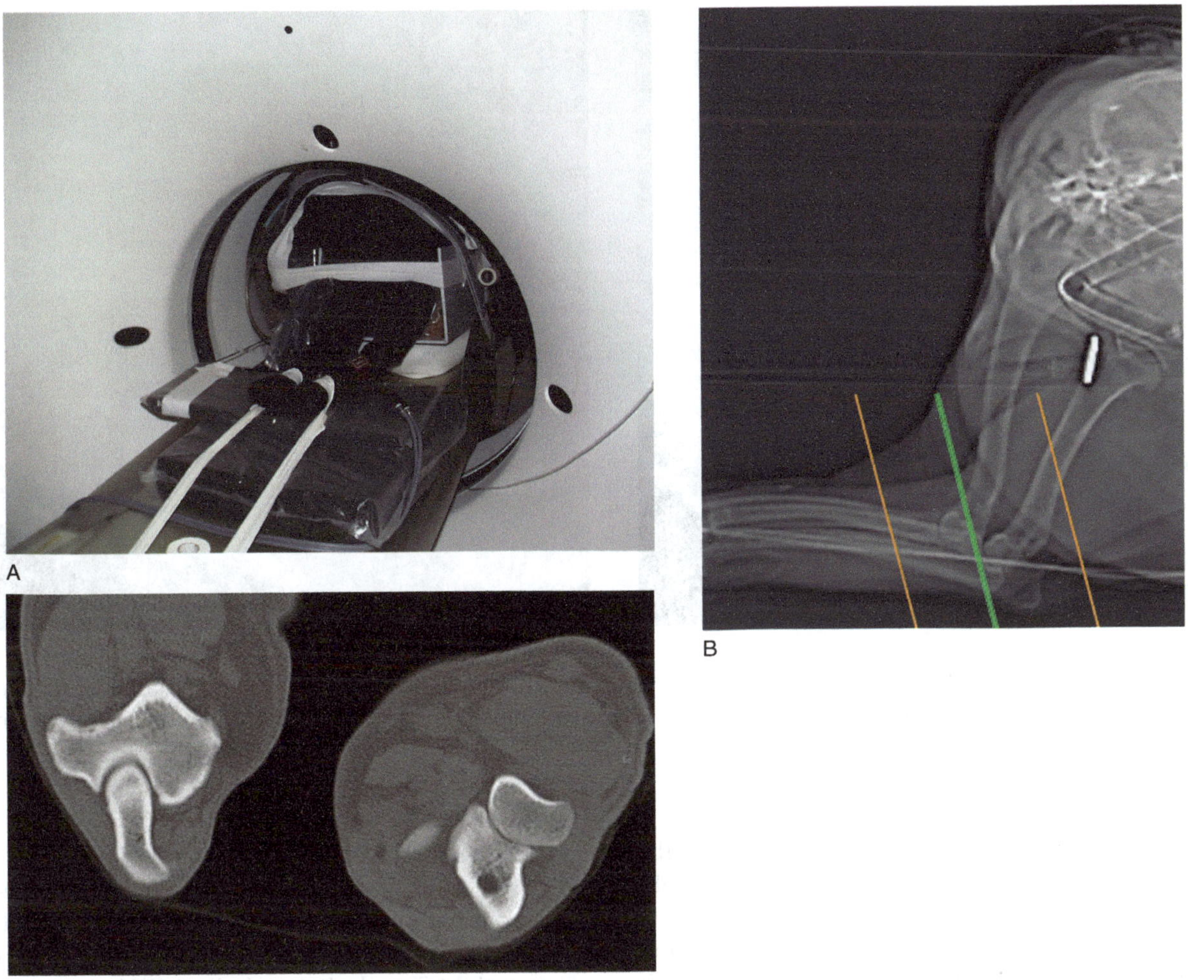

Figure 2.5 There are many ways to CT scan a canine elbow joint. (A) To avoid streak artifacts on elbow CT images emanating from the head and neck, the head is fixed in a laterally flexed position and the forelimbs are slightly elevated. (B) Lateral topogram illustrating the slightly tilted scan plane (colored lines) to avoid the presence of the head and neck in the scan plane without extreme flexion of the neck. (C) Resulting artifact-free elbow CT image.

to leave the DFOV sufficiently large to accommodate the anatomic area of interest within the DFOV over its entire length. Some reconstruction softwares are either unable to reconstruct orthogonal planes from tilted acquisitions or introduce image distortion (e.g. in Osirix 3.7). This can be remedied with additional software (macros).

The image reconstruction from helical scans with gantry tilt always requires a longer reconstruction time because the necessary mathematical interpolation is very complicated: the X-Y plane of the tilted gantry needs to be normalized to the X-Y plane of the moving patient table. In some CT scanners multiplanar reconstructions or helical acquisitions are not even possible with gantry tilt. The latest generations of CT scanners with 80 or more detector rows often do not have the costly mechanical gantry tilt. An isotropic image resolution can be achieved with any orthogonal image reconstruction so there is less of a need for this feature. For veterinary use with non-standardized patients and problems, gantry tilt remains a useful tool.

Slice thickness

General considerations (Figures 2.6, 2.9)

Slice thickness (synonym *slice width*) is arguably the single most important setting to select for a CT scan. Slice thickness is directly proportional to the magnitude of volume averaging (synonym *partial volume artifact*) and inversely proportional to the magnitude of image noise. Thus thick-slice CT images are blurry but contain little noise, whereas thin-slice images are sharp but noisy. There are several strategies to deal with this dilemma.

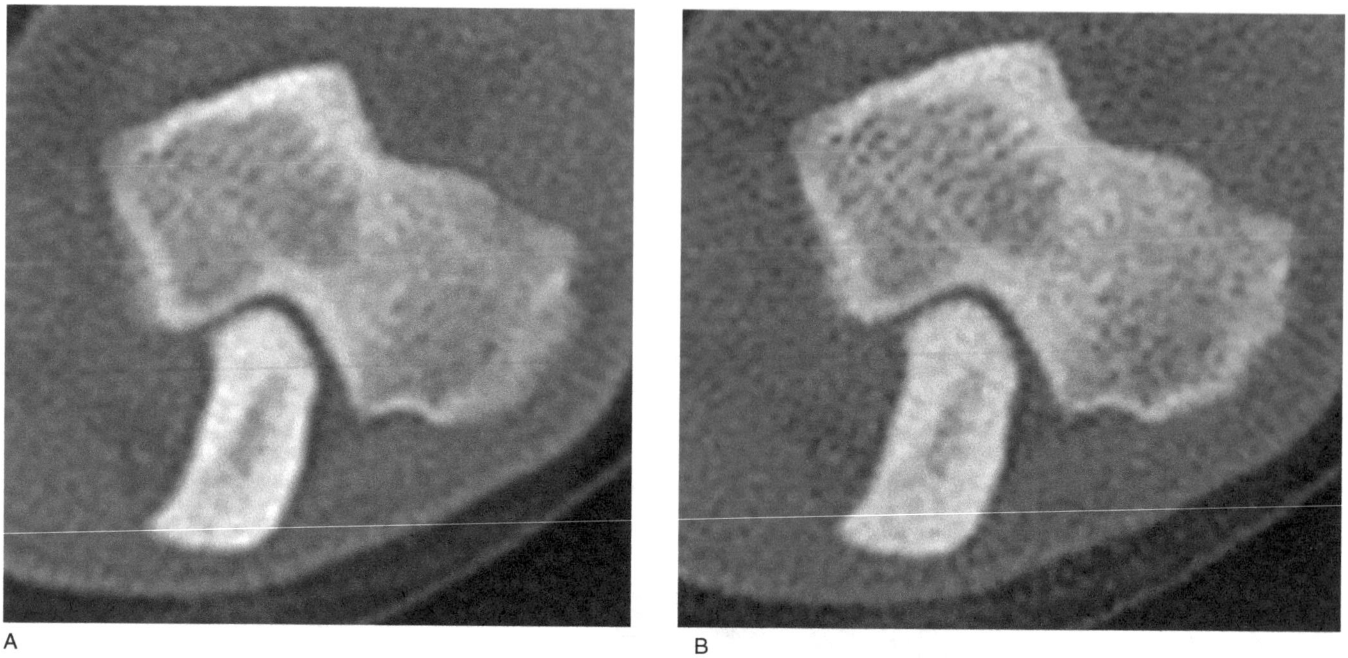

Figure 2.6 Canine elbow CT images acquired with (A) 2 mm and (B) 1 mm slice thickness and otherwise identical settings. The increased slice thickness results in more blur but less image noise. For orthopedic settings, the thin-slice image is preferable.

- Thin-slice images should be obtained with higher mAs settings to keep the noise at an acceptable level.
- Structures with a wide inherent object contrast, such as bone, nasal turbinates and lungs, should be viewed with wide window settings. Wide window settings suppress the visibility of noise. Therefore a higher noise level is tolerable as long as these image series are only reviewed with these window settings.
- Structures with a narrow inherent object contrast, such as the brain, spinal cord, liver and other soft tissue organs, require viewing with a narrow window setting, which enhances noise. Therefore a thicker slice width (3 to 5 mm) should be selected in most circumstances for these structures.
- Most CT users have a probably subconscious preference for sharp, thin-sliced images with wide window settings, because these are aesthetically more pleasing than blurry thick-slice images windowed narrowly to the tolerance level for image noise. It is important to select slice width and window width rationally and not intuitively.

Another limitation of thin-slice imaging is the limited coverage of the patient or the prolonged time to scan a defined area. The tube heat capacity is also limited, so it is not always possible to scan a large area with very thin slices. Helical and, in particular, helical multislice CT have vastly improved our ability to scan a large patient volume in a short time span with thinner slices. Selection of the appropriate slice interval in sequential CT and pitch in helical CT helps to find the optimal compromise in slice thickness selection.

Another artifact that can be minimized with thin-slice imaging is non-linear partial volume (*see* Chapter 4), which contributes to the streaks in the caudal fossa of the calvarium. By obtaining images with a thin slice width originally and then fusing the raw data into bigger sections, non-linear partial volume artifact is minimized and noise is reduced. Because of the binning of thin detectors, all thick-slice images in multislice CT are obtained as a fusion from smaller slices, and non-linear partial volume is reduced automatically.

Thick-slice images can be appropriate for specific purposes and the partial volume artifact can work favorably to achieve this. It is, for instance, not necessary to select the smallest slice width to detect pulmonary nodules. Due to the partial volume artifact and the large density differences in the lungs, a pulmonary nodule that is smaller than the slice width will still create a visible, albeit blurry, opacity. Therefore a 3 to 5 mm slice width is acceptable for lung metastasis screening in dogs and cats. A short thin-slice series can then be obtained as a follow-up.

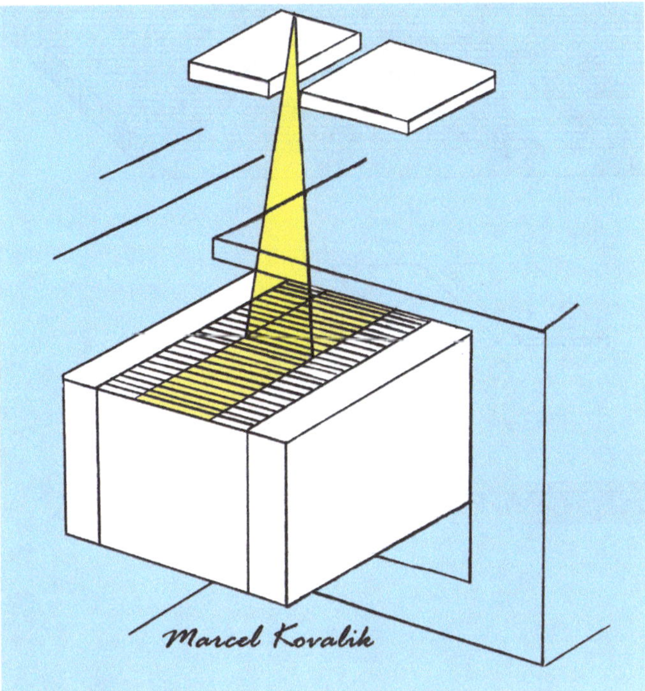

Figure 2.7 Illustration of a single-slice CT detector array. Two lead jaws restrict the X-ray beam exposure of the detector elements and thereby determine the slice thickness.

Slice thickness selection and detector design

Single-slice CT (Figure 2.7)

In a single-slice CT unit, submillimeter-thin and usually 10 mm long detector cells are aligned in a row in the X-Y plane of the gantry. The position of a mechanical collimator, made of two lead jaws, determines the exposed width of the detectors and thereby the slice thickness. Slice thickness cannot be modified retrospectively from raw data after the image acquisition in a single-slice CT unit.

Multislice CT (Figure 2.8)

In a multislice CT unit, several rows of detectors are lined up along the Z-axis of the gantry. The slice thickness is determined by the combination of detectors from which data are pooled together, a process called *binning*. It is possible to reconstruct CT images from the same acquisition both as thin- and thick-slice images. The ability to change the slice thickness retrospectively from the raw data is one of the major advantages of multislice CT. Dual reconstruction should be part of the standard protocol for almost all body parts with multislice CT.

A basic understanding of the detector alignment helps in selecting the appropriate slice thickness. Two design types exist. In an *unequal-detector-width design* only the central detectors are very thin and the detector width enlarges symmetrically peripherally. This design is cheaper and prevalent in older units and scanners with fewer detector rows. In an *equal-detector-width design* all detectors have a very small width (0.5–1 mm). This design is more expensive and prevalent in the newest generation of scanners with many detector rows. The mechanical collimator is used to determine the number of detector rows to be exposed.

A CT image sequence can only be reconstructed with slices of equal thickness. Therefore in an unequal-detector-width-design CT scanner, only certain binning combinations are numerically possible. The number in the multislice CT unit name (e.g. 'four-slice CT') usually corresponds to the maximum number of detector row combinations that can be binned together, not the number of detector rows, which is usually greater. For instance, a so-called 'four-slice scanner' usually has eight detector rows with two 1 mm, two 1.5 mm, two 2.5 mm and two 5 mm detectors. Possible binning combinations are then 4×2.5 mm, 4×5 mm, 2×10 mm and 1×20 mm. The outermost detector row can be partially collimated by the collimator, adding further binned slice thickness options of 2×0.5 mm, 4×1 mm, 4×8 mm.

Slice thickness and slice sensitivity profile (Figure 2.9)

Due to the fact that the focal spot of a CT unit is much smaller than the selected slice thickness, the X-ray beam in CT is not truly a slice but a wedge and is thus thinner at the isocenter of the gantry than at the detector level. The *slice sensitivity profile* expresses this relationship mathematically and states that the contrast resolution degrades towards the slice periphery. It is possible to reconstruct image data only from the center of the slice (*half-width-height-maximum*) and some manufacturers (e.g. Siemens) offer two different reconstruction options for each selected slice thickness: the thin-slice option reconstructs in half-width-height-maximum mode, which increases image resolution; and the thick-slice option reconstructs the whole slice width data, allowing the use of higher pitches in helical CT.

Slice interval (Figure 2.9)

The slice interval (synonym *slice increment*) is the interval at which CT images are acquired in sequential mode CT. In helical mode, data are obtained continuously, hence slice interval is not applicable here. The slice interval is selected in relation to slice width. As a

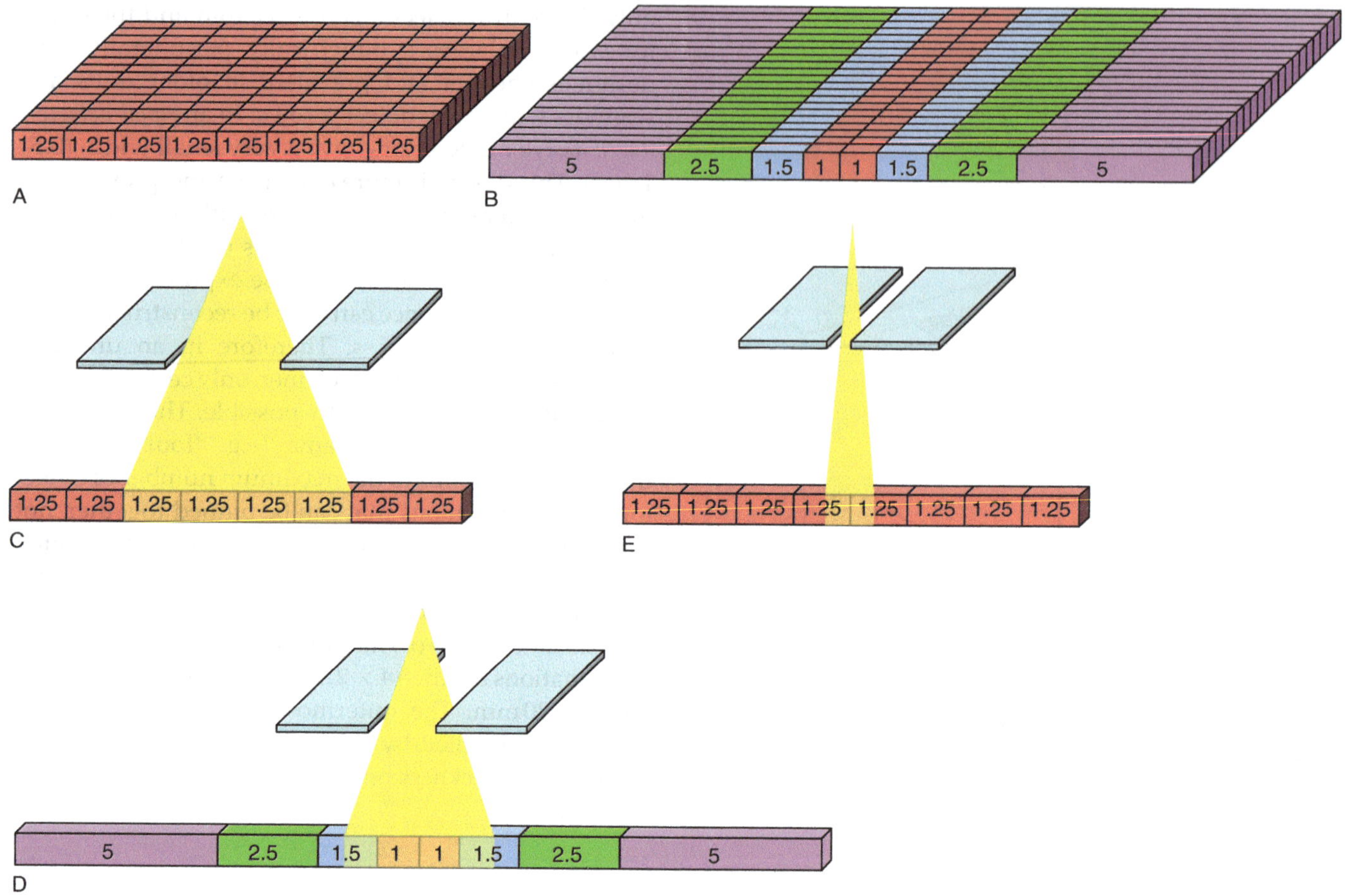

Figure 2.8 Multi-slice CT detector row design and collimation options. (A) Equal-width detector-row design with eight rows of 1.25 mm wide detectors. (B) Unequal-width detector-row design with rows of two each 1 mm, 1.5 mm, 2.5 mm and 5 mm wide detectors. This is the typical design of a 'four-slice' CT unit as only a maximum of four consecutive images can be reconstructed per tube rotation from these eight rows of detectors. (C) The collimator is used to determine the number of detector rows to be exposed in multislice CT. (D) In addition, the outermost pair of detectors can be partially collimated, resulting in more possible slice thickness options. In this case, four images of 1 mm slice thickness are generated. (E) The collimator can also be used to generate ultra-thin slice images if only the central detector pair is used. This will increase scan time as it does not use the full array of detectors.

default most units will preselect a slice interval equal to the slice width, ensuring a continuous image acquisition.

Continuous scanning is essential if the anatomy changes rapidly along the Z plane, which is the case for most body parts. However, some body parts, such as the nose, do not rapidly change their anatomic features along the Z plane. In older CT units, where tube heating is an issue it might then be better to obtain 1 mm thick images for maximal anatomic detail of the nose, but leave a 2 mm slice interval to not overload the tube. If continuous scanning is essential, such as for a metastasis check of the lungs, then helical mode should be considered.

For some body parts another compromise that can be made between limited tube heat capacity and optimal image detail is to obtain several small series of continuous slices and leave gaps between them. For instance for spinal CT the intervertebral disk spaces can be scanned continuously and gaps can be left over the vertebral bodies. Leaving a slice gap will always limit the ability to perform orthogonal reconstructions.

Overlapping scanning is rarely performed because of tube heat issues, but this might be useful if maximum image detail is required for a small area. Orthogonal reconstructions in particular will improve with overlapping images.

Sequential versus helical mode

In sequential CT (synonym *axial*) mode, a complete set of data is acquired from all angles of the tube position, resulting in optimal image resolution. In helical CT, the

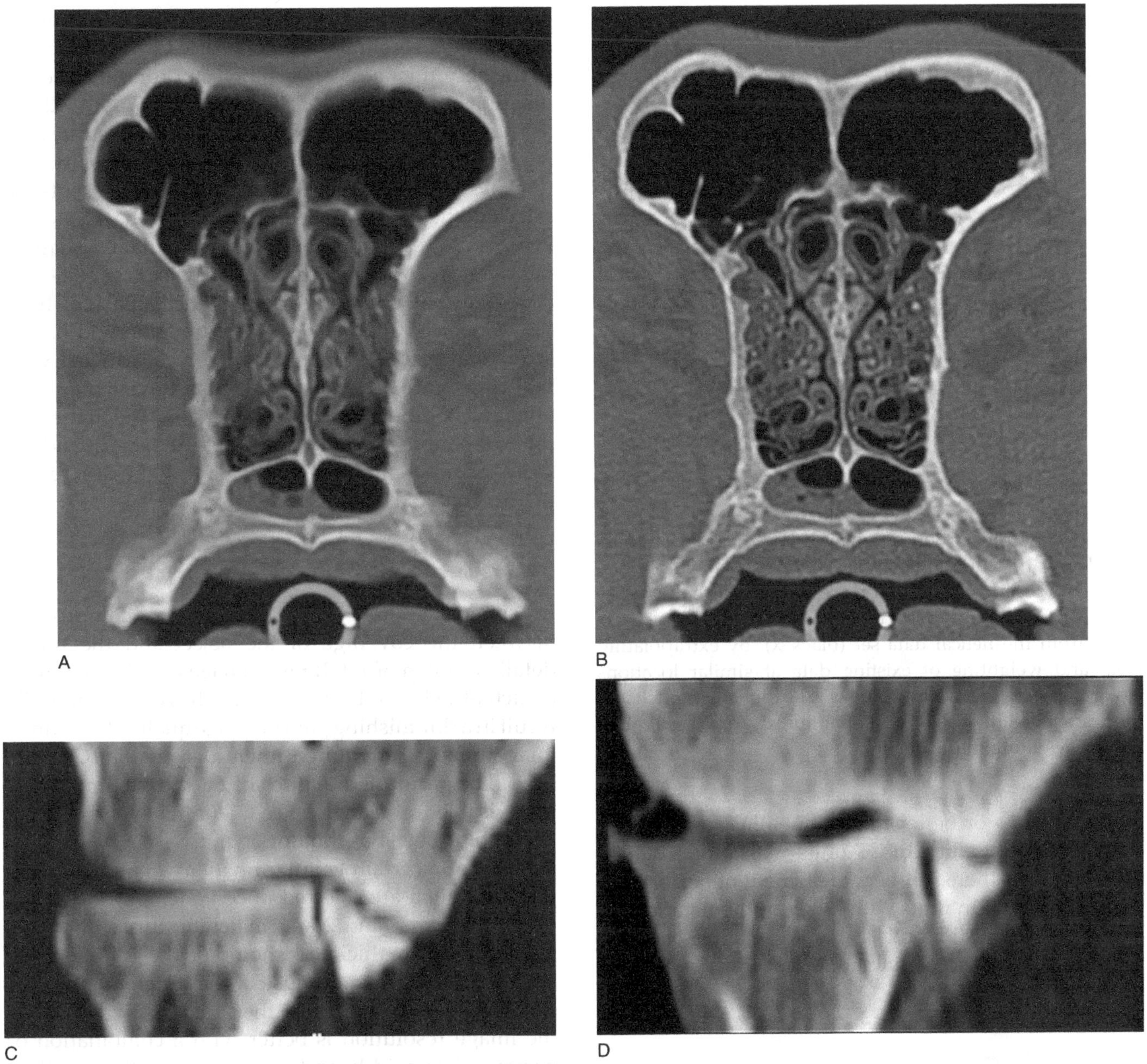

Figure 2.9 (A) The 5 mm slice thickness image of the nose reveals ambiguous features of the nasal turbinates due to partial volume related image blur. (B) The 1 mm thick image supports the diagnosis of bacterial rhinitis based on the presence of normal turbinate and secretion. Leaving a gap between thin slices is a better option than obtaining continuous thick slice images of mediocre quality. (C) Frontally reconstructed view of a canine elbow specimen obtained with sequential scanning and a 1 mm slice width and interval. (D) CT arthrography imaged sequentially with a 1 mm slice width and a 0.5 mm interval shows a smoother outline of the subchondral bone due to a reduction in stair step artifact (images courtesy of Andrew Gendler).

data represent a helix of data, and the incomplete data set has to be completed by mathematical guesses or interpolations. Therefore helical CT images have a lower image resolution than sequentially scanned CT images. In general, if maximum image detail is required, a sequential CT should be performed. However, there are other factors that influence image quality. Body parts with anticipated motion are preferentially scanned helically in any scanner, as the likelihood of occurrence of motion is lower during the shorter helical acquisition time. Also, the ability to perform interleaved image reconstructions helically and the fact that with a multislice CT there is data redundancy of each anatomic area can make helical

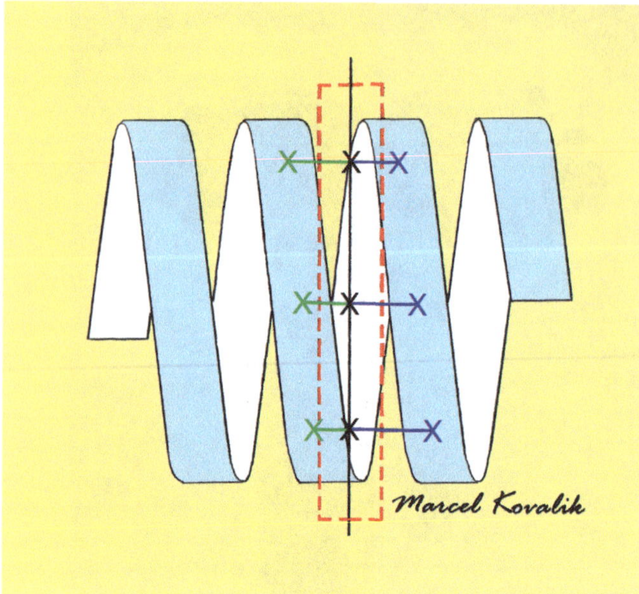

Figure 2.10 Illustration of a helical CT image reconstruction. Data are acquired as a helical set of volumetric data. The width of the helical band represents the slice thickness. The CT image (red box) is reconstructed in the transverse plane from the helical data set (black X), by extrapolating from and weighting of existing data at similar locations along the helix (green X and blue X). The higher the pitch, the more stretched the helix, the more imprecise are these calculations, resulting in image blur.

mode equal to or better than sequential scanning for overall image quality. In CT units with more than 16 detector rows, there is little more benefit of performing a sequential CT. In units with lower numbers of detectors, it is often still preferential to obtain head and spine images in sequential mode, but this needs to be tested.

Helical pitch

Introduction (Figure 2.10)

In helical CT, the patient moves through the gantry while parts of the gantry rotate around it. This results in a helical (synonym *spiral*) set of continuous data that represents the entire volume of the scanned area. The relationship between the table increment during one full gantry rotation and the slice thickness is expressed as the pitch, a unitless number. Pitch is directly proportional to image blur, therefore a highly pitched CT scan results in a very blurry image. In single-slice CT, the collimation and slice thickness are synonymous. In multislice CT, however, this is not the case, and pitch can be defined as the relation of table increment to the collimated width of all included detectors combined (*collimator pitch*, similar to single-slice CT) or in relation to the slice thickness of each detector (or binned combinations thereof, *detector pitch*) (Boxes 2.1 and 2.2).

The stretch of the helix in Figure 2.10 illustrates the magnitude of the pitch and its relationship to slice thickness. The width of the helical band represents the selected slice width or collimation width. A pitch of zero would result in a complete ring of data, a sequential CT scan. With a pitch of 1, the helix is stretched to a degree that after one rotation the table will have moved exactly by one slice or collimation width. The sequential plane CT image is then reconstructed with mathematical interpolations from available data obtained at other positions of the helix. The higher the pitch, the more stretched is the helical data set and the more incorrect are these mathematical guesses, resulting in a blurred image.

Pitch selection in single-slice CT (Figure 2.11)

In single-slice CT units the optimal compromise between the coverage of the object and the image detail is a pitch of 1.4. If more image detail is required, a pitch of 1 should be selected. Pitches of less than 0.75 result in a diminishing gain of image quality. If maximal image quality is required, then a sequential CT scan should be performed. A pitch of 2 is the maximum that is advisable for a single-slice CT unit; beyond this the image blur becomes too dominant.

To cover a certain length of patient area, slice thickness and pitch are selected in conjunction. Selecting a pitch between 1 and 2 and matching this with a corresponding slice thickness should be the guiding principle in this process. Because of the different effects of slice thickness and pitch on the slice sensitivity profile, the image resolution is better with a combination of narrow slice width and greater pitch than with a thicker slice and a smaller pitch, as long as the pitch does not exceed 2 and the mAs are sufficiently increased for the smaller slice width.

Pitch selection in multislice CT

In multislice CT units the manufacturers do not always specify which definition of pitch they use. However, this can be deciphered based on the suggested pitch numbers in their protocols. Detector pitches have relatively high numbers (3 to 8 in a four-slice unit), whereas the collimator pitch is a lower number (between 0.5 and 1.5 in a four-slice unit). As a guiding principle, the pitches in multislice CT can be comparatively higher

Box 2.1

$$\text{single-slice collimator pitch} = \frac{\text{table increment per } 360^\circ \text{ gantry rotation}}{\text{collimation width at isocenter}}$$

$$\text{multislice collimator pitch} = \frac{\text{detector pitch}}{\text{number of selected detectors or binned combinations}}$$

$$\text{multislice detector pitch} = \frac{\text{table increment per } 360^\circ \text{ gantry rotation}}{\text{detector width}}$$

Box 2.2 Examples

Single-slice CT:

- 2.5 mm slice width and 2.5 mm table increment = collimator pitch of 1
- 2.5 mm slice width and 5 mm table increment = collimator pitch of 2

Four-slice CT:

- 2.5 mm detector width and 7.5 mm table increment
  = detector pitch of 3
  = collimator pitch of 0.75
- 2.5 mm detector width and 10 mm table increment
  = detector pitch of 4
  = collimator pitch of 1

than in single-slice CT, because each detector scans the same patient data as the patient passes the gantry during the scan and the data redundancy is used to make more accurate interpolations during the image reconstruction.

The relationship between slice thickness and pitch selection is more complicated in multislice CT. In some CT designs, data from all locations at every angle can only be obtained with the use of specific pitches, and therefore the pitch is not freely selectable.

Helical image reconstruction interval (Figures 2.12 and 2.13)

In a sequential CT acquisition, each slice image is obtained separately at one specific location and cannot be modified retrospectively. In helical CT, the image data are acquired as a volume. As a result, a slice image can be reconstructed from any point within that volume. Therefore the interval at which images are to be reconstructed needs to be defined by the user in helical CT. It is critical to understand that changes in the helical image reconstruction interval (HIRI) do not affect the slice width. As a default, the CT units will preselect a HIRI that is equal to the selected slice width, resulting in a continuous set of images. Alternatively, one can use gaps between images. This is rarely used but may be advantageous for an initial and quick reconstruction of a contrast bolus imaging study. More commonly, interleaved (synonym *overlapping*) reconstruction is applied, which has several advantages. Because of the slice sensitivity profile, the contrast resolution in the slice periphery in the Z plane is reduced. Small lesions at the edge of the slice could be missed. By overlapping the slices, such lesions will then be in the center of another slice, enhancing their visibility. Equally, the partial volume artifact will be minimal in one particular slice where the lesion location exactly matches the slice location. Because the slice images are also overlapping in terms of acquisition time, any motion artifact will also be minimized by a smaller HIRI. Finally, multiplanar reconstructions are performed by using the total acquired DICOM images. If these images overlap, they are also used in an overlapping fashion in these reconstructed images, which greatly improves image quality.

The optimal compromise between data size-related matters (original image reconstruction and transfer time, storage space, computer capacity for multiplanar reconstruction of large DICOM series) and

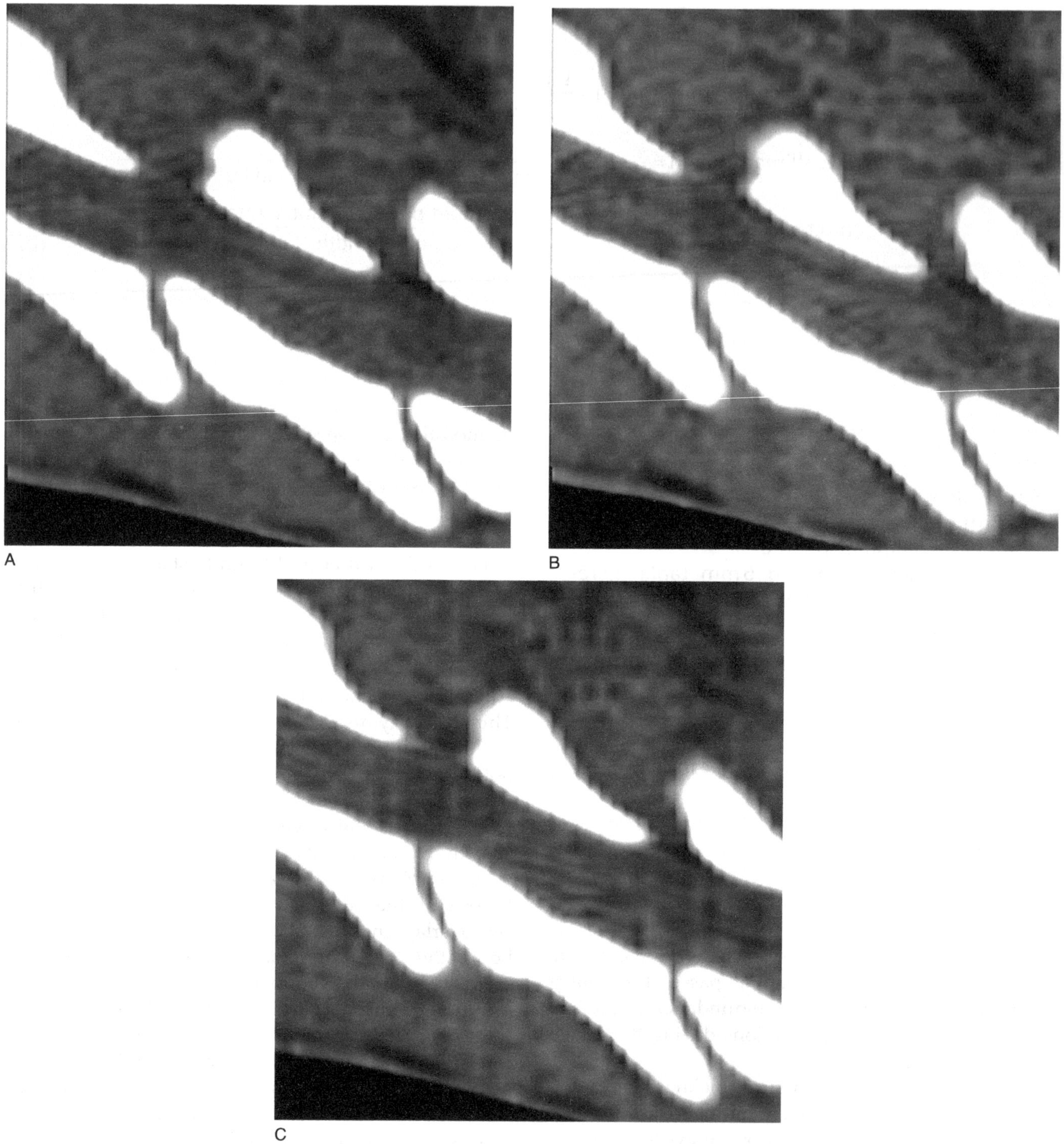

Figure 2.11 Examples of different pitch selections (otherwise identical settings) and their effect on image quality of sagittally reconstructed cervical spinal CT images acquired with a single-slice CT unit. (A) Sequential CT scan (pitch = 0). (B) Helical series with a pitch of 1 introduces slight image blur, reducing the visibility of the intervertebral disk. (C) Helical series with a pitch of 2 results in further blurring and loss of intervertebral disk definition.

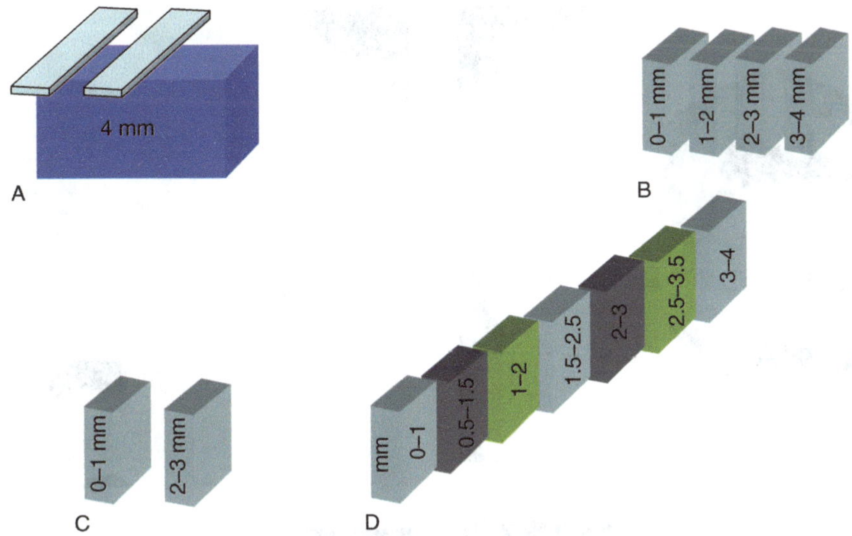

Figure 2.12 Illustration of the helical image reconstruction interval (HIRI). (A) A 4 mm long patient volume set of data has been acquired with a helical CT scan and a 1 mm slice collimation. (B) The default option on most CT scanners is to reconstruct images with a HIRI equal to the selected slice width. In this example this results in four 1 mm thick slice images spaced 1 mm apart, which is continuous image reconstruction. (C) Another option is to leave gaps between images, resulting in this example in two 1 mm thick images spaced 2 mm apart. (D) With interleaved reconstruction, images are reconstructed at an interval smaller than the slice width, in this example resulting in seven 1 mm thick images, spaced 0.5 mm apart. Interleaved image reconstruction increases image resolution for several reasons.

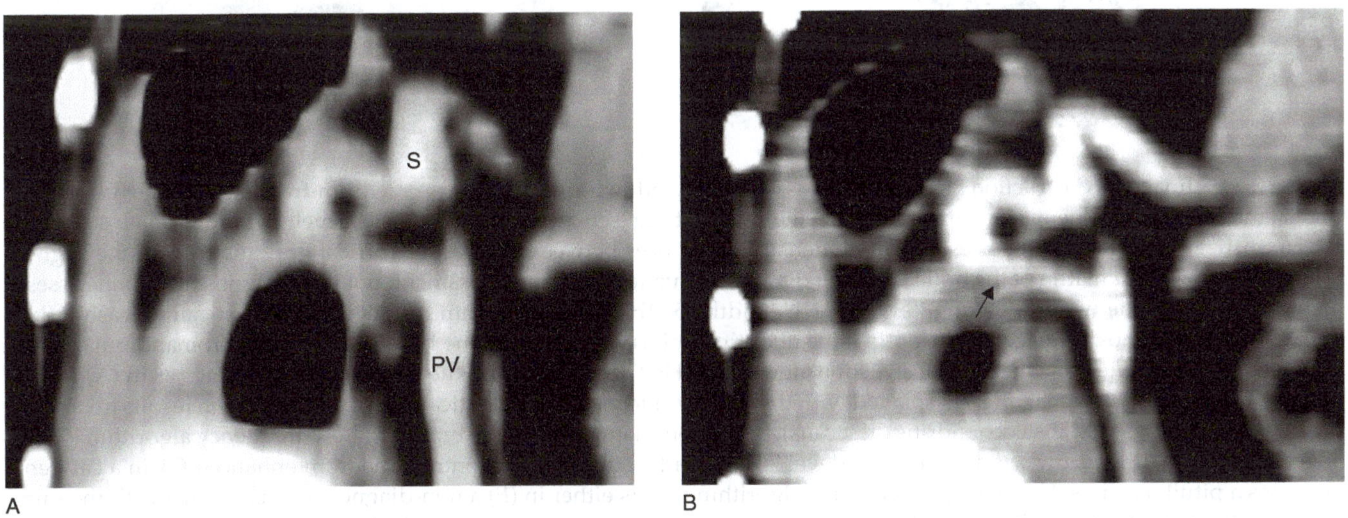

Figure 2.13 Two dorsal reconstructions of an abdominal vascular CT study with different HIRI and otherwise identical settings (3 mm slice width). (A) With a 3 mm HIRI the connection between the portal vein (PV) and the shunt vessel (S) is ambiguous. (B) With a 0.3 mm HIRI the connecting branch of the shunt vessel (arrow) is clearly visible.

image quality is a HIRI of half of the slice thickness and this can be applied to all helical CT protocols. With smaller intervals there is a diminishing gain of further image quality that is only occasionally justified.

Image reconstruction algorithm (Figure 2.14)

The image reconstruction algorithm (synonyms *filter, kernel*) is the mathematical method used to create a

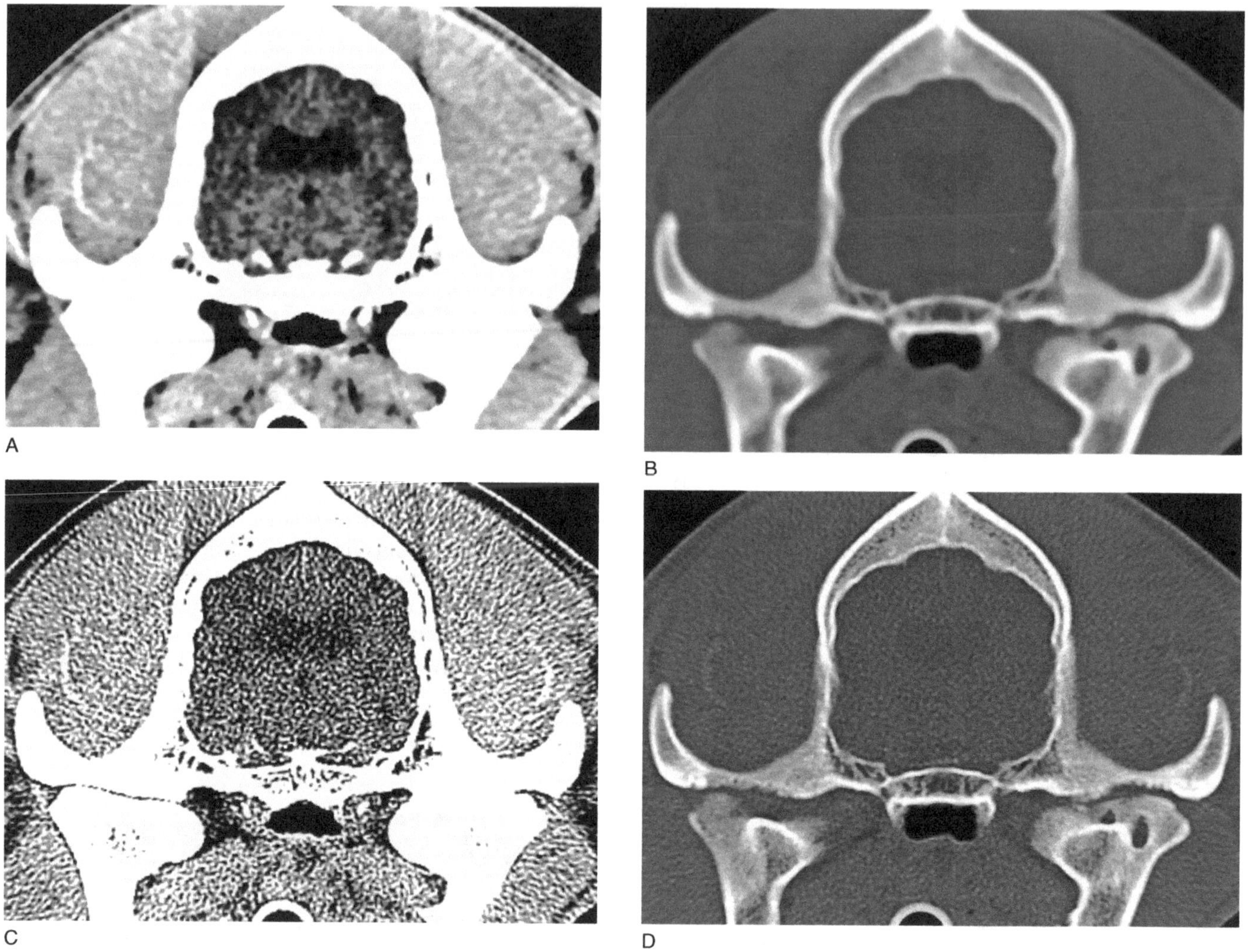

Figure 2.14 Image reconstruction algorithm and associated windowing choices. (A) A medium-frequency image reconstruction algorithm ('H40', Siemens) with a narrow window setting set at a tolerable noise level (window level 40/width 100 Hounsfield units [HU]) enhances the subtle density differences between the darker cortical gray matter and the slightly brighter central white matter of the brain. This is a diagnostic quality for brain assessment, but non-diagnostic for bone assessment. (B) With a wide window setting (level 300 HU, width 1500 HU) this algorithm results in an aesthetically pleasing (less noise) but non-diagnostic image for the brain and suboptimal blurry display of bone lesions in the temporomandibular joints (TMJ). (C) A high-frequency image reconstruction algorithm ('H60', Siemens) with the same window settings as in (A) results in a non-diagnostic noisy image. (D) Displayed with the wide window settings identical to (B), this algorithm results in optimal detail of bone lesions (TMJ osteochondritis dissecans), but is non-diagnostic for the brain. (E) Low-frequency algorithm ('H30', Siemens) image with narrow window settings (level 70 HU, width 170 HU) of a contrast-medium enhanced CT in a cat demonstrates a pituitary mass. Using a high-frequency algorithm results either in (F) a non-diagnostic noisy image with the same narrow settings or (G) an aesthetically pleasing image with wide window settings (level 60 HU, width 1000 HU) in which the contrast uptake remains invisible. High-frequency algorithm images are non-diagnostic for contrast medium uptake assessment regardless of window settings.

matrix image from projectional raw data via Fourier transformation. The spatial frequency of data sampling and various techniques of edge enhancement or smoothening are the main variables. The various manufacturers have different names and types of algorithm that are not exactly identical, but the basic principles are the same.

Low or *medium spatial frequency algorithms* ('smooth', 'standard', 'detail', low number kernels such as 'H30' in Siemens CT units) smoothen the image and thereby reduce visible image noise and improve contrast resolution. These algorithms should be used to display body parts with inherently small object contrast in which a narrow window setting is necessary to maximize the

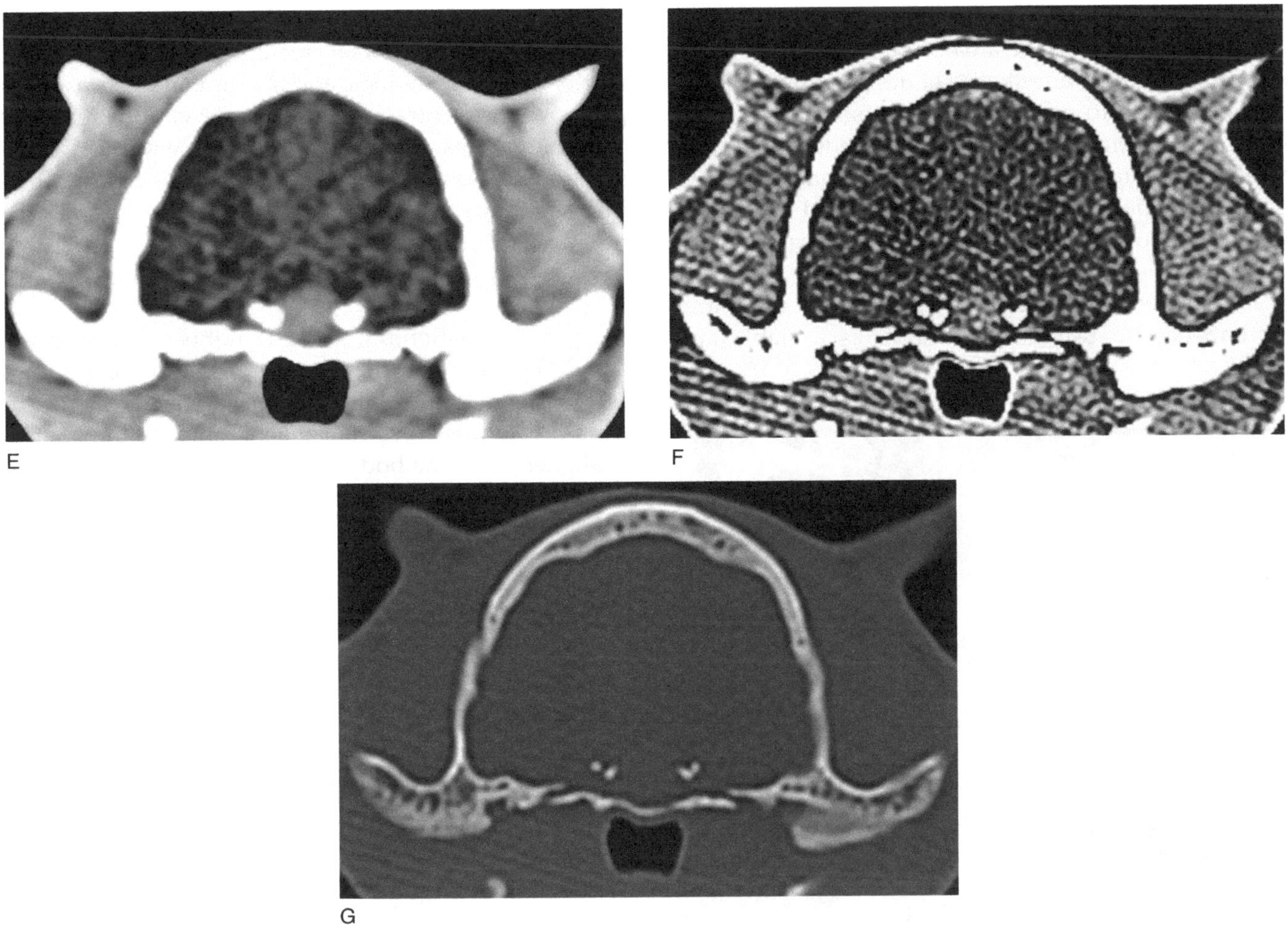

Figure 2.14 (*Continued*)

difference in grayness between tissues of close density values. This is the case for all soft tissue organs, in particular the brain, and all post-contrast studies. In some special algorithms the grain size of noise is reduced to allow better assessment of brain parenchyma.

High spatial frequency algorithms ('bone', 'lung', 'edge', high kernel numbers such as 'H60') increase image sharpness at the expense of increased noise. Edge enhancement can be part of the algorithm or selected separately. These algorithms should be used to display body parts with inherently wide object contrast, such as the lungs, bone and the nasal turbinates, in which a wide window setting is necessary to display the wide range of densities within the available grayscale of the monitor. The wide window settings will reduce the visibility of noise. For this reason, images that have been generated with a high-frequency reconstruction algorithm cannot be used diagnostically with a narrow window setting or for any assessment of intravascular contrast medium uptake.

Special hard and software combinations (Figure 2.15)

Many CT manufacturers offer specific imaging protocols that involve specific hardware and software settings combined, such as optimized high-resolution protocols. It often requires central positioning of the body parts. Because of the hardware used, such images can not then be retrospectively reconstructed from normal series.

Patient Set-Up

Patient direction and recumbency options (Figure 2.16)

The patient direction (head/tail first) and recumbency (ventral, dorsal, right or left) is specific for the each body part and discussed in detail in each organ-specific chapter.

Head-first or tail-first orientation of the patient should be guided by the area of interest in relation to the gantry and the anesthetic set up. To avoid artifacts it is preferable to orient the patient so that no anesthetic equipment passes through the gantry. Thus in a tail-first orientation the anesthetic equipment should be on the patient side, whereas with a head-first orientation it should be positioned on the opposite side of the gantry.

As a general rule, head CT is preferred in ventral recumbency, to use the mandibles as a stable and adjustable anchoring point; spinal CT should always be performed in dorsal recumbency to minimize motion artifacts; thoracic and abdominal CT is usually performed in ventral recumbency for various reasons; and extremities are performed in a wide range of positioning options to avoid other body parts in the imaging plane.

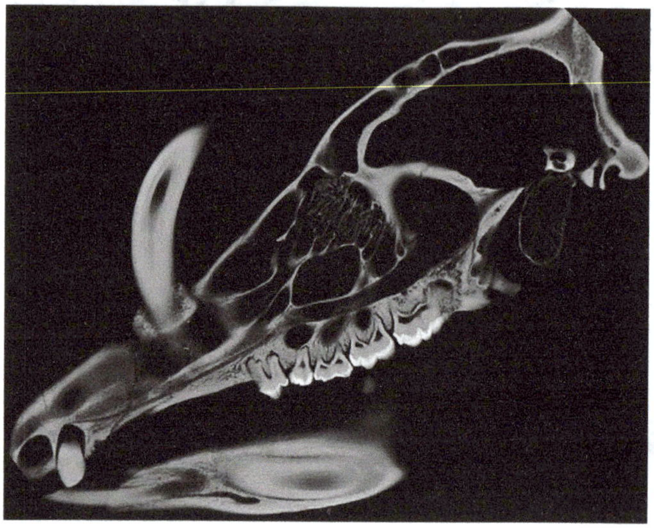

Figure 2.15 Sagittal ultra-high resolution image of a Babyrousa pig skull using a special collimator, small slice width and restricted scan field of view.

Patient positioning

For proper positioning, the laser lights of the scanner should be used and the patient aligned in height and symmetrically in all three planes. The table height should be adjusted so that the isocenter of the gantry is aligned with the body center and not to the area of interest in a peripheral area such as the spine. For head and spine imaging, a very precise alignment in the X-Y plane is crucial and worth the effort, even if multiplanar reconstruction can straighten out the patient virtually later. Radiolucent positional aids that hold the body part in a fixed orientation but allow positional adjustments are essential for this purpose. These can be commercially available troughs, blocks and Velcro bands, but in addition a range of polystyrene or other packing material can be helpful. Self-adhesive tape is also very useful. For thoracic and abdominal studies a roughly precise alignment is sufficient. For extremities, the degree of desired joint flexion needs to be considered. In very small animals, such as rodents and birds, other patient orientations can be used.

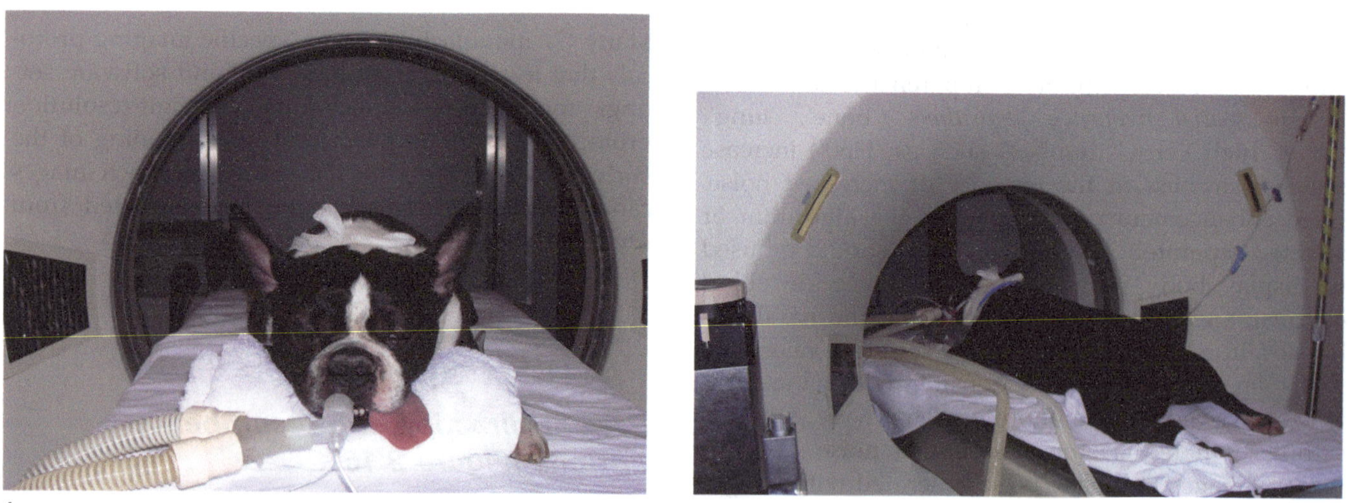

A B

Figure 2.16 (A) Optimally the anesthetic equipment does not cross the gantry, either in tail-first patient orientation with the equipment on the patient side or in head-first orientation with the equipment on the opposite side of the gantry. (B) In this set-up the anesthetic equipment crosses the gantry and will induce image artifacts.

Topogram preparation and selection

Before the CT scan, radiographic surveys are performed and used to plan the CT scan location. Manufacturers have different names for these views (topogram, scanogram, survey), and they can be obtained as dorsoventral, ventrodorsal, left or right lateral. For almost all applications two orthogonal topograms should be performed and used for planning. In some scanners (some Toshiba and Phillips units) only one topogram can be performed. The length and direction of the topogram are determined in the protocol and this must be anticipated in the patient set-up. The risk is that the topogram is too long or scans in a direction that pulls on the anesthetic equipment. To minimize this, it is advisable to start topograms in a position of maximum extension of the anesthetic equipment and program a table movement towards it during the topographic scan. At the end of the patient set-up the table position needs to be set to the zero position in most scanners.

Patient Restraint

Introduction

Due to the relatively high radiation dose, manual restraint by personnel is usually not an option for small animal CT, therefore a safe form of restraint for 1 to 20 min is required. With a CT table height of about 1 m, a fall from the table could have fatal consequences in a small animal patient and needs to be prevented.

General anesthesia

General gas inhalation anesthesia is the most common form of patient restraint for CT studies. It is extremely safe and controllable, provides a motionless patient and allows hyperventilation to induce apnea during thoracoabdominal CT studies. Injection anesthetic protocols, particularly with reversible agents, are gaining popularity for performing short CT studies of 1 to 10 min duration. This is particularly relevant for multislice CT, which allows for very quick scanning of the patient. The development of safe, short-term anesthetic protocols will play a major role for the full implementation of multislice CT in veterinary practice.

Alternative restraining options

Computed tomography imaging has been largely limited to patients under general anesthesia. Exceptions include very limited examinations performed under heavy sedation or on patients immobilized or unconscious due to pre-existing medical conditions. The immobility requirement was largely a function of prolonged imaging time and poor quality MPR images associated with single-slice CT systems. With the availability of 8- to 16-slice systems, isotropic imaging is possible and the quality of MPR images greatly improved. Imaging heads (i.e. nasal and bulla series) with isotropic systems no longer needs precise positioning because the original image set is not viewed, rather the reformatted transverse, dorsal and sagittal plane images form the basis of image analysis.

The challenges of restricting motion to make use of these additional features have been limiting. However, a new device attempts to take advantage of the typical behavior of ill cats to provide a clinically and image-supportive environment. Most dyspneic cats will preferably remain immobile with elbows abducted in sternal recumbency. Even open-mouth breathing cats have rapid, shallow breathing and rarely pant as violently as dyspneic canine patients. This natural behavior provides an opportunity to provide CT imaging of the head, neck and thorax with minimal movement in a physically restrictive device if appropriate clinically supportive aspects are addressed. The primary clinical supportive aspects are the need to provide oxygen and intravenous (IV) therapy without the build-up of inappropriate levels of moisture, heat and carbon dioxide.

The VetMouseTrap was designed to meet these and additional criteria (Table 2.1).

Table 2.1
Clinical and imaging criteria for patient restraint devices.

Clinical criteria	Imaging criteria
Oxygen access	No metal parts
Intravenous catheter access	No sharp edges
Non-heating	Symmetric in cross-section
Transparent to view patient	Movement restrictive
Low humidity	Low CT attenuation
Portable	Rugged
Quick patient removal	
Easily cleanable	
Symmetric end-to-end	
Secure closure	

The VetMouseTrap is made from transparent acrylic (Plexiglas), cut along the long axis into symmetrical top and bottom components (Figure 2.17). Additional 'leg' portions are glued to both ends to provide stability. Disk-shaped end plates seal the front and back of the bottom portion. A slit is cut into each disk end plate providing a notch for IV catheter lines entering either end of the device. The top portion has a half-circle-shaped disk end plate glued at a distance that provides an interlocking device when the top portion is placed on to the bottom portion. The slit in the top portion becomes a circular hole when the top portion is in place. This slit provides rapid placement or removal of the patient from the device without the need to disconnect the catheter from the source or patient. Holes in each bottom portion end-plate disk are appropriately

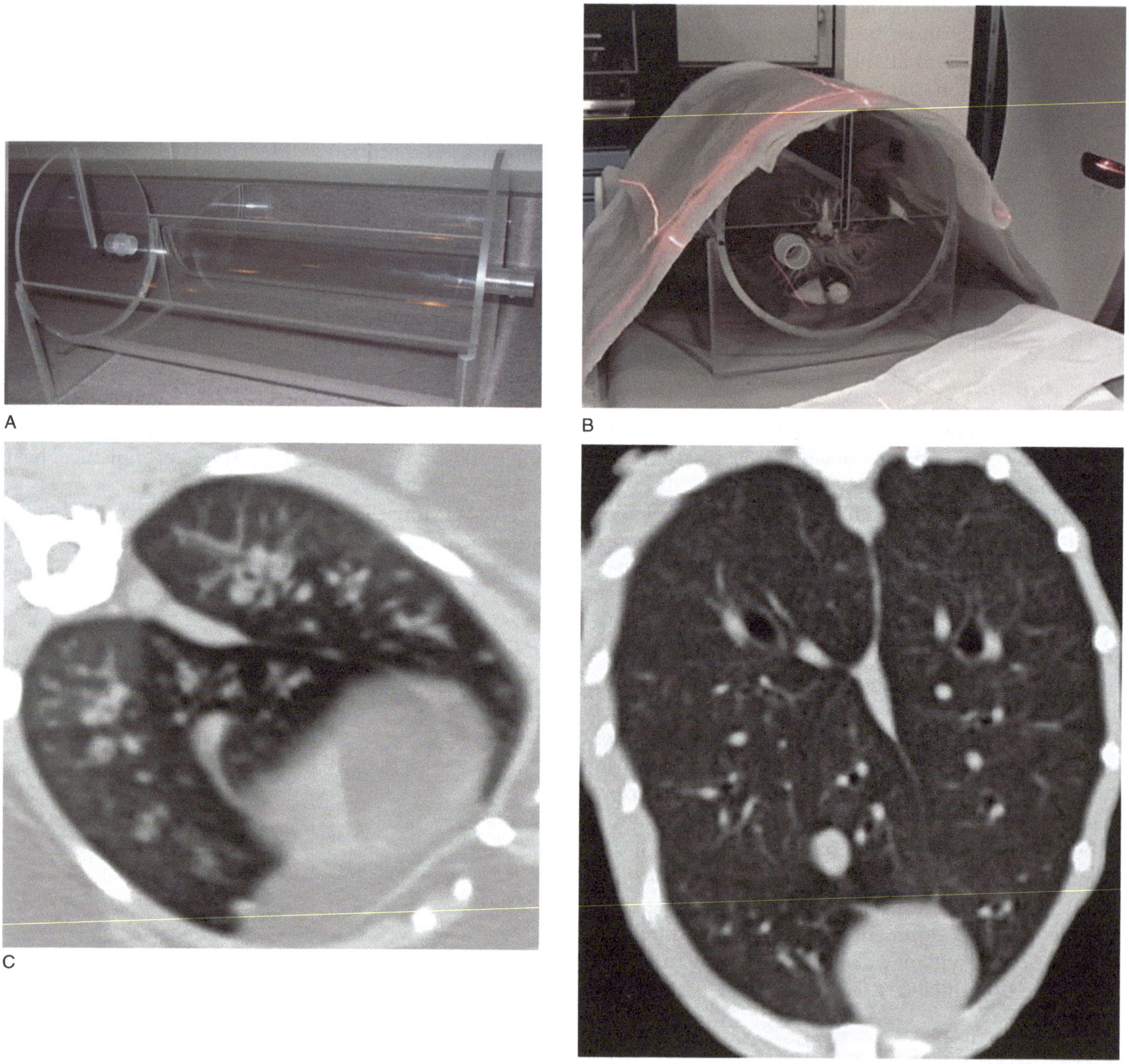

A B C D

Figure 2.17 (A) A VetMouseTrap device made of Plexiglas with ports for oxygen supply and exhaust. (B) A fully conscious cat positioned in a VetMouseTrap securely anchored to the CT table. (C) Originally acquired lung CT image, and (D) transverse plane reconstruction of the thorax using multiplanar reconstruction software.

sized for oxygen delivery or anesthesia tubing. Various sizes (both diameter and length) are available for different-sized patients.

The VetMouseTrap has been successfully integrated into an emergency medical practice using a 16-slice CT system and has shown improvements over conventional survey thoracic radiographs. Using the VetMouseTrap, survey CT imaging has provided improved head, upper airway, lung, pleural, mediastinal and diaphragm imaging. With IV iodinated contrast there is improved characterization of mass lesions, overall heart size evaluation, assessment of left ventricular wall thickness and identification of left atrial enlargement. Because the patients are not handled throughout the imaging, imaging is performed earlier in the clinical work-up than with radiographs.

Limitations of the device include its fixed size and the inability to totally restrict movement. While practical for many calm or ill canine patients, most dogs do not remain immobile within the device and continue to pace or dig. Dogs are also more prone to violent panting, making motion more of a limitation to head and chest imaging.

Additional devices should be developed to allow awake or minimally sedated imaging in dogs and cats. Current protocols exist for the imaging of sedated dogs and cats for portosystemic shunts, nasal disease and upper airway (virtual laryngoscopy and bronchoscopy) evaluation. Additional protocols and methodology may provide more advanced CT imaging, expanding the role of CT in clinical imaging.

Further Reading

Bushberg JT, Seibert JA, Leidholdt EM and Boone JM (2002) Computed tomography. In: Bushberg JT, Seibert JA, Leidholdt EM and Boone JM (eds) *The essential physics of medical imaging (2e)*, pp 327–72. Philadelphia, PA: Lippincott Williams & Wilkins.

Oliveira CR, Ranallo FN, Pijanowski GJ *et al.* (2011) The VetMouseTrap™: a device for computed tomographic imaging of the thorax of awake cats. *Vet Radiol Ultrasound* **52**: 41–52.

CHAPTER THREE

Principles of CT Image Interpretation

Jimmy Saunders and Tobias Schwarz

Basic CT Descriptive Terminology

Basic terminology

Terminology of location

- **Cranial (Cr)**: directed towards the cranium. It applies to the axial skeleton (head, neck, spine and pelvis) thorax, abdomen and the appendicular skeleton (proximal to the carpus/tarsus).
- **Caudal (Cd)**: directed towards the tail. It applies to the axial skeleton, thorax, abdomen and appendicular skeleton (proximal to the carpus/tarsus).
- **Distal (Di)**: directed away from the body. It applies to the appendicular skeleton.
- **Dorsal (D)**: directed towards the back for the axial skeleton, thorax and abdomen, and towards the head for the distal part of the appendicular skeleton (carpus/tarsus and distal extremities).
- **Lateral (L)**: directed away from the median plane towards the flank. It applies to the axial skeleton, thorax, abdomen, appendicular skeleton and tail.
- **Left (Le)**: directed to the left of the body. It applies to the axial skeleton, thorax and abdomen.
- **Medial (M)**: directed towards the median plane (midline). It applies to the axial skeleton, thorax, abdomen and appendicular skeleton.
- **Palmar (Pa)/Plantar (Pl)**: directed towards the tail. It applies to the distal appendicular skeleton (carpus/tarsus and distal extremities). The term 'palmar' is used for the forelimbs and 'plantar' for the hindlimbs.
- **Proximal (Pr)**: directed towards the body. It applies to the appendicular skeleton.
- **Right (Rt)**: directed to the right of the body. It applies to the axial skeleton, thorax and abdomen.
- **Rostral (R)**: directed towards the nose. It applies to the head.
- **Ventral (V)**: directed towards the belly. It applies to the axial skeleton, thorax and abdomen.

Terminology of direction

The terms *craniad, caudad, distad, dorsad, laterad, mediad, palmad, plantad, proximad, rostrad* and *ventrad* can be used to describe a direction or motion towards the equivalent location.

Scanning planes (Figures 3.1, 3.2 and 3.3)

The standard planes for scanning and reconstruction are:

- **transverse plane**
- **sagittal plane**
- **dorsal plane:** for the axial skeleton, thorax and abdomen
- **frontal plane:** for the appendicular skeleton. The plane cuts along the long axis of both front or hind limbs and is perpendicular to the transverse and sagittal planes.

The terms coronal and para-sagittal should not be used. The term dorsal should not be used for a plane for the appendicular skeleton. Equally, the term axial should not be used to avoid confusion with CT acquisition mode (axial versus helical).The term median may be used for a mid-sagittal plane.

Veterinary Computed Tomography, First Edition. Edited by Tobias Schwarz, Jimmy Saunders.

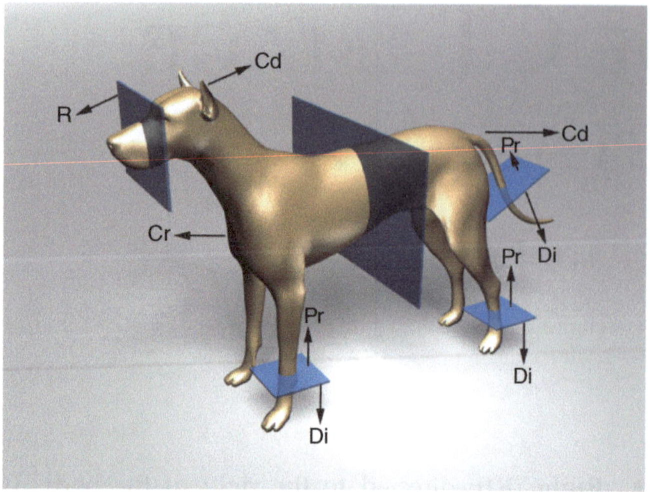

Figure 3.1 Terminology of location used in the transverse plane. Cd = caudal; Cr = cranial; Di = distal; Pr = proximal; R = rostral.

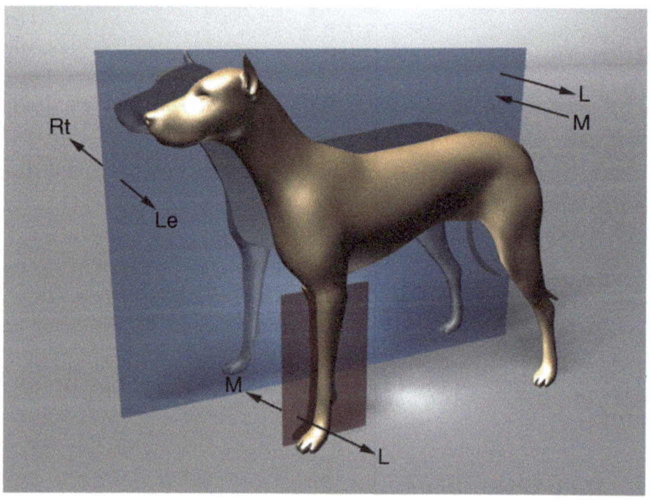

Figure 3.2 Terminology of location used in the sagittal plane. L = lateral; Le = left; M = medial; Rt = right.

Image orientation (Table 3.1, Figures 3.4, 3.5 and 3.6)

Transverse and frontal plane images of the right and left limb are viewed in a mirrored orientation. Recumbency-related orientation with the upper patient side at image top should only be used for viewing recumbency-relevant techniques (biopsy access) or pathology (relevant fluid–gas interfaces). Three-dimensionally reconstructed images should be oriented along the intended viewing perspective.

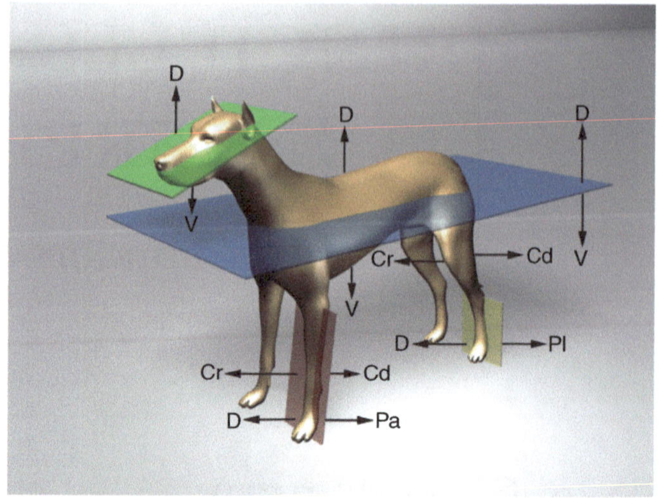

Figure 3.3 Terminology of location used in the dorsal (green and blue) and frontal (brown and yellow) planes. Cd = caudal; Cr = cranial; D = dorsal; Pa = palmar; Pl = plantar; V = ventral.

Image Labels

CT images come with a large amount of additional information displayed as text on the image periphery. It is useful to be familiar with the meaning of this displayed information. Usually the information is grouped into patient, institution and scanning parameters. Large amounts of text display can be distracting and the option of annotation-free display that most viewing software programs provide should be considered. For medical publications all text overlay should always be removed.

Tomographic Reconstruction: CT Numbers or Hounsfield Units

Computed tomography measures and computes the spatial distribution of the linear attenuation coefficient in each pixel, $\mu(x,y)$. However, this coefficient is a physical quantity, strongly dependent on the spectral energy used. Therefore it cannot be used as such for image interpretation and comparison. Instead these values are displayed relative to the attenuation of water. CT values characterize the linear attenuation coefficient of the tissue in each volume element relative to the attenuation value of water. The CT values of different tissues are therefore defined to be relatively stable and to a high degree independent of the

Table 3.1
Image orientation in the three planes.

Plane	Anatomical region	Orientation	Figure
Transverse	Thorax, abdomen, axial skeleton	• Patient right to image left • Most dorsal body part to image top	3.4A,B,C
Transverse	Appendicular skeleton	• Patient right to image left • Most cranial/dorsal extremity part to image top	3.4D,E
Dorsal	Thorax, abdomen, axial skeleton	• Patient right to image left • Most cranial/rostral body part to image top	3.5A,B
Frontal	Appendicular skeleton	• Patient right to image left • Most proximal extremity part to image top	3.5C
Sagittal	Thorax, abdomen, axial skeleton	• Most cranial/rostral body part to image left • Most dorsal body part to image top	3.6A,B
Sagittal	Appendicular skeleton	• Most cranial/dorsal extremity part to image left • Most proximal extremity part to image top	3.6C

X-ray spectrum. In honor of the inventor of CT, CT values (CT numbers) are specified in Hounsfield units (HU). The two terms can be used interchangeably. For an arbitrary tissue T with attenuation coefficient, the CT value is defined as:

$$\text{CT value} = (\mu_T - \mu_{water}) / \mu_{water} \cdot 1000 \text{ (HU)}.$$

On this scale, water has the value 0HU by definition. Air corresponds to a CT value of –1000HU since $\mu_T = \mu_{air} \cong 0$. In this book, the terms *dense* and *attenuating* are used interchangeably in combination with the terms *hypo-*, *iso-* or *hyper-* to describe normal or abnormal tissue density.

Digital Image Display: Windowing Techniques (Figures 2.14 and 4.16)

Once the CT images have been reconstructed, the image data must be conveyed to the radiologist for review and diagnosis. There are some basic post-processing techniques that are applied to all CT images.

CT images typically possess 12bits of gray scale, for a total of 4096 shades of gray. Electronic display devices such as computer monitors have the ability to display about 8bits (256 shades of gray). The human eye has a limited ability (30 to 90 shades of gray) and 6 to 8bits is considered sufficient for image display. In practice, the window level corresponds to brightness and the window width corresponds to contrast of a monitor display. Appropriate windowing is essential for diagnostic interpretation and should not be performed solely based on aesthetic criteria. The window level should be matched with the density level of the organ of interest. The window width needs to match the object contrast latitude. Structures with an inherently wide range of densities, such as the lungs or the nasal cavities (bone, soft tissue, air), need to be viewed with a wide window, and structures with a narrow contrast latitude (all soft tissues, in particular white/gray matter of the brain) need to be displayed with a narrow window width. Any assessment of intravenous contrast medium uptake in soft tissues also requires a narrow window setting for display. Image noise is most visible on narrow window settings. Since image noise depends on slice width and the selected image reconstruction algorithm, images acquired with certain settings require a specific windowing. Also the point spread effect needs to be considered when selecting the window width. Further particulars about windowing techniques are given in Chapter 2 in the section on image reconstruction algorithm and Chapter 4 in the section on point spread effect.

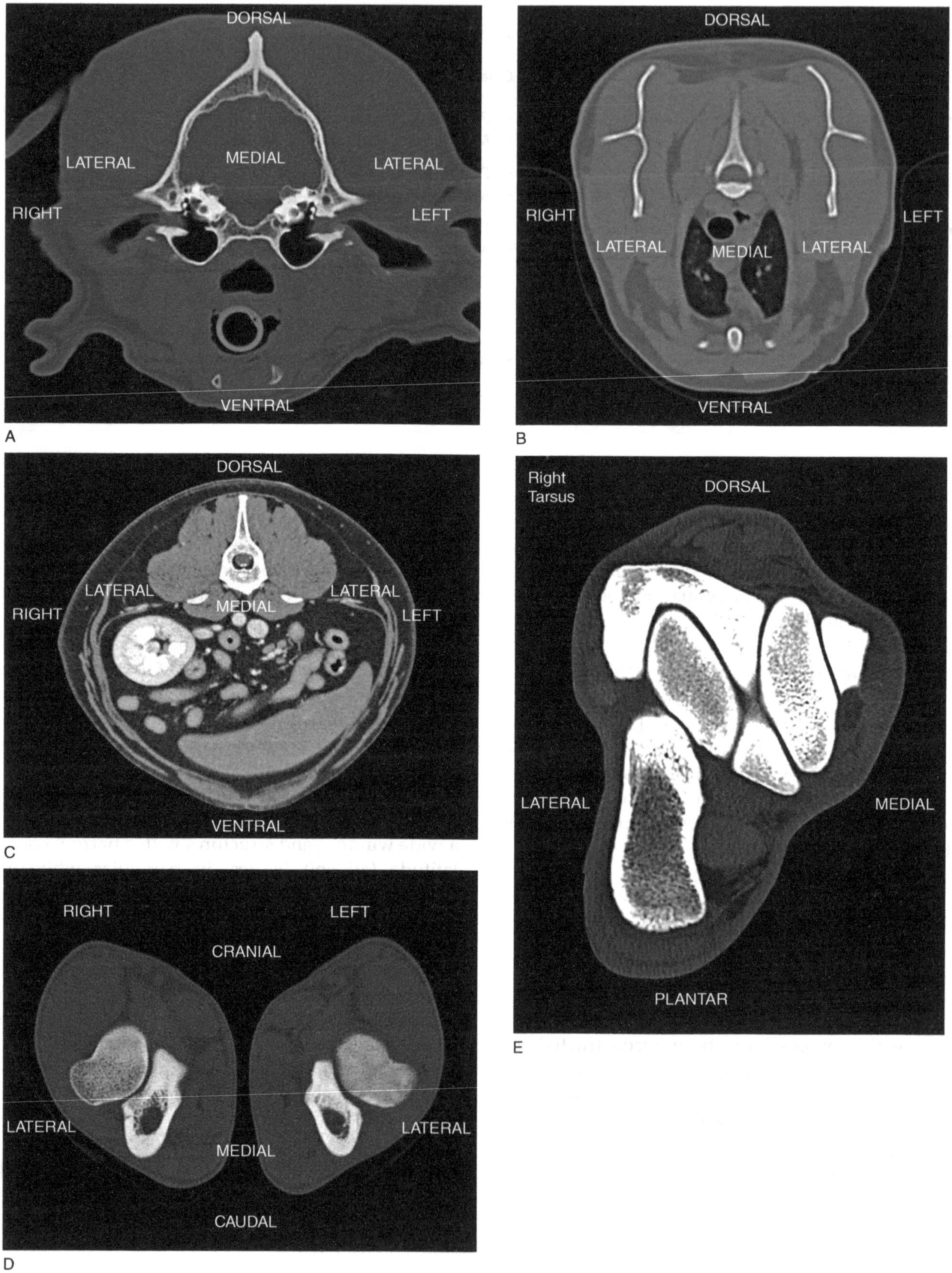

Figure 3.4 Transverse plane CT images. (A) Canine head, (B) feline thorax and spine, (C) canine abdomen and spine, (D) both canine elbows, (E) right equine tarsus.

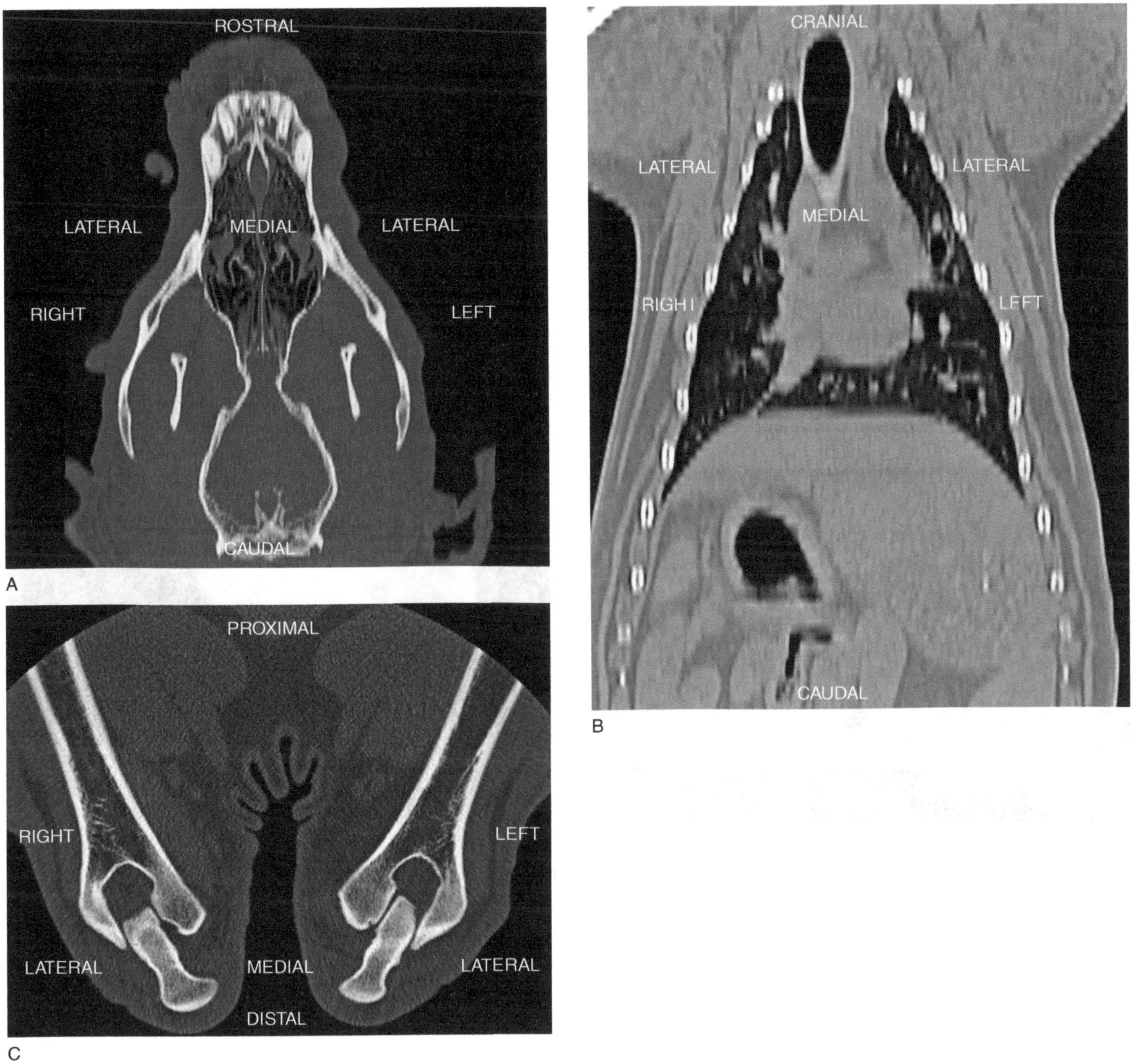

Figure 3.5 Dorsal and frontal plane CT images. (A) Canine head (dorsal), (B) canine thorax and cranial abdomen (dorsal), (C) both canine elbows (frontal).

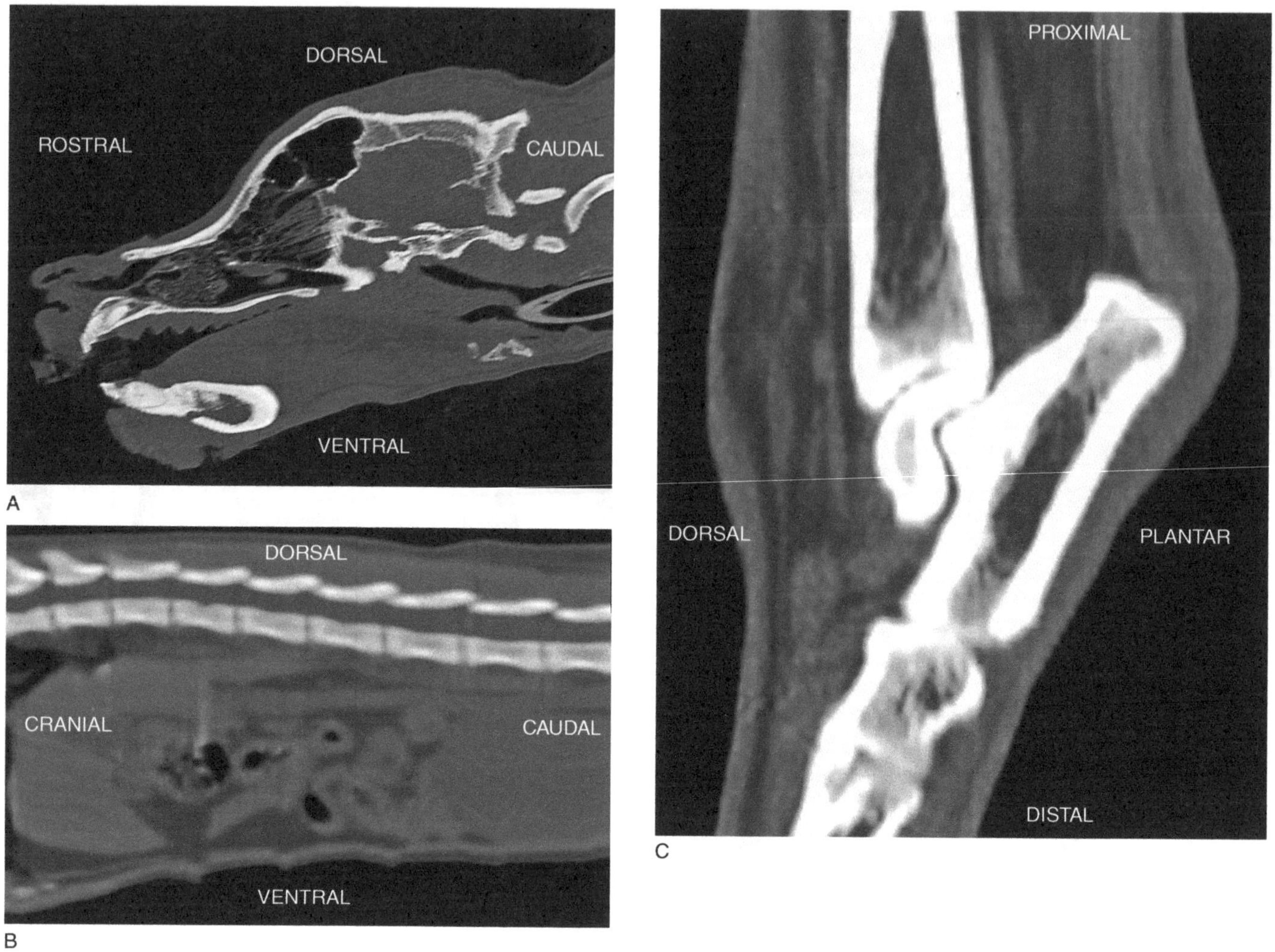

Figure 3.6 Sagittal plane CT images. (A) Canine head, (B) canine abdomen and spine, (C) canine tarsus.

CHAPTER FOUR

Artifacts in CT

Tobias Schwarz

Introduction

Artifacts are a common phenomenon in CT, which can result in severe image degradation. In veterinary practice some of those artifacts are particularly marked because of the variance in patient anatomy and the fact that older, less sophisticated CT units are frequently used. Most CT artifacts occur due to interactions between patient and machine, which are all subject to the laws of physics.

A diagnostic imaging artifact can be defined as an appearance on an image that is not representative of a structure within the patient. In CT, any discrepancy between the reconstructed values in the image and the true attenuation coefficient of the imaged object represents an artifact. If they are visible they are referred to as qualitative errors and if the image appears normal but CT attenuation measurements are incorrect these are quantitative errors. The concepts of *ray* and *view* are essential for the understanding of many CT artifacts. The X-ray intensity sampled by one detector to produce one signal represents a ray (synonym *projection*). The sum of the rays from all detectors sampled at a given moment represents one view. As the X-ray tube revolves around the patient, more views are taken. Most CT artifacts appear as streaks. This is due to the fact that a CT image is reconstructed as a matrix that is derived from multiple projections of attenuated X-rays. A matrix requires data input from *each* projection. Therefore any error or total attenuation that affects only one projection will be projected in those pixels that lay along the path of this projection. The filtered back projection, which is used for CT image reconstruction, will furthermore enhance streaks, since the error is filtered similarly to the true value. Also, the filtering and back projection involves some cancellations of negative and positive contributions along image lines. With perfect data, contributions from neighboring views combine to form the proper pixel reconstruction. Abruptly changing contributions from neighboring views, however, lead to incomplete cancellation, resulting in a streak. The CT reconstruction algorithm is extremely sensitive to any error that varies abruptly from ray to ray or view to view and is rather tolerant towards gradual changes. Widening of the display window can always reduce the visibility of streaks, but this is usually a very limited practical remedy, since narrow windowing is essential for evaluation of most soft tissue structures.

Geometrical Errors

Geometrical errors are caused by imperfect or inconsistent positioning of the x-ray beam in relation to the patient and geometrical inaccuracies that occur during the processing of image data. These errors are qualitative in nature.

Aliasing

Cause and appearance (Figures 4.1 and 4.2)

In diagnostic imaging *aliasing* refers to image artifacts caused by insufficient data sampling of a wave leading to data ambiguity. This principle is intuitively understandable in other imaging modalities such as ultrasound, where we are dealing with waves in the temporal domain. To understand aliasing in CT we have to grasp the concept of spatial frequency. Any object size can be expressed in its relation to the wavelength of a sine wave. Computation of data requires a sampling of discrete data and the frequency of sampling is essential for the true representation of the wave. A small object with a sharp edge must be expressed by a high-frequency wave (short wavelength) and proper representation of this wave requires

Veterinary Computed Tomography, First Edition. Edited by Tobias Schwarz, Jimmy Saunders.

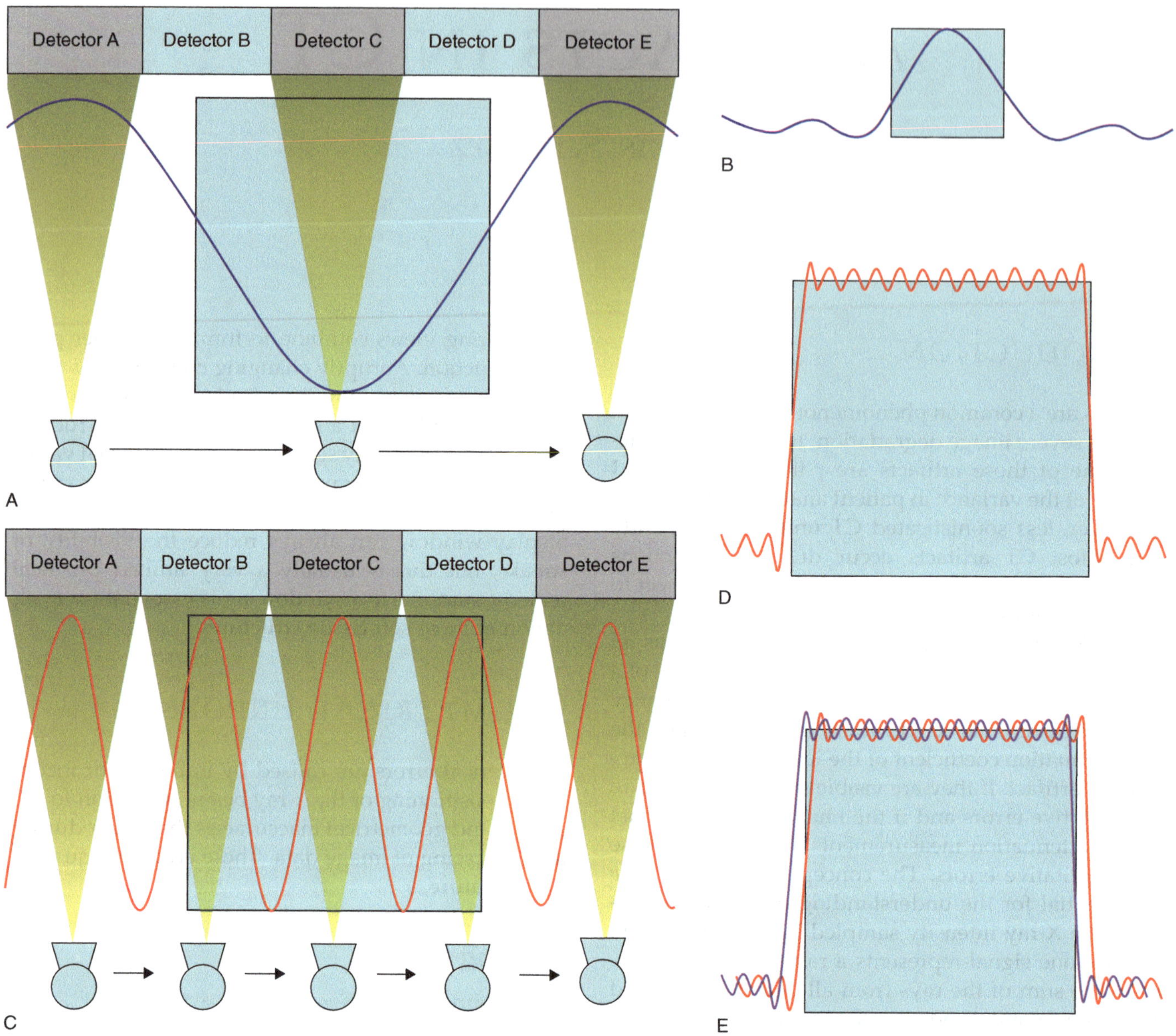

Figure 4.1 The concept of spatial frequency and aliasing can be illustrated on an imaginary CT scanner with a stationary set of detectors and a linearly moving, narrowly collimated X-ray tube exposing a cubic object. (A) If the X-ray tube emits radiation only at the level of every second detector, the sampling frequency (blue sinus wave) is low. (B) If the projectional attenuation data of this acquisition are expressed as a sinus wave (Fourier transformation) they will poorly represent the object with blurry margins, but no aliasing occurs. (C) If the X-ray tube emits radiation at each detector level once, the sampling frequency (red sinus wave) is higher. (D) With a higher sampling frequency, the geometrical shape of the object can be more accurately described mathematically in attenuation values expressed in sinus and cosinus waves. (E) However, the sharp edges of an object would require very high-frequency waveforms with at least two samples per detector width. If the sampling frequency is too low, then the exact location of the edge is ambiguous and could be expressed by two slightly shifted waveforms (red and pink sinus waves). Since in CT projections from all angles are used to create a matrix image, there is a random chance of mismatch of these data and a streak artifact occurs.

high-frequency sampling. The continuous wave of the pattern of X-ray intensities reaching the detector is sampled discretely by each detector to produce a set of signals representing one projection (= a ray). The entire array of detectors represents one view sample in the temporal domain. Consequently there are two types of aliasing: *ray aliasing* and *view aliasing*, which will be discussed separately.

Ray aliasing (synonym *projection aliasing*) occurs as a pattern of radial dark and bright streaks emanating

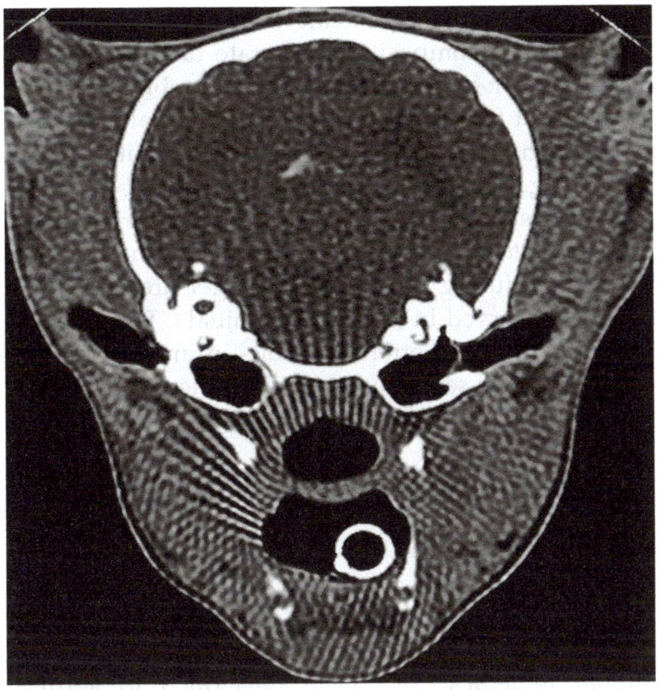

Figure 4.2 An example of ray aliasing with streaks emanating from the sharp margins of the tracheal tube and to a lesser degree the calvarium.

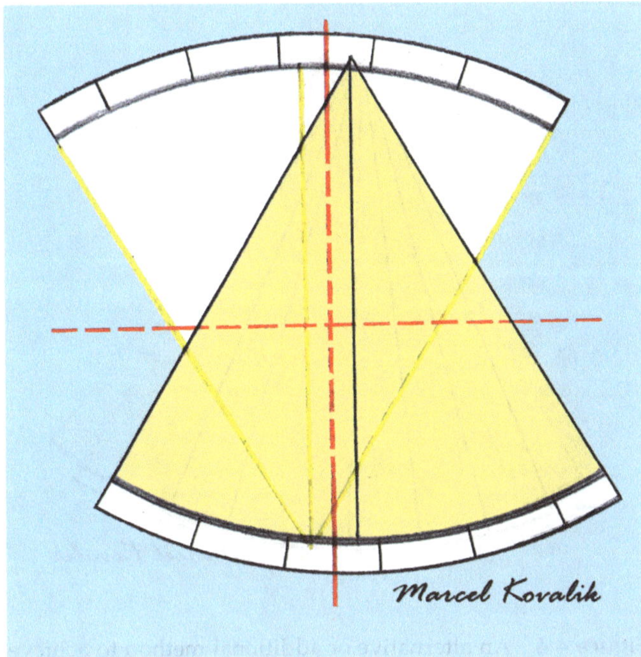

Figure 4.3 Illustration of a quarter-detector offset in a CT unit. Because the X-ray tube and detector array are offset by one-quarter of the detector width in the X-Y plane, the resulting eccentric motion of the tube/detector array pair results in the detector being sampled twice at two slightly different anatomic locations in the 0° and 180° position, fulfilling the Nyquist limit of two samples per detector width.

directly from a high-frequency object. Objects in the image cause the artifact, with sharp, well-defined edges that contain strong, high-frequency components, exceeding the Nyquist limit of the imaging system. The Nyquist theorem states that samples must not be further apart than two samples per wavelength, based on the highest-frequency component of the wave. The maximum frequency contained in a CT signal is limited by the focal spot size and the size of the detector cell. Mathematically it can be shown that at least two samples per detector width are necessary to prevent aliasing. In a fourth-generation CT scanner this is not problematic because each stationary detector receives a multitude of differently angled samples from the revolving X-ray tube. However, in a third-generation CT scanner the focal spot and detector cell are in a fixed relationship, as they both rotate around the patient. With only one sample per detector width, third-generation CT scanners would always undersample.

View aliasing (synonym *inter-view aliasing*) occurs as fine radial streaks in the image periphery only visible at a distance from highly attenuating objects. View aliasing is caused by an insufficient number of views per beam rotation. All ray samples at a given moment in time contribute to one view of an object, which will be represented as a streak in the image matrix composition. As the tube moves around the gantry more views are taken. The combined effect of many adjacent views will result in streak cancellation. If views are only taken at coarse intervals, this streak cancellation will be incomplete with an increasing degree in the image periphery.

Remedies (Figures 4.3 and 4.4)

The simplest way to suppress ray aliasing would be to increase the beam width, which would filter out high-frequency components. However, this would also sacrifice spatial resolution. Avoidance of high-frequency objects in the image should be attempted but is not always practical. In CT engineering two solutions have been applied to third-generation CT scanners. One is the so-called *quarter detector offset* (synonyms *quarter ray offset, quarter detector shift*) in which the center of rotation of the central beam is offset from the gantry isocenter by one quarter detector cell width. When the central detector is rotated 180° from the 0° starting point, a ray sample that is one-half detector width away from the original sample but otherwise similar will be collected, thereby gathering the required two samples per beam width. Another approach is the

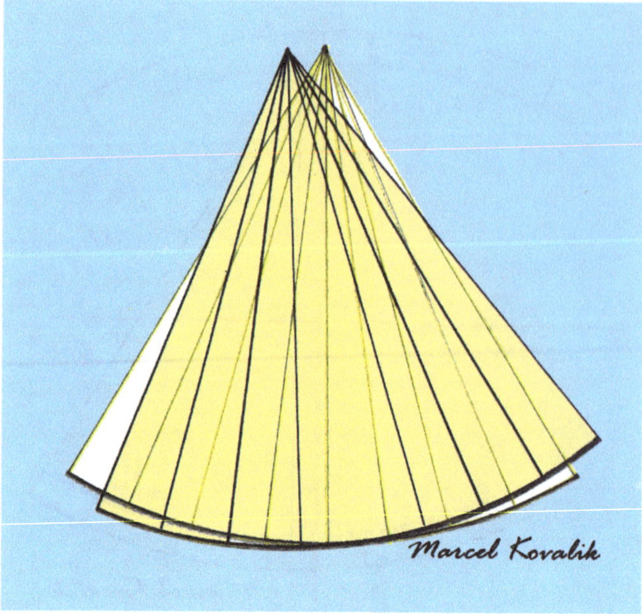

Figure 4.4 An alternative or additional method to achieve two samples per detector width in a third-generation CT scanner is the use of a dynamic focal spot, in which the focal spot is slightly shifted between views as the tube rotates around the patient.

so-called *dynamic focal spot* (synonym *focal spot wobble*), in which the X-ray focal spot is electrostatically or electromagnetically alternatively reflected between two positions of ray samples from consecutive views, thus achieving two samples per beam width.

Remedies against view aliasing include avoidance of high-density objects, which is often not practical, and increasing the number of views. This can be achieved in most CT units by simply increasing the tube rotation time. For example, in veterinary practice head scans are usually acquired under general anesthesia so that motion artifacts are negligible. Increasing the tube rotation time from 1 s to 2 s will reduce view aliasing without significantly increasing motion unsharpness.

Motion artifacts

Cause and appearance (Figure 4.5)

Motion artifacts in CT can occur as *streaks*, *blurring*, *ghosting* and *slice mismatch*. Commonly observed artifact-inducing motions include voluntary patient and respiratory movement, and involuntary cardiac and peristaltic motion. *Streaks* emanate from the edge of an abruptly moving and highly attenuating body part, whereas *blurring* occurs with more gradual motion patterns. In both cases the geometric inconsistencies between views violate a basic requirement of image matrix composition: accurate data input from *each* view. *Ghosting* describes a faint double margin of an object. It frequently occurs in abdominal CT, when a short abrupt movement occurs to a moderately attenuating organ margin, resulting in two object positions each consistent for a relatively large number of views. *Slice mismatch* occurs due to patient movement along the Z-axis during the scan of a larger area. It is frequently observed in cranial abdominal CT in patients with respiratory motion. It results in images that are spatially out of sequence, with doubling of some body parts and skipping of others.

Remedies

General comments

The problem of patient motion is a particular problem in veterinary patients because of their inherent uncooperativeness. Many different technological and operational remedies have been developed to address motion such as appropriate chemical patient restraint, adaptation of technical settings to minimize scan time and the use of motion correction software.

Technological remedies

Modern CT units have motion correction applications that can apply different technological solutions to patient motion. One obvious solution to the problem is to either scan or collect data from only a part of the tube revolution, a technique called *underscanning* (synonym *partial scan*). However, this also significantly decreases image resolution. The alternative technique is *overscanning*, where the tube rotates for about 400° for each image. This technique takes into account that the largest data discrepancy will be between the first and the last view because these are separated by the longest time span. By averaging the first few views with the repeated views, the averaged data of the first few views will be closer to the last projection. Another issue is the relationship between the motion direction and the tube position. Motion parallel to the central beam only minimally affects image quality, since the integration along the path does not change. For example, respiratory motion has its greatest amplitude along the Y-axis of the gantry for a patient in sternal or dorsal recumbence (up and down). Therefore, by starting thoracic scans with the tube in a 0° or 180° position, the first and the last views of the tube revolution, which are prone to the highest artifact magnitude, will be less affected and the overall motion artifact will be reduced. Scan modes for specific body parts in CT units often incorporate the optimal tube start position

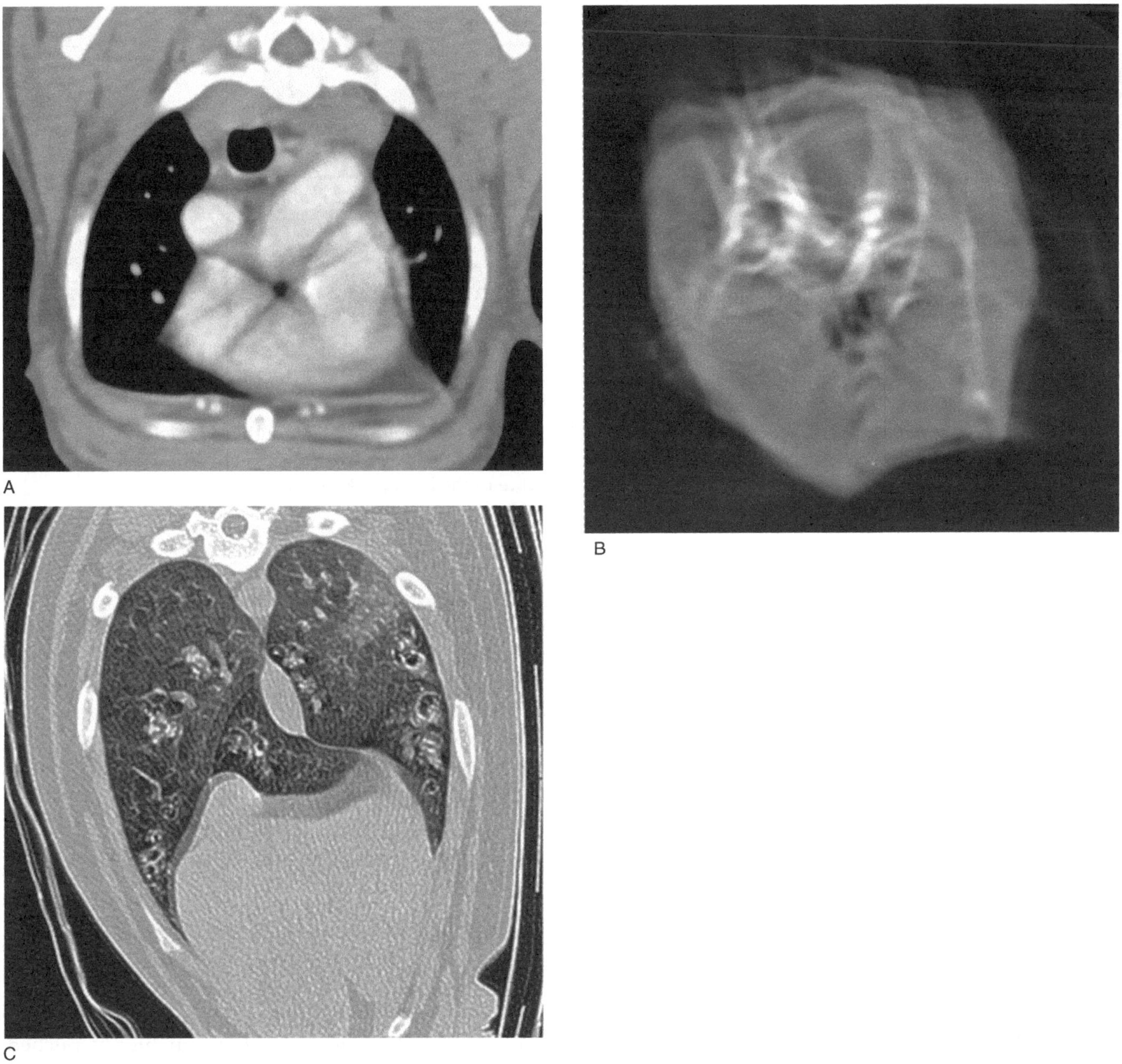

Figure 4.5 Motion artifacts in CT. (A) Streaks emanating from the heart base due to cardiac motion. (B) Blurring and streaks of a cat lifting its head during the scan. (C) Double lung margins, called ghost images, in a dog that is breathing during the scan.

and regional scanning protocols should therefore be planned within those scan modes. *Respiratory and cardiac gating* is a technique based on the fact that the time taken to acquire a complete set of projections is shorter than the entire cardiac or respiratory cycle. By acquiring the scan within the cycle period of minimal motion with the help of predictive algorithms, image quality can be improved. *Interleaved reconstructions* are another useful and simple technique to reduce the effect of motion. Helical CT acquires image data as a volume, which can be sliced at any interval. Although each image still represents a full tube rotation time span (such as 1 s), by reconstructing images at shorter intervals there will be a sufficient number of images that are exactly timed within the normal expiratory pause of a normally breathing animal and almost free of artifacts. Because of the lack of voluntary breath holding in animals, thoracic and abdominal CT examinations are a particular challenge in veterinary practice.

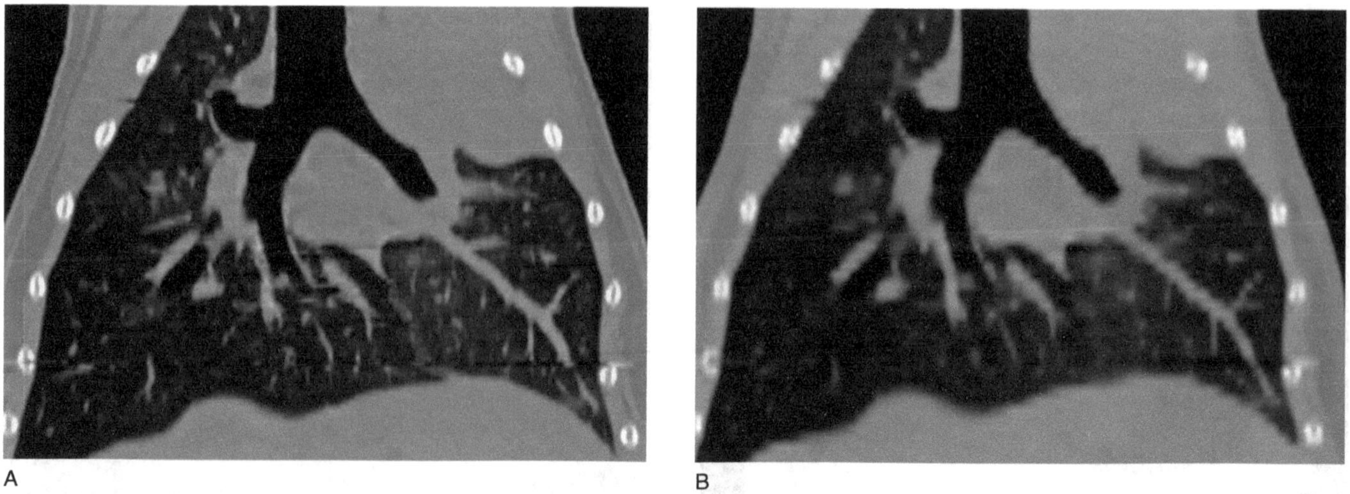

Figure 4.6 (A) Dorsal reconstruction of a thoracic CT scan obtained in a single-slice CT unit with a slice width of 1 mm and a pitch of 1. There is excellent image detail of lung and mediastinum. (B) Image from a repeat study with a pitch of 5 and otherwise identical settings. There is a noticeable image blur due to the high pitch factor.

Operational remedies

Minimizing scan time by using higher pitched helical CT settings is essential for motion artifact reduction in the thorax and cranial abdomen. General gas inhalation anesthesia allows induction of apnea in several ways.

- *Rigorous hyperventilation* prior to scanning with capnometer control. The CO_2 pressure should be less than 30 mm Hg in dogs and less than 25 mmHg in cats. This can then result in a 20 to 40 s period of apnea. There should be a minimal time delay (3 to 5 s) between the finish of hyperventilation and the start of the scan for not wasting the valuable apnea time span, but long enough for the anesthetist to safely leave the scanning room. A close co-ordination with the anesthetist and reduction to only essential personnel in the scanning room is essential to establish a safe and efficient protocol.
- *Bag-holding with the lungs inflated* with a long Bain breathing system, allowing the anesthetist to perform this maneuver protected from radiation behind a shield or in a different room. Extended lung inflation will reduce the cardiac output and this fact needs to be considered in patients with suspected cardiovascular diseases.
- *Drug-induced apnea* with neuromuscular blocking agents such as *atracurium*. The shortest-acting drugs last about 25 min, and the patient needs to be mechanically ventilated for this period under close supervision.

Thoracic and abdominal studies should always start at the level of the diaphragm and scan away from it. This way the area with the highest respiratory motion amplitude is scanned first, when the patient is still in respiratory pause. Spinal CT scans should always be acquired in dorsal recumbency so that the firmly anchored patient back does not move with the expanding thoracic bellows.

High pitch blurring (Figures 2.10 and 4.6)

Helical CT is a volume scanning procedure with the patient moving through the gantry and a continuously spinning X-ray tube. The image resolution of a helical CT scan depends on the chosen slice width and pitch (*see* Chapter 2). Image structures in highly pitched scans will appear blurred and indistinct. This artifact is the result of the non-planar geometry of helical image data requiring interpolation into planar image data sets. Interpolation is a weighted averaging of data from either side of the reconstruction plane with different weighting factors for each projection angle. By increasing pitch, the averaged data are sampled between more and more distant points within the scan volume, resulting in a loss of axial and azimuthal resolution. To avoid this blurring, the pitch should not exceed a value of 2 in a single-slice CT unit. In multislice CT, manufacturers often have pitches that are specifically matched to the detector selection and collimator pitch, and these should be used (*see* Chapter 2).

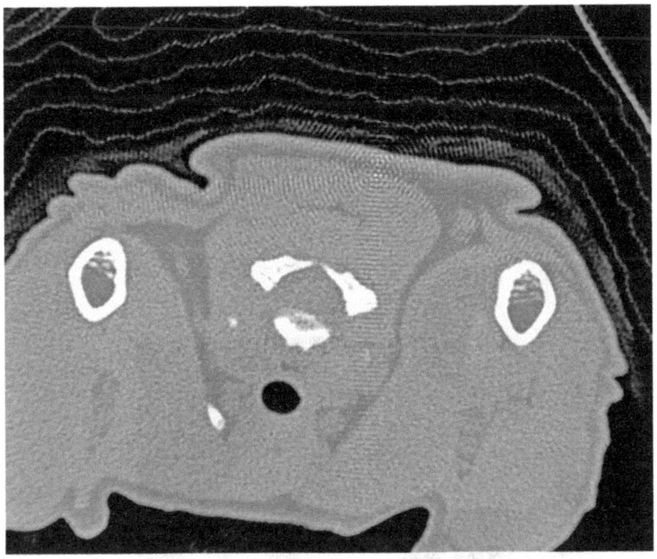

Figure 4.7 Windmill artifact with a 16-slice CT unit over a feline shoulder area. The distinct propeller-like pattern of lines over the image is due to the complex interpolation of image data in multislice CT.

Helical multislice CT artifacts

Windmill artifact (Figure 4.7)

The interpolation process from helical data with multiple detectors is complex. Data from different projections of different detectors are used and mapped together for the image formation. With higher pitches, these sections can become apparent as wedge-shaped compartments of the image, giving it the appearance of a propeller or windmill blades. This artifact is minimized by applying different types of image interpolation (z-filter interpolators) and using non-integer pitches in relation to the detector width.

Cone beam effect (Figure 4.8)

Due to the relatively small focal spot and relatively larger detector width, the X-ray beam in CT represents a wedge and not truly a slice. With multiple detectors this effect is even more accentuated and results in a cone-shaped beam form. A small lesion in the periphery of the scan field could then be partially included in one view and not in the opposing view. The conflicting density information leads to a streak formation. Cone beam effect is minimized by adapted forms of image reconstruction.

Stair step artifact (Figure 4.9)

Stair step-like margins of objects that are obliquely oriented along the Z-axis are commonly seen in multiplanar and three-dimensionally reformatted images created with wide slice collimation and interval. To remedy this effect collimation and increment should be less than the longitudinal dimension of the object. In helical CT units, interleaved slice reconstruction effectively minimizes this effect.

Zebra artifact (Figure 4.10)

Faint stripes parallel to the X-Y plane can be present in multiplanar and three-dimensionally reformatted CT images. Maximal intensity projections in particular are affected by this error. An algorithmic correction can be applied to remedy this artifact.

Partial volume effect

Cause and appearance (Figures 2.6, 2.9, 4.8 and 4.11–4.13)

The partial volume effect (synonym *volume averaging, partial volume averaging, partial volume artifact*) occurs if an object is only partially intruding, traversing obliquely or is smaller than the scanning plane. The effect can be noted as *blurring* of object margins, *erroneous attenuation measurements*, *pseudolesions* and *streaks*. Each detector generates its output signal based on its X-ray exposure, which is the result of the *mean* attenuation along the path of the beam. Plotting those attenuation measurements into a matrix and considering slice width, each volume element (voxel) represents a mean attenuation value for the used slice thickness. The true attenuation values of objects that are partially intruding, obliquely traversing or thinner than the slice width will be averaged with the attenuation values of neighboring structures. This averaging blurs sharp object margins, and if attenuation values are measured at such locations they will not be representative for either of the neighboring structures. A *pseudolesion* is the visible misrepresentation in such a case. Partial volume *streaks* are generated by the wedge-shaped geometry of the X-ray beam field as discussed in the section on cone beam effect. Partial volume is dependent on patient anatomy. Abrupt anatomical changes along the Z-axis will have the most dramatic partial volume effects.

Remedies

To remedy volume averaging it is essential to narrow the slice collimation as much as possible. This reduces the likelihood of partially intruding objects per se and

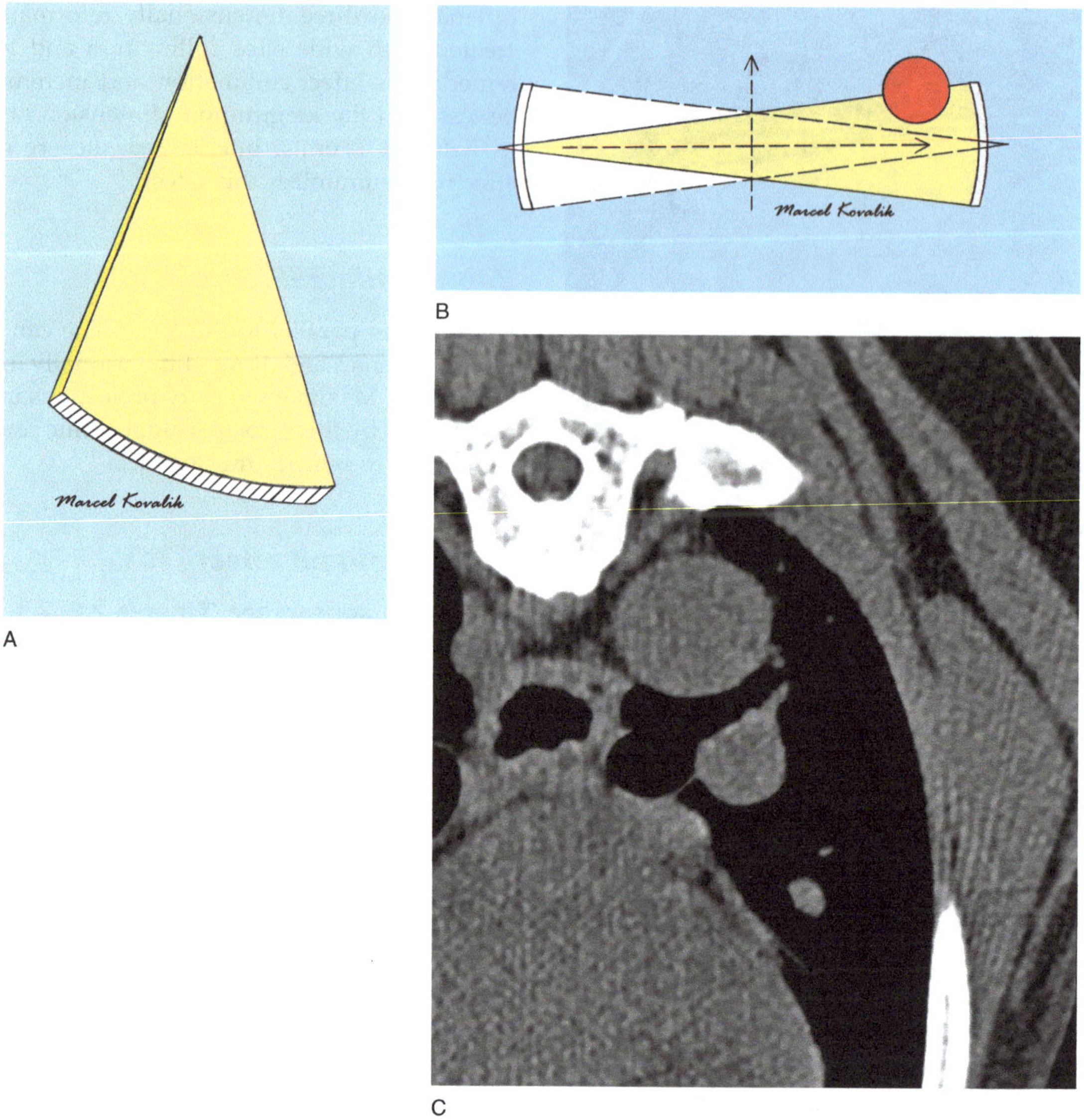

Figure 4.8 (A) The X-ray beam in a CT unit is not truly a slice, but a wedge. With multiple detectors, this shape more resembles a cone. (B) If an object (red circle) is located in the periphery of the scan field of view it may be partially included in one projection and not at all in the projection along the opposite direction. Contradictory density values for the same point cause a streak artifact, which can be seen with partial volume and cone beam truncation artifact. (C) Radiating streaks emanating from a canine rib in the lower right corner as a result of cone beam truncation and aliasing in a 16-slice CT unit.

also reduces the likelihood of streaks due to the narrower beam angle. There is a linear relationship between slice width and photon flux. Insufficient photon flux results in image noise, which is a major limitation of slice collimation in clinical practice Centering patients at the isocenter of the scanner reduces the likelihood of partial volume streaks. Changing patient positioning to avoid abrupt anatomical changes along the Z-axis should be considered but can be difficult to achieve.

Truncated view artifact (Figures 2.2 and 4.14)

This artifact (synonyms *out-of-field artifact, truncated projections, peripheral artifact*) is characterized by a bright rim along the image periphery and/or streaks originating from the area of structures outside the scan field of view (SFOV). The SFOV is the part of the gantry that is included in *each* view. Its size is limited by the length of the detector array, which dictates the

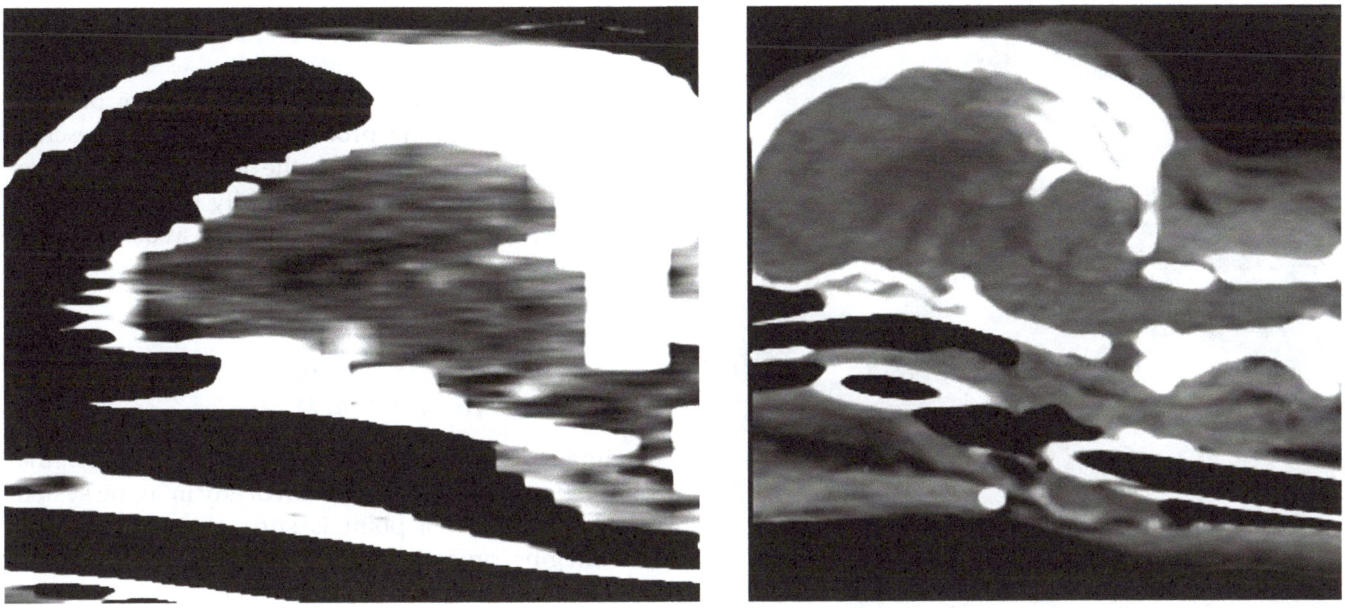

A B

Figure 4.9 (A) Sagittal reconstruction of a canine head obtained with 5 mm slice width and interval. All anatomic margins have a large step-like contour. (B) Sagittal reconstruction of another canine head with 1 mm slice width and interval has minimal stair step artifact.

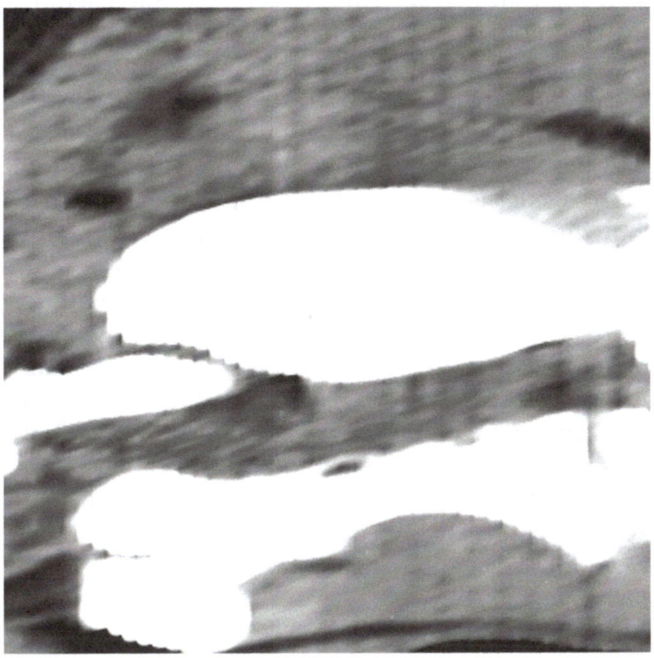

Figure 4.10 Sagittal CT image of the canine cranial cervical spine with vertically superimposed stripes, a so-called zebra artifact, caused by the helical image data interpolation.

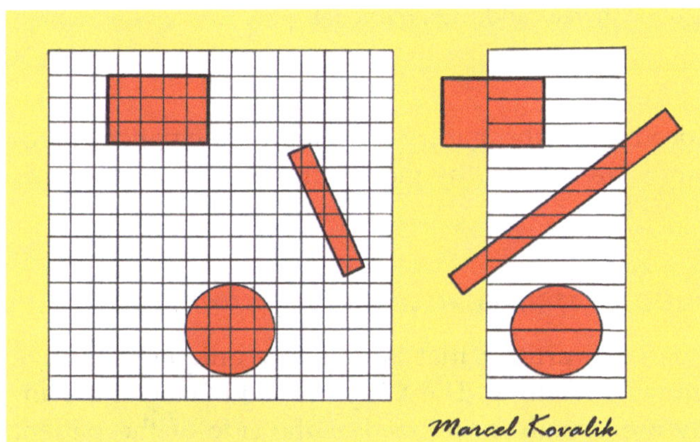

Figure 4.11 Display of three objects within a CT image on the left and their corresponding position when observing them from the perspective of the X-ray tube looking at the collimated detector cells on the right. The rectangular object on top protrudes partially into the width of three detectors. The thin rectangular object crosses obliquely through the scanning plane and causes volume averaging for seven detector cells. The round object is smaller than the slice width and causes partial volume for four detectors. Partial volume artifact will cause image blur in all three objects.

fan angle of the X-ray beam in a third-generation CT scanner. Structures outside the SFOV are attenuated only in some *truncated* views of the rotating X-ray beam, thus violating a basic assumption of the imaging system and resulting in streaks and misplaced attenuation values in the matrix. If the SFOV is elective it should always be chosen to exceed the patient diameter. Some CT scanners can enlarge their effective SFOV by an *asymmetric scanning* technique, where the periphery of the detector array is lined up with the

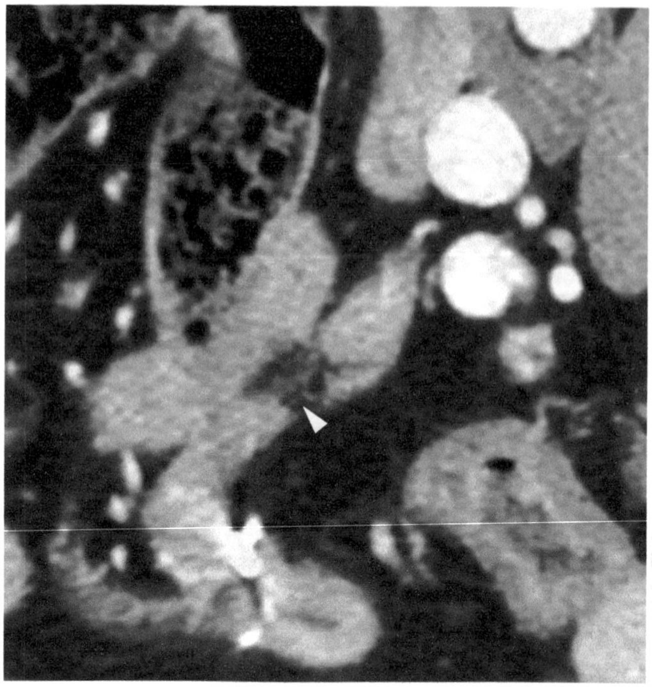

Figure 4.12 Close up of a CT image of the canine pancreas with a small hypodense area (arrowhead). This is a pseudolesion, the result of volume averaging between the edge of the pancreas and mesenteric fat.

isocenter of the gantry. Specific mathematical algorithms are applied by manufacturers to minimize this artifact.

Flipped gantry artifact (Figure 4.15)

This is an artifact that is probably unique to a large animal CT setting. The X-ray tube and detector assembly are usually positioned at the side of the patient table to ease access and minimize the necessary table motion. However, in CT units that are modified for standing horses, the patient is usually positioned from the opposite side of the gantry. Therefore the imaging plane is located far into the gantry, giving less access to the relevant anatomy in these already large animals. In some institutions the gantry was rotated and reinstalled. Apart from the fact that the side and direction designations are reversed, a detrimental artifact occurs on all multiplanar image reconstructions that manifests with thin streaks along the X-Y plane. This is related to the fact that each acquired image represents a slice with two sides on it. When rotating the gantry without further modifications, the slice order is reversed, but the internal orientation of each slice is not. A simple software adaptation is necessary to remedy this artifact.

Algorithm Distortions

These effects are not due to geometric or physical errors in the scanning process but are misrepresentation of density data due to the reconstruction algorithm. The effects are not necessarily undesirable, but their presence should be recognized to avoid misinterpretation of image data.

Point spread effect and blooming (Figures 4.16, 4.17, 4.18 and 4.22)

No image structure is absolutely faithful to the original object. Point spread is a function of any imaging system that defines how a point is spread out in space by the imaging process. In CT the point spread function is widest (making structures appear thicker) with a low-frequency algorithm protocol and low and narrow window settings. Such settings are commonly used for brain CT, making calvarial structures appear artificially thick. Objects appear artificially thin if imaged with a high-frequency algorithm and viewed with high and wide window settings. Such settings are commonly used in bone CT where bony walls may show artifactual bony thinning and lucencies. If the inherent object contrast is reduced, such as with a tympanic bulla filled with fluid instead of air, the spatial frequency of the object (bulla wall) decreases and the point spread is widened, showing an artifactual wall thickening, a finding that could lead to the misdiagnosis of bulla osteitis. A related artifact seen with highly concentrated contrast media is called *blooming*, where contrast-enhanced structures appear bigger than they really are (*see also* Chapter 5). Clinicians should be aware of this phenomenon and compare bone thickness only in similar image settings and with similar object contrast. The effect can be minimized by choosing a window width at least equal to the object contrast and a window level at the mean of object and background density.

Edge enhancement and rebound artifact (Figure 4.19)

Edge enhancement is a feature that can be applied in many CT units to make bony edges appear more sharp and dense. These edges will be surrounded by an artificial radiolucent halo (synonyms *rebound effect, Überschwinger effect*), which sometimes could be misinterpreted as a radiolucent lesion or prevent

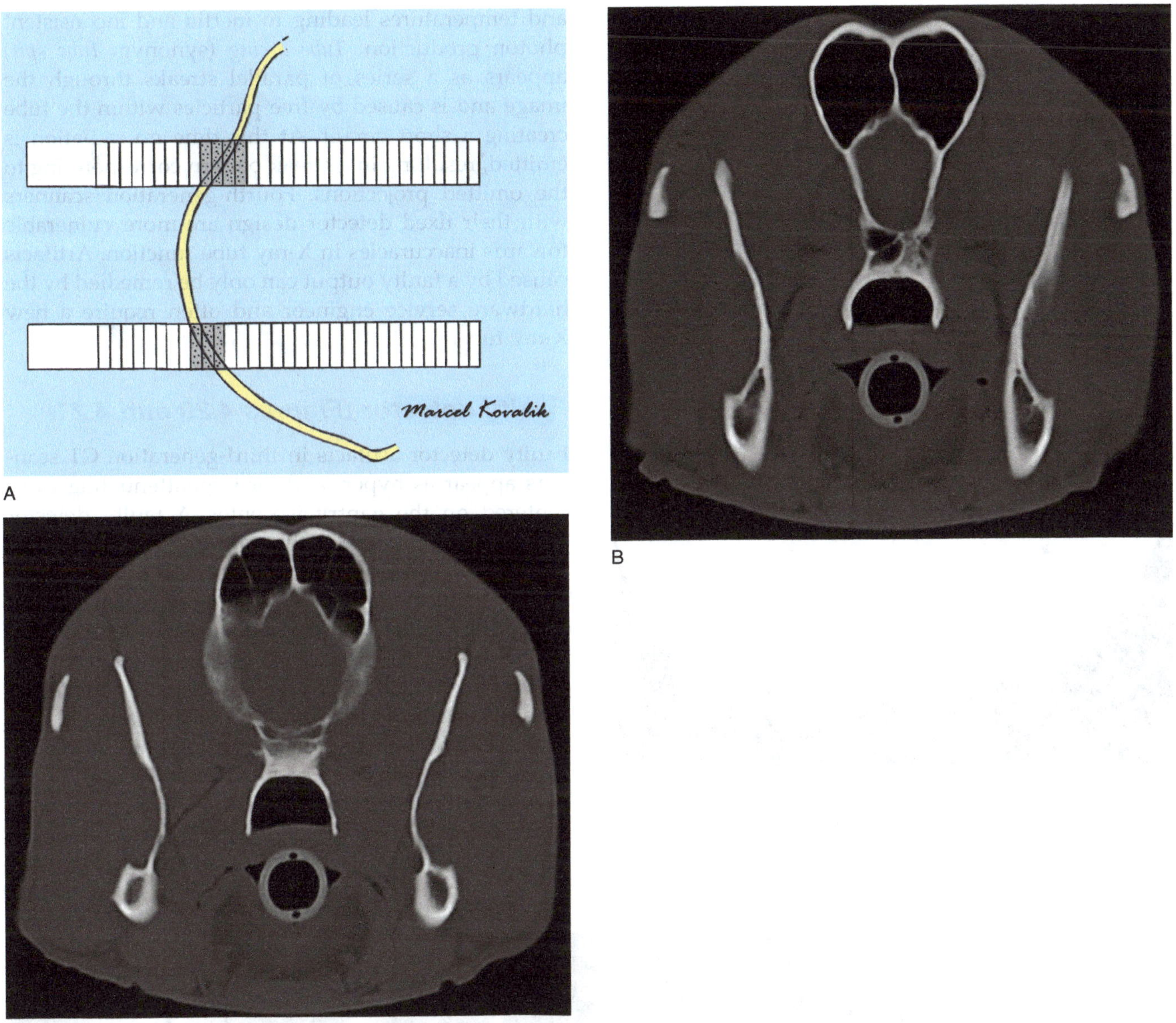

Figure 4.13 (A) Illustrated view of a canine skull half from dorsal (rostral on top) with two detector rows underneath. In the bottom detector row, three detectors are affected by partial volume (grayed). In the top detector row, four detectors are affected by partial volume, because the calvarium crosses the detector row in a more oblique orientation. This will result in more pronounced blur. (B) CT image at the level of the frontal lobe of the brain where the small calvarium is parallel to the Z plane, causing only moderate partial volume-related blurring. (C) Several millimeters caudally, the calvarium expands into the direction of the X-Y plane, causing a marked blurring of the bone margin.

interpretation of this area. This is clinically particularly relevant for interpretation of small and potential anatomic spaces such as the epidural, subdural and pleural space. It is therefore useful to document the use of edge enhancement and to select it only for appropriate purposes. In the absence of edge enhancement a phenomenon intrinsic to the physiology of human vision, the *Mach effect*, can create an illusion of similar nature. In this case the line should lose its virtual enhancement by blocking visualization of the adjacent structure.

Attenuation Measurement-Induced Artifacts

These artifacts are caused by errors made by producing or measuring the amount of X-ray beam attenuation.

Faulty output

Image blurring and streaks can be caused by off-focus radiation from within the X-ray tube, mechanical tube misalignment or tube rotor wobble. The shaft of the rotating anode is exposed to a very high rotation speed and temperatures leading to inertia and inconsistent photon production. *Tube arcing* (synonym *tube spit*) appears as a series of parallel streaks through the image and is caused by free particles within the tube creating a short circuit. At this time no radiation is emitted, resulting in a streak pattern corresponding to the omitted projections. Fourth-generation scanners with their fixed detector design are more vulnerable towards inaccuracies in X-ray tube function. Artifacts caused by a faulty output can only be remedied by the hardware service engineer and often require a new X-ray tube.

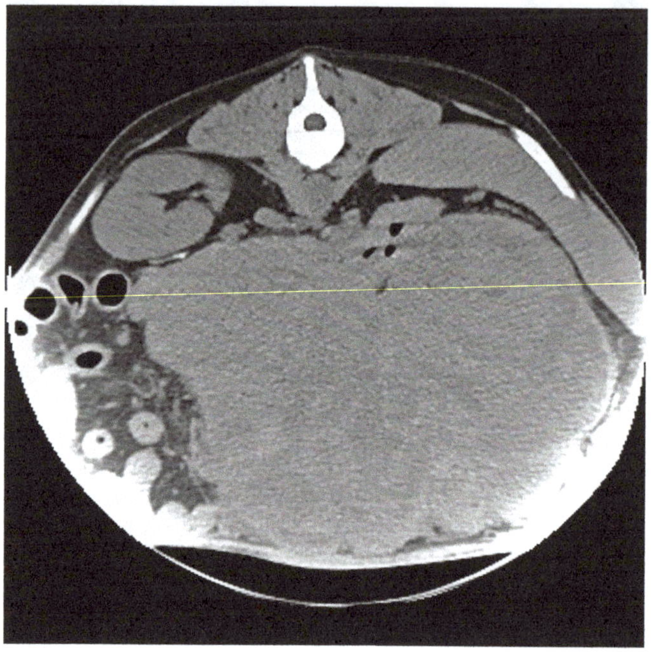

Figure 4.14 Truncated view artifact in a canine abdomen in which the ventral abdomen was not included in the scan field of view, resulting in a white rim in the lower image periphery.

Faulty detector (Figures 4.20 and 4.21)

Faulty detector artifacts in third-generation CT scanners appear as hyper- and/or hypoattenuating rings centered on the gantry isocenter. A faulty detector creates a ring because as the opposing X-ray tube and detector fan rotate around the patient, the ray between the tube and the faulty detector traces a tangent to a circle. The smaller the ring size, the more centrally the erroneous detector is located on the array. In fourth-generation CT units each view is defined by one detector and each X-ray tube position defines a ray of that view. Thus a single bad detector affects all projections of one view, which creates a much less severe and non-circular artifact. Erroneous detector output can have many reasons. Gas or solid-state detector elements emit a small thermally activated signal even without

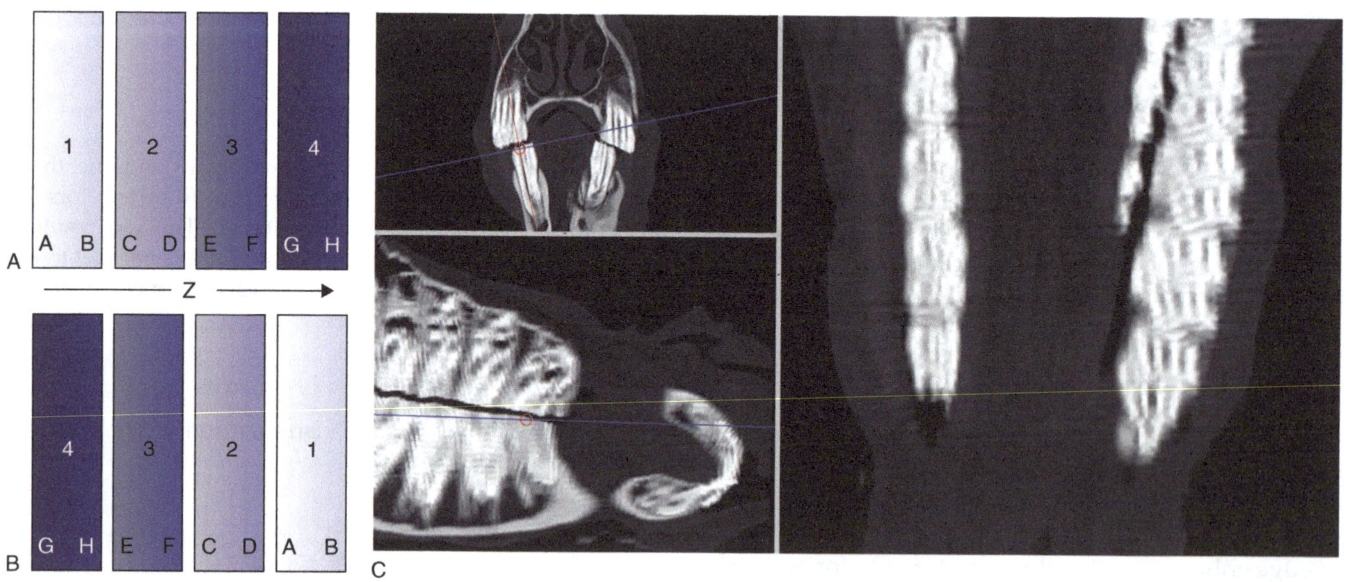

Figure 4.15 (A) Normal orientation of four consecutive image slices along the Z plane (Z). Each slice has two sides that are matched in orientation. (B) If the gantry is flipped without further modifications, the scanned images will align in the opposite order, resulting in normal transverse plane viewing, but they are not flipped themselves, resulting in mismatching slice sides. (C) Resulting streaks in the X-Y plane on orthogonal reconstructions of a horse head CT (image courtesy of Sarah Powell).

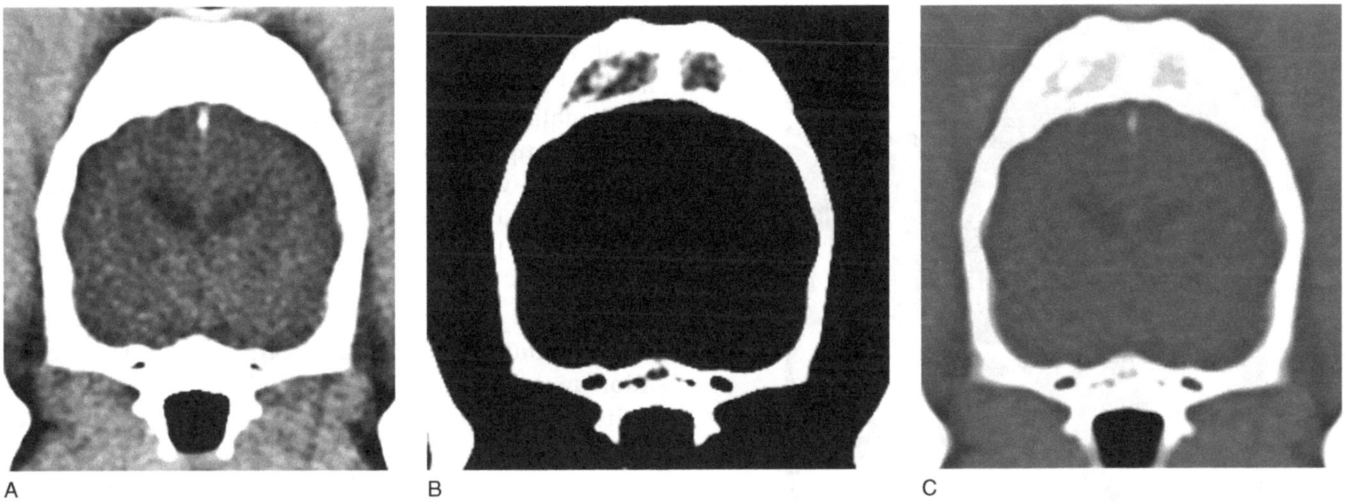

Figure 4.16 Apparent skull bone thickness of a dog with (A) 40/140 HU, (B) 400/140 HU and (C) 40/800 HU window level and width. Compared to (A), skull bones appear thinner if the window is set higher (B) or wider (C) due to a reduced point spread effect.

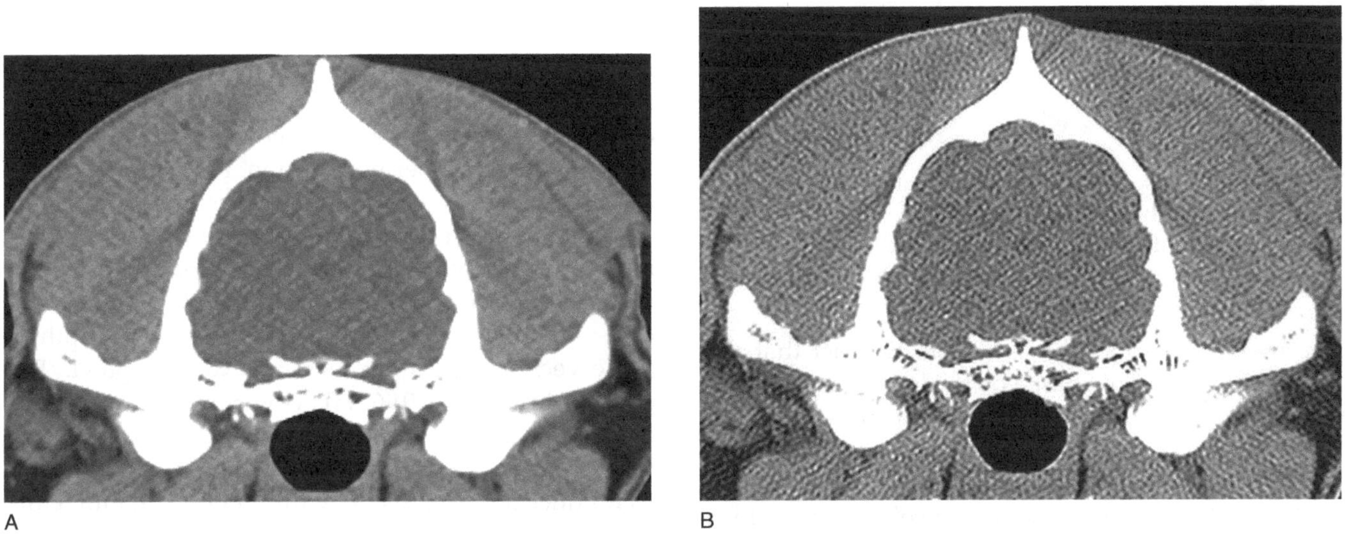

Figure 4.17 Apparent skull bone thickness of a dog with (A) a medium-frequency and (B) a high-frequency image reconstruction algorithm. Due to the edge-enhancing properties of the high-frequency reconstruction algorithm the skull appears thinner in (B).

any exposure to radiation (dark currents). The detector output signal must be proportional to the exposed radiation intensity to produce accurate attenuation measurements. With aging, however, the output linearity degrades. Many solid-state detectors also suffer from *hysteresis*, radiation damage induced by exposure history and recovery time. One important cause of hysteresis is *afterglow*, which refers to the tendency of scintillation crystals to emit light after irradiation has ceased. However, this does not result in a ring artifact but image distortion and loss of resolution, particularly noticeable at high tube rotation speed. To prevent detector-based artifacts, an air calibration of the CT unit should be performed daily and always after marked changes in room temperature have occurred. Before calling the service to fix a ring artifact it is worth recalibrating the CT unit, because in many instances this will eliminate the artifact.

Scatter

Scattered photons reduce image contrast and make structures appear/measure less dense than they really are by additively contributing to the exposure in conventional radiography and CT. In CT they also produce cupping and streaks because they introduce non-linear

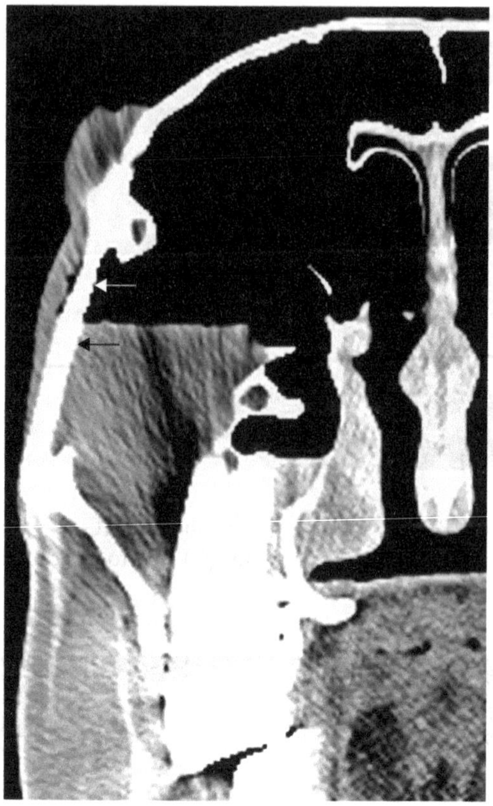

Figure 4.18 Close-up of a partially fluid-filled maxillary sinus in a horse. The lateral sinus wall appears thicker where bordered by fluid (black arrow) compared with air (white arrow). Low object contrast increases the point spread effect.

measurement errors. This is due to the fact that the attenuation values are based on the logarithm of radiation intensities, and adding the logarithm of scatter-based intensities results in an exponential rather than linear increase in value. Production of scattered photons is limited with pre-patient collimation, which restricts the exposed area of the patient. Scatter radiation reaching the detector can be effectively limited with post-patient collimation in a third-generation CT scanner similar to a grid in conventional radiology. Fourth-generation CT scanners are more prone to scatter artifacts because post-patient collimation is not possible. Software algorithms can be employed to reduce scatter-related artifacts.

High-density streaks

Cause and appearance (Figures 2.4 and 4.22)

Very dense matter like metals and minerals such as highly concentrated positive contrast media will create a starburst pattern of black and white streaks emanating from the object and widening towards the periphery (synonyms *metal or starburst artifact*). Such materials severely reduce X-ray transmission and may result in either no signal generated by the detector or a signal so small that it is below the recording range of the data processing system. As explained above, the matrix composition requires *some* data input from *each* projection. Otherwise a streak will be generated. Another visible side effect of zero-penetration can be an apparent hollow appearance of full-thickness high-density objects (see section below on beam hardening). High-density artifacts were particularly marked in older CT units in which the recording range for attenuation measurements was limited to 2000 Hounsfield units (HU). *Streaming* (synonym *streamlining)* consists of high-density streaks from vascular structures where non-enhanced and contrast-enhanced blood intertwines without homogeneously mixing. This is commonly seen in any vessel where contrast medium has not been passed through a capillary system yet.

Remedies (Figures 2.4 and 2.5)

Remedies include the removal or avoidance (patient positioning, gantry tilt) of high-density objects, the use of contrast media of lower concentration and increased kilovoltage for higher penetration. Reduction of high-density streaks is also the main reason why modern CT units have wider scales with up to 4096 HU. This limit, dictated by the 12-bit storage capacity of the CT values, has been furthermore expanded by an *extended CT scale technique* where the 12-bit storage depth is preserved but a scaling factor of 10 is applied. The extended range of 40 960 HU covers the density range of metallic implants (8000–20 000 HU) at the cost of lower contrast resolution. A variety of interpolation techniques has been used by different CT manufacturers to substitute the over-range values in attenuation profiles. Metals and minerals simultaneously also induce other artifacts such as beam hardening and partial volume.

Photon starvation (Figures 4.23 and 38.4A)

Serious streaking artifacts can occur in highly attenuating body parts such as the shoulders or thighs, where an insufficient number of photons reach the detector (synonym *noise-induced streaks*). When the X-ray beam is in a horizontal position the attenuation is greatest, resulting in a very noisy projection. The reconstruction process magnifies this noise, resulting in horizontal streaks. There is an inverse linear relationship between image noise and slice thickness. The effect of noise will therefore be more marked on thin-slice images. To remedy this situation a higher current is required and/

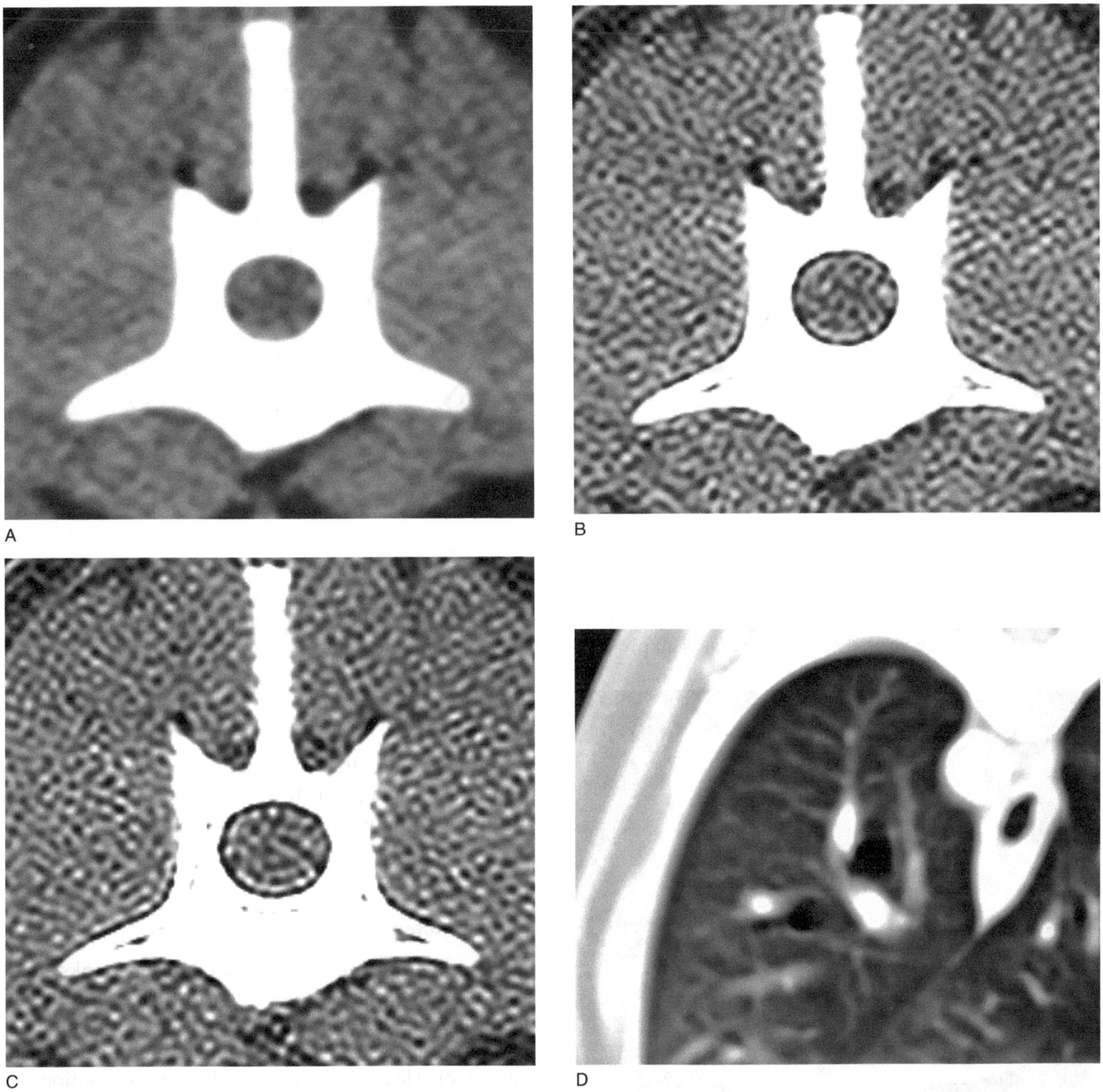

Figure 4.19 CT images with different image reconstruction algorithms and edge enhancement causing rebound artifact. (A) Canine lumbar spine CT reconstructed with a medium frequency algorithm ('detail', GE) which does not enhance edges. The content of the vertebral canal appears homogeneous, including its border with the vertebral wall. (B) High-frequency algorithm ('bone', GE) producing a black ring at the border between the vertebra and the content of the vertebral canal, and a white ring directly inside of it. This is a rebound artifact and should not be interpreted as a display of the epidural or subarachnoid space. (C) High-frequency algorithm with additional edge enhancement ('bone' and 'E2', GE) producing a more marked double rim. (D) Lung CT image demonstrating an artifactual black rim around the lungs mimicking a small pneumothorax.

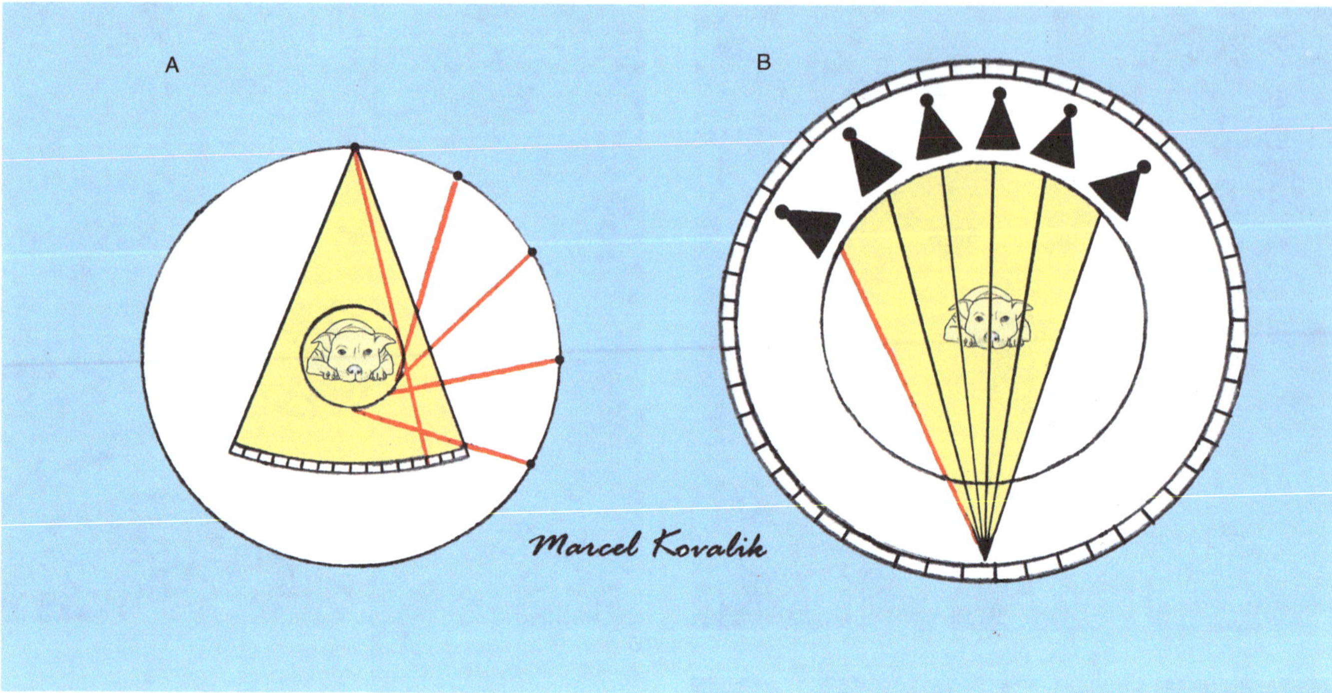

Figure 4.20 Effect of a faulty detector in different CT designs. (A) In a third-generation scanner, the ray between the tube and the faulty detector traces a tangent to a circle, creating a ring centered over the isocenter of the gantry. (B) In a fourth-generation scanner, a single bad detector affects all projections of one view and does not create a circular artifact.

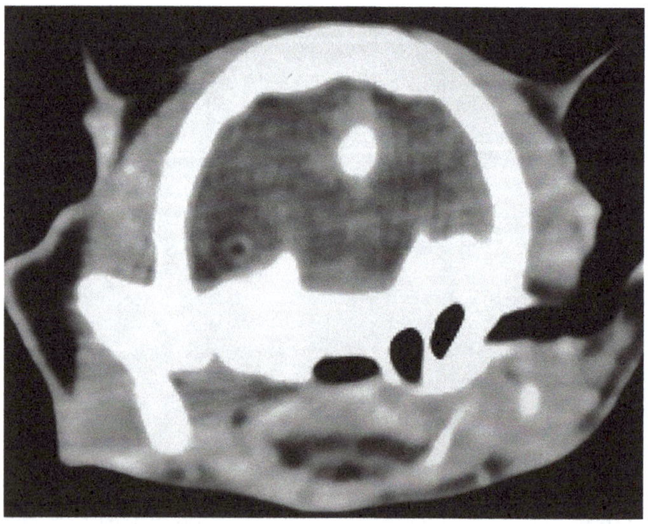

Figure 4.21 Small ring artifacts over the right temporal lobe of the brain in a cat.

or the slice thickness should be increased. To minimize patient exposure CT manufacturers have developed *automatic tube current modulation* to increase the current for selected projections only. Software correction algorithms can also be used. Careful and creative patient positioning is essential to combat those artifacts, such as by placing extremities out of the scanning plane for imaging studies of the trunk or bending the head for extremity imaging.

Energy Spectrum Effects

These are artifacts that arise from the inadequate measurement of changes in the energy spectrum of polychromatic radiation during patient transmission.

Beam hardening

Appearance and cause (Figure 4.24)

Beam hardening appears as dark bands or streaks adjacent to highly attenuating structures. It is particularly prominent in the brainstem and cerebellum between the temporal bones, where it is also called *interpetrosal lucency* or *Hounsfield bar*. Another manifestation of beam hardening is called *cupping*, where thick, dense objects, such as the head, can appear artificially radiolucent centrally. Beam hardening is caused by selective resorption of low-energy photons from the polychromatic X-ray beam by highly attenuating dense structures. In a thick, round, homogeneously dense object, the X-ray beam is continuously hardened as it penetrates the object from any angle during the X-ray tube rotation. Beams that only tangentially penetrate the object will be less hardened. Putting all attenuation measurements into a matrix will result in an object the peripheral density of which was derived from attenuation values of minimally and maximally hardened

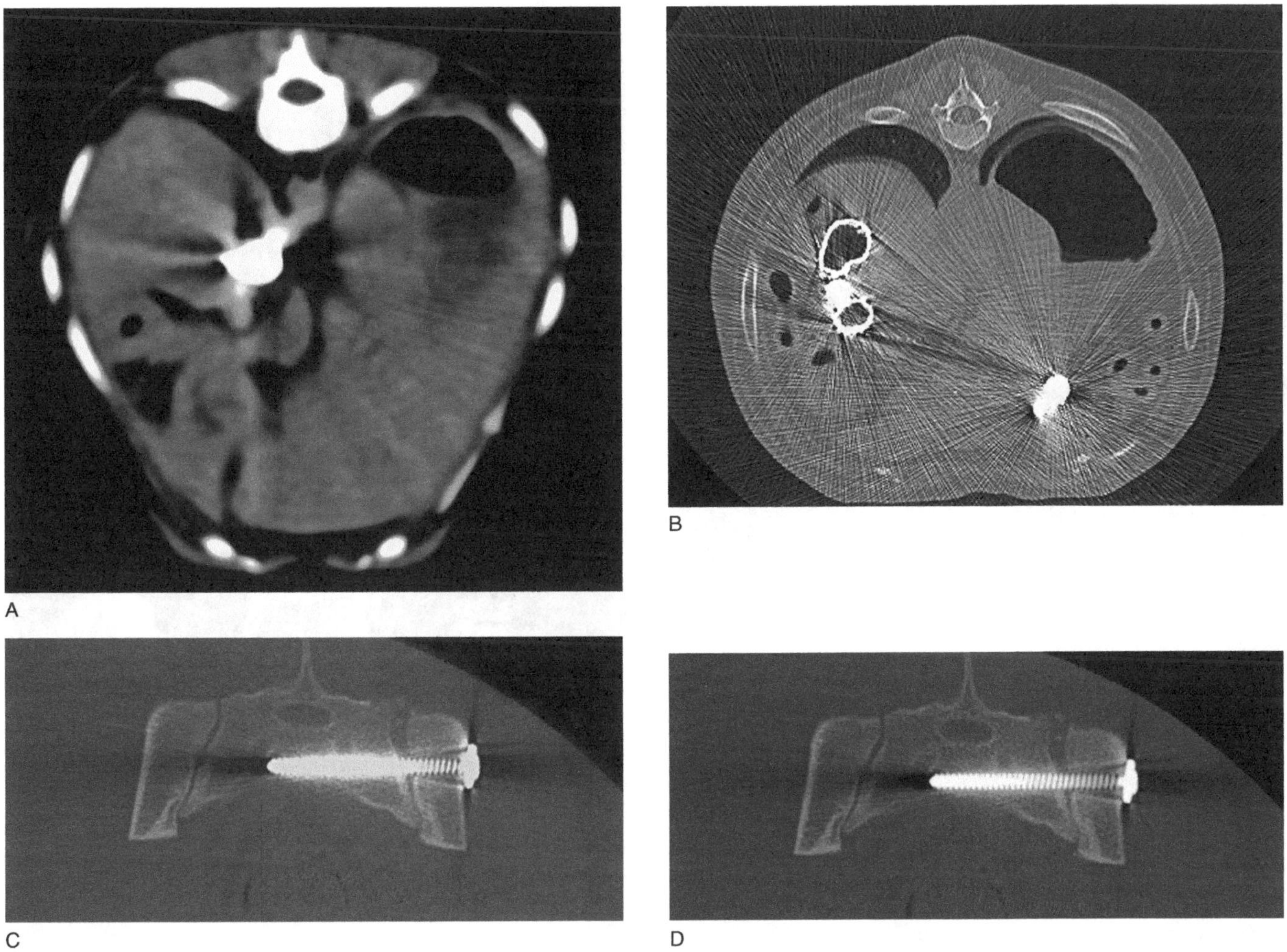

Figure 4.22 (A) High-density streak artifact and blooming emanating from the hepatic caudal vena cava due to injection via the saphenous vein creating only limited hemodilution of the iodinated contrast medium. (B) Streak artifacts emanating from different parts of the colon due to residual barium content after a gastrointestinal contrast study. (C) Streak artifacts and blooming emanating from the lag screw placed through the sacroiliac joint of a dog. (D) Reconstruction with an extended CT scale reduces the artifact magnitude.

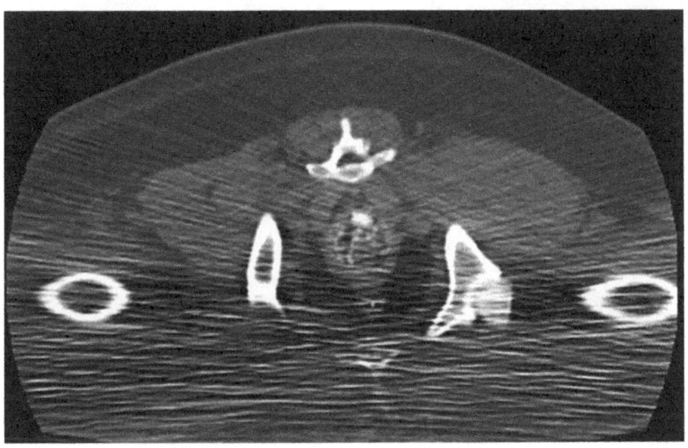

Figure 4.23 Photon starvation in a canine pelvis where the hind limbs have not been extended backwards. The selected mAs provides insufficient photon density only along the X-axis where the thighs contribute to additional patient thickness, resulting in horizontal streaks.

beams, whereas the object center density was only created by maximally hardened beams, making it appear artificially radiolucent. In other object shapes, beam hardening will create a streak, because of the attenuation value inconsistencies between differently angled views for the same pixel. Because beam hardening is responsible for neglect of tissue attenuation, it always makes affected areas darker than they should appear.

Remedies (Figure 4.25)

Beam hardening artifacts can be reduced by pre-patient beam filtration. In CT, bow-tie filters are used. The name derives from the cross-sectional profile of these filters, which is similar to the shape of a bow tie. Their purpose is to minimize cupping, by adding filtration

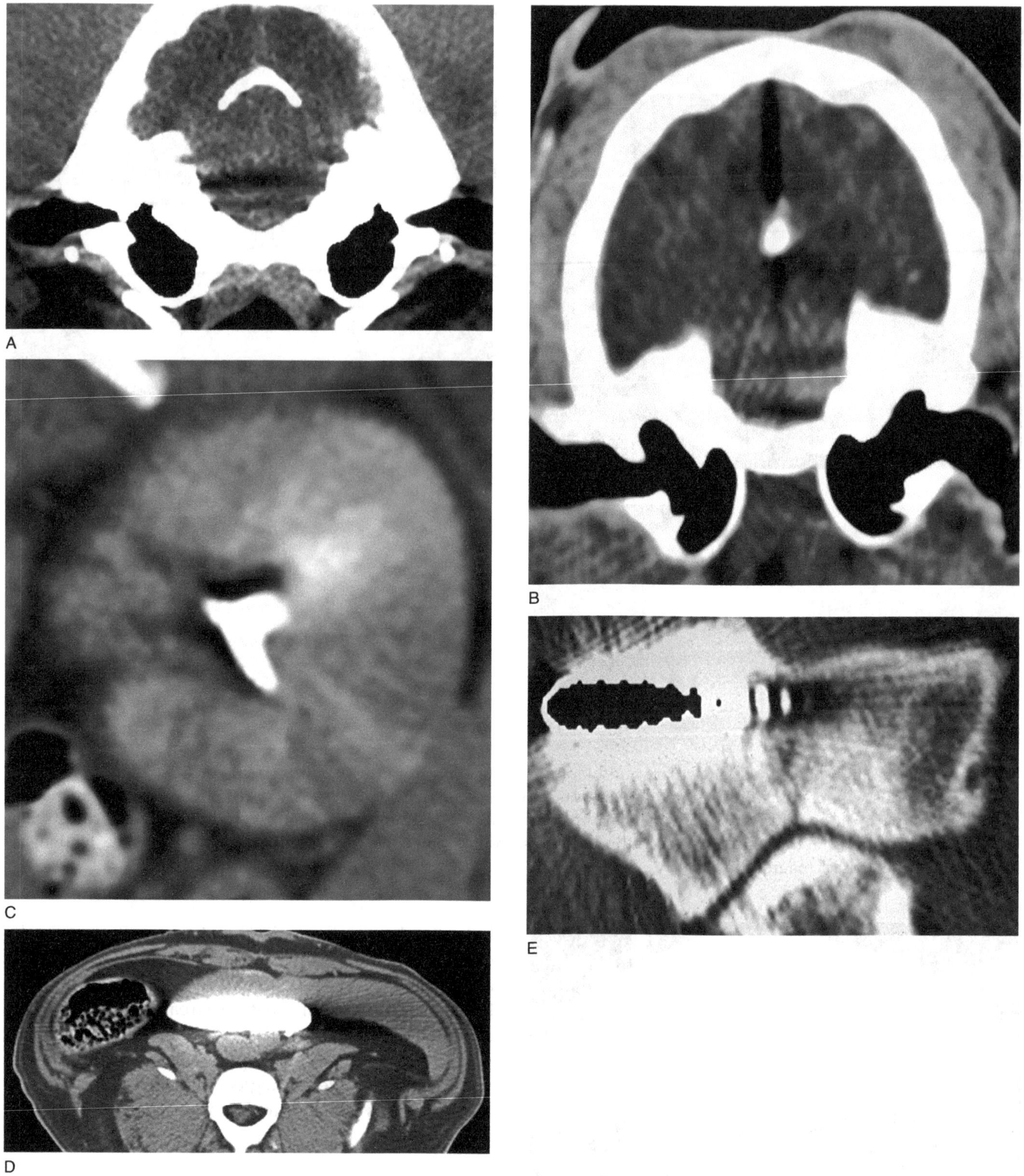

Figure 4.24 Different manifestations of beam hardening in CT. (A) Classical interpetrosal lucency in the caudal fossa of a dog brain between the petrous temporal bones (horizontal black streaks). (B) Between the tentorium cerebelli and the dorsal calvarium in a cat (vertical black streak). (C) Radiolucent halo around the contrast-enhanced renal pelvis. (D) Lateral to a contrast-medium enhanced urinary bladder in a dog (black horizontal streaks). (E) The ultimate form of cupping with zero penetration of X-ray beams through this metallic lag screw in a canine elbow, giving it an artificially hollow appearance.

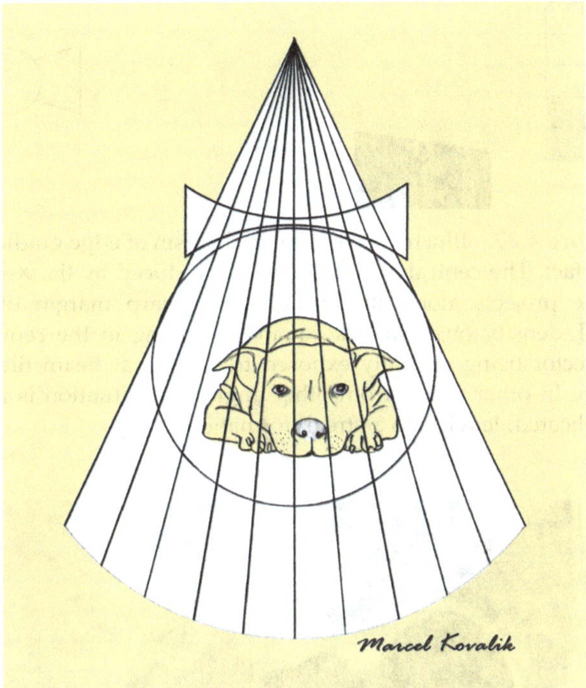

Figure 4.25 Illustration of a bow-tie filter in CT. The double concave shape of the filter compensates for the convex body shape of the patient, resulting in a homogeneous filtration of low energy photons throughout all parts of the patient anatomy. These filters are matched to human body parts and are not optimized for animals.

to peripheral beams. The shape and size of these filters is customized for different human body parts, which explains their limited effectiveness in animals of various sizes and shapes. The selection of a body region, which is usually required prior to scanning, may already incorporate the selection of a filter. Selecting the scan field of view may also be associated with filter selection. *Beam hardening is independent of slice thickness.* It cannot be completely remedied in clinical circumstances but it can be reduced by software using an iterative correction algorithm. Optimal filtration should be used by applying the appropriate SFOV and body region. Avoidance of highly attenuating structures by removing high-density objects, changing patient positioning and gantry tilt should always be explored.

Non-linear partial volume effect (Figure 4.26)

Non-linear partial volume artifacts appear as streaks emanating from high-density objects with abrupt margins along the Z-axis of the scanner, such as the petrous temporal bone. The petrous temporal bone is the densest bone of the body and has many bony protuberances that can partially protrude into the

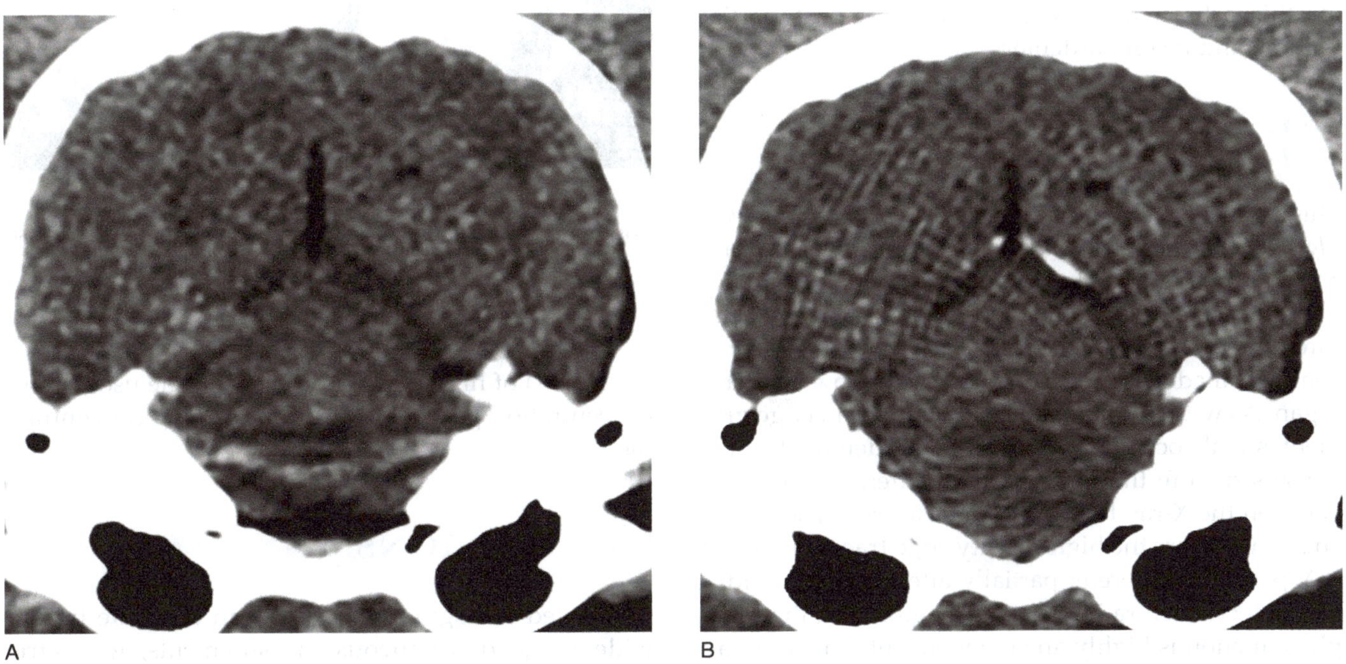

Figure 4.26 (A) Conventionally acquired CT image of the caudal fossa of a canine head with 5 mm slice width in a single-slice CT with mainly hypoattenuating streaks between the petrous temporal bones (horizontal) and between the tentorium cerebelli and the dorsal calvarium (vertical). (B) Image with 5 mm section thickness reformatted from the raw data of five slices of 1 mm thickness. There is marked reduction in artifact magnitude due to reduction of non-linear partial volume effect.

scanning plane causing partial volume. But since these protuberances are very dense, they also cause beam hardening, which distorts the attenuation values non-linearly resulting in streaks. Avoiding abrupt Z-axis changes in patient anatomy (removal of high-density objects, change of patient positioning or gantry tilt) should be considered but can be difficult to achieve. Narrowing the slice width is essential but problematic due to image noise that becomes particularly visible in the narrowly windowed images necessary for brain evaluation. A practical solution to this dilemma is *thick-section reformatting*, where image raw data of several contiguous thinly collimated slices are added to form a thick-section image. This effectively adds the number of photons contributing to image formation and thus decreases noise without reintroducing the non-linear partial volume artifact. The effect is related to the logarithmic function of image reconstruction. Whereas in conventional image reconstruction voxel density is calculated as the *logarithm of the sum* of the attenuation values, in a reformatted image each voxel density is calculated as the *sum of the logarithms* of attenuation values, resulting in a different numerical value. Thick-section reformatting software is incorporated in most modern CT units and the procedure takes less than a minute to perform. In multislice CT, where all thick-slice images are generated by binning of thin detectors, the advantages of thick-section reformatting are automatically included. Other remedies for this artifact are similar to those against partial volume and beam hardening.

Edge gradient streaks (Figures 4.27 and 4.28)

This artifact (synonyms *high-density edge gradient streak, edge gradient effect, air-contrast interface artifact*) appears as a streak emanating from and tracing along the direction of unusually straight edges of high-density structures in the X-Y plane, such as metallic objects or a contrast media–gas interface in a hollow visceral organ. As with non-linear partial volume, an edge gradient streak occurs due to beam hardening from a dense structure that only partially attenuates the ray between the X-ray tube and a detector cell. The difference is that here the high-density edge traces along the X-Y plane and thereby partially attenuates the width of a detector cell rather than its length. With that, this phenomenon is highly angle-dependent: only one ray of one view of the rotating X-ray beam may be affected and result in data inconsistency and thus a dark streak tracing along the direction of the edge. Remedies include removal or avoidance (patient positioning, gantry tilt) of high-density objects and the use of low-concentration gastrointestinal and urological contrast media.

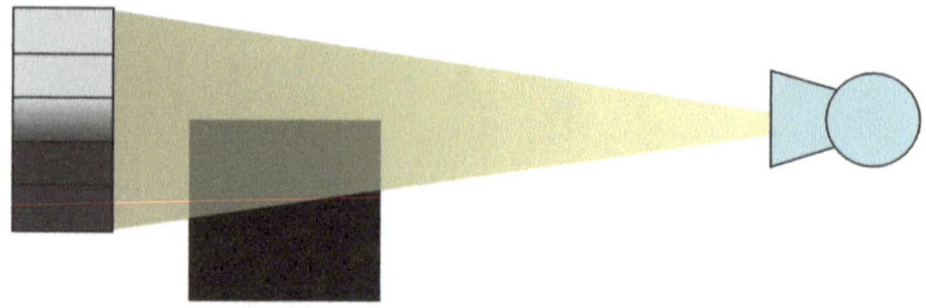

Figure 4.27 Illustration of the mechanism of edge gradient artifact. The central ray of one view produced by the X-ray tube projects along the straight and sharp margin of a high-density object (black square), resulting in the central detector being partially exposed to non-linear beam filtration. In other views from other angles this situation is not replicated, leaving to a streak formation.

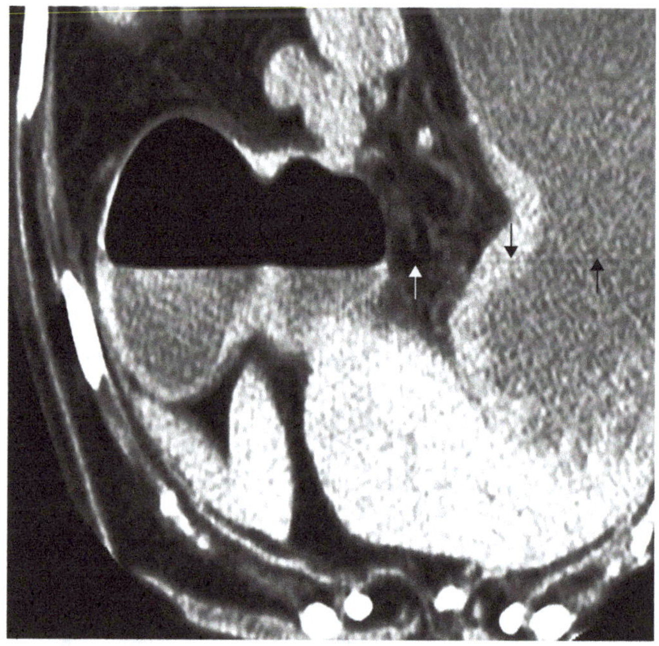

Figure 4.28 Fluid–gas interface in the pyloric antrum of a dog, with a faint streak emanating from it along its course (arrows) as an example of an edge gradient artifact.

Conclusions

Computed tomography artifacts can originate from a wide range of erroneous measurements, geometric assumptions and algorithmic distortions. Due to the image reconstruction as a matrix, most CT artifacts result in streaks. Remedies include various hardware and software engineering approaches and a number of operational solutions. In veterinary CT practice it is particularly important to understand the nature of these often detrimental artifacts to be able to apply the full range of operator-dependent remedies.

Further Reading

Barrett FB and Keat N (2004) Artifacts in CT: recognition and avoidance. *RadioGraphics* **24**: 1679–91.

Barthez PY, Koblik PD, Hornof WJ *et al.* (1996) Apparent wall thickening in fluid filled versus air filled tympanic bulla in computed tomography. *Vet Radiol Ultrasound* **37**: 95–8.

Hsieh J (2000) Image artifacts in CT. In: Goldman L and Fowlkes J (eds) (2000) *Categorical course in diagnostic radiology physics: CT and US cross-sectional imaging*, pp 97–115. Oak Brook: RSNA.

Joseph P (1981) Artifacts in computed tomography. In: Newton T and Potts D (eds) (1981) *Radiology of the skull and brain*, pp 3956–92. St Louis, MO: Mosby.

Link TM, Berning W, Scherf S *et al.* (2000) CT of metal implants: reduction of artifacts using an extended CT scale technique. *J Comput Assist Tomogr* **24**: 165–72.

Porat-Mosenco Y, Schwarz T and Kass PH (2004) Thick-section reformatting of thinly collimated computed tomography for reduction of skull-base-related artifacts in dogs and horses. *Vet Radiol Ultrasound* **45**: 131–5.

CHAPTER FIVE

CT Contrast Media and Applications

Rachel Pollard and Sarah Puchalski

Intravenous Contrast Medium Administration

Introduction

Intravenous contrast medium administration has become a routine procedure in veterinary CT studies. Contrast agents are administered through a catheter into a peripheral vein with the goal of enhancing the ability to see anatomic detail. An indwelling catheter is preferable to minimize the risk of extravasation of contrast medium, which would result in regional inflammation and tissue sloughing. Contrast enhancement occurs in two ways. First, contrast medium reaches an area through the blood vessels so that a major portion of tissue enhancement is a direct reflection of blood flow. Since most contrast agents are small particles, they freely diffuse across endothelial walls so that the second mechanism of enhancement is a reflection of vascular permeability.

Procedure for intravenous administration of contrast medium

The standard procedure for intravenous administration of contrast medium is given in Table 5.1.

Contrast agents

Iodinated contrast agents

Iodinated contrast agents are made up of iodine ions bound to sodium or meglumine salts, and are further subdivided into ionic and non-ionic agents based on their osmolality. The osmotic pressure exerted by a substance depends on the number of particles in solution. Since ionic contrast agents dissociate into two separate particles, they exert two to three times the osmotic pressure of non-dissociative, non-ionic agents. Ionic contrast agents are much more hypertonic (1900–2100 mOsm/kg) than non-ionic agents (290–900 mOsm/kg) or blood plasma (290 mOsm/kg). Traditional contrast agents consist of tri-iodinated monomeric benzene rings. One method of reducing osmolality involves creating a dimer by linking two tri-iodinated benzene rings. A list of commercially available ionic and non-ionic iodinated contrast agents is provided in Table 5.2.

The greater osmotic pressure exerted by ionic iodinated contrast agents is considered to be one of the main reasons why side effects are more common with these agents in comparison to non-ionic agents. Contrast agent reactions are classified as acute, delayed or systemic. Acute reactions are the most common and occur within the first hour following contrast agent administration. Acute reactions can be further subdivided into mild, intermediate and severe reactions. Mild reactions do not require intervention, while intermediate and severe reactions require the administration of medications and/or hemodynamic support. Adverse effects of ionic iodinated contrast agents in veterinary patients including vomiting, anxiety, hypotension, cardiac and respiratory arrest have been anecdotally described, with a mortality rate of 1 in 80 animals. Two studies looking at the incidence of heart rate and systolic blood pressure alterations associated with contrast medium administration in anesthetized dogs and cats found that ionic iodinated agents were more likely to cause physiologically significant alterations in blood pressure and heart rate than non-ionic agents. Severe contrast agent reactions appear to be rare in small animals undergoing CT and can manifest as profound hypotension or hypertension with bronchospasm as a result of ionic iodinated contrast administration. Delayed reactions have not been reported in veterinary patients, but in people typically involve skin rashes and occur after 1 hour but within 7 days of contrast agent administration. Systemic reactions are a

Veterinary Computed Tomography, First Edition. Edited by Tobias Schwarz, Jimmy Saunders.

Table 5.1
Standard procedure for administration of intravenous contrast in small animals and equine CT.

	Small animals	Equines
Application site	Mostly cephalic vein	Mostly jugular vein
Type/Agent	Iodine based, ionic or non-ionic	
Dose	600–880 mg iodine (I)/kg body weight (bw)*	
Administration rate	2 ml/s	
Injection mode	Manual or via power injector	
Scan delay	1–3 min after the contrast bolus is complete so as to allow contrast medium to reach the target organ	

*Most iodinated contrast agents range from 300–400 mg I/ml, which equates to a volume of approximately 2 ml/kg bw or 1 ml/lb.

Table 5.2
The iodine concentration and osmolality is shown for a variety of commercially available contrast agents.

	Iodine concentration (mg/ml)	Osmolality at 37°C (mOsm/kg water)
Ionic monomer		
Diatrizoate	370	2100
Iothalamate	400	2400
Ioxithalamate	380	2100
Metrizoate	350	1970
Ionic dimer		
Ioxaglate	320	577
Non-ionic monomer		
Iobitridol	350	915
Iohexol	350	823
Iomeprol	350	610
Iopamidol	370	774
Iopentol	350	810
Iopromide	350	774
Ioversol	350	790
Ioxilan	350	700
Non-ionic dimer		
Iodixanol	320	290
Iotrolan	300	290

separate category of contrast agent side effects related to chemotoxicity that encompass complications such as contrast-induced nephrotoxicity (CIN). Case reports describing CIN secondary to ionic iodinated contrast agent administration in one dog and one cat have been published.

Iodinated contrast agents are contraindicated in animals that are dehydrated. In many institutions, ionic iodinated agents are no longer in use. However, should the cost of non-ionic agents be prohibitive, care should be taken to avoid ionic iodinated agent administration in animals with heart disease or severe renal compromise.

Gadolinium contrast agents

Gadolinium-based contrast agents are typically used for magnetic resonance imaging (MRI). However, these agents are radiodense and can also be used to provide contrast enhancement for CT (Figure 29.1A). In people, gadolinium is used for CT under circumstances where iodinated contrast agents are contraindicated; however, high doses of gadolinium are needed to provide adequate enhancement (0.3 mmol Gd-DTPA/kg bw).

Gadolinium contrast agents have a lower rate of complications with an overall incidence of acute reactions (mild–severe) reported in 0.48–19.9% of people. More recently, a severe late adverse reaction to gadolinium contrast agents has been reported called 'nephrogenic systemic fibrosis'. This disease develops in people with end stage renal disease who receive gadolinium and results in necrotizing dermatitis and renal sclerosis 2–75 days following contrast medium administration. Very little information is present in the veterinary literature regarding adverse reactions to gadolinium contrast agents. Two recent reports described the incidence of adverse hemodynamic alterations (heart rate and blood pressure) caused by gadolinium agents to be less than the incidence seen with ionic iodinated agents and similar to what is seen with non-ionic iodinated agents in both dogs and cats.

Undesired effects of contrast agents

Streak and blooming artifacts

Streak artifacts are created when high-density material in the imaging plane results in marked attenuation of X-rays such that data are missed. This results in high- and low-density streaks overlying the image (Figure 5.1). Large quantities of intravascular contrast media can result in streak artifacts, particularly when the vessel into which contrast is injected is in the imaging field. Blooming refers to the blur of vascular margins and apparent increase in vessel diameter and is related to the altered point spread effect in high-density structures. To avoid these artifacts, one should carefully consider into which vein contrast agent will be injected for a given study. For example, a cephalic

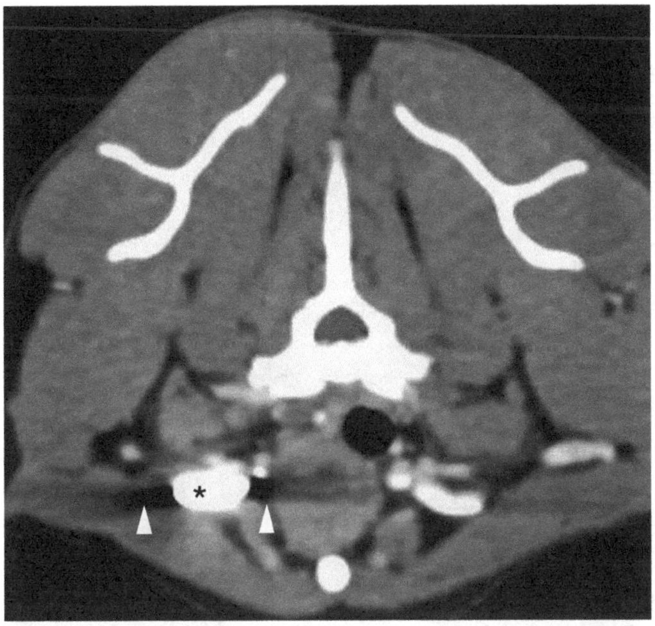

Figure 5.1 An example of a streak artifact. Contrast medium was injected into a catheter in the right cephalic vein and is highly concentrated in the axillary vein (asterisk). Black streaks are emanating from the high-density contrast material (arrowheads). This dog was imaged in ventral recumbency.

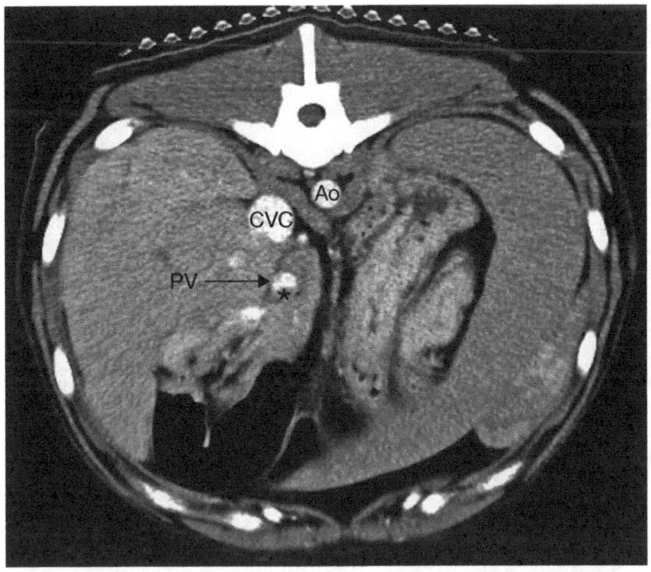

Figure 5.2 An example of streamlining artifact. Contrast agent is only seen filling a portion of the portal vein (PV). The ventral portion of the portal vein does not contain contrast medium (asterisk). Notice more uniform filling of the aorta (Ao) and caudal vena cava (CVC). This dog was imaged in dorsal recumbency.

catheter is preferable to a saphenous catheter when abdominal CT is performed to avoid streak artifact from the caudal vena cava. Contrast agent dilution (to a concentration of 175 mg I/ml) is an alternative method for decreasing contrast-associated streak artifacts.

Streamlining artifact

Streamlining is an artifact that results from non-uniform dispersal of an imaging agent within a vessel. This was first reported during portal scintigraphy but has also been described during CT portography in dogs (Figure 5.2). The result of streamlining is that contrast agent is segregated into discrete channels of portal flow (often the dependent aspect of the portal vein) and is consequently not delivered uniformly to the portal branches in the liver. This is a difficult artifact to eliminate and must simply be recognized as a potential complication of CT portography.

Equine Intra-Arterial Contrast Administration

Introduction

Contrast media improve the clinical utility of CT for the identification and characterization of soft tissue lesions, including tendons, ligaments and synovial structures. In most species, a total body systemic dose is given via an intravenous route. However, the systemic dose of contrast media in the horse has not been established. Generally, the equine systemic dose is extrapolated from humans or small animals, resulting in a large, unwieldy volume of contrast media. The large volume is difficult to deliver and may be prohibitively expensive. To circumvent these problems while benefiting from the technique, local delivery of contrast media via a regional artery can be employed in some clinically important anatomic locations.

Anatomical considerations

The most common use of intra-arterial contrast is for the evaluation of the distal extremity in equine lameness conditions.

The forelimb

In the forelimb, the median artery provides the major blood supply to the entire distal limb and foot. The median artery is accessible to puncture above the carpus by ultrasonographic guidance. At this level, the artery is several centimeters deep and adjacent to the flexor carpi ulnaris muscle and the flexor carpi radialis muscle. This level is recommended for

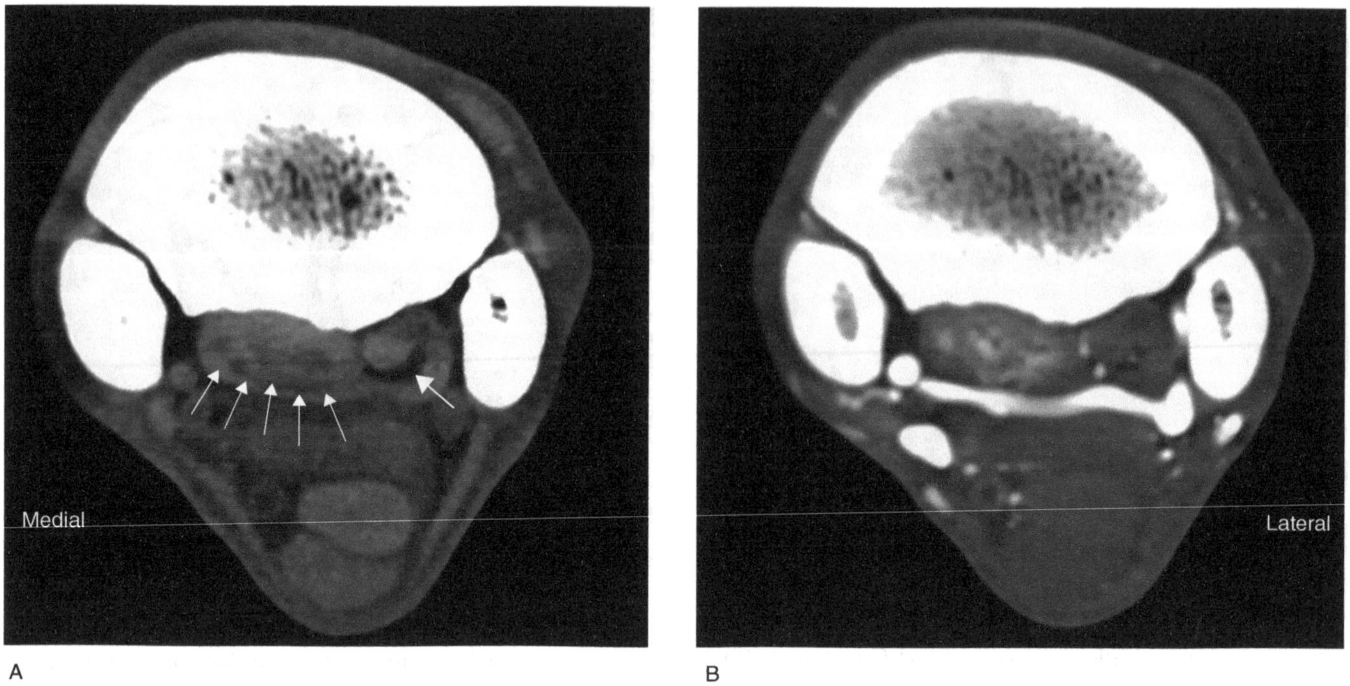

Figure 5.3 Paired CT images of the proximal suspensory (interosseous) ligament made before (A) and during an intra-arterial contrast medium infusion (B). The catheter was placed in the median artery proximal to the carpus. The medial head of the suspensory ligament is enlarged (small arrows). The normal fat-dense signal expected in the interosseous muscle (large arrow) has been lost and replaced by tissue of intermediate density to ligament and fat, likely fluid. The contrast study shows irregular enhancement in the medial head of the suspensory ligament.

evaluation of the soft tissue structures of the carpus, metacarpus (including the suspensory ligament) and digit (Figure 5.3). The median artery passes through the carpal canal and is bound by a retinaculum at the level of the carpus, giving off several branches but becoming the medial palmar artery at the level of the distal carpus/proximal metacarpus (Figure 5.4). The medial palmar artery supplies the entire foot via medial and lateral branches that divide in the metacarpal region. The medial palmar artery is easily accessible in the proximal metacarpal region; it is superficial and parallel to the skin surface. Proximally, catheter placement can be foiled by the carpal retinaculum, which will hamper advancement and arterial backflow. If the catheter is placed distally in the proximal metacarpal region, contrast streaming through the medial arteries can occur, resulting in only one side of the hoof receiving contrast medium.

The hindlimb

In the hindlimb the arterial supply is more complex. The cranial tibial artery and its branches supply the metatarsal region and digit with a lesser component arriving from the caudal tibial artery. The cranial tibial artery is accessible to ultrasound-guided puncture at the level of the distal crus/tarsocrural joint. It is most easily identified at the level of the lateral trochlear ridge of the talus (Figure 5.5). At this level it is closely associated with the lateral digital extensor tendon and the tarsocrural joint. The cranial tibial artery supplies the plantar, proximal metatarsus via the perforating tarsal artery. Catheterization at this level is recommended for evaluation of the proximal suspensory ligament and flexor tendons in the metatarsal region. The digit receives the majority, but not all, of its blood supply from the dorsal metatarsal artery conveniently located on the dorsolateral aspect of the third metatarsal bone. This artery can be punctured blindly or by ultrasonographic guidance.

Catheter placement

Procedure

Successful catheter placement is critical for the acquisition of a diagnostic contrast- enhanced CT study. For this reason, ultrasound guidance is recommended for all but a few arterial catheterization procedures. A higher frequency linear or less commonly a curvilinear ultrasound probe (7.5–12.5 MHz) is held with the scan plane parallel to the long axis of the blood vessel. In

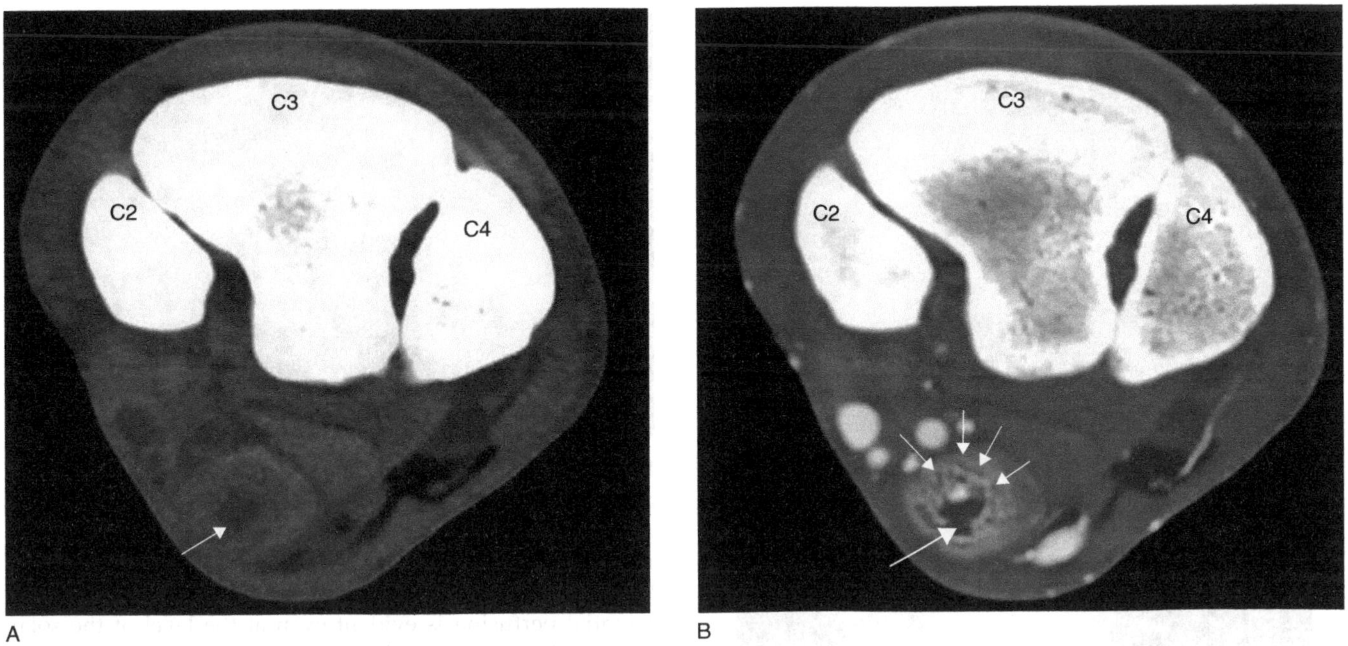

Figure 5.4 Paired CT images of the distal row of carpal bones and carpal canal made (A) prior to contrast medium administration and (B) during an intra-arterial infusion of contrast medium administered via the median artery. (A) There is a lesion in the superficial digital flexor tendon (arrow) that is hypodense prior to contrast medium administration and (B) shows a central, avascular core (large arrow) with a peripheral rim of new blood vessels (small arrows) after intravascular contrast medium has been administered. C2 = second carpal bone, C3 = third carpal bone, C4 = fourth carpal bone.

the forelimb, the arteries run in close proximity to the regional veins. The operator should take time to assess the blood vessels for the characteristic thick, hyperechoic arterial walls and pulsatile blood flow. Occasionally, color flow Doppler may be necessary to characterize blood flow and ensure its arterial nature. In the hindlimb, depending on the location, the arteries may be slightly distant from the veins. The cranial tibial artery is very close to the joint capsule of the tarsocrural joint and therefore adequate preparation of the skin surface and aseptic ultrasound probe handling techniques are recommended.

The importance of a single, clean, confident puncture of the superficial wall of the artery cannot be overstated. Furthermore, accidental puncture of the deep wall of the artery will result in marked vasospasm. Therefore, experience in ultrasound-guided procedures is helpful for successful completion of catheter placement. The catheter should be directed so that the tip is distal. Identification and tracking of the catheter and stylette tip from first perforation of the skin surface to initial contact with the arterial wall is valuable for optimal control. Once the superficial wall is punctured, the catheter and stylette should be fed distally into the artery and then the catheter should be advanced in a routine fashion. It is advantageous to watch these steps with ultrasound and it is often useful to have an assistant. An 18- to 20-gauge catheter is adequate. The length of the catheter depends on the depth of the artery. Generally, a 5–10 cm catheter is sufficient to be well seated (2 cm) within the artery. Once the catheter is placed, it should be attached to a three-way stopcock and flushed with heparinized saline. Suturing the catheter in place is recommended.

Complications associated with catheter placement

Common complications of catheter placement include placing the catheter in the regional vein, vasospasm and perivascular hematoma formation. When vasospasm occurs, no backflow of arterial blood will occur. In this event, the catheter is likely still useful. Observe the artery with ultrasound distally while flushing the catheter with saline to check its patency. Perivascular hematoma formation occurs with vascular trauma and generally resolves with minimal intervention. Catheter placement that is too distal in the medial palmar artery will result in contrast medium supplying only one side of the foot (distal to the lateral branch) or contrast streaming through either the medial or lateral digital arteries (Figure 5.6).

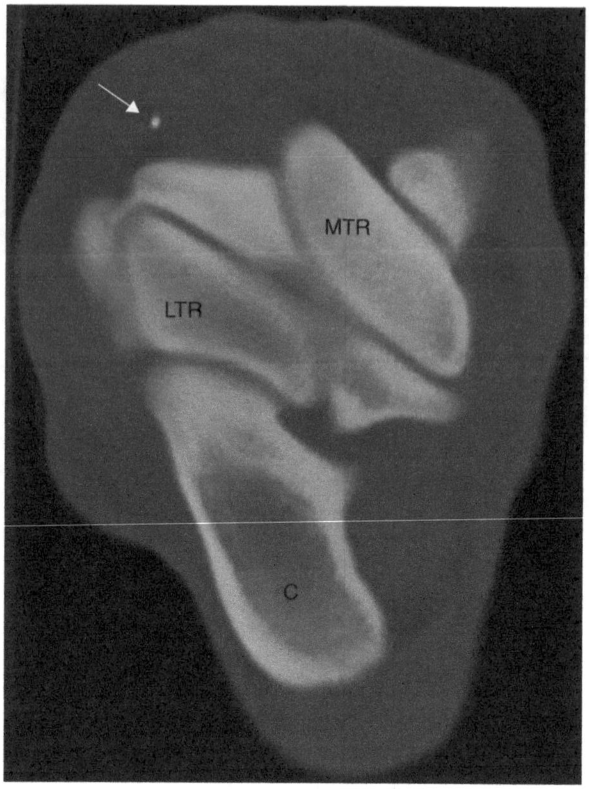

Figure 5.5 CT images of the distal tibia and proximal tarsus. The radiodense catheter is in the cranial tibial artery (arrow). This artery is accessible for puncture with ultrasonographic guidance. Care should be taken to use an aseptic technique as this artery is immediately superficial to the tarsocrural joint. C = calcaneus, LTR = lateral trochlear ridge of the talus, MTR = medial trochlear ridge.

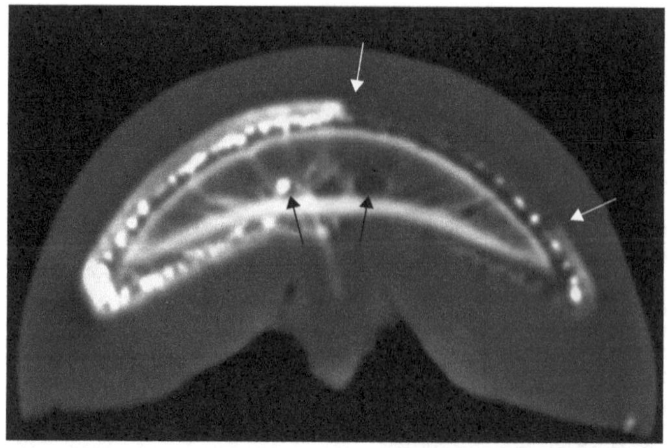

Figure 5.6 CT image of the distal phalanx during an intra-arterial contrast medium infusion administered via the medial palmar artery. Contrast streaming is present, resulting in differential perfusion of the limb. The region of lamina between the white arrows has decreased perfusion. The differential perfusion is evident even at the level of the solar canal and the proper palmar digital arteries (black arrows). This artifact of technique should not be confused with a clinically significant perfusion deficit as seen in laminitis and distal limb (artery) trauma.

Table 5.3
Standard procedure for administration of intra-arterial contrast medium in equine CT.

Application site	Forelimb: median or medial palmar/plantar artery Hindlimb: cranial tibial artery
Type/Agent	Iodine based, ionic or non-ionic
Dose	150–200 mg I/kg bw*
Concentration	150–200 (400) mg I/ml
Administration rate	2 ml/s
Injection mode	Manual or via power injector
Scan delay post start injection	5–10 s (contrast administered during the complete image acquisition)

Contrast medium administration

Iodinated (non-ionic or ionic) contrast medium is used in intra-arterial infusions. The iodine concentration should be 150–200 mg iodine/ml. Higher concentrations result in blooming artifact and therefore many contrast preparations will require dilution with normal saline to achieve the desired iodine concentration. An infusion rate of 2 ml/s is recommended, though rates ranging from 1 to 3 ml/s are adequate. These rates are best achieved by using a pressure injector or infusion pump. Generally, the dose is calculated based on the amount of time necessary to image the desired region. For example, a 50 s scan looking for soft tissue injury will require approximately 55 s or 110 ml at 2 ml/s. The total dose should not exceed the patient's calculated systemic dose, but this is rarely a concern. The standard procedure for intra-arterial administration in equines is described in Table 5.3.

The goals for contrast medium administration via an intra-arterial route are to identify and characterize soft tissue lesions, quantify blood flow or to perform a selective angiogram. The timing of the start of the contrast medium infusion should allow for influx and extravasation of contrast medium into the injured regions prior to the actual scan acquisition to better characterize soft tissue lesions. Five to 10 s is generally adequate. To quantify blood flow several images should be obtained prior to the arrival of contrast media to the region. This can be done with specialized

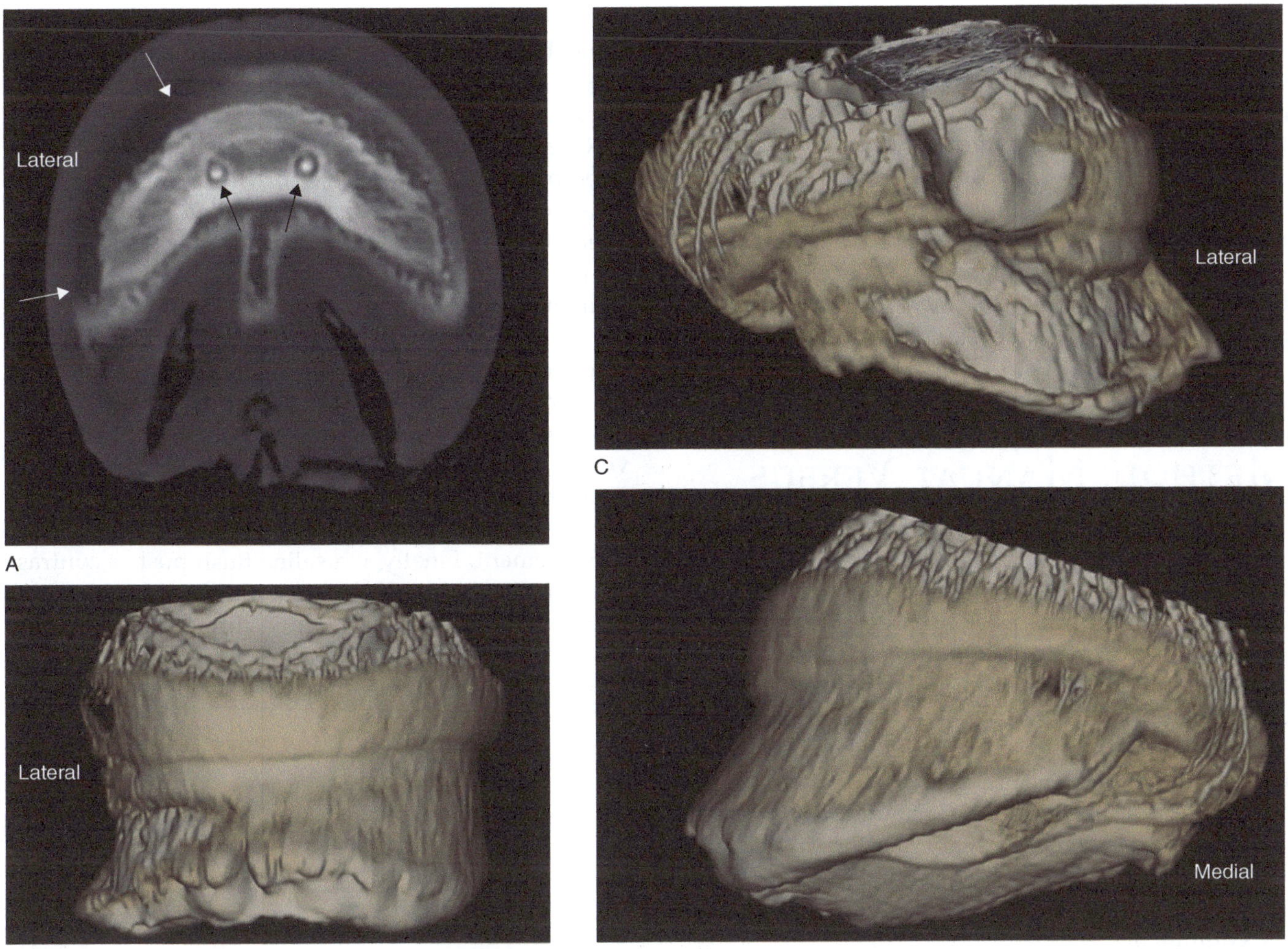

Figure 5.7 (A) Transverse and (B–D) volume-rendered CT images of a horse with severe chronic laminitis during an intra-arterial contrast medium infusion. There is differential perfusion of the laminae. The region between the white arrows has a complete perfusion deficit while the proper palmar digital arteries of the solar canal (black arrows) have symmetric blood flow. The bone of the distal phalanx has mottled opacity and an irregular surface consistent with the patient's clinical disease. (B) A dorsal view of the lamina shows the line of demarcation between avascular and perfused lamina. Compare the lateral (C) and medial (D) vascular pattern.

protocols and commercially available or proprietary software. In these protocols, the scanning will begin prior to the contrast infusion. To perform an angiogram for assessment of vascular patency in laminitis or distal limb trauma, the contrast medium infusion should begin at or just prior to the onset of scanning (Figure 5.7).

Undesired effects of contrast medium administration

Complications associated with contrast administration in horses have not been reported. Anecdotal experience would suggest that they appear to be infrequent and include transient elevations in blood pressure and heart rate, horses becoming 'light' under anesthesia and hives. Caution should be taken as with any species to ensure that contrast medium is only administered into the vascular space, not the subcutaneous tissues.

Interpretation of intra-arterial contrast studies

Interpretation of intra-arterial contrast-enhanced images requires a methodical approach with concurrent comparison to pre-contrast images. Contrast medium aids interpretation in several ways, most importantly by increasing lesion conspicuity. Contrast media can also help to characterize lesions, monitor healing over time and identify regions of hyperemia that may not be associated with frank fiber tearing. Tendon and ligament lesions are generally contrast enhancing via extravasation of contrast medium or by neovessel formation. Core lesions are frequently peripherally enhancing with an avascular center that, over time, changes to become a smaller lesion with central enhancement. Coupling contrast-enhanced soft tissue scanning and the widely known advantages of CT for bone imaging provides an excellent technique for complete evaluation of many anatomic regions implicated in equine lameness.

Contrast Administration Method: Manual Versus Power Injector

For standard CT image acquisition, contrast agents can be administered by hand or by use of an automated power injector. Power injection has certain advantages over hand injection, including uniform contrast agent delivery, optimal timing of delivery and reduced radiation exposure for associated personnel. When performing angiographic or perfusion/dynamic CT studies, a power injector is mandatory to ensure uniform contrast agent delivery, which will allow for assessment of rise times and other quantitative parameters. The downside to power injectors is the cost of the equipment.

Maximal injection rate is based on the viscosity and volume of contrast agent and the cross-sectional area of the catheter. In adult people, contrast agents are typically administered by way of power injector into a 20-gauge peripheral venous catheter at a rate of 4 ml/s. This results in a peak injection pressure as high as 300–325 psi. Although uncommon, rupture of the IV tubing can occur, resulting in loss of vascular access, extravasation of contrast and blood contamination of the area. Maximum injection rates should be adjusted to catheter size so as not to exceed 5 ml/s for a 20-gauge catheter, 3 ml/s for a 22-gauge catheter and 1.5 ml/s for a 24-gauge catheter with a maximal injection pressure of 150 psi.

The use of power injectors in veterinary patients has been sporadically reported. Many institutions will administer contrast agents by hand. When using power injectors for CT portography in dogs, injection rate and catheter size differ, ranging from 1 ml/s through an 18-gauge catheter to 5 ml/s through 18- to 20-gauge catheters. At our institution, catheter size is dictated by patient size varying from 18- to 24-gauge with a maximal injection rate of 2 ml/s used in an attempt to minimize hemodynamic effects related to rapid bolus administration. A rate of 2 ml/s into an 18-gauge catheter is used for arterial injections in horses.

Regardless of whether contrast medium is administered by hand or power injector, the use of saline flush must be considered. Saline flush will add the contrast agent that might have been retained in the catheter to the volume that reaches the patient. This will ultimately reduce the quantity and thereby the cost of contrast agent needed for a given examination. Depending on the capacity of the catheter, this saving may or may not be significant. Another benefit of using a saline flush is diminution of contrast pooling in the vessel into which it is injected. This will reduce streak artifact and would theoretically decrease the total dose required to achieve satisfactory systemic vascular enhancement. Finally, if a saline flush pushes contrast medium from peripheral to central vessels as a solid bolus there will be less dilution through mixing with blood, resulting in improved systemic vascular enhancement. Saline flush by hand is relatively

Table 5.4
Chapters with detailed description of CT contrast procedures.

Contrast procedure	Chapter: Small animals	Chapter: Equines
CT dacryocystography	14	
CT myelography	22	39
Biliary contrast medium excretion	29	
CT portography (transsplenic)	29	
CT gastro-enterography*	31	
CT urography	32	
CT vaginography	33	
CT lymphangiography	36	
CT arthrography	38	39

*Specific application of oral and rectal contrast medium applications (Figure 5.8). In some species, such as fish, oral and rectal applications of contrast medium can be performed successfully to demonstrate the presence of a mass and its effect on the coelomic viscera. This is particularly helpful in fish, because they do not have contrasting intracoelomic fat. Due to the time limitations in performing CT scans in anesthetized fish, the barium enema approach is preferred. It is very quick and easy to perform and provides filling of a long segment of intestines outlining a mass effect. The barium concentration should be kept very low (1–5% w/v suspension).

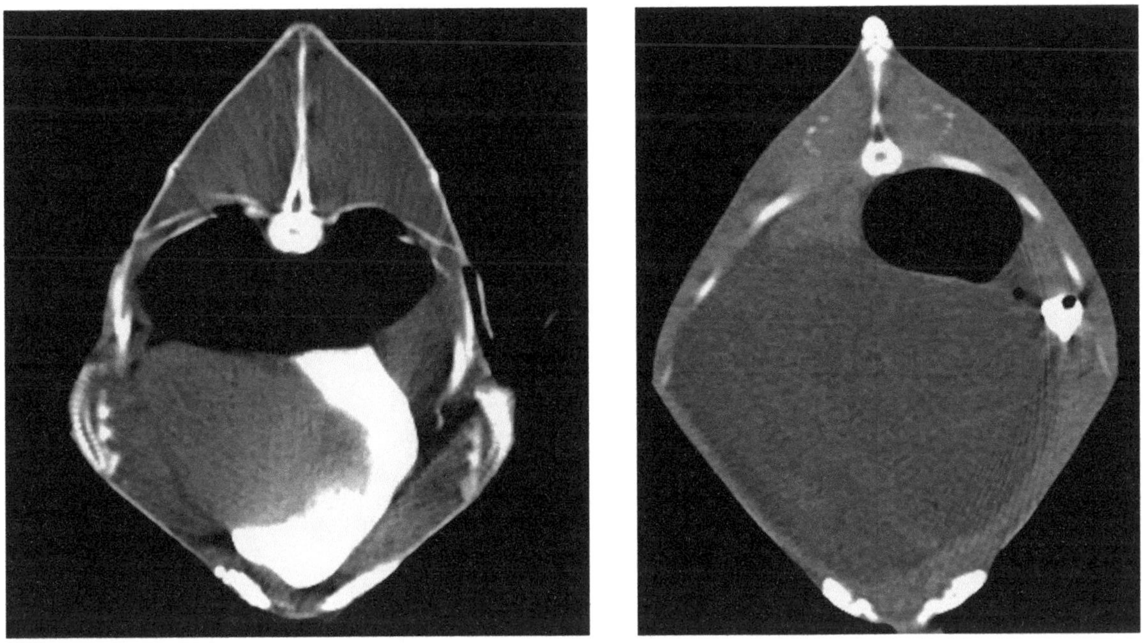

Figure 5.8 (A) Cranial coeloma of a sea bass where a low-concentration barium suspension was given into the stomach via a gastric tube prior to CT. The coeloma contains very little fat and a contrast study aided in localizing the stomach. (B) Koi carp with egg retention in which a rectal barium enema was performed immediately prior to CT. The contrast-enhanced colon is displaced to the left dorsal body wall by the retained eggs.

straightforward. Dual-syringe or two separate power injectors are necessary should saline flush follow contrast agent administration by this method.

Other Contrast Media Applications

The different contrast procedures are discussed in more detail in the chapters listed in Table 5.4.

Further Reading

Amaral JG, Traubici J, BenDavid G, Reintamm G and Daneman A (2006) Safety of power injector use in children as measured by incidence of extravasation. *Am J Roentgenol* **187**: 580–3.

Kruger EF, Puchalski SM, Pollard RE, Galuppo LD, Hornof WJ and Wisner ER (2008) Measurement of equine laminar blood flow and permeability by dynamic contrast enhanced computed tomography. *Am J Vet Res* **69**: 371–7.

Pollard RE and Pascoe PJ (2008) Severe reaction to intravenous administration of an ionic iodinated contrast agent in two anesthetized dogs. *J Am Vet Med Assoc* **233**: 274–8.

Pollard RE, Puchalski SM and Pascoe PJ (2008) Hemodynamic and serum biochemical alterations associated with intravenous administration of three types of contrast media in anesthetized dogs. *Am J Vet Res* **69**: 1268–73.

Pollard RE, Puchalski SM and Pascoe PJ (2008) Hemodynamic and serum biochemical alterations associated with intravenous administration of three types of contrast media in anesthetized cats. *Am J Vet Res* **69**: 1274–8.

Puchalski SM, Galuppo LD, Hornof WJ and Wisner ER (2007) Intraarterial contrast-enhanced computed tomography of the equine distal extremity. *Vet Radiol Ultrasound* **48**: 21–9.

Shuman WP, Adam JL, Schoenecker SA, Tazioli PR and Moss AA (1986) Use of a power injector during dynamic computed tomography. *J Comput Assist Tomogr* **10**: 1000–2.

Tateishi K, Kishimoto M, Shimizu J and Yamada K (2008) A comparison between injection speed and iodine delivery rate in contrast-enhanced computed tomography (CT) for normal beagles. *J Vet Med Sci* **70**: 1027–30.

CHAPTER SIX

Special Software Applications

Jennifer Kinns, Robert Malinowski, Fintan McEvoy, Tobias Schwarz and Allison Zwingenberger

Densitometry

The CT image is generated from a voxel-by-voxel matrix of CT numbers. These CT numbers can be read from the display and are typically given in Hounsfield units (HU). CT densitometry is concerned with a statistical description of the CT number for a particular tissue. For example, the mean CT number or the interquartile range of CT numbers for lung may be of interest. A basic requirement is that the tissue concerned must be separated or segmented from surrounding tissues. In some cases this can be done by placing hand-drawn regions of interest around the organ of interest. Alternatively, automated software segmentation can be used, allowing reproducible segmentation on large sequences of CT images. Software to perform these techniques is available from the CT manufacturers and may also be created using free and open source image analysis programs.

Bone mineral density

The mineral content of bone is of particular interest in human medicine for the detection and management of osteoporosis. There are limited, mainly research accounts of alterations in bone mineral density (BMD) in domestic animals. Traditionally BMD has been measured using dual-energy X-ray absorptiometry (DEXA). This technology dates back to the 1980s, but the dual energy principle for enhancing tissue contrast has found its way into a very recent development, dual-energy CT (DECT). DEXA measurements are based on the differential attenuation of a dual-energy X-ray beam by tissues, and because it is a projection technique its output in given as grams per square centimeter (g/cm^2). Conventional CT can perform a similar role and gives a volumetric bone mineral density (g/cm^3). A phantom, usually containing two types of attenuating material, must be included in the image if a reading in g/cm^3 is required. The change in CT number is linear with increasing BMD so significance can be attached to changes in CT number even without the use of a phantom.

Pulmonary densitometry

The lungs are readily segmented from surrounding tissues, and significant pathologies are associated with both increases and decreases in its attenuating properties. Diffuse disease such as fibrosis and multifocal diseases can be difficult to identify on CT or difficult to quantify. Pulmonary densitometry can provide a single figure that describes the attenuating properties of lung. It is used in humans for the assessment of pulmonary emphysema and has recently been used in a veterinary setting to describe changes associated with *Angiostrongylus vasorum* infection (McEvoy *et al.* 2009). In that report there was a strong correlation between pulmonary density and the actual worm burden. Here and in other situations there is a correlation between the measured density and the extent of disease or function impairment. Data from a densitometry study are shown in Figure 6.1. The steps required are an initial segmentation of the image so that only lung is retained. This can be done by a threshold technique based on CT numbers. The image data are then analyzed to quantify the number of voxels in the image at each particular CT number. The resulting data may

Veterinary Computed Tomography, First Edition. Edited by Tobias Schwarz, Jimmy Saunders.

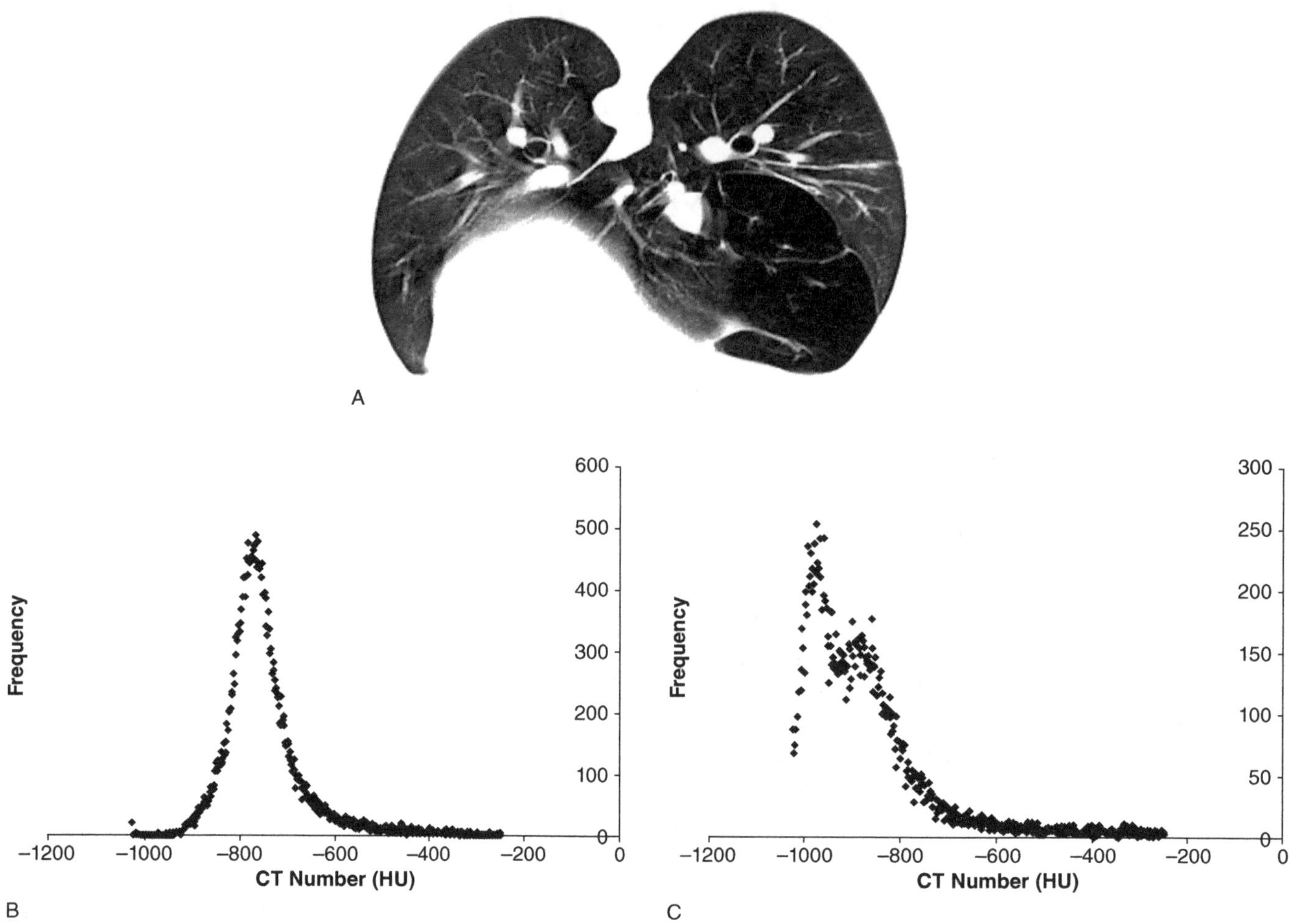

Figure 6.1 (A) Transverse CT image showing the results of segmentation. All tissues other than pulmonary parenchyma have been removed from the image. The threshold range was −1024 to −250 HU. This dog has extensive lobar emphysema. (B) Frequency plot from a normal canine thorax showing the number of voxels present for each CT number, indicating how the data are normally distributed. (C) Frequency plot from the dog in A. Note how the shape of the plot differs from normal. The mean CT number for this individual's lungs was −897 HU, while that for the age-matched normal control was −747 HU.

be plotted or descriptive statistics can be used to describe the data set.

Perfusion densitometry

Changes is CT number over time are seen in perfusion studies and are covered elsewhere in this text. The concept of relating CT number to a tissue feature (iodine concentration in this case) is the same as described here for densitometry. If the numerical results from densitometry studies are to be shared across imaging centers, then strict machine calibration is required. CT machines are typically calibrated to a water phantom but not to more or less attenuating materials. There can be a significant variation in CT number for a given tissue across different machines.

Automated Bolus Tracking

Principle

Bolus tracking refers to the technique where a CT scan is started automatically based on continuous attenuation measurements of target vessels. This software is available for all modern CT scanners under different names ('SmartPrep' on GE, 'CARE bolus' on Siemens, 'Trigger bolus' on Philips and 'Real Prep' on Toshiba units) and works similarly in all of them.

From the survey CT study a target vessel location is identified and a single slice image at this location is then obtained and the scanning is paused. The operator now selects a region of interest (ROI) over the target vessel. At this point personnel must leave the scanning room again, and the contrast medium is injected remotely via power injector. Contrast medium injection and CT scanning are started at exactly the same time, and this can be automated with modern power injectors and CT units. The single-slice CT scan is repeated over the same location at 3 to 4s intervals, while software reconstructs images and calculates density data from the ROI. When contrast medium arrives at the target vessel, the increased attenuation is either visually displayed as a graph and the operator starts the diagnostic CT scan (semi-automatic mode) or the diagnostic CT series is started completely automatically.

Recommendations for use

The proposed advantages of automated bolus tracking are convenience and maximum contrast enhancement of the target structure. The alternative for correct timing of start times for CT scans is to do a test bolus, which is time-consuming and laborious. Bolus tracking is a popular option for human patients, particularly with multidetector scanners in which scanning occurs so fast that it would be easy to miss a vascular phase without this technique.

Limitations

Automated bolus tracking has several marked disadvantages for veterinary patients unless the newest and most advanced software is available.

- Because of the considerable delay times between individual monitor scans and between monitor and diagnostic scans (3–4s), the short pure arterial phase (5–10s in most organs) is usually missed with this technique.
- If a dual-phase scan is performed, the start time for the second phase cannot be measured with this technology and needs to be guessed a priori when setting up the scan protocol. This is the most important phase in most applications (e.g. portal vein for shunts). Missing it would be detrimental to the study and the study cannot easily be repeated.
- Venous phase imaging should usually start between 20 and 40s post start injection. During this time period the animal should be manually hyperventilated for thoracoabdominal studies, so that it is in respiratory apnea during the scan. This is not possible with most anesthetic set-ups during a bolus tracking CT as the monitor scans occur at frequent intervals during this time. This increases the risk of motion artifacts for the most relevant structures of interest on top of missing the phase the software is designed to match.

CT Perfusion Imaging

Principle

CT is capable of capturing data about blood dynamics in tissues. Contrast medium travels through major blood vessels to capillary beds in the tissues. As it reaches these small vessels, a certain amount of contrast medium is transferred to the interstitial space by diffusion. Most tissues enhance proportionally to their vascularity, except the brain, which is protected by the blood–brain barrier.

CT measures tissue perfusion by collecting data on contrast enhancement in defined pixels over time. This can be accomplished with a dynamic CT scan with 1–3s continuous images for 1–3min during and after a constant rate contrast injection. Perfusion software then calculates the perfusion, or blood flow per unit volume of tissue, relative blood volume and permeability.

Software programs calculate these perfusion parameters and generate pixel maps to represent the degree of blood flow to each tissue in the image. These visual representations of the data can be very helpful in detecting subtle changes in perfusion, and may highlight a lesion that cannot be seen on the anatomic images.

Recommendations for use

Perfusion imaging is used extensively in human patients to investigate cerebrovascular disease such as acute stroke. The abnormal hemodynamics such as reduced blood volume and blood flow can help to evaluate the extent of tissue damage and likelihood of recovery (Figure 6.2). In cancer imaging, perfusion images can be used to evaluate the vascularity and its response to treatment such as chemotherapy or radiation therapy, which may be more accurate than a change in size. Perfusion imaging has been used to evaluate the liver in dogs with portosystemic shunts, the pancreas, nasal tumors and brain tumors. The liver requires unique perfusion measurements because of its dual blood supply from the portal vein and hepatic artery. The hepatic perfusion index can be calculated to describe the proportion of blood contributed by the hepatic artery to the total liver perfusion (Figure 6.3). This is normally approximately 25%. Dogs with portosystemic shunts have a higher hepatic perfusion index to compensate for reduced portal blood supply.

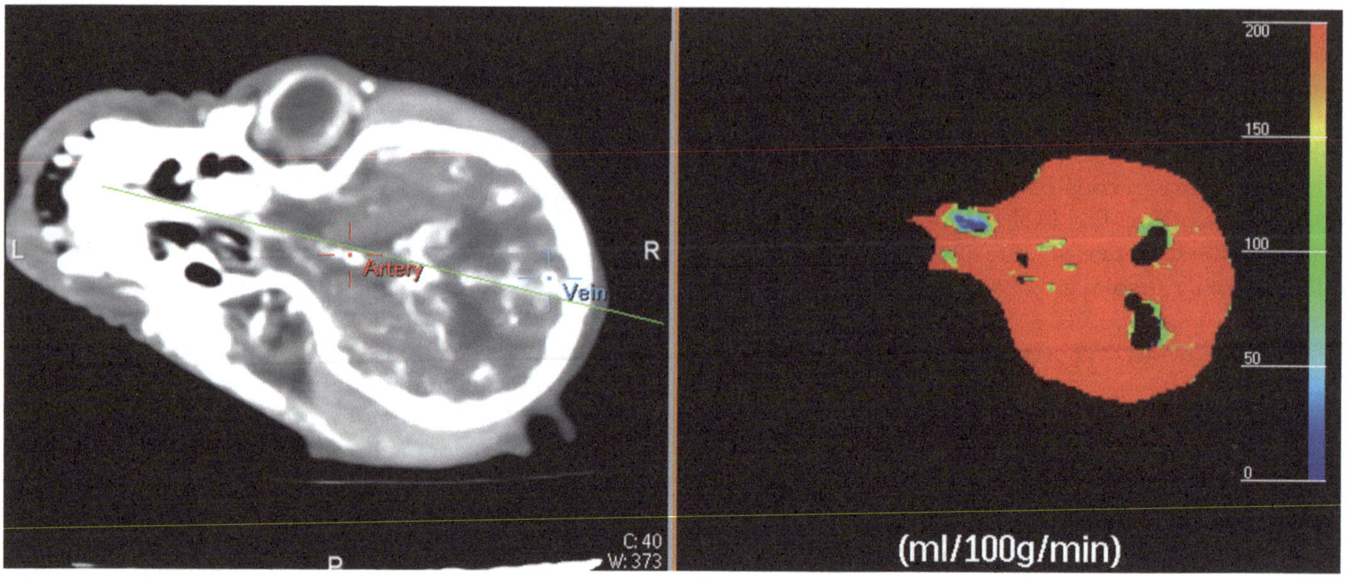

Figure 6.2 Calculated cerebral blood flow map of a dog with head trauma. There is an oval area of decreased perfusion in the olfactory lobe of the brain. This is much more apparent on the perfusion map than the corresponding hypodense area on the contrast-enhanced image.

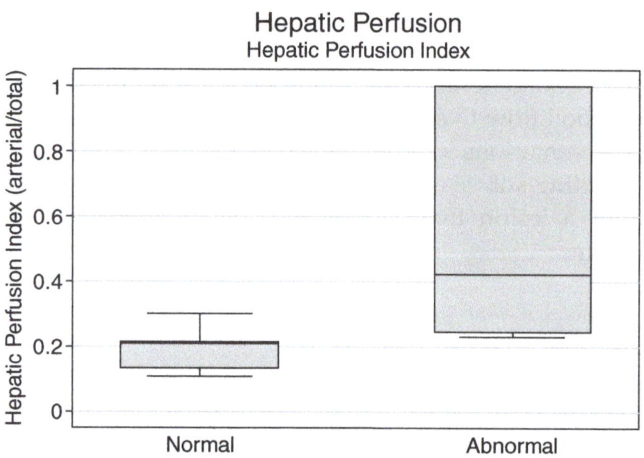

Figure 6.3 Box plot of the hepatic perfusion index in normal dogs compared to those with portosystemic shunts. Arterial perfusion is higher in dogs with reduced portal blood supply.

Limitations

The software generally uses either compartmental analysis, or deconvolution, to model the flow of contrast between tissues. Each of these models has advantages and both have been validated in various tissues. Deconvolution is less susceptible to image noise and is good for low-perfusion tumors where data are scarce. Compartmental analysis has been evaluated more thoroughly in organs with complex perfusion, such as the liver.

Multiplanar Reconstruction

Principle

CT images are acquired as transverse slices through the anatomy. The data are stacked along this axis to create a volume, and then re-sliced along the other planes to create sagittal, dorsal or oblique projections. This technique is simple and quick and does not require a powerful computer.

Recommendation for use

Multiplanar reconstruction (MPR) can be essential for the accurate evaluation of a CT scan of certain lesion types. It may also be necessary to provide measurements for surgical or interventional radiology planning, and it can often be helpful in delineating the lesion. Sagittal and dorsal plane reconstructions are standard, but oblique plane orientation may be necessary to delineate some lesions or anatomic structures.

Trauma to the axial or appendicular skeleton should be evaluated in multiple planes (Figure 6.4). Fracture lines may be difficult to delineate on transverse slices, but when seen in long axis are more easily interpreted. Luxations or subluxations, particularly of the spine, are most easily recognized when viewed on reconstructed images. Long-axis distance is very difficult to appreciate on transverse views. The intervertebral disk space,

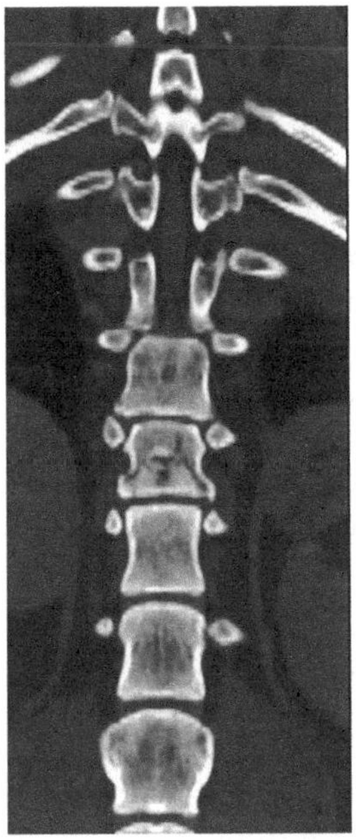

Figure 6.4 Dorsal plane reconstruction of the spine of a dog that was hit by a car. The 11th thoracic vertebra has a compression fracture and multiple fracture lines are visible.

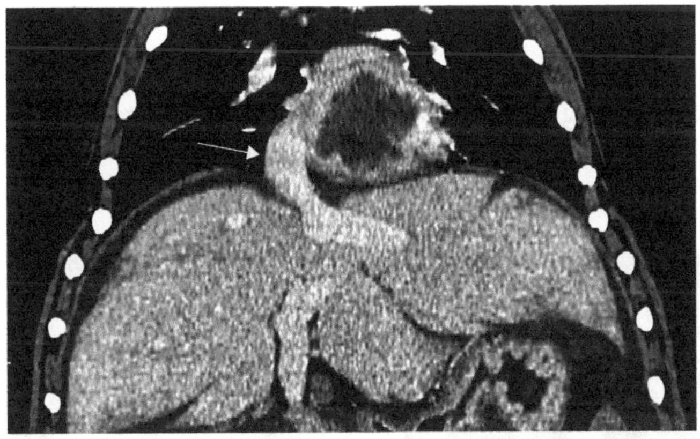

Figure 6.5 Dorsal plane reconstruction of the caudal thorax and cranial abdomen of a dog with a paraesophageal mass. The reconstruction allows visualization of caudal vena cava displacement (arrow).

for example, is most readily evaluated on sagittal plane image. Non-traumatic orthopedic cases also benefit from orthogonal evaluation. The orientation and extent of medial coronoid process lesions, for example, are better evaluated on sagittal reconstructions.

Mass lesions in any location are usefully evaluated by MPR. Long-axis lesion measurements are more easily obtained on reconstructed images. The surrounding anatomy is often best appreciated on more familiar sagittal or dorsal plane images. Multiplanar reconstruction may be necessary to determine the anatomic origin of a lesion. Fascial planes, vascular position and tract (such as trachea) orientation are better appreciated in long axis. Focal pulmonary lesions often require MPR to determine the lobar origin, by following the bronchus to that area of pulmonary parenchyma. Differentiation of pulmonary nodules from end-on vessels can also require orthogonal reconstruction.

Angiographic studies may also be evaluated by MPR (Figure 6.5). Determination of portosystemic shunt direction, the size of a thrombus or the extent of intravascular tumor invasion are best appreciated on multiplanar images.

Limitations

The quality of MPR is limited by the acquisition parameters. MPR images may have stair step artifacts. These can be limited by obtaining overlapping slices in helical acquisitions. The spatial resolution of sagittal and dorsal images is also reduced compared with transverse images due to data interpolation, so measurements made in these planes will be less accurate and the images may appear blurred. Acquisition with thinner slices will improve the quality of multiplanar reconstructions.

Curvilinear Reconstruction

Principle

Curvilinear reconstruction allows the operator to select a curved reconstruction plane that follows a structure of interest, such as a vessel (Figure 6.6). The process flattens out the structure and allows it to be displayed on a single image for direct viewing and more accurate measurements. This software function is not available in all multiplanar reconstruction programs and is typically offered as an add-on package.

Recommendation for use

If available, curvilinear reconstruction is best used to evaluate curved or tortuous anatomic structures that are not easily followed on sagittal, dorsal or oblique plane images. Single vessels can be followed in this way, allowing delineation of portosystemic shunt direction, the displacement of a vessel by a mass lesion or intravascular lesions. It can also be useful for flattening the dorsal plane image of the spinal cord.

Limitations

Curvilinear reconstruction can be difficult and time-consuming to use effectively. Software solutions that automate the segmentation and analysis processes are costly.

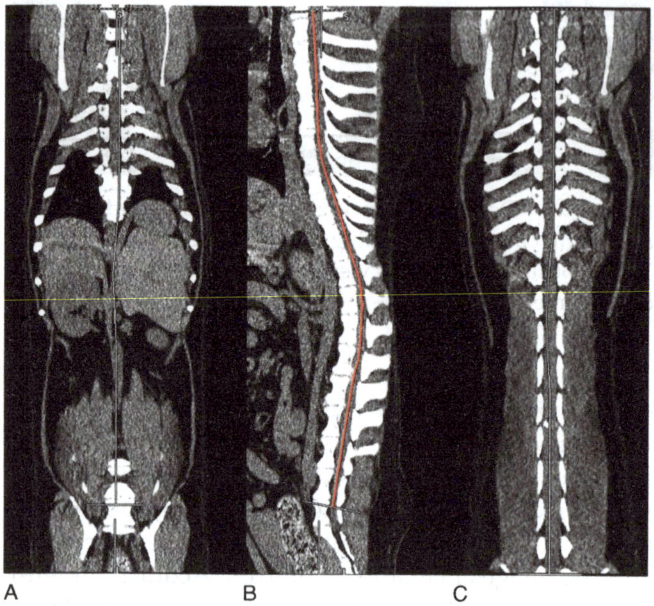

Figure 6.6 Curvilinear reconstruction of the spine of a dog. (A) Standard dorsal plane MPR. (B) Sagittal MPR with the curved line within the vertebral canal that is used for reconstruction. (C) The resulting flattened dorsal plane image of the spinal cord.

Paddle Wheel Reconstruction (Figure 6.7)

Reviewing transverse plane images of large volumes of thin-sliced thoracic CT studies is laborious and the image orientation does not match the anatomic orientation of the bronchovascular tree. Circularly oriented image reconstructions (reminiscent of the paddle wheels of old steam boats) pivoted around the carina elegantly solve this problem and provide better anatomic viewing conditions. As with any orthogonal reconstruction, the image quality largely depends on the original imaging parameters, namely slice width, pitch and helical image reconstruction interval. Most modern DICOM (digital imaging and communication in medicine) viewers offer circular reconstruction modes or it can be done manually from the sagittal reconstruction.

3D Reconstruction

Principle

Maximum intensity projection (MIP) depicts the maximum intensity that each ray encounters and displays this as a two-dimensional projection that can be rotated on any plane for three-dimensional evaluation.

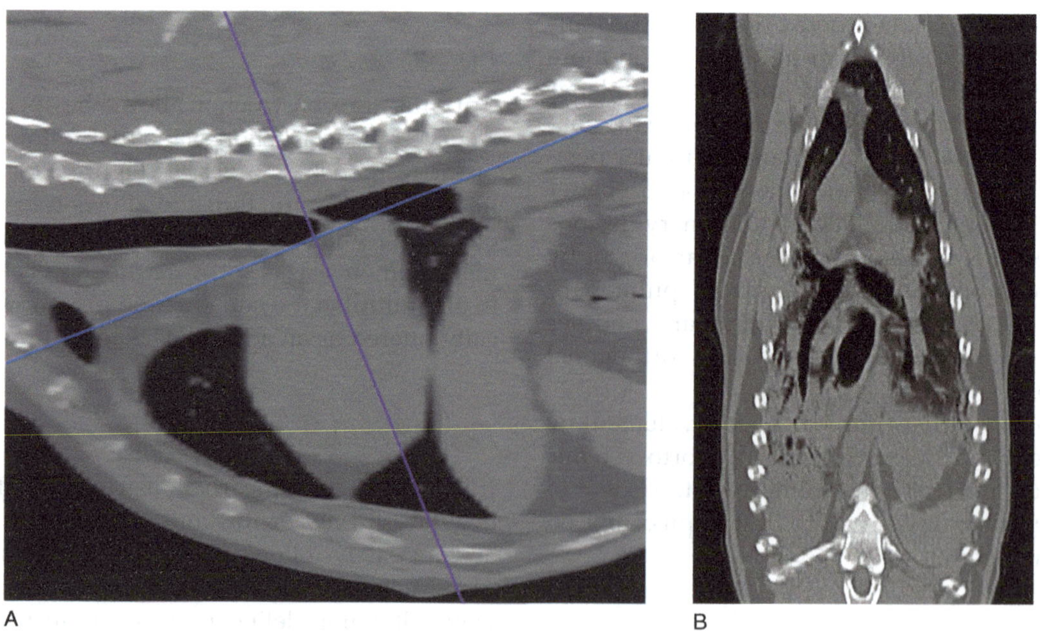

Figure 6.7 (A) Sagitally reconstructed thoracic CT image with superimposed purple and blue crossbars. The blue crossbar represents the selected paddle wheel reconstruction plane, which is pivoted over the carina. (B) Corresponding paddle wheel reconstruction image demonstrating the caudal bronchovascular structures displayed along their anatomic orientation.

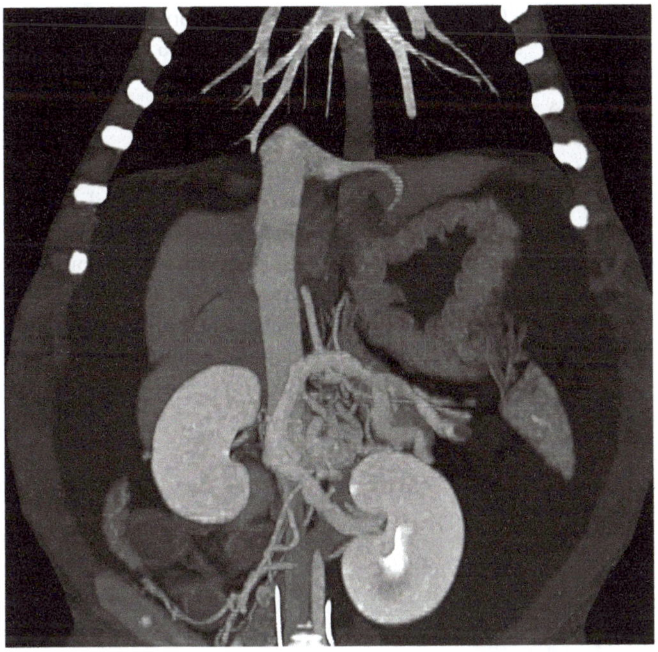

Figure 6.8 Maximum intensity projection image of the abdominal vasculature of a dog that presented with ascites. Multiple tortuous vessels are present cranial and axial to the kidneys.

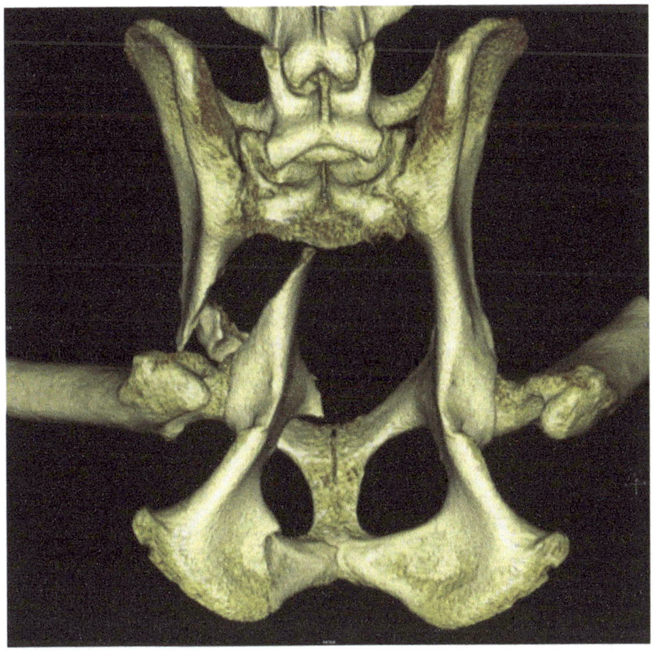

Figure 6.9 Volume rendered image of a comminuted pelvic fracture in a dog.

In volume rendering, each voxel is represented using opacity and color to give the resulting image a realistic appearance. The color ranges used can be customized by the user to create a variety of visual effects.

Recommendation for use

Maximum intensity projection reconstruction is most useful in evaluating contrast-enhanced vascular structures (Figure 6.8). As most surrounding structures are removed from the image automatically, the vessels can be more easily visualized than with standard multiplanar or 3D reconstructive techniques. It is most useful in assessing vascular structures for filling defects. A MIP projection of abdomen, for example, would allow evaluation for presence of portal system thrombi, and evaluation of the pulmonary arterial system with MIP would be useful for detection of pulmonary thromboemboli. MIP evaluation may also be used to improve the detection of pulmonary nodules.

Volume rendering is most useful for surgical planning and client communication. It should not be relied on for diagnosis due to the limitations of spatial and contrast resolution, and the inherent problem of superimposition. Orthopedic evaluation particularly benefits from 3D reconstruction. Planning of fracture repair can be improved by 3D visualization of the injury, particularly with complex lesions of the axial skeleton (Figure 6.9). Angular limb deformities can be assessed more accurately when presented in three dimensions. This is particularly true when multiple lesions are present, such as concurrent valgus and rotational deformities. Corrective surgery can be rehearsed in advance by creating physical rapid prototype models generated from the surface geometry of the reconstruction. Modeling from the 3D images allows evaluation of osteotomy orientation, for example, before the procedure is carried out on the patient. Three-dimensional reconstruction can also aid in planning for interventional procedures such as stent placement or shunt attenuation, although all necessary measurements should be acquired from transverse or MPR images.

Three-dimensional reconstruction has particular benefits when presenting information to clients. Lesions are much easier for the layperson to understand when visualized using this method. This applies not only to orthopedic lesions, but also to soft tissue mass lesions and vascular anomalies.

Limitations

The signal-to-noise ratio limits the quality of the volume-rendered image because structures that are separate anatomically may not be seen as such on the 3D image. In addition, a smoothing and shading algorithm is used to created the 3D image which can limit visualization of subtle lesions such as small non-displaced fractures. Thick slices will also limit the quality of the reconstruction and create a blocky appearance on the renderings. This can be minimized by using thinner slices or applying an image-smoothing process after the initial reconstruction. Real-time 3D reconstruction is very computer processor intensive and requires a high-end workstation to perform.

Reference

McEvoy FJ, Buelund LE, Strathe AB *et al.* (2009) Quantitative computed tomography evaluation of pulmonary disease. *Vet Radiol Ultrasound* **50**: 47–51.

Further Reading

Griffith JF and Genant HK (2008) Bone mass and architecture determination: state of the art. *Best Pract Res Clin Endocrinol Metab* **22**: 737–64.

Miles KA (2004) Brain perfusion: computed tomography applications. *Neuroradiology* **46** (Suppl 2): s194–200.

Miles KA (2003) Functional CT imaging in oncology. *Eur Radiol* **13** (Suppl 5): M134–8.

Peterson KL, MacLeod AG, Wisner ER, Larson RF and Pollard RE (2008) Quantitative assessment of blood volume, blood flow, and permeability of the brain of clinically normal dogs by use of dynamic contrast-enhanced computed tomography. *Am J Vet Res* **69**: 45–50.

Zwingenberger AL and Shofer FS (2007) Dynamic computed tomographic quantitation of hepatic perfusion in dogs with and without portal vascular anomalies. *Am J Vet Res* **68**: 970–4.

CHAPTER SEVEN

Digital Environment

Robert Malinowski

Picture Archive and Communication Systems

The picture archive and communication system (PACS) is the core of any modern digital radiology network. Ranging widely in size and complexity, PACS is a computer server (or series of servers) that functions as a central storage point for studies generated by imaging equipment. PACS indexes and organizes all of the incoming data, giving users the ability to search images by patient name, medical record number, modality, clinician and many other criteria. Images are viewable wherever they are needed, typically just seconds after they were acquired.

Once a study is stored on the PACS, the images can be viewed using several different methods. The most common approach is to use a dedicated image viewing workstation computer with high-resolution grayscale monitors. Using medical-grade monitors ensures that the images will be displayed accurately for a valid diagnostic interpretation. Another way to access images is via a web-based (often called thin-client) viewer, a common feature on many PACS solutions. Using a combination of viewers gives access to PACS both inside and outside the clinical environment.

PACS software gives radiologists and clinicians a powerful set of tools to display and manipulate images. In addition to the most common features (zoom, pan, windows/level, annotate), many PACS have advanced functionality available such as three-dimensional reconstruction, voice recognition, surgical planning/templating and electronic reporting.

PACS is essential for a filmless environment. With a proper PACS implementation and an adequate number of image viewing workstations, hard copy film can be completely eliminated. PACS gives instant access to any study, any time, anywhere.

DICOM

DICOM (digital imaging and communication in medicine) is a global standard created to facilitate the exchange of information between medical imaging devices. Much as JPEG images have become ubiquitous on digital cameras, DICOM is the most common image format for radiology equipment. DICOM is also a network communication protocol. Having a standard format in place ensures that one piece of equipment, regardless of vendor or modality type, will be able to communicate with others. Using DICOM-compliant equipment greatly simplifies the transfer of information to PACS, digital film printers and other devices.

DICOM files contain image data as well as information about the patient and the modality on which they were acquired. Single images, as well as ciné loops and sequences, can all be stored in DICOM files.

Three pieces of information are needed to ensure that DICOM devices can successfully communicate with one another:

- AE title: application entity, the name given to each modality on the network
- IP address: the unique numerical network identifier
- port number: the data port used to transmit information.

RIS/HIS (Figure 7.1)

Ideally, PACS is not installed as a stand-alone system but rather functions as one component of a tightly integrated system, uniting all electronic clinical systems to reduce errors and maximize efficiency. The exact functions vary between vendors, but in general

Veterinary Computed Tomography, First Edition. Edited by Tobias Schwarz, Jimmy Saunders.

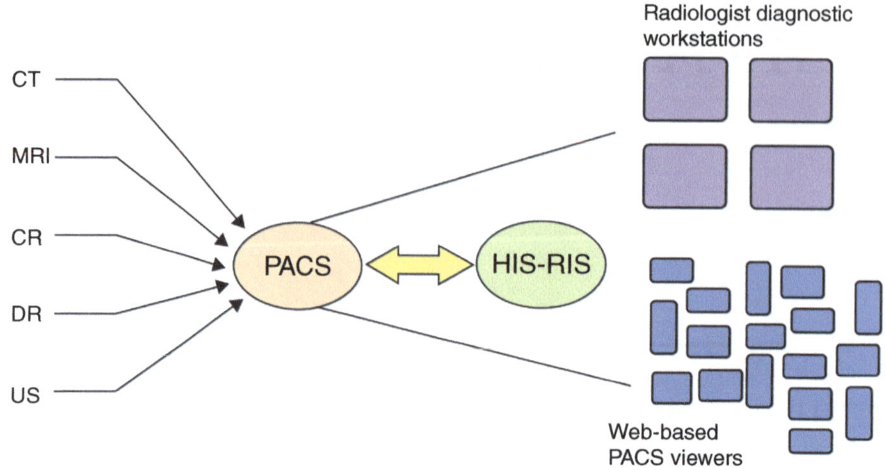

Figure 7.1 Typical structure of a digital radiology network.

the HIS (hospital information system) is used to register patients, schedule appointments and perform accounting operations. The RIS (radiology information system) may be part of the HIS or a completely separate system. It typically functions as the link connecting HIS and PACS, transferring patient information, study details and reports between the systems.

In a typical RIS/HIS/PACS workflow, an electronic order for a procedure is placed in the RIS using patient demographics supplied by the HIS. Once the order is approved, it is transferred to a work list, where it is accessible by the modality. The study is then selected on the modality and the procedure performed. Next, the images are evaluated and, if acceptable, are sent to the PACS. Finally, the order is closed on the RIS and charges are entered into the HIS. Work flows vary greatly between equipment vendors, but all are designed to reduce manual data entry and associated errors.

Transfer Speed

As CT technology continues to advance, the average file size of a study has increased. A thin-sliced or reconstructed series can easily generate thousands of images occupying several gigabytes of space. Special attention must be given to the design of the network infrastructure to ensure that these data can be transmitted in a timely manner. If these details are ignored, transfer times will be greatly increased and efficiency will suffer.

Ideally, all network switches and adaptors will utilize Gigabit Ethernet for maximum transfer rates. It is also advisable to place all radiology equipment (modalities, PACS, workstations, printers) on a separate VLAN (virtual local area network). This approach isolates DICOM traffic from the rest of the network and ensures that the system can operate at the highest possible speed. It also keeps all of the radiology equipment containing confidential patient information inaccessible to outside intruders, viruses and worms.

DICOM images can be compressed at the modality to reduce the amount of time it takes to transmit them across the network. Several compression types are available depending on the purpose of the final image and the desired file size.

Non-Proprietary Workstations

Many PACS vendors impose strict constraints on the type of hardware that can be used to run their software. While these guidelines are designed to keep the system running properly, they limit choice and typically result in the purchase of expensive workstations directly from the vendor. However, if a web-based viewer for the PACS is available, the hardware requirements are much less severe. The thin-client software will function on most recent computers, provided that processor, memory and browser requirements are met. However, due to the fact that standard definition monitors are usually used in this scenario, the images must be considered non-diagnostic only.

Another option is to install free or open-source DICOM viewing software, along with high-resolution monitors, and use the configuration for reading electronic films. Since DICOM is a standardized format and transmission protocol, this non-proprietary workstation will function as just another node on the DICOM network, capable of receiving and displaying studies.

CHAPTER EIGHT

CT Planning for Radiotherapy

Lisa J. Forrest

Introduction

Veterinary radiation oncology has followed its counterpart in the human field with advances in treatment planning and delivery. The introduction of three-dimensional treatment planning in the 1980s led to advances in equipment and software, which in turn led to the development of multileaf collimators, three-dimensional conformal radiotherapy (3DCRT) and intensity-modulated radiotherapy (IMRT). Many veterinary radiation oncology centers are upgrading their systems to advanced linear accelerators with 3DCRT and IMRT capabilities. These new systems are capable of precise shaping of dose distributions with the use of computer-controlled multileaf collimators (3DCRT, IMRT) that can also control the dose intensity (IMRT) to precisely achieve the plan prescription. The advances in conformal tumor therapy and conformal avoidance of critical structures adjacent to the tumor place increasing importance on precise daily dose delivery.

Principles of External Beam Radiotherapy

Radiotherapy is a clinical treatment modality where ionizing radiation is used to treat patients with malignant tumors. The goal of radiation therapy is to deliver a measured dose of radiation to a defined volume with minimal damage to surrounding normal tissue, resulting in eradication of the tumor. Radiation doses are measured in units of absorbed dose, Gray (Gy). A Gray is equal to 1 J/kg energy absorbed in tissue. In general, radiation doses are given in small daily fractions (Monday through Friday) to achieve the desired total dose over several weeks. Examples of fractionation schemes in veterinary radiation oncology include daily 2.5–3.2 Gy fractions for 15–20 treatments for a total dose of 48–50 Gy. Radiotherapy is useful in the treatment of localized tumors and can provide long-term local control with preservation of regional function. There are several principles that dictate the prescription of irradiation and therefore the management of cancer patients. Tumor staging, biologic behavior of specific tumor types and defining the goals of therapy are all important steps in the evaluation of a cancer patient, but are beyond the scope of this chapter.

Principles of Radiotherapy Treatment Planning

CT continues to be the imaging choice for radiotherapy treatment planning in human oncology. Once a diagnosis is obtained and radiotherapy is the treatment choice, patients will receive a radiotherapy planning CT or CT simulation. The patient will be imaged in the treatment position and immobilization devices such as head frames, masks, bite blocks and formable mattresses will be used. These immobilization devices ensure that the patient is in the same position for every delivered fraction of radiation. As the precision of radiotherapy delivery increases so does the importance of immobilization devices. Larger overall doses and dose per fraction are being delivered with equal importance placed on conformal avoidance of adjacent normal structures. The same devices are being used more and more in veterinary medicine (Figures 8.1 and 8.2).

The planning CT will be uploaded into the radiotherapy treatment-planning computer. The basics of radiotherapy planning are to identify the volumes that will be irradiated and sensitive structures within the radiation field on the CT image. These include:

Veterinary Computed Tomography, First Edition. Edited by Tobias Schwarz, Jimmy Saunders.

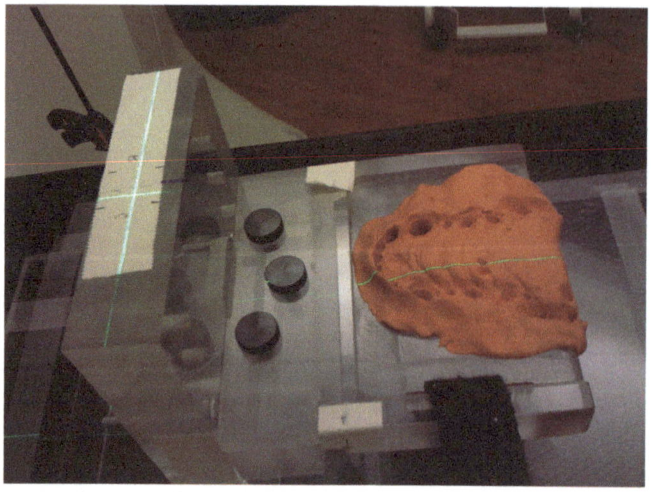

Figure 8.1 Bite block immobilization apparatus for treatment of a canine nasal tumor. Dental molding materials are mixed together and the dog's maxilla is pressed into the mold. The material hardens quickly and creates a reproducible patient set-up for radiotherapy.

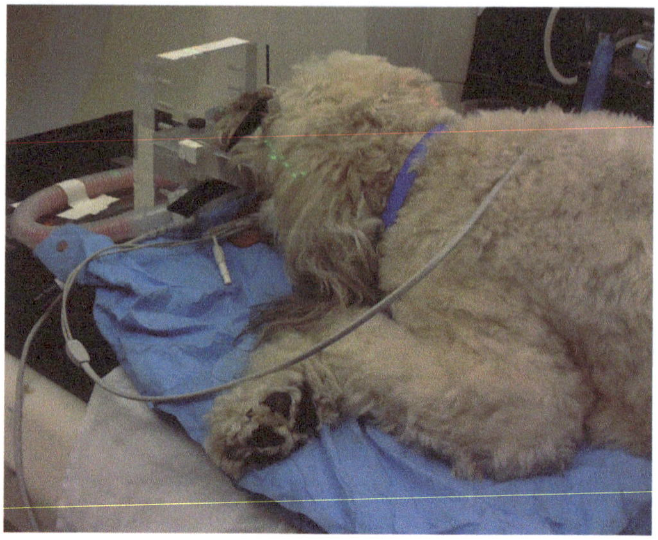

Figure 8.2 Dog with a nasal tumor placed in a patient-specific vacuum-formable mattress (blue) and bite block immobilization system (same system as Figure 8.1).

- the gross tumor volume (GTV)
- the clinical tumor volume (CTV)
- the planning tumor volume (PTV)
- the organs at risk (OAR).

The GTV is the tumor volume that can be identified on imaging, which can include CT, magnetic resonance imaging (MRI), positron emission tomography (PET) and/or other methods such as ultrasonography. The CTV is a margin beyond the visible tumor where microscopic tumor and tumor spread to lymph nodes or along facial planes is suspected. The PTV is a margin beyond the CTV to take into account errors in daily positioning and organ motion.

Reducing Set-Up Errors

CT is the optimal imaging modality for radiotherapy treatment planning because of the precise patient dimensions and patient electron density information, which are used by the treatment-planning computer software to accurately determine dose distribution in the tumor and surrounding tissues. Despite the better soft tissue resolution of MRI, this modality is used as an adjunct to CT rather than replacing it in radiotherapy treatment planning. This is because MRI does not image bone well, does not provide the electron density of tissues needed for dosimetry calculations, and because of the presence of intrinsic system-related and object-induced MR image distortions. Even if electron density information provides little change to dosimetry calculations, it is essential to image the patient in the treatment position. In the MR suite it is difficult to set patients up in the therapy position using mattresses and bite-block systems, which often contain ferromagnetic structures. Often dogs and cats are in dorsal recumbent position on radiofrequency coil, which is not an optimal treatment position. This makes it difficult to reproduce daily patient positioning during the course of therapy.

With the increased use of IMRT and the ability to achieve steep dose gradients between the PTV and OAR, the need for daily image guidance is essential. Many new treatment machines have on-board imaging capabilities. Some examples include an in-room CT scanner that shares the same couch as the linear accelerator; kilovoltage cone-beam CT where the X-ray tube is mounted on a retractable arm; and helical tomotherapy (HT), which was developed at the University of Wisconsin-Madison. HT combines a linear accelerator and a helical CT scanner where the linear accelerator rotates 360° around the patient as the patient is translated through the aperture creating a helical treatment beam. HT is an advanced form of conformal IMRT that also uses image verification to precisely deliver radiation to the desired target. Image-guided radiation therapy seeks to remove uncertainties associated with anatomical positioning at each treatment by acquiring images of the patient immediately prior to radiation beam delivery. The strategy of targeting sensitive normal structures for avoidance while effectively

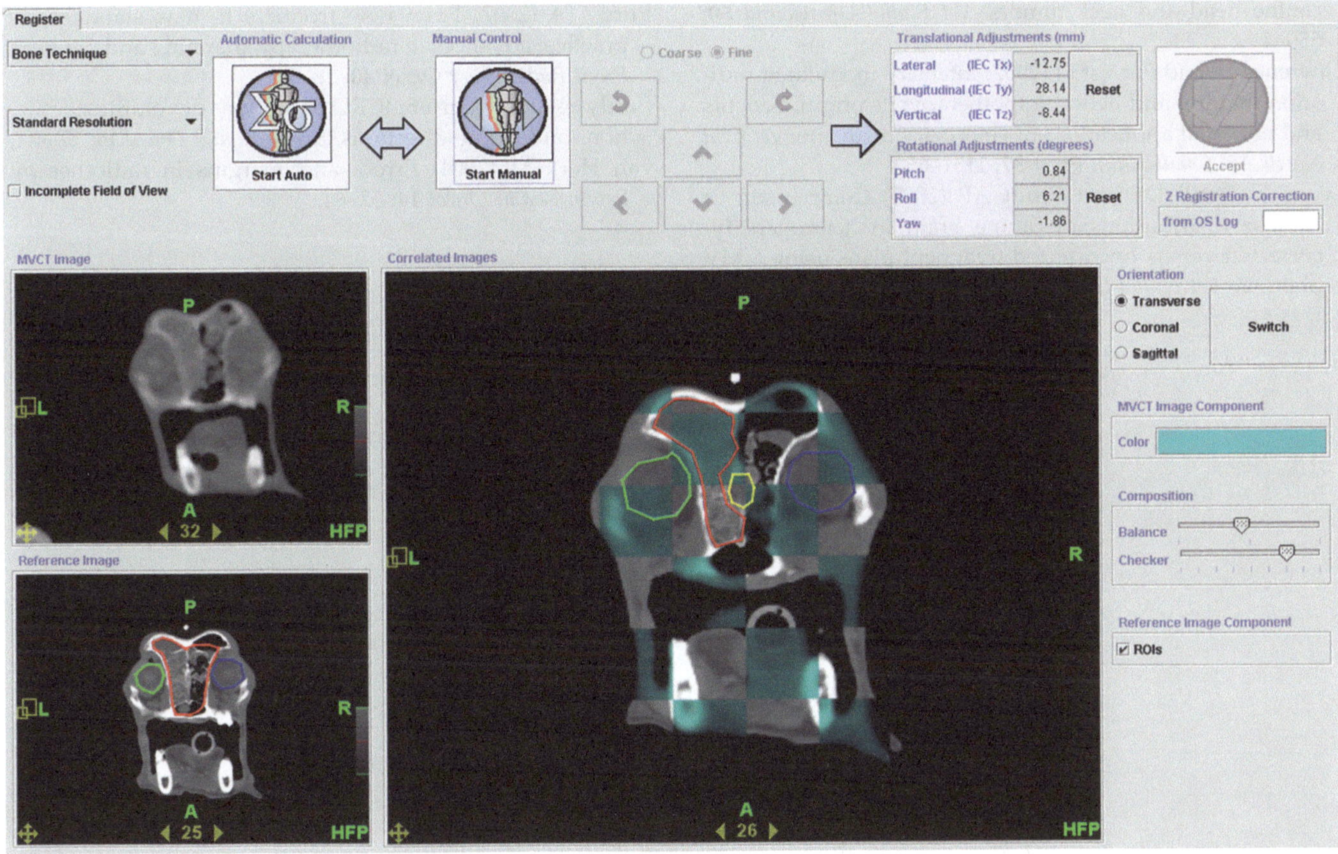

Figure 8.3 Typical image of the tomotherapy operator station showing alignment of the MVCT (top left) with the original planning kVCT (bottom left) of a dog treated with helical tomotherapy. In the correlated image (large image, right) the turquoise squares represent the MVCT image obtained prior to treatment and the grey areas represent the planning kVCT. The round light green and blue contours represent the left and right eyes, respectively. The yellow contour is the rostral brain and the red contour is the PTV. Note the positional changes in millimeters in the upper left of the image in six dimensions after alignment. The machine automatically will change vertical, longitudinal and roll changes.

treating arbitrarily shaped treatment volumes was not possible before the emergence of IMRT. HT acquires a megavoltage CT (MVCT; using the linear accelerator), which is aligned with the planning kilovoltage CT (kVCT) each day before treatment. Based on 3-D image alignment, patients are repositioned as necessary, in the lateral, longitudinal, vertical, pitch, roll and yaw dimensions after final registration of the images (Figure 8.3).

Summary

CT plays an important role in radiotherapy treatment planning and delivery. Accurate patient dose delivery is highly dependent on accurate patient data, which are best acquired with CT imaging. These data include body contour, outline, density of relevant internal structures, and the location and extent of the target volume and OAR. The most important information that is best obtained with CT is the delineation of target volume and surrounding structures with respect to the external body contour. This is essential for treatment planning and optimization of dose distribution.

Further Reading

Harmon J, Van Ufflen D and LaRue S (2009) Assessment of radiotherapy patient cranial immobilization device using daily on-board kilovoltage imaging. *Vet Radiol Ultrasound* **50**: 230–4.

ICRU (1993) ICRU Report 50: Prescribing, recording and reporting photon beam therapy. International Commission on Radiation Units and Measurements. Bethesda, MD.

Kent MS, Gordon IK, Benavides I, Primas P and Young J (2009) Assessment of the accuracy and precision of a patient immobilization device for radiation therapy in canine head and neck tumors. *Vet Radiol Ultrasound* **50**: 550–4.

Lawrence JA and Forrest LJ (2007) Intensity-modulated radiation therapy and helical tomotherapy: its origin, benefits and potential applications in veterinary medicine. *Vet Clin North Am Small Anim Pract* **37**: 1151–65.

Lyons J, Thrall DE and Pruitt AF (2007) Comparison of isodose distributions in canine brain in heterogeneity-corrected versus uncorrected treatment plans using 6 MV photons. *Vet Radiol Ultrasound* **48**: 292–6.

Purdy JA (2007) From new frontiers to new standards of practice: advances in radiotherapy, planning and delivery. *Front Radiat Ther Oncol* **40**: 18–39.

Purdy JA (2004) Current ICRU definitions of volumes: limitations and future directions. *Semin Radiat Oncol* **14**: 27–40.

van Herk M (2004) Errors and margins in radiotherapy. *Semin Radiat Oncol* **14**: 52–64.

CHAPTER NINE

Interventional CT

Tobias Schwarz and Sarah Puchalski

Introduction

Interventional radiology involves the use of imaging procedures for delivering different treatment options or obtaining diagnostic samples. CT has gained popularity in this field because it is cross-sectional and free of magnification errors. This allows precise localization and sizing for stenting and other procedures that are difficult to match with other modalities with the same accuracy. Compared to other imaging modalities, CT is also free of or less vulnerable to image degradation caused by artifacts such as scatter (radiography), gas and bone (ultrasound), mineral or metal (magnetic resonance imaging). The biggest restriction of interventional CT is the limited ability to perform real-time imaging due to the high radiation dose to the operator this would involve without the use of special equipment.

CT for Biopsy Procedures

Biopsy mode software applications in CT

Most modern CT scanners have a biopsy software application that can usually be added to the diagnostic protocol of the patient. It consists of short-ranging CT scans that can be quickly and easily repeated, designed for fast checks of biopsy device position. It is advisable to select a large display field of view to be able to see the full trajectory of the biopsy needle.

CT-guided biopsy procedures

CT guidance implies real-time imaging during the procedure. In most circumstances this can only be achieved with CT-fluoroscopy, a robotic arm device and appropriate personnel shielding. This advanced and often very specific technology has not been expanded to veterinary patients yet and is cost prohibitive at the moment.

Stereotactic CT brain biopsy devices have been developed and tested successfully on veterinary patients and are commercially available. The procedure has a high diagnostic yield, but is relatively time-consuming and has potentially serious side effects. It should only be used in experienced hands.

CT-assisted biopsies (Figures 9.1 and 9.2)

CT assistance implies that the biopsying device (including full-core biopsies and fine needle aspirates) is inserted in steps under CT monitoring. The actual biopsy relies on trajectory information obtained from the CT scan but it is not performed under real-time imaging guidance. In addition to general precautions there are three conditions that need to be met for a CT-assisted biopsy:

- The target should not be easily moveable. Because the final biopsy step is performed blindly, organs that would shift away under pressure cannot be biopsied safely. Therefore CT-assisted biopsy is not usually applicable for the abdomen.
- The anticipated path of the biopsy needle is entirely within the X-Y plane. Any deviation would make the procedure unsafe because further needle advancement could not be planned accurately.
- Expected side effects due to organ perforation are manageable.

In most clinical circumstances CT-assisted biopsies are elected if real-time imaging guidance modalities such ultrasound or fluoroscopy cannot be performed. This is usually the case for inaccessible body parts and organs such as lungs, mediastinum, head and spine.

Veterinary Computed Tomography, First Edition. Edited by Tobias Schwarz, Jimmy Saunders.

CT assisted biopsy procedure (Figure 9.3)

In general, a non-bulky biopsying needle device should be selected to ease the needle positioning and minimize artifacts. Biopsy guns with big metal housings cannot be used. For bone biopsies a Jamshidi needle or similar device should be available. The procedure is much easier and quicker if only fine needle aspirates are performed, but the procedural steps are similar:

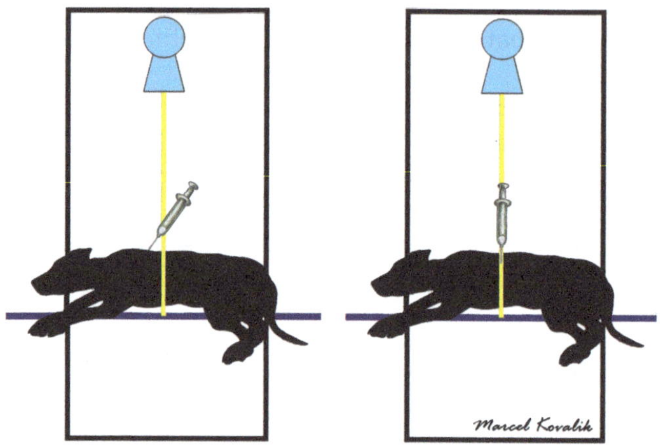

Figure 9.1 Needle positioning for CT-assisted biopsy. The situation on the left needs to be avoided as further needle advancement cannot be monitored predictably on transverse plane images. The needle should be perfectly aligned with the X-Y plane of the CT scanner, as shown on the right, with the help of the positional laser lights on the scanning unit.

- From the diagnostic CT scan, the area and anticipated access point is identified and surgically prepared.
- Also from the diagnostic CT scan at the exact intended biopsy level, the distance between the surface entrance point and a palpable landmark is measured, as well as the optimal biopsy path angle and depth towards vertical.
- The biopsy depth is then marked with a sterile permanent marker on the biopsy needle.
- The entrance point is measured from the landmark and marked on the patient.
- The needle is inserted into the entrance point just beyond the skin surface and secured in a sterile manner in the anticipated trajectory angle.
- The biopsy location needs to be at the laser light location and the laser light needs to be completely superimposed on the needle shaft.
- A biopsy scan is performed.
- Needle entrance location, trajectory angle and depth are checked on the biopsy CT scan.
- If errors occurred, the needle position is corrected, otherwise the needle is further advanced and in either case another biopsy CT scan is performed. Scans are repeated until the needle is in the correct position.
- The needle is inserted to the marked target depth and the biopsy procedure is performed.

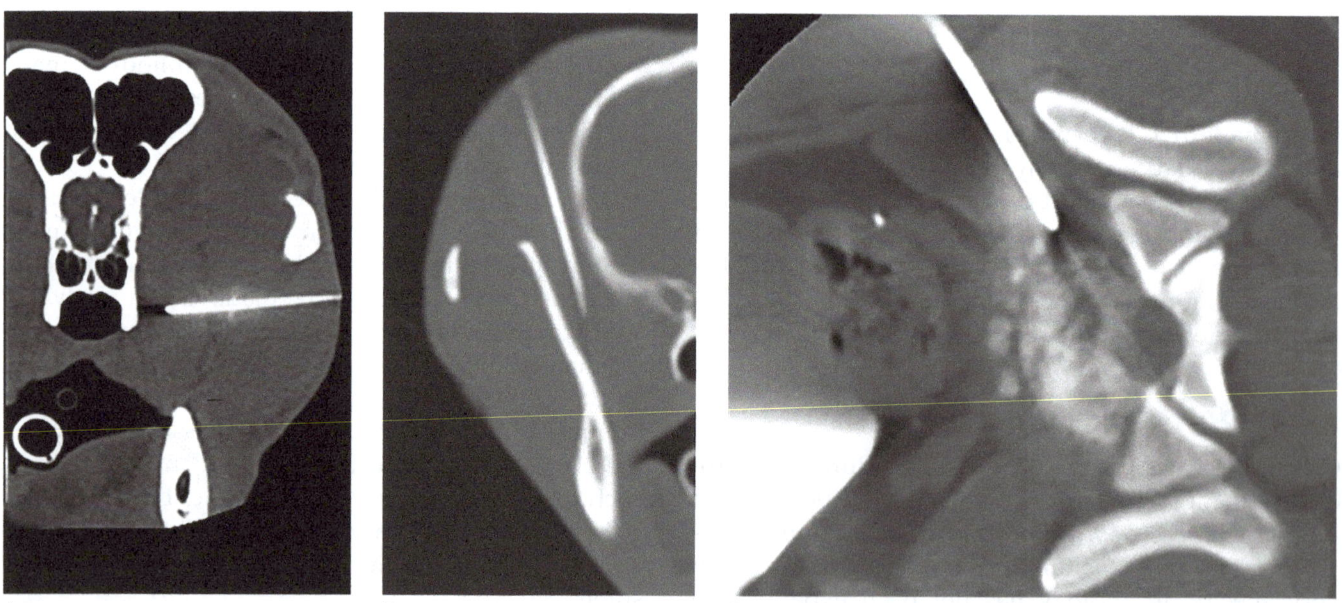

A B C

Figure 9.2 CT-assisted fine needle aspirates for otherwise inaccessible body parts. (A) Pterygoid muscle with a lateral approach ventral to the zygomatic arch. (B) Temporal muscle between the mandible and skull, dorsal access. (C) Lumbosacral disk space from ventrolateral in lateral patient recumbence.

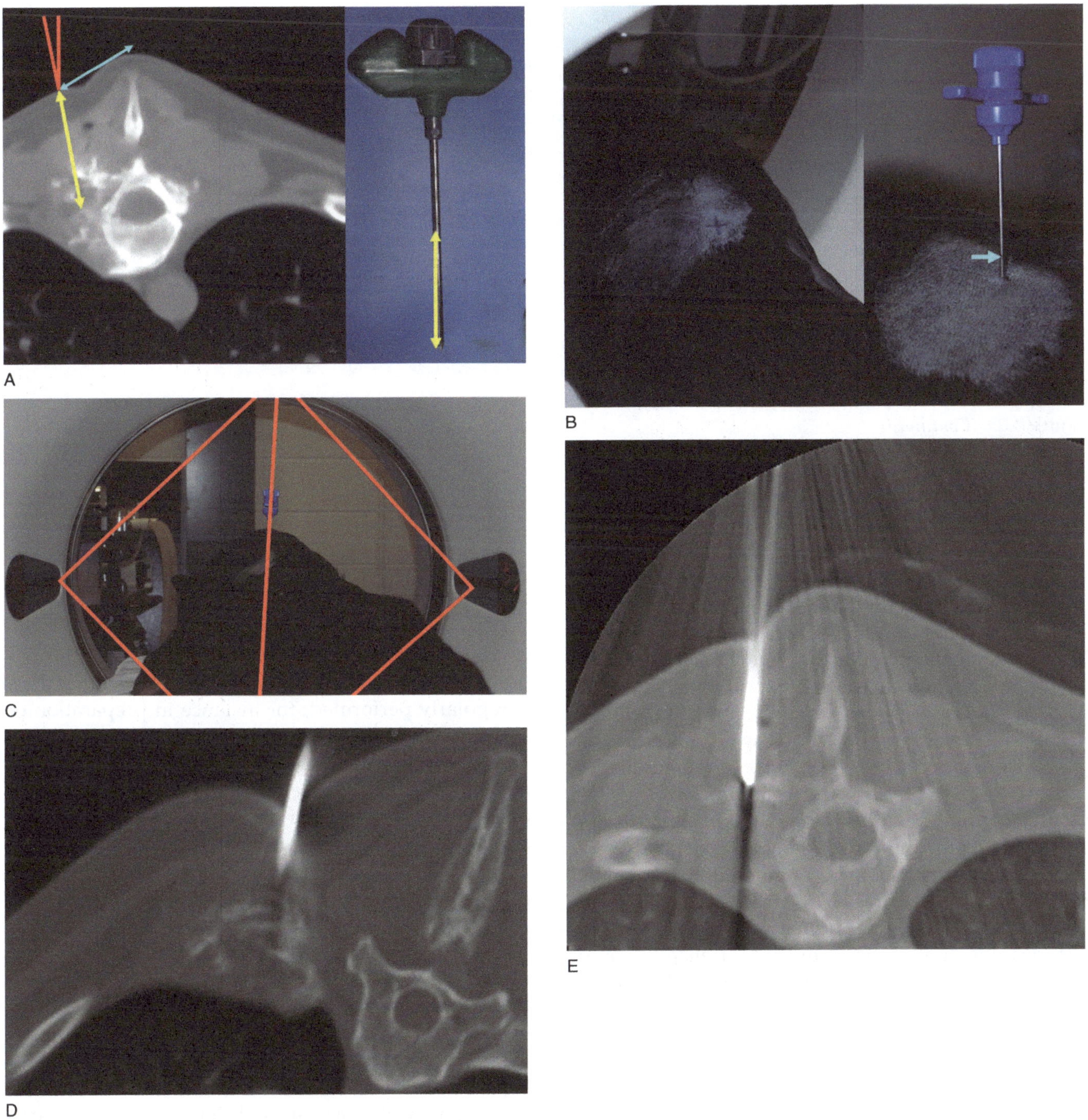

Figure 9.3 Procedural steps during a CT-assisted biopsy of a proliferative vertebral lesion in a dog using a Jamshidi needle. (A) Identify the optimal slice location for a biopsy from the diagnostic CT scan. On the CT image at that location, determine the biopsy path by measuring the surface distance of the entrance point to a palpable landmark (spinous process, magenta arrow), the angle of the path towards vertical (red open angle) and the length of the biopsy path within the body (yellow arrow). Mark up that length on the biopsy needle shaft. (B) Drive the CT table to the surgically prepared biopsy location level. Determine the biopsy entrance point by measuring the distance from the palpable landmark. Insert the biopsy needle superficially. The magenta arrow marks the anticipated biopsy path depth. (C) Using the side laser lights, ensure perfect alignment of the needle shaft with the X-Y plane. (D) Perform a biopsy CT scan to check needle position. (E) Advance or correct needle position accordingly and repeat biopsy CT scan. (F) Perform biopsy procedure and harvest material. Final diagnosis: disseminated blastomycosis.

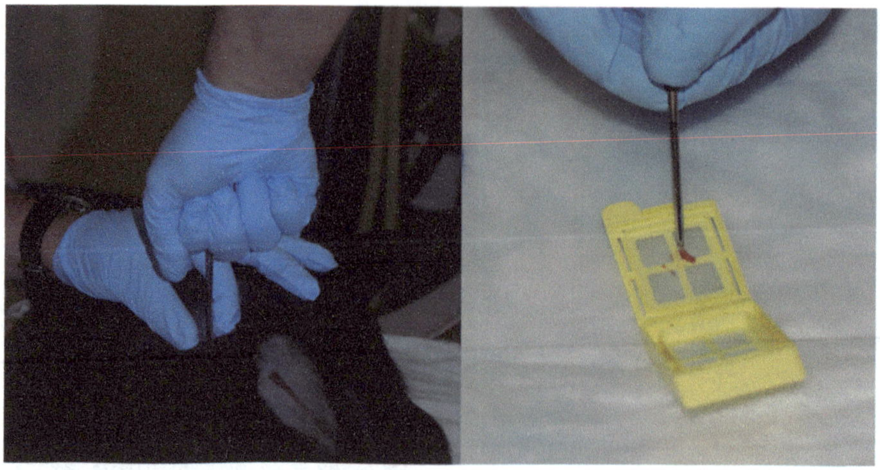

F

Figure 9.3 (*Continued*)

Particulars of thoracic biopsy procedures (Figure 9.4)

In the authors' opinion, only fine needle aspirates can be performed safely in the thorax with CT assistance. However, CT-assisted fine needle aspiration is arguably the most valuable imaging guided sampling procedure for the thorax as almost all organs can be reached safely. It is essential that the patient is scanned during the respiratory pause during all procedures to prevent organ shift between scans. Hyperventilation prior to biopsying is helpful to minimize the risk of pleural tearing. The needle cannot be advanced beyond the skin level during the preparatory stage and therefore the trajectory has to be more accurately planned for thoracic procedures. Fine needle aspirates with CT assistance can be performed with pulmonary trajectories for lung lesions or with transpulmonary trajectories to reach mediastinal structures. The needle needs to be connected to the suction device (syringe) in the initial set-up and should not be disconnected during the procedure, to prevent significant pneumothorax. It is not recommended to perform more than five pulmonary aspirates as the risk of developing significant pneumothorax increases after numerous lung punctures. It is normal to observe mild pneumothorax and pulmonary hemorrhage after the procedure and a post-biopsy scan should be performed 5 to 10 min afterwards. For this scan it is important to include the lesion site, and the highest and lowest points of the thorax to be able to monitor free pleural fluid and gas accumulation respectively. The post-biopsy scan should also be assessed diagnostically, as it often can reveal additional diagnostic features.

CT Monitoring of Stents and Other Devices (Figures 9.5, 24.7B and 26.18C)

CT can be used to obtain exact size and shape information for stenting and catheterization procedures. This is regularly performed, for instance in preparation of surgical procedures of intrahepatic portosystemic shunts. With CT-fluoroscopy this can be performed in real time. CT is also useful for follow-up monitoring of stenting devices, other permanent implants or accidentally dislodged intravascular material.

CT Assisted Embolization Techniques (Figure 9.6)

If radiopaque material is used for embolization procedures in various tissues, CT can be used to document the correct location of the embolizing material. With hepatic chemoembolization, an oil-based contrast medium is applied as part of the embolization process, increasing the cytotoxic drug concentration and dwell time. Due to its slow reticuloendothelial clearance the hepatic contrast enhancement can be used to monitor drug delivery, persistence and tumor necrosis.

CT-Monitored Cryoablation of Tumors (Figure 9.7)

CT has a high sensitivity to detect subtle density changes. Most soft tissues have density values

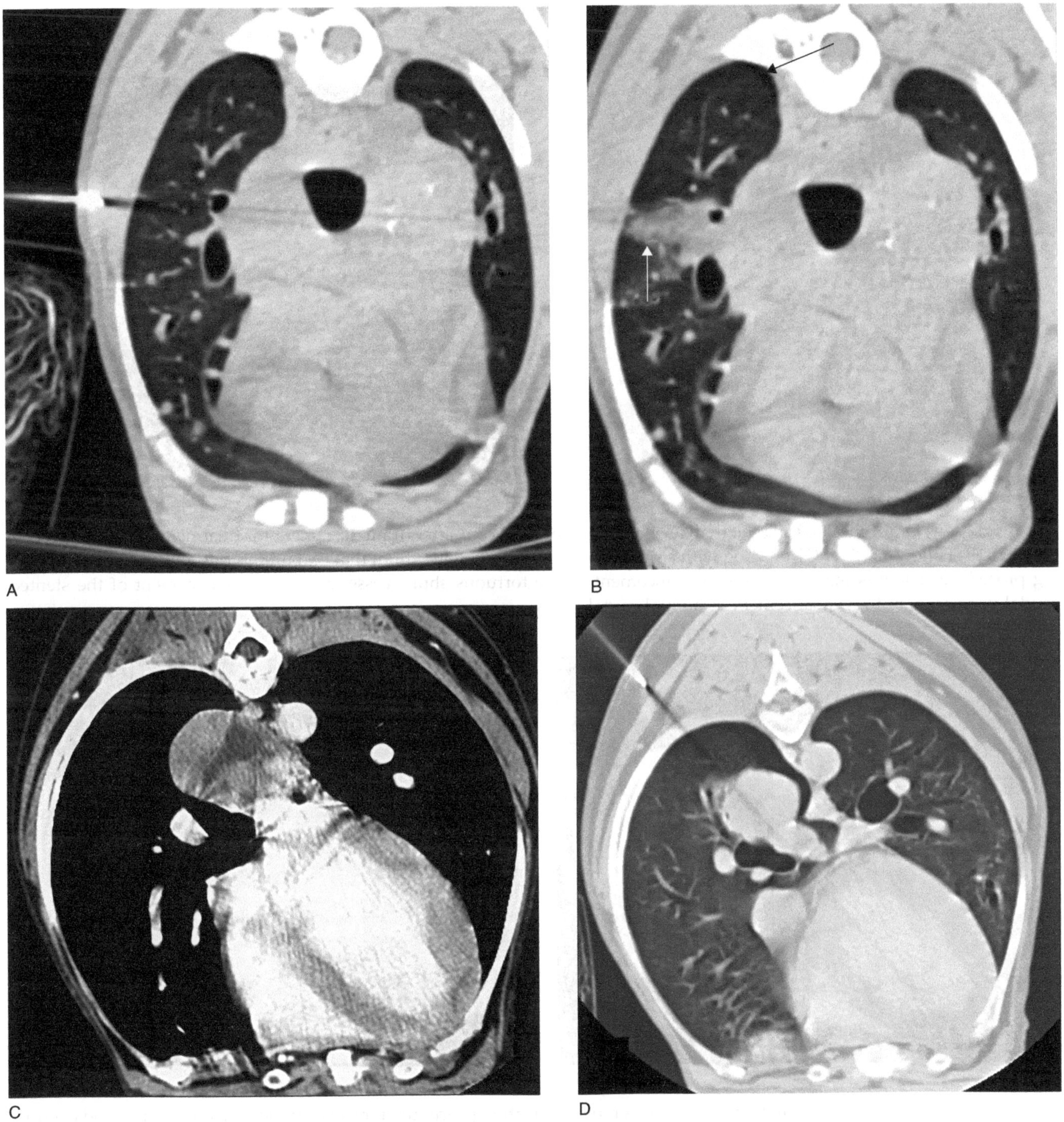

Figure 9.4 (A) Set-up for a transpulmonary CT-assisted fine needle aspirate of a perihilar mediastinal mass. (B) The post-biopsy scan reveals a small pneumothorax (black arrow) and pulmonary hemorrhage along the needle track (white arrow). (C) Diagnostic CT scan with a mass that could be pulmonary or mediastinal. (D) Biopsy-induced pneumothorax reveals the mass as pulmonary.

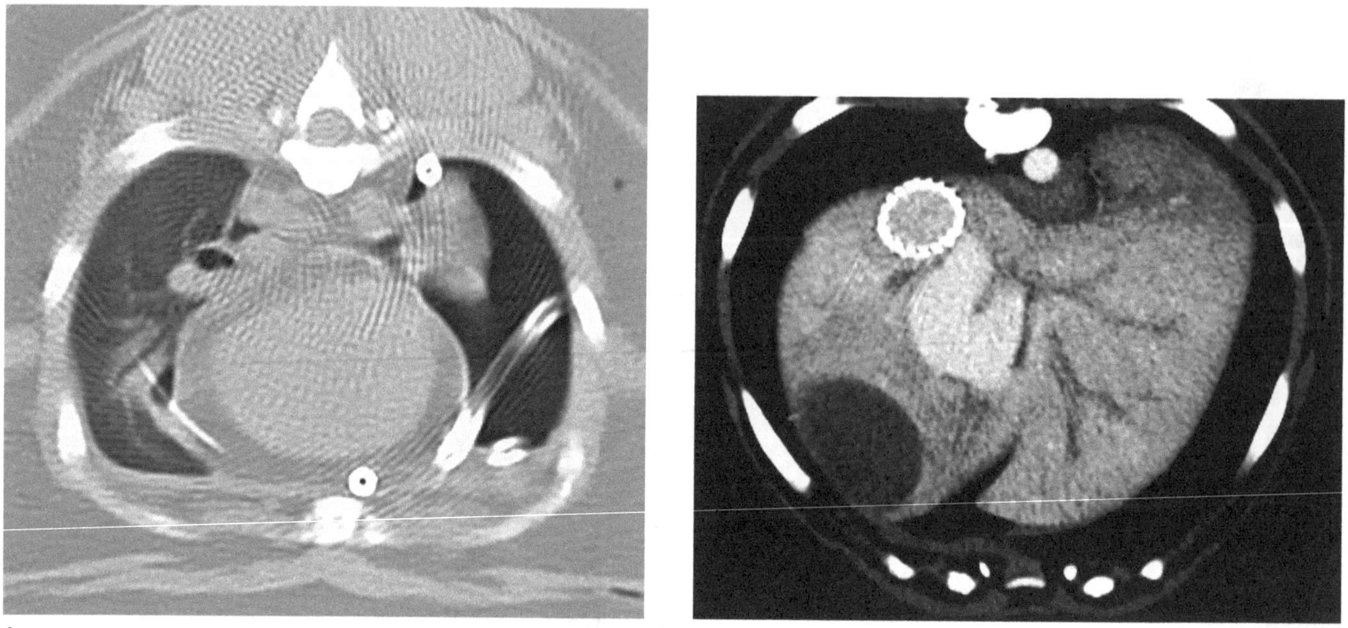

A B

Figure 9.5 (A) Drain check CT in a cat that developed a pneumothorax after drain placement for treatment of chronic pleural effusion. (B) Follow-up liver CT of a dog with a right-divisional intrahepatic shunt that had undergone an intravascular stenting procedure. There is marked contrast enhancement of the tortuous shunt vessel and mild enhancement of the stented caudal vena cava, but no enhancement of normal portal veins.

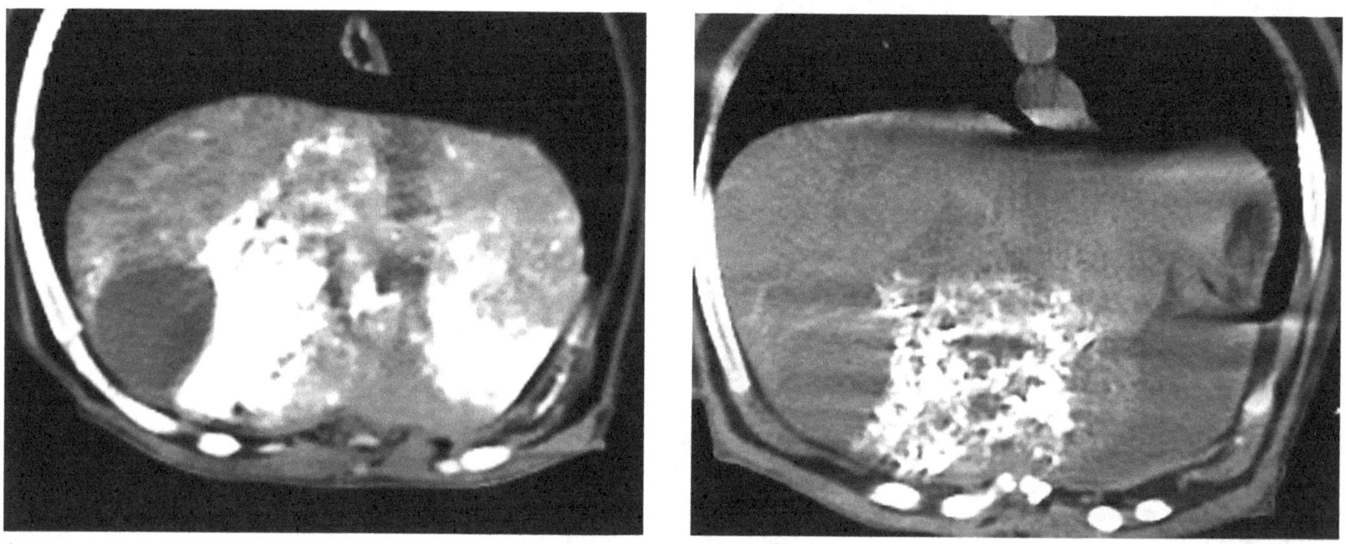

A B

Figure 9.6 CT images of a dog that underwent a chemoembolization procedure for a liver tumour using an oil-based contrast medium as one of the embolizing agents. (A) 30 days and (B) 60 days post-procedure contrast medium is still present and can be used to monitor the progression of neoplastic growth (images courtesy of Tom Cave).

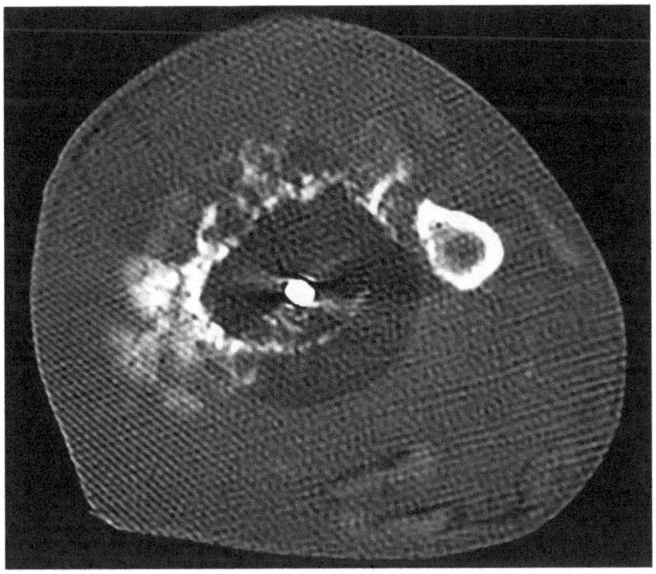

Figure 9.7 CT-monitored cryoablation procedure of a distal radial osteosarcoma in a dog. The frozen soft tissue around the central metallic cryoablation probe is hypodense, allowing exact sizing of the ice ball.

between 40 and 60 HU, which drop in the frozen state to 20 to 40 HU. This makes it an ideal monitoring device for cryosurgical procedures in which determination of the exact size and location of the ice ball is crucial for effective destruction of neoplastic lesions.

Interventional CT in Equines

In equine clinical medicine, CT-guided procedures are performed using the same principles as outlined for small animals. Regions where CT guidance can be particularly helpful are generally associated with foot lameness. CT imaging can be used to guide needle placement into lesions housed within the hoof capsule for the administration of medications such as biological agents (platelet-rich plasma, bone marrow extract supernatant, stem cells). Minimally invasive surgery can also be performed using CT guidance. Procedures such as debridement of osseous cyst-like lesion of the distal or middle phalanges or osteomyelitis of the distal phalanx can be performed with minimal disruption of the hoof capsule. Similarly, CT is very useful for preoperative planning. Using the CT scanner to provide external landmarks, which can be permanently affixed to the skin or hoof surface, is used to aid in implant placement for fracture repair and to minimize the size of hoof wall resections for the removal of subcapsular masses.

Further Reading

Moissonier P, Blot S, Devauchelle P *et al.* (2002) Stereotactic CT-guided brain biopsy in the dog. *J Small Anim Pract* **43**: 115–23.

Tidwell AS and Johnson KL (1994) Computed tomography-guided percutaneous biopsy in the dog and cat: description of technique and preliminary evaluation in 14 patients. *Vet Radiol Ultrasound* **35**: 445–6.

Vignoli M, Ohlert S, Rossi F *et al.* (2004) Computed tomography-guided fine-needle aspiration and tissue-core biopsy of bone lesions in small animals. *Vet Radiol Ultrasound* **45**: 125–30.

Vignoli M and Saunders JH (2011) Image-guided interventional procedures in the dog and cat. *The Vet J* **187**: 296–303.

Zekas LJ, Crawford JT and O'Brien RT (2005) Computed tomography-guided fine-needle aspirate and tissue-core biopsy of intrathoracic lesions in thirty dogs and cats. *Vet Radiol Ultrasound* **46**: 200–4.

CHAPTER TEN

Purchase Considerations

Victor Rendano Jr.

I used to worry about when the coffee would be ready; now I worry about whether or not I will have enough money to buy the coffee beans.

Victor Rendano VMD, MSc, DACVR, DACVR-RO

The majority of people who will read this chapter are those who depend on the financial success of the CT equipment, either directly via its usage or secondarily because of not only the cash flow it brings to other departments and the prestige, but also the increased referrals it brings to the overall entity. Initially, the CT equipment will need to be purchased, then upgraded, maintained or replaced. Depending on your situation, you may need to make all of the decisions or work to improve some of the decisions that have already been made for you.

There is no unequivocal right or wrong way to achieve financial viability. The major considerations for financial viability, however, include:

- the business plan
- the service contract
- case load considerations (Table 10.1).

Each option has its pros and cons, but the person who is ultimately responsible for the viability of the entity is ultimately responsible for making sure it is done correctly for that entity. Do everything in your power to get it right the first time, as some mistakes can be so costly to fix that they could imperil the financial viability of your entity.

Business Plan: Income versus Expenses, i.e. Profit or Loss

The business plan is a series of questions and answers. The questions are routine; the correct responses require someone to research the answers.

Most considerations in a business plan are estimates:

- what it will cost to buy or lease, maintain and replace the equipment
- what it will cost to outfit and use the space where the equipment is located
- what it will cost to maintain the staff to run the equipment
- what it will cost to have the ancillary equipment to use the CT unit, e.g. anesthetic equipment, monitoring devices, image storage software and hardware, heating and air conditioning.

To establish a rapport with you colleagues and clients, decisions need to be made about how you will let them know about this equipment and what it can do for them. Advertising, continuing education programs, reporting of findings and handling of referrals helps establish who you are, where you are, what you do and how you do it.

The number of answer permutations when buying CT equipment is endless. However, the methodical approach to obtain correct answers to these questions will be your road map to success. Buying equipment without researching what equipment will fit your needs, what the space requirements for that equipment are, what the heating and air conditioning requirements are, what the radiation safety requirements are, what the electrical needs are and how the equipment would be brought into or removed from the building will ensure you spend money needlessly, and you may never get the project to completion.

The number of permutations when letting others know about your equipment is finite. These interactions are influenced by the location of the CT facility and its alignment with other entities. Will you be a stand-alone imaging facility, part of a private practice group or associated with academia?

Whatever your work situation, the basic tenets of success are letting others know you have the equipment and what the equipment can do for their patients,

Veterinary Computed Tomography, First Edition. Edited by Tobias Schwarz, Jimmy Saunders.

Table 10.1
Major considerations for financial viability.

Business plan
• Location of the facility
• Stand-alone versus specialty group practice
• Interaction with primary care facilities
• Interaction with regional specialists
• Advertising
• New versus used equipment purchase
• Continuing education, training, personnel
• Business insurance
• Malpractice insurance
• Cost to develop site
• Cost to maintain site
• Transportation of the patient
Service contract
• Self-insured versus service contract
• PM contract
• Contract without tube replacement
• Contract with tube replacement
• Availability of repair and parts
• Same day, evening and weekend repairs
Case load considerations
• Number of cases
• Cost per case
• Income per study per case

e.g. the disease processes for which CT is most likely to add needed information. Cost-effectiveness, availability and diagnostic accuracy will then solidify its use if the regional resources are adequate to maintain this level of imaging.

Service Contract: All, Some or Nothing at All

You need to determine the part of your budget specifically available to buy or lease the equipment. You can then pursue vendors who can provide you with the equipment you can afford. Your objectives are to acquire better equipment than you can afford, at a price you can afford, with 'bumper-to-bumper' coverage 24 hours a day, seven days a week. The vendor's objectives are to sell you a piece of equipment that is within your budget and to adjust the value of the equipment downwards as you ask for more warranty services. Thus the art of negotiating becomes important in determining what equipment you acquire and how it will be maintained. Sometimes you get lucky: a desired piece of equipment becomes available on the market at a reduced price and you need to act immediately. However, the methodical approach to a service contract, independent of how much time you have to buy the equipment, will often be the corner stone of financial success, so you should not rush this part of the negotiation. If you self-insure, i.e. have no service contract, then you should have an agreement with a person or company who knows how to diagnose and repair the equipment on an as-needed basis. This is often an informal discussion with a summary letter thanking them for agreeing to help you maintain your equipment at a designated fee per hour or fee per call plus parts as mutually agreed.

If you choose to enter into a formal contract then you must make sure you understand exactly what you are getting for your money. The service contract will address the following issues:

- type of service
- rates for maintenance
- price for parts supplied by maintenance provider
- basic service to be performed by maintenance provider
- customer's duties
- reports of service
- performance of service
- limitation of service
- renewal
- termination
- indemnity and hold harmless
- insurance
- safe working environment
- disclaimer of warranty for products not manufactured by maintenance provider
- entire and binding agreement
- no waiver
- payment terms
- applicable law/dispute resolution
- arbitration
- waiver of subrogation.

If these issues read like 'legalese', it is because that is what they are. There is never a problem until there is a problem and once the parties pull out the contract to see 'exactly what it says', then they are closer to going to court for resolution, which means time, money and wasted energy.

Caseload Considerations: Fixed and Variable Costs of Doing Business

The day has come to do your first study. The number of cases you do and the fee per case will determine if you have enough money to buy the coffee beans for the amount of coffee you have to make. You put pen to paper. What should I charge to meet my financial obligations? You look at the cost sheet for keeping the equipment running. It costs you US$100 000 to secure the space, provide the needed utilities, purchase the anesthetic and monitoring equipment and a few holding cages, modernize the room, and purchase the CT equipment and image storage device. If you borrowed the money at 8% interest on a five-year note, your monthly payment would be $2027.

You calculate that your maintenance (cleaning, repairs to the room), insurance, taxes and utilities (electric, heating, telephone, water usage, etc.) for the space will be $650 per month.

Your service contract for routine preventative maintenance (PM) and unlimited telephone support is $500 per month without part replacement cost, so you should consider putting $50 per case into a reserve fund to cover catastrophic problems, e.g. tube replacement cost.

Therefore the monthly payment to the lender, the insurance, taxes, utilities and the maintenance contract are fixed costs, i.e. $3177 whether you image a case or not.

The technical help required to run the equipment will cost you $30 per case in an existing multi-specialty facility. If you are a stand-alone facility, your technical costs will vary depending on the employment agreement: fee per case, hourly fee or annual salary. General equipment costs such as anesthetic machine, monitoring equipment, etc., will cost you $100 per case. Front office support staff, paper supplies and advertisement for your service will cost you $38 per case. Your time to oversee the case, review the images, generate the report, and talk to the owner and the referring veterinarian should generate you $150 per case. These numbers add up to $318 per case in variable costs.

Most clients in my practice area will pay between $400 and $1000 for the CT study. If you select a target price of $600–700 per case per CT study, then you need to do 10 cases per month to meet the financial obligation (Table 10.2).

Table 10.2
Cost calculations worksheet.

Fixed costs per month	**Example**	**Practice figures**
• Equipment loan	$2207	
• Service contract	$500	
• Taxes, utilities, insurance	$650	
• *Total: monthly fixed cost*	*$3177*	
Non-fixed costs per month	**Example**	**Practice figures**
• Technical help per case	$30	
• Non-technical support	$38	
• Fund for part replacement	$50	
• Professional services	$150	
• General equipment costs (anesthesia, monitoring, etc.)	$100	
• *Total: per case*	*$368.00*	
Cost per case worksheet	**Example**	**Practice figures**
6 cases per month	6 cases	
$3177 fixed cost	$3177	
$368/case non-fixed	$2208	
	Total: $5385	
	$5385/6 = $897.50	
10 cases per month	10 cases	
$3177 fixed cost	$3177	
$368/case non-fixed	$3680	
	Total: $6857	
	$6857/10 = $685.70	

As you do more cases your profit margin will increase. As you do less your costs will need to decrease perhaps by your answering the telephone, doing the study yourself without technical support or discontinuing the maintenance contract, otherwise you will need to subsidize the CT service with cash flow from other services. If you do not decrease costs you will go out of business.

The fee you charge the client per CT study can be increased if you offer additional services while using this unit, e.g. you scan more than one area, you scan an area prior to and after contrast medium administration, you do a CT guided biopsy. The additional fees combined with the base fee will influence the number of cases you need to do per month for financial viability; usually, the base number will be four or five per month.

There are also peripheral considerations for handling a case that will also need to be considered. If you are a stand-alone imaging center, you will need to orchestrate everything: admitting the pet, ensuring the pet is stable for anesthesia, overseeing catheter placement and anesthesia, housing, recovery and discharge.

These efforts will be an additional revenue stream for you. If you are part of a specialty group, you will need to decide who will do the patient care before and after the patient is in the CT suite and who will monitor the pet while the CT scan is being done. Who receives these fees will also determine the potential profitability of having a CT scanner.

Usually, there is wild enthusiasm about purchasing the CT scanner. It has almost become a 'must have' piece of equipment. However, there is concern when one begins to consider the cost of having a CT scanner, and then there is the pride and usually jubilation of owning the CT scanner. The equipment allows us to do the best we can as imagers for our patients, and at the end of the day that, in my opinion, is the ultimate reward.

May you have an abundance of the best coffee beans and share your coffee generously.

CHAPTER ELEVEN

NASAL CAVITIES AND FRONTAL SINUSES

Jimmy Saunders and Tobias Schwarz

IMAGING PROTOCOL

See Table 11.1.

CT: ANATOMY AND NORMAL VARIANTS

Nasal cavities and paranasal sinuses in carnivores

The nasal cavities are surrounded bilaterally by the incisive, nasal, maxillary, lacrimal, zygomatic, palatine, vomer, presphenoid and ethmoid bones (Figure 11.1). They extend from the nostrils rostrally to the cribriform plate and nasopharynx caudally. The cribriform plate is a sieve-like partition between the nasal and cranial cavities that is perforate by ± 300 foramina (<1.5 mm in diameter) serving for the passage of olfactory nerve bundles (Figure 11.2E). On CT, the integrity of the cribriform plate is best evaluated on dorsal planes.

The right and left cavities are separated by a nasal septum (cartilaginous and membranous rostrally, ossified caudally) that appears commonly curved on CT in its rostral part in cats and brachycephalic dogs.

The caudal half of the nasal cavities is largely filled by the ethmoidal turbinates (Figure 11.2B, 11.2C) that attach caudally to the cribriform plate and are covered by the orbital lamina of the ethmoid bone. The ethmoidal turbinates are so extensive that they also invade the lower part of the frontal sinuses (Figure 11.2C). They are composed of four long endoturbinates (I to IV) and six small ectoturbinates (1 to 6) (Figure 11.2B). The difference between the two groups is based on their location. Each ethmoidal element possesses a basal bony leaf, which attaches to the orbital lamina of the ethmoid bone.

The rostral half of the nasal cavities lodges the dorsal and ventral nasal conchae, which are usually referred to as nasal turbinates (Figure 11.2A). The dorsal nasal turbinate is a smooth, curved plate that arises from the nasal bone as an extension of the first endoturbinate. The ventral nasal turbinate is thick but short and occupies the rostral two-thirds of the nasal cavity. It arises from the maxilla as an extension of the second endoturbinate, which breaks up to form many longitudinal scrolls, greatly enlarging the covering mucosa, which is richly vascularized. The ventral turbinate is continued rostrally by the alar fold. The nasal turbinates restrict the air flow. Variations in the structure of the ethmoidal turbinates are commonly observed on CT.

Four narrow nasal passages, the nasal meati, are present between and along the turbinates (Figure 11.2C). The dorsal nasal meatus is a passage between the dorsal nasal turbinate and the dorsal wall of the nasal cavity; the middle nasal meatus lies between the dorsal and ventral nasal turbinates; the ventral nasal meatus is located between the ventral nasal turbinate and the floor of the nasal cavity; the common nasal meatus is a longitudinal narrow space bounded between the nasal septum and the turbinates, and it communicates with the three other meati. The nasopharyngeal meatus extends from the dilated caudal portion of the ventral nasal meatus to the choana and opens into the nasal portion of the pharynx.

The paranasal sinuses of the dog consist of the frontal sinuses, the maxillary recesses and the nasal fundus. All communicate with the nasal cavities. The frontal sinuses are composed of three compartments (rostralis, medialis, lateralis) from which the rostral

Veterinary Computed Tomography, First Edition. Edited by Tobias Schwarz, Jimmy Saunders.

Table 11.1
CT imaging protocol (intravenous contrast study: standard protocol; *see* Chapter 5).

Series	Pre- and post-contrast*	Bone
Decubitus	Ventral	
Scan margins	Nostrils ⟷ C2	
Voltage (kVp)	100–120	
Current (mAs)	100–120 (250: skull)	
Tube rotation time (s)	0.8	
Slice width (mm)	1.25	
Sequential slice interval (mm)	1.25	
Kernel frequency	Medium	High
Window level (HU)	+80	+400
Window width (HU)	200	2500

*Intravenous contrast studies are not mandatory for diagnosis in the majority of cases. They may be useful to better define the mucosa in selected cases or for biopsy guidance.

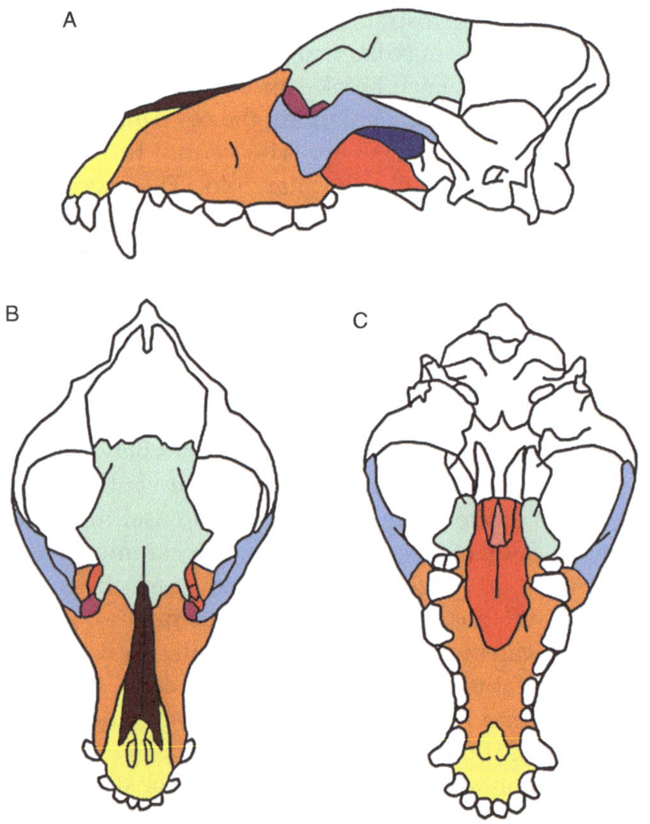

Figure 11.1 (A) Lateral, (B) dorsal and (C) ventral views of the canine skull. The bones surrounding the nasal cavities and frontal sinuses are colored. Incisive bone (yellow), lacrimal bone (purple), maxillary bone (orange), nasal bone (brown), palatine bone (red), presphenoid bone (dark blue), vomer bone (pink), zygomatic bone (sky blue), frontal bone (green).

compartment is further subdivided in three compartments (medialis, intermedius, lateralis), which drain separately into the nasal cavity via the ethmoidal meati. The lateral compartment of the rostral frontal sinus is the largest and occupies much of the frontal bone, including the zygomatic process (Figure 11.2D). The frontal crest separates the right and left frontal sinuses from each other.

Feline anatomical specificities
The rostral half of the nasal cavities lodges the dorsal conchae and the short, but very thick, ventral conchae. The ethmoturbinates are more strongly developed in cats compared with dogs and invade the lower part of the frontal sinuses. The frontal sinuses are not divided into compartments and are significantly bigger in male cats, giving them their characteristic head shape. The maxillary recess is very small. In contrast to dogs, who only have a nasal fundus, cats do have a true sphenoidal sinus with a curved septum. A curved nasal septum is a normal feature in cats.

Disease Features

In dogs, sinonasal neoplasms and fungal rhinitis represent ±75% of chronic nasal disease, while chronic non-specific rhinitis and foreign body rhinitis are responsible for ±20% of nasal disorders. Nasal neoplasia and chronic rhinosinusitis represent ±70% of chronic nasal disease in cats.

Malformation/Developmental

Dermoid cyst/Meningiocele

Dermoid sinus is a failure of separation of the neural tube and cutaneous ectoderm during embryonic development resulting in a tract extending from the skin into the subcutaneous tissues.

CT features (Figure 11.3)

- Abnormal development of the pre-nasal space.
- Tract starts on the midline of the nasal planum and runs along the nasal septum.
- Possible extension of the tract into the brain/cranial vault causing cerebral abscesses or recurrent meningitis.
- Contrast medium can help to better define the direction of the tract and improve visualization of strongly enhancing cerebral lesions.

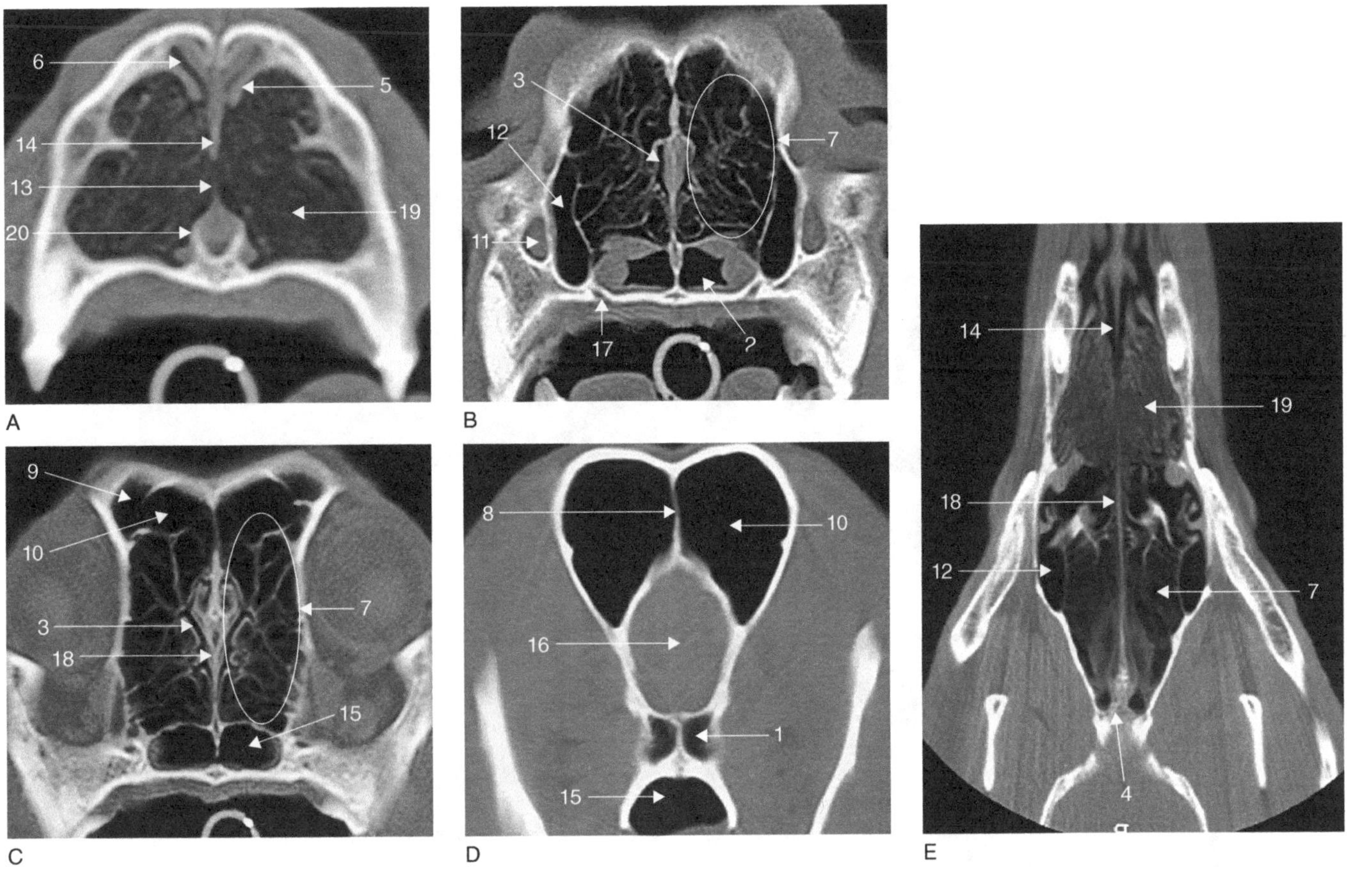

Figure 11.2 (A–D) Transverse CT images of the nasal cavities and frontal sinuses in the normal dog at the level of: (A) Triadan 06 (illustrating the region rostral to the maxillary recesses), (B) the maxillary recesses (illustrating the middle part of the nasal cavities), (C) Triadan 10 (illustrating the region between the maxillary recesses and the frontal sinuses) and (D) the frontal sinuses. For the facility, these four regions will be used in this chapter to determine the level at which the figures were obtained. (E) Dorsally reconstructed CT image. 1 = nasal fundus; 2 = nasopharyngeal meatus; 3 = common nasal meatus; 4 = cribriform plate; 5 = dorsal nasal concha; 6 = dorsal nasal meatus; 7 = ethmoturbinates; 8 = frontal crest; 9 = frontal sinus (lateral compartment); 10 = frontal sinus (medial compartment); 11 = infraorbital canal; 12 = maxillary recess; 13 = middle nasal meatus; 14 = nasal septum (cartilaginous); 15 = choana; 16 = olfactory bulb of the brain; 17 = palatine canal; 18 = perpendicular lamina of the ethmoid bone; 19 = ventral nasal concha; 20 = ventral nasal meatus.

Inflammatory

Nasal polyps

Nasal polyps are an uncommon cause of nasal obstruction in the young (6-24 months) cat. Their precise etiopathogenesis is still obscure even if development secondarily to chronic inflammation has been suggested. Polyps within the nasal cavity are very rare in dogs and are usually unilateral.

CT features (Figure 11.4)

- Soft-tissue opacification of the nasal cavity that replaces the normal turbinate pattern.
- Osteolysis is rarely identified (in contrast to tumors and cryptococcosis).
- Local turbinate destruction, unilateral (dog).

Non-specific rhinitis

Non-specific rhinitis includes lymphoplasmocytic, eosinophilic and hyperplastic rhinitis based on the predominant inflammatory cell pattern and the stage of the disorder. Affected animals show a disruption of the mucociliary clearance system with consequent stasis of secretions, mucosal congestion, edema and hyperplasia, creating an ideal microenvironment for bacterial proliferation. The underlying etiopathogenesis of non-specific rhinitis has still to be elucidated.

CT features (Figure 11.5)

- Distribution of the lesions: diffuse, localized or random; bilateral > unilateral.
- Increased density of the nasal passages and/or frontal sinuses due to mucosa swelling/infiltration

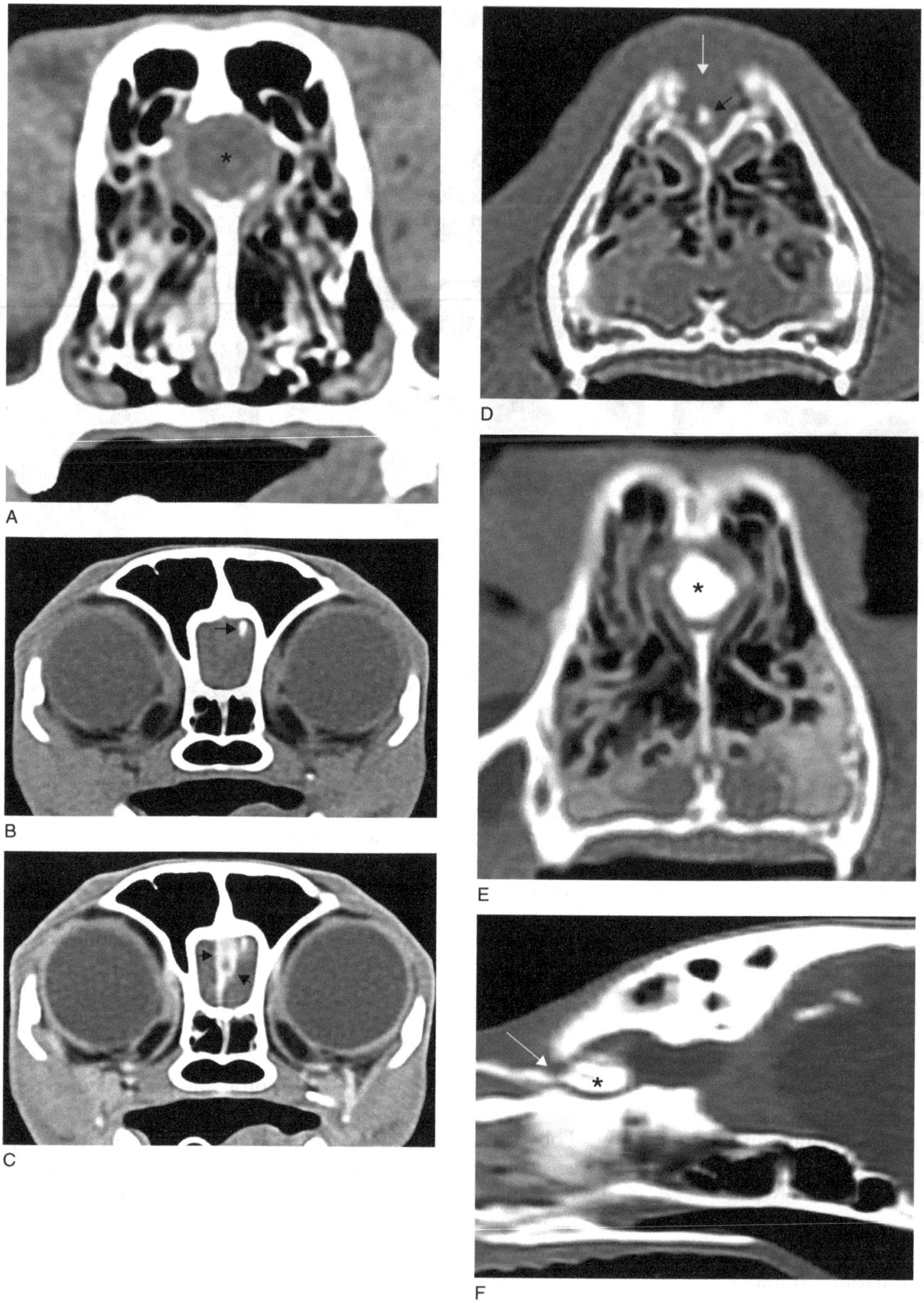

Figure 11.3 Adult cat with a dermoid cyst. (A) Post-contrast (IV) transverse CT image (mid-nasal cavities) shows a rounded soft tissue density (asterisk) in the dorsal third of the nasal septum. (B) Pre-contrast transverse CT image (frontal sinuses) shows a small hyperdensity (arrow) in the left olfactory lobe. (C) Post-contrast CT image (same level as B) shows a markedly contrast enhancing mass in the middle part of the olfactory lobe (arrows). (D) CT fistulogram (rostral nasal cavities) shows a dorsal opening of the nasal planum (white arrow) and a small contrast density within it (black arrow). (E) CT fistulogram (same level as A) shows contrast accumulation within the previously described mass (asterisk). (F) Sagittally reconstructed CT-fistulogram shows an opening into the cribriform plate (arrow) and contrast accumulation in the olfactory lobe (asterisk).

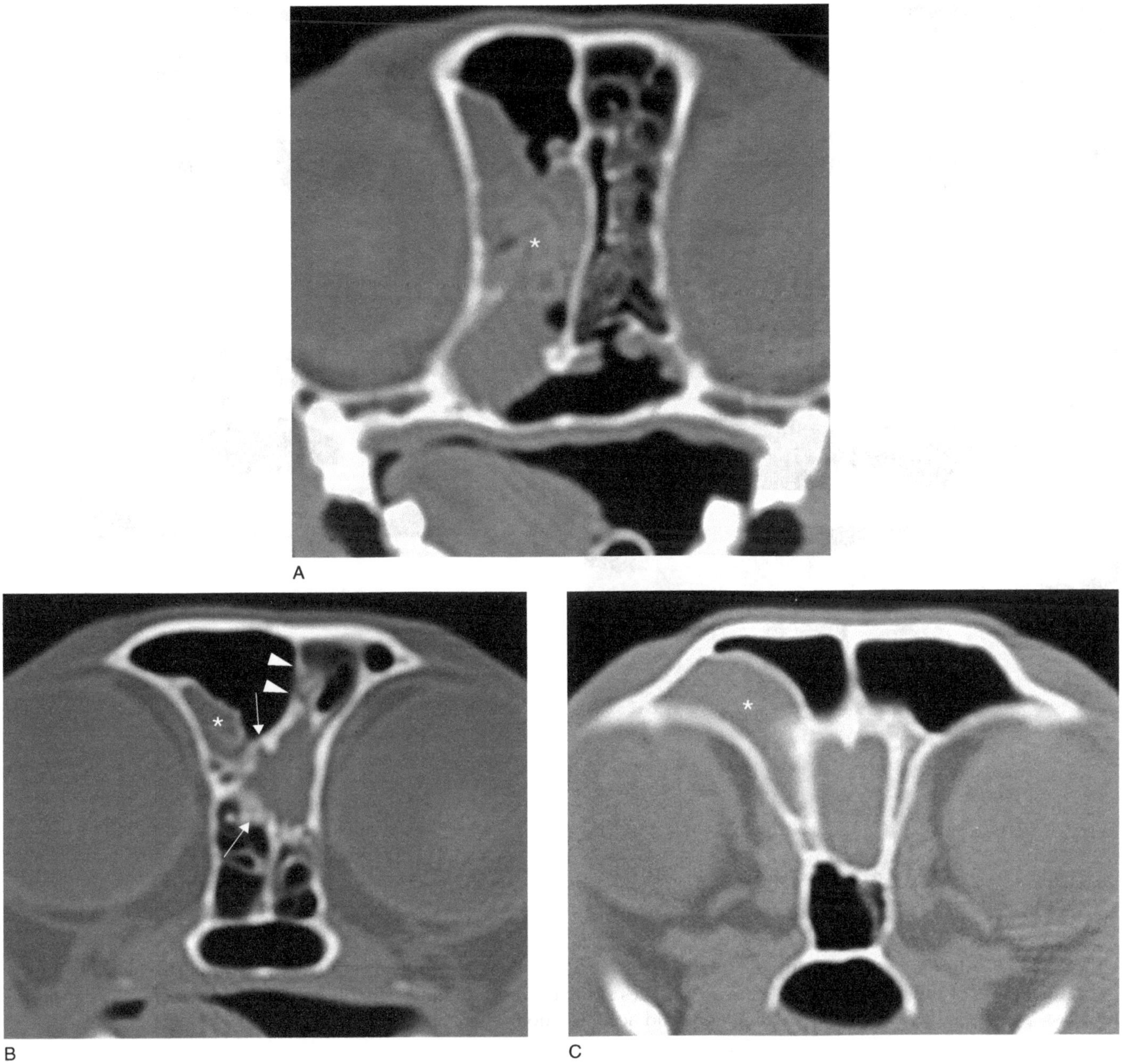

Figure 11.4 Transverse CT images of a young cat with a nasal polyp. (A) The right nasal cavity is obliterated by soft tissue density (asterisk). Remnants of the ethmoturbinates are still visible. The nasal septum is displaced to the left. (B) There is malformation of the cribriform plate (arrows) and a small amount of fluid in the right frontal sinus (asterisk). The frontal crest is deviated to the left (arrowheads). (C) The right frontal sinus is divided into a medial and a lateral compartment. The latter is filled with fluid (asterisk).

by inflammatory cells and fluid accumulation (pus, mucus, hemorrhage).

- Mild to moderate bone loss (turbinates, facial bones, hard palate). Less severe compared to most nasal neoplasia and fungal rhinitis.

Infectious

Fungal rhinitis

In Europe and North America, canine fungal rhinitis is nearly exclusively due to *Aspergillus fumigatus*.

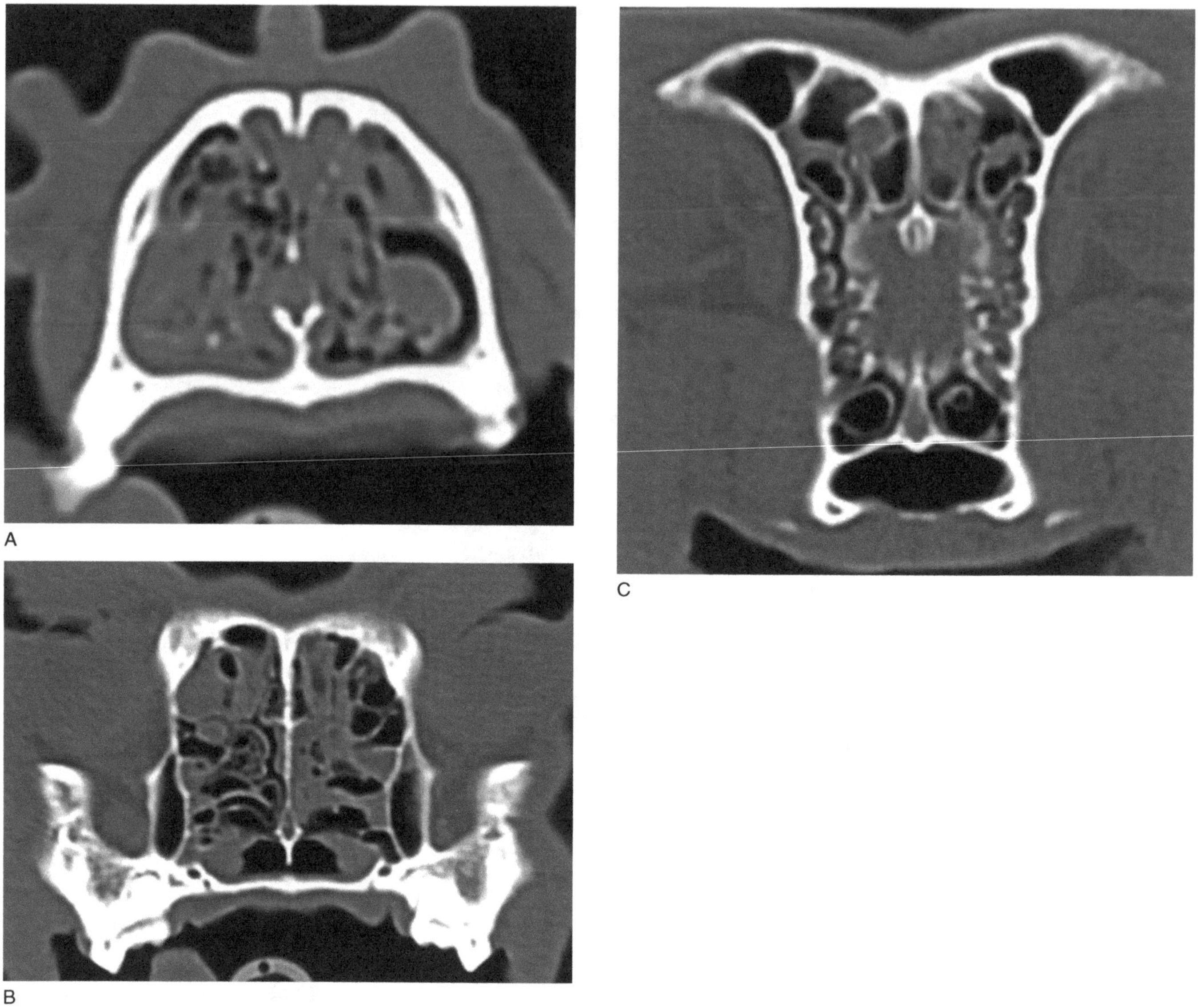

Figure 11.5 Adult dog with non-specific rhinitis. Transverse CT images at the level of (A) the rostral, (B) the mid and (C) the caudal parts of the nasal cavities. The nasal cavities show diffuse, randomly distributed bilaterally increased density of the nasal passages due to mucosal swelling and fluid accumulation. There are no bone lesions.

Sinonasal aspergillosis is far more common in dogs than in cats and is characterized by the formation of superficial mucosal fungal plaques within the nasal cavity and/or frontal sinus in otherwise healthy animals. The fungus does not invade beneath the level of mucosal epithelium but incites a severe chronic inflammatory response. This colonization and invasion of the nasal mucosa by *Asp. fumigatus* causes a destructive rhinitis often accompanied by bone reaction (frontal sinus osteomyelitis), presumably due to an endotoxin responsible for the turbinate necrosis.

Cryptococcosis (*Cryptococcus neoformans, C. gattii*) occurs frequently in Australia but it has also been reported in New Zealand and the west of North America. Unlike other systemic mycoses, Cryptococcosis is more common in cats than in dogs. Patients with cryptococcosis may be presented with involvement of the nasal cavity and/or nasal planum (nasal form) only, with a more extensive nasal cavity disease and local spread (nasal + local form) or with cutaneous tissue, ocular/central nervous system or body cavities organ involvement (nasal + disseminated form).

Other fungal agents have sporadically been reported to cause rhinitis, such as *Asp. nigrans, Asp. nidulans, Asp. flavus, Asp. niger* and *Penicillium* species in dogs. Hyalohyphomycosis and phaeohyphomycosis are reported in cats.

CT features

- Canine sinonasal aspergillosis (Figures 11.6 and 11.7):
  - moderate to severe cavitary destruction (hyperlucency) of the turbinates with presence of a variable amount of abnormal soft tissue in the nasal passages
  - non-specific thickening of the mucosa adjacent to the inner surface of bones of the frontal sinus, maxillary recess and nasal cavity
  - bone changes: thickened reactive bone and/or destruction of thin bone structures (frontal crest, cribriform plate, medial border maxillary recess).

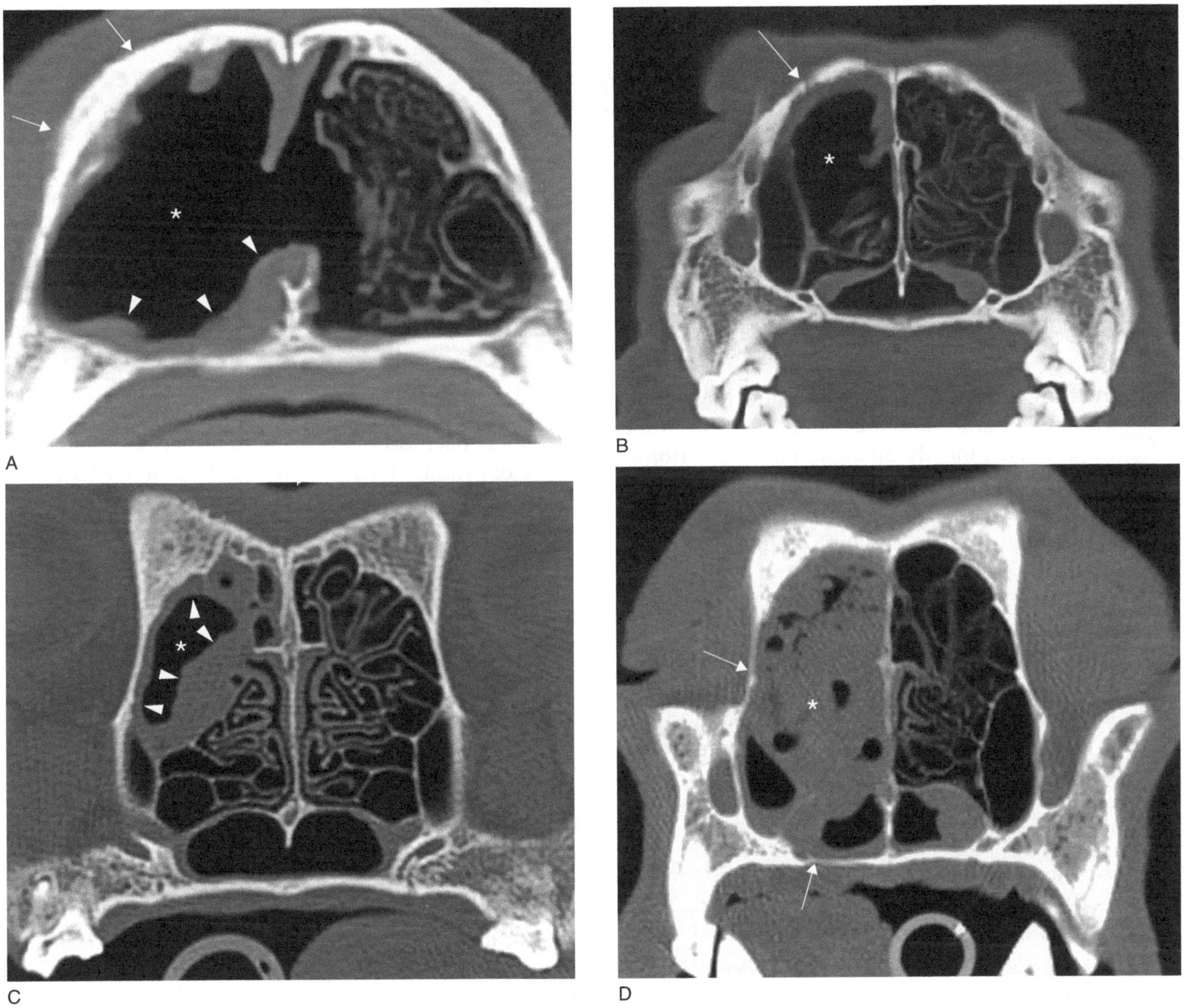

Figure 11.6 Transverse CT images show the nasal cavities in four dogs with nasal aspergillosis. (A) There is complete destruction of the nasal turbinates on the right side (asterisk) with extension to the contralateral side through the nasal septum. The nasal mucosa is thickened ventrally (arrowheads). The maxilla is thickened on the right side (arrows). (B) There is severe destruction of the nasal turbinates in the right nasal passage (asterisk). There is mucosal thickening dorsally and medially, and maxilla bone reaction (arrow). (C) There is partial destruction of the ethmoturbinates in the dorsolateral aspect of the right nasal cavity (asterisk). There is mucosal thickening surrounding the destroyed area (arrowheads). (D) There is a large amount of soft tissue/fluid density in the right nasal cavity (asterisk). There is severe turbinate destruction. The palatine bone and the maxilla are thinned (arrows).

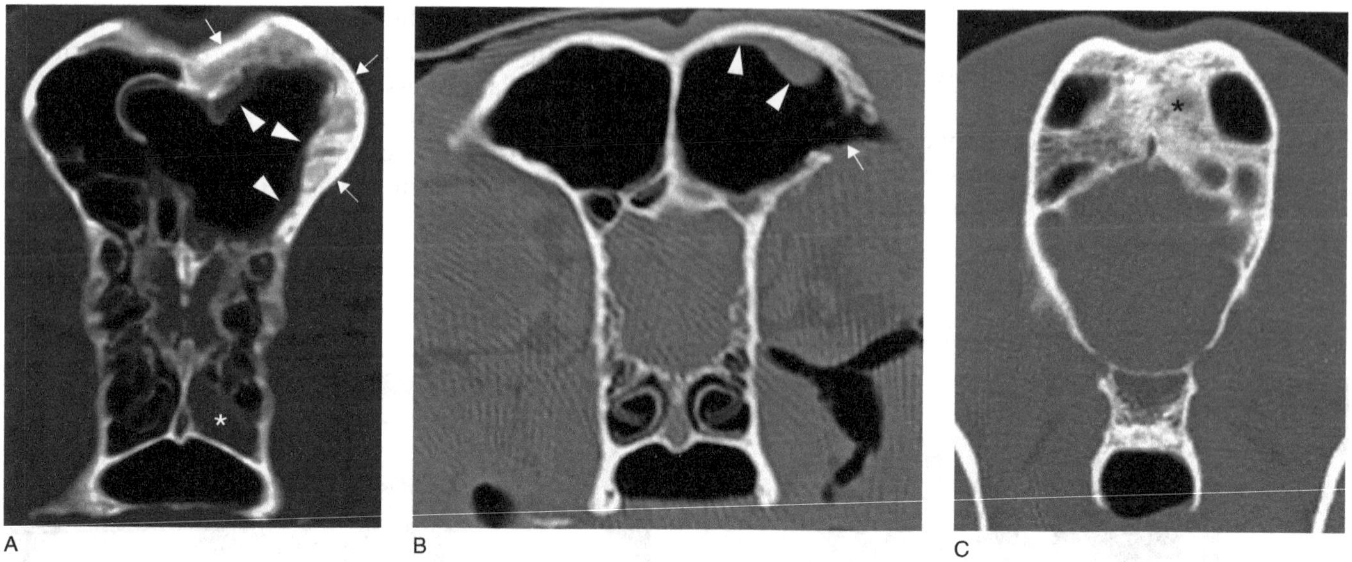

Figure 11.7 Transverse CT images of the frontal sinuses in dogs with nasal aspergillosis. (A) There is hyperostosis of the lateral wall of the left frontal sinus (arrows) with a rim of soft tissue along the inner surface of the bone (arrowheads). There is lysis of the frontal crest. Abnormal soft tissue is present in the nasal fundus (asterisk). (B) There is lysis of the lateral aspect of the left frontal bone (arrow) and rim of soft tissue along the dorsal aspect of the sinus (arrowheads). (C) There is increased density, hyperostosis, of the frontal bone (asterisk).

- Feline fungal rhinitis (Figures 11.8 and 11.9):
  - variable amount of abnormal soft tissue in the nasal cavity, mostly bilateral and in the dorsal extranasal soft tissues
  - turbinate lysis, variable in severity
  - lysis of hard palate, nasal septum, frontal bone or cribriform plate
  - fluid/soft tissue density in the frontal sinus and/or nasopharynx
  - non-specific contrast medium enhancement
  - regional lymphadenopathy
  - extension of the process to the central nervous system (via cribriform plate or systemic) (*see* Chapter 19).

Parasitic rhinitis

Nasal parasites are rare in dogs and cats. *Cuterebra* spp. (arthropod) and *Linguatula serrata* (arthropod) have been reported in both species. *Eucoleus boehmi* (nematode) and *Pneumonyssoides caninum* (arthropod) have been specifically reported in dogs and *Mammomonogamus* (nematode) in cats.

CT features

- Have not been reported.
- Anticipated features on CT:
  - in most cases, normal CT examination
  - increased density of the nasal cavity due to mucosal thickening
  - in exceptional cases, facial deformation.

Bacterial rhinitis

No single bacterium has been identified as a potential cause of primary bacterial rhinitis. Secondary bacterial infection is common in dogs with chronic nasal disease and explains the transient response to antibiotics seen in some dogs. This accumulation of bacterial organisms in dogs with chronic nasal disease could result from mucus trapping and decreased nasal mucosal defense mechanisms.

Dental rhinitis

Periapical infections of the upper teeth may result in a purulent nasal discharge if the infection extends to the nasal mucosa. A dental rhinitis may also be due to an abnormal tooth growth, e.g. an impacted tooth.

CT features (Figure 11.10)

- Localized increased nasal density, possibly associated with turbinate destruction.
- Periapical infection; *see* Chapter 12.

Traumatic

Foreign body rhinitis

Foreign body rhinitis is more frequent in dogs, particularly hunting dogs, than in cats. The sneeze reflex is in most cases an effective way of expelling foreign material from the nose. However, sometimes a foreign body

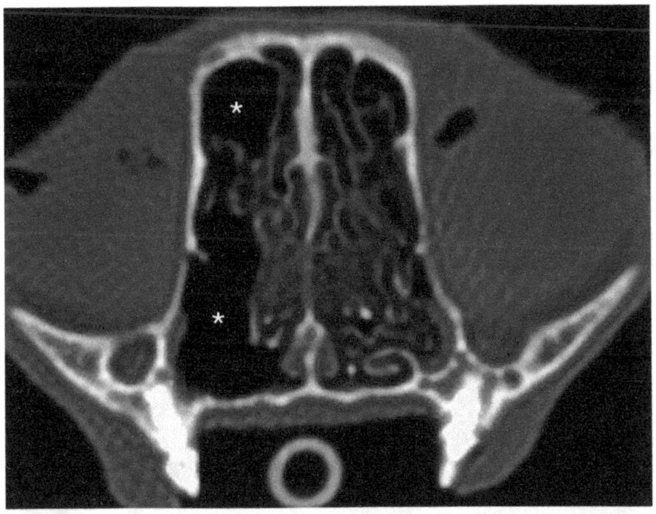

A

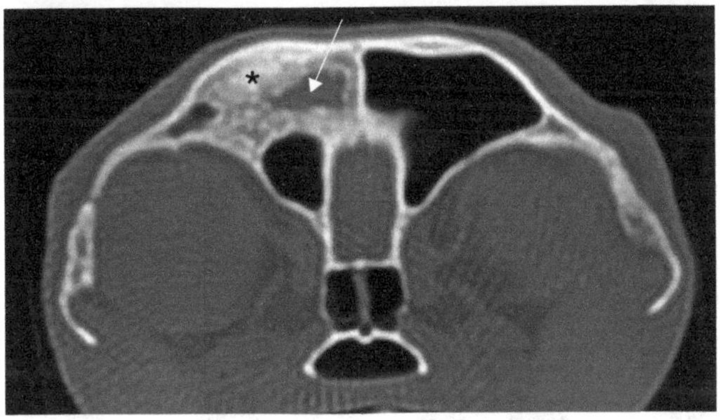

B

Figure 11.8 Adult cat with cryptococcosis. (A) Transverse CT image shows severe destruction of the turbinates in the lateral half of the right nasal cavity (asterisks). (B) Transverse CT image shows severe hyperostosis of the right frontal bone (asterisk), the sinus is filled with soft tissue/fluid density (arrow).

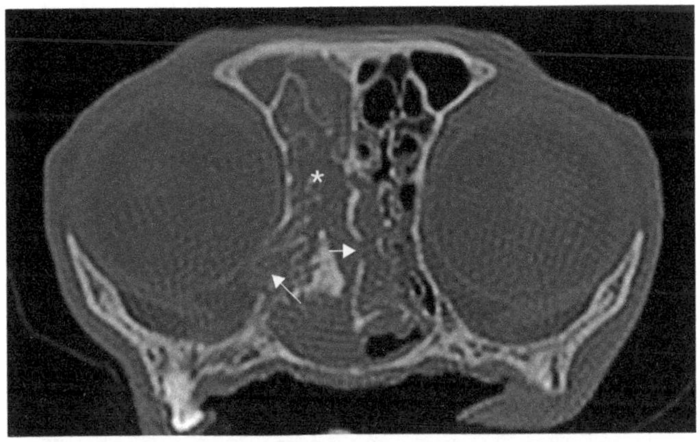

A

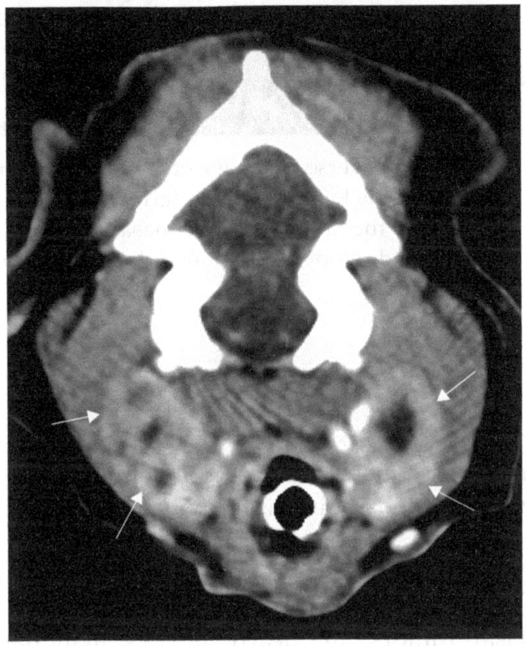

B

Figure 11.9 Adult cat with cryptococcosis and retropharyngeal lymphadenopathy. (A) Transverse CT image shows complete obliteration of the right nasal cavity (asterisk) with extension through the ventral half of the nasal septum into the left nasal cavity (short arrow) and through the frontal bone in the direction of the orbit (long arrow). Remnants of ethmoturbinates are visible and a mineralization is present in the right nasal cavity. (B) Post-contrast transverse CT image shows strong contrast enhancement of both retropharyngeal lymph nodes (arrows) with central hypodense areas, consistent with necrosis.

can become lodged in the nasal turbinates and cause local chronic inflammation, possibly accompanied by secondary aspergillosis.

The most commonly reported foreign bodies are wooden sticks and grass awns. Less commonly fishhooks, bullets and needles may be found in the nasopharynx or oropharynx.

CT features (Figure 11.11)

- Foreign bodies have different densities, ranging from low (wood) to very high (metallic) and are non-contrast enhancing.
- CT appearance pattern depends of size, hydration, composition of surrounding tissues and the presence of inflammatory response.
- Unilateral, localized turbinate destruction surrounding the foreign body.

Traumatic rhinitis

Traumatic rhinitis in dogs is caused by depression fractures, bony sequestra and subsequent osteomyelitis. Most fractures are caused by dog bites or blunt trauma.

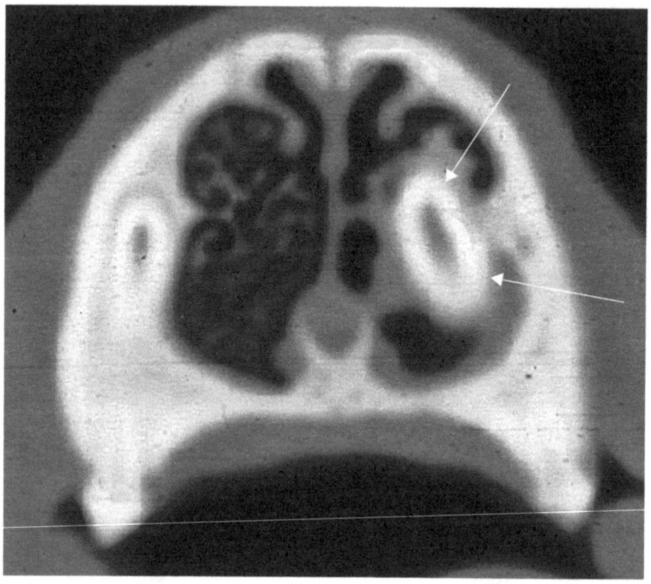

Figure 11.10 Transverse CT image of a young dog with an impacted tooth in the left nasal cavity (arrows). A rim of soft tissue surrounds the tooth and the nasal turbinates are destructed. On endoscopy, aspergillus colonies were visible around the tooth.

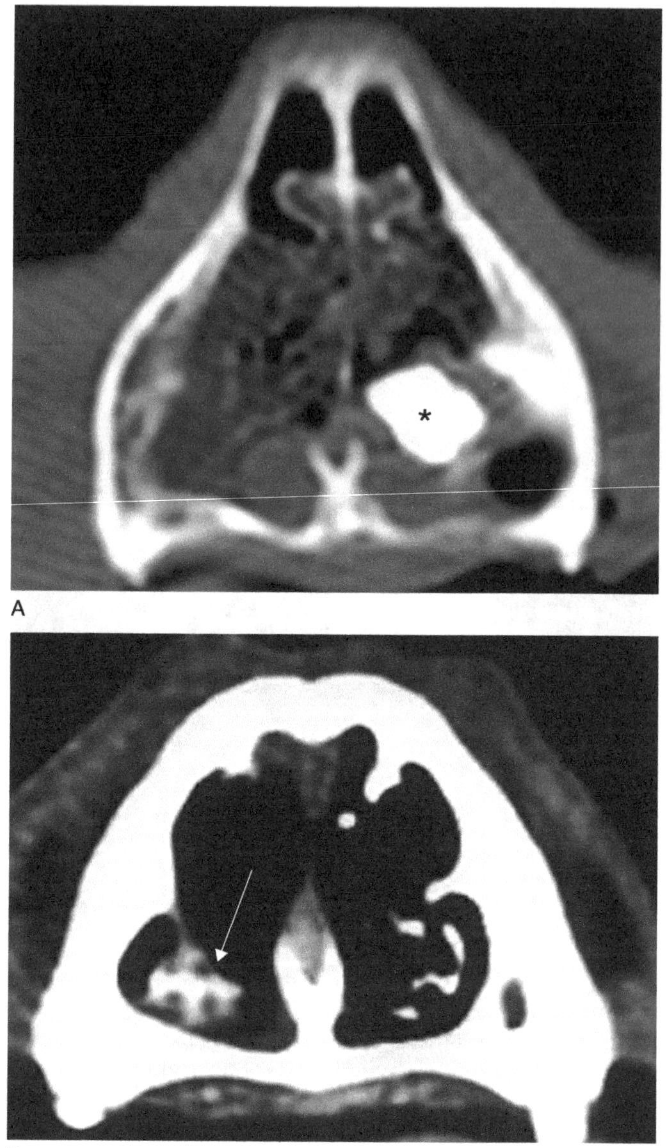

Figure 11.11 Foreign body rhinitis in the rostral part of the nasal cavities in two patients. (A) Transverse CT image shows a hyperdense, rounded structure (asterisk) surrounded by a rim of soft tissue. There is destruction of the nasal turbinates ventrally. (B) Transverse CT image shows a linear hyperdense structure in the rostral aspect of the right nasal cavity (arrow). A grass awn was retrieved on endoscopy.

CT features (Figure 11.12)

- Fracture, sequestrum or osteomyelitis.
- Increased density in nasal cavities.

Sinonasal neoplasms

Sinonasal tumors are nearly always malignant in both dogs and cats. In dogs, tumors may be epithelial (adenocarcinoma, undifferentiated carcinoma, squamous cell carcinoma) or mesenchymal (osteosarcoma and chondrosarcoma) in origin. In cats, lymphoma and epithelial neoplasms are the most common tumor types. Next to these types, more than 20 other malignant tumor types have been reported in the nasal cavity with only a few case reports of benign processes.

Sinonasal tumors most commonly start in one nasal cavity (rarely in the frontal sinus) and progressively invade the entire nasal cavity, the frontal sinus, the orbital region or, through bone, the contralateral nasal cavity, the oral cavity or the central nervous system. Distant metastases are rare. Nasal lymphoma originates from nasal tissue, shows a predominance of B-cells and is generally restricted to the nasal cavity.

In dogs, sinonasal tumors seem to correlate with the nasal length and thus with the amount of surface area that is exposed to environmental carcinogens. Therefore, dolicho- and mesaticephalic dogs have a higher risk of developing sinonasal neoplasia than the open-mouth breathing brachycephalic dogs, which are then more prone to lower respiratory tract disorders.

Some neoplasms arising from the face (e.g. squamous cell carcinoma of the nasal plane, osteosarcoma, multilobular tumor of bone) may extend into the nasal

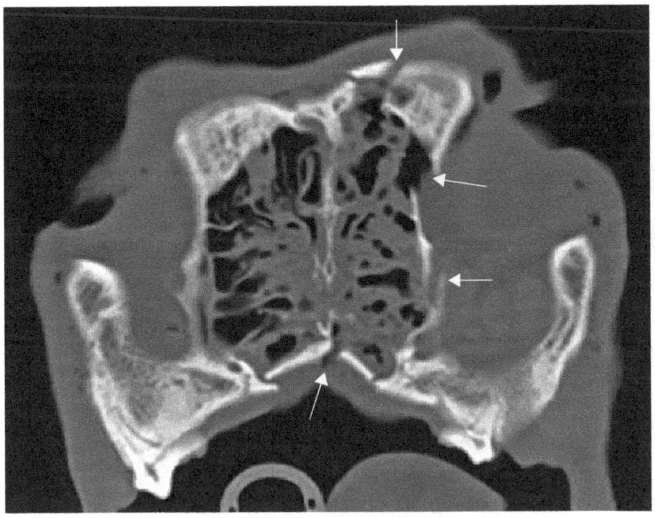

Figure 11.12 Transverse CT image in an adult dog with traumatic rhinitis shows multiple fractures of the maxilla, zygomatic and frontal bones (arrows). There is a diffuse, bilateral (left > right) increase in density of the nasal passages due to mucosa swelling and fluid accumulation.

cavity. These neoplasms should be differentiated from the typical 'nasal' neoplasms because of different treatment options. Other structures included in the nasal cavities such as the infraorbital nerve may also show tumoral processes.

CT features (Figures 11.13–11.17)

- Presence of a space-occupying mass; mostly the convex surface of the mass is visible.
- Process may be uni- or bilateral. It starts in one nasal cavity, usually caudally, but may extend in the other cavity or causes deviation of the nasal septum.
- Destruction of the ethmoid bones and bone surrounding the nasal cavities.
- Turbinate destruction, variable depending on the stage and aggressiveness of the disease process.
- Contrast study is not usually needed for diagnosis but may help to differentiate a mass from its surrounding fluid. A moderate to severe enhancement is usually seen.
- Hamartoma: calcified mass.
- Fluid in the nasal sinuses.

Idiopathic chronic rhinitis

This disorder is likely the consequence of a complex progression of microbial, physiological, anatomical, and immunological interactions. Feline herpesvirus type 1 has been suggested as an important pathogen for initiating factor acute rhinitis following acute viral cytolysis during a bout of acute severe rhinitis is related to this disorder.

Idiopathic chronic rhinitis is perpetuated by recurrent bacterial infection, an exuberant inflammatory response, permanent or cumulative destruction of nasal epithelium and bony turbinates following chronic reactivation of virus from the trigeminal ganglia into nasal tissue.

CT features (Figure 11.18)

- Soft-tissue opacification of the nasal cavity and frontal or sphenopalatine sinuses.
- Lysis of nasal and frontal bones.
- Turbinate destruction.
- Asymmetry of the cribriform plate.

Further Reading

De Rycke LM, Saunders JH, Gielen IM, van Bree HJ and Simoens PJ (2003) Magnetic resonance imaging, computed tomography and cross sectional anatomy of the normal canine nasal cavities and paranasal sinuses in the mesaticephalic dog. *Am J Vet Res* **64**: 1093–8.

Ketaki K, Reichle JK, Fischetti AJ and Goggin JM (2009) Computed tomographic findings of fungal rhinitis and sinusitis in cats. *Vet Radiol Ultrasound* **50**: 65–8.

Lefebvre J, Kuehn NF and Wortinger A (2005) Computed tomography as an aid in the diagnosis of chronic nasal disease in dogs. *J Small Anim Pract* **46**: 280–5.

Losonsky JS, Abbott LC and Kuriashkin IV (1997) Computed tomography of the normal feline nasal cavity and paranasal sinuses. *Vet Radiol Ultrasound* **38**: 251–8.

Reetz JA, Mai W, Muravnick KB, Goldschmidt MH, Schwarz T (2006) Computed tomographic evaluation of anatomic and pathologic variations in the feline nasal septum and paranasal sinuses. *Vet Radiol Ultrasound* **47**: 321–7.

Saunders JH, van Bree H, Gielen I and de Rooster H (2003) Computed tomography in dogs with chronic nasal disease. *Vet Radiol Ultrasound* **44**: 409–14.

Saunders JH, Zonderland JL, Clercx C *et al.* (2002) Computed tomographic findings in 35 dogs with nasal aspergillosis. *Vet Radiol Ultrasound* **43**: 5–9.

Windsor RC and Johnson L (2006) Canine chronic inflammatory rhinitis. *Clin Tech Small Anim Pract* **21**: 76–81.

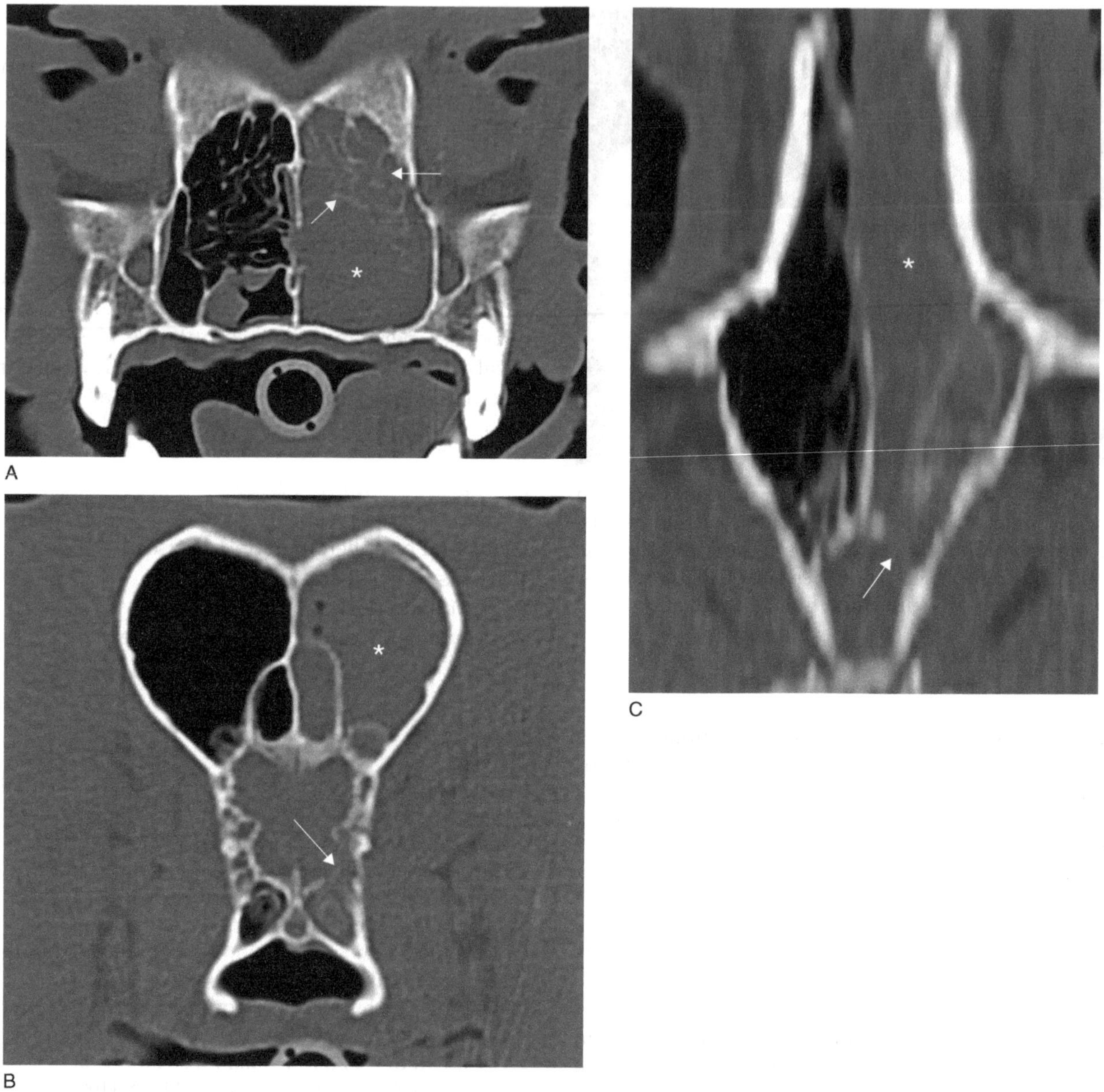

Figure 11.13 Adult dog with nasal adenocarcinoma. (A) Transverse CT image shows a completely obliterated (asterisk) left nasal cavity. The ethmoturbinates are destroyed in the ventral part of the cavity while some are intact dorsally (arrows). The maxillary recess is filled. (B) Transverse CT image shows the left frontal sinus completely filled with fluid/soft tissue (asterisk). There is suspicion of cribriform plate destruction ventrally (arrow). (C) Dorsally reconstructed CT image confirms cribriform plate lysis (arrow). The mass extends over the entire length of the left nasal cavity (asterisk) and slightly into the right cavity.

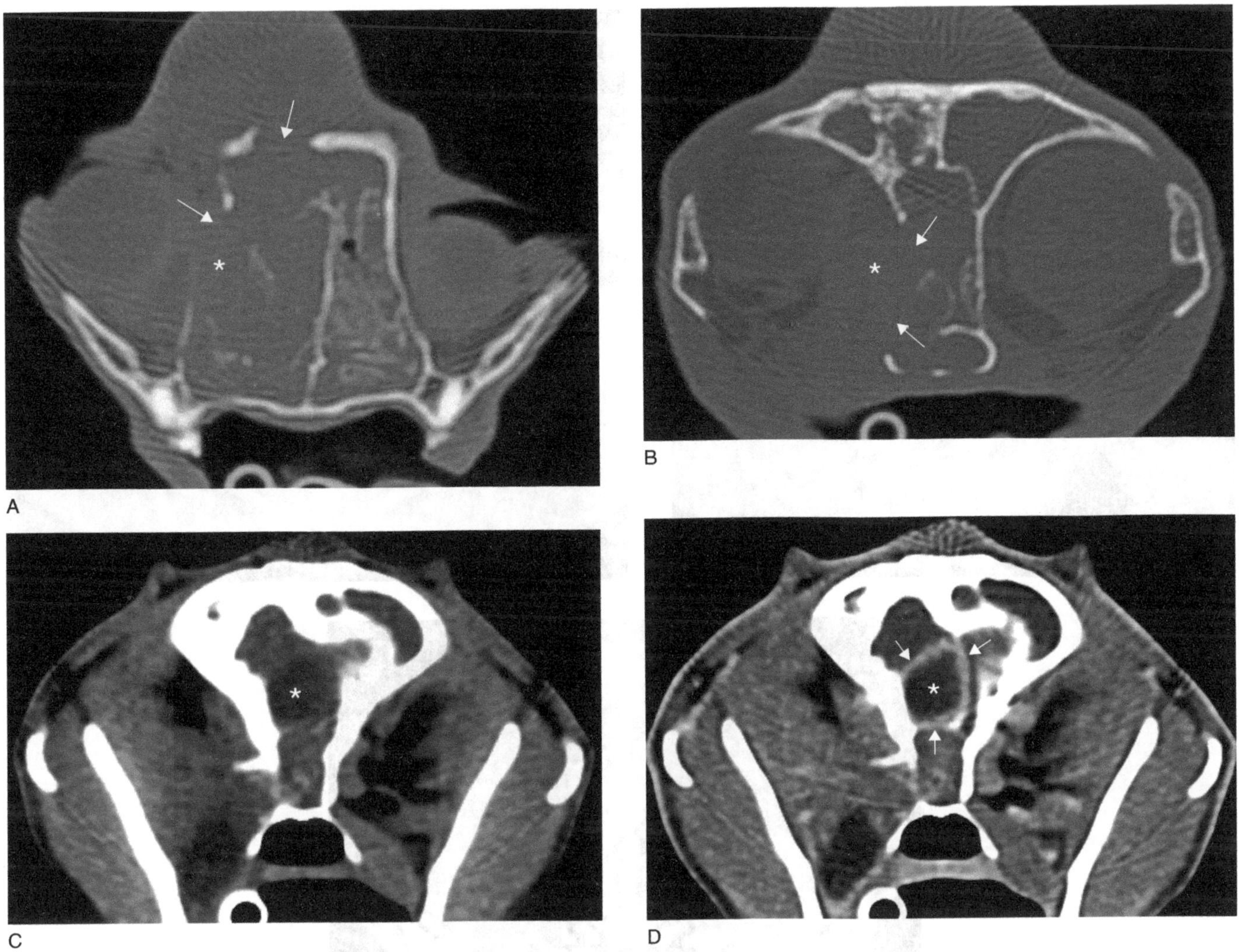

Figure 11.14 Adult cat with nasal adenocarcinoma with cystic extension into the brain. (A) Transverse CT image shows severe soft tissue swelling with complete obliteration of both nasal cavities. A mass is present on the right side (asterisk) and displaces the nasal septum to the left. The turbinates are destroyed on the right side. There is severe destruction of the right maxilla (arrows). (B) Transverse CT image shows a mass invading the caudal nasal cavities and peri-orbital tissues (asterisk). There is complete lysis of the right frontal bone and cribriform plate (arrows). Both frontal sinuses are filled. (C) Pre-contrast transverse CT image shows a hypodense area within the olfactory lobe (asterisk). (D) Post-contrast transverse CT image at the same level shows cyst wall enhancement (arrows) surrounding the non-enhancing cystic lumen (asterisk).

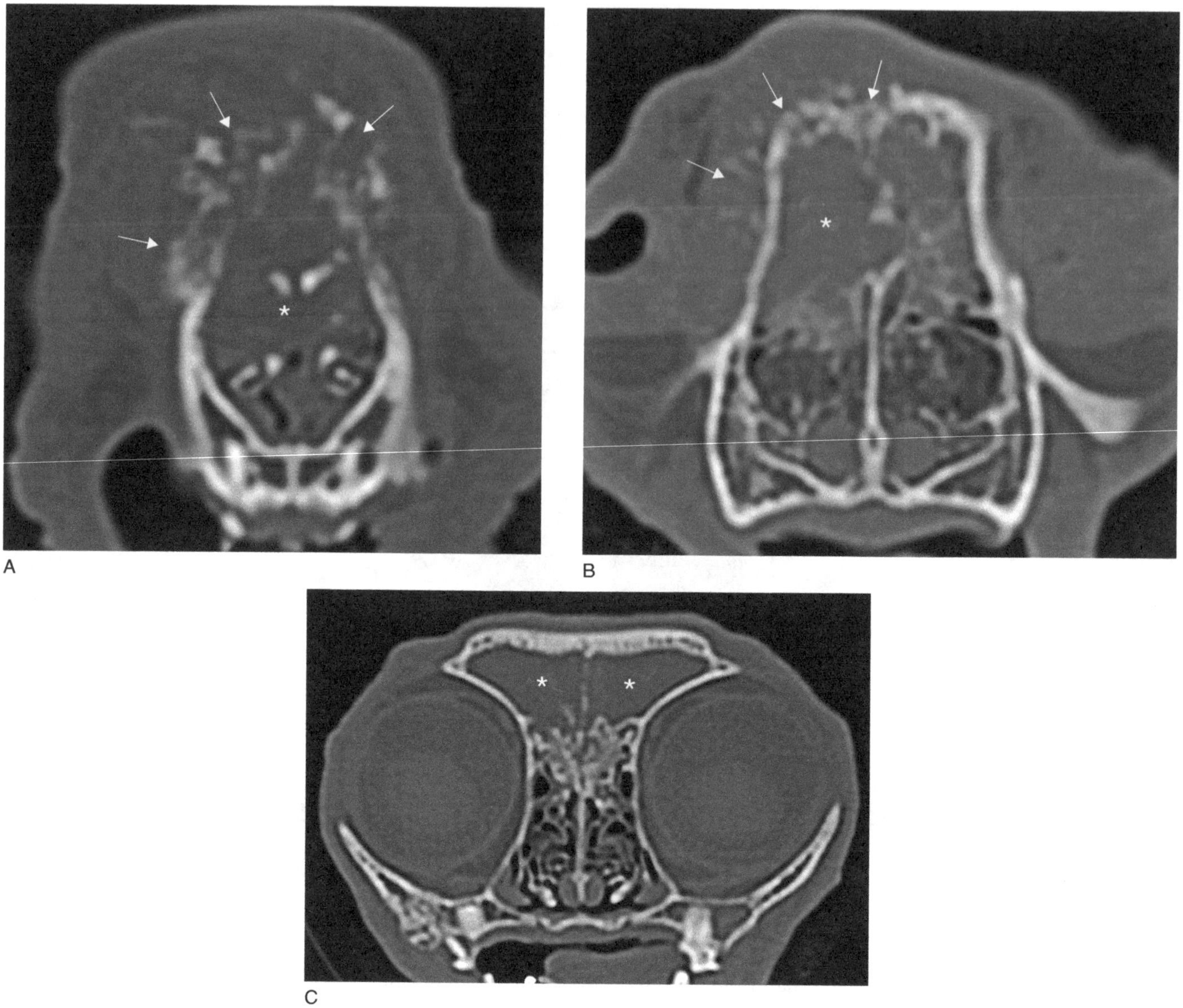

Figure 11.15 Adult cat with nasal hemangiosarcoma. (A) Transverse CT image shows rostral obliteration of the nasal cavities (asterisk), nasal turbinate destruction, nasal bone destruction and exuberant periosteal reactions (arrows). (B) Transverse CT image shows a mass (asterisk) in the dorsal half of the right nasal cavity with turbinate destruction. The nasal septum is destroyed dorsally and the process extends to the left nasal cavity. Spiculated periosteal reactions are visible at the dorsolateral aspect of the maxilla (arrows). (C) Transverse CT image shows the frontal sinuses completely filled with fluid (asterisks) while the ventral aspect of the nasal cavities appears normal.

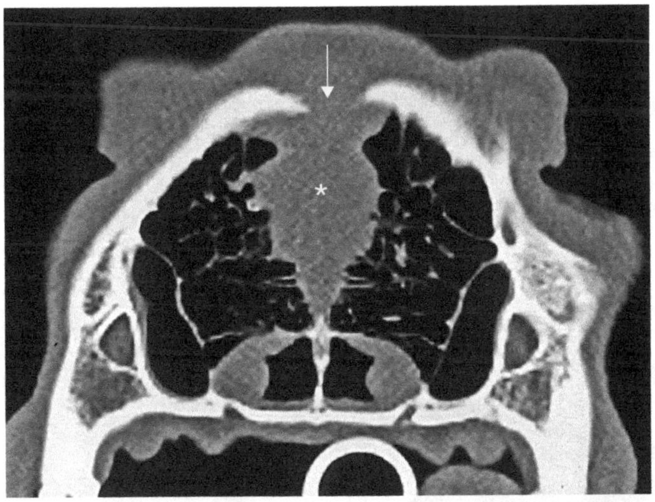

A

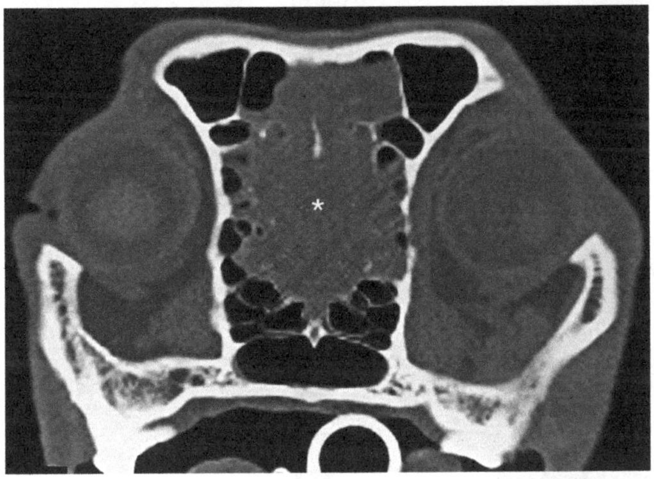

B

Figure 11.16 Adult dog with nasal septum neoplasia. (A) Transverse CT image shows a triangular-shaped soft tissue density located on the midline of the nasal cavities at the normal location of the nasal septum (asterisk). There is destruction of the nasal bone in the midline of the nasal planum (arrow). (B) Transverse CT image shows destruction of the nasal septum and ethmoturbinates by a large soft tissue density mass located in the middle of the nasal cavities (asterisk).

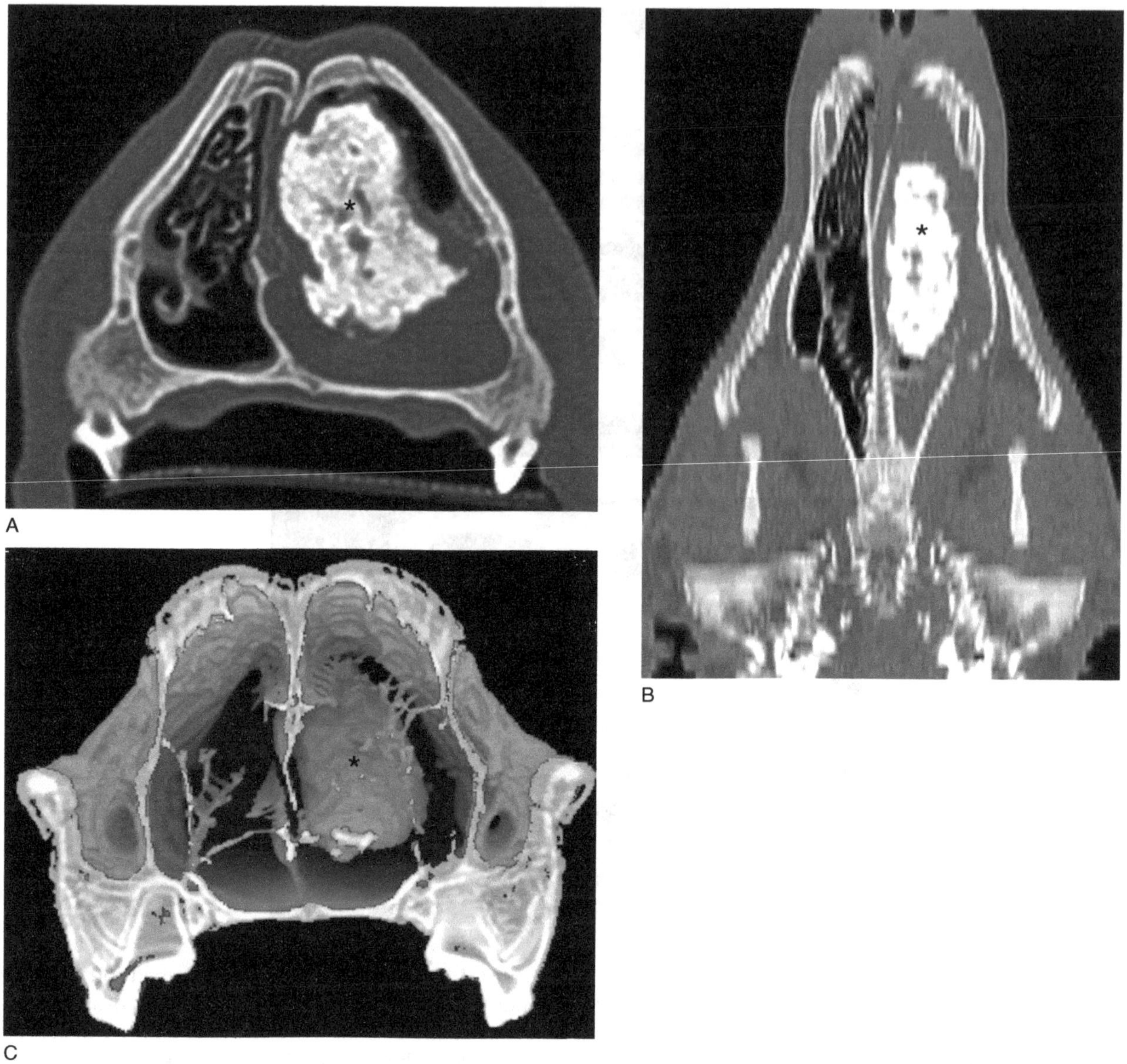

Figure 11.17 Adult dog with osseous hamartoma. (A) An osseous mass (asterisk) surrounded by fluid is visible in the rostral part of the left nasal cavity. The nasal septum is deviated towards the right. (B) Dorsally reconstructed CT image shows the osseous mass filling the left nasal cavity over almost its entire length. (C) Volume rendering shows the previously described mass (asterisk).

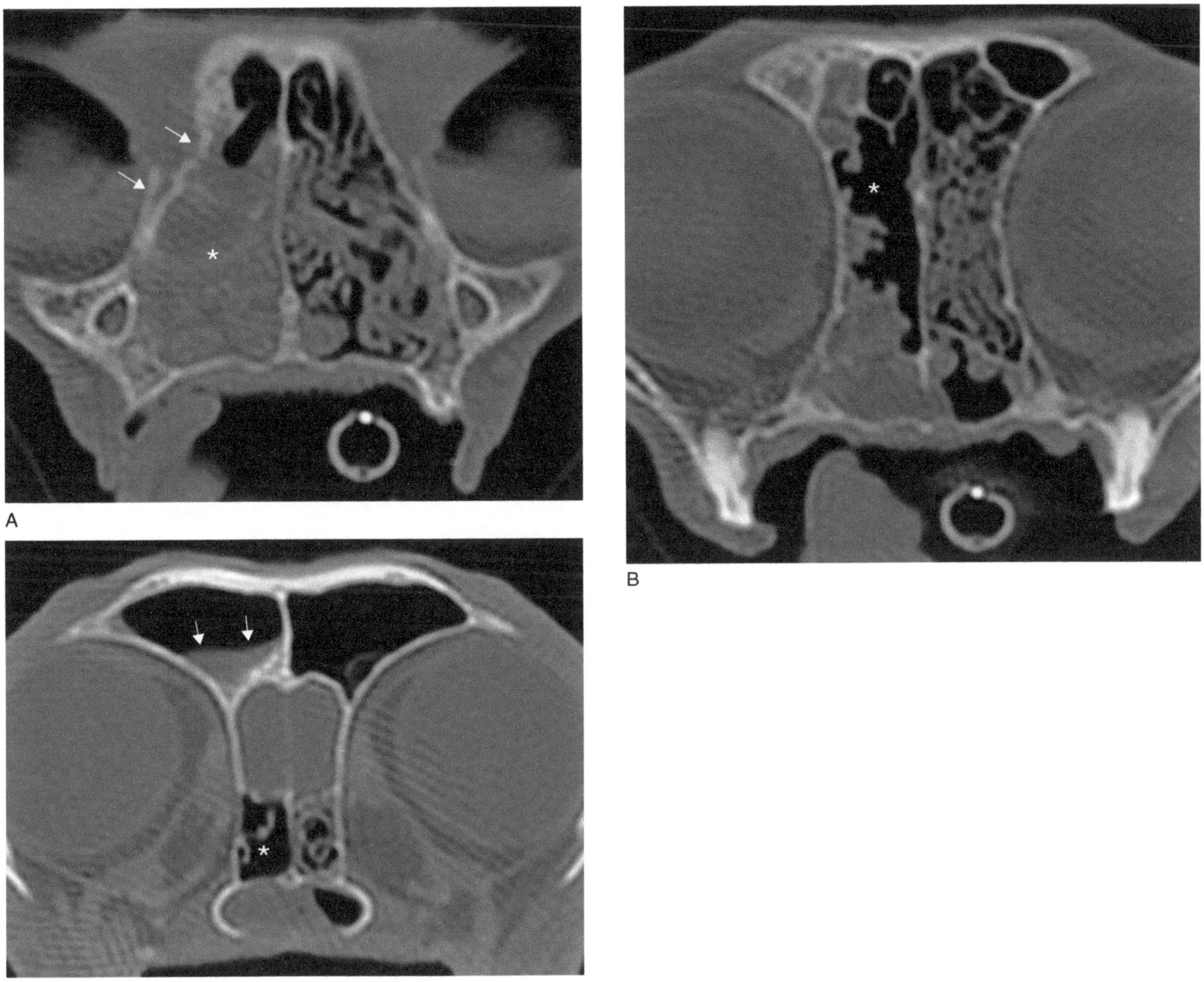

A

B

C

Figure 11.18 Adult cat with idiopathic chronic rhinitis. (A) Transverse CT image shows almost complete filling of the right nasal cavity (asterisk). There is lysis of the right maxilla laterally (arrows). Mucosal thickening of the turbinates is present in the left nasal cavity. (B) Transverse CT image shows extensive ethmoturbinate destruction in the right nasal cavity (asterisk). Some remnants of turbinates along the outer wall are present with a thickened mucosa/fluid. The right side of the nasopharynx is filled with soft tissue density. Diffuse mucosal thickening is present in the left nasal cavity. (C) Transverse CT image shows a fluid level (arrows) in the right frontal sinus, turbinate destruction in the right sphenoidal sinus (asterisk) and partial filling of the nasopharynx.

CHAPTER TWELVE

Oral Cavity, Mandible, Maxilla and Dental Apparatus

Lisa J. Forrest and Tobias Schwarz

Imaging Protocol

See Table 12.1.

CT: Anatomy and Normal Variants

Oral cavity

In both dogs and cats the oral cavity contains the teeth and the tongue and is further divided into the vestibule and the oral cavity proper. The vestibule is external to the teeth and gums and internal to the lips and cheeks. It opens via the oral fissure between the lips, rostral. A space on either side, which is caudal to the last molars, provides free communication between the rostral vestibule and the oral cavity proper. The parotid and zygomatic salivary ducts open into the dorsocaudal part of the vestibule. The parotid duct opens on a small parotid papilla, which is located in the cheek opposite to the maxillary fourth premolar tooth in dogs and in the cat opens opposite the maxillary third or fourth premolar teeth.

The dorsal margin of the oral cavity proper is the hard palate and a small part of the adjacent soft palate; the lateral and rostral margins are the dental arches and teeth; the floor or ventral margin is the tongue and reflected mucosa beneath the tongue. The tongue occupies the ventral portion of the oral cavity that contains muscles and surrounding layers of fat (Figure 12.1). It is important to position the tongue as symmetrical as possible, which can be challenging with anesthetic equipment placement. If specific lesions in other areas are assessed, it is useful to move the tongue away from the area of interest to prevent silhouetting of gum and lingual tissue. The ducts of the sublingual and mandibular salivary glands open under the body of the tongue. When the mouth is closed the tongue fills the oral cavity. The incisive papillae where the incisive duct opens are caudal to the maxillary central incisor teeth. These paired ducts extend through the palatine fissures to connect the nasal cavity to the oral cavity.

The soft palate continues caudal from the hard palate as the separation between the naso- and oral-pharynx, and passes just caudal to the last maxillary molar in mesaticephalic breeds. Whereas in extremely brachycephalic breeds the hard palate/soft palate junction is more than 1 cm caudal to this transverse level. The soft palate is long in dogs and may be overlong in brachycephalic breeds leading to obstruction of air passage. In the average dog the soft palate is 6 cm long, 3 cm wide and 0.5 cm thick. The thickness gradually enlarges to 1 cm at the middle to caudal third, after which it thins to a concave border at its caudal end.

The palatine tonsil is located within the tonsillar fossa on the dorsolateral oropharyngeal wall and can occasionally be identified due to a small air bubble in this fossa. All the soft tissues of the soft palate and pharynx wall are strongly contrast enhancing (Figure 12.2).

Mandible

The mandible is similar in the dog and cat. It articulates with the skull via the temporomandibular joint (TMJ; *see* Chapter 13) and is fused rostrally via the mandibular symphysis. The mandibular symphysis contains a fibrocartilage pad rostrodorsally

Veterinary Computed Tomography, First Edition. Edited by Tobias Schwarz, Jimmy Saunders.

Table 12.1
CT imaging protocol (intravenous contrast study: standard protocol; *see* Chapter 5).

Series	Pre- and post-contrast	Bone	Open mouth	Mandibular traction
Decubitus	Ventral			
Special positioning	N/A		Open mouth maximally with radiolucent mouth gag	Tie hindlegs to one table end, tie mandible (loop around canines) to other table and under tension (*see* Figure 13.1)
Rostral scan margin	Incisors			Molars
Caudal scan margin	Medial retropharyngeal lymph nodes		Tympanic bullae	
Scan direction	Rostral or caudal			
Voltage (kVp)	120			
Current (mAs)	130			
Tube rotation time (s)	1 or 2			
Slice width (mm)	5	1	2	1
Sequential slice interval (mm)	5	1	2	1
Kernel frequency	Medium	High	Medium	High
Window level (HU)	+100 (post-contrast: +80)	+500	A: +80 B: +500	+500
Window width (HU)	150 (post-contrast: 200)	3000	A: 200 B: 3000	3000

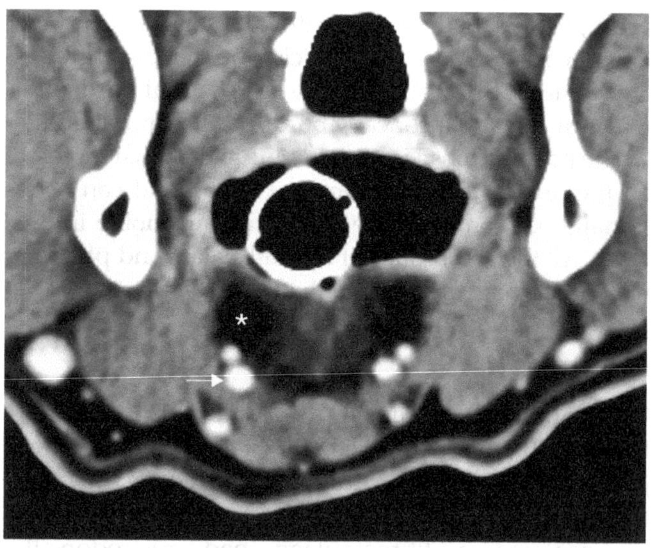

Figure 12.1 Transverse post-contrast CT image of the tongue base shows prominent hypodense layers of intermuscular fat laterally and ventrally (asterisk). The contrast-enhanced tongue vessels (arrow) serve as landmarks.

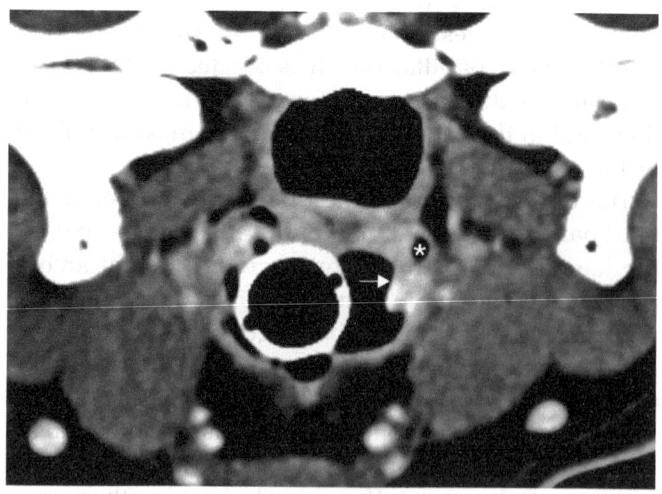

Figure 12.2 Transverse post-contrast-enhanced CT image of a canine oropharynx. Ventral to the soft palate the contrast-enhancing palatine tonsil (arrow) partially protrudes from its tonsillar fossa, also containing a small air bubble (asterisk).

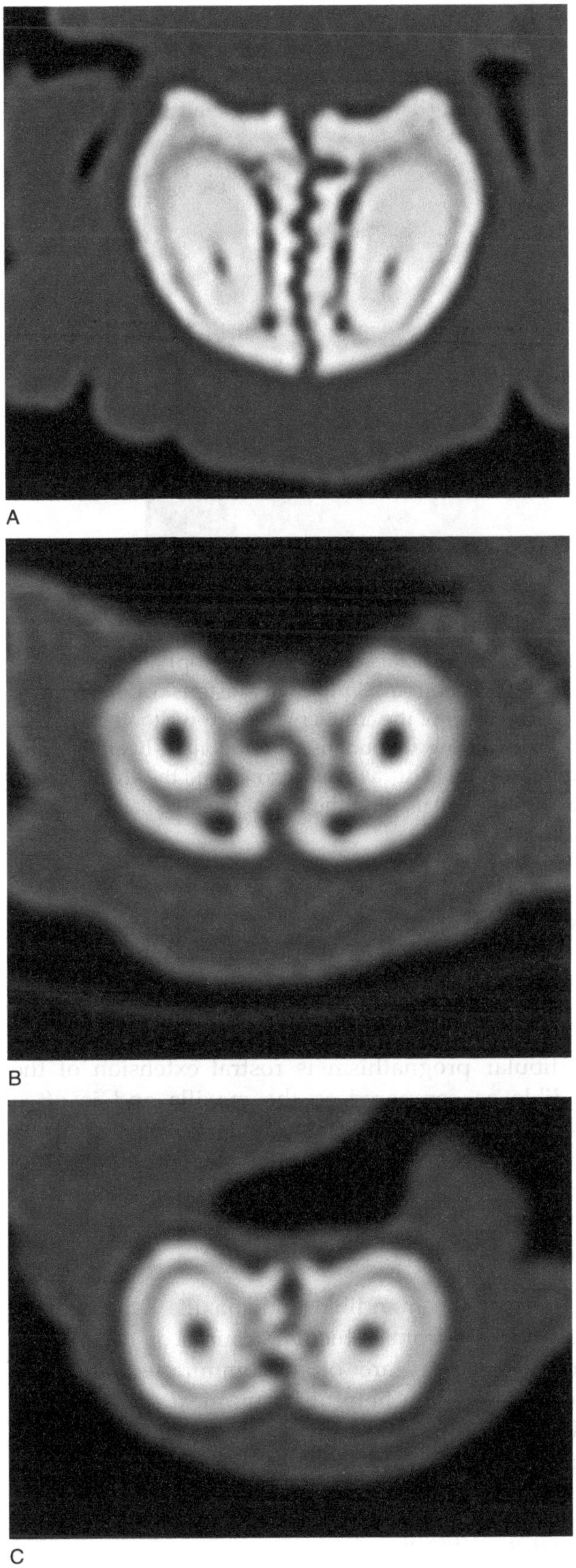

Figure 12.3 Transverse CT image of the normal mandibular symphysis with interdigitating bony rugosities in (A) a normal dog, (B) a normal cat and (C) a cat with impingement of its left coronoid mandibular process lateral to the zygomatic arch. The mandibular symphysis in (C) remains aligned, ruling out symphyseal laxity as the cause of impingement.

(synchondrosis) and cruciate ligaments caudoventrally (syndesmosis), giving it the required rigidity and flexibility for the uneven mandibular movements during mastication. On CT images the interdigitating bony rugosities supporting the ligamentous structures are well visible. In case of abnormal mandibular position (TMJ luxation, coronoid impingement), the symphyseal surfaces can be angled, but should not separate lateromedially or dorsoventrally (Figure 12.3).

Maxilla

The maxilla is similar in the cat and dog. Different breeds of cats and dogs will have different cephalic indices resulting in ranges from short, broad heads (brachycephalic breeds) to normal, medium heads (mesocephalic breeds) and long, narrow heads (longicephalic breeds).

Teeth (Figure 12.4)

Adult dogs and cats have a full set of 42 and 30 teeth respectively (*see* Box 12.1). For a dental CT examination, it is important to be able to identify the correct number and location of individual roots for each tooth. The dental anatomic nomenclature is somewhat different in orientation and naming. The modified Triadan dental numbering system has been developed for unequivocal tooth identification across veterinary species and should be applied in CT reports.

Box 12.1 Canine and feline dental anatomy

Canine adult dental chart	***Feline adult dental chart***
3I-1C-4P-2M	3I-1C-3P-1M
3I-1C-4P-3M	3I-1C-2P-1M

Dental anatomic orientations

Mesial/Distal	Towards/away from midline of dental arch
Coronal/Apical	Towards/away from the tooth crown
Palatal or Lingual	Towards hard palate (maxillary teeth) or tongue (mandibular teeth)
Buccal or Labial	Towards the cheek (back teeth) or lips (front teeth)

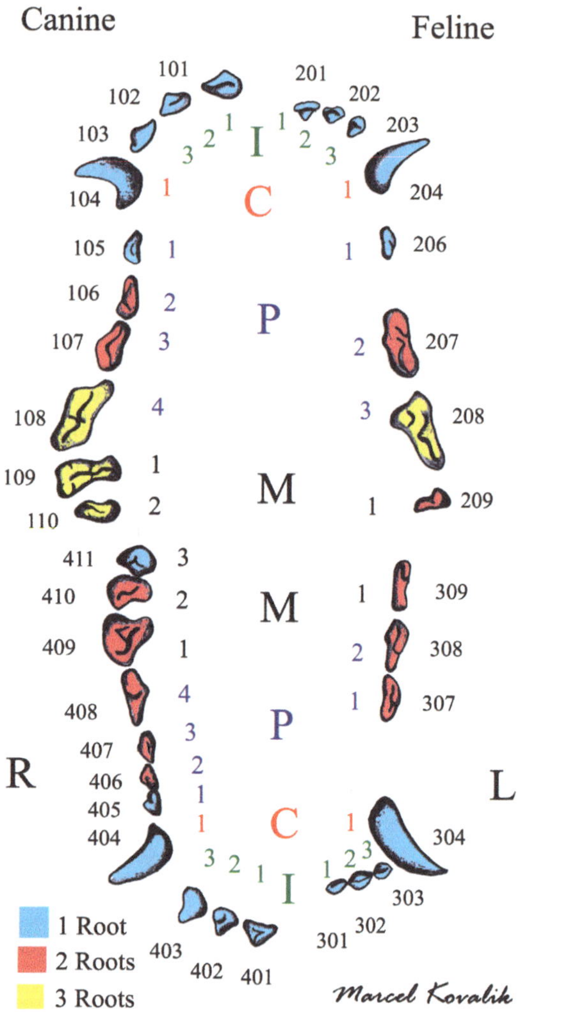

Figure 12.4 Triadan (outside teeth) and traditional anatomic chart (inside teeth) of the canine (left) and feline (right) dental nomenclature of the permanent teeth. The root numbers for each tooth are color coded.

In thin-sliced bone algorithm CT images it is possible to identify all relevant dental and periodontal anatomic structures (Figure 12.5). Due to the curved shape of the roots and the peculiar dental alignment it is essential to account for and follow each dental root on subsequent images.

Non-Dental Diseases

Malformation/Developmental

Mucopolysaccharidosis (MPS)

Radiographic skeletal changes in cats with MPS VI include epiphyseal dysplasia, generalized osteoporosis, pectus excavatum, and vertebral and skull changes.

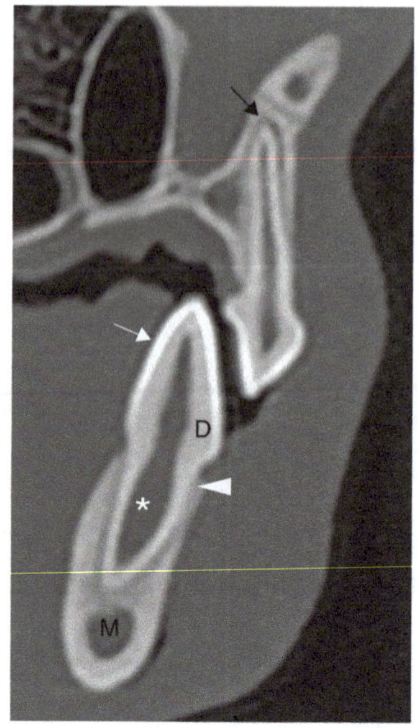

Figure 12.5 Dental CT anatomy of the carnassial teeth. Depicted are the distal root of 208 (P^4, top) and the mesial root of 309 (M_1, bottom). Pulp cavity (asterisk), dentine layer (D), enamel layer of the crown (white arrow), tooth root apex with surrounding hypodense periodontal ligament and hyperdense lamina dura (black arrow), and the alveolar crest (arrowhead), demarcating the top of the alveolar socket.

CT features

Specific skull changes seen on CT include shortened dimensions to the incisive and maxillary bones.

Prognathism

Mandibular prognathism is rostral extension of the mandible as compared to the maxilla and is often present in bulldog breeds. Maxillary prognathism is rostral extension of the maxilla as compared to the mandible.

Trauma

Fractures of the mandible and maxilla can occur in dogs and cats from vehicular trauma or other head trauma. Fractures are often comminuted and 3-D reconstructions are helpful for surgical planning. CT is also helpful to monitor fracture healing and callus formation (for TMJ dislocation and fractures, *see* Chapter 13).

CT features (Figure 12.6)

- Malalignment of mandible or maxilla.
- Bone fragments separated from either the maxilla or mandible.

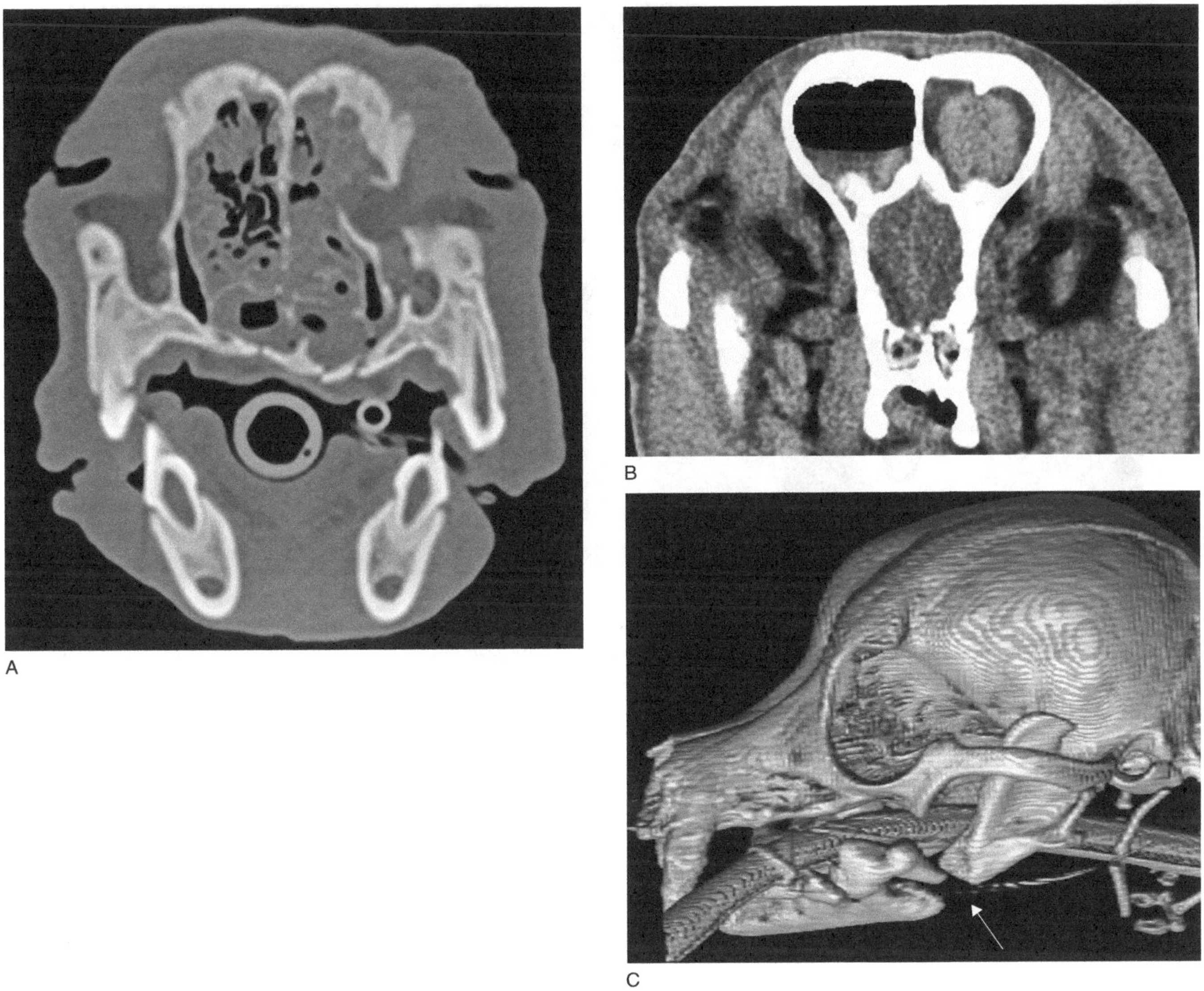

Figure 12.6 (A) Transverse CT image of a dog with head trauma demonstrating multiple nasal, maxillary and palatine fractures, and (B) bilateral frontal sinus effusion with a large hyperdense hematoma in the left frontal sinus. (C) Three-dimensional MIP reconstruction of a dog skull with a view of the left mandible with a comminuted fracture involving the 309 tooth (arrow).

- Adjacent soft tissue swelling with or without hyperdense hematoma formation.
- 3-D reconstruction and/or sagittal and dorsal plane reconstructions assist interpretation
  - 1 mm slice thickness through the oral cavity is necessary for quality reconstructions.

Infection and inflammation

Oral and lingual abscesses

Oral or lingual abscess formation can occur in dogs as a result of chewing on sharp sticks that can break and lodge in the oral cavity or the tongue base. More commonly, such lesions are seen in the pharyngeal walls and retropharyngeal space (*see* Chapter 18).

CT features (Figure 12.7)

- Fluid density mass in the tongue, oral or pharyngeal wall that is hypodense in comparison to oral mucosa.
- Rim contrast enhancement of the mass.
- Foreign body remnants may or may not be visible. Wood is usually not or barely visible on CT images.
- Enlarged medial retropharyngeal lymph nodes (*see* Chapter 17).

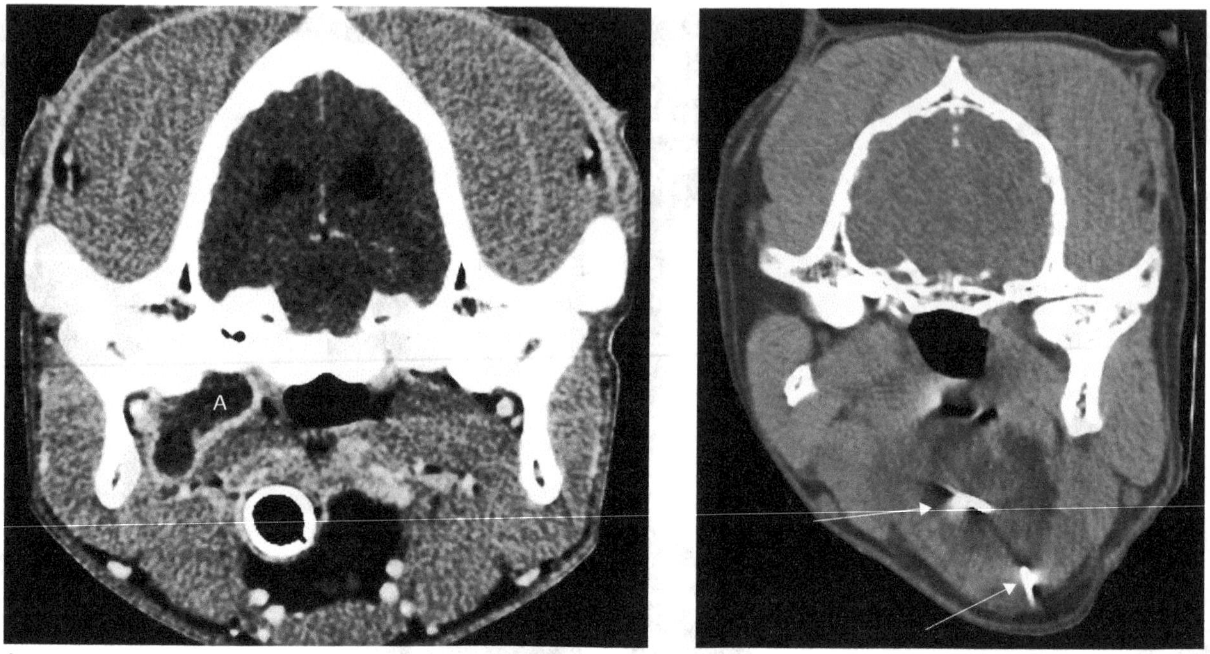

Figure 12.7 (A) Transverse post-contrast CT image of a dog with an orally penetrating foreign body abscess medial to the right temporomandibular joint with a hypodense cavity (A) and a contrast-enhancing rim. (B) Transverse CT image of a cat with two needle pieces (arrows) in the tongue base and surrounding soft tissue swelling.

Tonsillitis

Tonsillitis is a relatively common disease in dogs and leads to uni- or bilateral swelling of the palatine tonsils with protrusion from the tonsillar fossa. CT images may reveal moderate swelling and homogeneous contrast enhancement, as well as mild lymphadenopathy.

Osteomyelitis

Infections of the maxilla or mandible can occur secondary to penetrating trauma, bite wounds and fractures.

CT features

- Bone lysis
  - focal
  - moth eaten.
- Bone proliferation can be variable
  - palisading
  - spiculating
  - expansile.
- Bone medullary changes
  - low-density areas
  - trabecular coarsening and focal cortical erosions.
- Soft tissue thickening
  - lack of contrast enhancement can indicate necrotic tissue.

Craniomandibular osteopathy

See Chapter 16.

Neoplasia

Mandibular and maxillary tumors

Approximately 6% of all canine and 3% of all feline cancers occur in the oral cavity. Squamous cell carcinoma commonly occurs in the mandible and maxilla of both dogs and cats. Tumors that occur in the dog but rarely in the cat include fibrosarcoma, malignant melanoma, osteosarcoma, chondrosarcoma and tumors of the periodontal ligament (epulides, see below). Fibrosarcomas in large breed dogs are histologically often low-grade yet biologically high-grade aggressive tumors. Primary bone tumors are often highly osteolytic and to a lesser extent osteoproductive, but typically only affect one bone. Oral soft tissue neoplasia can invade adjacent bones and cause osteolysis and periosteal reaction, which is usually not confined to one bone. It may be possible to distinguish these two tumor groups based on monostotic/polyostotic behavior; however, the CT features of specific tumor types are not pathognomonic.

*CT features (**see also** Chapter 13)*

- Squamous cell carcinoma (Figures 12.8 and 13.13)

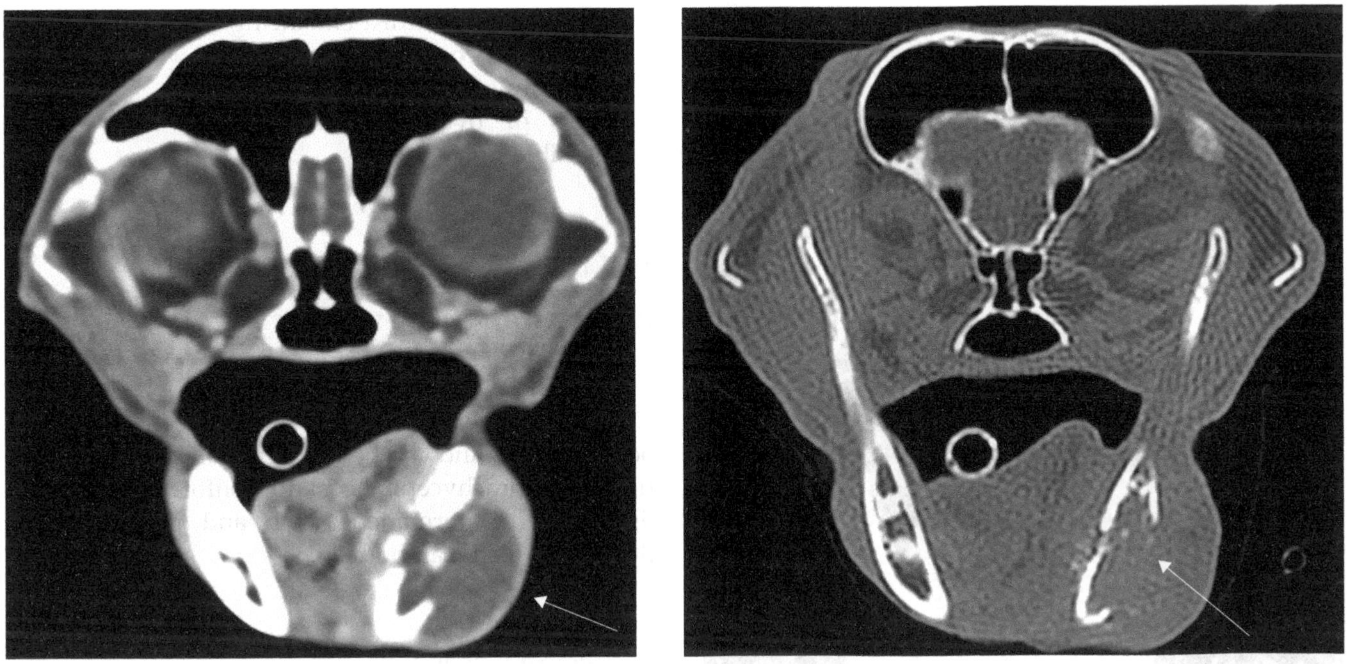

A B

Figure 12.8 Transverse (A) post-contrast and (B) bone algorithm CT images of a cat with a squamous cell carcinoma of the left mandible. Note the soft tissue mass effect and bony lysis of the left mandible (arrow).

  - canine: rostral mandible, variable bony lysis, rare metastatic spread
  - feline: mandible or maxilla, bony sclerosis and lysis, heterogeneous contrast enhancement and spread to local lymph nodes is common; other common sites include sublingual and maxillary locations.
- Fibrosarcoma (Figure 12.9)
  - often have bony involvement.
- Malignant melanoma (Figure 12.10)
  - variable bone lysis
  - often metastasis to regional lymph nodes and lungs.
- Osteosarcoma (Figure 13.13)
  - monostotic
  - usually highly osteolytic
  - varying degrees of periosteal reaction.
- Chondrosarcoma
  - monostotic
  - usually highly osteolytic and osteoproductive
  - varying degrees of periosteal reaction.
- Bone marrow neoplasia
  - focal (plasmacytoma) or diffuse (multiple myeloma)
  - highly osteolytic, punch-out lesions
  - locally invasive
  - usually lack of periosteal reaction.
- Multilobular osteochondrosarcoma (Figure 13.13)

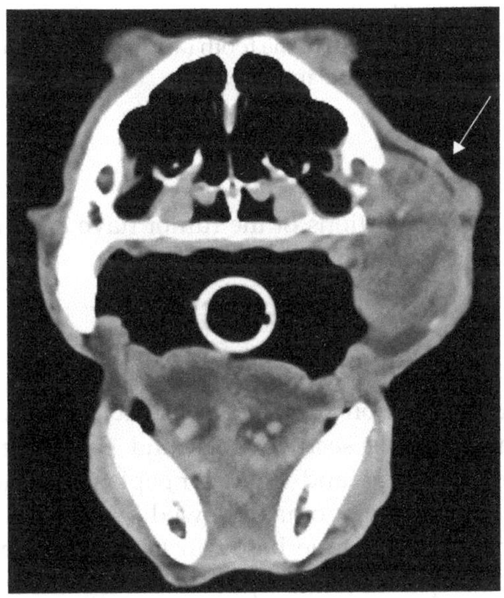

Figure 12.9 Transverse post-contrast CT image of a dog with left maxillary fibrosarcoma. Note the maxillary soft tissue mass with adjacent lysis and tooth loss (arrow).

  - often arise from the temporo-occipital area of the skull, although involvement of the mandible, maxilla and hard palate have been reported
  - margins are well defined and little bony lysis is present

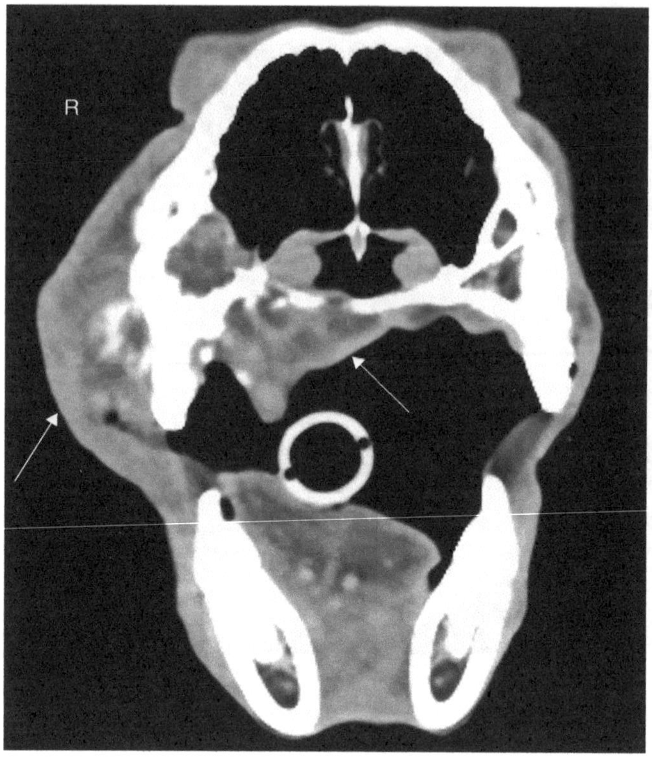

Figure 12.10 Transverse post-contrast CT image of a dog with right maxillary malignant melanoma has a soft tissue density mass with inhomogeneous contrast enhancement on buccal and palatal sides of the tooth (arrows), with bony lysis of the right hard palate and maxilla.

- central portions of the tumor have a characteristic coarse granular density.

Palatal, tonsillar and lingual neoplasia

The most common tumor of the soft palate is lymphoma, which is seen in dogs and cats. The most common tonsillar and lingual neoplasia in dogs is squamous cell carcinoma, followed by other types of carcinoma. The tongue base can be a site of ectopic thyroid neoplasia (*see* Chapter 18). Most oral neoplasias are locally very invasive to other soft tissues and bone, and have a high rate of regional metastases. CT is excellent for exact lesion localization, margination and assessment of metastatic spread. An open-mouth CT series is best to prevent silhouetting with neighboring soft tissues.

CT features (Figure 12.11)
- Thickened, contrast-enhanced soft tissue neoplasia.
- Irregularly contrast-enhancing, can have non-enhancing core.
- Local muscle infiltration.
- Lysis of hyoid, mandibular and other bones possible.

Dental Diseases

Malformation/Developmental

Abnormal tooth number and position

Congenital absence or supernumerary teeth frequently occur in dogs and can be identified on CT. In association with brachycephalic skull conformation, malalignement of permanent teeth and persistence of deciduous teeth can be seen.

Dental cystic lesions

Dentigerous cysts arise from proliferation of the reduced enamel epithelium in association with an unerupted tooth crown. They are most commonly seen around the first premolars in brachycephalic dogs. The cyst can continue to grow, destroy mandible or maxilla and lead to nasal obstruction or mandibular fracture. Radicular cysts develop from the tooth root and can become equally expansile.

CT features (Figure 12.12)
- Fluid-filled cyst in rostral maxilla or mandible, surrounding premolar tooth crown (dentigerous cyst) or root (radicular cyst).
- Thin cyst lining, can be contrast-enhancing.
- Compression atrophy of neighboring bony structures.
- Possible pathologic fracture.

Dental fractures, extractions and endodontic treatment

Dental fracture lines usually follow distinct patterns of dental anatomy. The canine tooth can be impacted into the nasal cavity. Exposed pulp will become necrotic and dentine will cease to build up. Root fragments can be assessed for any reaction in the surrounding tissues. Endodontic material is radiopaque and treated pulp cavities can be assessed for complete filling and late reactions. However, the beam hardening and high-density streak artifacts caused by this material can hamper proper assessment.

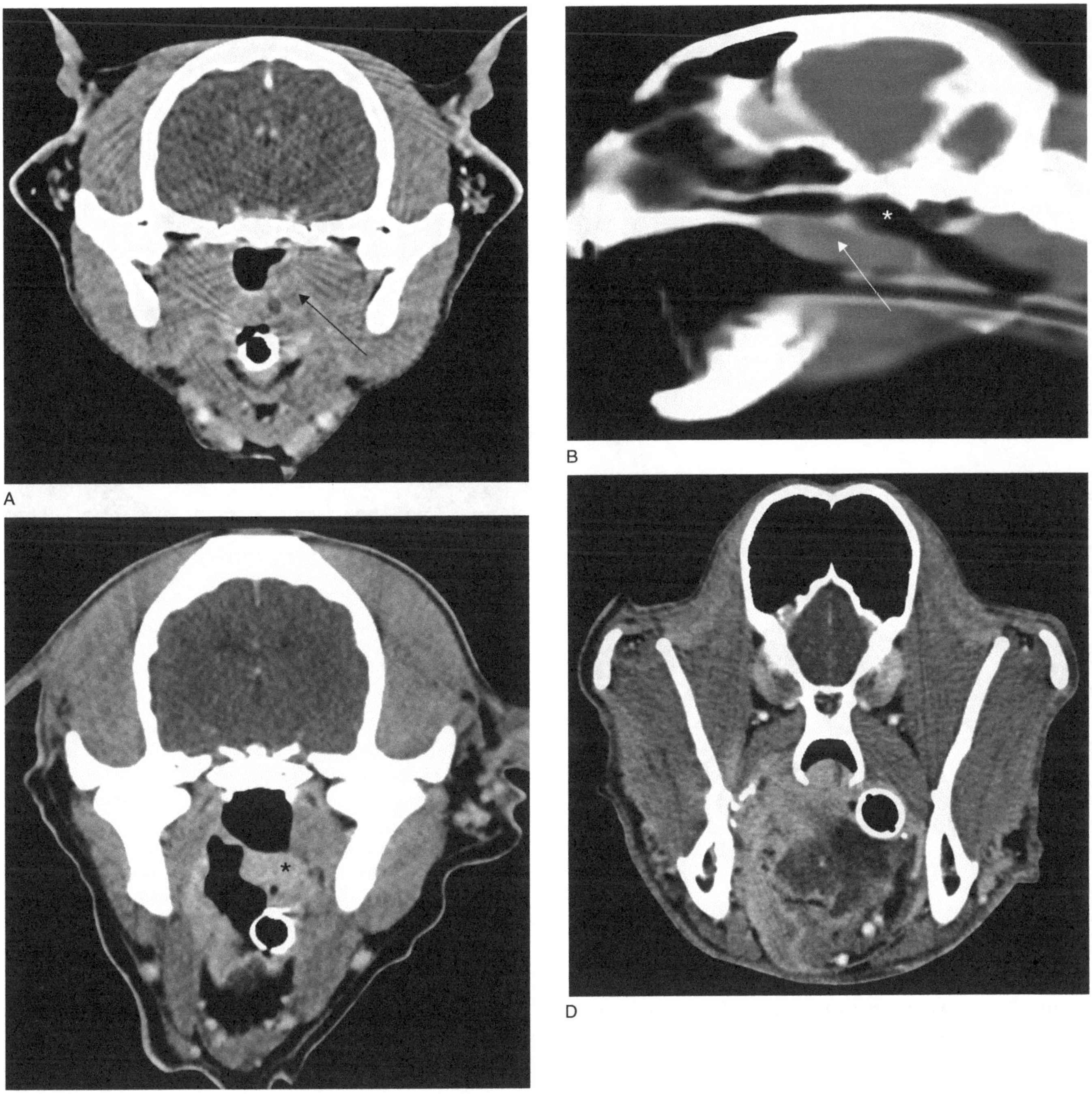

Figure 12.11 Transverse post-contrast CT images of (A) a cat with lymphoma. Note the nasopharyngeal soft tissue swelling (black arrow) and (B) the thickened soft palate (white arrow) and narrowed nasopharynx (asterisk) on reconstructed sagittal image. (C) A dog with a homogeneously contrast-enhancing left tonsillar squamous cell carcinoma (asterisk). (D) A dog with a tongue carcinoma. The mass is irregularly contrast enhancing with a non-enhancing core and is displacing the soft palate.

CT features (Figure 12.13)

- Fissure lines through the tooth are well visible with thin-sliced technique.
- Reactive periodontal bone loss in case of infection.
- Presence of root remnants possible.
- Radiopaque material in pulp cavity in case of endodontic treatment.
- Impaction can dislodge the canine tooth into the nasal cavity, where it can serve as a nidus for fungal rhinitis in dogs (*see* Figure 11.10).

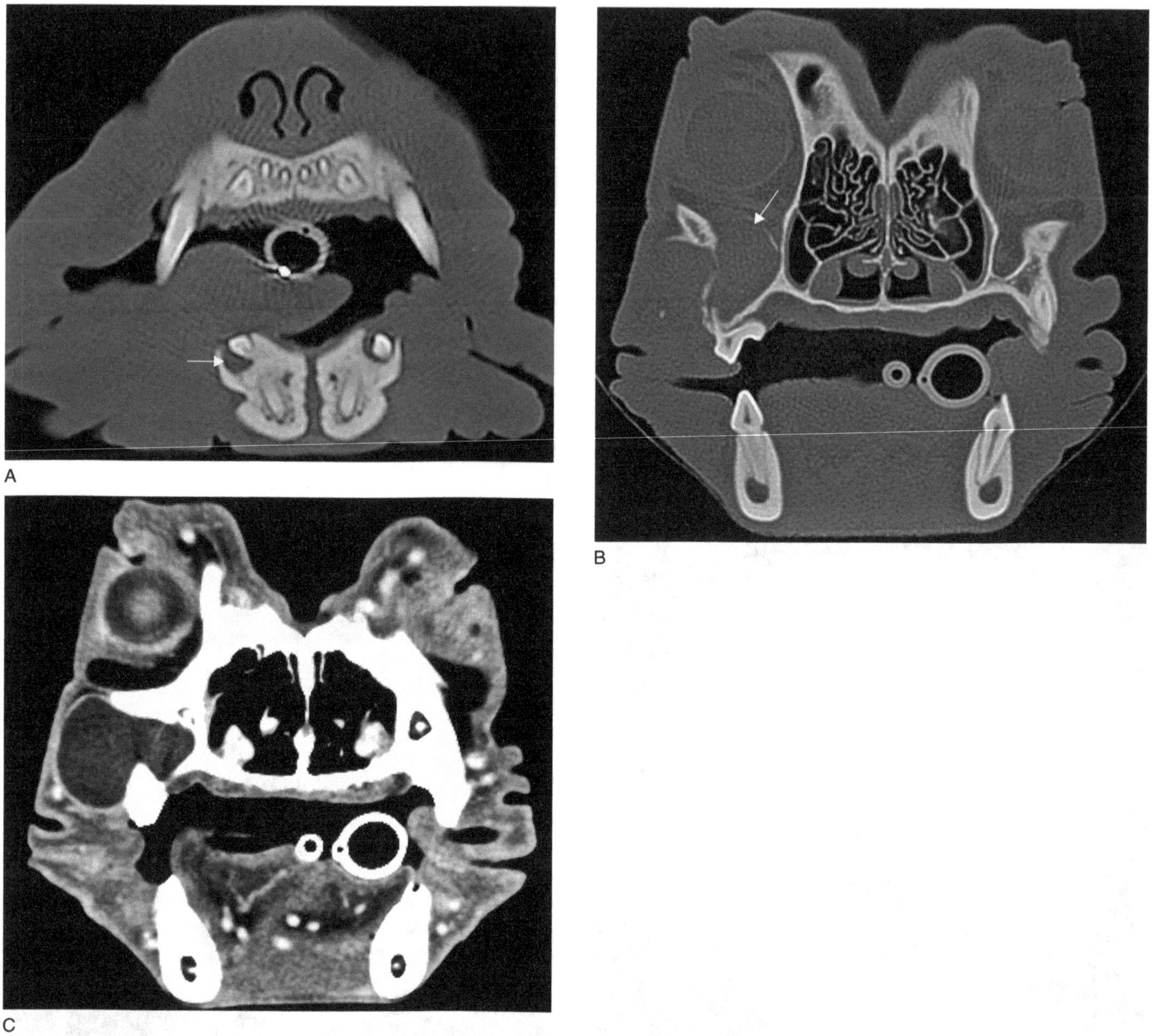

Figure 12.12 (A) Transverse CT image of a small dentigerous cyst (arrow) in both rostral mandibles in a bulldog encroaching the unerupted P_1. (B) Apical cyst of 109 (M^1) in a boxer dog that expands into the orbital cavity with a thin bony rim (arrow). (C) Transverse post-contrast CT image shows the non-enhancing nature of the cyst fluid.

Caries, pulpitis, tooth root infection, periodontitis

Caries, cavitary loss of tooth crown material due to bacterial infection, is relatively uncommon in dogs and cats. Larger lesions can be readily identified on CT images. If the pulp cavity has been infected (pulpitis) due to trauma or ascending tooth root infection, the pulp chamber may contain gas and over time become enlarged due to the cessation of dentine lay-down. The hallmark feature of a tooth root infection is lysis of the root apex and the surrounding alveolar bone. In periodontitis, diffuse osteolytic and osteoproductive changes of the alveolar socket can be seen. Root resorption can frequently be observed in feline odontoclastic resorptive lesions in older cats.

CT features (Figure 12.14)

- Odontolytic crown defect in caries.
- Gas in pulpal chamber is a sign of an exposed and infected pulp.
- Thinning of the tooth wall indicates non-vital tooth due to previous pulpitis.

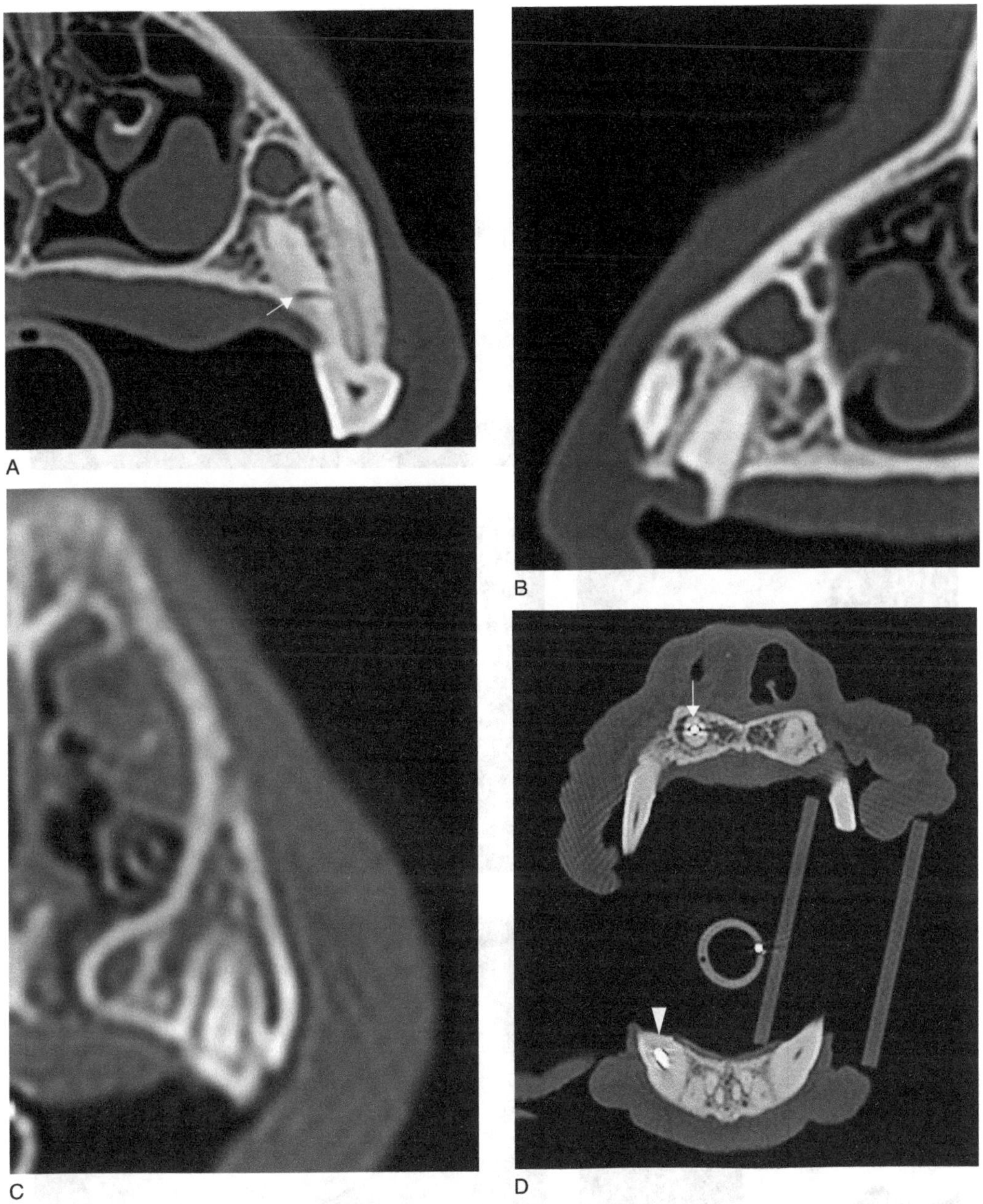

Figure 12.13 Transverse CT images of patients with tooth fracture. (A) A horizontal root fracture (arrow) of 208 (P^4). (B) Root remnants of a recently incompletely extracted 109 (M^1) in a dog and (C) a 204 (C^1) with a crown fracture in a cat sustained 6 years earlier without evidence of reactive changes (image courtesy of Casey Jarrett). (D) 103 (I^3; arrow) and 404 (C_1; arrowhead) in a dog with mineral-dense endodontic filling material, causing high-density streak artifacts.

- Apical budding with an osteolucent bone socket indicates tooth root infection. Fistulation into the nasal or orbital cavity or external facial swelling are further possible complications.
- Diffuse loss of periodontal bone and irregular periosteal reaction can be observed in severe periodontitis.
- Lack of a radiolucent dental ligament, dental neck erosion and root resorption can be seen in feline odontoclastic resorptive lesions.

Periodontal and odontogenic neoplasia

Epulides (previously described as adamantinomas) are benign gingival proliferations originating from the periodontal ligament that are common in dogs and rare in cats. Fibromatous and ossifying epulides do not invade the underlying bone, whereas acanthomatous epulides are locally aggressive and do invade underlying bone. Odontogenic tumors originate from the dental lamina and are rare in dogs and cats.

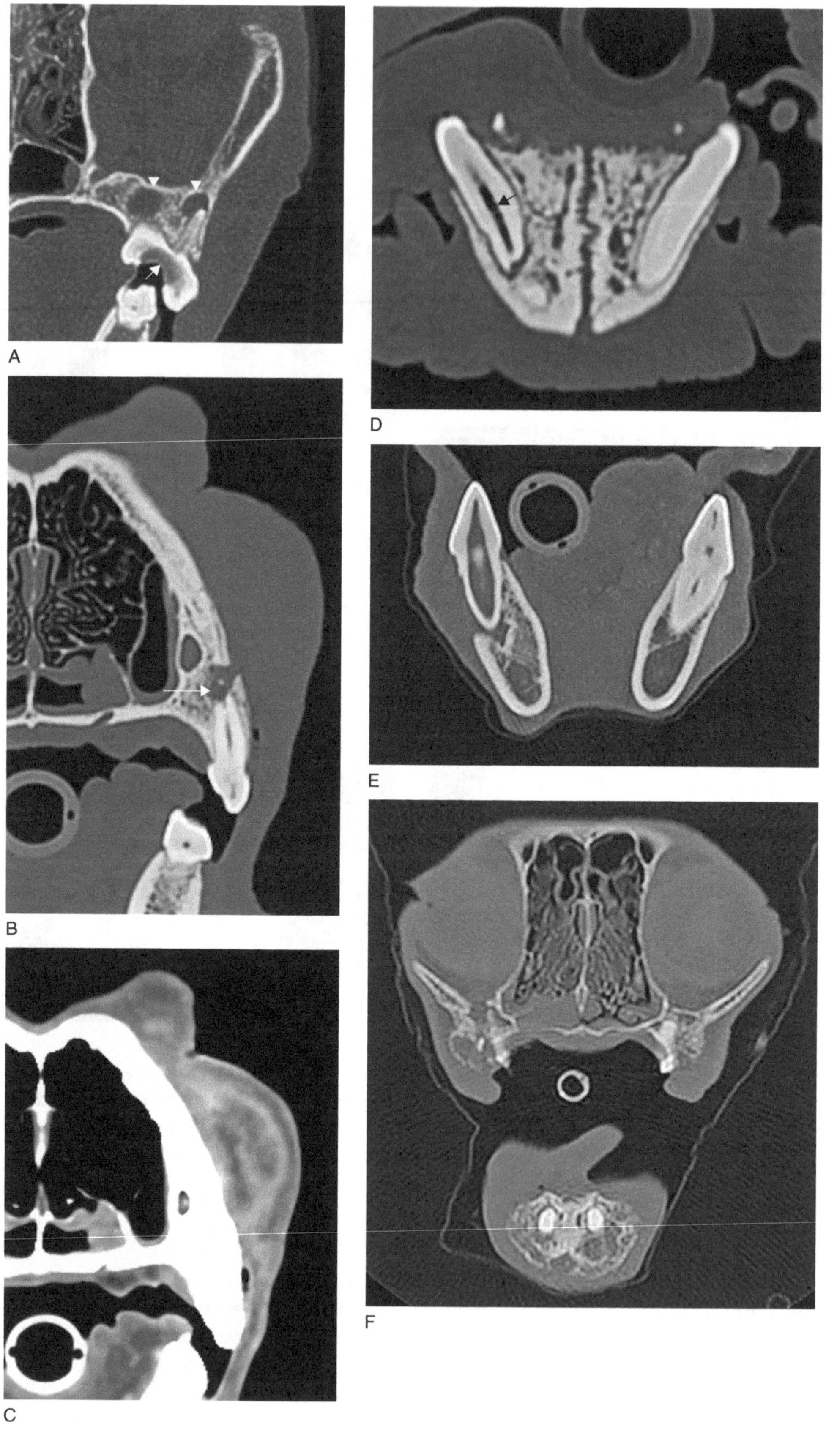
A
B
C
D
E
F

Figure 12.14 (A) CT image of 209 (M^1) in a dog with a large crown defect due to caries (arrow) and osteolucent periapical lucencies around two visible roots (arrowheads). (B) Caudal root of 208 (P^4) in a dog with a periapical osteolucent abscess (arrow) cavity communicating with a large external infraorbital soft tissue swelling, which on (C) contrast-enhanced CT shows rim enhancement with a non-enhancing abscess cavity. (D) 404 (C_1) in a dog with pulpal gas (arrow) indicating a non-vital tooth. (E) Mesial root of 408 (M_1) in a dog with chronic tooth root infection and a non-vital pulp. Compared to 308, the tooth wall is thinned. (F) Combination of marked lytic and productive periodontal bone changes in a cat with severe chronic periodontal disease.

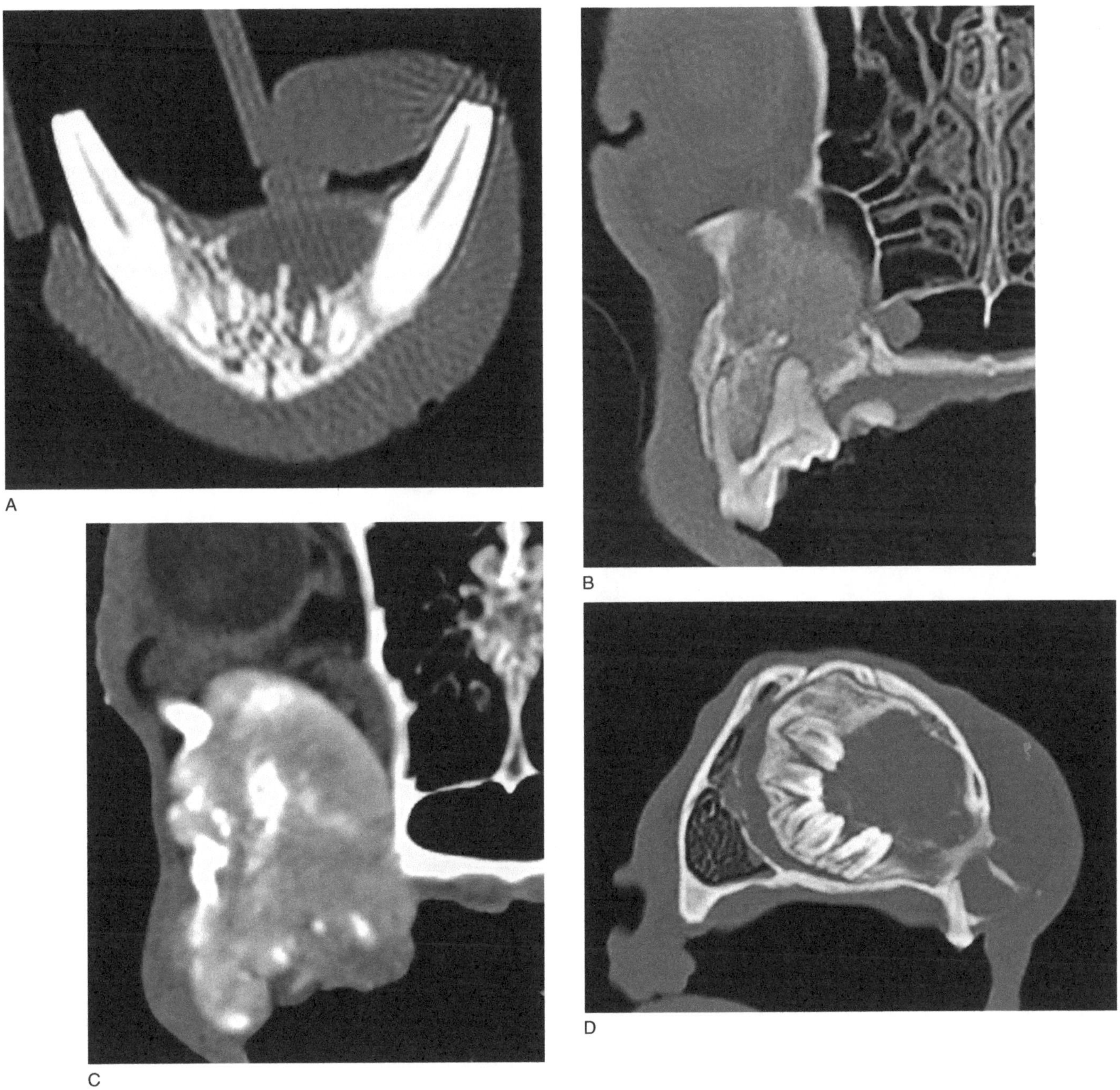

Figure 12.15 (A) Acanthomatous epulis in a dog. The soft tissue mass is locally invasive and destructive to the mandibular symphysis. (B) Pre-contrast bone algorithm image of a cementifying fibroma around 109 (M^1). This tumor arises from the periodontal ligament and produces mildly dense cementum. (C) Post-contrast study of the same dog shows marked irregular contrast enhancement. (D) Compound odontoma in a 9-month-old dog. Notice the expansile cystic nature of the mass containing teeth.

Inductive odontogenic tumors such as compound odontomas produce a large amount of stroma, whereas non-inductive types such as ameloblastoma do not. Odontomas are benign but expansile masses that include enamel and dentin structures within the mass.

CT features (Figures 12.15, 13.10D)

- Epulis
  - soft tissue mass adjacent to dental arcade
  - usually marked contrast enhancement, but often similar to normal strong gingival and labial contrast enhancement
  - subtle irregular periosteal reaction and osteolysis in acanthomatous epulis
  - exclusively new bone formation in benign ossifying epulides possible
  - differentiation between benign and aggressive epulides and determination of tumor margin remains difficult with CT.
- Odontogenic neoplasia
  - always involve dental structures
  - dental structures within the mass as hallmark of odontoma.

Further Reading

Fayad LM, Carrino JA and Fishman EK (2007) Musculoskeletal infection: role of CT in the emergency department. *RadioGraphics* **27**: 1723–36.

Floyd MR (1991) The modified Triadan system: nomenclature of veterinary dentistry. *J Vet Dent* **8**: 18–19.

Gendler A, Lewis JR, Reetz JA and Schwarz T (2010) Computed tomographic features of oral squamous cell carcinoma in cats: 18 cases (2002–2008). *J Am Vet Med Assoc* **236**: 319–25.

George TF and Smallwood JE (1992) Anatomic atlas for computed tomography in the mesaticephalic dog: head and neck. *Vet Radiol Ultrasound* **33**: 217–40.

Hudson JA, Montgomery RD, Hathcock JT and Jarboe JM (1994) Computed tomography of craniomandibular osteopathy in a dog. *Vet Radiol Ultrasound* **35**: 94–9.

Seiler G, Rossi F, Vignoli M, Cianciolo R, Scanlon T and Giger U (2007) Computed tomographic features of skull osteomyelitis in four young dogs. *Vet Radiol Ultrasound* **48**: 544–9.

CHAPTER THIRTEEN

Temporomandibular Joint and Masticatory Apparatus

Tobias Schwarz

Imaging Protocol

See Chapter 12.

CT: Anatomy and Normal Variants

Temporomandibular joint (TMJ)

In dogs and cats the TMJ is a condylar synovial joint formed by the mandibular condyle and the fossa mandibularis of the squamous part of the temporal bone with a ventrally extending retroarticular (synonym *retroglenoid*) process and a small tubercle extending from the rostral fossa margin. The TMJ acts as a hinge joint to open and close the mouth, but there is also a small degree of transverse motion to allow the shearing action of the carnassial teeth.

In CT the bony components of the joint can be seen in great detail. There are some shape variations of different parts of the mandibular condyle in dogs. The mandibular condyle completes ossification relatively late, so that its margins can appear irregular in up to 12 months old dogs (Figure 13.1). In cats the condyle is more uniformly cylindric (Figure 13.2). There is an unnamed fossa in the rostrolateral aspect of the condyle in the dog that can be pronounced in some breeds. Details of soft tissue components are poorly delineated. The TMJ disk is not visible.

Mandibular symphysis

The mandibular symphysis can be considered as the third joint of the jaw that works synergistically with both TMJs during mastication. Its elastic properties allow an unequal hinge and transverse motion of the TMJs required for the shearing action of the carnassial teeth. Further details are given in Chapter 12.

Masticatory muscles (Table 13.1)

Disease Features

Malformation/Developmental/Degenerative

Canine TMJ dysplasia

This congenital malformation of the TMJ exists in two forms (*see* Box 13.1).

CT features (Figure 13.3)

- Curved to S-shaped condyle and fossa.
- Various shapes or absence of the retroarticular process.
- Stronger medial inclination of joint angle.
- Mandibular condyle subluxation possible.

Temporomandibular degenerative joint disease and osteochondrosis

Degenerative joint disease of the TMJ is sometimes suspected in dogs with pain on mastication/reluctance to chew in the absence of other dental and masticatory pathology, when CT imaging features suggest irregular joint margins and abnormal joint laxity. Occasionally when mineralized joint mice are seen with a matching defect in the articular surface, osteochondrosis is suspected.

Veterinary Computed Tomography, First Edition. Edited by Tobias Schwarz, Jimmy Saunders.

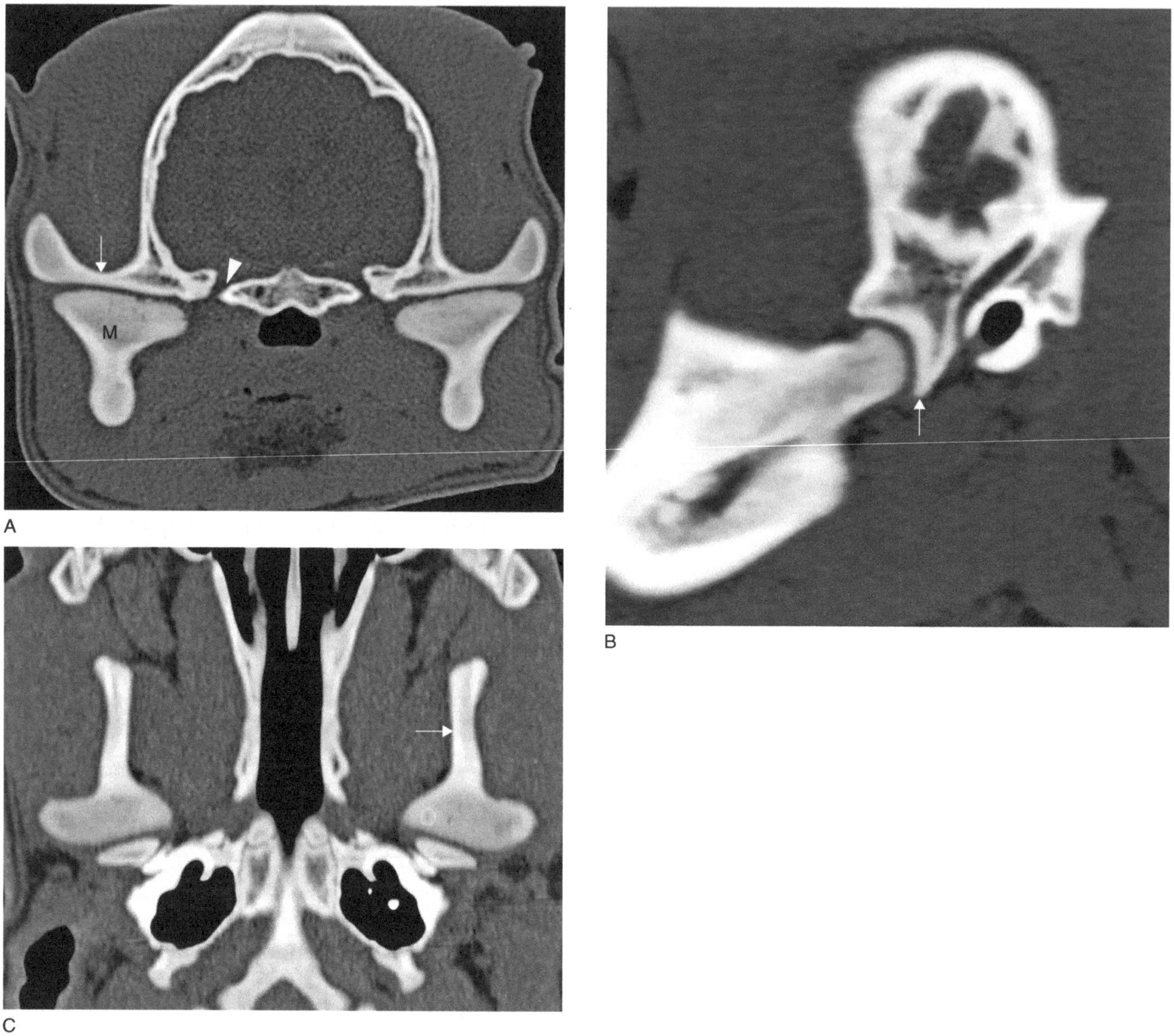

Figure 13.1 Normal TMJ of a 6-month-old dog. (A) Transverse CT image with the irregularly marginated condyle of the mandible (M) and the mandibular fossa of the temporal bone (arrow). The oval foramen is at the same level (arrowhead). (B) Sagittal image demonstrating the joint congruency and the retroarticular process (arrow). (C) Dorsally reconstructed image demonstrating joint congruency and the coronoid process (arrow) of the mandible.

CT features (Figure 13.4)

- Irregular bony articular margins.
- Subluxation on mandibular traction view.
- Cystic defects in mandibular condyle.
- Mineralized joint mice with matching bony defects.

Dislocation and trauma

Dislocation

TMJ dislocation can either be complete (luxation) or partial (subluxation). It is usually seen as consequence of head trauma and open jaw lock. In most cases the mandibular condyle luxates rostrad. Subluxation can be associated with dysplastic and/or degenerative changes leading to excessive joint laxity.

CT features

- Luxation (Figure 13.5)
  - empty mandibular fossa, usually rostrally displaced condyle
  - dental malocclusion and mandibular shift
  - associated with open jaw lock:

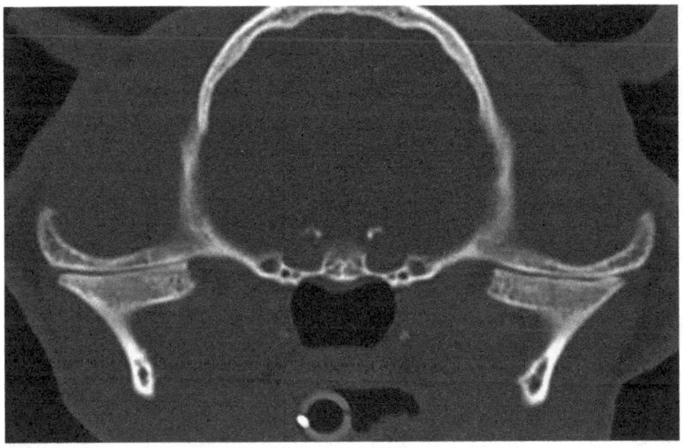

Figure 13.2 Normal feline TMJ with a more cylindrical mandibular condyle.

Box 13.1 Canine TMJ dysplasia

A Luxating form

Excessively flat mandibular condyle and fossa and absent retroarticular process. This very rare form can be associated with TMJ subluxation, luxation and open jaw lock in dogs.

B Chondrodystrophic malformation

Excessively curved mandibular condyle and fossa, misshapen retroarticular process. This is commonly seen in chondrodystrophic breeds and is without clinical consequences.

Table 13.1
Anatomic details of the canine and feline muscles of mastication.

Name	Origin	Insertion	Function	Fiber type	Innervation
Temporal	Temporal fossa and zygomatic arch	Medial and lateral aspect coronoid process of mandible	Jaw closer	2M	Mandibular nerve
Masseter	Zygomatic arch	Lateral, ventral and caudal aspect mandibular ramus	Jaw closer	2M	Mandibular nerve
Medial pterygoid	Pterygoid fossa	Medial and caudal aspect angular process of mandible	Jaw closer	2M	Mandibular nerve
Lateral pterygoid	Pterygoid fossa	Medial TMJ	Medial TMJ translation	2M	Mandibular nerve
Digastricus	Occipital bone	Caudoventral mandible	Jaw opener	2A	Mandibular and facial nerves

  - contralateral to locked coronoid process in dogs
  - usually ipsilateral to locked coronoid process in cats.
- Subluxation (Figure 13.3)
  - best demonstrated by mandibular traction CT (see protocol)
  - sagittal reconstruction most helpful
  - signs of underlying degenerative joint disease or dysplasia may be visible.

Open jaw lock

Open jaw lock is a rare emergency in dogs and cats. Usually, but not always, the condition is caused by the coronoid process of one mandible being dislodged laterally to the zygomatic arch. As a consequence, one TMJ is also dislocated partially or completely (contralateral in dogs, ipsilateral in cats). Etiologic theories include excessive TMJ or mandibular symphysis laxity, pterygoid muscle spasm, old depression fractures or malformation of the zygomatic arch.

CT protocol

- Whenever possible, the CT should be performed in the open jaw lock position.
- A post-contrast series is very helpful to identify local inflammation caused by friction of current or previous coronoid displacement.
- A post-reduction series is helpful to ensure normal TMJ articulation.

CT features (Figure 13.6)

- Unilateral lateral coronoid process displacement lateral to zygomatic arch.

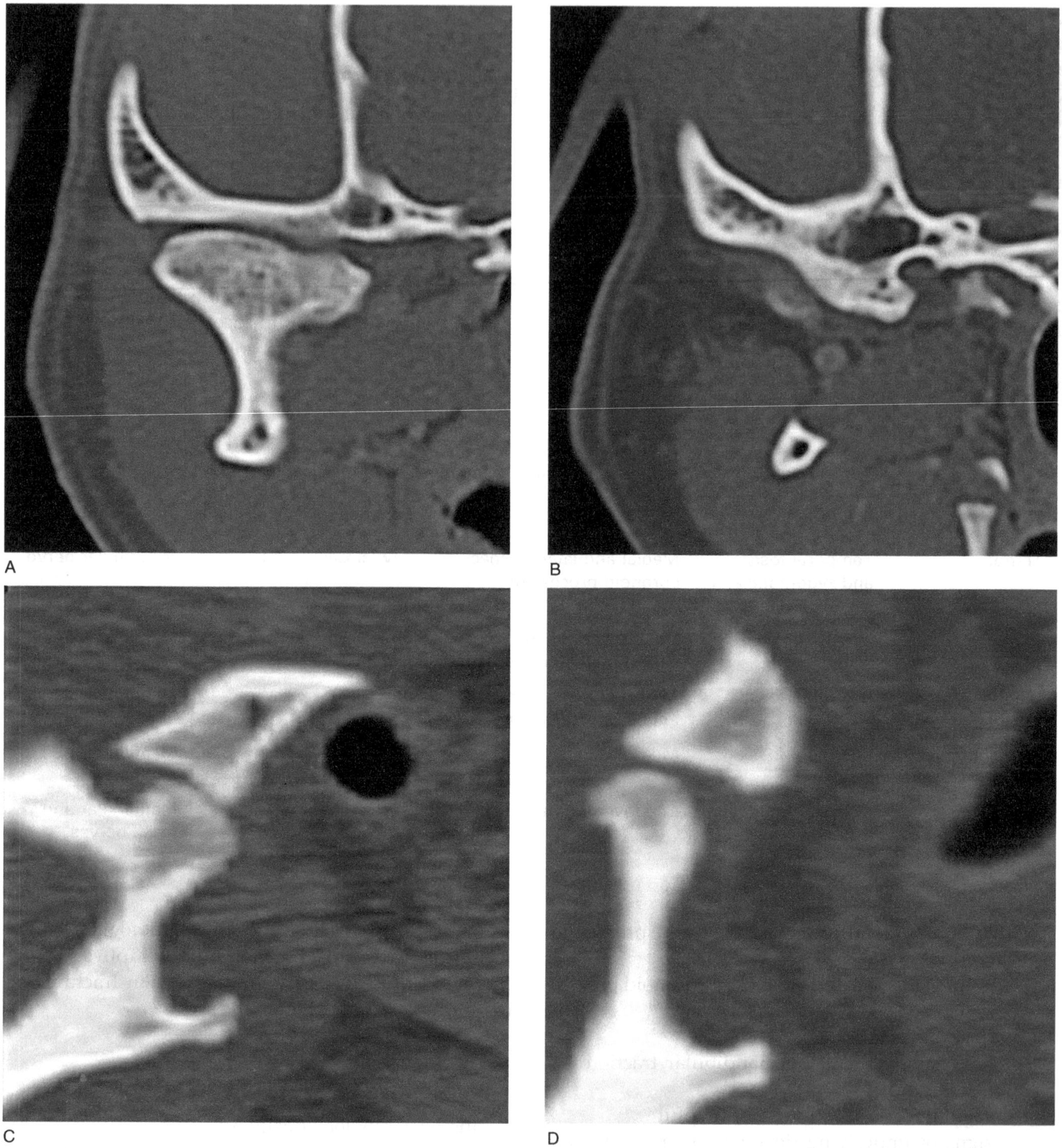

Figure 13.3 TMJ of a beagle with (A) abnormally curved surfaces of both articulating bones and (B) a very pronounced retroarticular process. This type of TMJ dysplasia is common in chondrodystrophic dog breeds and may not be clinically relevant. (C) Sagittal image of a dysplastic TMJ in a dog with masticatory pain. The articular surfaces are flat, there is no retroarticular process and the mandibular condyle is subluxated caudally. (D) Under applied traction the same mandibular condyle subluxates rostrally, indicating abnormal joint laxity.

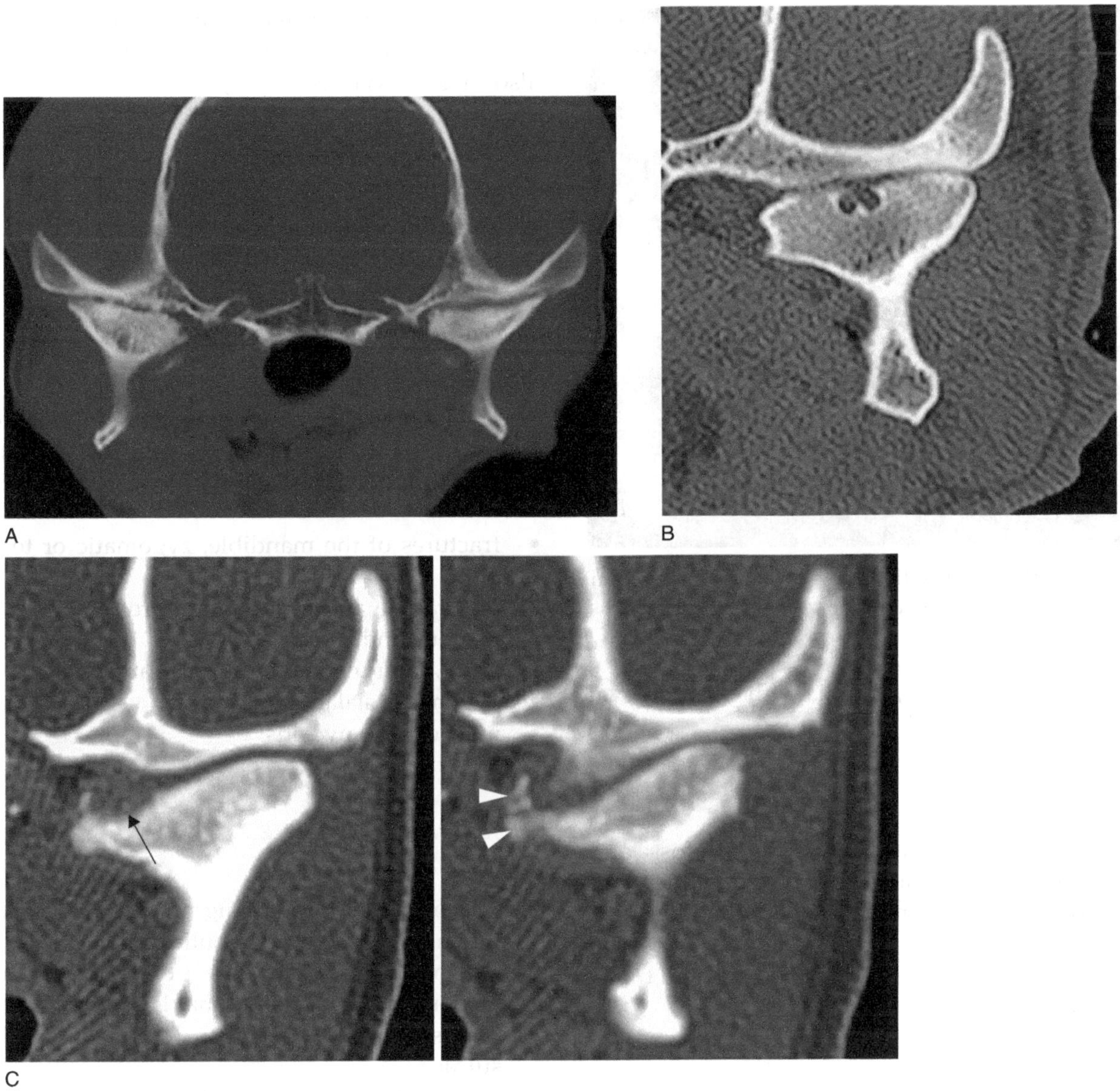

Figure 13.4 Imaging features of three dogs with masticatory pain. (A) Bilateral irregular bony joint margins of the TMJ and adjacent sclerosis, consistent with DJD. (B) Subchondral bone cyst in the mandibular condyle. (C) Subchondral bone defect (arrow) and corresponding free bone fragments in the medial TMJ (arrowheads). The latter two cases are consistent with osteochondrosis.

- Ipsi- (cats) or contralateral TMJ dislocation (partial or full).
- Rim enhancement of masseter musculature adjacent to previously or currently displaced coronoid process.

Jaw drop

This is a rare clinical syndrome seen in dogs that cannot actively close their mouth, but the jaw is not locked. It requires a bilateral flaccid mandibular nerve paralysis seen in conditions such as idiopathic trigeminal neuropathy, lymphoma or juvenile masticatory myositis (see below). Rare differentials include meningioma, rabies and botulism.

CT features (Figure 13.7)

- Marked bilaterally symmetrical masticatory muscle atrophy.
- Bilateral CT imaging features of the trigeminal nerve with neuropathy or lymphoma have not been reported.
- Chronic slow-growing bilateral trigeminal nerve neoplasia could reveal enlarged contrast-enhancing

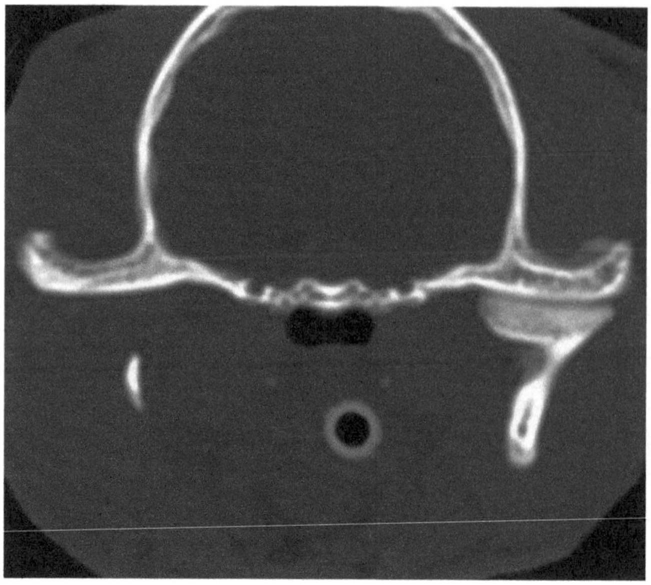

Figure 13.5 Rostral luxation of the right mandibular condyle in a cat resulting in an empty mandibular fossa.

trigeminal nerve roots/ganglia with enlarged oval foramina (bone atrophy).

TMJ fractures

Fractures involving the mandibular condyle, fossa and retroarticular process are an occasional consequence of head trauma and are often associated with other fractures of the mandible and zygomatic arch. Most are oriented in a sagittal plane and are best seen on transverse plane images.

CT features (Figure 13.8)

- Incomplete non-displaced fissure or fracture with usually displaced lateral condyle or fossa fragment; fossa is often comminuted.
- Retroarticular process fractures are often in transverse plane orientation, best seen on sagittal plane images.

TMJ ankylosis

This is a condition occasionally seen in outdoor cats with a history of confirmed or suspected old trauma. The cats are unable to open their mouth, and have varying degrees of fibrosis and new bone formation around one or both TMJs. The condition is thought to be the end stage of traumatic hemarthrosis, possibly secondary to a fall from a height. If the condition is unilateral, then a condylectomy is possible, whereas cats can usually not masticate properly post bilateral condylectomy. Mass lesions arising from the TMJ can also cause ankylosis.

CT features (Figure 13.9)

- Irregular new bone formation around TMJ.
- Irregular joint surfaces, mineralized particles in joint.
- Limited joint extension.

False TMJ ankylosis

This is defined as an abnormal joint immobility due to extra-articular lesions that restrict the movement of the TMJ. Such lesions can include:

- fractures of the mandible, zygomatic or temporal bone
- old trauma and insinuating fibrosis
- osseous and soft tissue masses
- aural, pharyngeal, retroorbital abscesses
- zygomatic sialadenitis
- masticatory myositis
- tetanus.

CT features (Figures 12.7, 13.10–13.12, 14.4, 14.5, 14.19)

- Osseous lesion impinging on coronoid process of the mandible in open mouth position.
- Osseous masses can have a defect in surface corresponding to mandible that is sawing into mass.
- Periosteal reaction along impinged mandibular surface.
- Post-contrast, open mouth position CT scan can reveal impinging soft tissue enhanced mass or contrast-enhanced reactive soft tissue between impinging bones.

Infection and inflammation

Masticatory muscle infection and abscessation

Infection and abscess formation of the masticatory muscles are seen in dogs as a result of oral and pharyngeal traumatic lacerations, with or without a migrating foreign body penetrating the retro-orbital space or mandibular area or salivary glands. External injuries and bite wounds leading to masticatory and periaural abscesses are seen in dogs and cats.

Cellulitis, sialadenitis and otitis externa/media can spread into surrounding masticatory muscles.

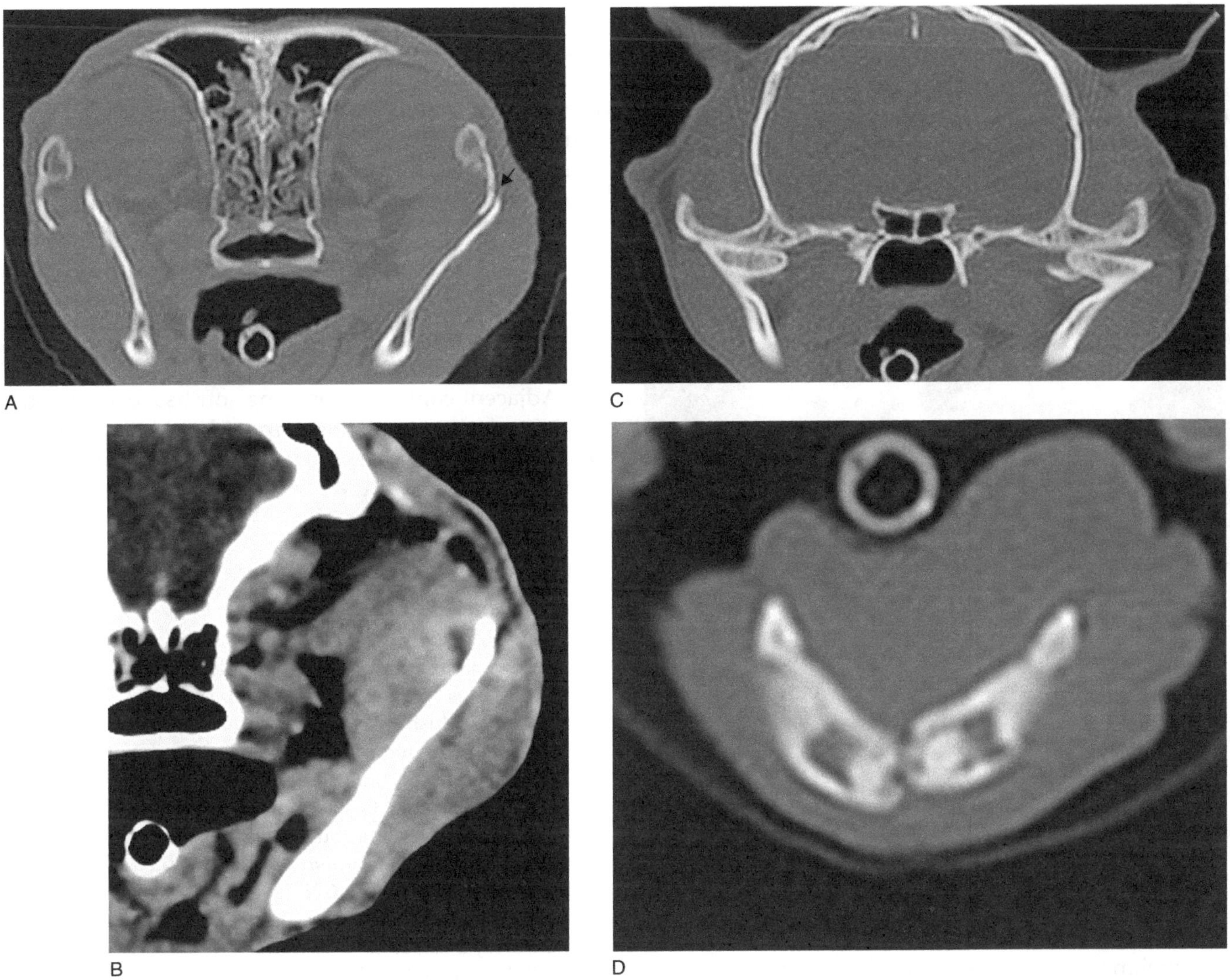

Figure 13.6 Transverse CT images of a cat with open jaw lock. (A) The coronoid process of the left mandible is dislocated and locked lateral to the zygomatic arch (arrow). (B) Post-contrast images show masseter muscle enhancement with central necrosis indicating chronic friction. (C) There is ipsilateral rostral subluxation of the mandibular condyle and (D) the mandibular symphysis is subluxated. Mandibular symphyseal laxity is the most likely cause of jaw lock in this cat. Compare with Figure 12.3C.

CT features (Figures 12.7 and 13.11)

- Marked local soft tissue swelling with a post-contrast contrast-enhanced rim and a large non-enhancing core.
- Abscess capsule shape reflects gravitational propensity.
- Radiodense foreign body.
- Patchy muscular contrast enhancement in case of infectious spread.
- Mandibular or medial retropharyngeal lymphnode enlargement.

Canine masticatory myositis

This is an immune-mediated disorder in which dogs develop auto-antibodies against type 2M muscle fibers, which are exclusively found in the masticatory muscles (the digastricus muscle with 2A fibers remains unaffected). It is predominantly seen in large breed, young to middle-aged dogs that present initially with pain on yawning or mastication and later on with restricted jaw opening and masticatory muscle atrophy.

There is a juvenile form of masticatory myositis seen in Cavalier King Charles spaniel puppies with bilateral

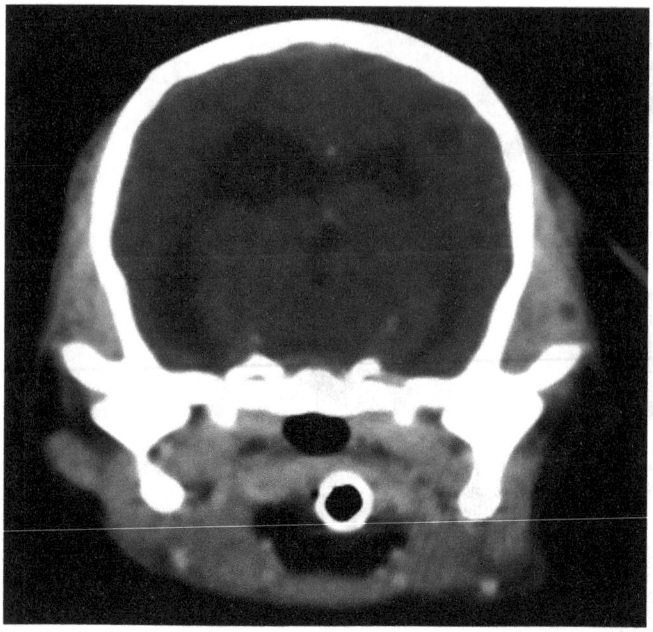

Figure 13.7 Severe generalized masticatory muscle atrophy in a 4-month-old Cavalier King Charles spaniel with atypical masticatory myositis presenting with jaw drop.

masticatory muscle atrophy. This poorly understood condition results in jaw drop (see above).

Definitive diagnosis requires biopsy, for which CT can be particularly helpful to avoid unaffected or necrotic areas.

CT features (Figures 13.7 and 13.12)

- Swelling and/or atrophy of masticatory muscles.
- Patchy muscular contrast enhancement in swollen muscles, can have non-enhancing core.
- Restrictive jaw opening in absence of osseous restrictive lesions.
- Mild mandibular or medial retropharyngeal lymphadenopathy.
- Juvenile masticatory myositis is characterized by marked bilaterally symmetric muscle atrophy.

Neoplasia

Neoplasia involving the TMJ is rare in dogs and cats. These are often fast-growing, aggressive tumors with marked osteolytic tendencies, which in the case of primary bone tumors are confined to one bone. Multilobular osteochondrosarcoma (synonyms *chondroma rodens, multilobular tumor of bone*) is a predominantly proliferative bone tumor that can arise from the bones of the TMJ. Other tumors in the vicinity of the TMJ can cause false ankylosis (*see* above and Chapter 12).

CT features (Figure 13.13)

- Osteolysis of TMJ or parts of it.
- Irregular periosteal reaction.
- Adjacent contrast-enhancing soft tissue swelling.
- Mass lesion restricting coronoid process motion.
- Mandibular and/or medial retropharyngeal lymphadenopathy.

Further Reading

Dickie AM, Schwarz T and Sullivan M (2002) Temporomandibular joint morphology in the Cavalier King Charles spaniel. *Vet Radiol Ultrasound* **43**: 260–6.

Mayhew PD, Bush WW and Glass EN (2002) Trigeminal neuropathy in dogs: a retrospective study of 29 cases (1991–2000). *J Am Anim Hosp Assoc* **38**: 262–70.

Meomartino L, Fatone G, Brunetti A, Lamagna F and Potenta A (1999) Temporomandibular ankylosis in the cat: a review of seven cases. *J Small Anim Pract* **40**: 7–10.

Pitcher GDC and Hahn CN (2007) Atypical masticatory muscle myositis in three cavalier King Charles spaniel littermates. *J Small Anim Pract* **48**: 226–8.

Platt SR, McConnell JF, Garosi LS, Ladlow J, De Stefani A and Shelton GD (2006) Magnetic resonance imaging in the diagnosis of canine inflammatory myopathies in three dogs. *Vet Radiol Ultrasound* **47**: 532–7.

Reiter AM (2004) Symphysiotomy, symphysiectomy, and intermandibular arthrodesis in a cat with open-mouth jaw locking – Case report and literature review. *J Vet Dent* **21**: 147–58.

Reiter AM and Schwarz T (2007) Computed tomographic appearance of masticatory myositis in dogs: 7 cases (1999–2006). *J Am Vet Med Assoc* **231**: 924–30.

Schwarz T, Weller R, Dickie AM, Konar M and Sullivan M. (2002) Imaging of the canine and feline temporomandibular joint: a review. *Vet Radiol Ultrasound* **43**: 85–97.

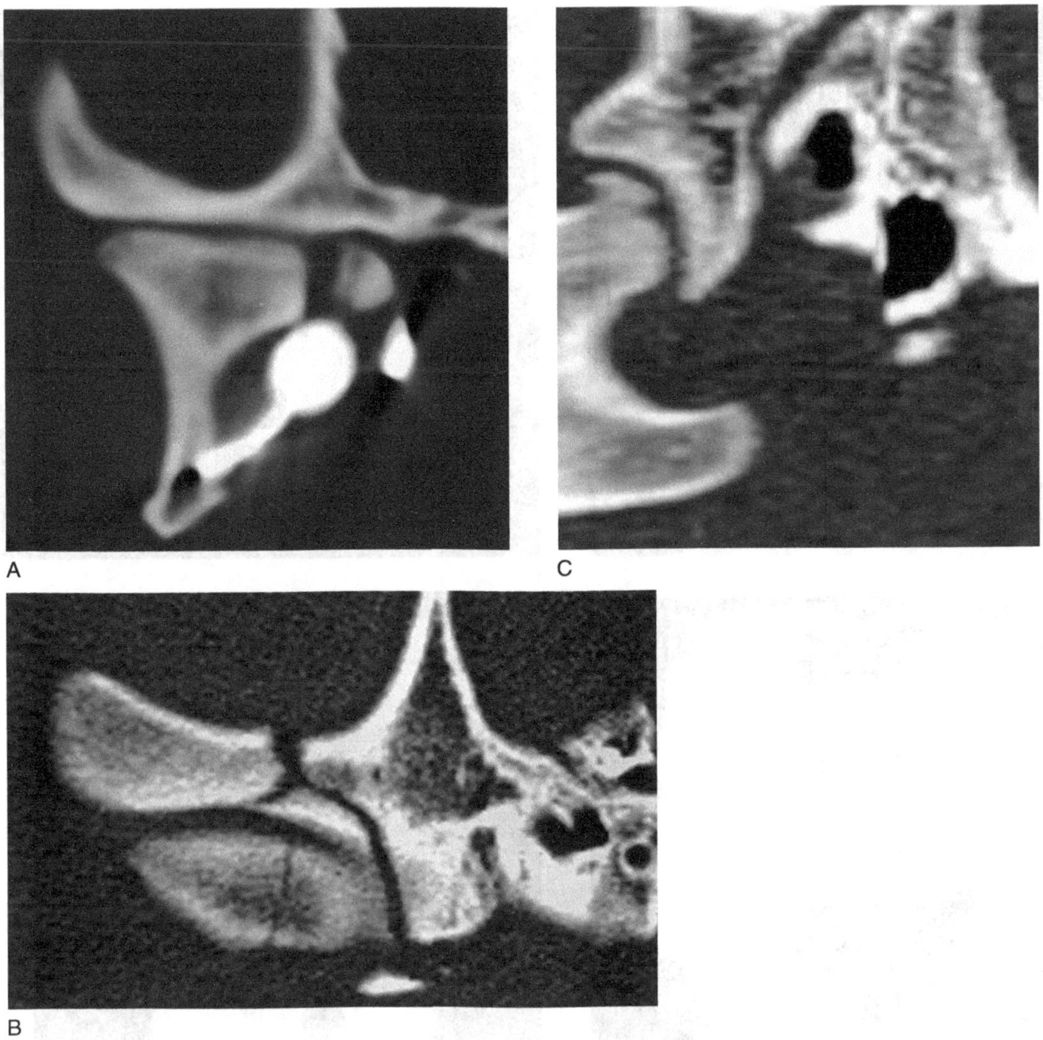

Figure 13.8 Features of TMJ fractures in dogs. (A) Sagittal fracture of the medial mandibular condyle compartment due to a penetrating metal foreign body (hunting arrow tip). (B) Comminuted fracture of the mandibular fossa and fissure of the mandibular condyle. (C) Dorsally oriented chip fracture of the mandibular condyle.

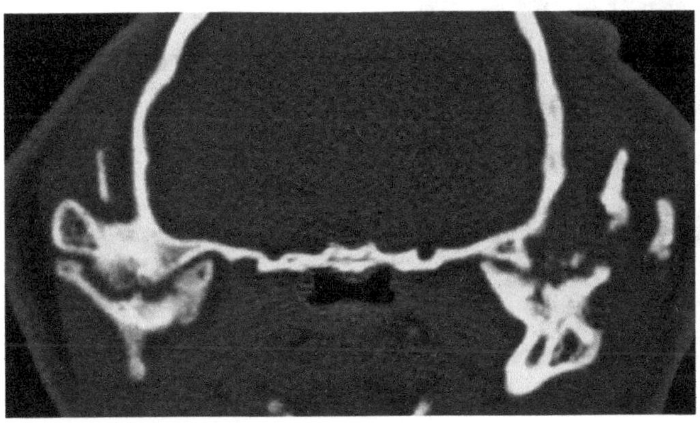

Figure 13.9 Bilateral TMJ ankylosis in a cat with complete loss of normal joint surfaces.

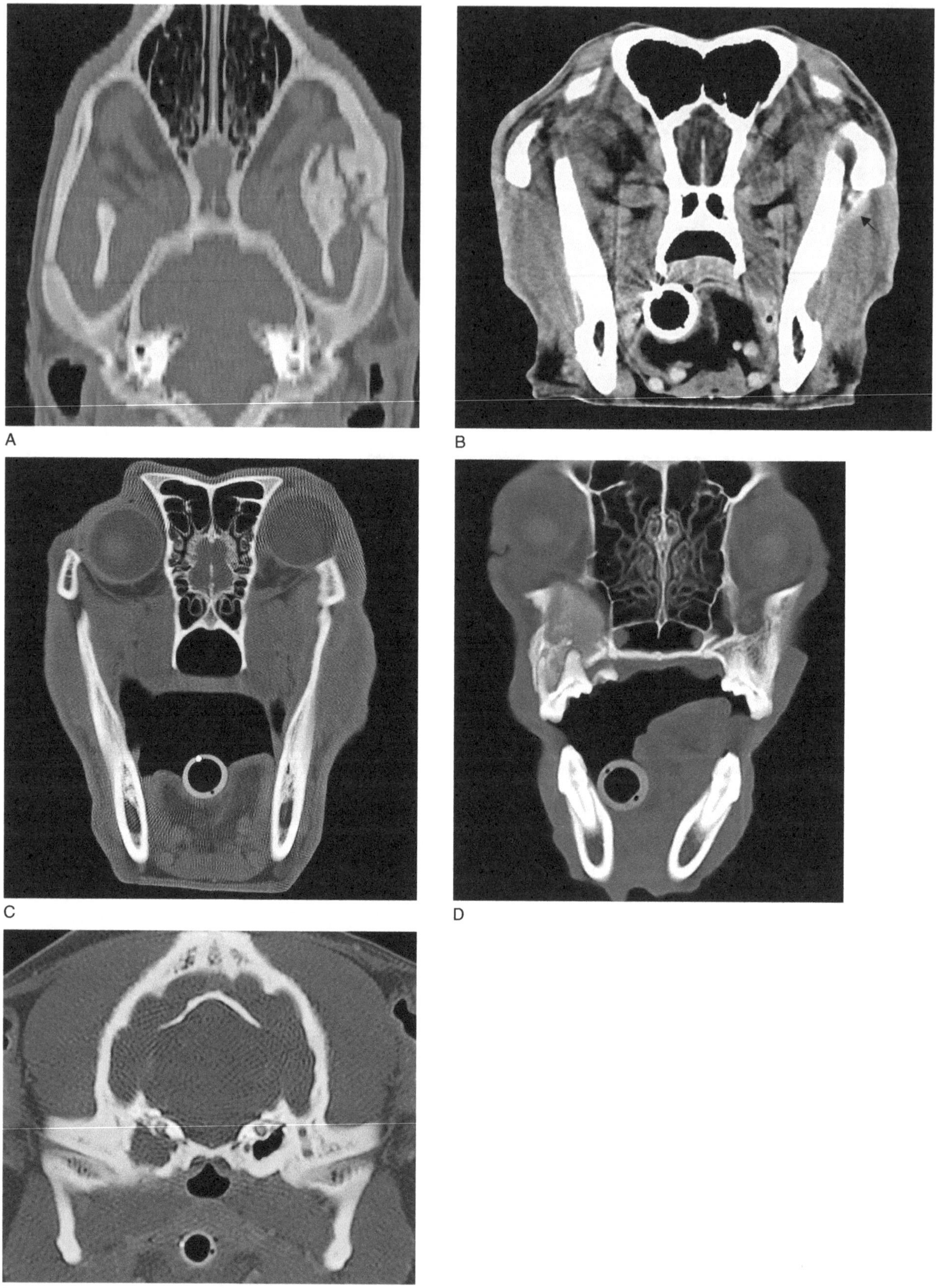

A B C D E

Figure 13.10 Features of false TMJ ankylosis in dogs resulting inability to fully open their mouth. (A) Dorsal plane image of a fused fractured left zygomatic arch and mandibular coronoid process (image courtesy of Massimo Vignoli). (B) An old depression fracture or malformation of the left zygomatic arch leading to a kissing lesion with the coronoid process of the mandible, focal masseter muscle contrast enhancement (arrow) and (C) coronoid process impingement on the zygomatic arch on the open-mouth CT. (D) A cementifying fibroma arising from the M^1 periodontal ligament restricting rostral motion of the coronoid process of the right mandible. (E) An expansile cholesteatoma of the right middle ear restricting the right TMJ.

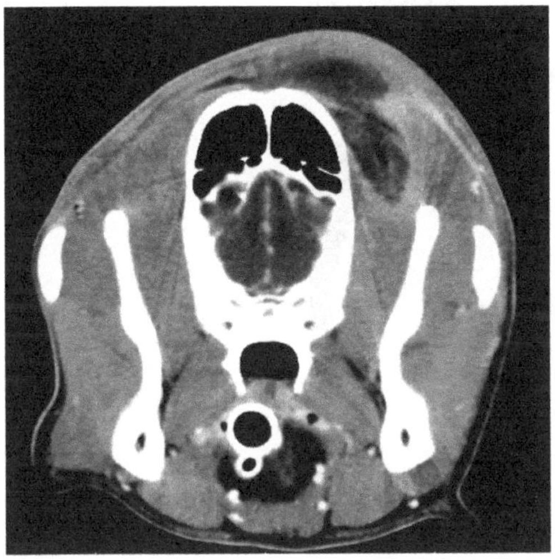

Figure 13.11 Left temporal muscle abscess from a bite wound in a dog with contrast-enhancing rim and non-enhancing content. The ventral propensity of the abscess material also causes impingement of the coronoid process of the left mandible.

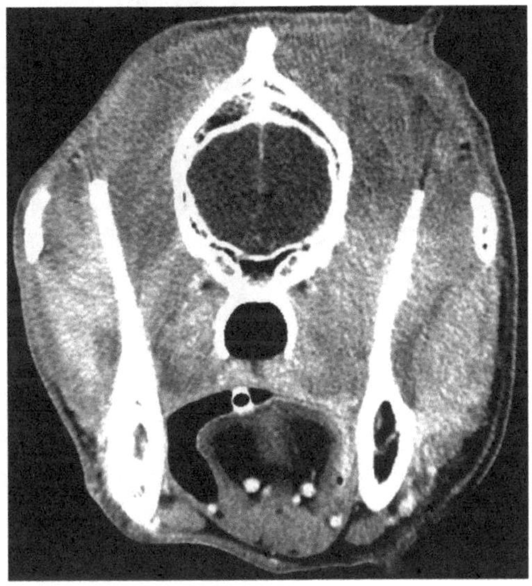

Figure 13.12 Post-contrast image of a dog with chronic active masticatory myositis. There is right temporalis muscle atrophy, left temporalis, masseter and bilateral pterygoid muscle swelling with patchy areas of contrast enhancement.

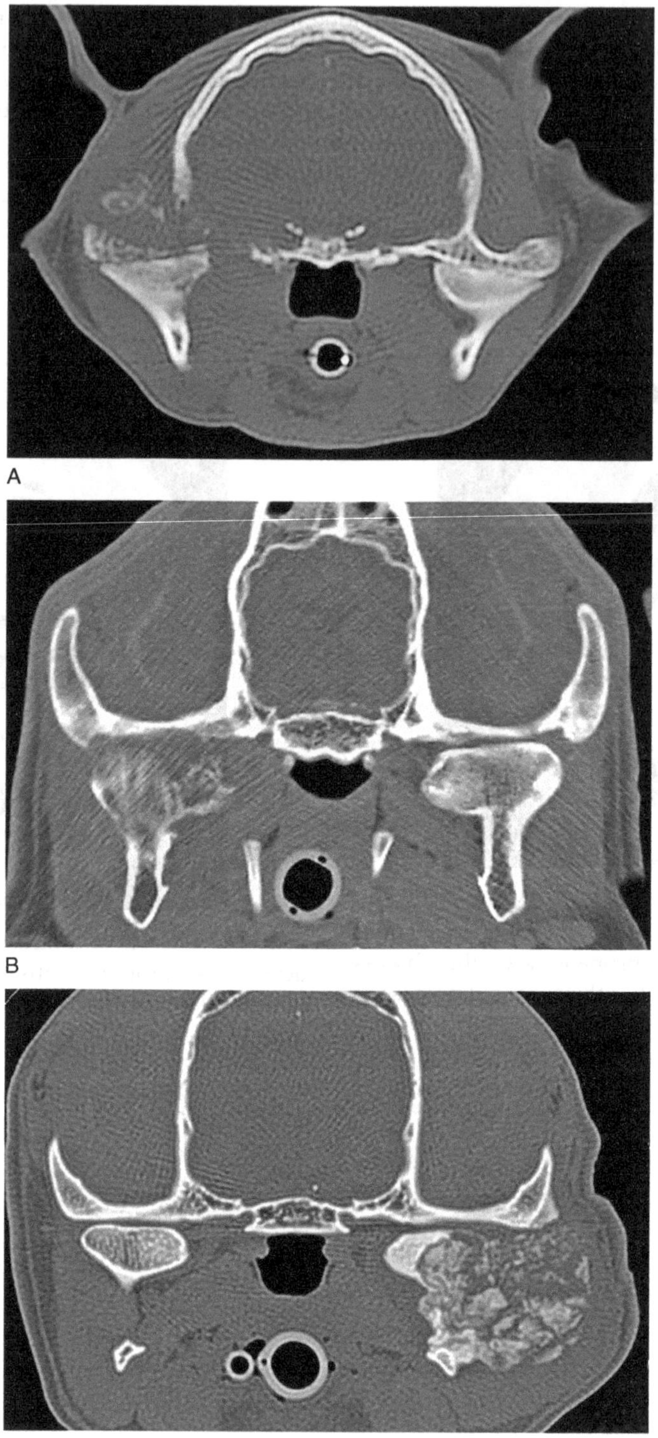

A

B

C

Figure 13.13 Neoplasia affecting the TMJ in a cat and two dogs. (A) An aggressive squamous cell carcinoma in a cat with marked osteolysis of the right calvarium, mandibular fossa and condyle. (B) Aggressive osteosarcoma in a dog causing osteolysis exclusively in the right mandible. (C) A multilobular osteochondrosarcoma arising from and invading the left mandibular condyle causing ankylosis of the TMJ.

CHAPTER FOURTEEN

Orbita, Salivary Glands and Lacrimal System

Susanne Boroffka (orbita), Sophie Dennison, Tobias Schwarz and Jimmy Saunders

Imaging Protocol

See Table 14.1.

The Orbita

CT: anatomy and normal variants

The eye is located in the orbit and consists of two parts that are embedded in orbital fat and other soft tissues: the ocular globe and the ocular adnexa. The optic nerve connects the eye with the brain.

The orbit is mainly osseous and six bones (frontal, lacrimal, maxillary, zygomatic, palatine and sphenoid) form its margin. The variation in the shape and size of the skull in different breeds is considerable. For example, brachycephalic breeds have a much shallower bony orbit than dolicho- or mesaticephalic breeds.

The ocular globe consists of the intraocular structures and conjunctivae. The lens is a hyperdense, poorly delineated oval structure, and the anterior chamber and vitreous are hypodense. The ciliary body and posterior chamber are not visible, whereas the iris may be visible as a very thin line anterior to the lens. The optic disk may be seen as a small, round, hyperdense rim with a hypodense core. Sclera, choroid and retina form a well-defined ring enhancement after contrast medium injection, but cannot be differentiated from one another. The ocular adnexa consist of the seven extraocular muscles, the eyelids and the nasolacrimal apparatus. Six extraocular muscles originate in the vicinity of the optic foramen at the apex of the orbital cone, the seventh arises from a small depression in the palatine bone.

The optic nerve is divided in four regions. The optic nerve originates from the optic chiasma (intracranial part), passes through the optic canal/foramen with the internal ophthalmic artery and vein (intracanalicular part) to enter the orbit (intraorbital part) and join the retina (intraocular part). The optic nerve is surrounded by cerebrospinal fluid within the optic nerve sheath.

The oculomotor, trochlear, abducens and ophthalmic branch of the trigeminal nerves, the anastomotic branch of the external ophthalmic artery and orbital venous plexus pass through the orbital fissure and supplies the ocular adnexa. The low attenuation of the orbital fat facilitates the identification of the optic nerve, extraocular muscles, zygomatic gland and medial pterygoid muscle. The fascial structures of the orbit, the bulbar sheath (vagina bulbi) and the periorbital sheath cannot be identified.

Feline anatomical specificities
The feline orbit is only slightly larger than the globe. The bony floor consists of only a small part of maxillary bone holding the last molar teeth. The extraocular muscles and zygomatic salivary gland are small.

Veterinary Computed Tomography, First Edition. Edited by Tobias Schwarz, Jimmy Saunders.

Table 14.1
CT imaging protocol (intravenous contrast study: standard protocol; *see* Chapter 5).

Series	Pre- and post-contrast	Bone	Dorsal oblique post contrast
Decubitus	Ventral		
Special positioning	Hard palate parallel with table		43–45° from plane parallel to skull base
Scan margins	Rostral to eyelids ⟷ Medial retropharyngeal lymph nodes		Rostral orbita ⟷ Rostral tympanic bullae
Voltage (kVp)	120		
Current (mAs)	100		
Tube rotation time (s)	1–2		
Slice width (mm)	3	1	
Sequential slice interval (mm)	3	1	
Kernel frequency	Medium	High	Medium
Window level (HU)	+80–100	+500	+100
Window width (HU)	150–200	3000	150

Disease features

Malformation/Developmental: Anophthalmos and microphthalmos

True anophthalmos is due to failure of the optic vesicle to form and occurs very rarely. In secondary anophthalmos the optic vesicle starts to develop but stops or degenerates, leaving the fetus/young animal with only residual ocular tissue. In microphthalmos a small globe is present within the orbital soft tissue. In young animals that fail to develop, whose eyes becomes phthisical or who lose an eye due to trauma and/or inflammation, orbital development will be markedly reduced.

CT features

- True anophthalmos: absence of ocular tissue, extraocular muscles and lacrimal glands and ducts.
- Secondary anophthalmos: residual ocular tissue, extremely small eyes.
- Microphthalmos: abnormally small globe, extraocular muscles and lacrimal glands.
- Orbital asymmetry (if unilateral), reduced size of the bony orbital wall and zygomatic arch.

Endophthalmitis and panophthalmitis

Endophthalmitis is an inflammation of the intraocular cavities affecting both anterior and posterior ocular segments. Extension of the inflammation to the three layers of the globe is called panophthalmitis.

Endophthalmitis is mostly septic and induced by bacteria, virus or fungi entering the eye through the ocular blood supply, the cerebrospinal fluid and optic nerve, or by perforation of the cornea, conjunctiva and/or sclera. Endophthalmitis may also be caused by a direct ocular 'trauma'. In this case it may be septic (corneal ulceration/perforation, lens-induced, intraocular surgery, ocular trauma, primary neoplasia) or aseptic (cataract, ruptured lens capsule, retained native lens material, toxic agents). Feline infectious peritonitis may be a cause in the cat.

CT features (Figures 14.1 and 14.2)

- Deformation of the globe.
- Retinal detachment.
- Strong heterogeneous contrast enhancement and thickening of the intraocular structures and scleroretinal rim.
- Loss of definition of the extraocular muscles and fat if orbital cellulitis ensues.
- Foreign material may be identified depending on its attenuation properties.

Orbital cellulitis and abscessation

Cellulitis, inflammation/infection of the orbital fat, is commonly caused by trauma, foreign bodies, extension of sinusitis, bone sequestration and tooth root abscesses, periodontal or endodontic disease. Also hematogeneous, transscleral or transmucosal (conjunctiva, oral, nasal) injury or disease may result in inoculation of the orbital space with infectious organisms. An orbital cellulitis may be diffuse or may

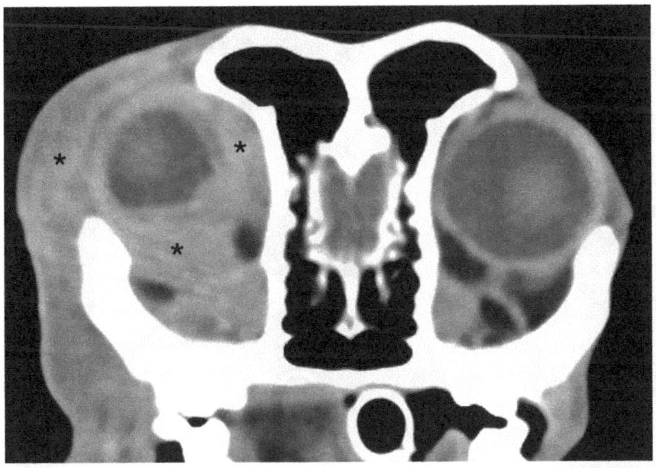

Figure 14.1 Adult dog with pyogranulomatous orbital cellulitis. Post-contrast transverse CT image shows whispy and heterogeneous contrast-enhancing soft tissue surrounding the right globe (asterisks) with associated exophthalmos. Extraocular muscles cannot be identified clearly due to obliteration of the orbital fat (image courtesy of the Department of Surgical and Radiological Sciences, UC Davis).

produce a focal mass lesion that should be differentiated from a neoplasia. Cellulitis may result in an orbital abscess or zygomatic sialoadenitis.

Foreign bodies commonly penetrate the orbital cavity via the facial skin or oral cavity, resulting in inflammation, infection and abscessation with exophthalmus.

CT features (Figures 14.3 and 14.4)

- Rostral displacement of the globe (exophthalmos) and/or of the eyelids.
- Diffuse loss of definition of the extraocular muscles and optic nerve through obscuration of the periorbital and orbital fat.
- Diffuse heterogeneous contrast enhancement of the orbital soft tissues or mass lesion in the orbit that enhances either homogeneously (i.e. pseudotumor) or with ring contrast enhancement (i.e. abscess).
- Foreign bodies may be seen sufficiently dense (metal, bone, glass, stone) or as a filling defect surrounded by contrast-enhanced tissue (wood, plastic).
- Fungal cellulitis, such as aspergillosis, has been associated with bone lysis.
- Hypodense area around the root(s) of affected teeth with possible widening of the pulp cavity. Sclerosis of the surrounding maxillary bone of the affected tooth/teeth.

Extraocular polymyositis

Uni- or bilateral extraocular polymyositis is a rare, immune-mediated inflammatory myopathy affecting mostly young female dogs. Golden retrievers, Doberman and Springer spaniels seem predisposed.

CT features (Figure 14.5)

- Acute polymyositis
  - bilateral rostral displacement of the globes with retraction of the upper eyelids (exophthalmos)
  - bilateral, symmetrical thickening of the optic nerve and/or extraocular muscles
  - loss of definition of the extraocular muscles, optic nerve and periorbital fat
  - strong and heterogeneous contrast enhancement of the extraocular muscles
  - thickening may be followed up to intracranial optic nerve with contrast enhancement of the meninges.
- Chronic polymyositis
  - caudal displacement of the globe (enophthalmos)
  - atrophy of the optic nerve and extraocular muscles.

Masticatory/Eosinophilic myositis (*see also* Chapter 13)

Masticatory/eosinophilic myositis predominantly affects large breed dogs with a predisposition for young German shepherd dogs, Weimaraners, Shetland sheepdogs, labrador and golden retrievers. It affects the temporal, masseter and pterygoid muscles, and is bilateral in most cases. Cellular and humoral-mediated destruction of type IIM myofibers is thought to be the causative factor. It has not been reported in cats.

CT features in acute masticatory/eosinophilic myositis

- Acute masticatory/eosinophilic myositis
  - bilateral displacement of the globes rostrally (exophthalmos)
  - swelling of the temporal, masseter, and pterygoid muscles
  - heterogeneous contrast enhancement of the affected muscles
  - third eyelid protrusion
  - swelling of the eyelids.
- Chronic masticatory/eosinophilic myositis
  - bilateral caudal displacement of the globe (enophthalmos)
  - atrophy of the temporal, masseter and pterygoid muscles.

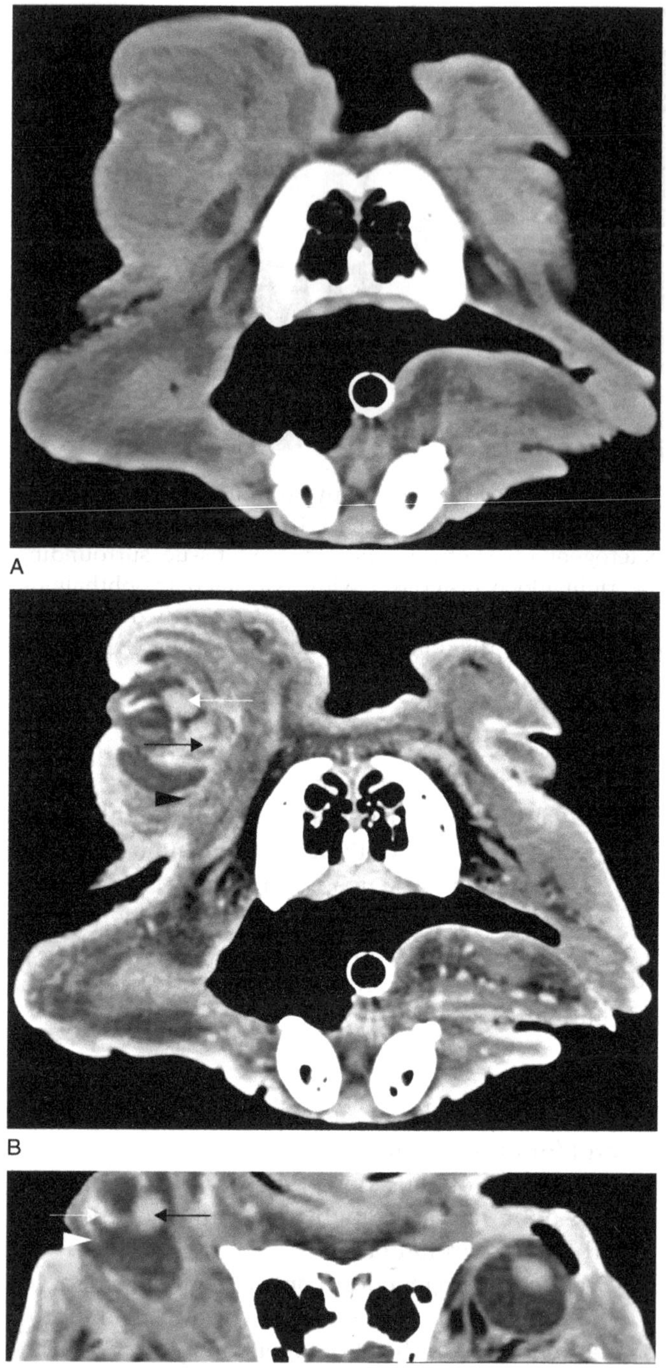

Figure 14.2 Adult dog with severe right-sided panuveitis caused by a cat scratch. (A) Transverse CT image shows a severe soft tissue swelling surrounding the right globe with associated exophthalmos. (B) Post-contrast transverse CT image shows a severely deformed right globe and the lens is luxated (white arrow). There are several contrast-enhanced linear structures within the vitreous representing a detached retina (arrowhead) and vitreous membranes (black arrow). No bony involvement is noted. (C) Post-contrast dorsal-oblique reformatted CT image shows the whispy, ill-defined and heterogeneous contrast-enhancing soft tissues surrounding the severely deformed right globe with associated exophthalmos. The extraocular muscles and optic nerve cannot be identified due to obliteration of the orbital fat and inflammation tissue. The iris (white arrow) is severely thickened and contrast enhancing due to iritis. The lens (black arrow) is displaced posterior and medial. Part of the detached retina is visible at the lateral aspect (arrowhead).

Optic neuritis

Optic neuritis is an inflammation of one or both optic nerves and may be a primary disease or secondary to systemic central nervous system disorder. Causes are idiopathic, systemic mycosis, canine distemper, feline infectious peritonitis, neoplasia, granulomatous-meningo encephalitis or toxoplasmosis.

CT features

- In most cases, the orbital structures, including the optic nerve, appear normal.
- Thickening of the optic nerve with contrast enhancement of the optic nerve sheath may be visible.

Cystic orbital disease

Orbital cysts (*see also* Dacryops below)

Orbital cysts may arise from any epithelial or glandular tissue within the orbit and/or surrounding tissue, such as lacrimal gland, gland of the nictitating membrane, zygomatic salivary gland or mucosa of the paranasal sinus, conjunctiva or nasolacrimal apparatus. Causes are trauma, blocked salivary ducts and/or infection.

CT features (Figure 14.6 – salivary cyst)

- Enlargement of the affected gland or tissue.
- Space-occupying, often peripherally contrast-enhancing (ring enhancement), cystic structure containing non-enhancing fluid.
- Possible loss of definition of the extraocular muscles and fat.

Trauma

Traumatic proptosis of the globe

In proptosis, the globe is displaced rostrally, either through forces displacing the globe itself or through orbital hemorrhage and edema caused by forward stretching of the orbital tissues. Brachycephalic animals are predisposed.

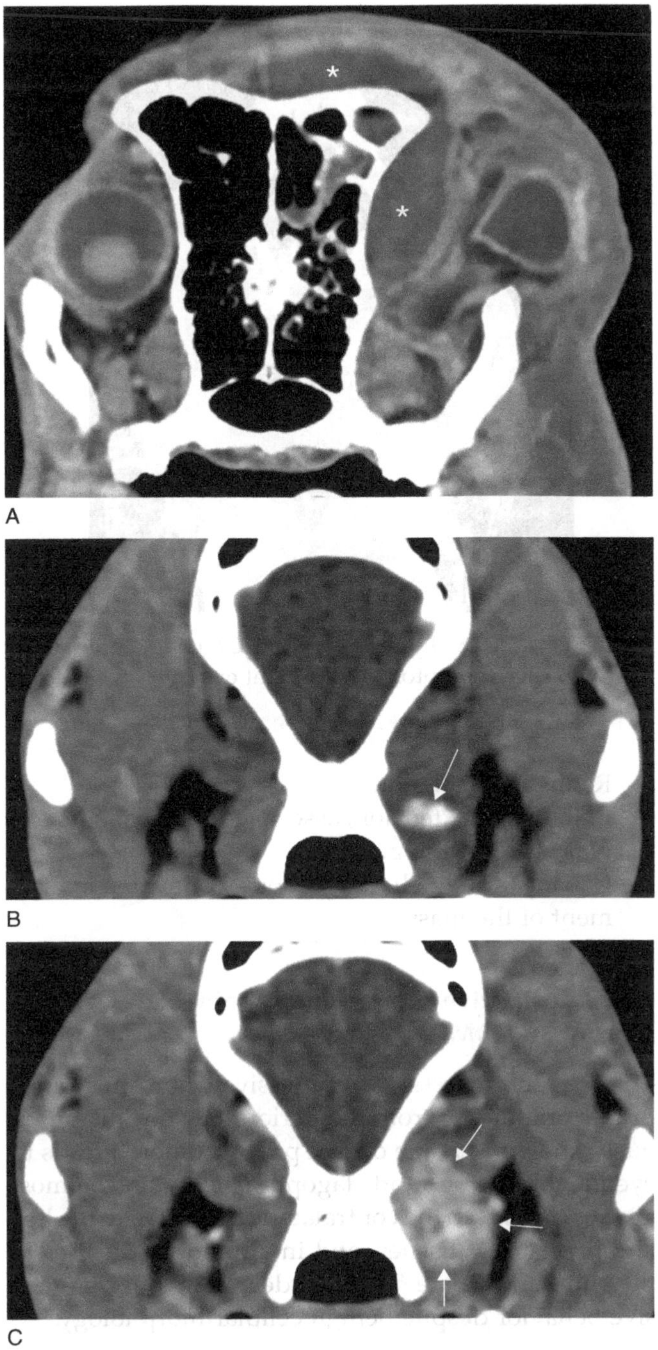

Figure 14.3 Adult dog with orbital foreign body and secondary abscessation. (A) Transverse CT image shows a large left orbital abscess extending to the temporal muscle (asterisks), causing marked exophthalmos. (B) Orally penetrated very dense (glass material) foreign body (arrow) in the left pterygoid muscle causing swelling and (C) enhancement post contrast (arrows) (image courtesy of Björn Åblad).

CT features (Figure 14.7)

- Rostral displacement of the globe beyond the bony orbital rim with entrapment of the eyelids, asymmetry.

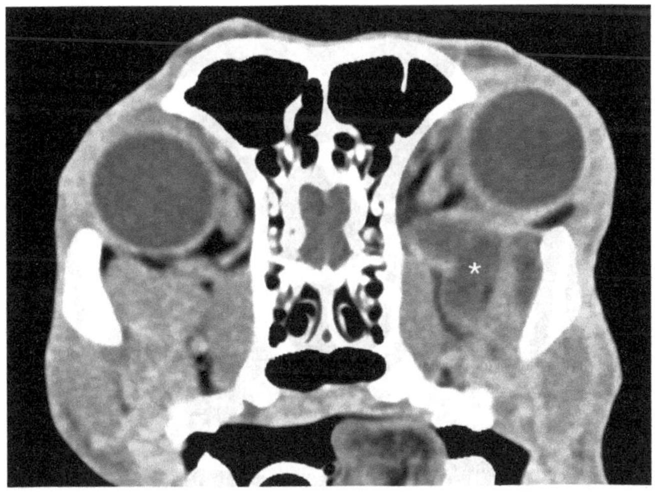

Figure 14.4 Adult dog with a zygomatic sialoadenitis with sialocele and/or abscess formation. Post-contrast transverse CT shows an enlarged, fluid-filled and septated left zygomatic gland (asterisk). Note the ring enhancement of the more dorsal aspect of the gland.

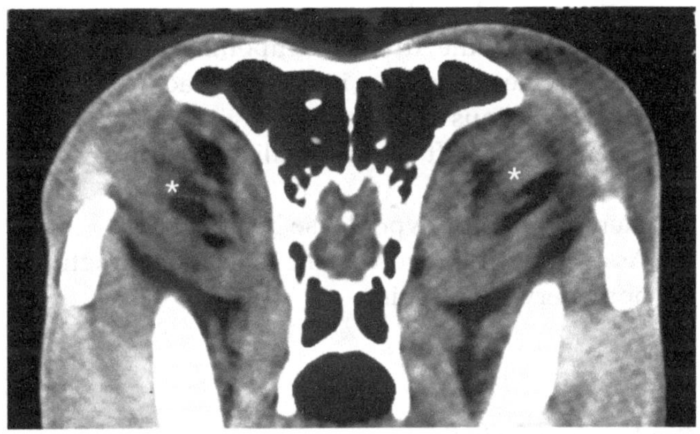

Figure 14.5 Adult dog with extraocular myositis. Transverse CT image shows bilaterally ill-defined symmetrical swelling of ocular muscles (asterisks) with obliteration of the orbital fat.

- Mass effect caudal to the globe with disintegration of the normal orbital anatomy.

Orbital fractures

Fractures of the frontal, temporal and zygomatic bones may occur after head trauma and may cause exophthalmos or enophthalmos, strabismus, orbital and periocular hemorrhage, and facial asymmetry. Fractures involving the paranasal sinus may cause orbital emphysema with crepitus.

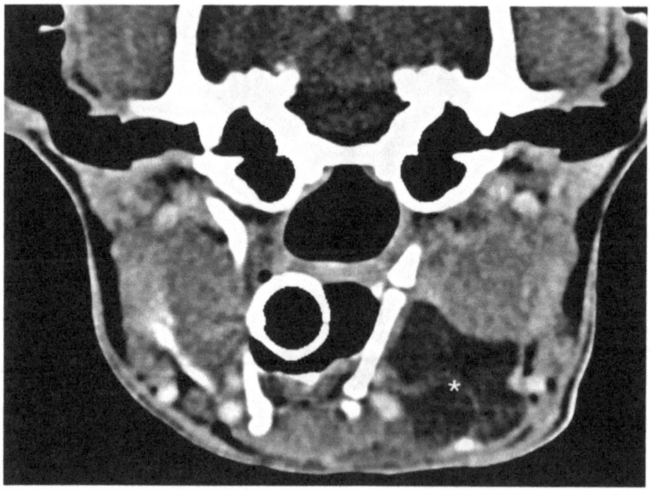

Figure 14.6 Transverse CT image. A salivary cyst (asterisk) arising from the left sublingual gland that extends to the cranioventral neck (ranula).

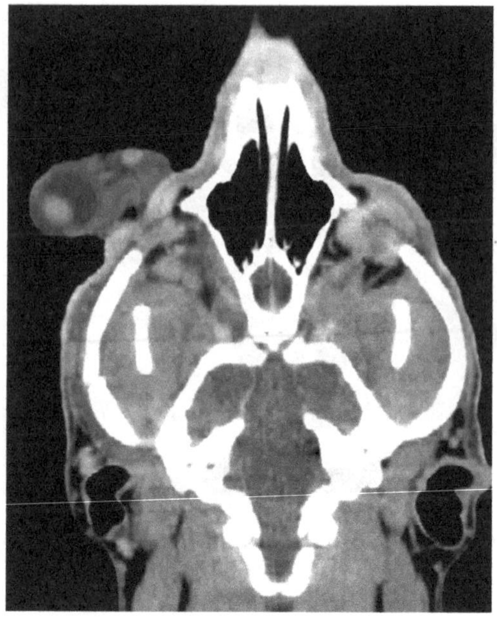

Figure 14.7 Dorsally reconstructed CT image in an adult dog with severe proptosis of the right eye.

CT features (Figure 14.8)

- Rostral or caudal displacement of the globe.
- Mass effect caudal to the globe with disintegration of the normal orbital anatomy.
- Fractures of the frontal, temporal and/or zygomatic bone, including infraction fractures of the paranasal sinus and/or nasal cavity.
- Extension of soft tissue swelling, gas in the soft tissues.
- Identification of hyperdense hemorrhage.
- Assessment of involvement of ocular structures, optic nerve and brain.

Neoplasia

Ocular neoplasia

Intraocular neoplasia may mimic or induce ocular inflammatory disease also causing hyphema and/or secondary glaucoma. Ocular tumors most commonly arise from the iris and ciliary body, and less frequently from the conjunctiva, including the nictitating membrane, the cornea or the choroidea. In dogs, primary and secondary intraocular tumors occur in equal frequency. The most frequent primary intraocular tumor is iridociliary melanoma, which usually occurs unilaterally. Other uveal tumors are adenomas or adenocarcinomas. Lymphosarcoma is the most common metastatic ocular tumor in dogs and cats and may occur uni- or bilaterally. Extraocular extension rarely occurs.

CT features (Figure 14.9)

- Intraocular mass lesion arising from the intraocular structures.
- Buphthalmos if secondary glaucoma occurs.
- Retinal detachment.
- Extraocular extension, associated distorsion or displacement of the globe.
- Usually strong, homogeneous contrast enhancement of the mass.

Feline restrictive orbital myofibroblastic sarcoma (FROMS)

This is a rare, aggressive, progressively fibrosing tumor in cats originating from the periorbital subcutis previously known as feline orbital pseudotumor. It leads to eyelid thickening and lagophthalmus and almost always extends to the contralateral eye, often to the lips and other facial tissues, and in a minority of cases to the gums and palate. The disorder shows quite aggressive behavior despite benign cellular morphology.

CT features (Figures 14.10 and 14.11)

- Loss of retrobulbar fat layers with diffuse soft tissue proliferation.
- Scleral and episcleral thickening of the eyeball.
- Ex- or enophthalmos eyelid thickening.
- Moderate contrast enhancement of the altered structures.
- Lysis of the bony structures adjacent to the orbit.

Orbital neoplasia

In dogs and cats more than 90% of orbital tumors are malignant and regional infiltration, including the

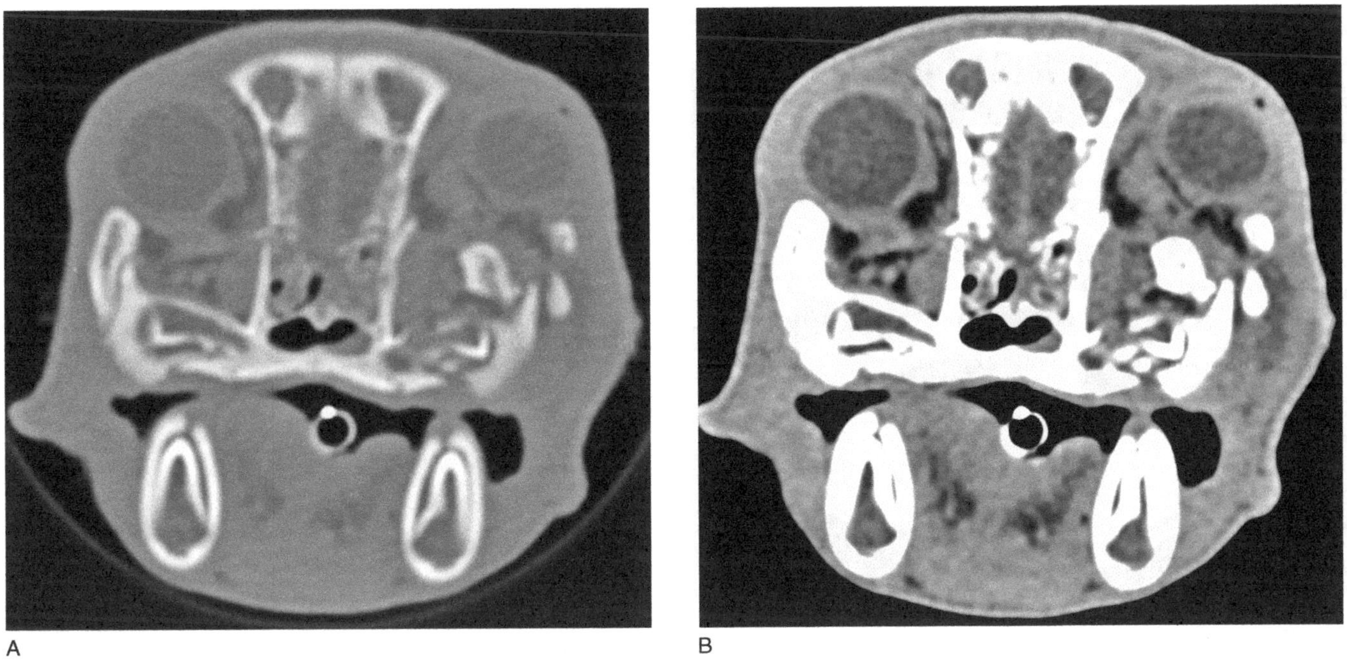

Figure 14.8 Three-month-old dog with multiple fractures involving the orbit. (A) Transverse CT image shows a complex fracture involving the frontal, lacrimal, maxillary, palatine and zygomatic bones. (B) Transverse CT image (same level as A) shows the left globe dorsally displaced by the bone fragments originating from the zygomatic arch and surrounding hematoma.

central nervous system, is seen very often. Various types of orbital tumor have been reported with osteosarcoma, mast cell tumor, reticulum cell sarcoma, fibrosarcoma and neurofibrosarcoma being the most common canine primary tumors. In cats, squamous cell sarcoma occurs most often. Nasal tumors may also invade the orbit via destruction of the thin medial orbital wall.

Optic nerve tumors include neurofibrosarcoma, glioma and meningioma. Optic nerve sheath meningioma may be osteolytic and invade the surrounding tissues.

CT features (Figures 14.12–14.16)

- Space-occupying mass lesion with well-defined borders within the orbit.
- Homogeneous or heterogeneous contrast enhancement of the mass lesion.
- Rostral or caudal displacement of the globe with or without indention.
- Displacement of the extraocular muscles and optic nerve.
- Often definition of the orbital fat and soft tissues is preserved.
- Tumor extension into the surrounding soft tissues and/or paranasal sinuses (lysis of the medial bony orbital wall and/or zygomatic bone).
- Enlargement and heterogeneous contrast enhancement of the mandibular lymph nodes.
- Optic meningiomas: expansile, partially mineralized soft tissue mass posterior to the eye that can be tracked to the optic nerve. There is often significant bone atrophy of the orbital wall and optic canal.

The Salivary Glands

CT: anatomy and normal variants

The salivary glands can be seen on CT, but the normal papillae and ducts are not visualized. Salivary glands are normally strongly contrast enhancing structures, rendering them well visible (Figure 14.17).

- The zygomatic gland is located in the pterygopalatine fossa lateral to the pterygoid muscle origin and has an irregular trapezoid shape.
- The mandibular gland is the biggest salivary gland, located caudally to the mandibular ramus and is oval.
- The parotid gland surrounds the external ear canal ventrally, is dorsally adjacent to the mandibular gland and has the shape of the croissant. It can be difficult to differentiate its margins from the mandibular gland.
- The sublingual gland is small and difficult to identify on CT. It is located at the caudal level of the mandible between the tongue base and the

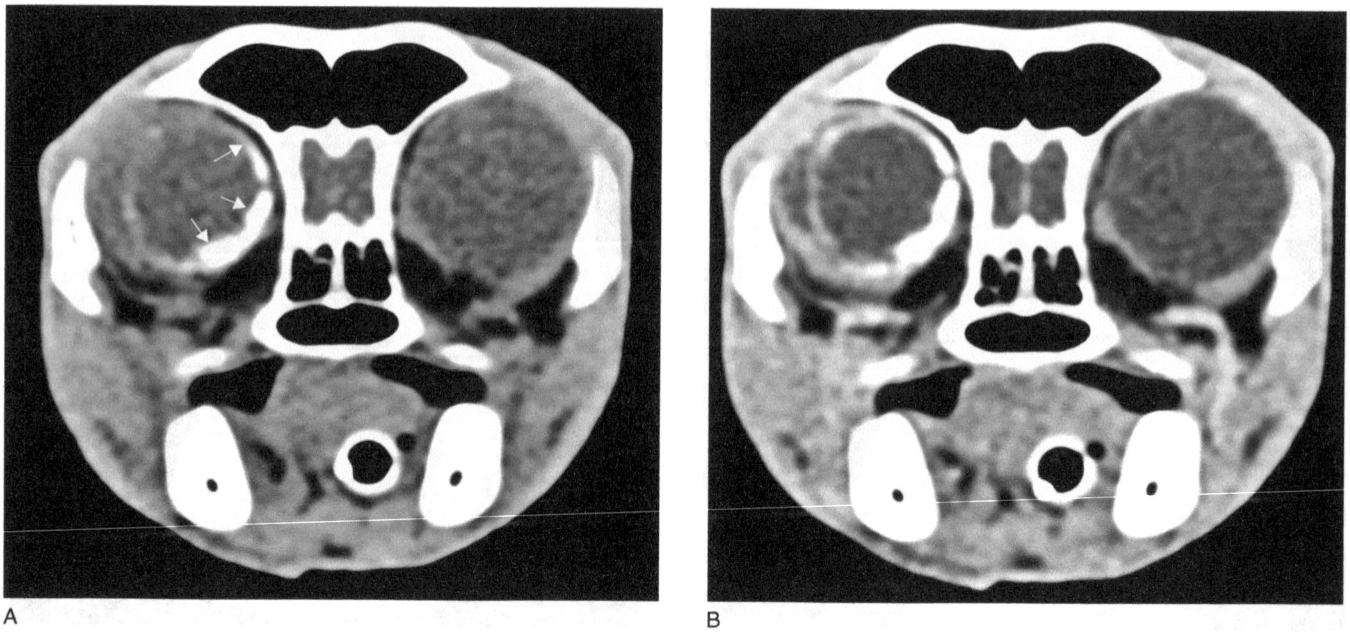

Figure 14.9 Adult cat with intraocular melanoma. (A) Transverse CT image shows a hyperdense intraocular mass lesion (arrows) most pronounced at the ventromedial aspect of the globe. (B) Post-contrast transverse CT image shows marked contrast enhancement of the mass.

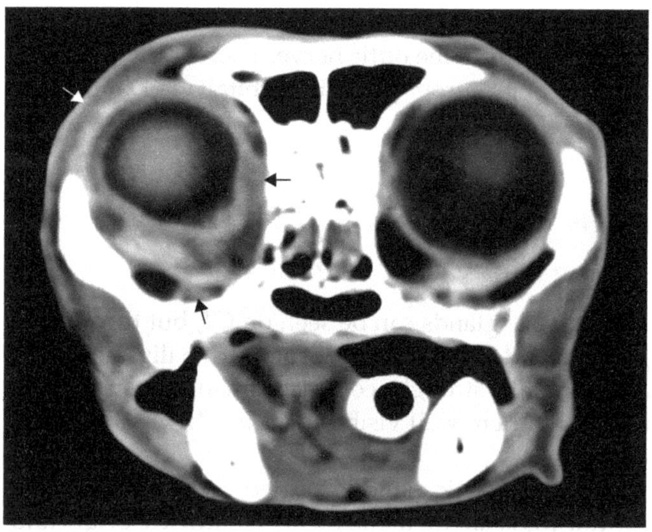

Figure 14.10 Adult cat with feline restrictive orbital myofibroblastic sarcoma. Post-contrast transverse CT image shows strong contrast-enhancing orbital soft tissue proliferation restricting the right globe (arrows).

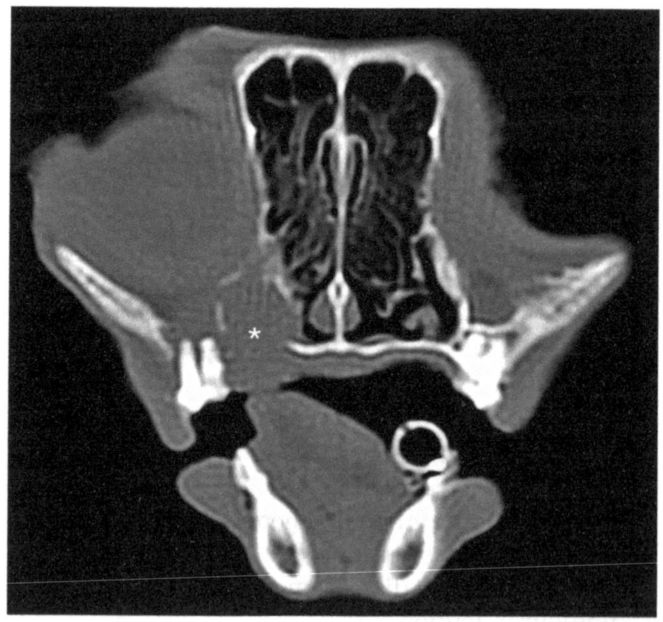

Figure 14.11 Adult cat with feline restrictive orbital myofibroblastic sarcoma. Transverse CT image shows extensive nasal and palatal osteolysis (asterisk). Note the left eye has been removed surgically.

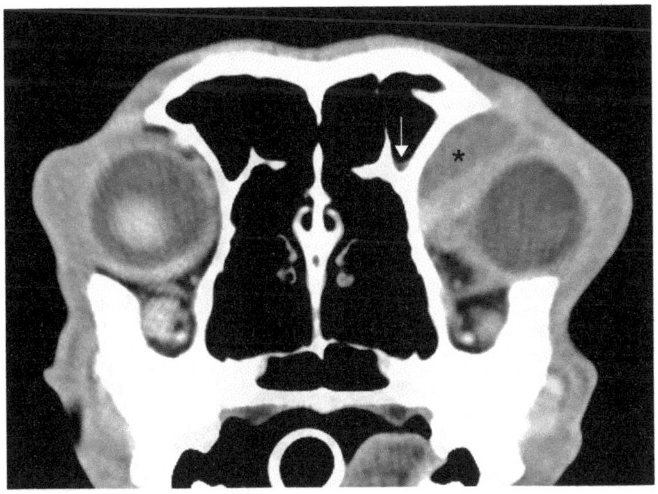

Figure 14.12 Adult dog with orbital anaplastic sarcoma. Post-contrast transverse CT image shows an ill-defined and mildly heterogeneously contrast-enhancing focal soft tissue mass (asterisk) dorsomedial and caudal to the eye, causing mild left-sided exophthalmos. The mass is adjacent to the frontal bone cortex and there is a small accumulation of fluid within the dependent frontal sinus (arrow).

mylohyoideus muscle, which attaches at medial aspect of both mandibles to suspend the ventral floor of the oral cavity. The sublingual gland has mono- and polystomatic compartments that cannot be differentiated without sialography.

Disease features

Inflammation/Infection

Salivary gland enlargement in limbic epilepsy (hypersialosis)

This is an idiopathic, poorly understood condition characterized by hypersalivation, enlarged painful mandibular salivary glands, retching, vomiting and behavioral abnormalities that respond to phenobarbitol treatment.

CT features

- Symmetrically enlarged mandibular salivary glands.
- Absence of other salivary gland abnormalities.

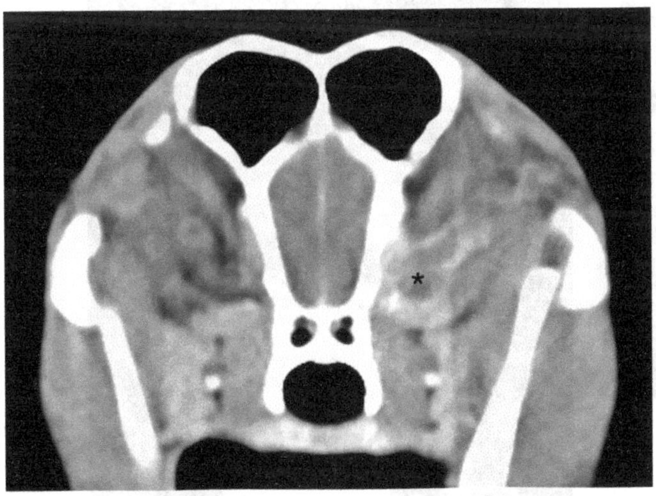

A

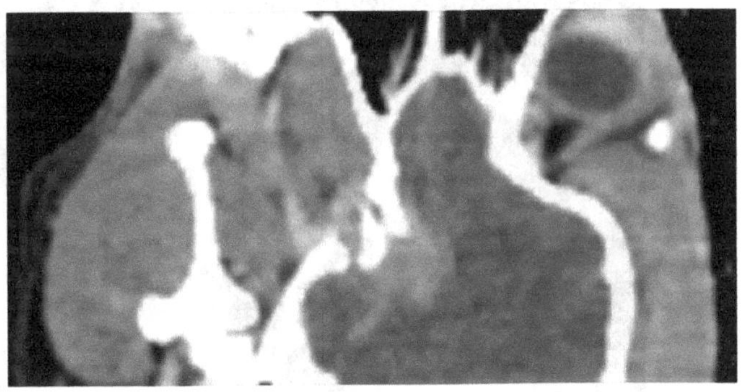

B

Figure 14.13 Adult dog with intracranial meningioma extending via the optic canal, orbital fissureand rostral alar foramen into the orbit. (A) Post-contrast CT image shows a wispy, ill-defined and heterogeneous contrast-enhancing mass lesion just caudal to the globe (asterisk). (B) Dorsal-oblique reformatted CT image shows the extension towards and through the rostral alar foramen, orbital fissure and optic canal towards the left base of the brain at the level of the pre-sphenoid and basisphenoid bones (image courtesy of the Department of Surgical and Radiological Sciences, UC Davis, USA).

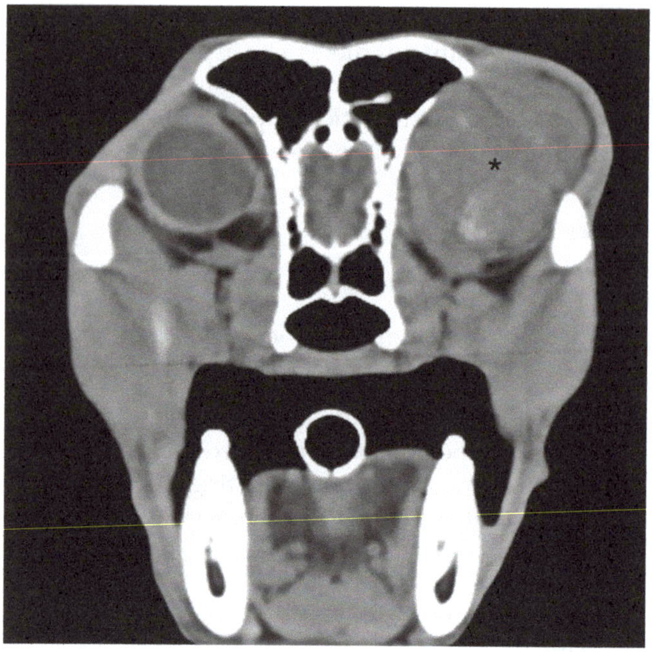

Figure 14.14 Adult dog with optic meningioma. Transverse CT image shows a large partially mineralized optic meningioma (asterisk), causing exophthalmos and adjacent bone atrophy.

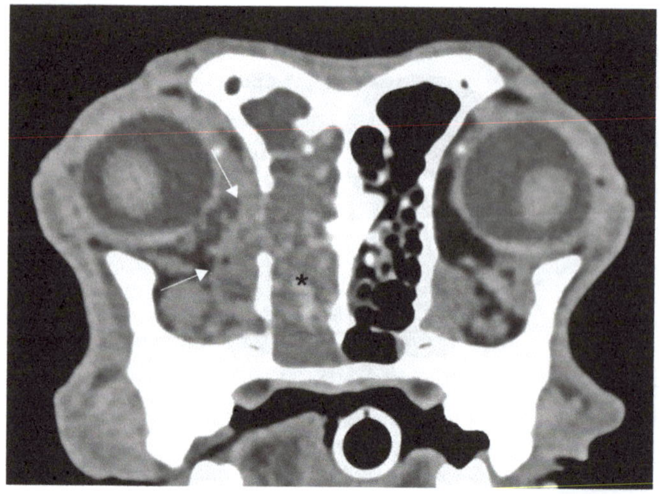

Figure 14.16 Adult dog with nasal and orbital adenocarcinoma. CT image shows a large heterogeneous contrast-enhancing, ill-defined soft tissue mass occupying the majority of the right nasal cavity (asterisk). There is destruction of the frontal bone of the orbit (arrows). The mass lesion extends to the ventromedial aspect of the orbital space causing mild right-sided exophthalmos (image courtesy of the Department of Surgical and Radiological Sciences, UC Davis, USA).

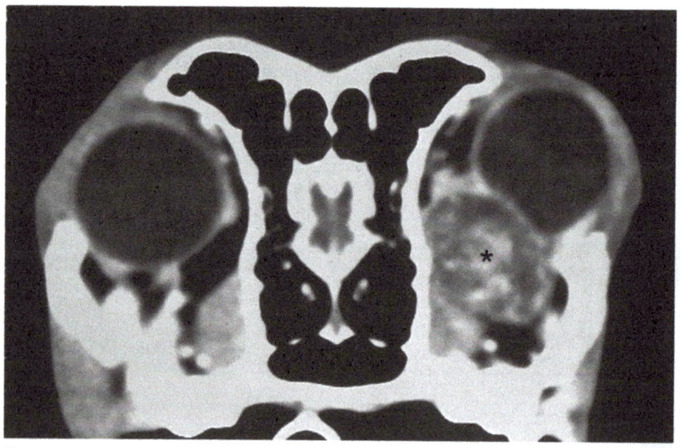

A

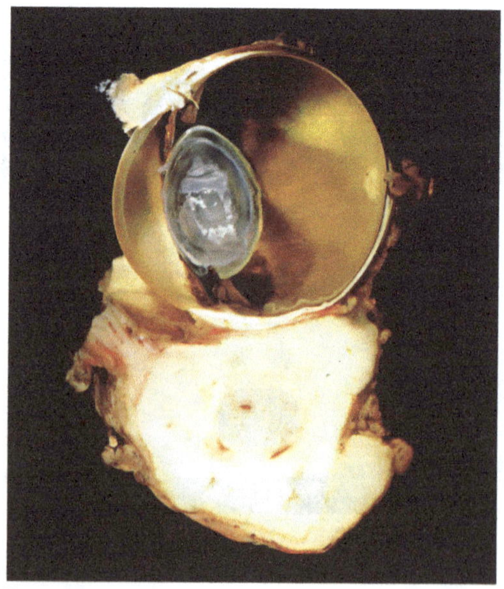

B

Figure 14.15 (A) Post-contrast transverse CT image of an irregularly contrast-enhancing nictitating gland carcinoma (asterisk) causing indention of the globe and exophthalmos. (B) Corresponding photograph of the enucleated eye.

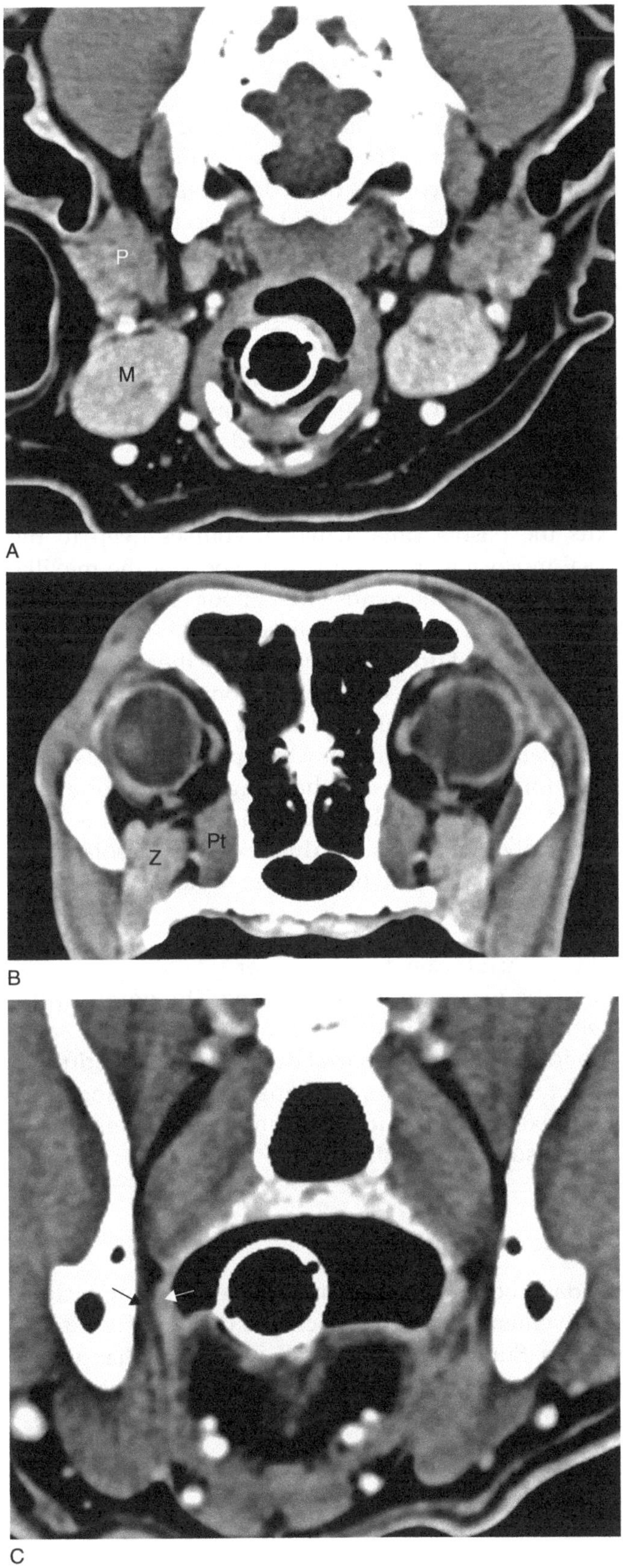

Figure 14.17 Contrast-enhanced transverse CT images of the normal canine salivary glands. (A) The parotid gland (P) surrounds the ventral ear base. Ventral to it is the large mandibular gland (M). (B) The zygomatic gland (Z) is located laterally to the pterygoid muscle orgin (Pt) in the rostroventral aspect of the orbital cavity. (C) The sublingual gland (white arrow) is located between the tongue base and the myelohoid muscle attachment (black arrow) at the medial mandible.

Sialolithiasis

Concretions in the salivary glands and/or ducts can occasionally be seen on CT images. They can be incidental or be related with an obstructive sialocele formation.

CT features (Figure 14.18)

- Sialoliths are usually only slightly hyperdense and can be difficult to identify on CT.
- If parenchymal, usually in center of gland.

Sialadenitis and abscessation

Inflammation of the salivary glands is occasionally seen in dogs secondary to tooth root infection (zygomatic gland), penetrating injuries or extension of infectious processes in the proximity of the gland. In sialadenitis there is often inflammation of the neighboring masticatory muscles.

CT features (Figure 14.19)

- Diffuse loss of silhouette of the salivary gland.
- Diffuse or patchy increase in attenuation in neighboring muscles and fat.
- Abscesses may or may not have demarcated contrast-enhancing rim.

Sialocele/Sialoadenitis

A sialocele is a swelling of connective tissue consisting of collected mucin due to a ruptured salivary gland duct usually caused by local trauma in the case of mucus extravasation phenomenon, and an obstructed salivary duct usually due to sialolithiasis in the case of a mucus retention cyst. Most commonly the sublingual glands are affected by this condition and the cyst extends to the ventral neck, giving the animal a frog-like neck shape (hence the name *ranula*).

A zygomatic sialoadenitis is an inflammation of the zygomatic salivary gland. Depending on the severity of the disease there may be ocular involvement.

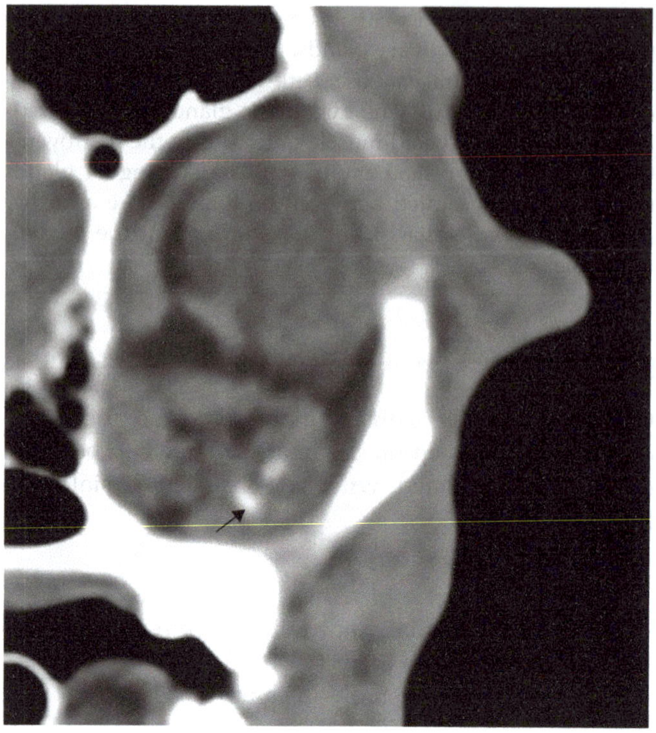

Figure 14.18 Transverse CT image. Close-up of a left canine zygomatic gland containing two mineral concretions (arrow). This was an incidental finding.

Immune-mediated, secondary to trauma, systemic or localized infection are discussed etiologies.

CT features (Figures 14.4 and 14.6)

- Enlargement (cystic fluid-distended sac) of the salivary gland.
- Obstructive sialoliths may be visible on pre contrast CT.
- Possible loss of definition of the extraocular muscles and fat.
- Strong contrast enhancement of the affected gland or tissue with possible ring enhancement (abscess formation and/or mucocele).

Neoplasia

Primary salivary gland neoplasia is very rare in dogs and cats and usually manifests as a non-painful swelling. Soft tissue tumors such as fibrosarcoma can infiltrate the salivary glands.

CT features (Figure 14.20)

- Irregularly contrast-enhancing masses originating from a salivary gland.
- Absence of normal gland in question.
- Can be difficult to differentiate from other soft tissue neoplasia.

Lacrimal System

CT: anatomy and normal variants

The lacrimal system is composed of secretory and excretory portions. The secretory portion produces lacrimal fluid and consists of the lacrimal gland, superficial gland of the third eyelid and accessory lacrimal glands. The excretory portion, or nasolacrimal drainage system, consists of the upper and lower lacrimal puncta, dorsal and ventral lacrimal canaliculi, and the nasolacrimal duct. Dogs do not have a distinct lacrimal sac. The dorsal and ventral canaliculi conjoin in dogs. The proximal 50% of the nasolacrimal duct is encased within an osseous canal contained within the lacrimal and maxillary bones, extending from the lacrimal foramen to the level of the conchal crest. Once the duct exits the nasolacrimal canal, it courses deep to the nasal mucosa along the medial aspect of the maxilla, terminating on the ventrolateral floor of the nasal vestibule at the inferior lacrimal punctum.

In meso- and dolichocephalic dogs, the nasolacrimal duct courses more or less horizontally through the nasolacrimal canal and nasal mucosa, parallel to the hard palate. However, brachycephalic animals with facial foreshortening may have right-angled or acute-angled deviation of the duct. This angulation is most commonly evident as the duct exits the nasolacrimal canal, and may cause obstruction to flow.

Feline anatomical specificities
Cats have a distinct lacrimal sac. The dorsal and ventral canaliculi converge at the lacrimal sac to form the nasolacrimal duct. The nasolacrimal duct courses in cats as in mesocephalic dogs in all except the most severely brachicephalic cats, such as Persians.

Disease features

CT dacryocystography is needed to prove or exclude involvement of the nasolacrimal duct in the disease process. Survey and intravenous contrast-enhanced CT are necessary to evaluate periductal tissue involvement.

Malformation/Developmental

Brachycephalic nasolacrimal duct obstruction

Obstruction to nasolacrimal duct flow occurs in brachycephalic breeds of dog and cat due to facial foreshortening. This causes angulation of the nasolacrimal duct, typically as it exits the nasolacrimal canal, and is commonly a bilateral condition.

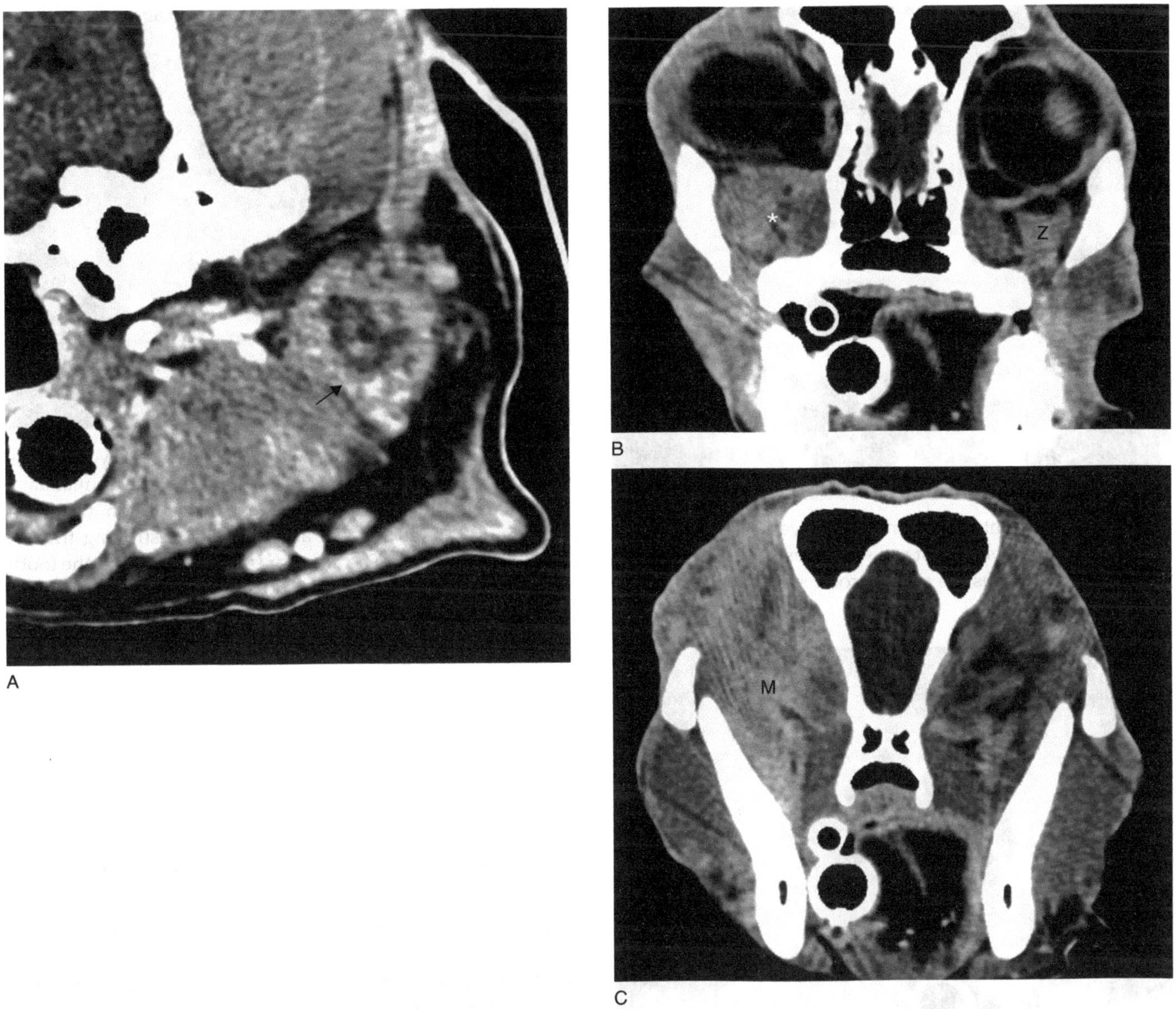

Figure 14.19 Transverse CT images. (A) A left parotid gland abscess with marked rim enhancement (arrow) and a non-enhancing purulent center. (B) A right zygomatic gland inflammation (asterisk) leading to swelling and loss of clear margin of the gland (compare to normal left zygomatic gland, Z) as well as (C) diffuse infiltration of masticatory muscles (M).

CT features

- Dacryocystography:
  - abnormal nasolacrimal duct course
  - obstruction to flow of contrast medium at site of abnormal angulation.

Congenital imperforate nasolacrimal duct

Congenital malformation resulting in non-patency of the nasolacrimal duct.

CT features

- Dacryocystography: obstruction to flow of contrast.

Infection/Inflammation

Chronic dacryocystitis

Inflammation or infection results in alterations in duct diameter, most commonly dilatation. Dacryocystitis occurs in association with nasolacrimal duct obstruction, including foreign body obstruction (plant awns or seeds are most frequently reported). Stagnation of tears permits overgrowth by microorganisms. Dacryocystitis has also been described in cats suffering from feline herpes virus.

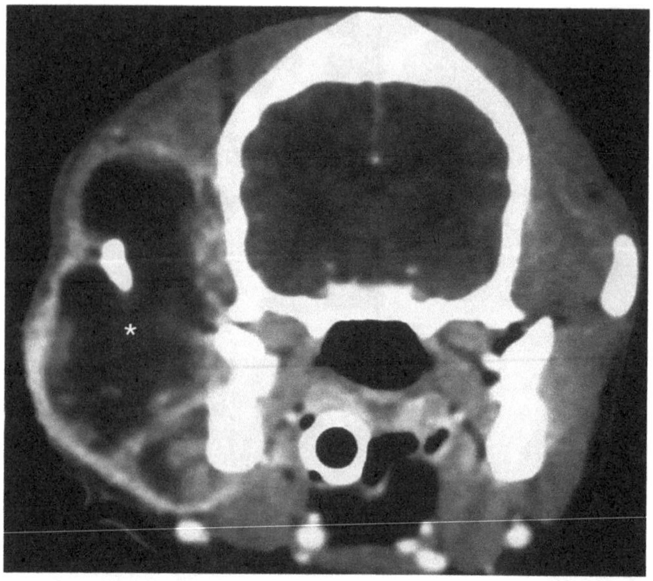

Figure 14.20 Contrast-enhanced transverse CT image of a dog with a large cystic right masseter muscle sarcoma (asterisk) that also invades the right parotid salivary gland.

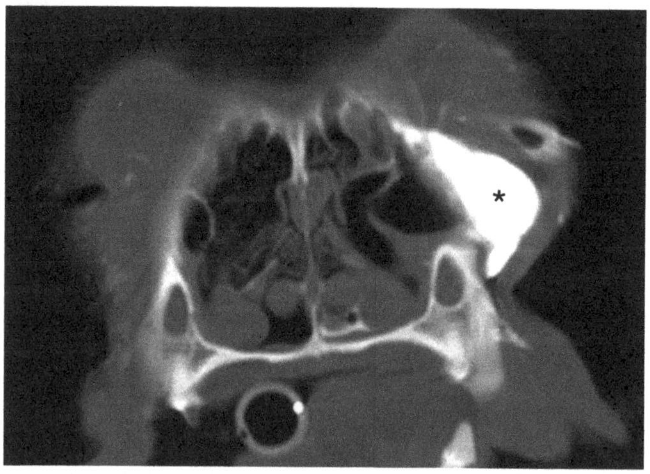

Figure 14.21 Contrast-enhanced transverse CT image of an adult dog with dacryocystitis. There is lysis of the left maxillary bone and the nasolacrimal duct is severely distended with contrast medium (asterisk).

CT features (Figure 14.21)

- Foreign material may be identified within the nasolacrimal duct depending on its attenuation properties.
- Periductal osteolysis.
- Dacryocystography:
  - dilatation of the nasolacrimal duct evident
  - obstruction to flow of contrast medium secondary to accumulation of cellular debris
  - foreign material may be identified as a filling defect within the nasolacrimal duct.

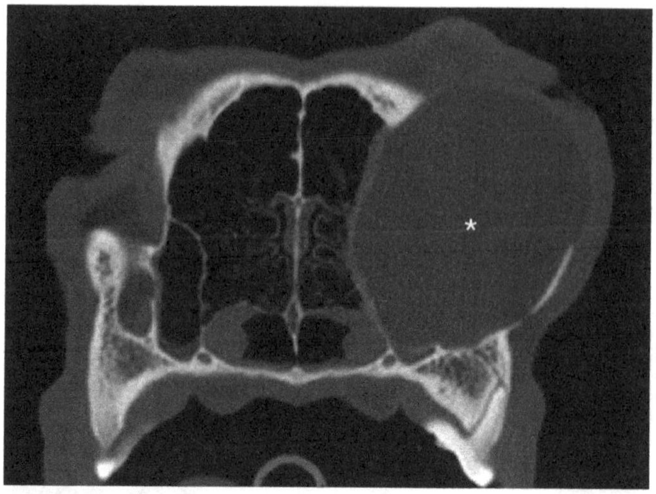

Figure 14.22 Adult dog with left-sided dacryops. This transverse CT image at the level of the third maxillary premolar tooth shows a large expansile lesion (asterisk) destroying the left maxilla and partially destroying the left ethmoid turbinates. The alveolar bone surrounding the tooth is within normal limits and no maxillary bone periosteal reaction is evident. The lesion is filled with fluid dense material that did not contrast enhance.

Dacryops

Cyst formation due to congenital ectopic lacrimal or salivary gland tissue or as a sequel to acquired traumatic disruption or inflammation. The expansile lesion progresses over time causing local destruction and malformation. Cysts may form anywhere along the nasolacrimal duct, and location has been suggested to be indicative of the ectopic tissue source. The position of the cyst will dictate which adjacent structures are affected.

CT features (Figure 14.22)

- Dacryocystography:
  - space-occupying, often peripherally contrast-enhancing, cystic structure containing non-contrast-enhancing fluid
  - dilatation of the duct proximal to the cyst and obstruction to flow if non-communicating with the duct
  - contrast may occasionally fill the lesion if there is communication with the duct.
- Non-aggressive destruction of surrounding osseous structures depending on location (turbinates, nasal/lacrimal/maxillary bone).

Damage secondary to non-lacrimal system disease processes

Damage to the nasolacrimal duct may occur secondarily to facial trauma, nasal tumor invasion or dental disease, most commonly involving the second and third maxillary pre-molars. Damage may result in impingement and subsequent obstruction to flow, erosion of the duct itself or laceration due to adjacent fracture or soft tissue damage.

CT features

- Primary pathology identified in the region of the nasolacrimal duct.
- Dacryocystography: nasolacrimal duct involvement demonstrated following dacryocystitis
  - obstruction to flow
  - leakage out of contrast medium from nasolacrimal duct into surrounding tissues.

Further Reading

Attali-Soussay K, Jegou JP and Clerc B (2001) Retrobulbar tumors in dogs and cats: 25 cases. *Vet Ophthalmol* **4**: 19–27.

Bell CM, Schwarz T and Dubielzig RR (2011) Diagnostic features of feline restrictive orbital myofibroblastic sarcoma. *Vet Pathol* **48**: 742–50.

Boroffka SAEB and Voorhout G (1999) Direct and reconstructed multiplanar computed tomography of the orbits of healthy dogs. *Am J Vet Res* **60**: 1500–7.

Boroffka SAEB, Verbruggen A-M, Grinwis GCM, Voorhout G and Barthez PY (2007) Assessment of ultrasonography and computed tomography for the evaluation of unilateral orbital disease in dogs. *J Am Vet Med Assoc* **230**: 671–80.

Duvoisin B, Zanella FE and Sievers KW (1998) Imaging of the normal and pathological orbit. *Eur Radiol* **8**: 175–88.

Penninck D, Daniel GB, Brawer R and Tidwell AS (2001) Cross-sectional imaging techniques in veterinary ophthalmology. *Clin Tech Small Anim Pract* **16**: 22–39.

Ramsey DT, Marrtta SM, Hamor RE *et al.* (1996) Ophthalmic manifestations of dental disease in dogs and cats. *J Am Anim Hosp Assoc* **32**: 215–24.

CHAPTER FIFTEEN

External, Middle and Inner Ear

Randi Drees

Imaging Protocol

See Table 15.1.

CT: Anatomy and Normal Variants (Figure 15.1)

External ear

The external ear varies greatly in shape and size between dog breeds. The pinna is shaped by the auricular cartilage, which is penetrated by a multitude of blood vessels. It forms several folds at its base and then gains tubular shape to form the external ear canal with the medially adjacent annular cartilage. The annular cartilage attaches to the osseous external auditory meatus formed by the petrous temporal bone. The annular and auricular cartilages are not always seen as separate entities on CT images. The lateral segment of the external ear canal is vertically oriented and purely cartilaginous supported; the medial segment is 45° oriented and has cartilaginous and osseous support. The auricular muscles attach at the base of the ear. The small, separate scutiform cartilage serves as attachment for several medial auricular muscles and is located superficially to the auricular fat pad. Spaniel breeds tend to have narrow external ear canals; evaluation of ear canal stenosis has been performed with canalograms in standard radiography. In chondrodystrophic breeds, mineralization of the auricular and annular cartilage can be seen as a normal variant on CT images.

Middle ear

The tympanic membrane spans the entrance to the tympanic cavity. It separates the external from the middle ear and is not always seen on CT images. The middle ear is contained within the petrous temporal bone and is comprised of the air-filled tympanic bulla containing the three auditory ossicles (malleolus, incus and stapes). The malleolus is the largest of the three bones and its lateral aspect is embedded in the dorsal aspect of the tympanic membrane. The incus articulates laterally with the malleolus and medially with the stapes, the innermost ossicle. The stapes joins the fibrocartilaginous ring covering the vestibular (oval) window, connecting to the inner ear. Due to their small size, the ossicles can only be seen as separate structures on thinly collimated or high-resolution CT images. Dorsomedially, the auditory (Eustachian) tube connects the middle ear to the nasopharynx. This canal can be seen on CT images if filled with contrast material.

The tympanic bulla is round to ovoid in shape; breed variations of more flattened bullae as seen in the Cavalier King Charles spaniel occur. The facial nerve (cranial nerve VII), sympathetic innervation of the eye and the parasympathetic innervation of the lacrimal gland are closely associated with the middle ear.

Inner ear

The inner ear is enclosed within the petrous temporal bone dorsomedially to the middle ear. The endolymph is contained within the membranous labyrinth, consisting of the semicircular ducts, utricle, sacculus, endolymphatic and cochlear duct. The membranous labyrinth is embedded in the bony labyrinth, consisting of the perilymphatic chamber (vestibulum), three semicircular canals and their respective ampulla, the spiral cochlea and the vestibular aqueduct. Due to the small size, there is limited visibility of the structures of the inner ear and their location in the petrous temporal

Veterinary Computed Tomography, First Edition. Edited by Tobias Schwarz, Jimmy Saunders.

Table 15.1
CT imaging protocol (intravenous contrast study: standard protocol; *see* Chapter 5).

Series	Pre- and post-contrast	Bone	Canalogram
Decubitus	Ventral		Lateral, side to evaluate up
Special positioning	Place forelegs caudal to scan field		
Scan margins	Rostral margin of temporomandibular joint ←→ Mid C1		
Voltage (kVp)	120		
Current (mAs)	100	130	100
Tube rotation time (s)	≤ 1		
Slice width (mm)	1–2	1	
Sequential slice interval (mm)	1–2	1	
Kernel frequency	Medium	High	Medium
Contrast medium application site	N/A		External ear canal
Contrast medium type	N/A		Iodinated, non-ionic
Contrast medium dose	N/A		2–5 ml (400 mg I/ml)
Contrast medium injection mode	N/A		Manual
Scan delay post start contrast injection	N/A		1 min
Window level (HU)	+250	+500	+100
Window width (HU)	50	3000	150

bone on CT images. Thinly collimated slices or high-resolution CT can enable visualization of the cochlea and vestibular aqueduct, other structures usually remain poorly visualized.

Feline anatomical specificities
The lateral segment of the external ear canal is vertically oriented and purely cartilaginously supported; the medial segment is horizontally oriented and has cartilaginous and osseous support. In the cat this segment has an approximately 90° angle. The feline tympanic bulla has one or more septa, incompletely dividing the tympanic cavity into a dorsolateral and ventromedial portion.

CT Disease Features

Malformation/Developmental

External ear canal atresia

External ear canal atresia is a rare congenital condition in which the external ear canal is absent or separated into a lateral and medial compartment. Trauma can lead to acquired occlusion of the external ear canal. Ceruminous secretions accumulating medial to the occlusion site can form a large fluid-filled pocket. Bullous effusion can occur sequentially.

CT features (Figure 15.2)

- Blind-ending, air-filled external auditory canal separated by a soft tissue membrane from the commonly fluid-filled medial portion of the external ear canal or complete obliteration of the external ear canal.
- Possibly fluid-dense material in the tympanic cavity.
- Possible thickening of the tympanic bulla.

Trauma

Soft tissue injury to the external ear commonly occurs with bite wounds; aural hematoma is a common complication. Fractures of the cranium or mandible can involve the tympanic bulla or petrous temporal bone. Fissure lines or fracture fragments can be identified on CT and aid treatment recommendation and planning.

CT features

- Severed soft tissue-dense structures in the aural region.
- Sharply marginated fracture lines or fragments.

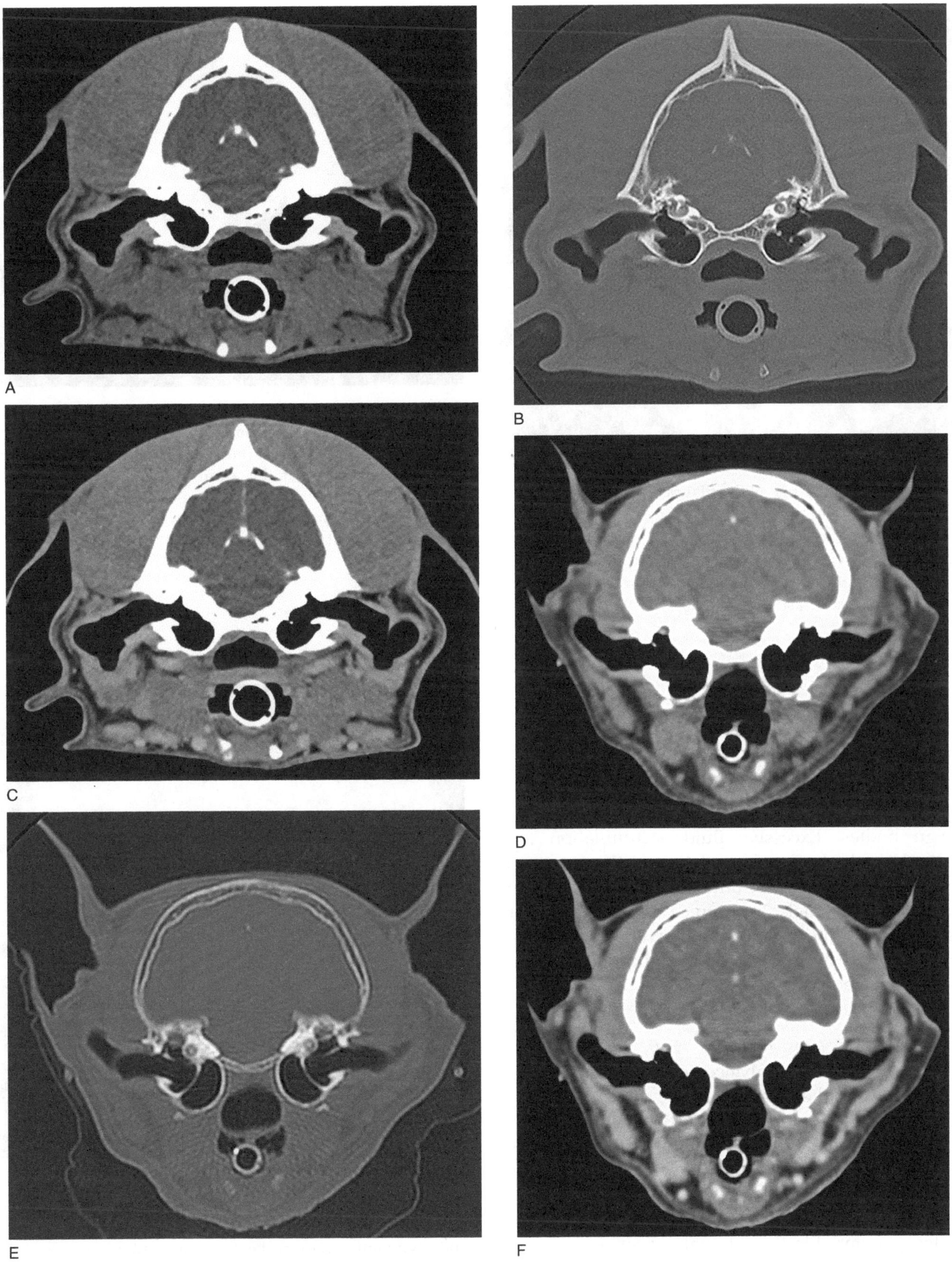

Figure 15.1 Transverse CT images of a normal dog: (A) soft tissue window, (B) bone window, (C) post-contrast soft tissue window; and of a normal cat: (D) soft tissue window, (E) bone window, (F) post-contrast soft tissue window.

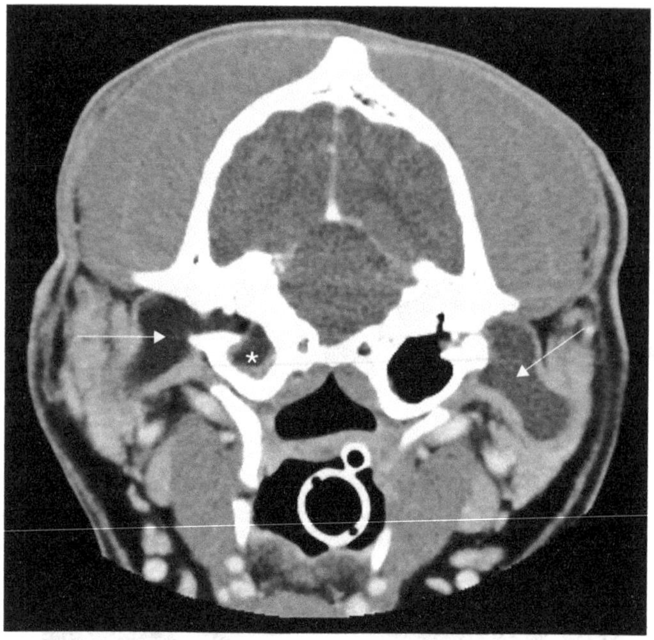

Figure 15.2 Adult dog with bilateral external ear canal atresia. Post-contrast transverse CT image shows both external ear canals (arrows) and the right tympanic cavity (asterisk) filled with non-enhancing soft tissue-dense material. The lining of the external ear canals and the right tympanic cavity are contrast enhancing.

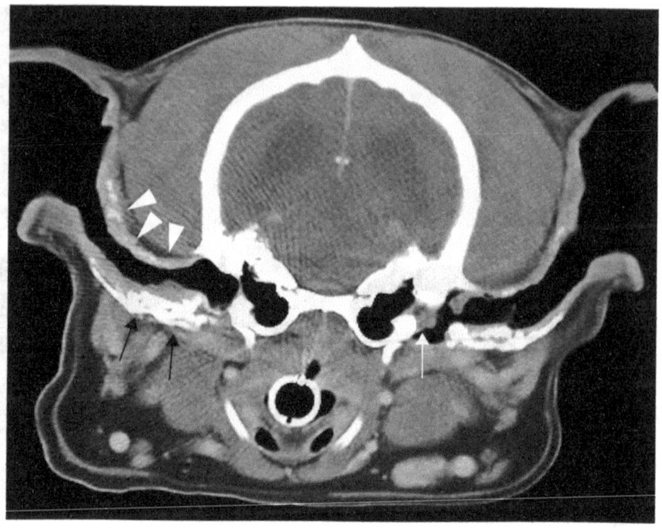

Figure 15.3 Adult dog with chronic otitis externa. Post-contrast transverse CT image shows the ear canal lining thickened and contrast enhancing (arrowheads) and extensive mineralization of the aural cartilages (black arrows). Mildly contrast enhancing soft tissue-dense material is adjacent to the left tympanic membrane, consistent with inflammatory proliferation (white arrow).

Infection/Inflammation

Otitis externa

Inflammation of the external ear canal results from infection, allergic and hypersensitivity reactions, or mechanical irritation of the ear canal by parasites or foreign bodies. Excessive fluid accumulation and swelling can limit visual inspection of the ear canal. Idiopathic or hyperplastic otitis has been described in young cocker spaniels. In chronic cases increased soft tissue volume due to soft tissue swelling, excessive cerumen production and exudate collection can lead to ear canal stenosis.

CT features (Figures 15.3 and 15.4)

- Increased contrast enhancement of the thin lining of the external ear canal in acute cases.
- In chronic cases, increased thickness and folding of the ear canal lining with increased contrast enhancement. Overall subjective narrowing of the external ear canal.
- Increased amount of non-enhancing soft tissue-dense material in the external ear canal.
- Mineralization of the auricular and annular cartilages in chronic cases.

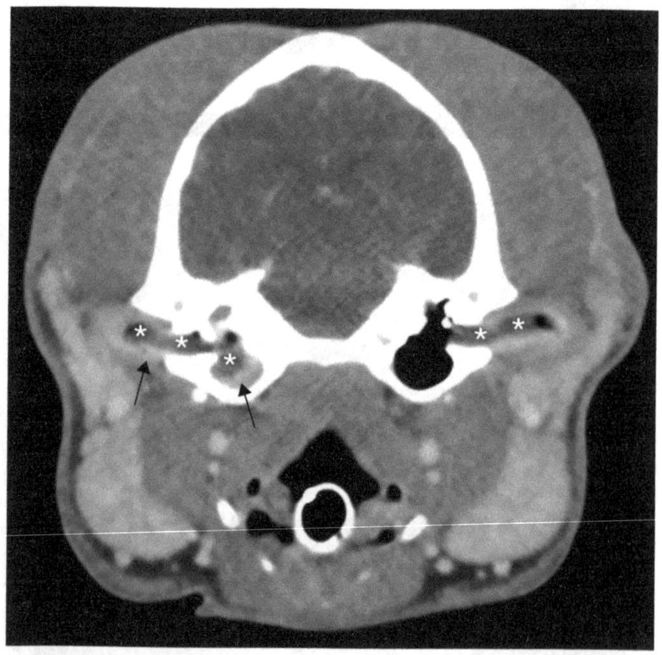

Figure 15.4 Adult dog with acute right otitis media and bilateral otitis externa. Post-contrast transverse CT image shows fluid-dense, non-contrast-enhancing material in the right tympanic cavity and external ear canal (asterisks) bilaterally, enhancement of the lining of the tympanic bulla and external ear canal (arrows).

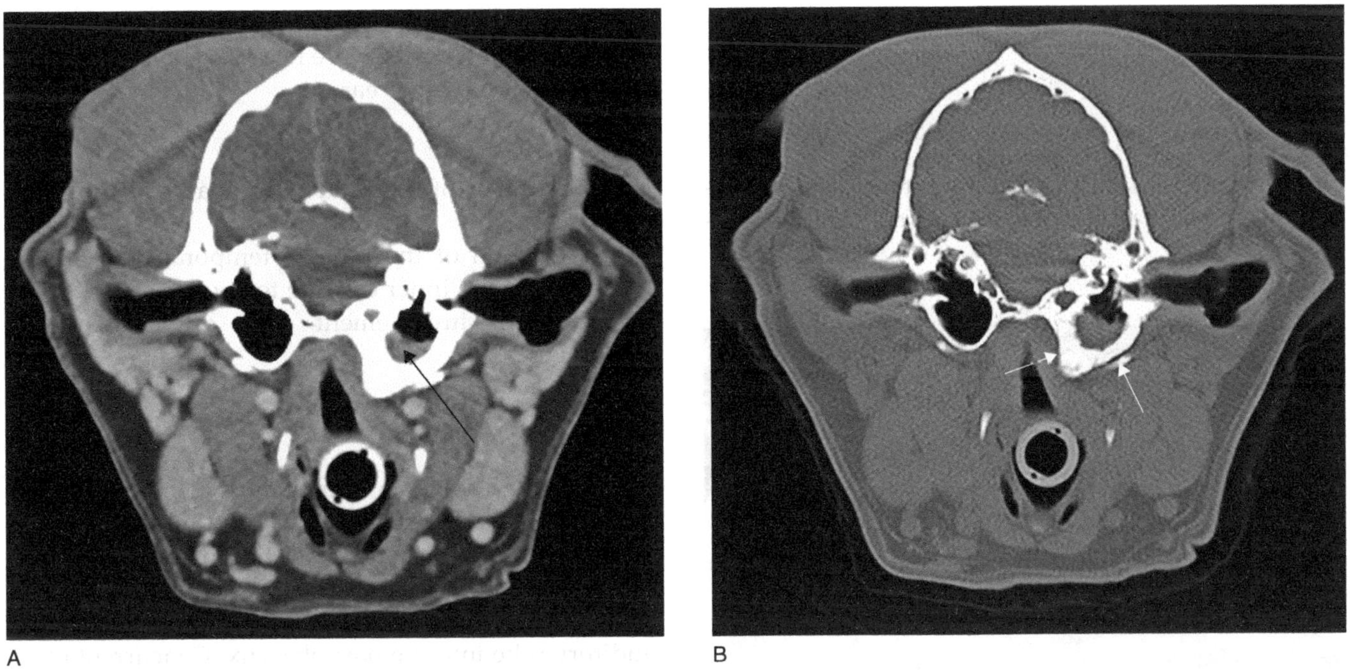

Figure 15.5 Adult dog with chronic left otitis media. Post-contrast transverse CT image shows (A) accumulation of non-contrast-enhancing soft tissue-dense material (arrow) in the tympanic cavity and (B) true sclerosis and thickening of the tympanic bulla (arrows) indicating chronicity.

- Foreign bodies such as grass awns can be difficult to detect if they are of similar density to the surrounding soft tissues.

Otitis media

Inflammation of the middle ear results from extension of external ear disease, hematogeneous spread, aspiration of pharyngeal contents through the auditory tube or functional disease of the auditory tube. Dysfunction of the auditory tube is thought to be the cause for bulla effusion in cats with sinonasal disease. In acute to subacute cases of otitis media, fluid is present in the tympanic cavity. In chronic cases inspissation of fluid and increased tissue proliferation are common. Osteitis of the tympanic bulla is commonly present in chronic cases. However, the wall of a fluid-filled tympanic bulla may appear artificially thickened on CT images. To avoid misdiagnosis of osteitis, acquisition of thin slices with high-frequency image reconstruction algorithm and evaluation with appropriate window settings are essential. Chronic aggressive disease can lead to osteolysis. Integrity of the tympanic membrane is often difficult to evaluate on CT images and can be determined by positive-contrast canalograms. Intracranial extent with involvement of the brainstem has been described.

CT features (Figures 15.4 and 15.5)

- Accumulation of fluid or, if inspissated, soft tissue- to mineral-dense material within the tympanic cavity.
- Possible contrast enhancement of the lining of the tympanic bulla.
- In chronic cases with marked fibrous proliferation, contrast enhancement of the contents of the tympanic cavity.
- Sclerosis and thickening and possible lysis of the tympanic bulla in severe and chronic cases.
- Accumulation of contrast medium in the tympanic bulla post canalogram with disruption of the tympanic membrane.

Otolithiasis

Otolithiasis has been described in dogs with external or middle-ear disease, vestibular disease or without evidence of current ear disease. Formation of the stones is thought to be due to mineralization of necrotic material resulting from current or previous otitis media. Care must be taken not to confuse auditory ossicles with otoliths.

CT features (Figure 15.6)

- Small mineral-dense foci usually adherent to the wall of the gas- or fluid-filled tympanic cavity.

- Possible associated focal thickening of the tympanic bulla.

Otitis interna

Otitis interna is usually caused by extension of inflammation or neoplasia of the middle ear. Thinly collimated CT images acquired with high-frequency image reconstruction algorithm are necessary to evaluate the structures of the inner ear.

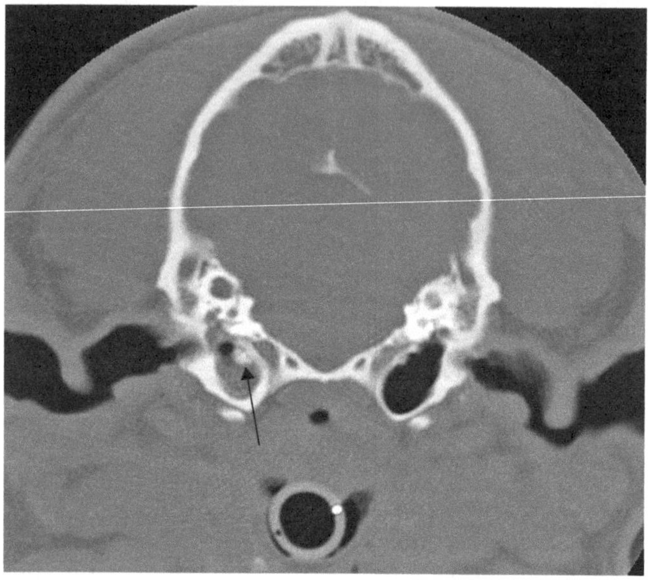

Figure 15.6 Adult cocker spaniel with chronic right otitis media with otholithiasis. Transverse CT image shows otholiths (arrow) that can persist after resolution of bulla effusion.

CT features

- Obliteration of the fluid-filled spaces of the inner ear.
- Destruction of the petrous temporal bone in the region of the inner ear due to neoplasia.
- Brainstem involvement seen on post-contrast images.

Inflammatory polyps

Inflammatory polyps originate most commonly in the tympanic bulla, less commonly in the auditory tube or nasopharynx of cats, and consist of inflammatory and epithelial cells. They can occur uni- or bilateral and are able to grow into the external ear canal or through the auditory tube into the nasopharynx. Concurrent otitis externa or media can be present, dependent on location of the polyp. Suggested causes are ascending infection or congenital. This disease is more commonly seen in cats aged 1–5 years without gender predilection. Polyps are seen with low incidence in dogs.

CT features (Figure 15.7)

- Soft tissue-dense mass, arising within the tympanic bulla, auditory tube or nasopharynx, possibly extending into the external ear canal or nasopharynx.

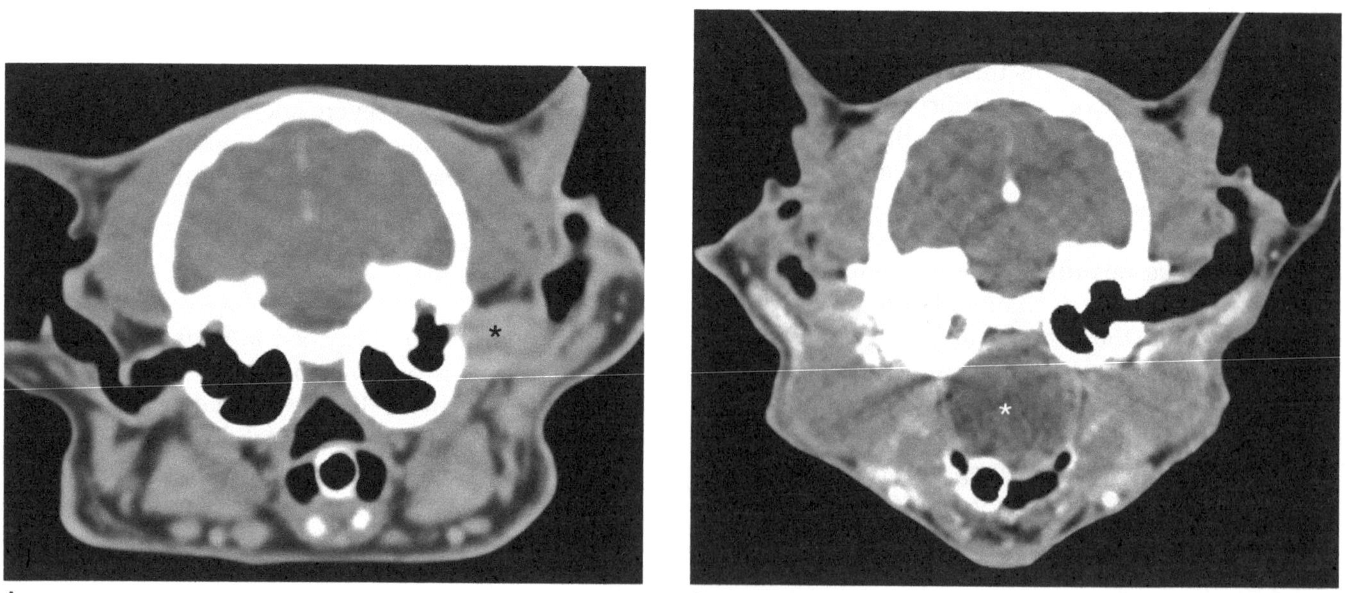

A B

Figure 15.7 Post-contrast transverse CT images in two different cats with inflammatory polyps. (A) Maine Coon cat with a polyp (asterisk) in the left external ear canal showing strong contrast enhancement. (B) Siamese cat with a nasopharyngeal polyp (asterisk) that obliterates the nasopharyngeal lumen and shows poor central and strong rim enhancement.

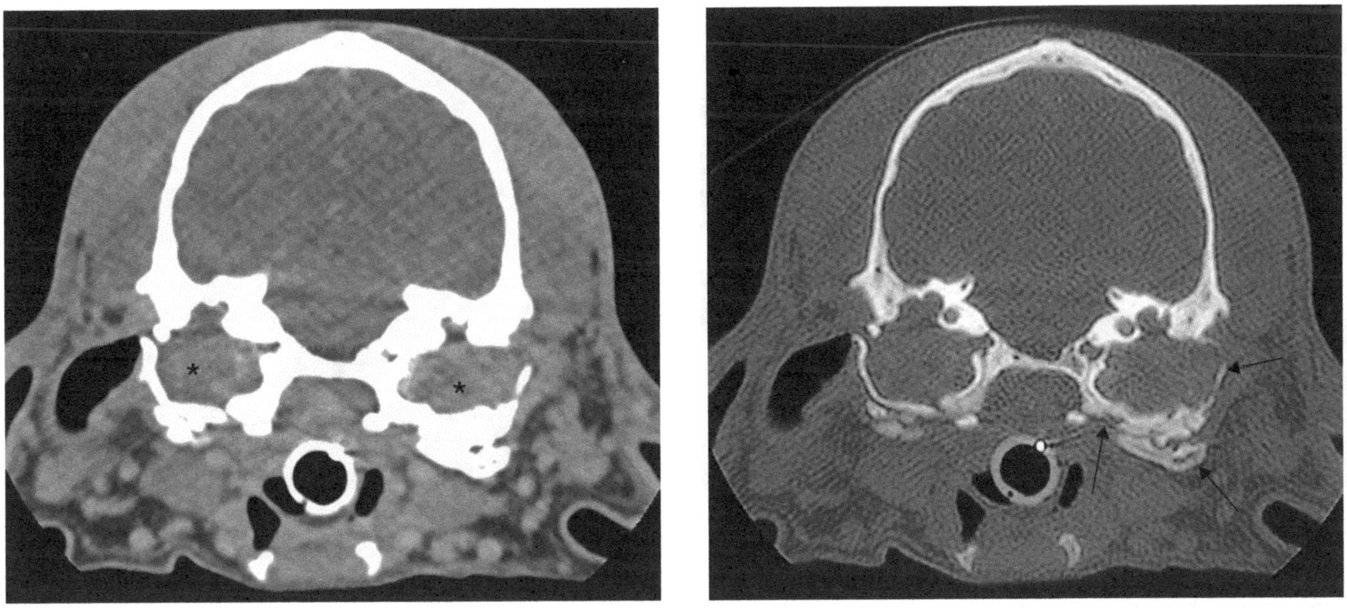

Figure 15.8 Adult dog with bilateral aural cholesteatoma. Transverse CT images show (A) both tympanic cavities filled with mildly and heterogeneously contrast-enhancing soft tissue-dense material (asterisks) and (B) the tympanic bullae that are expanded and have a mixed lytic and proliferative pattern (arrows).

- Usually strong homogeneous contrast enhancement or poor central enhancement with strong rim enhancement.

Neoplasia

Aural cholesteatoma

Aural cholesteatomas are epidermoid cysts forming, usually bilaterally, in the middle ear adjacent to the tympanic membrane. The etiology of those cysts in dogs is presumably acquired and secondary to chronic otitis media. Retraction of the tympanic membrane or migration of squamous epithelium leads to formation of a cyst in the middle ear, which contains keratin and/or sebaceous material that causes a mild to severe inflammatory response of the surrounding tissues. Severe cases can present with difficulty in opening the mouth and vestibular disease. Congenital inclusion of a squamous epithelium cyst behind the intact tympanic membrane can occur as a developmental defect with similar consequences.

CT features (Figure 15.8)
- Concurrent increase of soft tissue and commonly mineral-dense material in the tympanic cavity and external ear canal.
- Affection of the bony structures is variable from no involvement to marked lytic and proliferative changes, that can extend to the temporomandibular joint.

Other neoplasia

Cats are more commonly affected by malignant auricular tumors compared with dogs. Squamous cell carcinoma, malignant histiocytoma, mast cell tumor, sebaceous adenoma and papilloma commonly affect the pinna and external ear canal. Bones of the skull can be affected by primary bone tumors such as osteosarcoma, chondrosarcoma or less commonly benign tumors such as osteomas.

CT features (Figure 15.9)
- Mass effect to the soft tissues, potentially obliterating the external ear canal with auricular tumors.
- Squamous cell carcinoma in cats commonly causes lysis of the adjacent bony structures.
- Mixed lytic and proliferative lesions with primary bone tumors of the skull.

Further Reading

Barthez PY, Koblik PD, Hornof WJ, Wisner ER and Seibert JA (1996) Apparent wall thickening in fluid filled versus air filled tympanic bulla in computed tomography. *Vet Radiol Ultrasound* **37**: 95–8.

Detweiler DA, Johnson LR, Kass PH and Wisner ER (2006) Computed tomographic evidence of bulla effusion in cats with sinonasal disease: 2001-2004. *J Vet Int Med* **20**: 1080–4.

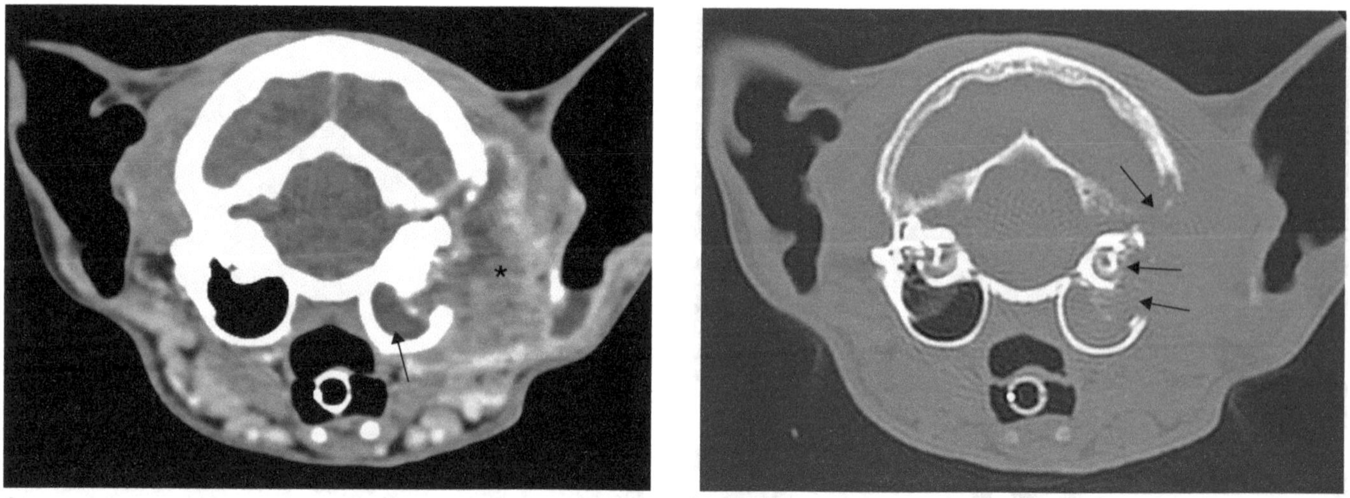

Figure 15.9 Adult cat with squamous cell carcinoma. Transverse CT images show (A) a large ill-marginated heterogeneously contrast-enhancing soft tissue-dense mass (asterisk) obliterating the left external ear canal, secondary accumulation of fluid-dense, non-enhancing material in the tympanic cavity (arrow) and (B) bone lysis of the tympanic bulla, inner ear structures and temporal bone (arrows).

Doust R, King A, Hammond G *et al.* (2007) Assessment of middle ear disease in the dog: a comparison of diagnostic imaging modalities. *J Small Anim Pract* **48**: 188–92.

Garosi LS, Dennis R and Schwarz T (2003) Review of diagnostic imaging of ear diseases in the dog and cat. *Vet Radiol Ultrasound* **44**: 137–46.

Hardie EM, Linder KE and Pease AP (2008) Aural cholesteatoma in twenty dogs. *Vet Surg* **37**: 763–70.

Russo M, Covelli EM, Meomartino L, Lamb CR and Brunetti A (2002) Computed tomographic anatomy of the canine inner and middle ear. *Vet Radiol Ultrasound* **43**: 22–6.

Seitz SE, Losonsky JM and Marretta SM (1996) Computed tomographic appearance of inflammatory polyps in cats. *Vet Radiol Ultrasound* **37**: 99–104.

Ziemer LS, Schwarz T and Sullivan M (2003) Otolithiasis in three dogs. *Vet Radiol Ultrasound* **44**: 28–31.

CHAPTER SIXTEEN

Calvarium and Zygomatic Arch

Federica Morandi

Imaging Protocol

See Table 16.1.

CT: Anatomy and Normal Variants

The calvarium, or roof of the skull, is formed by the frontal, parietal and part of the occipital bones. The zygomatic arch is formed by the zygomatic process of the temporal bone in the caudal half and by the zygomatic bone in the rostral half. Skull shapes are traditionally classified as dolichocephalic (long, narrow-headed, such as the collie), mesaticephalic (heads of medium proportion, such as the beagle) and brachycephalic (short, wide-headed, such as the Boston terrier). Cranial length (measured as the distance between the junction of the nasofrontal sutures and the external occipital protuberance) is much longer in dolichocephalic compared with mesaticephalic and brachycephalic breeds. Cranial width (the widest interparietal distance), however, does not vary significantly among the three skull shapes. Many brachycephalic dogs have a more dome-shaped appearance of the cranium than dolichocephalic or mesaticephalic breeds. The flat bones of the calvarium are connected via fibrous joints called sutures. Widened, open skull sutures and the fontanel (between the frontal and parietal bones) can be seen in animals with congenital hydrocephalus, not necessarily in association with clinical signs (Figure 16.1).

CT Disease Features

Malformation and developmental diseases

Occipital dysplasia (keyhole malformation)

The normal foramen magnum is located ventrally between the occipital condyles and provides an opening for passage of the spinal cord. The normal foramen magnum is round to ovoid, with a diameter similar to that of the vertebral canal. Occipital dysplasia refers to the abnormal dorsal extension of the foramen magnum secondary to abnormal development of the occipital bone. It is most common in miniature and toy breed dogs, and can be identified in animals that show no clinical signs.

CT features

- Abnormal dorsal extension of the foramen magnum, which assumes a keyhole shape (Figure 16.2).
- 3-D reconstructions can facilitate evaluation of the lesion.

Occipital bone malformation (Chiari I-like)

Occipital bone malformation, with underdevelopment of the occipital bone, results in a smaller than normal caudal fossa and can lead to overcrowding of the caudal fossa, with resulting herniation of the cerebellum and medulla oblongata and obstruction of cerebrospinal fluid flow, in turn leading to hydrocephalus

Veterinary Computed Tomography, First Edition. Edited by Tobias Schwarz, Jimmy Saunders.

Table 16.1
CT imaging protocol (intravenous contrast study: standard protocol; *see* Chapter 5).

Series	Pre- and post-contrast
Decubitus	Ventral
Scan margins	Upper molar 1 → Caudal aspect of the first cervical vertebra
Voltage (kVp)	120
Current (mAs)	130
Tube rotation time (s)	1
Slice width (mm)	5 (medium to large dogs); 2 (small dogs and cats)
Sequential slice interval (mm)	5 (medium to large dogs); 2 (small dogs and cats)
Kernel frequency	Sharp (high); reformat with standard (medium) if post-contrast series is acquired
Window level (HU)	+350 (post-contrast: +35)
Window width (HU)	2800 (post-contrast: 300)

and syringomyelia. This syndrome is termed Chiari I-like malformation, and is most common in the Cavalier King Charles spaniel, but has also been reported in other brachycephalic breeds. The severity of the abnormalities is variable, and there does not appear to be good correlation between the severity of the anatomical abnormalities and the presenting clini-

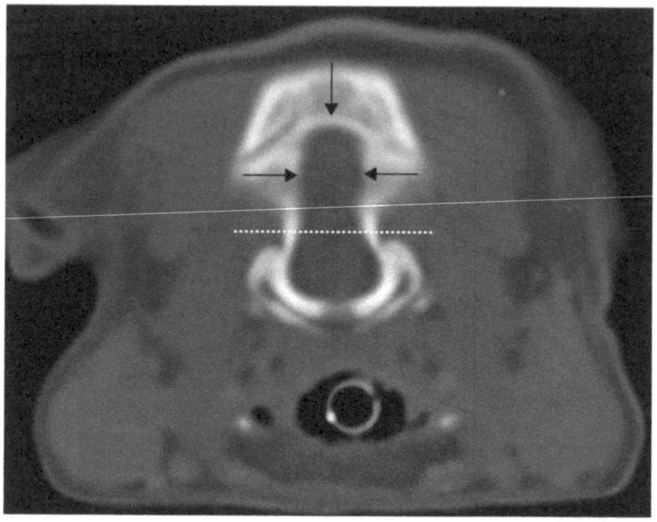

Figure 16.2 Transverse CT image of a one-year-old Shi-Tzu shows the elongated, keyhole shape appearance of the foramen magnum (arrows). The dotted line indicates the approximate normal dorsal extension of the foramen magnum.

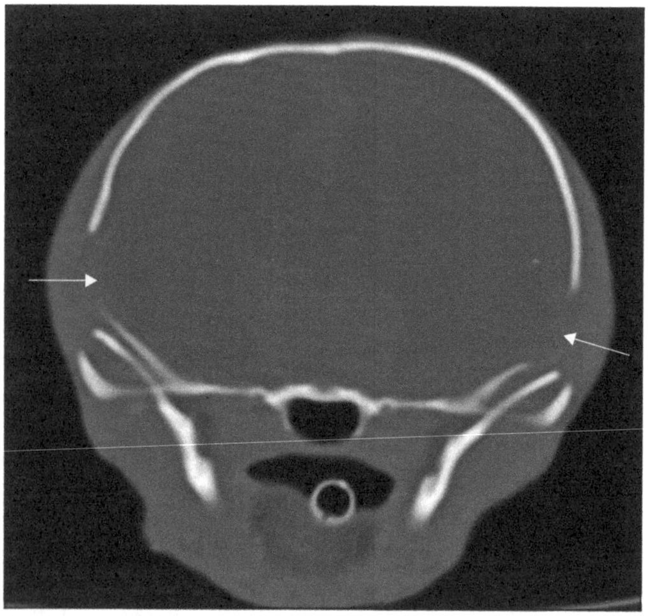

A

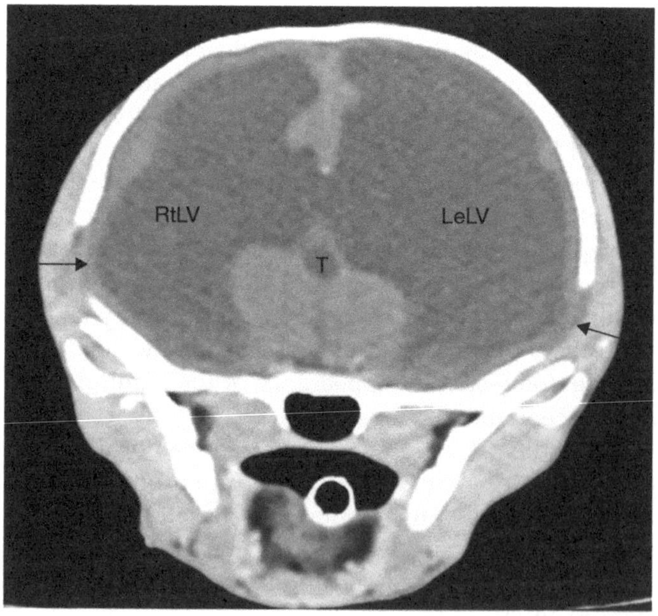

B

Figure 16.1 Two-year-old Yorkshire terrier with severe congenital hydrocephalus. (A,B) Transverse CT images show the open, wide suture between the parietal and temporal bones (arrows). RtLV = right lateral ventricle; LeLV = left lateral ventricle; T = third ventricle.

cal signs. Because many of the abnormalities associated with Chari I-like malformation affect soft tissue structures, they are best evaluated with MRI. Linear, area and volume measurements of the cranial cavity and caudal fossa have been calculated using CT in normal dogs, and they may be used for comparison with dogs with suspect occipital bone malformation.

CT features

- CT images reformatted in the sagittal plane can help in determining the presence of cerebellar herniation into the spinal canal.
- 3-D reconstructions can help in evaluating abnormal morphology of the occipital bone.
- Hydrocephalus and syringomyelia are best seen on soft tissue windows.

Trauma

Head trauma in small animals can be caused by motor vehicle accidents, falls, kicks, bites and gunshot wounds. CT is superior to radiography in evaluating the skull for possible fractures, and it offers the additional advantage of allowing simultaneous assessment of the brain for possible injuries. CT readily identifies pneumocephalus and acute hemorrhage; brain edema and contusions can also be identified, however, it is best documented using MRI. In traumatized and potentially unstable animals, CT has the additional advantage of short examination time compared with MRI, and may be obtained using only sedation in a neurologically compromised animal.

CT features

- Displaced fractures are readily identified; multiplanar and 3-D reconstructions can help in defining displacement (Figure 16.3).
- Open fractures can result in air accumulation inside the cranial vault (pneumocephalus) (Figure 16.4).
- Fractures of the zygomatic arch are often associated with temporomandibular joint fractures and/or luxations.
- Acute hemorrhage is hyperdense; chronic hemorrhage (within 1–2 weeks) becomes iso- to hypodense and may be more difficult to identify, especially in the absence of a significant mass effect. In addition to intraparenchymal hemorrhage, the following are possible.
  - Epidural hemorrhage/hematoma:
    - accumulates in the potential space between the dura and inner surface of the skull; often found in the temporoparietal region secondary to tearing of the middle meningeal artery by a fracture fragment
    - acute epidural hemorrhage/hematoma appears as a biconvex, well-defined, hyperdense mass between the inner surface of the skull and the underlying, displaced dura and brain.
  - Subdural hemorrhage/hematoma:
    - accumulates in the potential space between the dura and the pia/arachnoid
    - acute subdural hemorrhage/hematoma appears as a hyperdense, crescent-shaped mass lesion conforming to the inner margin of the skull
    - because of the close association with the inner skull margin, and because bone and hyperdense blood may have the same pixel density on a narrow window, care must be taken not to mistake subdural hemorrhage/hematoma for thickening of the skull.
  - Subarachnoid hemorrhage:
    - accumulates in the subarachnoid space, mixing with cerebrospinal fluid, and is often associated with cortical contusions
    - acute subarachnoid hemorrhage causes increased density of the sulci and fissures.
  - Acute interventricular hemorrhage/hematoma can sometimes be identified as increased density or a hyperdense mass in one or both lateral ventricles.
- Brain contusions occur commonly after head trauma and consist of heterogeneous area of hemorrhage, edema and necrosis, often in the superficial gray matter.
  - Initial findings include faint and ill-defined hypodense areas interspersed with small regions of hyperdense acute hemorrhage.
  - Contusion with predominant edema and necrosis can become more evident a few days after the initial trauma, as hypodense areas with associated mass effect.

Infection/Inflammation

Osteomyelitis/Sequestra

Osteomyelitis of the calvarium and zygomatic arch occurs most commonly secondary to penetrating wounds and foreign object penetration, and may be a complication of trauma. If a fractured bone fragment is cut off from blood supply a sequestrum will develop. Sequestra may be septic (a complication of chronic osteomyelitis) or sterile.

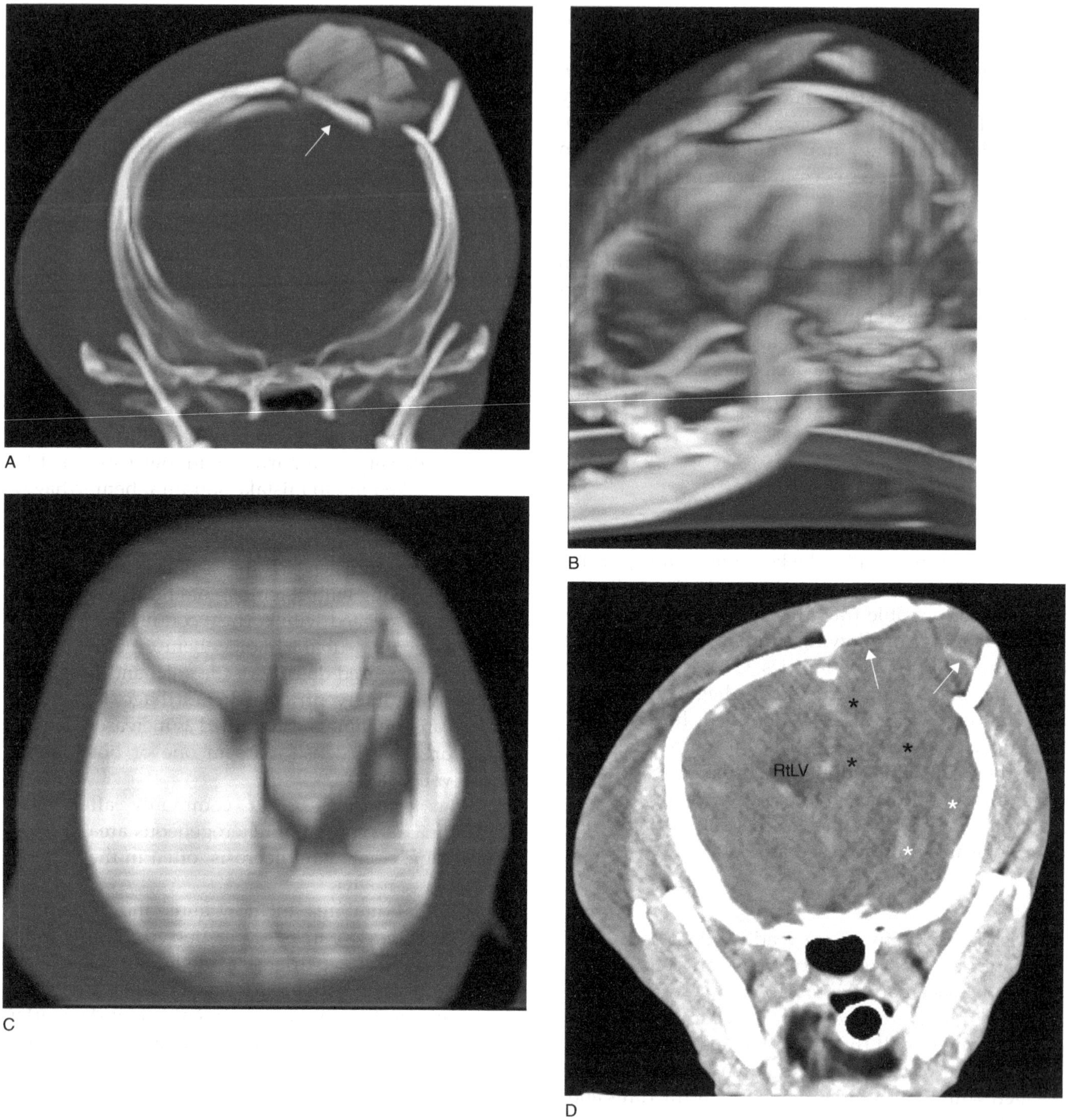

Figure 16.3 Nine-year-old Chihuahua that was kicked in the head by a horse 3 hours prior to imaging. Maximum intensity projection (MIP) (A) transverse, (B) parasagittal and (C) dorsal images show a comminuted fracture involving the dorsal aspect of the left parietal bone, with extension to the midline suture (arrow). The majority of the fragments are displaced laterally and dorsally, but one fragment is depressed, compressing brain parenchyma. Notice also the severe soft tissue swelling at the fracture site. (D) Post-contrast transverse CT image at the level of the mid-brain shows patchy areas of increased (white asterisks) and decreased (black asterisks) density within the left cerebral hemisphere, with obliteration of the left lateral ventricle, and displacement and partial loss of meningeal enhancement in the area of the fracture (arrows), suggesting partial herniation of brain tissue into the fracture defect. RtLV = right lateral ventricle.

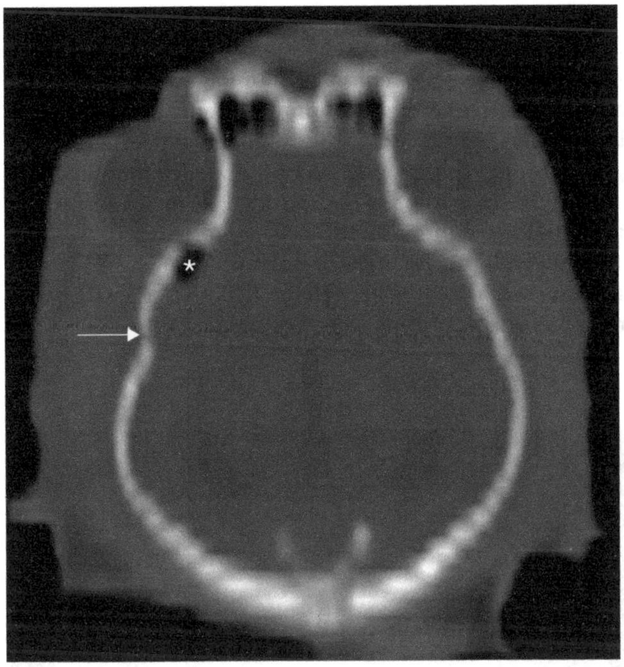

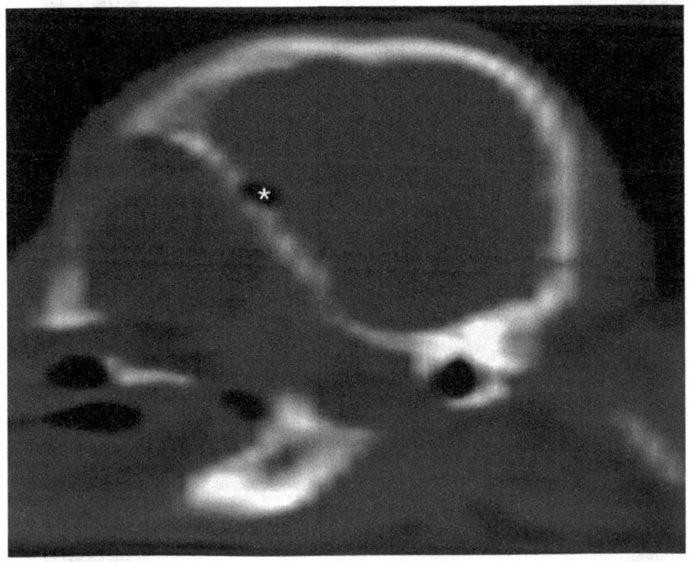

A B

Figure 16.4 Adult Yorkshire terrier that fell 8 feet down the stairs the day before. Maximum intensity projection (MIP) (A) dorsal and (B) sagittal images show the axially deviated right frontoparietal bone, indicating a depressed fracture (arrow). A gas pocket is visible just inside the margin of the frontal bone (asterisk) indicating pneumocephalus (other skull fractures, including fractures at the level of the frontal bone and sinus, were also present, but are not visible on these images).

CT features

- Aggressive lysis and periosteal proliferation of the affected bones.
- A sequestrum will appear as a sharply defined, hyperdense fragment of bone without evidence of associated lysis and/or production (Figure 16.5).
- Contrast administration may highlight a draining tract documenting communication with the sequestrum or foreign object.

Craniomandibular osteopathy

A benign proliferative bone disease of unknown etiology that occurs mainly in terrier breeds (especially West Highland White terriers), but also occasionally in Labrador retriever, Doberman pinscher and bullmastiff. Autosomal recessive inheritance is documented in West Highland White terriers, therwise the etiology is unknown. The disorder affects young (3- to 8-month-old) dogs and involves the mandible, tympanic bulla, calvarium and petrous temporal bone. Bone proliferation stops when skeletal maturation is completed. CT is useful to assess the presence and degree of temporomandibular joint ankylosis.

CT features (Figure 16.6)

- Smooth, benign osseous thickening of the mandible, tympanic bulla, petrous temporal bone and calvarium.
- No underlying lysis.
- Occasionally, changes resembling hypertrophic osteodystrophy have been concurrently described in long bones and ribs.
- CT is especially helpful in determining the location of the new bone production with respect to the temporomandibular joints.

Calvarial hyperostosis in bullmastiffs

Calvarial hyperostosis is a benign bone disease of the skull recently described in bullmastiffs; it is similar to craniomandibular osteopathy in dogs and infantile cortical hyperostosis in people. Affected animals are skeletally immature and present with painful osseous swelling of the skull, lymphadenopathy, eosinophilia and pyrexia.

CT features

- Smooth, benign osseous thickening of the calvarium due to periosteal proliferation of the frontal, parietal and occipital bones, without abnormalities of the mandibles.

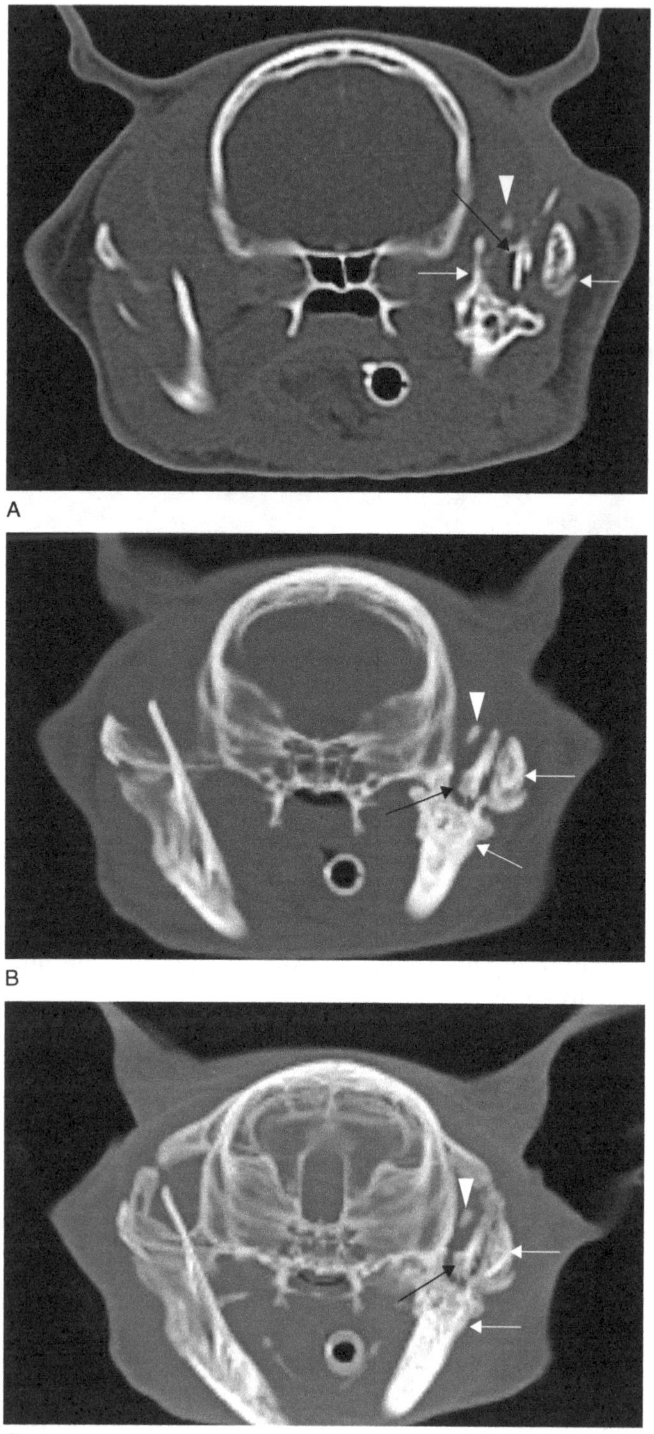

Figure 16.5 Adult cat with a two-year history of draining tract below the left pinna. (A) Transverse and (B,C) MIP transverse images show chronic malunion fracture of the left zygomatic arch and vertical ramus of the left mandible (white arrows). A large, sharply outlined separate osseous fragment representing a portion of the vertical ramus of the mandible (black arrow) is not included in the callus and is surrounded by faint radiolucency, representing a sequestrum; a second, much smaller fragment (arrowhead) is also observed medial to the largest one. Both sequestra were removed at surgery. (B) is slightly caudal to (C).

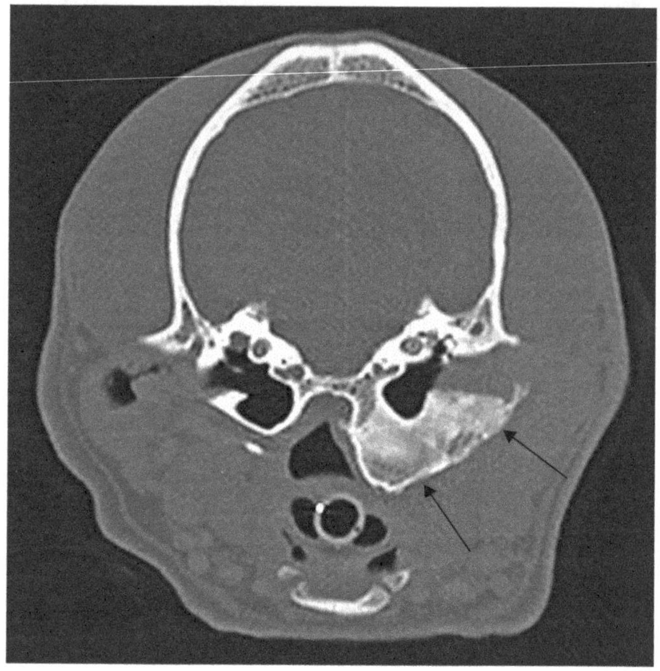

Figure 16.6 One-year-old West Highland White terrier with previously active unilateral craniomandibular osteopathy. Transverse CT image shows chronic smooth bone proliferation along the tympanic bulla (arrows) (image courtesy of Randi Drees).

- Occasionally periosteal thickening of the diaphysis of long bones has also been reported, without metaphyseal involvement.

Neoplasia

Multilobular tumor of bone

Multilobular tumor of bone (also called multilobular osteochondrosarcoma, MLO, chondroma rodens and multilobular osteoma) is a rare tumor of the skull of older, large breed dogs. The neoplasm has a predilection for the calvarium and zygomatic arch; it has also been reported at the level of the orbit, maxilla, mandi-

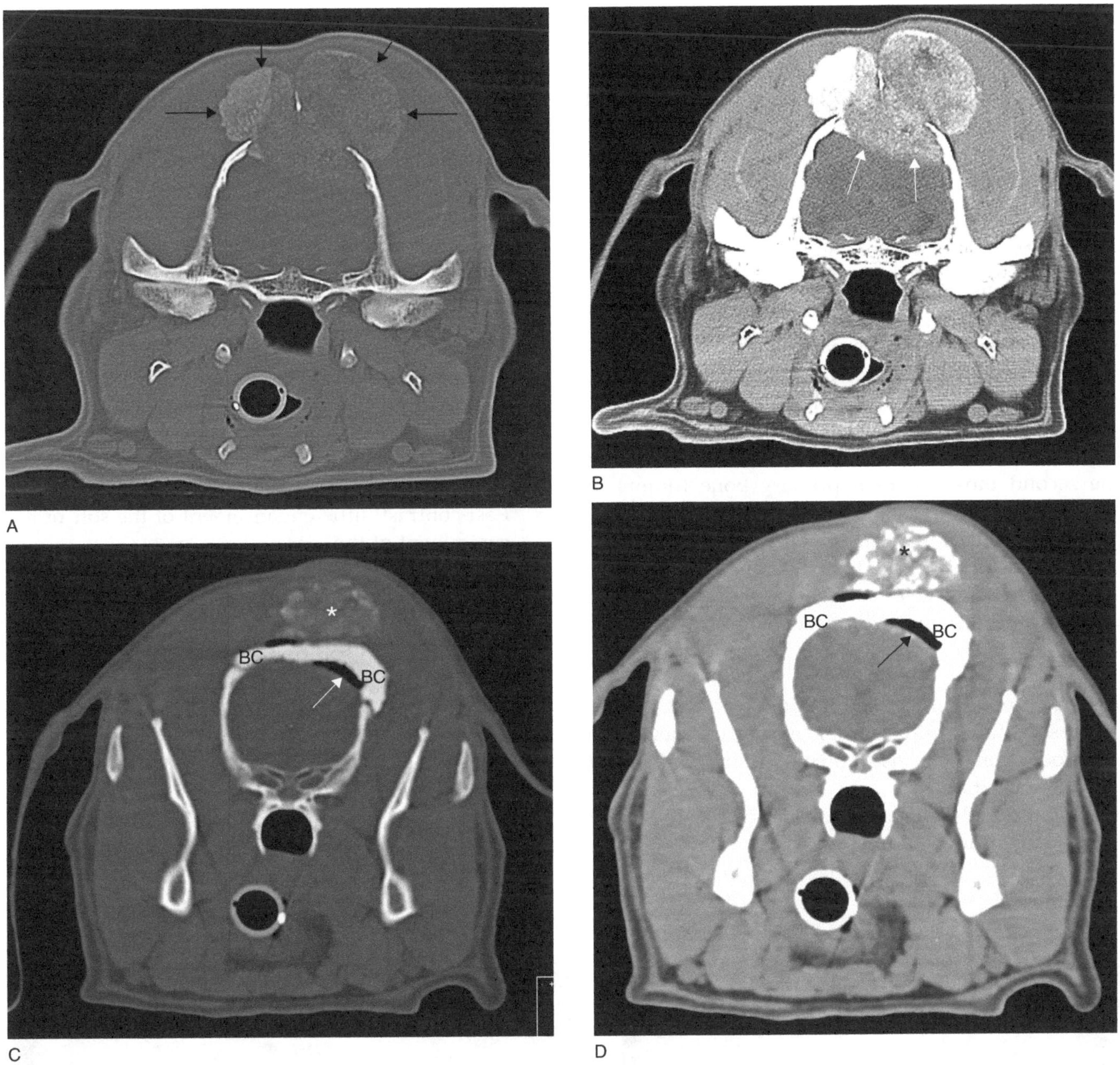

Figure 16.7 Adult dog with multilobular tumor of the calvarium. (A,B) At presentation, transverse CT images show a mass with typical fine granular appearance (black arrows), and invasion into the cranium with brain compression (white arrows). (C,D) Transverse CT image obtained one year after the initial tumor removal. The tumor has recurred (asterisk) dorsal to the bone cement layer (BC) that was placed to provide mechanical coverage to the brain. Notice the persistent pneumocephalus (arrow).

ble and tympanic bulla. Histologically, multilobular tumor of bones consists mostly of multiple oval to irregularly shaped islands of osseous, cartilaginous or ossifying cartilaginous tissue separated from adjacent island by fibrovascular septa. These tumors often invade the cranial vault and compress, but do not invade the brain. About 50% of dogs experience local recurrence after surgical excision, alone or in combination with radiotheraphy; metastases can occur.

CT features (Figure 16.7)

- Round to ovoid mass with coarse, non-homogeneous granular mineral density.

- Typical stippled or fine granular appearance best visible using a bone window display.
- Underlying lysis of the calvarium/zygomatic arch.
- Compression and displacement of the brain and meninges.
- Post-contrast: variable, but usually mild enhancement of the soft tissue component of the mass.

Osteosarcoma, chondrosarcoma

Osteosarcomas are the most common primary bone tumors of the skull, with up to 37% reportedly arising from the cranial vault. Compared with osteosarcomas of the appendicular skeleton and facial bones, osteosarcomas of the cranial vault tend to be predominantly productive. They occur most commonly in middle-aged to older, large breed dogs. Chondrosarcomas are the second most common primary bone tumors in dogs; their imaging characteristics can be very similar to osteosarcomas, featuring a combination of aggressive destructive and productive changes, but sometimes they can have smoother margination than osteosarcomas. A biopsy is needed to achieve histologic diagnosis.

CT features (Figures 16.8 and 16.9)

- Osseous mass with aggressive pattern of new bone production that may contain granular areas of mineralization.
- Usually well-defined margins for osteosarcomas of the calvarium.
- May compress the brain without invading it.
- May show more significant aggressive lysis at the level of the zygomatic arch.
- Post-contrast: usually mild enhancement of the soft tissue component of the mass.

Osteoma

Osteomas are benign, slow-growing tumors that have well-defined, smooth margins, and may arise from the calvarium, zygomatic arch, mandible or sinuses.

CT features

- Solid, very dense mass with little to no underlying lysis.
- If centered over the calvarium they may grow eccentrically and compress the brain without invading it.
- Post-contrast: little enhancement of the soft tissue component of the mass.

Soft tissue neoplasia

The most common soft tissue tumor of the zygomatic and calvarial regions, especially in cats, is squamous cell carcinoma; soft tissue sarcomas and mast cell tumors are also possible.

CT features (Figure 16.10)

- Large soft tissue mass with associated variable, aggressive lysis of underlying osseous structures.

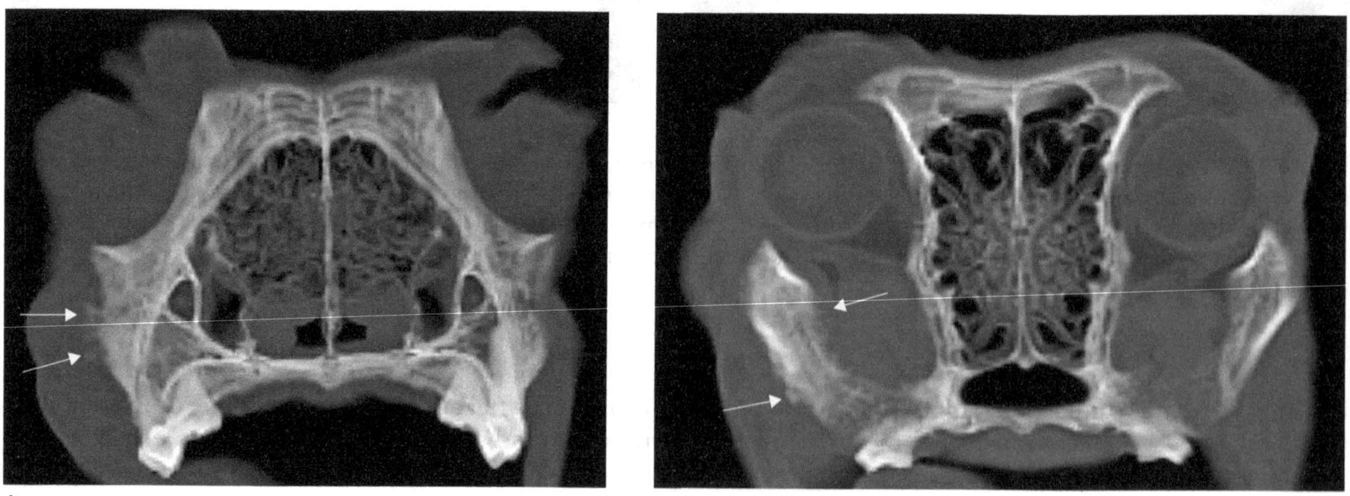

A B

Figure 16.8 Adult dog with osteosarcoma. Maximum intensity projection (MIP) transverse CT images of maxilla and zygomatic arch show irregular, speculated, aggressive periosteal reaction (arrows) at the level of the right maxilla and zygomatic arch, with associated soft tissue swelling. (A) is slightly rostral to (B).

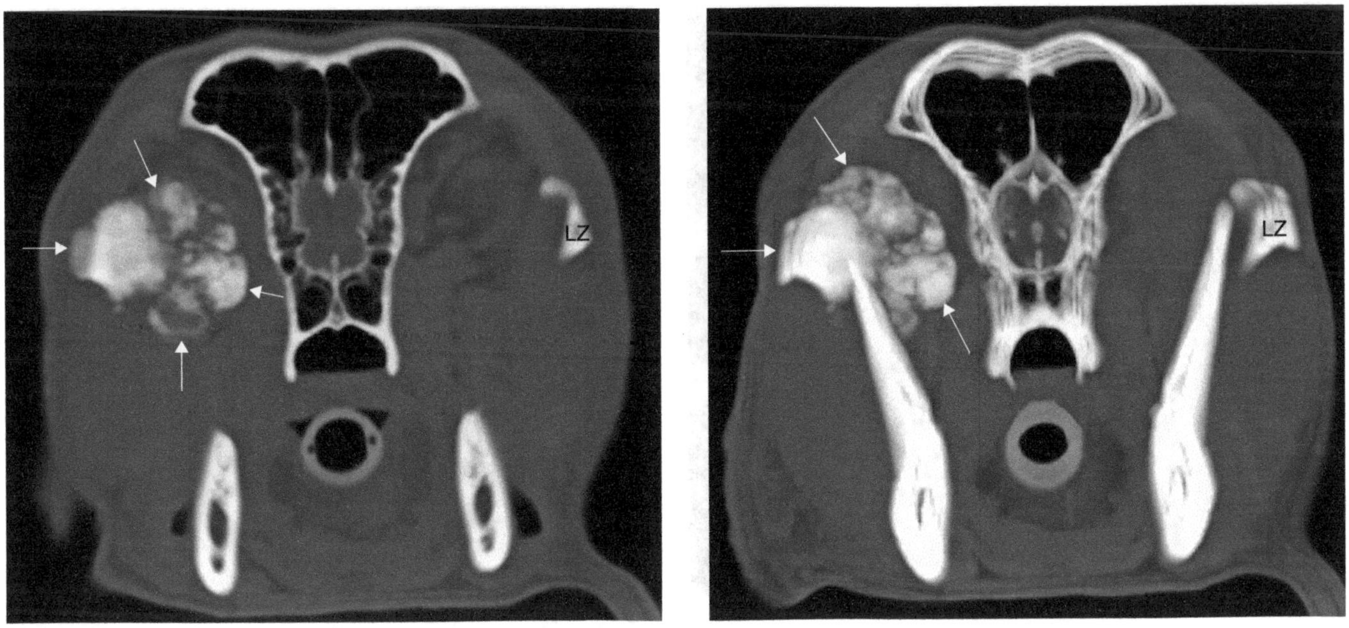

A B

Figure 16.9 Adult dog with chondrosarcoma. (A) Transverse and (B) MIP transverse CT images of the zygomatic arch with right exophthalmos show a large, productive osseous mass arising from the right zygomatic arch (arrows). The mass has smooth margins and a lobulated, popcorn-like appearance. LZ = left zygomatic arch.

- Very little associated new bone production.
- If periosteal new bone production is visible, it has usually aggressive pattern.
- Amorphous mineralizations may be present within the soft tissue mass.
- Post-contrast: variable, usually mild, enhancement of the soft tissue component of the mass.

Further Reading

Bar-AM Y, Pollard RE, Kass PH and Verstraete FJ (2008) The diagnostic yield of conventional radiographs and computed tomography in dogs and cats with maxillofacial trauma. *Vet Surg* **37**: 294–9.

Forrest LJ (2007) Cranial and nasal cavities: canine and feline. In: Thrall DE (ed.) *Textbook of veterinary diagnostic radiology (5e)*, pp. 119–41. St Louis, MI: Saunders Elsevier.

Garcia-Real I, Kass PH, Sturges BK and Wisner ER (2004) Morphometric analysis of the cranial cavity and caudal cranial fossa in the dog: a computerized tomographic study. *Vet Radiol Ultrasound* **45**: 38–45.

Hatchcock JT and Newton JC (2000) Computed tomographic characteristics of multilobular tumor of bone involving the cranium in 7 dogs and zygomatic arch in 2 dogs. *Vet Radiol Ultrasound* **41**: 214–7.

McConnell JF, Hayes A, Platt SR and Smith KC (2006) Calvarial hyperostosis syndrome in two Bullmastiffs. *Vet Radiol Ultrasound* **47**: 72–7.

Seiler G, Rossi F, Vignoli M, Cianciolo R, Scanlon T and Giger U (2007) Computed tomograpic features of skull osteomyelitis in four dogs. *Vet Radiol Ultrasound* **48**: 544–9.

Thomas WB (1999) Noneoplastic disorders of the brain. *Clin Tech Small Anim Pract* **14**: 125–47.

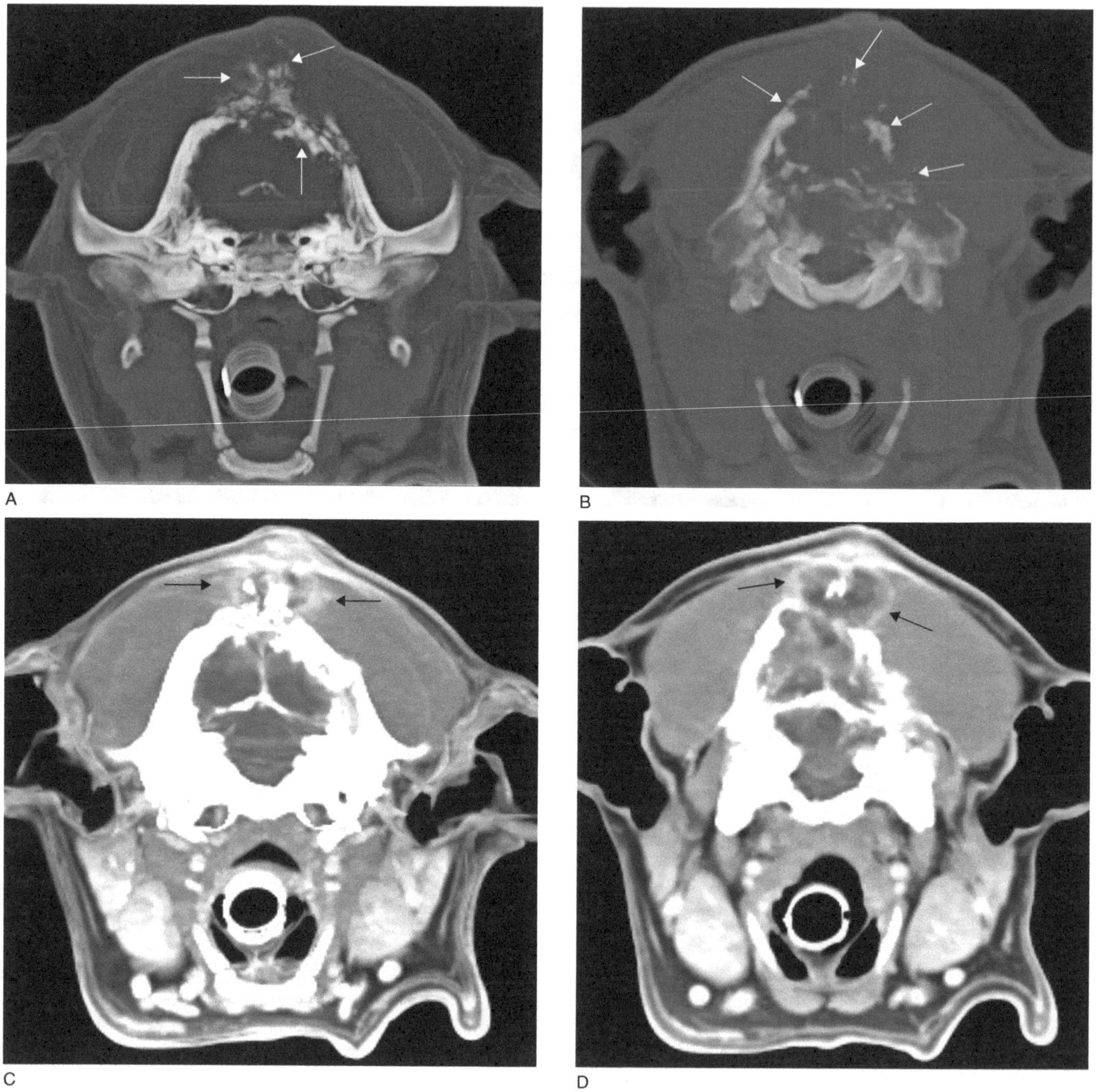

Figure 16.10 Adult dog with fibrous histiocytoma. Maximum intensity projection (MIP) transverse CT images of the caudal skull (A,B) show an extensive destructive mass associated with the dorsal aspect of the calvarium, with lysis of the occipital and parietal bones (arrows) (lysis of the temporal and frontal bones was also noted but is not depicted on these images), and (C,D) heterogeneous contrast enhancement. The mass invades the brain case with ventral displacement of the brain but without conclusive evidence of invasion of brain parenchyma.

CHAPTER SEVENTEEN

Lymph Nodes of Head and Neck

Olivier Taeymans

Imaging Protocol

See Table 17.1.

CT: Anatomy and Normal Variants

Mandibular lymph nodes (Figure 17.1)

Generally two to three mandibular lymph nodes (up to five) are very superficially located on the caudoventral aspect of the angular process of both mandibles, along both sides of the facial vein and rostral to the mandibular salivary gland. They measure about 1–2 cm in length in dogs. The afferent vessels come from the entire head, except the tongue, pharynx, larynx and ear. The efferent vessels lead to the medial retropharyngeal lymph node.

Parotid lymph node

A single parotid lymph node, measuring about 1 cm in dogs and 5 mm in cats, is located caudoventral to the temporomandibular joint. Its caudal half is covered by the parotid salivary gland, and therefore almost never discernable when normal (Figure 17.5). Its afferent vessels are related to the vast draining area of the mandibular node and also arise from the parotid gland and the ear. The efferent vessels lead to the medial retropharyngeal lymph node.

Medial and lateral retropharyngeal lymph nodes

Medial retropharyngeal lymph node (Figure 17.2)

This measures 3–4 cm in length in dogs. It is located on the dorsolateral aspect of the pharynx, caudal to the digastric muscle and ventrolateral to the longus capitis muscle. Its craniolateral border is in contact with the mandibular salivary gland. The afferent vessels are directed from the draining area of both parotid and mandibular lymph nodes, the cranial aspect of the esophagus and trachea (including the thyroid gland), and almost the entire neck musculature. The efferent vessels drain into the truncus trachealis.

Lateral retropharyngeal lymph node

This is only present in about 30% of dogs, where it is very small. It is almost always present in cats and similar in size to the medial node. It is superficially located between the ear base and the wing of C1. Its afferent vessels arise from the parotid salivary gland, and the external ear. The efferents lead to the medial retropharyngeal node.

Superficial and deep cervical lymph nodes

Superficial cervical nodes (prescapular lymph nodes) (Figure 17.3)

These are usually paired, located cranial to the supraspinatus muscle, in between the neck musculature, and measure up to 4 cm in length in dogs. They are composed of two dorsal and a smaller ventral node in cats, in which they also are more deeply located. Afferent vessels are derived form the cutaneous tissues of the head, neck and ears, the entire front leg and the cranial thorax. Efferent vessels lead to the truncus trachealis, thoracic duct or external jugular vein.

Deep cervical nodes

The cranial deep cervical node is present in 30% of dogs. It is small (1–6 mm), and located cranial to the thyroid gland. It is absent in cats.

Veterinary Computed Tomography, First Edition. Edited by Tobias Schwarz, Jimmy Saunders.

Table 17.1
CT imaging protocol (intravenous contrast study: standard protocol; *see* Chapter 5).

Series	Pre- and post-contrast
Decubitus	Dorsal
Special positioning	Front legs caudally retracted
Scan margins	Last molars ←→ Cranial T1
Voltage (kVp)	120
Current (mAs)	160
Tube rotation time (s)	1 or 2
Slice width (mm)	3
Sequential slice interval (mm)	3
Kernel frequency	Medium
Window level (HU)	+50 (post-contrast: +100)
Window width (HU)	250 (post-contrast: 300)

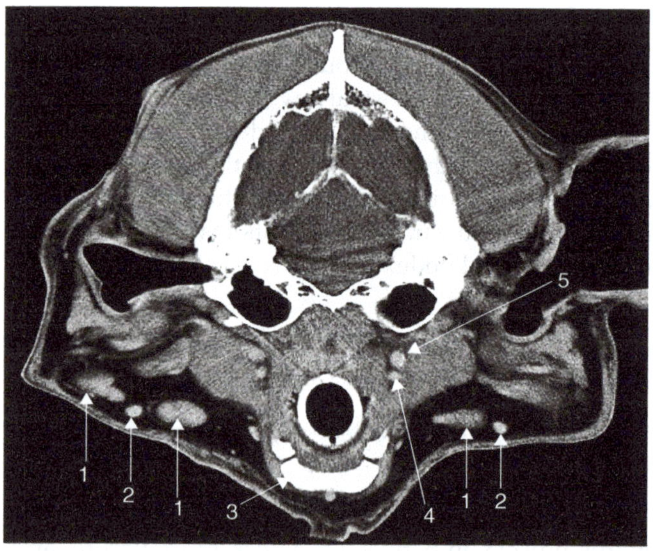

Figure 17.1 CT anatomy of the mandibular lymph nodes in a dog. Post-contrast transverse CT image obtained caudal to the angular processes of both mandibles. 1 = mandibular lymph nodes; 2 = linguofacial vein; 3 = basihyoid bone; 4 = facial artery; 5 = external carotid artery.

The middle deep cervical node is rarely present in dogs and cats. It is located along the mid-portion of the trachea, and is similar in size to the cranial deep cervical node.

The caudal deep cervical node is present in 30% of dogs. It is larger than the cranial and middle nodes, and is located ventral to the trachea, underneath the sternothyroid and sternohyoid muscles at the thoracic inlet. It is composed of multiple smaller nodes in cats.

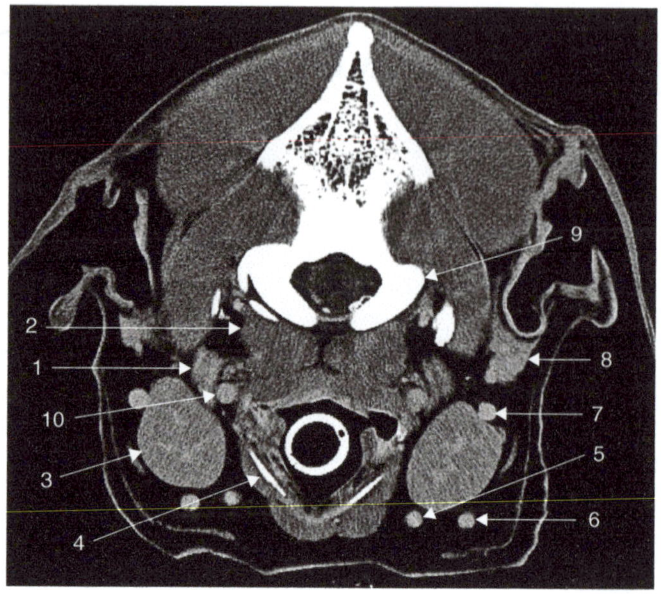

Figure 17.2 CT anatomy of the medial retropharyngeal lymph nodes in a dog. Post-contrast transverse CT image obtained caudal to the digastric muscles and caudal to the mandibular lymph nodes. 1 = right medial retropharyngeal lymph node; 2 = longus capitis m.; 3 = right mandibular salivary gland; 4 = thyroid cartilage; 5 = lingual vein; 6 = linguofacial vein; 7 = retromandibular vein; 8 = parotid salivary gland; 9 = occipital condyle; 10 = external carotid artery.

Disease Features

Neoplasia/Inflammation/Infection (Figures 17.4–17.6)

Differentiation between lymphoma, metastatic disease, reactive lymph nodes and infection cannot be made with certainty on CT, as there is a large overlap in appearance of these different conditions. However, some trends may be observed, as shown in Table 17.2.

Further Reading

Hayashi T, Tanaka R, Taira S, Koyama J, Katsura K and Kobayashi F (2003) Non-contrast-enhanced CT findings of high attenuation within metastatic cervical lymph nodes in patients with stage I or II tongue carcinoma during a follow-up period. *Am J Neuroradiol* **24**: 1330–3.

Pombo F, Rodriguez E, Caruncho MV, Villalva C and Crespo C (1994) CT attenuation values and enhancing characteristics of thoracoabdominal lymphomatous adenopathies. *J Comput Assist Tomogr* **18**: 59–62.

Wisner ER, Seibert JA and Katzberg RW (1998) Quantitative methods for indirect CT lymphography. *Vet Radiol Ultrasound* **39**: 110–16.

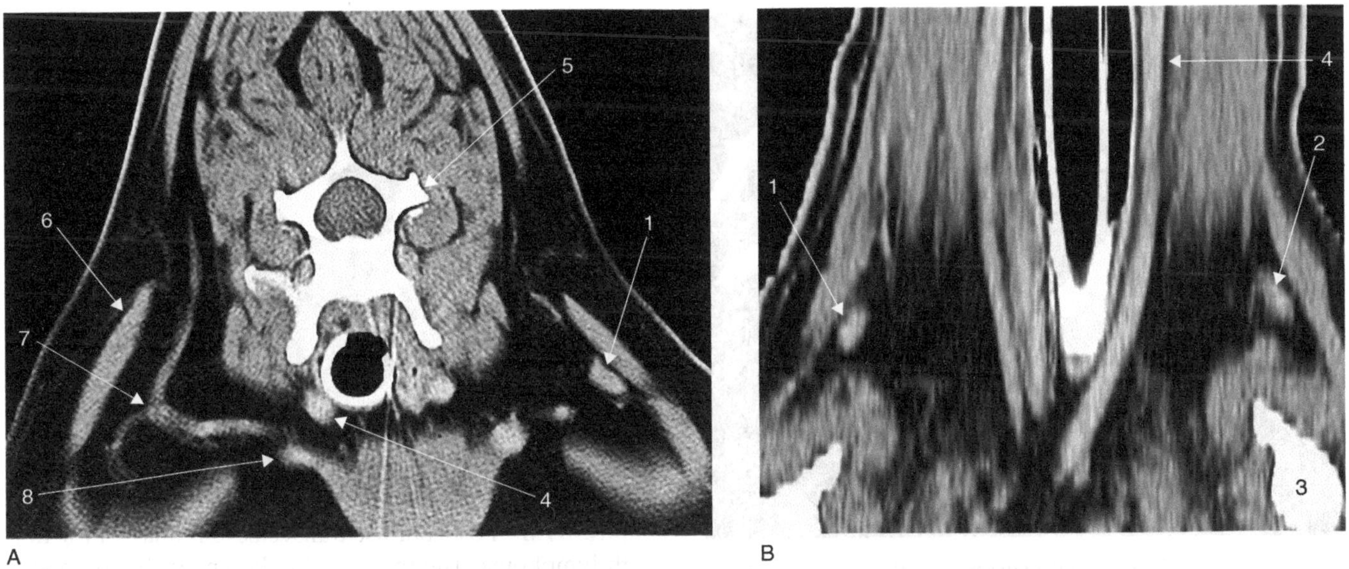

Figure 17.3 (A) Post-contrast transverse CT image and (B) dorsally reconstructed CT image of the superficial cervical lymph nodes in a dog. 1 = left superficial cervical lymph node; 2 = right superficial cervical lymph node; 3 = right humeral head; 4 = right common carotid artery; 5 = C6; 6 = right cleidomastoid muscle; 7 = right cephalic vein; 8 = right internal jugular vein.

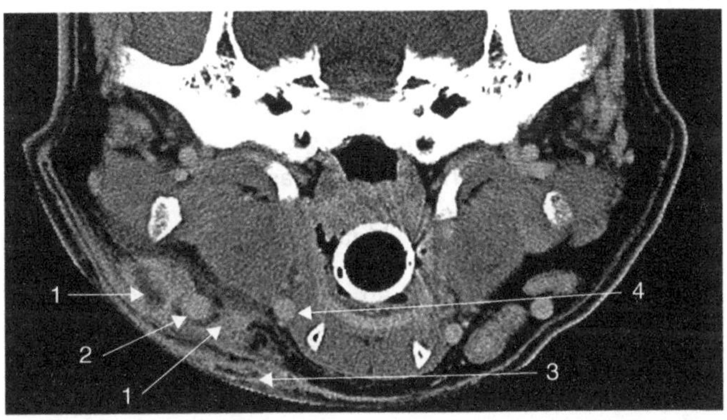

Figure 17.4 Transverse CT image in a dog with chronic subcutaneous cellulitis. The right mandibular lymph node is suppurative, likely from a non-retrieved foreign body. 1 = right mandibular lymph node; 2 = right linguofacial vein; 3 = steatitis, phlegmonous reaction; 4 = right lingual vein.

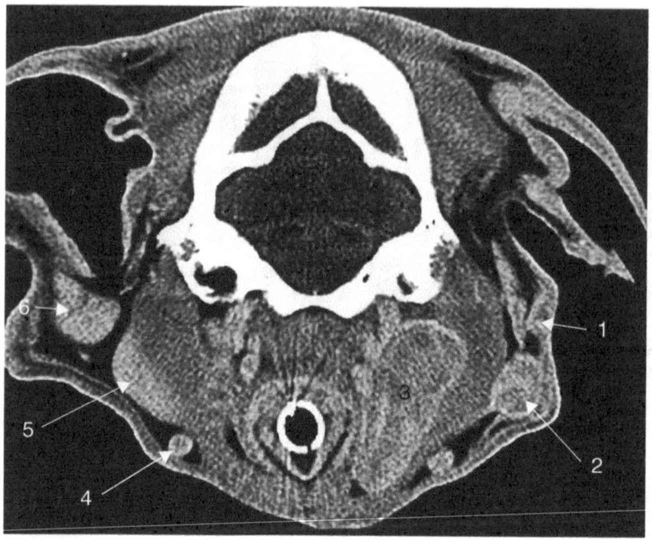

Figure 17.5 Adult cat with seruminal gland carcinoma in the left external ear canal with regional metastatic disease in the parotid and medial retropharyngeal lymph nodes. Transverse CT image shows the caudal aspect of the tumor (1). 2 = metastatic left parotid lymph node; 3 = metastatic left medial retropharyngeal lymph node; 4 = right external jugular vein; 5 = caudal aspect of the right mandibular salivary gland; 6 = right parotid salivary gland.

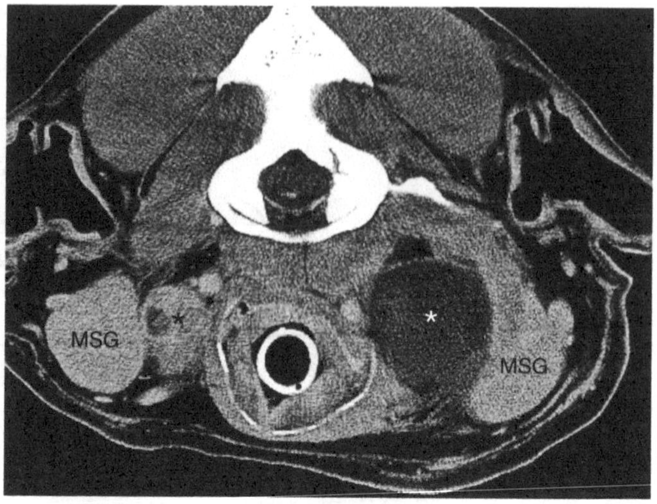

Figure 17.6 Post-contrast transverse CT image in a dog with lymphoma. The medial retropharyngeal lymph nodes are bilaterally severely enlarged (asterisks). The left node is almost completely hypodense due to liquefaction. The mandibular salivary glands (MSG) (left > right) are bilaterally displaced.

Table 17.2
CT features of normal and diseased lymph nodes.

	Normal	Reactive	Metastatic	Lymphoma	Abscess
Pre-contrast HU	30–50	50–60	50–60	60–100	30–50
Post-contrast HU	120–150	100–120	120–150	70–150	70–150
Shape	Oblong	Mildly rounded	Mildly rounded	Rounded	Rounded
Size	Normal	Mildly increased	Mildly increased	Moderately increased	Moderately increased
Homogeneity pre-contrast	Homogeneous	Homogeneous	Heterogeneous	Large hypodense areas	Central hypodense area
Homogeneity post-contrast	Homogeneous	Mildly heterogeneous	Heterogeneous	Large hypodense areas	Central hypodense area

CHAPTER EIGHTEEN

Pharynx, Larynx and Thyroid Gland

Olivier Taeymans and Tobias Schwarz

Imaging Protocol

See Table 18.1.

CT: Anatomy and Normal Variants

Pharynx

The nasopharynx is cranially delimited by the choanae and bilaterally bounded by both hamulus pterygoideus (Figure 18.1). Its ventral demarcation consists of the soft palate. Both the choanae and nasopharynx should be patent and gas-filled. The tongue base is located in the rostroventral part of the oropharynx and the soft palate forms its dorsal margin. Its lumen is generally collapsed, except when the patient is intubated. The pharynx extends to the level of the axis.

Auditory (Eustachian) tube

The auditory tube is normally collapsed and not visible on CT. The tube exits the tympanic bulla rostromedially via a short bony canal and continues rostrally as a musculotubular canal, entering the dorsolateral nasopharynx via a small ostium at a level just caudal to the pterygoid hamulus process (Figure 18.2).

Larynx

The hyoid apparatus vaults the caudal aspect of the pharynx. Its large stylohyoid bones attach to the styloid process of the temporal bones via a small fibrocartilageneous tympanohyoideum that runs along the cranioolateral aspect of the tympanic bullae. Distally the stylohyoid bones articulate with the epihyoid bones that articulate with the ceratohyoid bones. The stylohyoid and epihyoid bones are almost equal in length. A single basihyoid bone interconnects both ceratohyoid bones on the ventral aspect of the hyoid apparatus. The thyrohyoid bones connect the whole hyoid apparatus to the larynx (Figure 18.3). The remainder of the larynx is composed of the epiglottis, the large thyroid cartilage with the medially located arytenoid cartilage, and the caudally located cricoid cartilage (Figure 18.4).

Thyroid gland (Table 18.2)

The thyroid gland is composed of two separate lobes. In a few large breeds of dog an isthmus connects the caudal aspect of both lobes (Figure 18.5). Both lobes are oblong and span the dorsolateral aspect of the trachea from the first to the eighth tracheal ring. On CT, the lobes are hyperdense compared with the surrounding soft tissues due to their natural high iodine content. In dogs, the right lobe is slightly more cranially located than the left lobe. The cranial and caudal thyroid arteries and veins can be recognized after intravenous contrast injection (Figure 18.6). Normal parathyroid glands cannot be seen on CT.

> **Feline anatomical specificities**
> The pharynx extends to the level of C3 and the larynx is longer than in the dog.

Disease Features

Malformation/Developmental

Nasopharyngeal stenosis

Nasopharyngeal stenosis is a rare condition consisting of an obstruction of the nasopharynx as a consequence of scar tissue formation caudal to the choanae, above the soft palate. Causes of scar tissue include chronic inflammation, local trauma, congenital malformation, surgery or a space-occupying lesion.

Veterinary Computed Tomography, First Edition. Edited by Tobias Schwarz, Jimmy Saunders.

Table 18.1
CT imaging protocol (intravenous contrast study: standard protocol; *see* Chapter 5).

Series	Pre- and post-contrast	Bone
Decubitus	Dorsal	
Special positioning	Front legs caudally retracted	
Scan margins	Last molars ←→ Cranial C3 (bone) or C5 (soft tissue)	
Voltage (kVp)	120	
Current (mAs)	160	
Tube rotation time (s)	1 or 2	
Slice width (mm)	3	1
Sequential slice interval (mm)	3	1
Kernel frequency	Medium	High
Window level (HU)	+220	+400
Window width (HU)	120	2500

CT features (Figure 18.7)

- Circumferential narrowing of the nasopharynx by a contrast-enhancing or non-enhancing soft tissue membrane or band that may extend caudally over several millimeters.
- Dorsal displacement of the soft palate.
- Fluid accumulation in the nasal passages with or without destructive rhinitis; possible fluid accumulation in the tympanic bullae.
- Possible concurrent anomalies such as choanal atresia.
- An orifice may or may not be present in the stenosis.

Hyoid bone malformations

Laryngeal collapse may be detected in brachycephalic breeds as a result of brachycephalic airway syndrome, creating an increased negative pressure during inspiration. Laryngeal cartilages become deformed from this chronic negative pressure, weaken and collapse. In young brachycephalic dogs with laryngeal collapse, a defect in cartilage structure is suspected. Morphological congenital abnormalities of the hyoid bones have been reported once in a miniature poodle (Kang *et al.* 2008).

CT features

- Laryngeal collapse as a result of brachycephalic syndrome shows a symmetrically reduced laryngeal diameter.
- Morphologic congenital abnormalities have been reported as an asymmetric hyoid apparatus, best identified on 3-D reconstructions.

Thyroid goiter

Goiter refers to a non-neoplastic, non-inflammatory enlargement of the thyroid gland as a result of insufficient thyroid hormone synthesis in a functional hypothalamus-hypophysis-thyroid axis. This condition is rare in dogs, and has not been described in cats, although an enlarged adenomatous gland is sometimes referred to as a goiter. Goiter in dogs may result from congenital hypothyroidism or may be diet or drug-induced.

CT features

- No features have been reported.
- Anticipated features on CT:
  - diffuse increased size with a homogeneous parenchyma
  - decreased density in iodine deficiency and a normal density in the other etiologies.

Thyroid cysts

Thyroid cysts are very rarely reported and need to exceed a few millimeters to show on CT. Ultimobrachial duct cysts are reported in the thyroid parenchyma of dogs. Cysts have also been observed in canine primary hypothyroidism. Pseudocysts, not lined by epithelium may be more common e.g. as a consequence of neoplasia when the tumor outgrows its vascular supply. The majority of thyroid cysts are considered incidental. However, intravenous contrast is needed to differentiate cysts from enlarged parathyroid glands on CT.

CT features (Figure 18.8)

- Rounded, well-defined hypodense structure (±30 HU) of variable size within the thyroid parenchyma that may deform the thyroid lobe.

Infection/Inflammation

Nasopharyngeal polyps

Nasopharyngeal polyps are benign, pedunculated masses believed to originate from the middle ear or auditory tube lining, expanding into the nasopharynx and external auditory canal. They typically consist of myxomatous to dense fibrous connective tissue, covered by squamous epithelium. It is the most common nasopharyngeal disease of younger cats and has been reported once in a dog.

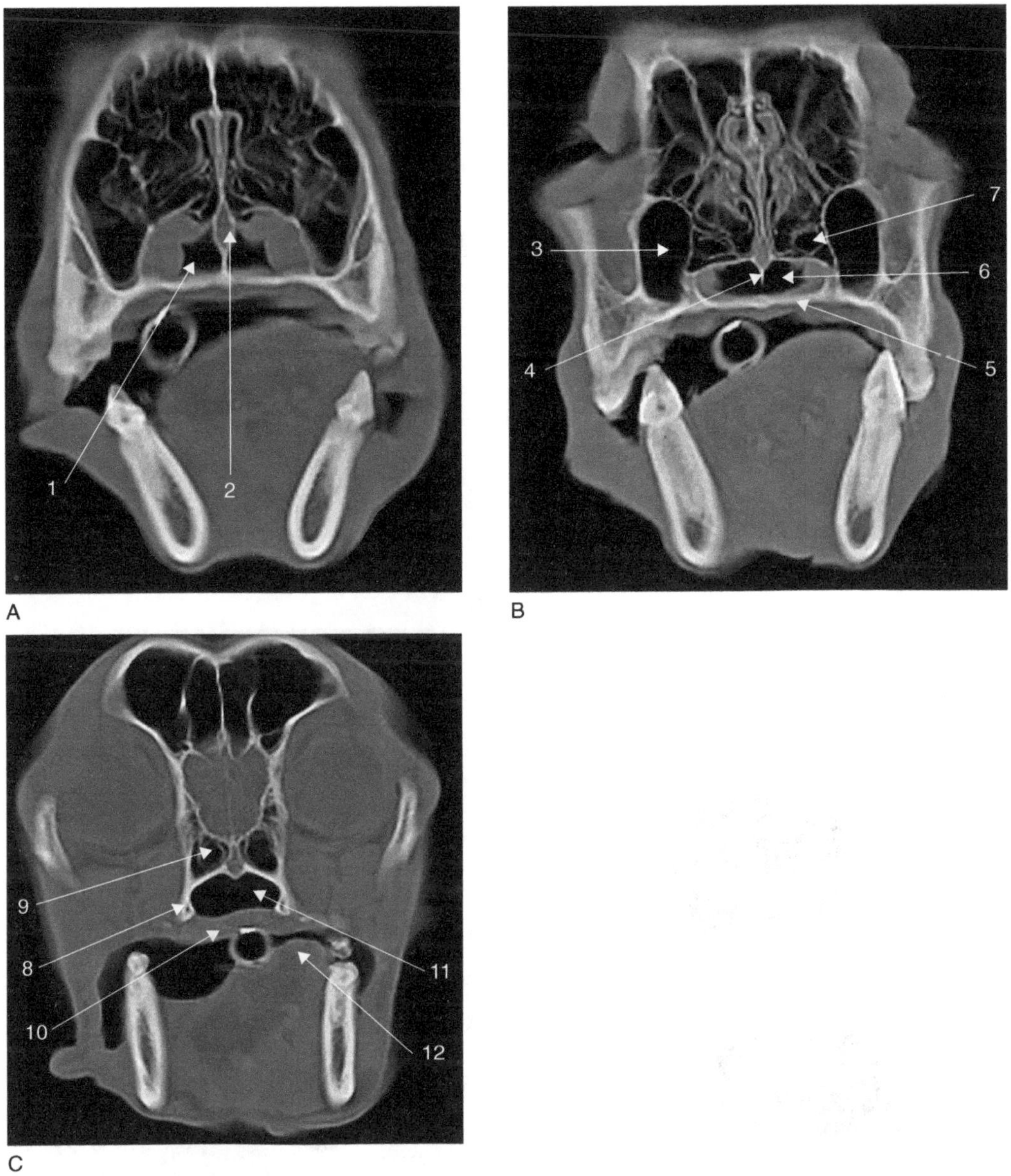

Figure 18.1 (A–C) CT anatomy of the nasopharynx in a dog. 1 = right nasopharyngeal meatus; 2 = vomer bone; 3 = maxillary recess; 4 = spina nasalis caudalis; 5 = palatine bone; 6 = choanae; 7 = endoturbinae IV; 8 = hamulus pterygoideus; 9 = ethmoidal labyrinth (sinus sphenoidalis); 10 = soft palate; 11 = nasopharynx; 12 = oropharynx with tongue base.

CT features (Figure 18.9)

- Homogeneous soft tissue density in tympanic bulla, nasopharyngeal area and/or auditory tube.
- Osseous thickening of affected tympanic bulla and possibly petrous temporal bone.
- Post-contrast: moderate (ring-like) enhancement.

Canine hypothyroidism

Canine hypothyroidism is related to a primary thyroid gland abnormality in more than 95% of the cases and this may result from idiopathic follicular atrophy or lymphocytic thyroiditis.

CT features

- No CT features have been reported.
- Anticipated features on CT:
  - the gland will show a decreased density and increased heterogeneity due to decreased iodine content (as iodine-containing follicles are gradually replaced by connective tissue)
  - a gradual decrease in size of the gland over time will be observed.

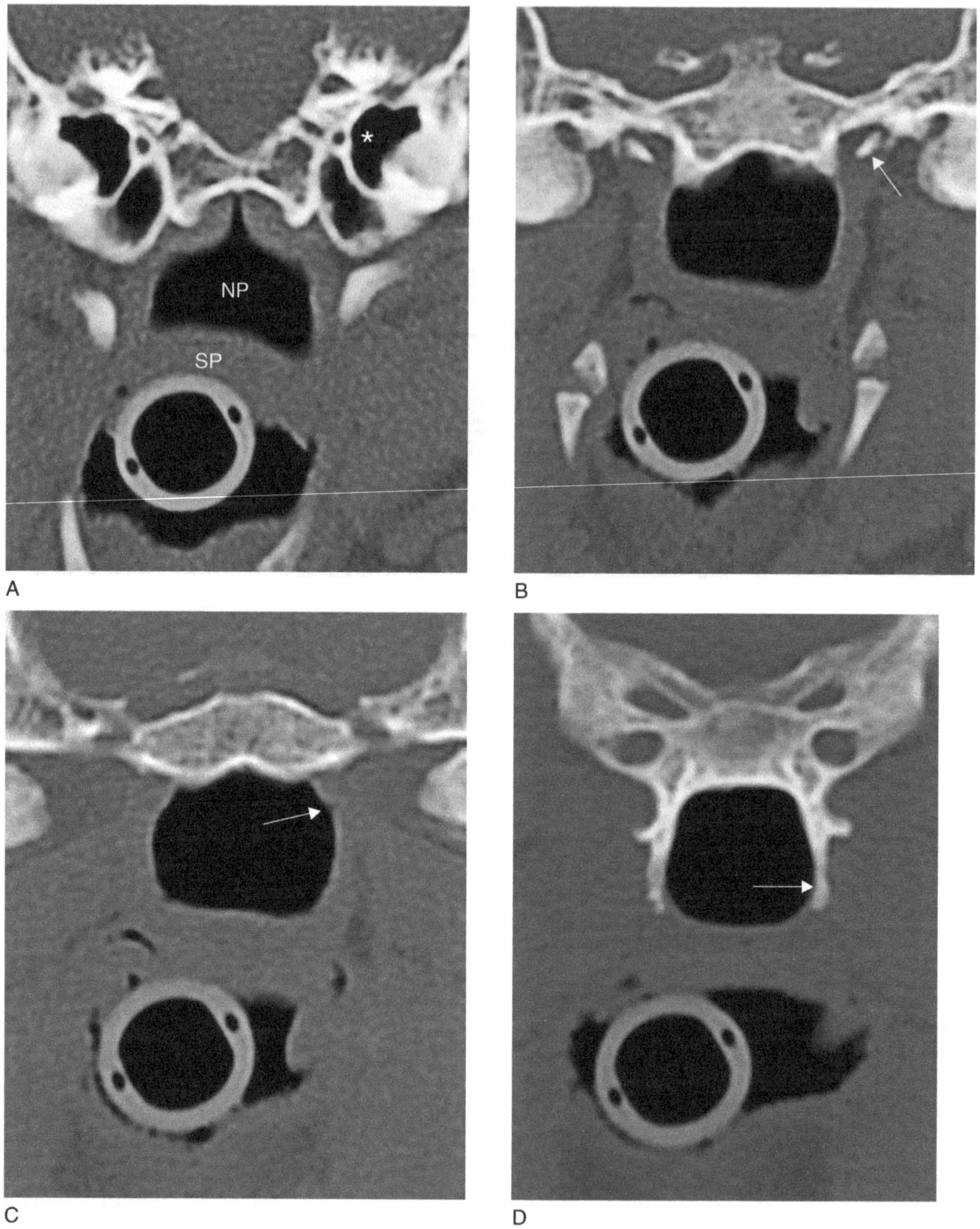

Figure 18.2 Location and course of the canine auditory tube from caudal to rostral in 3 mm intervals. (A) Rostral aspect of the tympanic bulla (asterisk). NP = nasopharynx; SP = soft palate. (B) Muscular process of the temporal bone (arrow) demarcating the ventrolateral musculotubular canal wall of the auditory tube. (C) A small indentation in the dorsolateral nasopharyngeal wall marks the pharyngeal ostium of the auditory tube (arrow). (D) Directly rostral to the ostium is the bony landmark of the pterygoid hamulus (arrow).

Trauma

Pharyngeal foreign body

Most commonly reported pharyngeal foreign bodies are wooden sticks in medium to large breed dogs. These usually penetrate the pharyngeal lining, as do fishhooks and needles. Non-penetrating foreign bodies such as grass awns may be found in the nasopharynx or oropharynx.

CT features (Figure 18.10)

- Foreign bodies have different densities, ranging from low (wood: –150 to +150 HU) to very high (metallic) and are non-contrast enhancing.

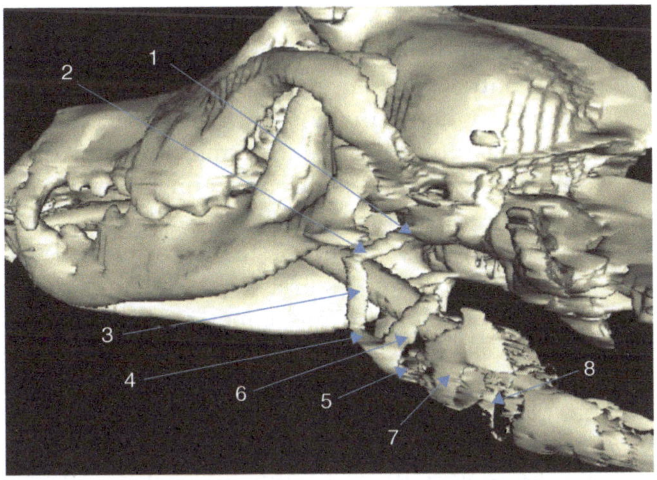

Figure 18.3 3-D surface-rendered (SR) reconstruction of the hyoid apparatus in a dog. 1 = tympanohyoideum; 2 = stylohyoid bone; 3 = epihyoid bone; 4 = ceratohyoid bone; 5 = basihyoid bone; 6 = thyrohyoid bone; 7 = thyroid cartilage; 8 = cricoid cartilage.

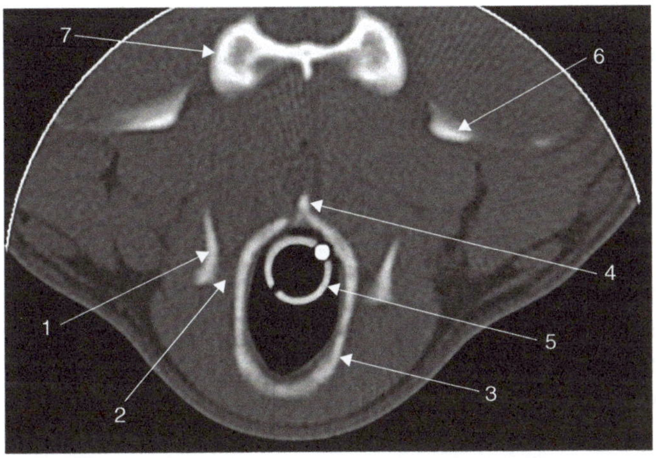

Figure 18.4 CT anatomy of the larynx in a dog. 1 = caudal horn of the thyroid cartilage; 2 = cricothyroid joint; 3 = cricoid cartilage; 4 = lamina cricoideae; 5 = tracheotube; 6 = wings of C1; 7 = body of C2.

- Often located in the facial planes in an area from C1 to C4.
- Foreign bodies are moderately well defined and surrounded by enhancing soft tissue swelling, fluid pockets and sometimes gas.
- Regional lymphadenopathy is often present.
- With chronic penetrating foreign bodies, fistulous tracts can often be seen in conjunction with granuloma, cellulitis or abscess formation. The fistula walls are contrast enhancing, while the lumen is hypodense.

Fractures/Luxations of the hyoid apparatus

CT is excellent at detecting laryngeal wall lesions, superior to most other imaging modalities. Hyoid fractures are most often the result of bite wounds, but may also result from road traffic accidents, gunshot wounds or shearing injuries by being shaken by the neck. Laryngeal collapse as a result of trauma is rare.

Table 18.2
Anatomic details of the canine and feline thyroid gland.

Thyroid	Canine	Feline
Precontrast attenuation (HU)	108	123
Postcontrast attenuation (HU)	169	169
Volume	Body weight: 30 kg = 1150 mm^3	
Parenchyma	Homogeneous	Homogeneous
Shape	Ovoid – triangular	Ovoid
CrCd location	C2–C4	

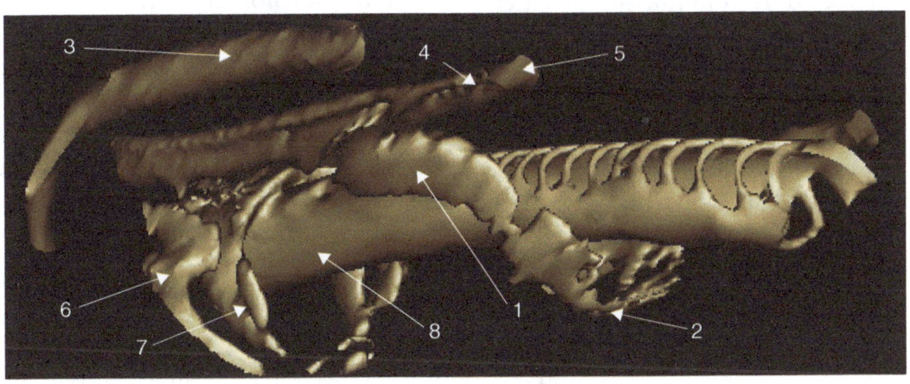

Figure 18.5 3-D SR reconstruction of the thyroid gland and surroundings in a large breed dog. Left is cranial for this patient. 1 = left thyroid lobe; 2 = isthmus; 3 = left external jugular vein; 4 = left internal jugular vein; 5 = left common carotid artery; 6 = thyroid cartilage; 7 = cricoid cartilage; 8 = tracheotube. The tracheal rings are not displayed on this window setting.

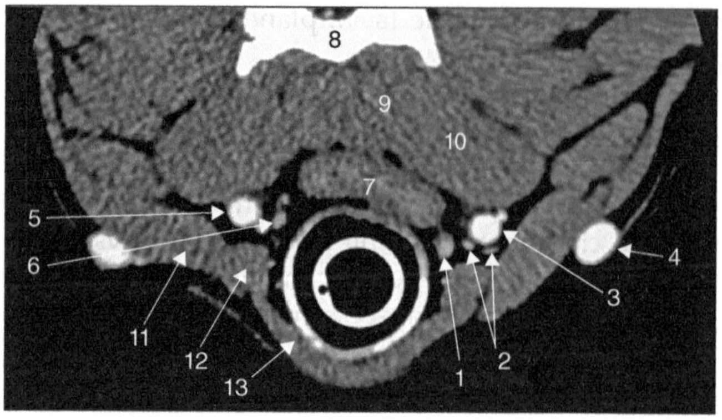

Figure 18.6 CT anatomy of a canine thyroid and its surroundings. 1 = cranial aspect of left lobe; 2 = left cranial thyroid vein; 3 = left internal jugular vein; 4 = left external jugular vein; 5 = right common carotid artery; 6 = right cranial thyroid artery; 7 = esophagus; 8 = C2; 9 = longus colli muscle; 10 = longus capitis muscle; 11 = sternocephalic muscle; 12 = sternothyroid muscle; 13 = sternohyoid muscle.

CT features (Figure 18.11)

- Discontinuity in the hyoid apparatus results in asymmetry of the larynx.
- Concomitant soft tissue swelling and possible gas pocket accumulations.
- Possible soft tissue defects/drain tracts.
- Regional lymphadenopathy.

Neoplasia

Thyroid neoplasia

Thyroid neoplasia in cats is in 99% of cases due to adenomas or adenomatous hyperplasia. In 70% of these, bilateral involvement of the lobes can be detected. Adenomas in cats are functional and result in hyperthyroidism.

In dogs, clinically detected thyroid masses are carcinomas in 90% of cases. These are twice as likely to be unilateral as bilateral, and they are large and fast growing. Carcinomas are non-functional in 90% of the cases and therefore do not result in hyperthyroidism. Functional adenomas are even less common. Since canine thyroid tumors are almost always non-secreting, thyroid masses will usually only be detected after gaining a size large enough to cause mechanical obstruction of the surrounding structures. Ectopic thyroid tissue located anywhere from the base of the tongue to the base of the heart can become neoplastic (Figure 18.12). Predisposed breeds for carcinomas are boxers, golden retrievers and possibly beagle hounds.

CT features (Figure 18.13)

- Large, inhomogeneous, soft tissue mass with moderate contrast enhancement. Hypodense areas (necrosis or hemorrhage) alternated with hyperdense zones (normal parenchyma, areas of dystrophic mineralization or dense connective tissue).
- Carcinomas are often locally aggressive with an increased rate of local tissue invasion (blood vessels, muscles, nerves, trachea, esophagus) with increased tumor size. Carcinomas also more often contain areas of dystrophic mineralization.
- The lungs are the primary site of metastatic spread after local invasion of the thyroid veins. Subsequent CT of the thorax is strongly recommended. Other sites of metastatic spread include the regional lymph nodes, kidneys, spleen, liver, bone and spine.

Pharyngeal neoplasia

Pharyngeal neoplasia is related to oral neoplasia (*see* Chapter 12). The most common oropharyngeal neoplasias are malignant melanoma, squamous cell carcinoma and fibrosarcoma in dogs, and lymphoma in cats.

Laryngeal neoplasia

Primary neoplasia of the larynx occurs uncommonly in small animals. The most common canine laryngeal tumors reported are carcinoma and rhabdomyoma in dogs, and lymphoma and squamous cell carcinoma in cats.

CT features (Figure 18.14)

- Laryngeal tumors are asymmetric intramural tumors with intraluminal and possible extraluminal extension of the mass, creating varying degrees of laryngeal obstruction. CT provides adequate assessment of tumor involvement in the perilaryngeal structures and tumor margins.
- Inhomogeneous soft tissue mass with moderate contrast enhancement. Often central hypodense areas of necrosis or hemorrhage.
- Lysis of the hyoid bones can be seen.

Reference

Kang H, Lee H, Kwak H, Kim N and Lee K (2008) Imaging diagnosis – congenital structural hyoid bone abnormalities in a dog. *Vet Radiol US* **49**: 357–9.

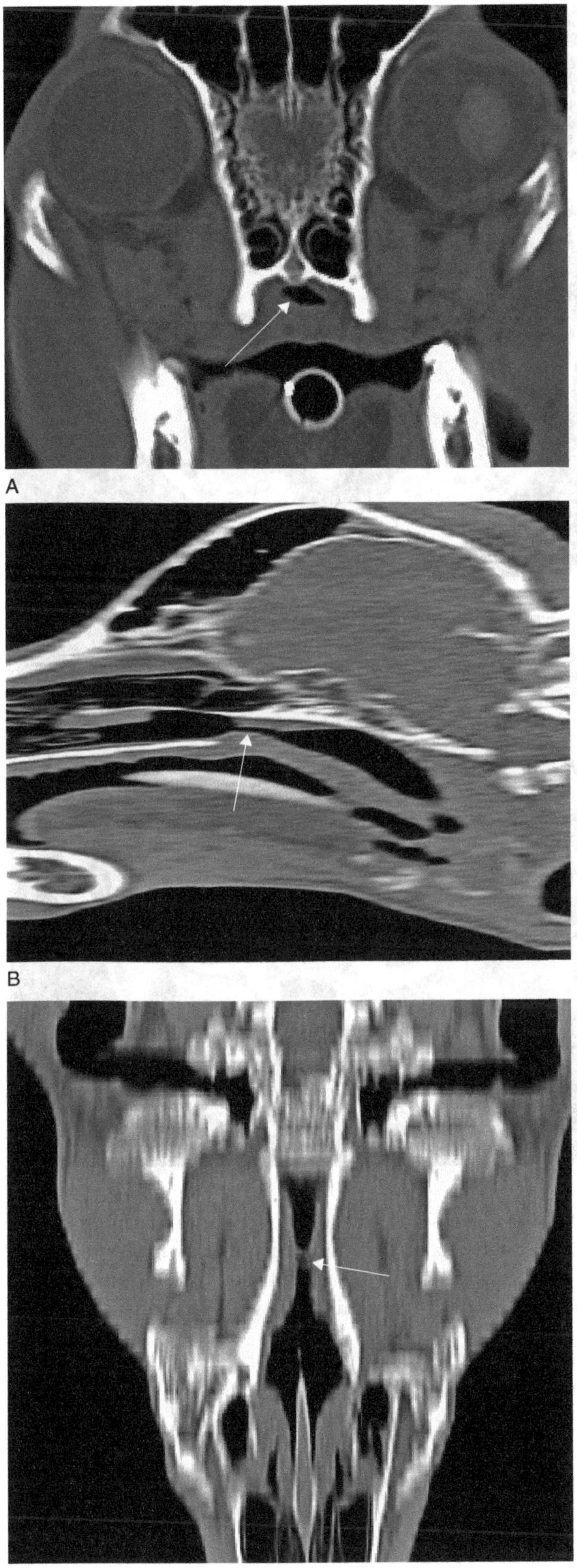

Figure 18.7 Adult dog with nasopharyngeal stenosis. (A) Pre-contrast transverse, and reconstructed (B) sagittal and (C) dorsal CT images show a circumferential narrowing of the nasopharynx (arrow) with presence of an orifice, caudal to the choanae. Note the dorsal displacement of the soft palate on the sagittal image.

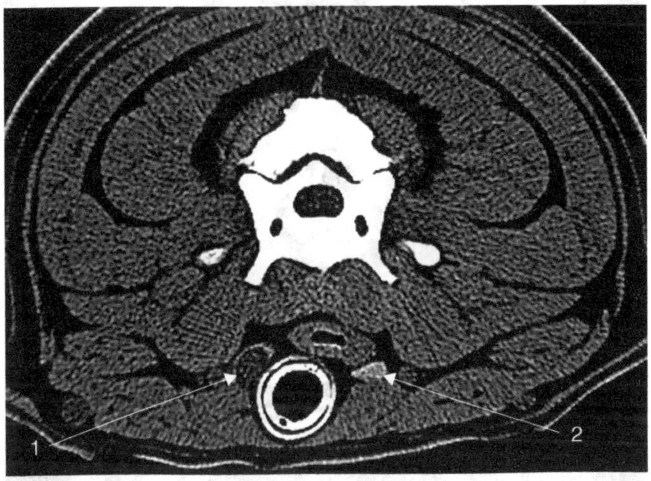

Figure 18.8 Adult dog with thyroid cyst. Transverse CT image shows (1) the right thyroid lobe containing a homogeneous hypodense (30 HU) cyst, measuring 1 cm in diameter. Normal thyroid parenchyma surrounds the cyst. The normal left thyroid lobe (2) shows a pre-contrast attenuation value of 115 HU.

Further Reading

Allen HS, Broussard J and Noone K (1999) Nasopharyngeal diseases in cats: a retrospective study of 53 cases (1991–1998). *J Am Anim Hosp Assoc* **35**: 457–61.

Cole LK and Samii V (2007) Contrast-enhanced computed tomographic imaging of the auditory tube in mesaticephalic dogs. *Vet Radiol Ultrasound* **48**: 125–8.

Drost WT, Mattoon JS, Samii VF, Weisbrode SE and Hoshaw-Woodard SL. Computed tomographic densitometry of normal feline thyroid glands. *Vet Radiol Ultrasound* **45**: 112–16.

George TF and Smallwood JE (1992) Anatomic atlas for computed tomography in the mesaticephalic dog: head and neck. *Vet Radiol Ultrasound* **33**: 217–40.

Nicholson I, Halfacree Z, Whatmough C, Mantis P and Baines S (2008) Computed tomography as an aid to management of chronic oropharyngeal stick injury in the dog. *J Small Anim Pract* **49**: 451–7.

Phillips DE, Radlinsky MG, Fischer JR and Biller DS (2003) Cystic thyroid and parathyroid lesions in cats. *J Am Anim Hosp Assoc* **39**: 349–54.

Taeymans O, Schwarz T, Duchateau L *et al.* (2008) Computed tomographic features of the normal canine thyroid gland. *Vet Radiol Ultrasound* **49**: 13–9.

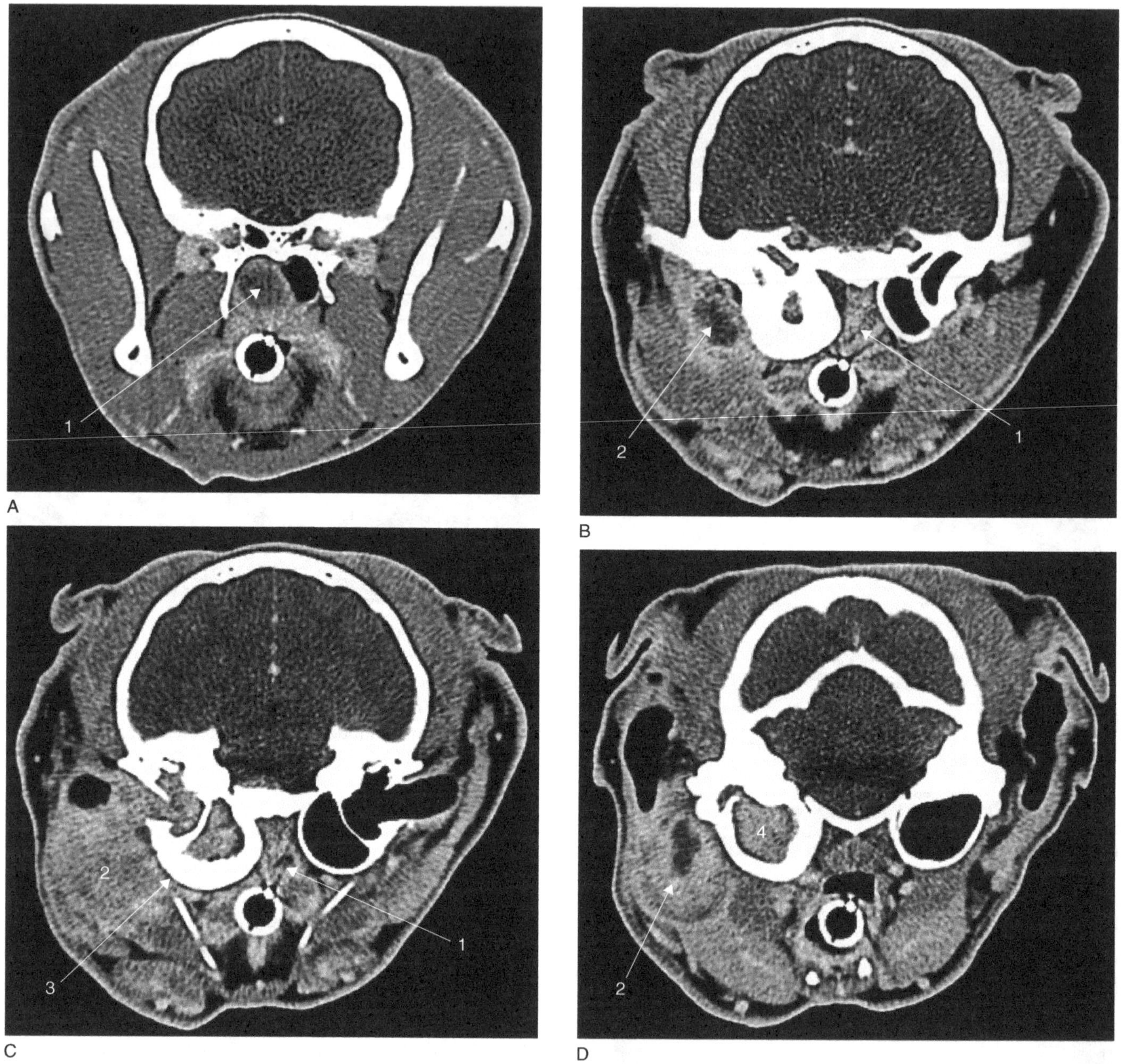

Figure 18.9 One-year-old cat with nasopharyngeal polyp. Post-contrast transverse CT images show a large nasopharyngeal polyp in the right nasopharyngeal area. Images are from rostral (upper left) to caudal (lower right). 1 = multi-lobulated nasopharyngeal soft tissue masses with peripheral ring-like enhancement; 2 = multi-lobulated soft tissue masses with peripheral ring-like enhancement in the auditory tube; 3 = marked thickening of the right tympanic bulla wall; 4 = soft-tissue mass in the right tympanic bulla.

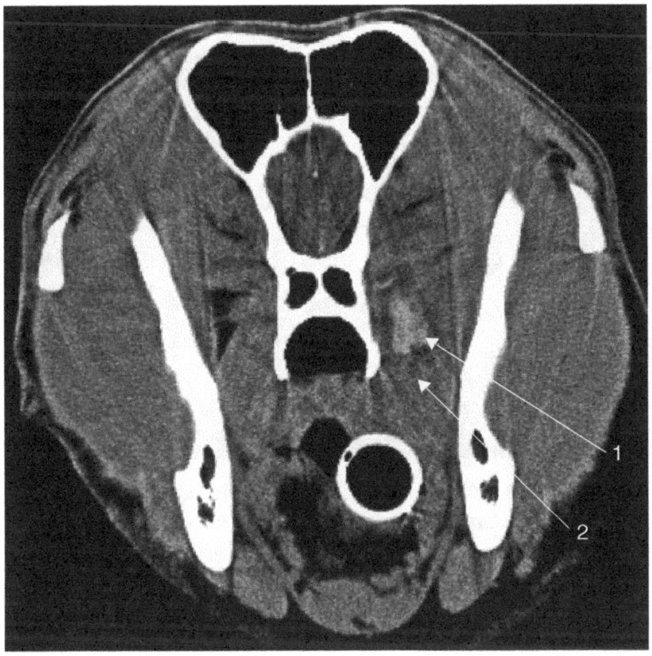

A

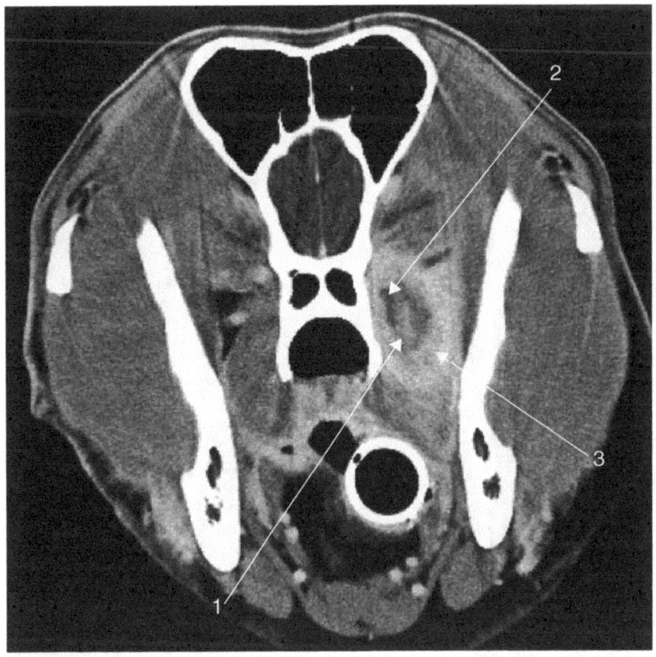

B

Figure 18.10 (A) Pre- and (B) post-contrast transverse CT images of a wooden foreign body in the left retropharyngeal tissues. 1 = foreign body (110 HU on both images); 2 = surrounding abscess (50 HU pre-contrast/100 HU post-contrast); 3 = abscess wall (65 HU pre-contrast/155 HU post-contrast).

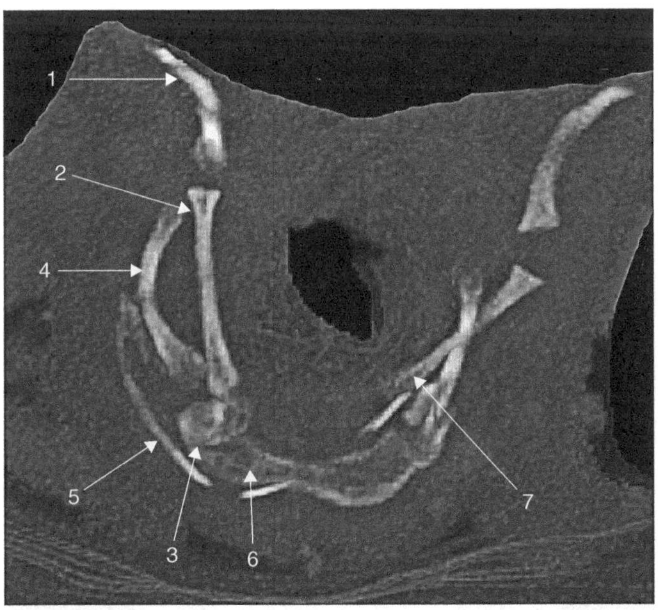

A

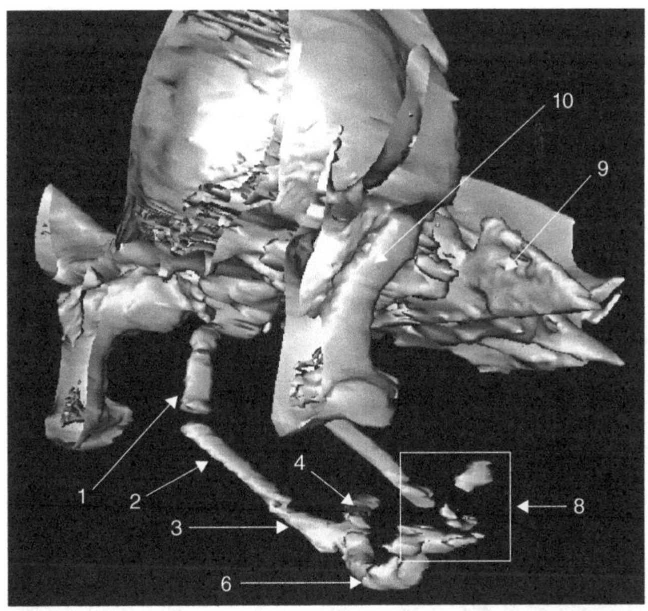

B

Figure 18.11 (A) Craniocaudal 3D-MIP reconstructed CT image of the hyoid apparatus of a dog that was hit by a car two days ago. Left on the image is on the patient's right. The left epihyoid bone is medially displaced as a consequence of a luxation in between the epihyoid and ceratohyoid bones. (B) Left cranioventral–right caudodorsal oblique 3-D SR reconstruction of the hyoid apparatus of a dog suffering from a gunshot wound. Left is cranial for the patient. Comminuted fractures are noted at the level of the left ceratohyoid and thyrohyoid bones. The left epihyoid bone is displaced caudally as a consequence of a luxation between the epihyoid and ceratohyoid bones. 1 = right stylohyoid bone; 2 = right epihyoid bone; 3 = right ceratohyoid bone; 4 = right thyrohyoid bone; 5 = thyroid cartilage; 6 = basihyoid bone; 7 = medially displaced left epihyoid bone; 8 = fractured left ceratohyoid and thyrohyoid bones; 9 = transverse process of C1; 10 = left mandibular ramus.

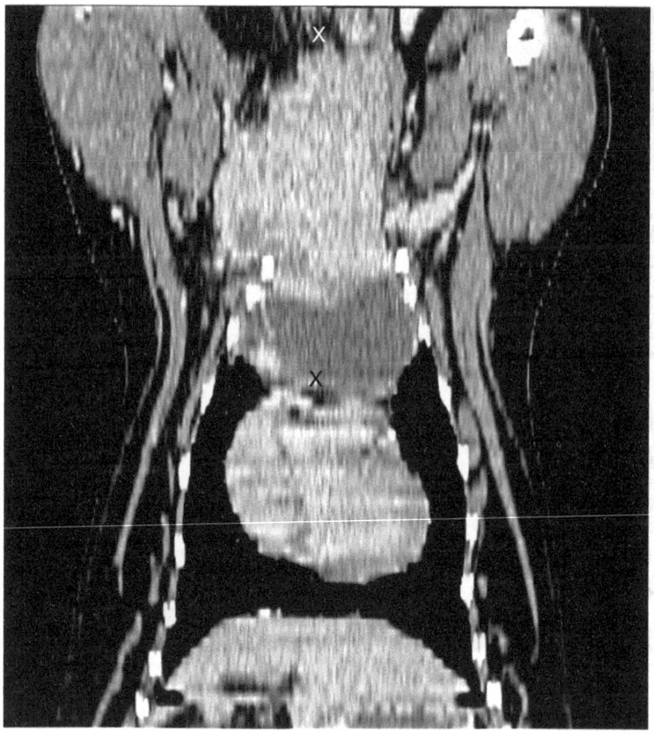

Figure 18.12 Adult dog with neoplastic ectopic thyroid tissue. Post-contrast MPR dorsal reconstructed CT image shows a moderately enhancing soft tissue mass (45 HU pre-contrast, 130 HU post-contrast) ventral to the trachea, located cranial to the thoracic inlet (white cross) and expanding caudally to the level of the heart base (black cross). Note its caudal cystic component (16 HU).

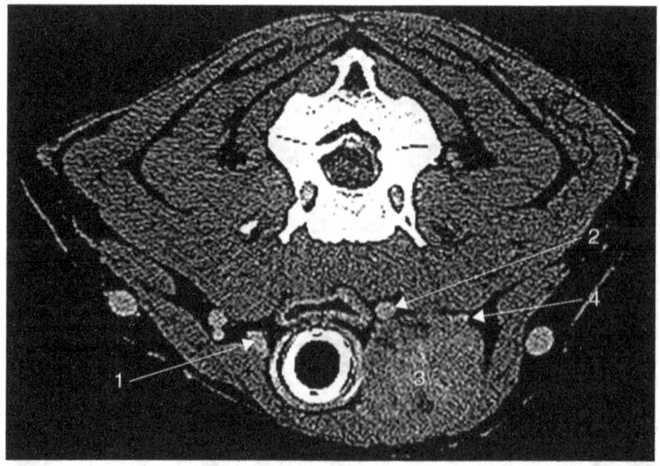

Figure 18.13 Adult dog with thyroid carcinoma. Post-contrast transverse CT image shows a mass-effect on the left side, displacing the trachea and left common carotid artery to the right. No local tissue invasion was detected. 1 = normal right thyroid lobe; 2 = left internal carotid artery; 3 = enlarged and heterogeneous left thyroid lobe; 4 = left internal jugular vein.

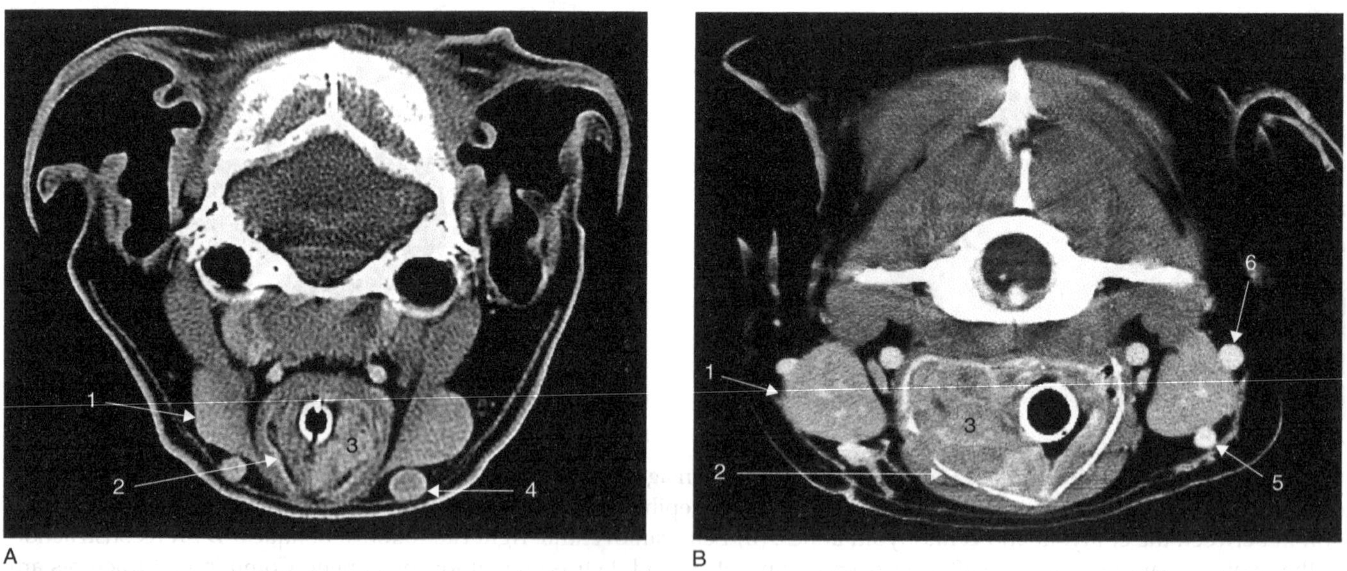

Figure 18.14 Post-contrast transverse CT images of laryngeal masses. (A) Squamous cell carcinoma of the larynx with intra-luminal extension in a cat. (B) Round cell tumor (suspected plasma cell) of the larynx with intra-luminal extension in a dog. Note the focal lysis of the right side of the thyroid cartilage. 1 = right mandibular salivary gland; 2 = thyroid cartilage; 3 = laryngeal mass; 4 = left external jugular vein; 5 = left linguofacial vein; 6 = left retromandibular vein.

CHAPTER NINETEEN

Brain

Silke Hecht

Imaging Protocol

See Table 19.1.

CT: Anatomy

General

Based on embryologic development, the brain can be subdivided into prosencephalon (forebrain: telencephalon and diencephalon), mesencephalon (midbrain) and rhombencephalon (hindbrain: metencephalon and myelencephalon). The anatomic subdivision of the brain is summarized in Table 19.2.

Identification of specific structures of the brain is aided by familiarity with their anatomic relationships to surrounding osseous structures and cerebrospinal fluid-filled spaces. The brain is contained within the cranial cavity of the skull, which is formed by the ethmoid, presphenoid, basisphenoid, occipital, parietal, temporal and frontal bones. While the roof of the cavity remains largely undivided, the base is divided into three fossae (Figure 19.1A). The rostral fossa extends from the cribriform plate to the level of the optic canals and contains the olfactory bulbs and the rostral parts of the cerebral hemispheres. The middle fossa extends from the optic canals to the petrosal crests and contains the pituitary gland, temporal and parietal lobes of the cerebral hemispheres (Figure 19.1B). The caudal fossa extends from the caudal limit of the pituitary fossa to the foramen magnum and contains the mesencephalon, pons, medulla and cerebellum. Additional useful osseous landmarks include the falx cerebri separating the two cerebral hemispheres, the tentorium cerebelli separating cerebellum and cerebrum, the dorsum sellae turcicae, the chiasmatic sulcus and various bony foramina and canals (*see also* Chapters 16, 20 and 21).

The brain is surrounded by cerebrospinal fluid in the subarachnoid space. The ventricular system consists of the paired lateral ventricles, third ventricle, mesencephalic aqueduct and the fourth ventricle. Cerebrospinal fluid, gray matter and white matter differ in density and can be distinguished when a narrow window width is used (cerebrospinal fluid ±5–10 HU; white matter ±25–30 HU; gray matter: ±35–50 HU).

Following intravenous administration of contrast medium, intracranial structures outside the blood–brain barrier, such as the pituitary gland, choroid plexus and blood vessels, show contrast enhancement, while normal brain parenchyma does not enhance.

Disease Features

General

Many different disorders of the brain may result in similar CT findings, and familiarity with signalment and pertinent history are crucial when evaluating CT images. Intracranial lesions may be extra-axial (i.e. originating outside actual brain parenchyma) or intra-axial (i.e. originating from brain parenchyma). Differential diagnoses for extra-axial lesions include neoplastic (e.g. meningioma), inflammatory (e.g. meningitis) and traumatic lesions (e.g. epidural hematoma). Differential diagnoses for solitary intra-axial lesions include hematoma, cyst, abscess/granuloma, infarct and neoplasia. Although inflammatory brain diseases usually appear as multifocal lesions, solitary masses may be encountered on occasion. Differential diagnoses for multifocal brain lesions include inflammation, infarcts, metabolic/toxic/nutritional encephalopathies and some intracranial neoplasms. Contrast enhancement of a lesion indicates vascularization and disruption of the blood–brain barrier.

Concurrent findings in brain disease

Pathologic sequelae associated with brain disease include mass effect, vasogenic edema, brain herniation,

Veterinary Computed Tomography, First Edition. Edited by Tobias Schwarz, Jimmy Saunders.

Table 19.1
CT imaging protocol (intravenous contrast study: standard protocol; *see* Chapter 5).

Series	Pre- and post-contrast	Dorsal plane (following post-contrast scan)*
Decubitus	Ventral	Dorsal
Special positioning	N/A	Dorsal recumbency, head flexed 90°
Slice orientation	Transverse (perpendicular to hard palate)	Dorsal (parallel to hard palate)
Scan margins	Cribriform plate ⟵⟶ Atlas	Parietal bones (dorsal) ⟵⟶ hard palate/base of skull (ventral)
Voltage (kVp)	130	
Current (mA)	150	
Tube rotation time (s)	1	
Slice width (collimated, mm)	3–5**	1–2
Sequential slice interval (mm)	3–5**	1–2
Kernel frequency	Standard	
Window level (HU)	Soft tissue: +30 Bone: +600	
Window width (HU)	Soft tissue: 200 Bone: 2000	

*Dorsal and sagittal reconstructed imaging is routinely performed and does not require additional image acquisition. Additional image acquisition with dorsal slice orientation can be performed to evaluate integrity of the cribriform plate or in cases where partial volume averaging and beam hardening artifacts interfere with evaluation of the caudal fossa on transverse images.
**Software of some CT units allows summation of raw data from thinly collimated slices (1 mm) to reformat thick-section (5 mm) images. This technique significantly improves image quality and may be considered in cases where artifacts hamper evaluation of the caudal fossa.

Table 19.2
Brain anatomy.

Brain subdivision	Major derivates	Lumen
Telencephalon	Cerebral cortex (hemispheres)	Lateral ventricles
	Basal nuclei Limbic system	
Diencephalon	Epithalamus Thalamus Hypothalamus	Third ventricle
Mesencephalon	Tectum Tegmentum Cerebral peduncles	Mesencephalic aqueduct
Metencephalon	Pons	Fourth ventricle
	Cerebellum	Fourth ventricle
Myelencephalon	Medulla oblongata	Fourth ventricle

hydrocephalus and hemorrhage. Cerebral necrosis is occasionally seen in animals with seizures.

Mass effect

Space-occupying lesions within the cranial vault (e.g. tumor or edema) are commonly associated with a mass effect, even if the underlying lesion itself cannot be delineated.

CT features
- Shift of the falx cerebri (Figure 19.2).
- Compression of the ventricular system.

Vasogenic edema

Damage to brain capillaries results in leakage of fluid into the extracellular space, which migrates along the white matter fiber tracts.

CT features (Figure 19.2)
- Extensive hypodense area, often exhibiting mass effect.

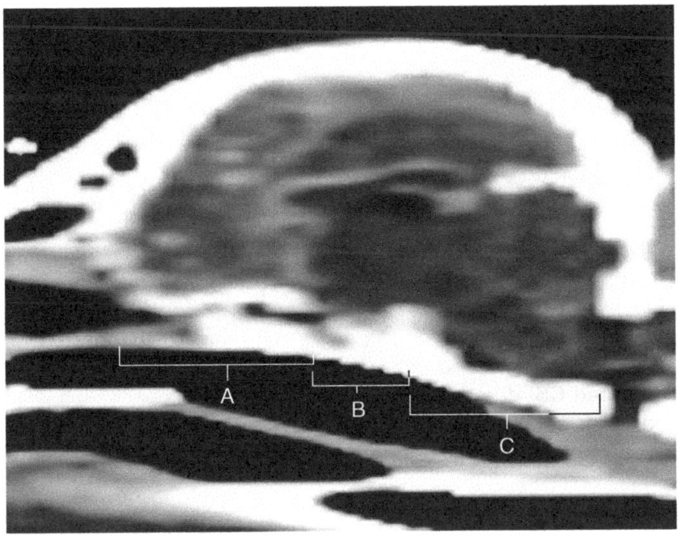

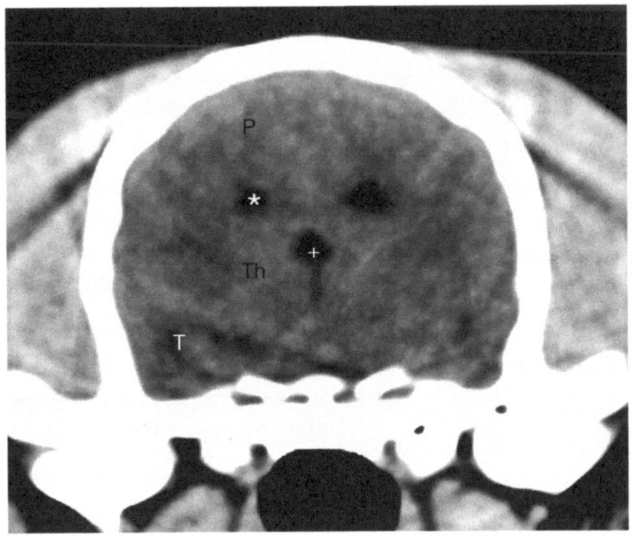

A B

Figure 19.1 CT anatomy of the canine brain. (A) Sagittally reconstructed CT image illustrating location of rostral (A), middle (B) and caudal fossa (C). (B) Transverse CT image at the level of the middle fossa showing lateral (asterisk) and third (+) ventricles, thalamus (Th), parietal (P) and temporal (T) lobes.

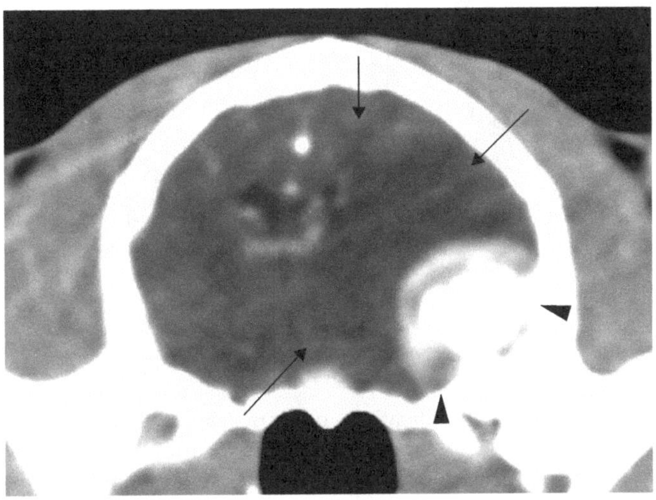

Figure 19.2 Adult cat with meningioma. Post-contrast transverse CT image shows a large intracranial extra-axial mass (arrowheads). Extensive hypodense area associated with the left cerebral hemisphere resulting in midline shift of the falx cerebri is consistent with vasogenic edema and mass effect (arrows).

- Post-contrast: underlying lesion may show enhancement while edema remains hypodense.

Brain herniation

Increase in intracranial pressure (e.g. due to an intracranial mass) can lead to compression and displacement of brain parenchyma.

CT features

- Evaluation best performed on sagittal reconstructions.
- Foramen magnum herniation: herniation of the caudal portion of the cerebellum into and through the foramen magnum.
- Caudal transtentorial herniation: displacement of portions of the cerebral cortex (or cortices) ventral to the tentorium cerebelli.

Hydrocephalus

Hydrocephalus is defined as abnormal accumulation of cerebrospinal fluid within the cranium, which can be classified in various ways (Table 19.3).

CT features

- Dilatation of one or more ventricles and/or dilatation of the subarachnoid space (Figure 19.3).
- Potential additional findings dependent on etiology: congenital anomalies, intracranial mass, traumatic lesions.

Note: Diagnosis of clinically significant hydrocephalus can be challenging. Ventriculomegaly and ventricular asymmetry are common findings in asymptomatic animals and may or may not represent a clinically significant change. Additionally, brain atrophy is an expected finding in older animals. Therefore, especially mild ventricular and/or subarachnoid space dilation should be judged in light of clinical presentation.

Table 19.3
Classification of hydrocephalus.

Hydrocephalus	Subclassification	Definition
Location	Internal	Ventricular system
	External	Subarachnoid space
Etiology	Obstructive	Blockage of CSF flow
	Non-obstructive	Compensatory (decreased volume of brain parenchyma; hydrocephalus *ex vacuo*) Decreased resorption or increased production of CSF (very rare)
	Congenital	
	Acquired	
Pressure	Hypertensive	Increased pressure within dilated CSF-filled space
	Normotensive	Normal pressure within dilated CSF-filled space
Morphology	Communicating	Communication between ventricular system and subarachnoid space
	Non-communicating	No communication between ventricular system and subarachnoid space

CSF = cerebrospinal fluid.

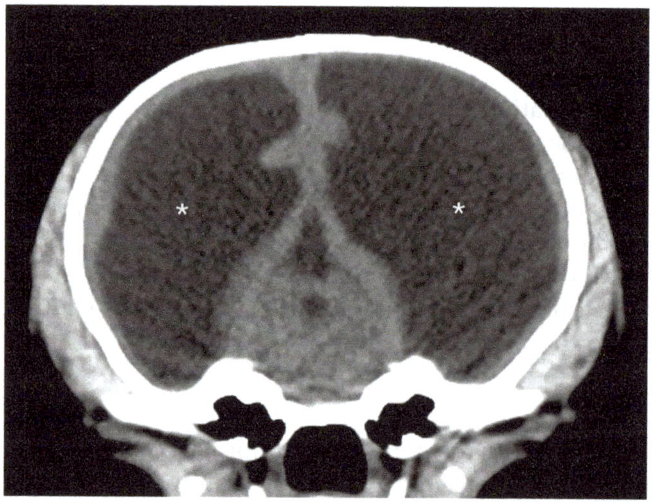

Figure 19.3 Yorkshire terrier with congenital hydrocephalus. Transverse CT image shows severe dilatation of the lateral ventricles (asterisks).

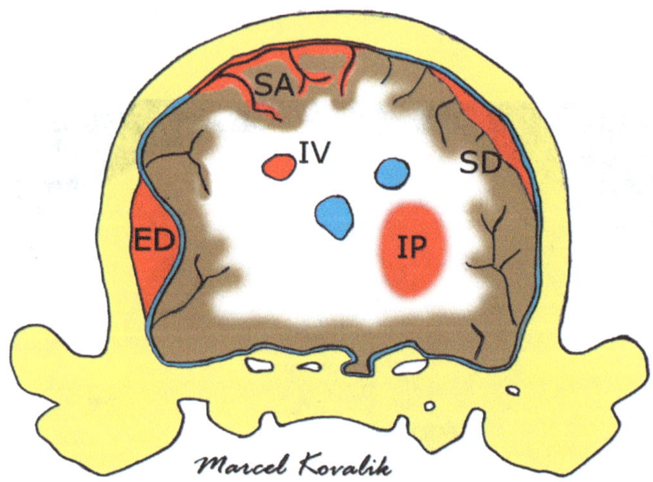

Figure 19.4 Classification of intracranial hemorrhage. Schematic transverse image illustrates location and appearance of epidural (ED), subdural (SD), subarachnoid (SA), intraparenchymal (IP) and intraventricular (IV) hematoma.

Intracranial hemorrhage

Intracranial hemorrhage can be classified based on location as epidural, subdural, subarachnoid, intraparenchymal or intraventricular (Figure 19.4). Epidural, subdural and subarachnoid hemorrhages are typically associated with trauma, while intraparenchymal hemorrhage may occur secondary to a variety of conditions including vascular malformation, coagulopathy, neoplasia and parasite migration. Intraventricular hemorrhage may be associated with trauma or extension of intraparenchymal hemorrhage into the ventricular system.

CT features

- Epidural hemorrhage: peripheral focal biconvex mass that may cross dural folds such as falx cerebri and tentorium cerebelli, but not sutures.
- Subdural hemorrhage: peripheral crescent-shaped collection of blood which may cross suture lines but is limited by the falx and tentorium.
- Subarachnoid and intraventricular hemorrhages: admixture of blood and cerebrospinal fluid; potential separation of fluid into hemorrhagic and non-hemorrhagic strata or formation of thrombi.

Table 19.4
Intracranial hemorrhage.

Time after hemorrhage	Events	Density
Immediately	Hematoma forms heterogeneous mass consisting of red blood cells, white blood cells, platelet clumps and serum	40–60 HU
Early hours	Formation of meshwork of fibrin fibrils and globin molecules; clot retraction	60–80 HU
Days	Further clot retraction; serum extrusion and vasogenic edema	80–100 HU in center, with hypodense halo
Weeks	Breakdown of globin molecules	Density decreases 0.7–1.5 HU/day from periphery to center
Weeks/months	Digestion of blood degradation products by macrophages	Resolution of hematoma or persistence of hypodense area

- Intraparenchymal hemorrhage: intra-axial mass lesion(s) of variable size and density.
- Attenuation properties of intracranial blood are determined by the aggregation of globin molecules in the hematoma, i.e. density varies with age of the hematoma (Table 19.4).
- Possible concurrent findings dependent on etiology: brain edema, intracranial mass, traumatic osseous changes (fractures).

Cerebral necrosis

Necrosis of hippocampus, piriform lobes and other areas of the cerebral cortex have been described in dogs and cats with seizures. It may not be possible to determine whether brain changes found on CT and/or histopathology represent the underlying cause or the result of seizures.

CT features
- Bilaterally symmetric hypodense areas associated with hippocampus, piriform lobes or other areas of the cerebral cortex without mass effect.
- Post-contrast: variable enhancement.

Malformation/Developmental

Congenital and developmental anomalies are frequently diagnosed in dogs but are rare in cats.

Congenital hydrocephalus

Congenital hydrocephalus is most commonly seen in toy and brachycephalic breed dogs.

CT features
- Dilatation of the ventricular system of variable severity (Figure 19.3).

Hydranencephaly/Porencephaly

In hydranencephaly there is lack of development and/or near complete destruction of the neocortex. Porencephaly appears as cavities in the cerebrum due to cell destruction or failure of development.

CT features
- Hydranencephaly: reduction of size of one or both cerebral cortices to a thin mantle surrounding a large, centrally located cavity.
- Porencephaly: cavitary areas associated with brain parenchyma which may communicate with subarachnoid space and/or ventricles.

Meningo-/encephalo-/meningoencephalocele

These disorders are uncommon in small animals.

CT features
- Protrusion of brain tissue and/or meninges through a calvarial defect.

Intracranial intra-arachnoid cysts

These anomalies arise from splitting/duplication of the arachnoidea in early embryonic development. Quadrigeminal cistern cysts dorsal to the quadrigeminal plate are most common, but cerebellomedullary

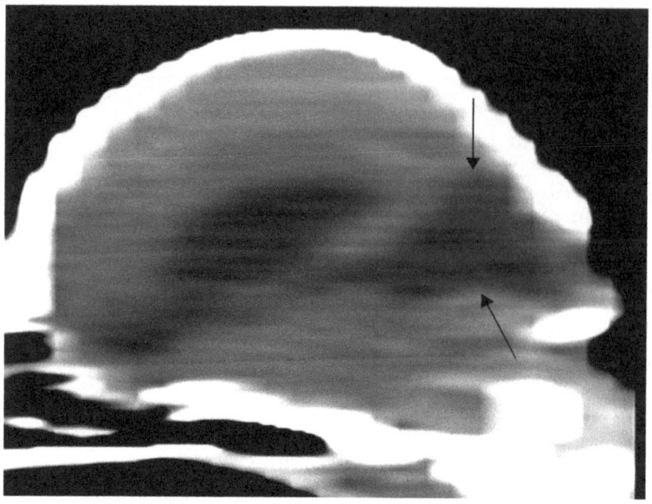

Figure 19.5 Yorkshire terrier with a quadrigeminal cistern cyst. Sagittal reconstructed CT image shows a large hypodense structure associated with the caudal cranium (arrows), with resultant compression of the cerebellum. Hydrocephalus is also visible.

cistern cysts have also been reported. Quadrigeminal cysts are of variable clinical significance and may be incidental.

CT features

- Well-circumscribed areas in specific locations containing fluid isodense to cerebrospinal fluid.
- Compression of occipital lobes and/or cerebellum.
- Sagittal reconstruction is useful in establishing cyst location and size (Figure 19.5).

Chiari-like malformation and syringomyelia

A disorder similar to Chiari type I malformation in humans has been reported in dogs. Cavalier King Charles spaniels are most commonly affected, but the disease is seen in a variety of breeds and can be found in symptomatic and asymptomatic animals.

CT features

- Sagittal reconstruction is most useful.
- Crowding of the caudal fossa with compression and, in severe cases, herniation of the cerebellum into or through the foramen magnum.
- Additional findings: hydrocephalus, focal 'kink' of the cranial aspect of the spinal cord, hypodense areas associated with spinal cord parenchyma (syringohydromyelia).

Cerebellar hypoplasia

Cerebellar hypoplasia can occur secondary to in utero/perinatal viral infection (most commonly parvovirus) or as a primary developmental defect.

CT features

- Small size of the cerebellum indicated by increased cerebrospinal fluid around the cerebellum and extending into the folia.
- CT diagnosis can be difficult in mild cases.

Dandy-Walker malformation

The primary abnormality in this group of congenital disorders is partial or complete absence of the cerebellar vermis and cystic dilation of the fourth ventricle. Additional abnormalities may be present.

CT features

- Enlarged caudal fossa filled with an enlarged fourth ventricle.
- Small size/partial absence of cerebellum.
- Hydrocephalus.

Trauma

CT is considered an excellent modality to assess patients with head trauma because it is fast and accurate in the evaluation of bony structures and intracranial hemorrhage.

Acute trauma

CT features

- Intracranial hemorrhage.
- Brain edema, mass effect, brain herniation.
- Skull fractures.

Chronic trauma

CT features

- Intracranial hemorrhage.
- Skull fractures (Figure 19.6).
- Meningeal and brain parenchymal changes compatible with meningoencephalomyelitis/brain abscess (Figure 19.6).
- Parenchymal brain defects with compensatory cerebrospinal fluid filling (hydrocephalus *ex vacuo*).

Inflammation

Inflammatory brain diseases can affect brain parenchyma (encephalitis), meninges (meningitis) or both

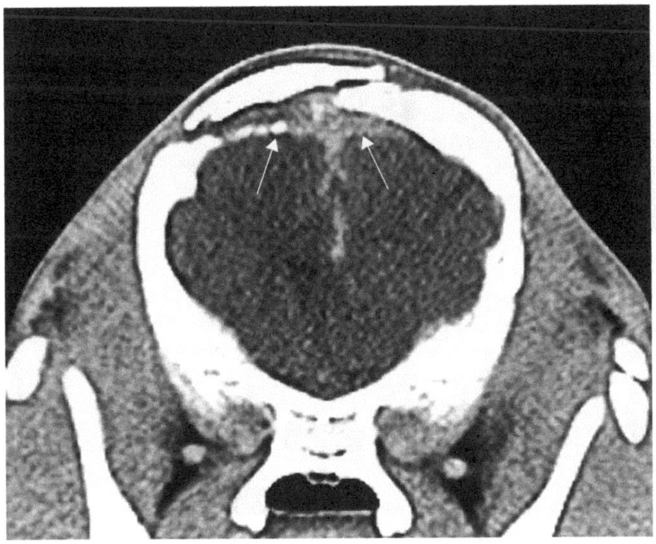

Figure 19.6 Puppy with bacterial meningitis 2 weeks following bite wounds to the head. Post-contrast transverse CT image shows skull fractures and extensive meningeal enhancement (arrows).

(meningoencephalitis), and can be subdivided into infectious inflammatory and non-infectious inflammatory disorders. These diseases may or may not cause changes detectable with CT.

Canine distemper virus encephalitis

The two most common clinical forms of distemper encephalitis are acute encephalitis in young dogs and chronic encephalitis in adult dogs.

CT features

- Focal or multifocal hypodense lesions:
  - post-contrast: uniform or ring enhancement.
- Predilection for white matter.
- May be associated with edema and mass effect.

Feline infectious peritonitis virus encephalitis

Neurological signs are generally associated with the dry form of feline infectious peritonitis, which results in pyogranulomatous inflammation of leptomeninges, choroid plexus, ependyma and brain parenchyma.

CT features

- Post-contrast: enhancement of ventricular lining, choroid plexus and meninges.
- Hydrocephalus.

Bacterial meningoencephalitis

Mechanisms of bacterial infection of the central nervous system include hematogeneous spread, contiguous infection from adjacent structures (inner ears, cribriform plate, sinuses, eyes and vertebrae), direct inoculation (trauma, bite wound and surgery) and migration of foreign bodies or aberrant parasites. In addition to meningitis and meningoencephalitis, central nervous system infection may result in focal parenchymal abscesses or empyema in subdural or epidural locations.

CT features

- Meningitis (Figure 19.6):
  - meningeal thickening
  - post-contrast: contrast enhancement.
- Encephalitis:
  - hypodensity of brain parenchyma
  - post-contrast: +/- enhancement.
- Abscess/empyema:
  - hypodense mass(es)
  - post-contrast: ring enhancement, usually associated with edema/mass effect.

Fungal meningoencephalitis

Several fungal infections have been reported to affect the central nervous system, including cryptococcosis, phaeohyphomycosis, blastomycosis, histoplasmosis, aspergillosis and fusariosis.

CT features

- Very variable.
- Solitary or multifocal parenchymal lesions with associated mass effect:
  - post-contrast: variable contrast enhancement.
- Meningeal, ependymal and choroid plexus enhancement.
- Extension outside the cranial vault possible (Figure 19.7).

Parasitic meningoencephalitis

Parasitic meningoencephalitis in dogs and cats is caused by aberrant migration of parasites such as *Dirofilaria*, *Baylisascaris*, *Cuterebra*, *Taenia*, *Ancylostoma*, *Toxascaris* and *Angiostrongylus*.

CT features

- Focal or multifocal parenchymal lesions
  - post-contrast: peripheral contrast enhancement.
- Intraparenchymal hemorrhage.
- Meningeal enhancement.

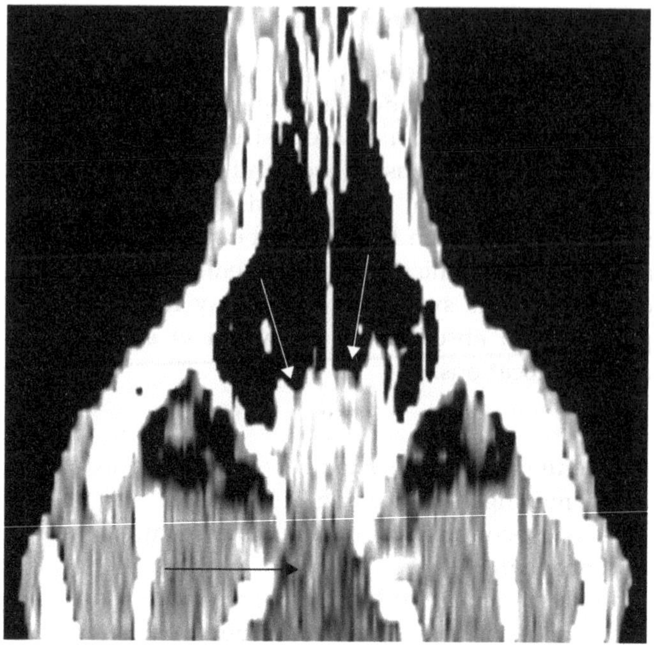

Figure 19.7 Labrador retriever with fungal encephalitis (blastomycosis). Post-contrast dorsally reconstructed CT image shows a homogeneously enhancing mass associated with the olfactory bulbs, extending through the cribriform plate into the caudal nasal cavity (white arrows). Midline shift of the falx cerebri (black arrow) is consistent with mass effect due to brain edema.

Protozoal meningoencephalitis

Protozoal meningoencephalitis may be caused by *Toxoplasma* and *Neospora* infection in dogs and *Toxoplasma* infection in cats.

CT features

- Variable.
- Focal or multifocal parenchymal lesions.
- Post-contrast: mild contrast enhancement.

Granulomatous meningoencephalitis and necrotizing meningoencephalitis

Granulomatous meningoencephalitis is an inflammatory central nervous system disorder of uncertain etiology, which can affect any breed but most often occurs in young to middle-aged toy breed dogs. Necrotizing meningoencephalitis is of uncertain cause and is characterized by cavitary necrosis in the neuroparenchyma. The disease was initially described in pugs ('pug dog encephalitis'), but similar disorders have since been reported in other small breeds. A distinct form of necrotizing meningoencephalitis described mainly in Yorkshire terriers has been termed 'necrotizing leukoencephalitis'.

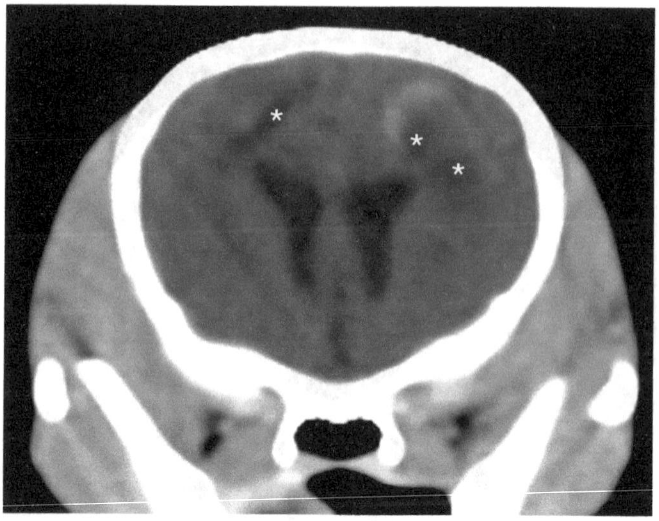

Figure 19.8 Adult Yorkshire terrier with necrotizing meningoencephalitis/leukoencephalitis. Transverse CT image shows numerous hypodense lesions (asterisks) in both cerebral hemispheres with mild to moderate peripheral contrast enhancement.

CT features

- Disseminated granulomatous meningoencephalitis:
  - post-contrast: multiple foci of ill-defined contrast enhancement involving parenchyma and meninges
  - possibly associated with edema and mass effect.
- Focal granulomatous meningoencephalitis:
  - isodense or hyperdense mass
    - post-contrast: variable contrast enhancement
  - possibly associated with edema and mass effect.
- Necrotizing meningoencephalitis/necrotizing leukoencephalitis (Figure 19.8)
  - multifocal hypodense lesions
    - post-contrast: variable contrast enhancement
  - commonly associated with hydrocephalus
  - necrotizing leukoencephalitis typically affects cerebrum and brainstem, while necrotizing meningoencephalitis is usually confined to cerebrum.

Cerebrovascular

The term 'cerebrovascular diseases' refers to all disorders in which there is an area of brain transiently or permanently affected by ischemia or bleeding and/or in which one or more blood vessels of the brain are primarily impaired by a pathological process. While intracranial aneurysms and cerebrovascular malformations play only a minor role in veterinary medicine, acute vascular events (stroke, infarct) are relatively common.

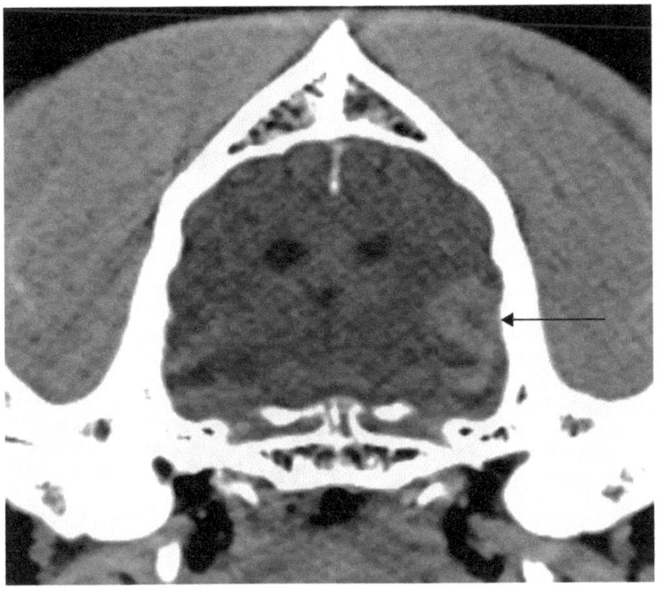

Figure 19.9 Adult dog with acute hemorrhagic infarct due to rupture of a cerebrovascular hamartoma. Transverse CT image prior to contrast medium administration shows a bilobed hyperdense mass within the left temporal lobe (arrow).

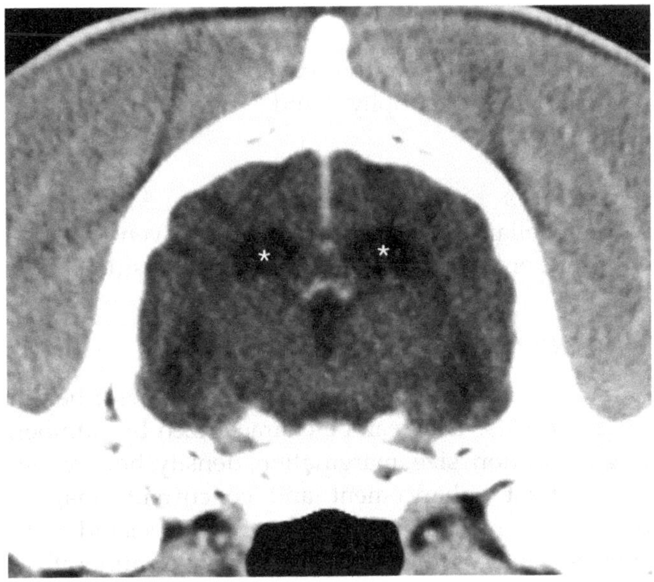

Figure 19.10 Adult dog with ceroid lipofuscinosis. Post-contrast transverse CT image shows ventriculomegaly (asterisks) and dilatation of cerebral sulci, consistent with brain atrophy.

Ischemic stroke

Ischemic strokes can be categorized according to anatomical site, size, age, pathology and etiology (e.g. atherosclerosis, hypertension, chronic renal disease, septic or neoplastic thromboemboli, idiopathic). Territorial infarcts most commonly affect the rostral cerebellar artery, followed by the middle cerebral and the rostral cerebral artery. Lacunar infarcts, unlikely to be detected on CT due to their small size, most commonly affect the caudal perforating arteries, followed by striate arteries (and others).

CT features

- Dependent on size and location of affected vessel and time elapsed between infarct and CT.
- Acute ischemic stroke:
  - slight decrease in density and subtle mass effect due to edema (3–6h after onset of signs)
    - post-contrast: peripheral enhancement (24h to 1 week after infarction).
- Chronic ischemic stroke:
  - increasingly sharp margination of infarcted area with ultimate loss of parenchymal volume.

Hemorrhagic stroke

Hemorrhagic stroke can be classified according to anatomical site, size, age and etiology (e.g. intracranial neoplasia, coagulopathies, parasite migration, cerebral vascular malformation, idiopathic).

CT features (Figure 19.9)

- Dependent on etiology, size and location of intracranial hemorrhage, and time elapsed between vascular event and CT.

Metabolic, nutritional, toxic and degenerative

A variety of conditions is summarized in this group. CT examination may show subtle changes or may be normal.

Metabolic, nutritional, toxic

Examples for diseases in this group include lysosomal storage diseases, mitochondrial encephalopathies, hepatic encephalopathy, thiamine deficiency and myelinolysis.

CT features

- Bilaterally symmetric hypodense lesions in the area of thalamic/deep gray matter nuclei without mass effect:
  - post-contrast: no contrast enhancement.
- Brain atrophy (ventriculomegaly, enlarged cerebral and cerebellar sulci) (Figure 19.10).

Degenerative

Examples of degenerative encephalopathies include neuroaxonal dystrophy and cerebellar cortical abiotrophy.

CT features

- Cerebellar and/or cerebral atrophy (ventriculomegaly, enlarged cerebral and cerebellar sulci).

Neoplasia

Numerous intracranial tumors have been described in dogs and cats. They can be characterized by number, origin, location, size, margination, density, homogeneity, contrast enhancement and concurrent imaging findings (ventriculomegaly, changes associated with cranium and/or meninges, hemorrhage, mineralization, mass effect, edema, cystic or necrotic component, etc.).

Meningeal tumors

Meningiomas originate from the meningeal lining of the brain and are the most common brain tumors in dogs and cats. Other tumor types that can affect the meninges include disseminated histiocytic sarcoma, lymphoma, granular cell tumor and metastases.

CT features

- Meningioma (Figure 19.2)
  - extra-axial rounded or plaque-like smoothly marginated mass in broad-based contact with underlying bone
  - usually single, can be multiple
  - isodense or hyperdense to brain parenchyma, mineralization or cystic component possible
    - post-contrast:
      - usually strong and homogeneous enhancement
      - may show 'dural tail sign' (linear enhancement extending along meninges adjacent to the mass)
  - may be associated with brain edema, mass effect, hyperostosis (cat > dog) or pressure atrophy of adjacent bone.
- Other meningeal neoplasms
  - variable, may mimic meningiomas.

Glial tumors

Glial tumors (astrocytoma, glioblastoma multiforme, oligodendroglioma) typically appear as single intra-axial lesions.

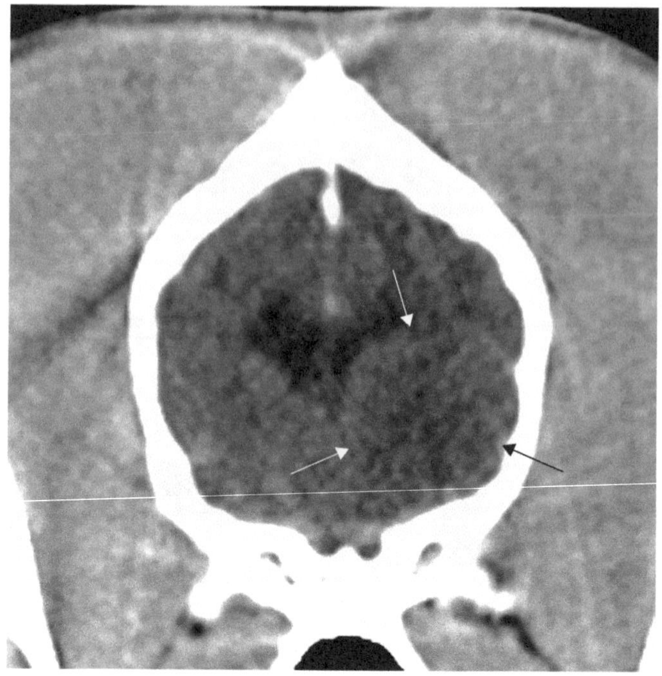

Figure 19.11 Boxer with poorly differentiated glioma. Post-contrast transverse CT image shows an indistinct intra-axial non-enhancing hyperdense mass involving left piriform lobe, parietal lobe and thalamus (arrows). Compression of the left lateral ventricle is consistent with mass effect.

CT features (Figure 19.11)

- Variable in appearance, ranging from an ovoid or amorphous mass to a diffuse infiltrate with distinct to poorly defined margins.
- Hypodense, isodense to hyperdense on pre-contrast images.
- Post-contrast:
  - enhancement ranging from none to strong
  - uniform, non-uniform and ring-enhancing patterns
  - concurrent brain edema and/or hemorrhage possible.

Ventricular tumors

Choroid plexus tumors originate from the choroid plexus within the ventricular system and predominantly occur in the third and fourth ventricle. Other ventricular tumors include ependymomas and meningiomas.

CT features (Figure 19.12)

- Variable sized rounded or lobulated mass associated with the ventricular system:
  - post-contrast: usually strongly contrast enhancing mass.

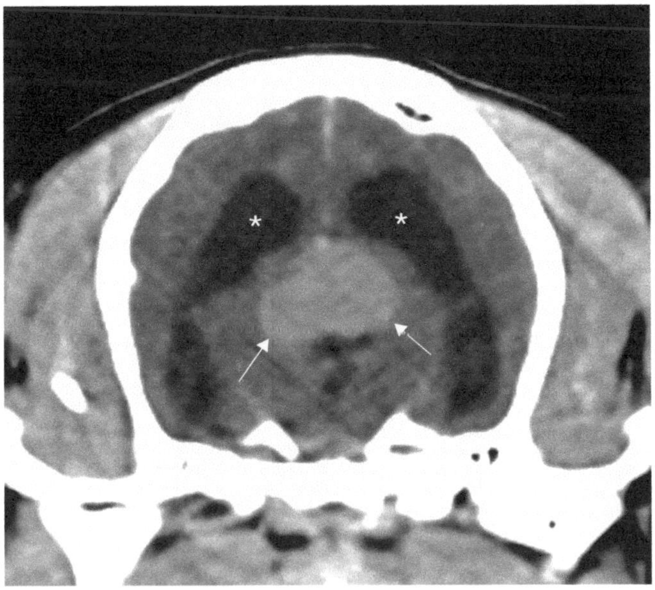

Figure 19.12 Pug with ventricular tumor (choroid plexus papilloma, presumptive). Post-contrast transverse CT image shows a rounded homogeneously enhancing mass arising from the third ventricle (arrows) with associated hydrocephalus (asterisks).

- Additional masses (metastases) common in choroid plexus carcinomas.
- Concurrent hydrocephalus common.

Other primary brain tumors

Numerous other neoplasms have been reported to affect the brain in dogs and cats including epidermoid /dermoid cysts, hamartomas, medulloblastomas, lymphoma, disseminated histiocytic sarcoma and granular cell tumors.

CT features

- Intracranial epidermoid and dermoid cyst
  - post-contrast: hypodense cerebellar mass with peripheral ring enhancement.
- Hamartomas
  - variable, may be associated with hemorrhage (Figure 19.9).
- Medulloblastoma
  - hypodense cerebellar mass
    - post-contrast: mild to strong contrast enhancement
  - may be associated with cysts and/or hemorrhage.
- Lymphoma, disseminated histiocytic sarcoma and granular cell tumors
  - very variable
  - intra- or extra-axial single or multiple mass(es)
  - may involve meninges
  - may extend beyond cranial vault
  - post-contrast: usually strongly enhancing.

Metastases

Many primary tumors including hemangiosarcomas and carcinomas have the potential for spread to the brain.

CT features

- Multiple round to ovoid lesions associated with brain parenchyma and/or meninges
  - post-contrast: usually strong enhancement, ring-enhancement possible.
- Often with associated brain edema.
- Hemangiosarcoma metastases may be associated with hemorrhage.

Central nervous system-associated tumors

Pituitary tumors, trigeminal nerve sheath tumors, nasal tumors and tumors of the skull may compress or invade brain parenchyma. These tumors are discussed in Chapters 11, 16, 20 and 21.

Further Reading

De Rycke LM, Gielen IM, Van Meervenne SA, Simoens PJ and van Bree HJ (2005) Computed tomography and cross-sectional anatomy of the brain in clinically normal dogs. *Am J Vet Res* **66**: 1743–56.

Kraft SL and Gavin PR (1999) Intracranial neoplasia. *Clin Tech Small Anim Pract* **14**: 112–23.

Parizel PM, Makkat S, Van Miert E, Van Goethem JW, van den Hauwe L and De Schepper AM (2001) Intracranial hemorrhage: principles of CT and MRI interpretation. *Eur Radiol* **11**: 1770–83.

Porat-Mosenco Y, Schwarz T and Kass PH (2004) Thick-section reformatting of thinly collimated computed tomography for reduction of skull-base-related artifacts in dogs and horses. *Vet Radiol Ultrasound* **45**: 131–5.

Summers BA, Cummings JF and de Lahunta A (1995) *Veterinary neuropathology*. St Louis, MI: Mosby.

Thomas WB (1999) Nonneoplastic disorders of the brain. *Clin Tech Small Anim Pract* **14**: 125–47.

Tidwell AS and Jones JC (1999) Advanced imaging concepts: a pictorial glossary of CT and MRI technology. *Clin Tech Small Anim Pract* **14**: 65–111.

Tucker RL and Gavin PR (1996) Brain imaging. *Vet Clin North Am Small Anim Pract* **26**: 735–58.

CHAPTER TWENTY

Pituitary Gland

Silke Hecht and Tobias Schwarz

Introduction

The pituitary gland is intimately associated with the brain, and some pituitary diseases (masses and hemorrhage) may result in neurologic symptoms indistinguishable from primary brain disorders. Therefore, evaluation of the pituitary gland is routinely performed as part of a CT examination of the brain. Specific indications for a specific CT examination of the pituitary gland include endocrinopathies such as pituitary-dependent hyperadrenocorticism in dogs and insulin-resistant diabetes mellitus/acromegaly in cats. Suprasellar extension indicating gross enlargement of the gland is easily identified on a routine brain CT scan without modification of imaging parameters. If further evaluation of a normal-sized pituitary gland is desired, or if dynamic studies are pursued for diagnosis and surgical planning of pituitary microadenomas, the scanning protocol has to be modified accordingly.

Imaging Protocol

In many instances the pituitary gland is evaluated in the frame of a brain CT study (transverse images and subsequent multiplanar/sagittally reconstructed images; *see* brain CT protocol, Chapter 19). Table 20.1 specifies imaging parameters for a CT examination targeted at the pituitary gland. Several different protocols for the dynamic examination of the canine and feline pituitary gland have been described. Three sample protocols for dynamic studies are listed here, but parameters may require modification dependent on the equipment available.

CT: Anatomy

General

The pituitary gland (hypophysis cerebri) is located within the hypophyseal fossa of the basisphenoid bone. The rostral boundary of the fossa is formed by the tuberculum sellae and rostral clinoid processes, and the caudal border is formed by the dorsum sellae and caudal clinoid processes (Figure 20.1). Due to the resemblance of this anatomic area to a Turkish saddle it is often referred to as 'sella turcica'. During embryonic development, Rathke's pouch arising from the primary oral cavity becomes closed and it remains as a small cavity (Rathke's cleft) between the anterior and posterior lobes of the pituitary gland.

The pituitary gland consists of two embryologically distinct components:

- The adenohypophysis develops from a dorsal invagination of ectoderm from the oral cavity and is comprised of three parts (parts distalis, pars intermedia and pars tuberalis). The blood supply of the adenohypophysis is provided by a venous portal system in which the primary capillary network of the hypothalamus is connected with a secondary capillary network forming the sinusoids of the adenohypophysis.
- The neurohypophysis develops from an invagination of neural ectoderm from the hypothalamus. It is continuous with the hypothalamus dorsally, contains a central cavity formed by an outpouching of the third ventricle, and is more or less centrally located within surrounding adenohypophyseal tissue. Unlike the adenohypophysis the neurohypophysis has a direct arterial blood supply.

Veterinary Computed Tomography, First Edition. Edited by Tobias Schwarz, Jimmy Saunders.

Table 20.1

CT Imaging protocol for the pituitary gland.

Series	Standard examination pre- and post-contrast	Dynamic CT examination (dog)**	Dynamic CT examination (cat)***	Helical CT examination (dog)****
Decubitus	Ventral			
Slice orientation	Transverse (perpendicular to skull base)			
Scan margins	Rostral clinoid process ←→ dorsum sellae	Initial scan to identify maximum size of pituitary gland: rostral clinoid process ←→ dorsum sellae		Tuberculum sellae ←→ dorsum sellae
Serial images		9–11 images at same table position (largest size of pituitary gland)	Images at same table position every 5–7 s for a total of 5 min	One helical scan before and 8 helical scans during and after bolus injection
Voltage (kVp)	110–130	120		
Current (mA)	100–150	220	100	63
Tube rotation time (s)	1–3	2.8–4.5	2	1.5
Interscan time (s)	N/A	9.5–11.2	3–5	16–26
Slice width (collimated, mm)	1–2	2		1
Sequential slice interval (mm)	1–2	N/A		
Kernel frequency	Standard		Bone	Standard
Pitch	N/A			2
Helical image reconstruction interval	N/A			0.5
Contrast medium application site	Peripheral vein	Saphenous vein	Cephalic vein	Peripheral vein
Contrast medium type	Iodine based			
Contrast medium dose	800 mg I/kg bw	760 mg I/kg bw	0.5 ml/kg bw (370 mg I/ml)	700 mg I/kg bw
Contrast medium injection mode	Manual	Manual (rapid injection)	Automated (150 psi; 5 ml/s)	Manual (rapid injection)
Scan delay post start contrast injection	None	First scan initiated 5 s after start of injection	Onset of injection timed to acquisition onset of third dynamic image	None
Window level (HU)	A*: +80 B*: 240	+80	+200	+80
Window width (HU)	A*: +250 B*: 250	250	1000	250

*Use of two different window settings to evaluate the brain-pituitary gland edge (A) and the bone-pituitary gland edge (B), respectively, improves accuracy in pituitary gland size measurements.
**Van der Vlugt-Meijer (2004).
***Tyson (2005).
****Van der Vlugt-Meijer (2007).

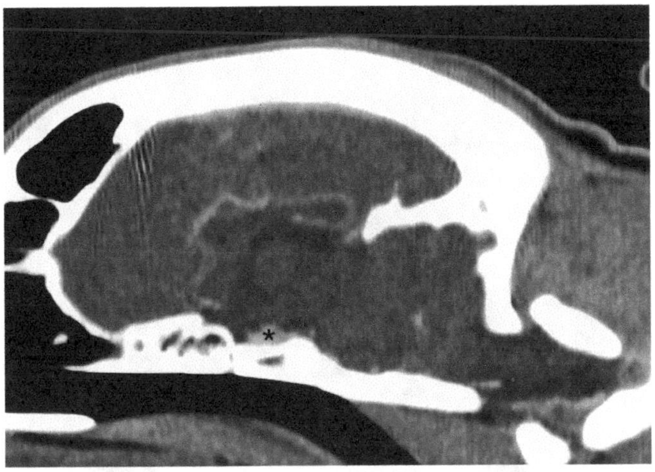

Figure 20.1 CT anatomy of the normal canine pituitary gland. Sagittally reconstructed post-contrast image illustrates location of the pituitary gland (asterisk) in the pituitary fossa bordered rostrally by the tuberculum sellae and caudally by the dorsum sellae with the caudal clinoid process.

The pituitary gland is surrounded by a venous circle formed by the venous sinuses laterally and the intercavernous sinuses rostrally and caudally. It is in close proximity to several components of the central nervous system, including hypothalamus, optic chiasm, mamillary bodies and cranial nerves III, IV, Va and VI.

Specific CT features and measurements

Mean pre-contrast attenuation values of the normal canine pituitary gland are approximately 50 HU in the central and 70 HU in the peripheral parts. Following intravenous administration of iodinated contrast medium, the gland is characterized by rapid and strong contrast enhancement. If a dynamic study is performed, initial central enhancement of the gland followed by complete homogeneous or ring enhancement is commonly observed. The reason for the early central neurohyphophyseal enhancement ('pituitary flush') is the direct arterial blood supply compared to the delayed enhancement of the adenohypophysis through the portal blood supply (Figure 20.2). Degree and timing of maximum contrast enhancement vary with contrast medium dose, speed of injection and individual factors. In cats, maximum enhancement has been reported to occur between 14 and 50 s from the onset of contrast medium injection. In dogs, maximum enhancement of the central and peripheral parts has been reported to occur 0–28 s and 14–70 s following maximum enhancement of the maxillary artery, respectively.

The pituitary gland is best measured following contrast medium administration. The gland measures approximately 10 x 7 x 5 mm (length x width x height) in normal dogs and 5.2 x 3.1 mm (width x height) in normal cats. To address variations in pituitary gland size between dogs of different sizes and breeds the pituitary gland height-to-brain ratio (P:B ratio) was introduced:

$$\text{P:B ratio} = \frac{\text{Pituitary gland height (mm)} \times 100\ \text{mm}}{\text{Brain area (mm}^2\text{)}}$$

The P:B ratio allows distinction of enlarged (PB ratio > 0.31) from non-enlarged (PB ratio ≤ 0.31) pituitary glands. It may be useful as an objective standard to compare different patients or different examinations of the same patient over time.

Anatomic variants and pitfalls

Pseudo pituitary masses in cats (Figure 20.3)

In cats, the prominent dorsum sellae may mimic a pituitary mass on transverse images. Comparison of pre- and post-contrast images, and comparison of transverse images to sagittally reconstructed images helps to identify this pitfall.

Empty sella in dogs (Figure 20.3)

Herniation of the subarachnoid space into the pituitary fossa with apparent complete lack or reduced size of the hypophysis can be associated with endocrine disturbances in humans. In one MRI study 11/370 dogs (3%) had a small or missing hypophysis (Konar *et al.* 2008). Ten of these dogs had no clinical signs of endocrinopathy, and it was concluded that empty sella may be an occasional incidental variant in dogs.

> **Note:** Care must be taken not to confuse an empty sella with a cyst or cystic mass occupying the pituitary fossa.

Disease Features

Malformation/Developmental

Rathke's cleft cyst

Rathke's cleft cyst is a cystic malformation of Rathke's cleft. This is a very uncommon finding in dogs; it may be associated with pituitary dwarfism or may be asymptomatic.

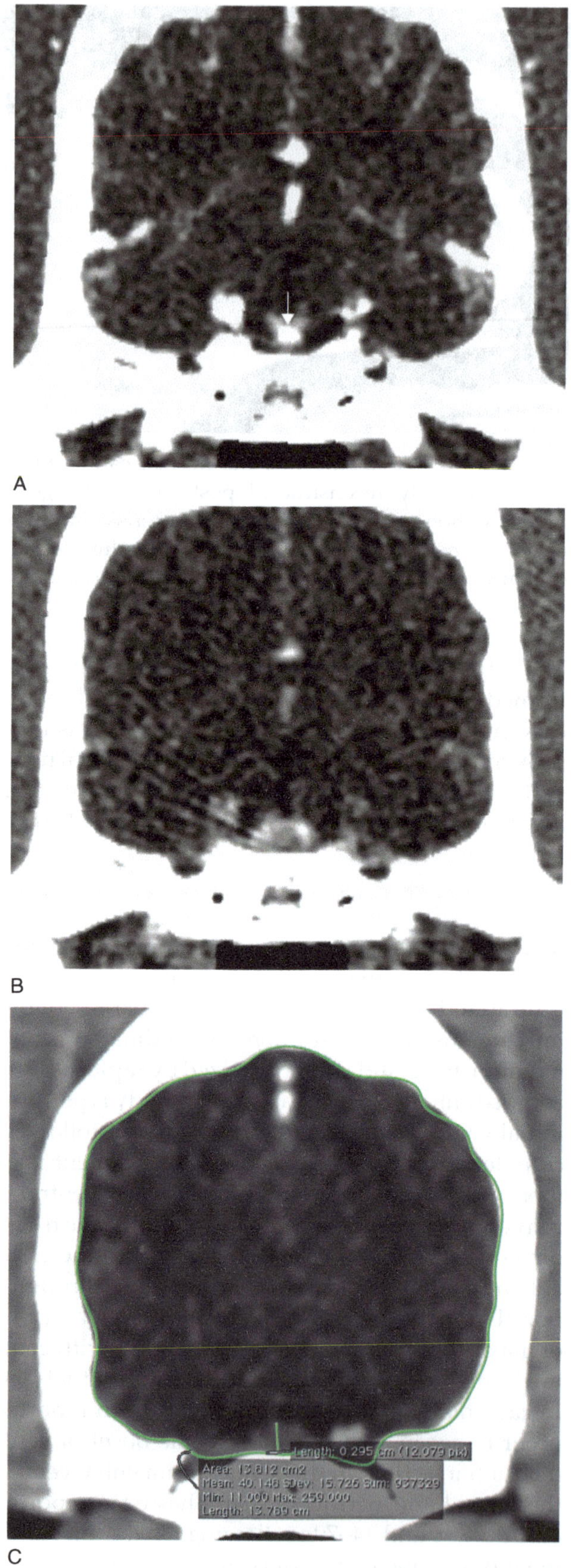

Figure 20.2 (A) Transverse dynamic post-contrast images demonstrating normal enhancement of the pituitary gland with an initial central contrast enhancement (pituitary flush, arrow) representing the arterial blood supply of the neurohypophysis and (B) subsequent homogeneous enhancement of the entire pituitary gland. (C) Pituitary brain ratio in a normal dog with a pituitary height of 3 mm and a corresponding cross-sectional brain area of 1360 mm^2 (P : B ratio 0.21).

CT features

- Well-circumscribed rounded to ovoid hypodense structure within and possibly extending dorsal to the pituitary fossa
  - post-contrast: ring enhancement possible.
- Can be difficult to differentiate from empty sella.

Vascular

Pituitary apoplexy-like disease in dogs

This syndrome is uncommon in dogs and may result from sudden infarction or hemorrhage in a normal pituitary gland or, more commonly, a pituitary tumor.

CT features

- Inhomogeneous pituitary mass with necrotic and/or hemorrhagic areas (diagnosis made based on combination of clinical and imaging findings).

Neoplasia

Pituitary macrotumors

Pituitary adenomas are fairly common in dogs but rare in cats. Pituitary adenocarcinomas are rare.

CT features

- Suprasellar extension of the pituitary gland/pituitary mass of variable size, homogeneity and margination (Figures 20.4 and 20.5).
- Adenoma, invasive adenoma and carcinoma have similar imaging features.
- Osseous involvement and presence of metastases are consistent with carcinoma (Figure 20.6), but metastases are rarely found on imaging.
- Concurrent findings (hemorrhage, hydrocephalus, brain edema, mass effect) possible and similar to other extra-axial brain tumors (*see* Chapter 19).

Pituitary microtumors

A diagnosis of a pituitary microtumor is usually made by exclusion in dogs with pituitary-dependent hyper-

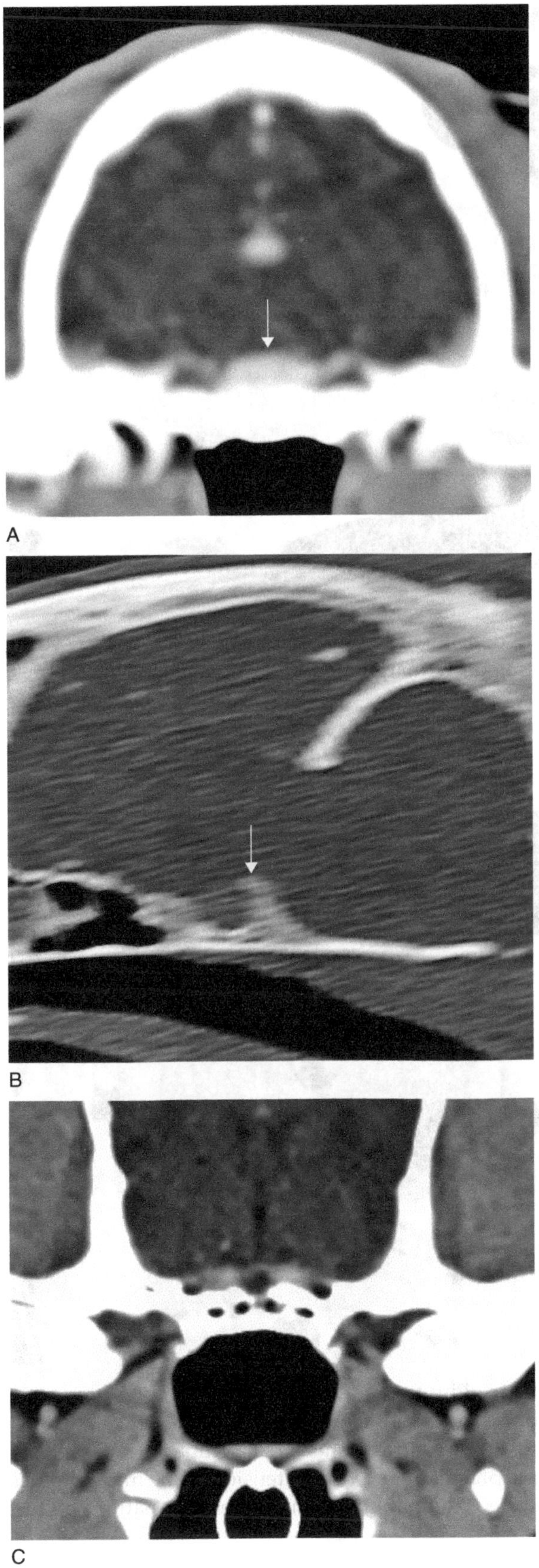

Figure 20.3 Pitfalls in pituitary imaging. (A) In cats, the prominent dorsum sellae may mimic a pituitary mass on transverse images (arrow). (B) Evaluation of a corresponding sagittally reconstructed image reveals a normal size pituitary gland bordered caudally by the dorsum sellae (arrow). (C) A hypodense non-contrast-enhancing canine pituitary gland consistent with an empty sella, an incidental finding.

adrenocorticism if no pituitary macrotumor is identified on imaging. Dynamic CT studies can identify an absent or displaced pituitary flush and indirectly suggest the presence of a microtumor. If further characterization is required (e.g. for surgical planning) a dynamic study is typically performed.

CT features

- Conventional CT scan: often normal, possibly mild enlargement of pituitary gland.
- Dynamic CT scan: displacement of neurohypophyseal flush (Figure 20.7).

> **Note:** A normal pituitary CT study (conventional and dynamic) does not rule out pituitary-dependent hyperadrenocorticism.

Craniopharyngiomas and suprasellar germ cell tumors

These are tumors arising in the suprasellar region which have been reported in both dogs and cats. Craniopharyngioma is a benign neoplasm that is derived from epithelial remnants of the oropharyngeal ectoderm of Rathke's pouch. Suprasellar germ cell tumors occur in the same location and are histologically characterized by the presence of several different cell types and positive staining for alpha-fetoprotein. Both tumor types occur in young adult to middle-aged animals, are often very large and grow along the ventral aspect of the brain.

CT features (Figure 20.8)

- Very large masses associated with the ventral aspect of the brain
  - post-contrast: usually strong enhancement of variable homogeneity.
- Osseous involvement and extension into pharynx, nasal cavity and tympanic bullae possible.
- Craniopharyngiomas have both solid and cystic areas and often have a stalk-like shape.

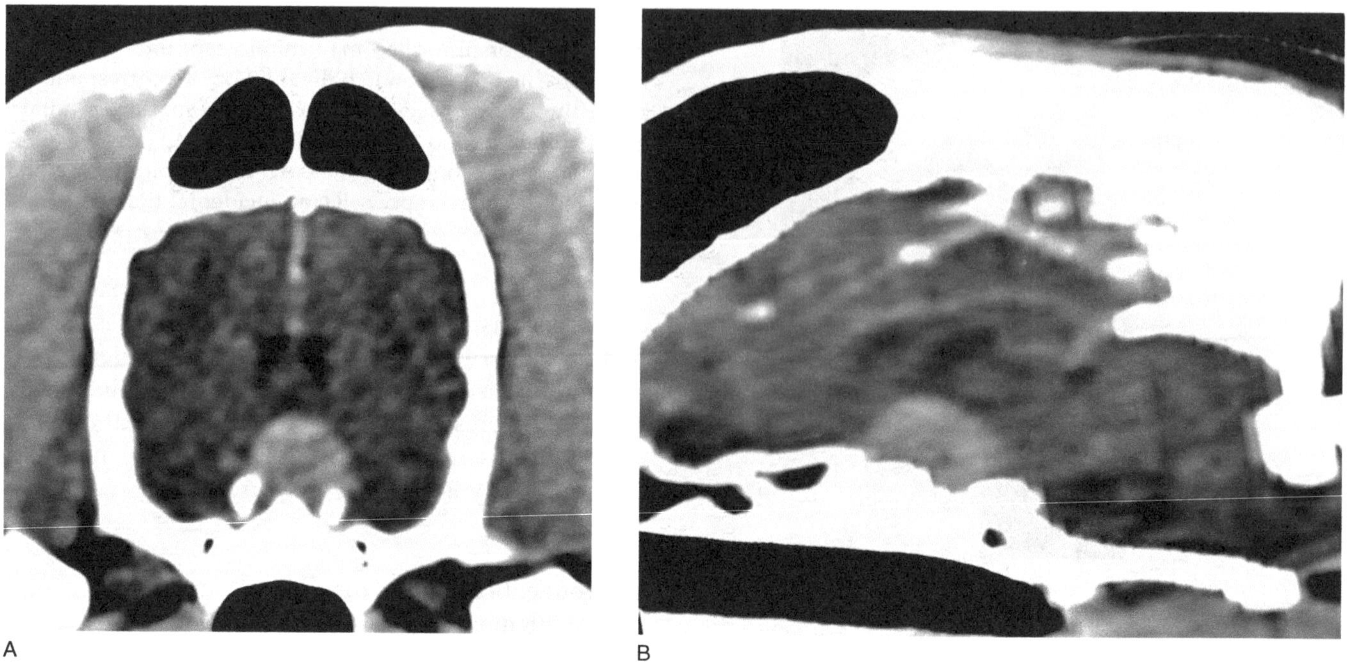

Figure 20.4 Pituitary macroadenoma in a dog presented with pituitary-dependent hyperadrenocorticism. (A) Transverse and (B) sagittally reconstructed post-contrast CT images show a large, smoothly marginated and homogeneously contrast enhancing extra-axial mass extending dorsally from the pituitary fossa.

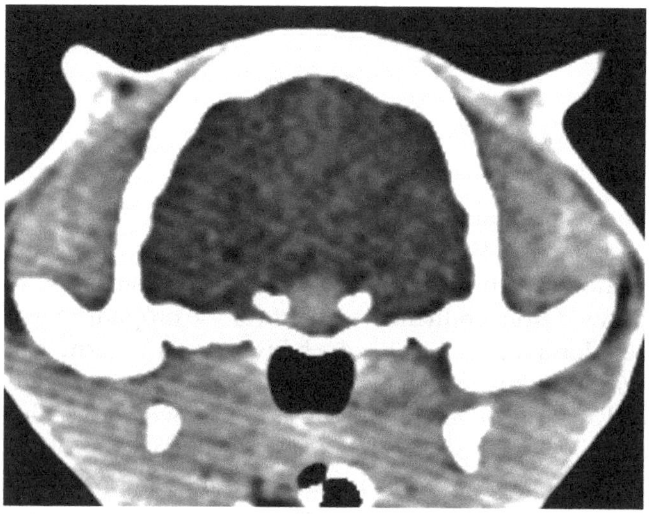

Figure 20.5 Pituitary tumor (macroadenoma, presumptive) in a cat presented with therapy resistant diabetes mellitus and acromegaly. On post-contrast transverse CT image there is a round, well circumscribed and homogeneously contrast enhancing mass extending from the pituitary fossa dorsally.

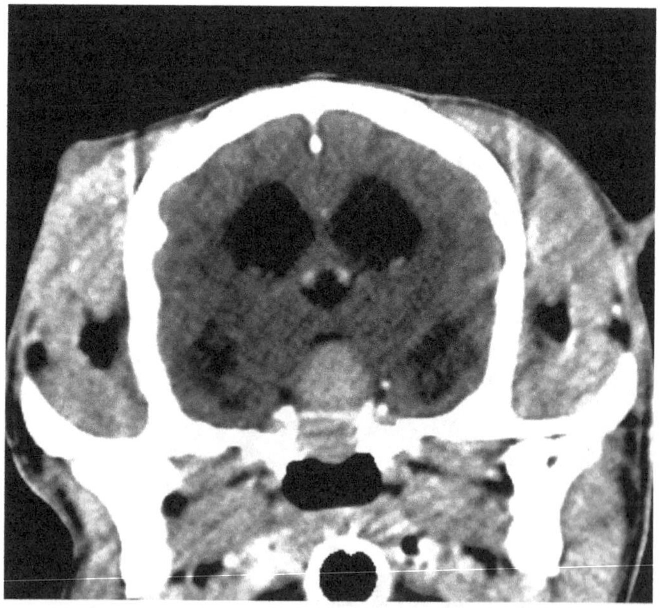

Figure 20.6 Pituitary adenocarcinoma in a dog presented for blindness and vestibular signs but no evidence of endocrinopathy. Post-contrast transverse CT image shows a lysis of the basisphenoid bone with extension of the mass into the nasopharynx, compatible with aggressive nature of the tumor.

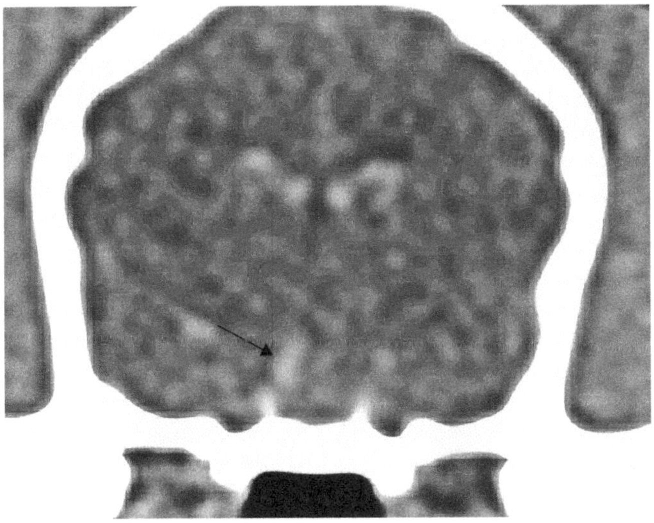

Figure 20.7 Dynamic contrast-enhanced transverse CT study in a dog with pituitary adenoma. Early arterial phase images demonstrate lateral displacement of the pituitary flush (arrow).

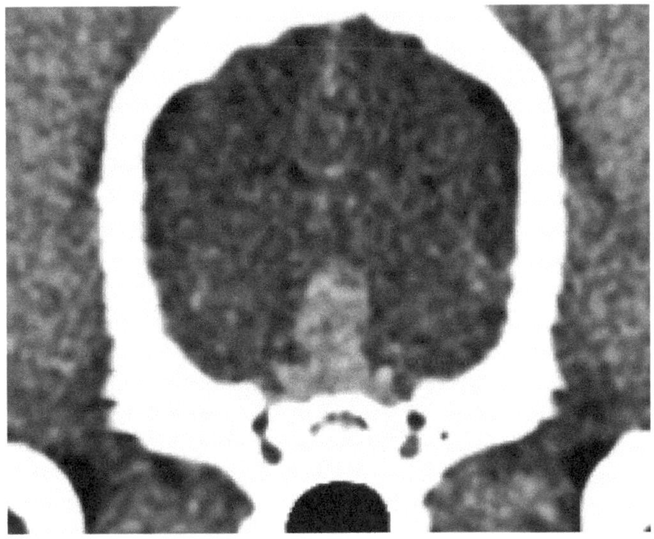

Figure 20.8 Transverse CT image shows a stalk-like contrast-enhancing mass arising from a canine pituitary gland consistent with a craniopharyngioma. Other pituitary masses should also be considered.

References

Konar M, Burgener IA and Lang J (2008) Magnetic resonance imaging features of empty sella in dogs. *Vet Radiol Ultrasound* **49**: 339-42.

Tyson R, Graham JP, Bermingham E, Randall S and Berry CR (2005) Dynamic computed tomography of the normal feline hypophysis cerebri (Glandula Pituitaria). *Vet Radiol Ultrasound* **46**: 33–8.

Van der Vlugt-Meijer RH, Meij BP and Voorhout G (2007) Dynamic helical computed tomographic evaluation of the pituitary gland in healthy dogs. *Vet Radiol Ultrasound* **48**: 118–24.

Van der Vlugt-Meijer RH, Meij BP and Voorhout G (2004) Dynamic computed tomographic evaluation of the pituitary gland in healthy dogs. *Am J Vet Res* **65**: 1518–24.

Further Reading

Auriemma E, Voorhout G and Barthez PY (2007) Determination of optimal window width and level for measurement of the canine pituitary gland height on computed tomographic images using a phantom. *Vet Radiol Ultrasound* **48**: 113–17.

Bertolini G, Rossetti E and Caldin M (2007) Pituitary apoplexy-like disease in 4 dogs. *J Vet Intern Med* **21**: 2151-7.

Hasegawa D, Uchida K, Kobayashi M *et al*. (2009) Imaging diagnosis – Rathke's cleft cyst. *Vet Radiol Ultrasound* **50**: 298–300.

Love NE, Fisher P and Hudson L (2000) The computed tomographic enhancement pattern of the normal canine pituitary gland. *Vet Radiol Ultrasound* **41**: 507–10.

Pollard RE, Reilly CM, Uerling MR, Wood FD and Feldman EC (2010) Cross-sectional imaging characteristics of pituitary adenomas, invasive adenomas and adenocarcinomas in dogs: 33 cases (1988–2006). *J Vet Intern Med* **24**: 160–5.

CHAPTER TWENTY-ONE

Cranial Nerves and Associated Skull Foramina

Laurent Couturier

Imaging Protocol

See Table 21.1 and Figures 21.1–21.3.

CT: Anatomy and Normal Variants

The anatomy of the cranial nerves and associated skull foramina is one of the most complex in the body. Some of the 12 cranial nerves are of greater clinical importance than others, especially in the dog. The cranial nerves are of soft tissue density, making them impossible to visualize on CT images; they can be visualized with MRI, because of the higher contrast resolution on MR images. Nevertheless, CT allows detailed identification of the skull foramina and thus allows indirect visualization of the emergence of cranial nerves from the skull base.

The normal anatomy with corresponding skull foramina is shown in Table 21.2.

Feline anatomical specificities

Cats do not have an alar canal and the maxillary branch of the trigeminal cranial nerve exits through the foramen rotundum on the ventral aspect of the skull. In dogs, the maxillary branch of the trigeminal cranial nerve exits through the foramun rotundum on the dorsal aspect of the skull base before joining the alar canal and exiting through the rostral alar foramen on the ventral aspect of the skull base.

CT Disease Features

Trauma

Trauma to the skull can modify the normal anatomy of skull foramina and distort the pathway of cranial nerves.

CT features

Images reconstructed with bone algorithms allow identification of small fractures of the base of the skull and particularly fractures affecting the skull foramina. Displaced fractures or associated hematoma can compress cranial nerve pathways.

Infection/Inflammation

Infectious diseases adjacent to skull foramina

Diseases such as otitis interna, middle-ear disease and abscesses in the soft tissues surrounding the head, or grass awn migration can result in focal osteitis of the skull bones, close to or involving the skull foramina and compressing a nerve pathway as a result.

CT features

- Bone lysis, and eventual secondary sclerosis, can be a sign of osteomyelitis, generally associated with soft tissue swelling and/or mass effect
  - one example is severe otitis media and secondary osteomyelitis of the petrous part of the temporal bone, which can distort and compress the facial and vestibulocochlear nerves. Clinically, the disease can progress from head tilt to unilateral paralysis of the facial cranial nerve.
- Post-contrast:
  - diffuse uptake of iodine in the soft tissues adjacent to the facial canal for example

Veterinary Computed Tomography, First Edition. Edited by Tobias Schwarz, Jimmy Saunders.

- if a fistula is identified it must be followed to delineate the margins of the lesion, looking for grass awn migration in particular.

Idiopathic neuritis

Neuritis of the optic, trigeminal and facial cranial nerves has been described in dogs and can be uni- or bilateral (especially for trigeminal neuritis with the clinical presentation of 'dropped jaw').

CT features

- Neuritis of the trigeminal cranial nerve is indirectly identified due to bilateral masticatory muscle atrophy.
- No lesion is identified on skull foramina since idiopathic neuritis does not result in significant cranial nerve enlargement.
- Post-contrast: Contrast enhancement has been described in the normal and abnormal CN V on MRI and can also be seen on CT. Asymmetrical contrast enhancement is suggestive of pathology.

Neoplasia

Neoplasia can affect cranial nerves primarily or compress them secondarily. All types of primary or secondary brain tumors can compress the pathway of cranial nerves. Most of the cranial nerve tumors are intradural extramedullary tumors. Their histological characteristics include malignant features in most

Table 21.1
CT imaging protocol (intravenous contrast study: standard protocol; *see* Chapter 5).

Series	Pre- and post-contrast	Bone
Recumbency	Ventral	
Scan margins	Cribriform plate → Occiput	
Voltage (kVp)	120	
Current (mAs)	250	
Tube rotation time (s)	0.5	
Slice width four-slices helical CT	4 × 1 mm	
Kernel frequency	Medium	High
Collimator pitch	0.75	
Helical image reconstruction interval	0.8	
Window level (HU)	+35	+200
Window width (HU)	100	2000

Table 21.2
Cranial nerves and corresponding skull foramina in the dog.

	Dog		
	Origin	Skull entrance foramen	Skull exit foramen
Olfactory CN I	Olfactory mucosa	Cribriform plate	Cribriform plate
Optic CN II (Figure 21.4B)	Diencephalon	Optic canal	Optic canal
Oculomotor CN III (Figure 21.4B)	Mesencephalon	Orbital fissure	Orbital fissure
Trochlear CN IV (Figure 21.4B)	Mesencephalon	Orbital fissure	Orbital fissure
Trigeminal CN V	Metencephalon		
Ophthalmic branch (Figure 21.4B)		Orbital fissure	Orbital fissure
Maxillary branch (Figure 21.2A)		Foramen rotundum	Rostral alar foramen
Mandibular branch (Figure 21.2B)		Foramen ovale	Foramen ovale
Abducens CN VI (Figure 21.4B)	Myelencephalon	Orbital fissure	Orbital fissure
Facial CN VII (Figures 21.1 and 21.3)	Myelencephalon	Internal acoustic meatus then facial canal	Stylomastoid foramen
Vestibulocochlear CN VIII (Figures 21.1 and 21.3)	Myelencephalon	Internal acoustic meatus	–
Glossopharyngeal CN IX	Myelencephalon	Jugular foramen	Tympano-occipital fissure
Vagal CN X	Myelencephalon	Jugular foramen	Tympano-occipital fissure
Accessory CN XI	Myelencephalon	Jugular foramen	Tympano-occipital fissure
Hypoglossal CN XII	Myelencephalon	Hypoglossal canal	Hypoglossal canal

CN = cranial nerve.

cases. The term malignant peripheral nerve sheath tumor or MPNST (neurofibroma/neurofibrosarcoma, neurilemoma and schwannoma/neurinoma) is now used to include all types of malignant tumor involving nerve sheaths.

Of the cranial nerves, MPNST most commonly involves the trigeminal nerve, producing signs of unilateral trigeminal nerve dysfunction (e.g. unilateral masticatory muscle atrophy – temporalis and/or masseter). Brainstem compression by a neurofibroma thought to be of cranial nerve origin, and by a trigeminal neurofibrosarcoma/schwannoma, has been reported in dogs. Lymphosarcoma occasionally affects cranial nerves in dogs and cats, and may extend intracranially. Myelomonocytic neoplasia of the trigeminal nerves, resulting in a dropped mandible and symetrical atrophy of the masticatory muscles, has also been described in this species. Various tumors of the ear canal, including squamous cell carcinoma, ceruminous adenocarcinoma and fibrosarcoma, as well as osteosarcoma of the skull, may involve the facial nerve or one of its branches. Neurofibromas involving the vestibulocochlear nerve are very rare. Cranial nerve function may be altered by compression from meningiomas lying on the calvarial floor (plaque-like meningiomas).

CT features (Figures 21.2–21.4)

- Enlargement of the cranial nerve pathway or nucleus, which can sometimes be directly identified, especially on post-contrast CT images, or indirectly because of enlarged skull foramina.

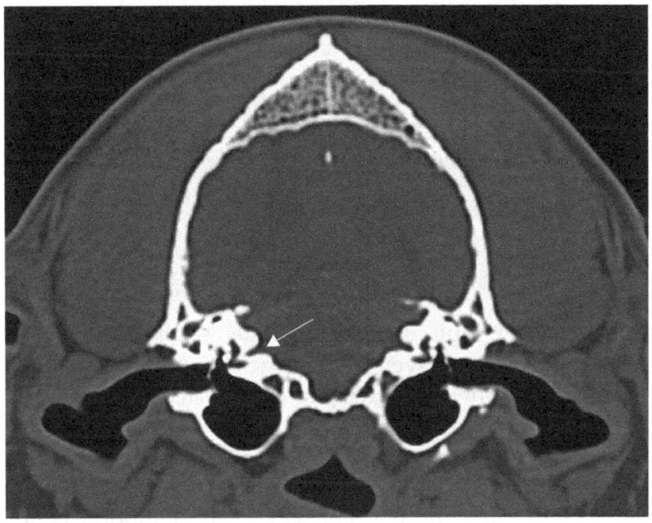

Figure 21.1 Transverse CT image at the level of the vestibule and semicircular canals in a normal dog. Note the normal appearance of the internal acoustic meatus (arrow), where the vestibulocochlear and facial cranial nerve enter together before the facial cranial nerve penetrates the facial canal in the petrosal part of the temporal bone.

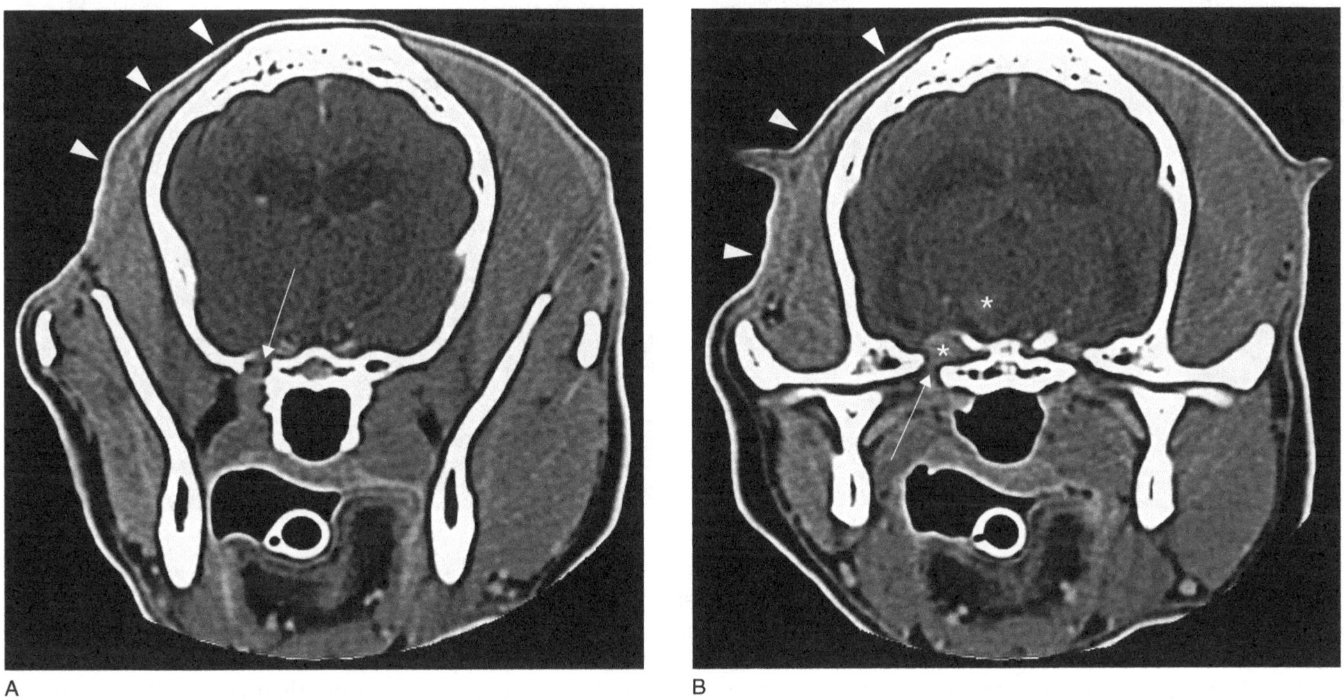

Figure 21.2 Adult dog with right trigeminal nerve sheath tumor. (A) Transverse CT image shows an enlarged rostral alar foramen (arrow) due to enlarged maxillary branch of cranial nerve V and a severe ipsilateral atrophy of the temporalis muscle (arrowheads). (B) Transverse CT image slightly caudal to A shows a right trigeminal nerve sheath tumor (asterisks) with suspected enlarged mandibular branch of cranial nerve V and secondarily enlarged oval foramen (arrow). There is severe ipsilateral atrophy of the temporalis muscle (arrowheads).

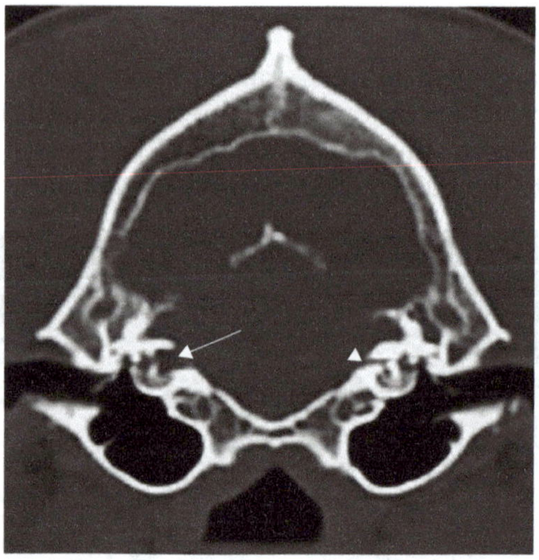

Figure 21.3 Adult dog with isolated right-sided facial nerve paralysis. Transverse CT image shows enlarged right facial canal (arrow) secondary to a suspected nerve sheath tumor of the right facial cranial nerve. Note the normal appearance of the contralateral facial canal just dorsal to the vestibule (arrowhead). The facial canal has an S-shaped pathway through the petrosal part of the temporal bone, making its identification difficult within the petrosal bone (image courtesy of Dr Ariel Cohen-Solal, Belgium).

- A mass can also been identified in intra- or extra-axial locations and its CT characteristics depend on the histologic type of the tumor. Mass effect on cranial nerve nuclei or pathways can explain the clinical signs of the patient.
- The mass can be hypo-, iso- or hyperdense on pre- and post-contrast images, depending on its attenuating and histological properties.

Further reading

Bagley RS, Wheeler SJ, Klopp L *et al.* (1998) Clinical features of trigeminal nerve-sheath tumor in 10 dogs. *J Am Anim Hosp Assoc* **34**: 19–25.

Couturier L, Degueurce C, Ruel Y, Dennis R and Begon D (2005) Anatomical study of cranial nerve emergence and skull foramina in the dog using magnetic resonance imaging and computed tomography. *Vet Radiol Ultrasound* **46**: 375–83.

Mayhew PD, Bush WW and Glass EN (2002) Trigeminal neuropathy in dogs: a retrospective study of 29 cases (1991–2000). *J Am Anim Hosp Assoc* **38**: 262–70.

Pettigrew R, Rylander H and Schwarz T (2009) Magnetic resonance imaging contrast enhancement of the trigeminal nerve in 42 dogs without evidence of trigeminal neuropathy. *Vet Radiol Ultrasound* **50**: 276–8.

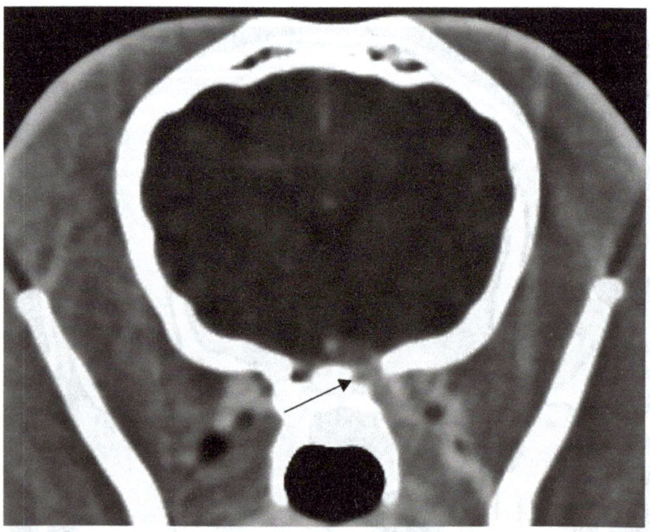

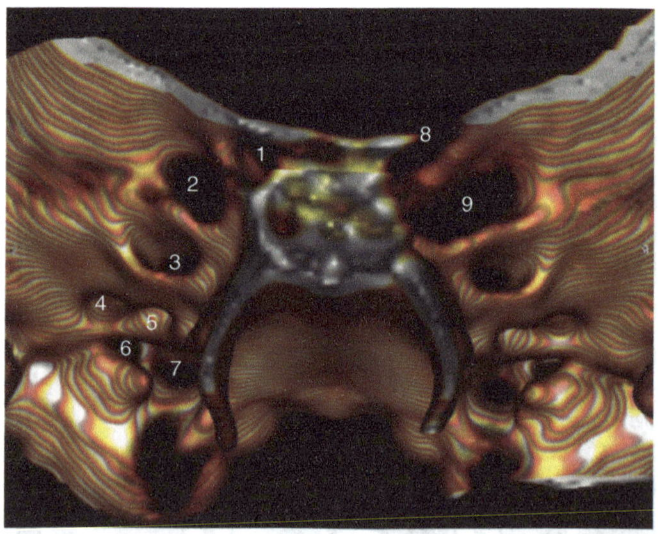

Figure 21.4 Adult dog with lymphoplasmocytic lymphoma with asymmetrical distribution. The dog was presented for acute left-sided blindness and exophthalmos. (A) Post-contrast transverse CT image at the level of the optic canal shows left-sided enlarged optic canal (arrow) secondary to an optic cranial nerve tumor. There is diffuse uptake of contrast medium in the left optic nerve tract. The contralateral optic cranial nerve area has a normal appearance. (B) 3-D reconstructed CT image of an isolated sphenoid bone. All the oculomotor nerves (oculomotor-trochlear-trigeminal ophthalmic branch – abducens cranial nerve in the orbital fissure and optic cranial nerve in the optic canal) are enlarged and there is secondary optic canal and orbital fissure enlargement on the left side. 1 = optic canal, 2 = optical fissure, 3 = rostral alar foramen, 4 = oval foramen, 5 = caudal alar foramen, 6 = musculotubal canal, 7 = foramen lacerum, 8 = enlarged optic canal, 9 = enlarged orbital fissure.

CHAPTER TWENTY-TWO

Vertebral Column and Spinal Cord

Gabriela Seiler, Jennifer Kinns, Sophie Dennison, Jimmy Saunders and Tobias Schwarz

Imaging Protocol

See Tables 22.1, 22.2.

CT: Anatomy and Normal Variants

Vertebral column (Figure 22.1)

The vertebral column consists of a large number of vertebrae firmly but not rigidly joined together. The vertebrae conform to a common pattern that can be further distinguished into five vertebral regions (abbreviation and number of vertebrae): cervical (C7), thoracic (T13), lumbar (L7), sacral (S3) and caudal (Cd variable). A typical vertebra consists of a massive vertebral body surmounted by an arch. The vertebral body is broadly cylindrical, somewhat flattened on its dorsal surface, convex cranially and concave caudally. The arch consists of two upright pedicles and a lamina joining them, forming the vertebral canal around the spinal cord. The bases of the pedicles are notched and when successive bones articulate, these notches combine to outline intervertebral foramina, the opening through which both the spinal nerves and the vessels that supply the structures within the vertebral canal pass. The vertebrae carry region specific processes, such as the spinous, articular and transverse process. Interbreed variations have been described in the morphology of the atlas and dimensions of vertebrae in general.

There are two sets of joints between vertebrae:

- synovial joints between the articular processes
- cartilaginous joints (intervertebral disks) between the vertebral bodies.

The intervertebral disk consists of a central nucleus pulposus (semi-fluid tissue) and a peripheric annulus fibrosus (fibrous tissue). These disks make an appreciable contribution to the articulated column in the normal animal but show consistently degenerative changes with advance in age, commonly causing back trouble. This normal joint pattern is modified in the cranial region where the atlanto-occipital and atlanto-axial joints allow free movement of the head, and in the pelvic region where sacral fusion occurs. Ligaments in the occipito-atlanto-axial region mainly ensure the stability between vertebrae and no intervertebral disk is present between these vertebrae.

In addition to the joints, three long ligaments extend along substantial portions of the spine. The dorsal longitudinal ligament runs along the floor of the vertebral canal from the axis to the sacrum, the ventral longitudinal ligament follows the ventral aspect of the vertebrae from the mid-thoracic region to the sacrum and the (supraspinous) common ligament runs over the summits of the spinous processes of the thoracic and lumbar vertebrae. The common ligament has a cranial continuation in the dog, but not in the cat, which attaches to the spinous process of the axis.

Typical CT density values for structures and lesions in the vertebral canal are listed in Table 22.3.

Meninges and spaces (Figure 22.2)

Epidural space

The epidural space contains fat and the venous sinuses. At the level of the intervertebral disk space the ventral venous sinuses are paired and exit from either side via the intervertebral foramen. The sinuses merge on the midline as they travel through the spinal canal, con-

Veterinary Computed Tomography, First Edition. Edited by Tobias Schwarz, Jimmy Saunders.

Table 22.1
CT imaging protocol (intravenous contrast study: standard protocol; *see* Chapter 5).

Series	Pre-contrast	Bone
Decubitus	Dorsal	
Special positioning	**Cervical spine**: elevate head to maintain extension; tape limbs caudally **Thoracolumbar spine**: tape limbs cranially; align gantry tilt with C3/4 of L3/4 intervertebral disk **Lumbosacral**: align gantry tilt with L7-S1 intervertebral disk	
Scan margins	**Cervical**: occipitoatlantal joint ←→ T2 vertebral body **Thoracolumbar**: cranial T2 vertebral body ←→ L4 vertebral body **Lumbosacral**: L4 verterbral body ←→ S3 vertebral body	
Voltage (kVp)	120 100	
Current (mAs)	200	
Tube rotation time (s)	1	
Slice width (mm)	1–2	
Sequential slice interval (mm)	1	
Kernel frequency	Medium	High
Window level (HU)	+100	+500
Window width (HU)	300	3000

Table 22.2
CT myelography.

Series	CT myelography (Figure 22.2)
Access site	Cervical (cisternal): occiput–C1 Lumbar: L5–L6 or L4–L5 (larger dogs)
Scan margin	If following conventional myelography, include two vertebral bodies cranial and caudal to region of interest for improved multiplanar reconstructions
Contrast medium application site	Lumbar or cervical myelogram injection
Contrast medium type	Non-ionic, monomeric, iodinated contrast medium only
Contrast medium dose	60 mg I/kg bw (0.2 ml/kg of 300 mg I/ml) Maximum dose: 135 mg I/kg bw (0.45 ml/kg of 300 mg/ml) or 20 ml iohexol
Contrast medium injection mode	Manual
Scan delay post start contrast injection	As soon as possible
Side effects	Post-myelogram seizures: increased risk with cisternal injection (> lumbar injection) and larger volumes of contrast medium. Iatrogenic brainstem injury (for cisternal injection)
Undesired effect	Accidental epidural injection can be recognized as the contrast medium will track along the nerve roots at each intervertebral foramen
Additional comment	CSF samples (cisternal easier) should be collected prior to contrast medium injection, as the contrast medium alters the differential cell count within 24 h and can affect the growth of bacteria in culture

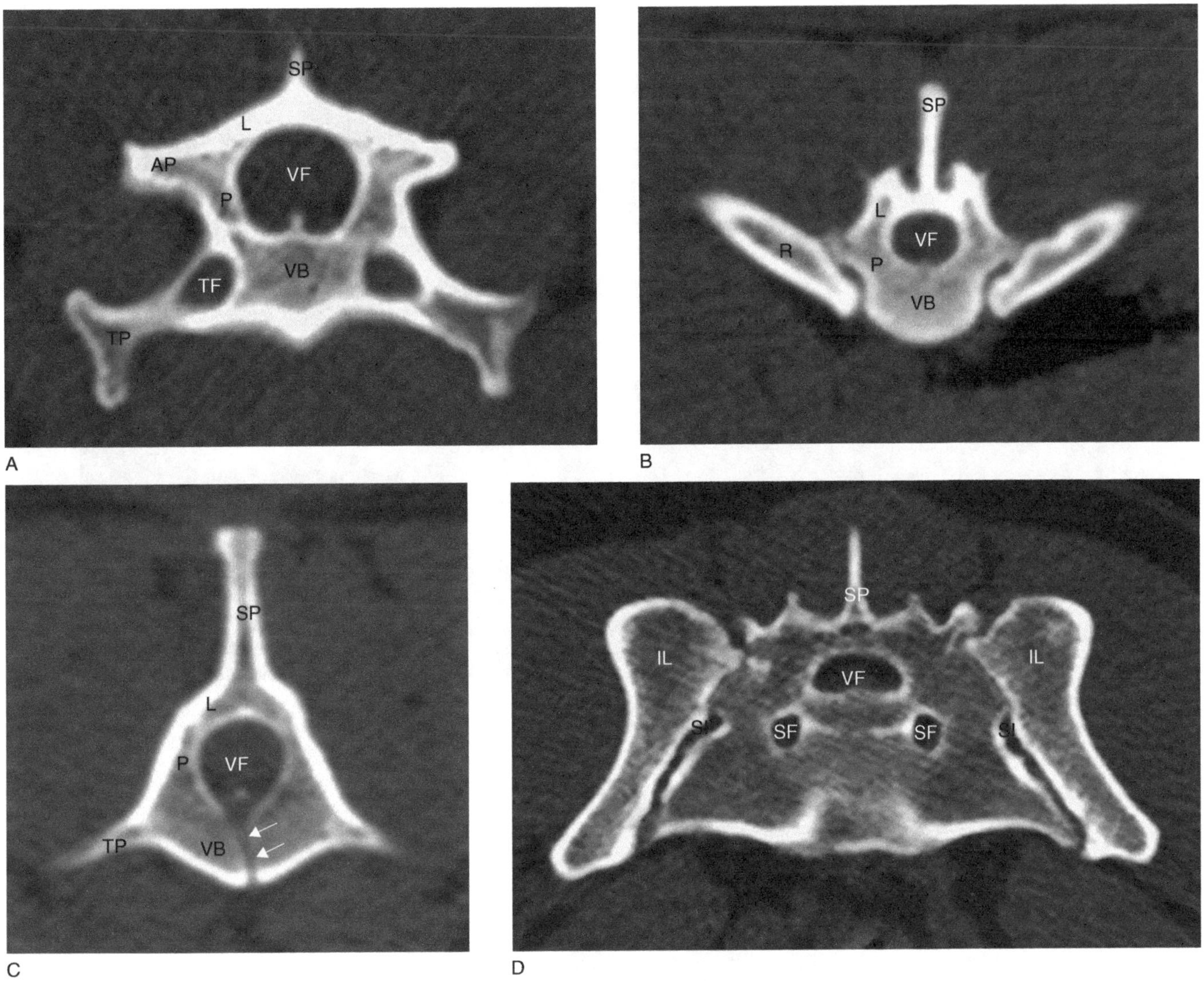

Figure 22.1 Transverse CT images of a normal dog. (A) Cervical vertebra (C6). (B) Thoracic vertebra. (C) Lumbar vertebra (L2) with nutrient foramina (arrows). (D) Sacrum and sacroiliac joint. AP = articular process; IL = ilium; L = vertebral lamina; P = vertebral pedicle; R = ribs; SF = sacral foramen; SI = sacro-iliac joint; SP = spinous process; TF = transverse foramen; TP = transverse process; VB = vertebral body; VF = vertebral foramen.

Table 22.3
Typical density values for structures in the vertebral canal.

Tissue	Density (HU)
Fat	–100
Spinal cord*	+40
Ligaments	+50
Hematoma	+100
Vertebral cortical bone	+1000

*No signal gray/white matter distinction.

necting with the basivertebral venous sinuses. There are no valves within these venous sinuses thus flow directionality may vary. Arteries course along the lateral, dorsal and cranially ventral aspects of the spinal cord.

Subdural space

This is a potential space created by lacerations of the dura border cell layer post mortem. Intra vitam it is not usually imaged unless contrast medium is inadvertently injected into it during a myelographic study.

Subarachnoid space

The subarachnoid space contains cerebrospinal fluid (CSF) and surrounds the spinal cord. The space is located between the arachnoid cells adhered to the dura mater and the pia mater, which is tightly adhered to the spinal cord. The spinal cord is suspended in the subarachnoid space through the denticulate ligament.

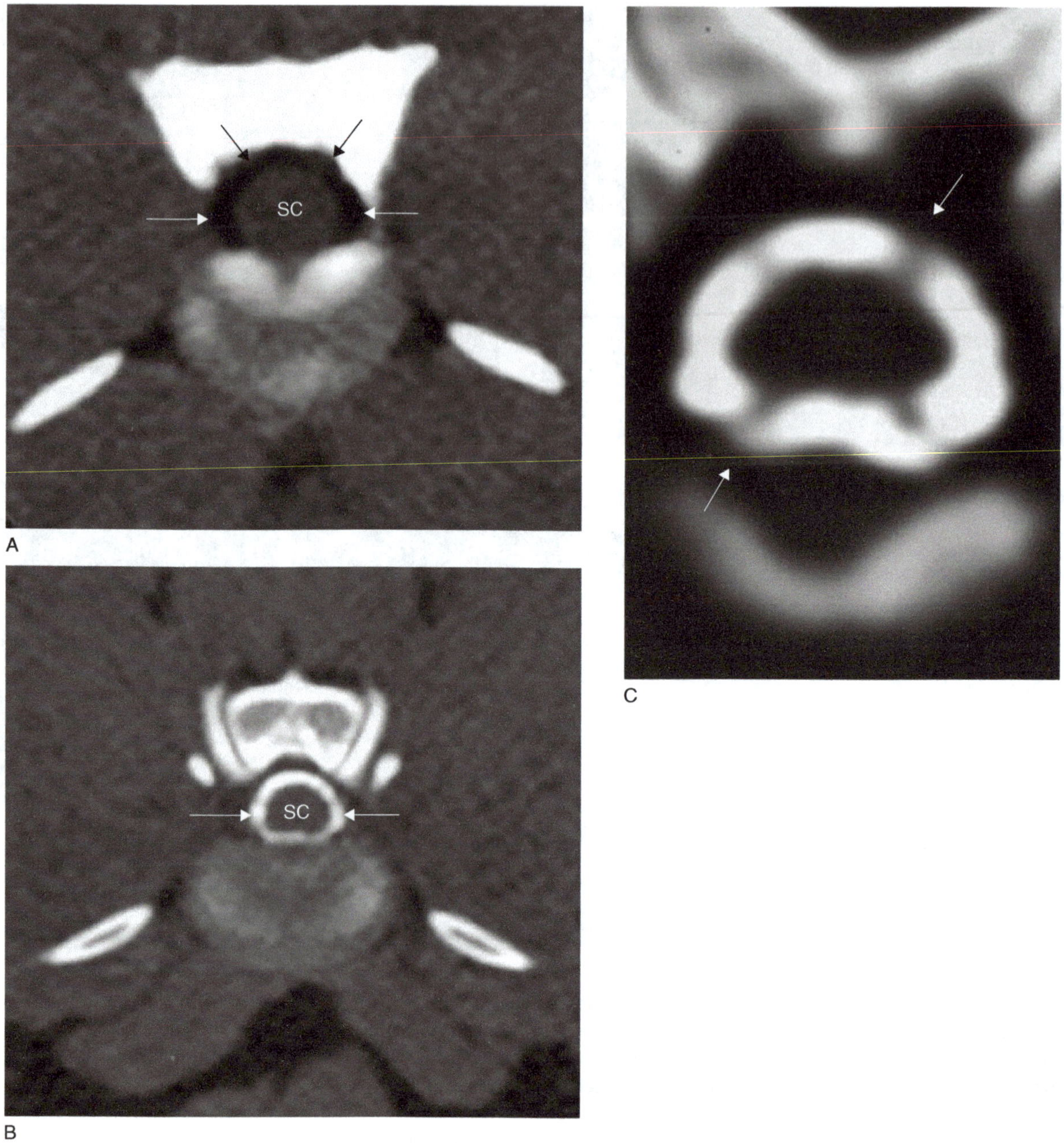

Figure 22.2 Normal dog (L3–L4 intervertebral disk space). (A) Transverse CT image shows the epidural fat (arrows), which is hypodense to the spinal cord. (B) Transverse CT myelogram shows the hyperdense (compared with spinal cord) contrast medium (arrows) within the subarachnoid space. (C) Transverse CT myelogram shows the nerve roots (arrows). SC = spinal cord.

Spinal cord (Figure 22.2)

Spinal cord segments become comparatively more cranial with respect to their corresponding vertebral body number as one moves caudally. The cord ends at approximately the level of L5 vertebral body, although the exact location of the terminal spinal cord varies according to the size of the animal. In general, the spinal cord terminates further cranially in large dogs than in small dogs. The cervical and lumbar intumescences are 'swellings' or enlargements of the spinal cord that correspond to the segments contributing to the brachial (C6–T1) and lumbosacral (L4–S1) plexi. These should not be mistaken for pathologic spinal cord swelling.

Nerve roots (Figure 22.2)

Nerve roots leave the spinal canal via intervertebral foramen and are named according to the exit location.

C1 to C7 nerve roots exit from the intervertebral foramen cranial to their respective vertebral body, C8 nerve roots exit caudal to the C7 vertebral body, and nerve roots caudal to C8 exit caudal to their respective vertebral body.

Cauda equina

The position of the end of the thecal sac and the beginning of the cauda equina is variable and ranges from L6 to the sacrum; in small breed dogs and cats it tends to be more caudally located than in large breed dogs. On transverse CT images the thecal sac presents as a round, soft tissue-dense structure in the center of the vertebral canal. It gradually becomes more dorsally located and the paired nerve roots can be seen as round opacities along its ventrolateral margins (Figure 22.3A). The nerve roots extend laterally until they exit the intervertebral foramina. The cauda equina is surrounded by a large amount of epidural fat and should be positioned symmetrically within the vertebral canal (Figures 22.3B, 22.3C). Within the intervertebral foramina the nerve roots are surrounded by fat as well. The lumbosacral disk is flat or dorsally convex and sometimes bulges slightly into the vertebral canal, which is not clinically relevant if no impingement of the cauda equina is present.

Many subclinical CT abnormalities of the lumbosacral spine are known in older dogs. Findings such as vertebral canal or foraminal bone proliferation, loss of epidural or foraminal fat, intervertebral disk bulging, degenerative articular process joint disease, disk mineralization and dural ossification should therefore always be correlated with clinical signs.

Disease Features (Table 22.4)

Malformation/Developmental

Atlantoaxial subluxation

Atlantoaxial subluxation is mostly congenital, rarely traumatic. Small breed dogs (Yorkshire terriers, Chihuahuas, miniature poodle) are more commonly affected but the disorder may be seen in cats and in large breed dogs. Predisposing factors include incomplete ossification of the atlas, aplasia, malangulation, hypoplasia of the odontoid process (dens) of the axis, failure to the ligaments that maintains the odontoid process in position or a traumatic fracture of the odontoid process.

CT features (Figure 22.4)

- Increased width of the space between the odontoid process and intercentrum of the atlas.
- Congenital:
  - odontoid process of the axis absent, hypoplastic or dysplastic. May be accompanied by an occipito-atlantoaxial malformation. An abnormally dorsal dens angulation can cause spinal cord bruising
  - incomplete ossification of the atlas
  - in case of failure of ligaments, the dens tends to protrude dorsally in the spinal cord.
- Traumatic:
  - fracture of the odontoid process.

Cavitary disease

Hydromyelia, syringomyelia and hydrosyringomyelia are referred to as cavitary conditions. They refer to dilatation of the central canal, cavitation of the cord parenchyma or a combination of the two respectively. Hydromyelia may be congenital or acquired but is often an incidental finding. The acquired form can result from a compressive lesion more cranially within the spinal cord or within the brain. It can also be induced during myelography if contrast medium is injected directly into the central canal (Figure 22.5A). Syringomyelia has been reported in association with occipitocervical malformation syndrome. Syringohydromyelia results when the cavitations communicate with the central canal.

CT features (Figure 22.5B)

- Hypodense central canal may be evident within the spinal cord.
- CT myelography:
  - contrast–filled, dilated central canal with hydromyelia
  - contrast-filled cavitations if syringohydromyelia.
- Syringomyelia not easily diagnosed on CT.

Cervical spondylomyelopathy

Caudal cervical spondylomyelopathy or wobbler syndrome is a general term to describe different causes of congenital or acquired vertebral canal stenosis in several large and giant breed dogs such as the Doberman pinscher and Great Dane. A large variety of lesions with different proposed etiologies have been attributed to this condition. Clinical signs result from extradural compressive myelopathy of the cervical spine. Compression can arise from vertebral

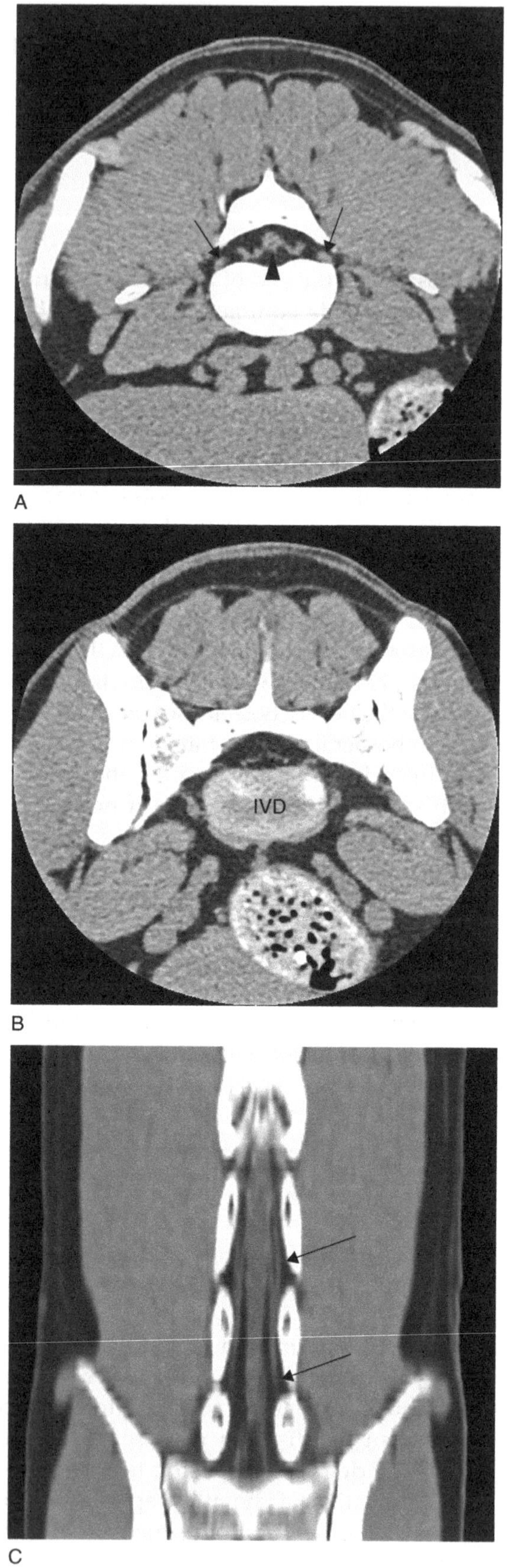

Figure 22.3 Normal canine lumbosacral region. (A) Transverse CT image (caudal L6) shows the thecal sac visible as a round, soft tissue-dense structure in the center of the vertebral canal (arrowhead). Several nerve roots accompany the thecal sac bilaterally on its ventrolateral aspect. The segmental nerve roots can be seen entering the intervertebral foramina (arrows). All nerve roots of the cauda equina are surrounded by hypodense fat. (B) Transverse CT image (lumbosacral disk space) shows the nerve roots much thinner but still surrounded by hypodense fat and symmetrically distributed in the vertebral canal. The dorsal aspect of the intervertebral disk (IVD) is flat. (C) Dorsally reconstructed CT image shows the nerve roots of the cauda equina (arrows) well outlined by epidural fat.

malformation, vertebral malalignment, hypertrophy of the ligamentum flavum, hypertrophied or malformed articular processes or bulging of the fibrous annulus. Spinal cord compression may be static or dynamic.

CT protocol

Dynamic images can be acquired to evaluate the effect of extension and flexion on the spinal cord. The study is then acquired with the animal in lateral recumbency and the neck secured in flexion or extension. This is possible even in very large dogs, but the legs must be secured caudally. The effect of traction may also be evaluated with the dog in standard dorsal recumbency using weighted maxillary traction.

CT features

- Vertebral body malformations such as flattening of the cranioventral border or 'thickening' of the dorsal arch of the lamina.
- Protrusion of bony structures into the vertebral canal (Figure 22.6A).
- Abnormally positioned vertebral bodies (such as craniodorsal tilting).
- Narrowed or collapsed intervertebral disk spaces.
- Intervertebral foraminal stenosis.
- Articular process abnormalities.
- Spondylosis deformans.
- Protrusion of soft tissue-dense material into the vertebral canal at the level of the intervertebral disk space.
- Dorsal ligament hypertrophy (Figure 22.6B).
- Thickening and bulging in the region of the ligamentum flavum (Figure 22.6C).
- Atrophy and/or deformity of the spinal cord.

Table 22.4
Differential diagnosis for spinal disorders (toxic disorders not included).

	Most common disorders	Less common disorders
Malformation/ Developmental	Atlantoaxial subluxation/dysplasia Cavitary disorders (syringo(hydro)myelia) Cervical spondylomyelopathy Congenital vertebral malformations Osteochondromatosis Sacral osteochondritis dissecans Spinal cord arachnoid cyst	Epidermoid cyst Hereditary myelopathy Meningomyeloceles Pilonodal (dermoid) cyst Sacrocaudal dysgenesis Intravertebral disk herniation (Schmorl's node) Tethered cord syndrome Osteochondromatosis
Trauma	Dural tear Spinal fracture/luxation Spinal cord hematoma/ hemorrhage	Brachial plexus avulsion myelopathy Gunshot injury Sacrocaudal injury Traumatic disk injury
Inflammatory and infectious	Discospondylitis Meningomyelitis	Cauda equina neuritis Foreign body migration Spinal epidural empyema
Degenerative	Articular process joint arthrosis/Intraspinal articular cysts Degenerative disk disease Degenerative lumbosacral stenosis Degenerative myelopathy Dural mineralization	Cervical fibrotic stenosis Leukodystrophies Lysosomal storage disease Sacroiliac joint pain
Neoplastic	Primary or secondary neoplasia	Extradural lipomatosis
Vascular	Ascending myelomalacia Fibrocartilaginous embolism	Ischemic neuromyopathy Neurogenic claudication Traumatic feline ischemic myelopathy Vascular malformation
Miscellaneous	Disseminated idiopathic skeletal hyperostosis (idiopathic)	Calcinosis circumscripta (idiopathic) Hypervitaminosis A (nutritional) Diagnostic, radiation, surgical injury (iatrogenic) Peridural scar (iatrogenic) Thiamine deficiency (nutritional)

Congenital vertebral malformations

Congenital vertebral anomalies/malformations are due to an anomalous vertebral development in the embryo. They include alterations in vertebral shape and number. Bulldogs, pugs and Boston terriers are most commonly affected. Most of these malformations are asymptomatic but severe neurological signs may occur. Common disorders include transitional vertebra, hemivertebra (wedge-shaped vertebra), butterfly vertebra, block vertebra or spina bifida. A transitional vertebra has characteristics of two adjacent vertebral regions such as having one rib, transverse process or sacral wing). A lumbosacral transitional vertebra may lead to asymmetry of the lumbosacral junction and increased stress on the intervertebral disk, predisposing it for degenerative lumbosacral stenosis in dogs. It is a component of the lower back pain syndrome and, in most severe cases the cauda equina syndrome particularly in working dogs.

CT features

- Hemivertebra (Figure 22.7A)
  - wedge-shaped vertebra, the degree of failure formation is variable, most common at mid-thoracic level
  - spinal angulation (scoliosis, kyphosis or lordosis).
- Block vertebra
  - two or more vertebrae are fused.
- Spina bifida (Figure 22.7B)

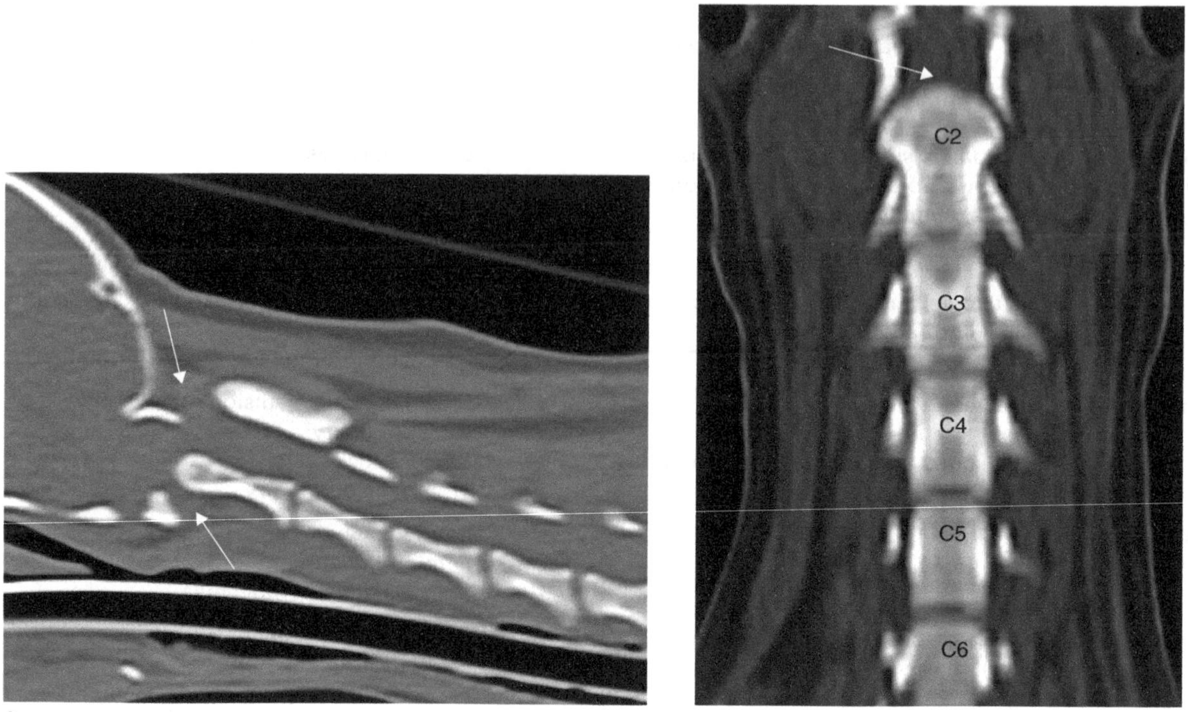

A B

Figure 22.4 14-month-old Chihuahua with congenital atlanto-axial subluxation. (A) Sagittally reconstructed CT image shows dorsal displacement of the second cervical vertebra (C2) (arrows). (B) Dorsally reconstructed CT image shows the absence of the dens of the axis (arrow).

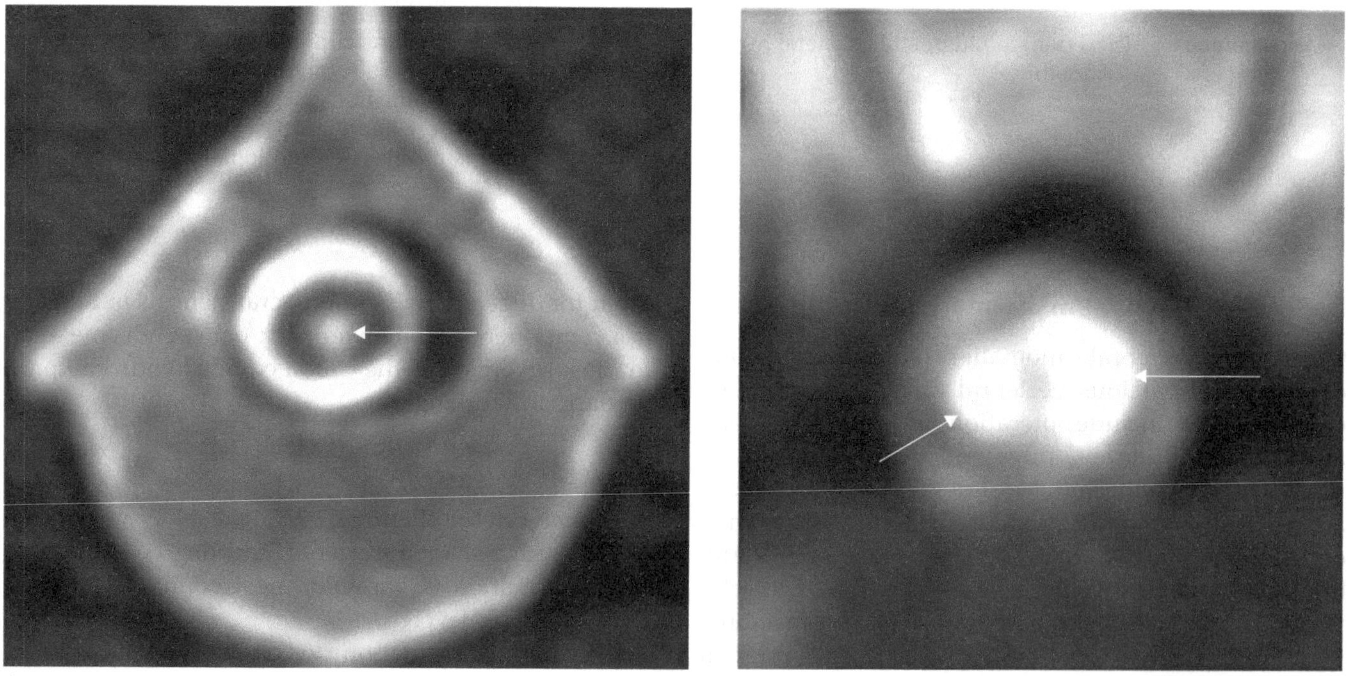

A B

Figure 22.5 Adult dogs with cavitary disorders. (A) Transverse CT myelogram shows contrast medium (arrow) within a mildly dilated central canal (canalogram). (B) Transverse CT myelogram shows contrast medium filling cavitations (syringomyelia) within the spinal cord (arrows).

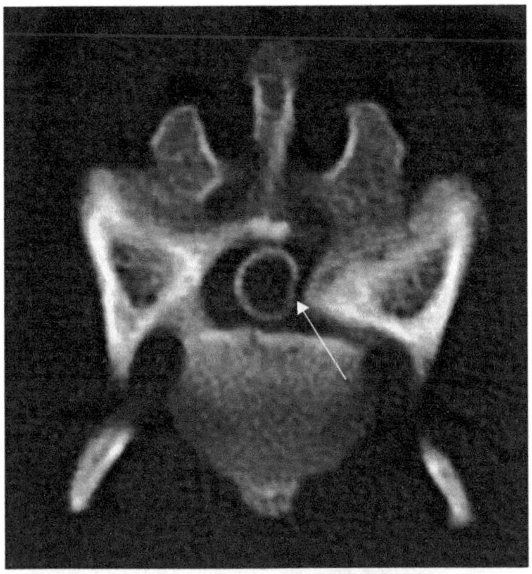

A

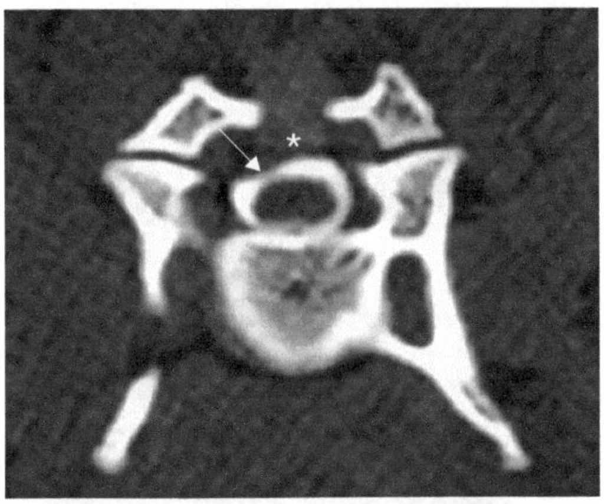

B

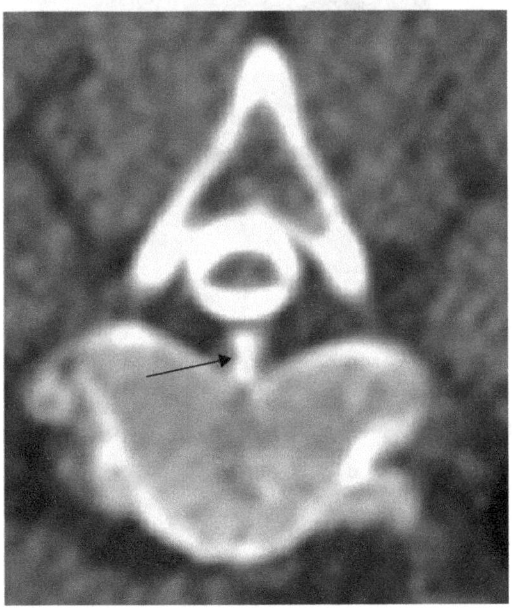

C

Figure 22.6 Three different dogs with cervical spondylopathy of different origin. (A) Transverse CT myelogram of the caudal cervical spine in an adult bullmastiff that presented with progressive asymmetric neuropathy. There is compression of the spinal cord (arrow) due to vertebral malalignment and an enlarged, degenerative articular process (image courtesy of N. Nelson, Ohio State University). (B) Transverse CT myelogram shows a ventral displacement of the spinal cord due to dorsal ligament hypertrophy (asterisk). The contrast medium in the subarachnoid space is thinned dorsally on the right side (arrow). (C) Transverse CT image shows a dorsal displacement of the spinal cord due to ligamentum flavum hypertrophy (arrow).

  - defect in the dorsal arch resulting in a split spinous process
  - CT-myelogram: meningocele.
- Butterfly vertebra
  - widened vertebral body with partial or complete longitudinal split
  - adjacent vertebral bodies abnormally shaped due to adaptation
  - dorsal reconstruction: longitudinal cleft through the body of a vertebra and a funnel shape at the ends.
- Transitional vertebra (Figure 22.7C)
  - asymmetry of the lumbosacral junction
  - additional transverse processes on the first sacral vertebra or joint transverse process of a lumbar vertebra with the ilial wing.

Osteochondromatosis (multiple cartilaginous exostoses)

Osteochondromatosis, a form of skeletal dysplasia, shows expansile bony lesions that usually arise from the osteochondral junction of bones. It results from an abnormal differentiation of cartilage cells during endochondral ossification and growth usually stops at skeletal maturity. The disease affects typically the costochondral rib junction, less frequently the metaphyses of long bones and the vertebrae, where it can cause spinal cord compression. Neoplastic transformation may occur.

CT features (Figure 22.8)

- Bone attenuating mass(es) of variable density with a thin, dense cortex and central low-density cancellous bone.
- Lesion may appear active (homogeneous, smoothly marginated) or inactive (irregular, poorly marginated).
- May invade the vertebral canal.

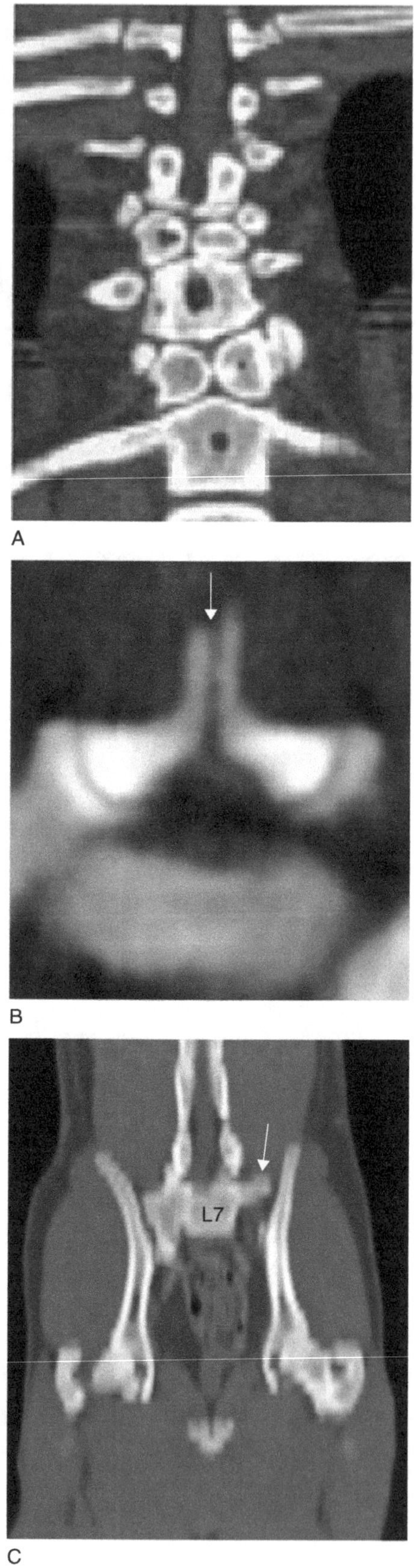

Figure 22.7 Three different dogs with vertebral malformations. (A) Dorsally reconstructed CT image of a young dog shows multiple butterfly vertebrae (arrows). (B) Transverse CT image of a young dog with spina bifida shows a split of the dorsal vertebral arch (arrow). (C) Dorsally reconstructed CT image of an adult dog with a transitional lumbosacral vertebra shows L7 forming a transverse process on the left (arrow), whereas the right side articulates with the ilium, forming a second 'sacral wing'.

Osteochondritis dissecans of the sacrum

Osteochondrosis of the cranial endplate of the sacrum has been described mainly in the German shepherd dog. Since the fibers of the fibrous annulus of the lumbosacral disk attach on the endplate in the region of the osteochondritic fragment, the disease usually leads to disk herniation and cauda equina compression at a young age. The caudal endplate of the seventh lumbar vertebra may also be affected.

CT features (Figure 22.9)

- Focal defect in the cranial endplate of the sacrum, surrounded by a sclerotic area in the vertebral body – usually lateralized.
- Osteochondral fragment may be craniodorsally displaced.
- Lumbsacral disk herniation.

Subarachnoid cyst

Subarachnoid cysts are focal enlargements of the subarachnoid space. They are not true cysts as they lack an epithelial lining. In dogs they are an uncommon finding and may cause spinal cord compression. The etiology is unknown but as most cases present at an early age a congenital origin is likely. Small breeds are more commonly affected in the thoracic area and large breeds in the cervical area. Rottweilers are overrepresented, suggesting a heritable component.

CT features (Figure 22.10)

- CT myelography with cisternal injection required for diagnosis
  - contrast filled focal enlargement of the dorsal subarachnoid space
  - varying degrees of spinal cord compression.

Trauma

Dural tear

Blunt trauma may cause tearing of the dura, leading to loss of CSF from the subarachnoid space.

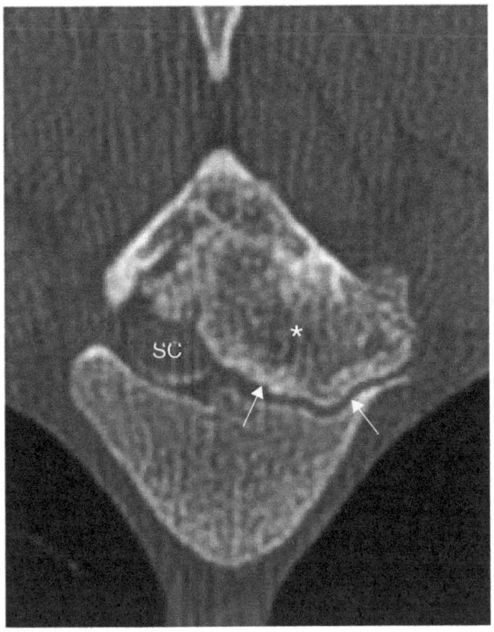

Figure 22.8 Adult dog with an osteochondroma. Transverse CT image shows bone proliferation (asterisk) originating from the dorsal arch and growing ventrally to invade the left half of the vertebral canal. The mass distorts the left dorsal aspect of the vertebral body (arrows). The spinal cord (SC) is compressed and displaced to the right.

CT features (Figure 22.11)

- Vertebral fracture or dislocation often present in association.
- CT myelography required for diagnosis
  - leakage of contrast from the subarachnoid space at the site of injury
  - contrast leakage may be extradural or intramedullary.

Spinal cord trauma

Blunt trauma that is sufficient to cause fracture or dislocation of the vertebral column is also likely to damage the spinal cord. Forces may also cause cord contusion with little bony disruption. Hemorrhage within the subdural or epidural space can result in extradural compression of the spinal cord.

CT features (Figure 22.12)

- Vertebral fracture or dislocation often present in association.
- Hyperdense material around the cord consistent with epidural or subdural hematoma.
- Focal hyperdensity within the cord consistent with contusion.
- Hypodensity within the cord due to edema.

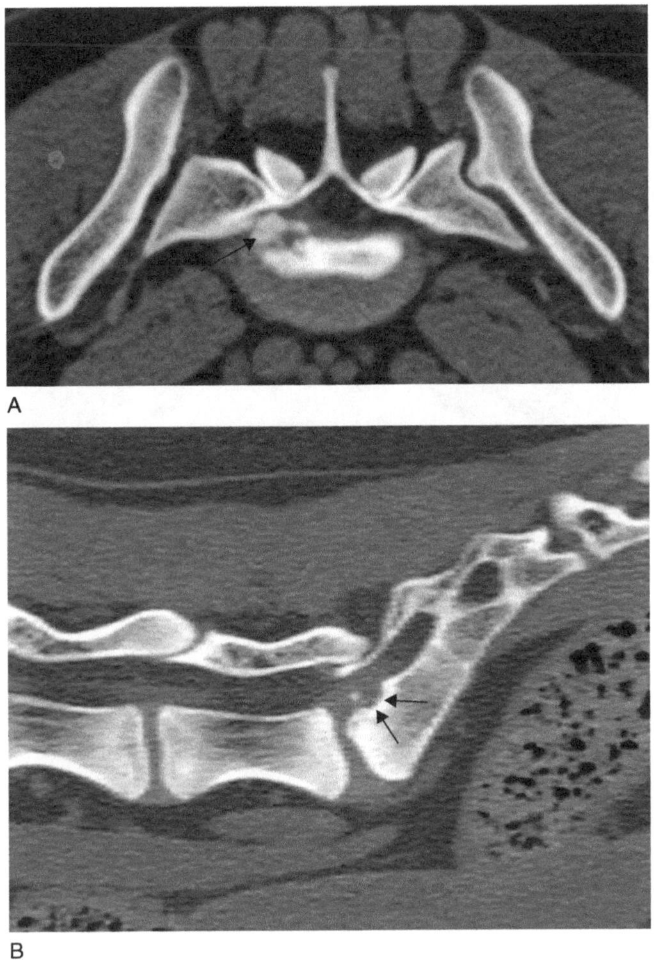

Figure 22.9 Young dog with osteochondritis dissecans of the sacrum. (A) Transverse CT image shows a separated bone fragment (arrow) at the dorsal aspect of the first sacral vertebral body on the right aspect. (B) Dorsally reconstructed CT image shows a separate bone fragment at the craniodorsal aspect of the first sacral vertebra in front of a bone defect (arrows).

- Intravenous contrast medium not necessary but CT myelography useful to rule out dural tear.

Vertebral fractures and sacroiliac luxation

Spinal fractures and/or luxations are the result of vehicular injury in around 65% of cases and affect the lumbar vertebrae more frequently. Other causes of injury include animal attacks or falling from a height. Patients must be positioned very carefully to reduce the risk of fracture displacement. Fractures of the caudal lumbar vertebrae or sacrum may lead to injury or compression of the cauda equina. Avulsion of the nerve roots of the cauda equina is a serious complication of tail fractures. CT is essential to determine fracture/spine stability by evaluating the integrity of

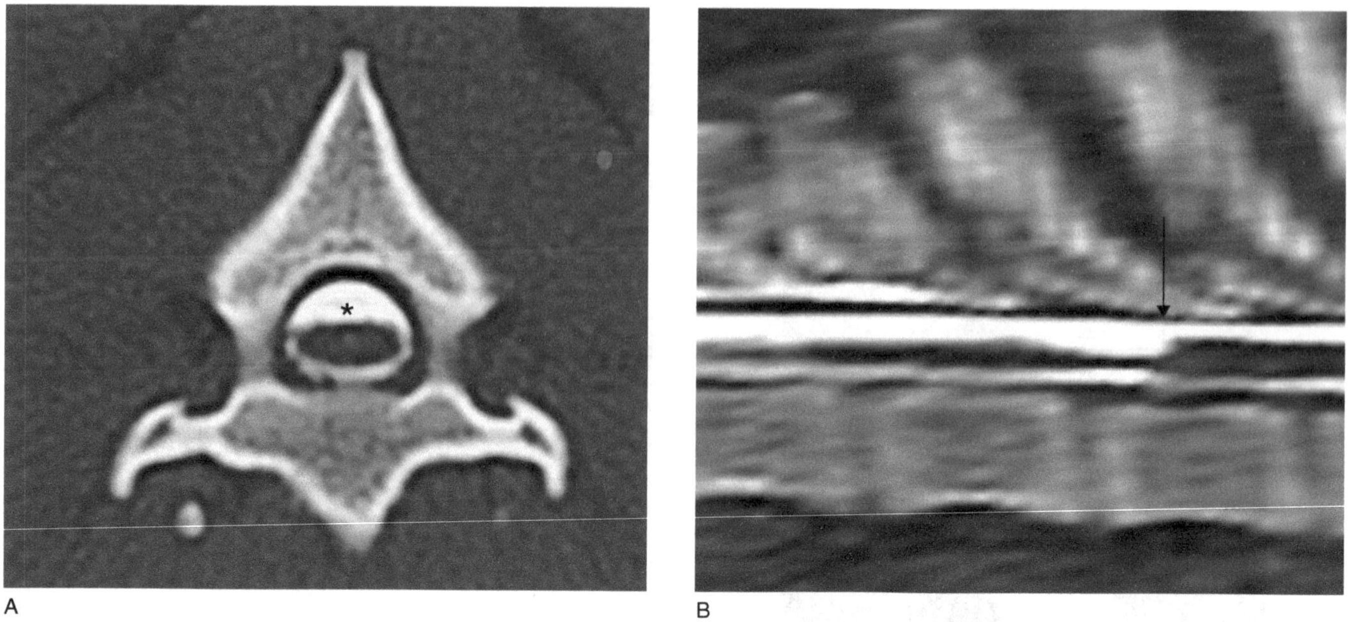

Figure 22.10 Subarachnoid cyst. (A) Transverse CT myelogram image shows a symmetric dilatation of the dorsal contrast column (asterisk). (B) Sagittally reconstructed CT myelogram shows the transition zone (arrow) between the dilated (cyst) and the normal dorsal contrast column.

the intervertebral disk, articular process and vertebral body. A three-compartment model has been proposed to evaluate fracture stability.

CT features (Figure 22.13)

- Epiphyseal slip fracture in young animals with often minimal displacement.
- Compression fracture (burst fracture); shortening of vertebral body.
- Displacement of bone fragments into the vertebral canal.
- Subluxation of the lumbosacral junction, sacroiliac or dorsal articular facet joints.
- Poor delineation of the nerve roots is a sign for nerve root injury or compression caused by hemorrhage.
- CT allows accurate 3-D description of vertebral or sacral fractures as well as sacroiliac luxations.

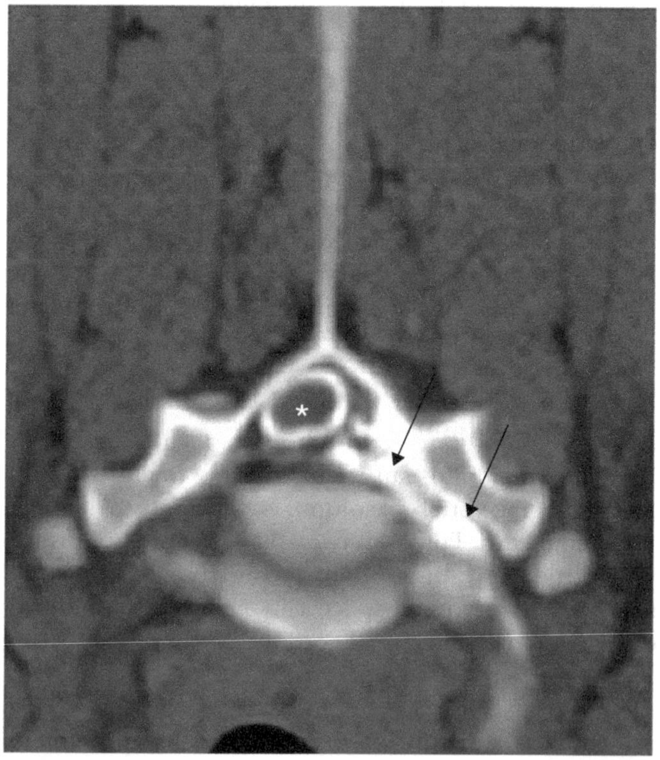

Figure 22.11 Adult dog with dural tear. Transverse CT myelogram shows leakage of contrast medium from the subarachnoid space to the extradural space (arrows). The spinal cord is medially displaced (asterisk).

Infection/Inflammation

Discospondylitis

Discospondylitis is an inflammatory condition centered on the intervertebral disks and involving the vertebral end plates and adjacent bone of both adjacent vertebral bodies. Large breed dogs are most commonly affected. The disease may be caused by *Staphylococcus intermedius*, *Streptococcus sp.*, *Escherichia coli* or *Brucella*

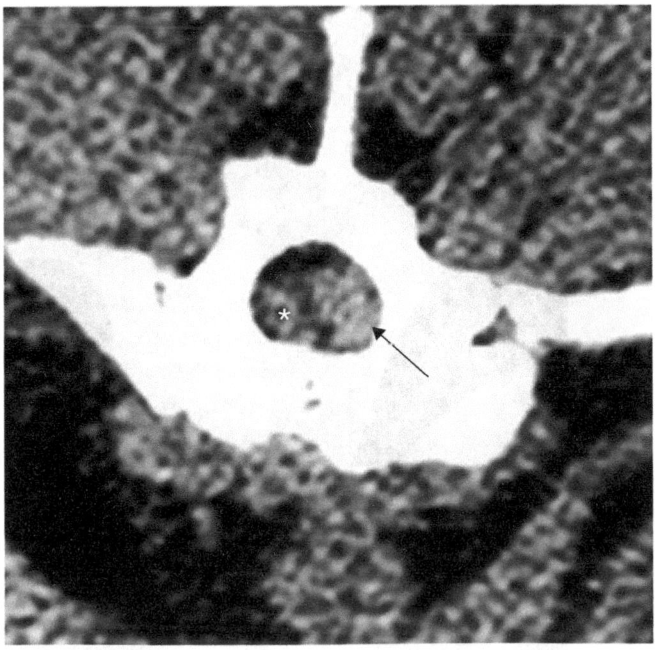

Figure 22.12 Spinal cord trauma in an adult dog. Transverse CT image shows hyperdense material on the left side of the vertebral canal (arrow). The spinal cord is displaced laterally (asterisk).

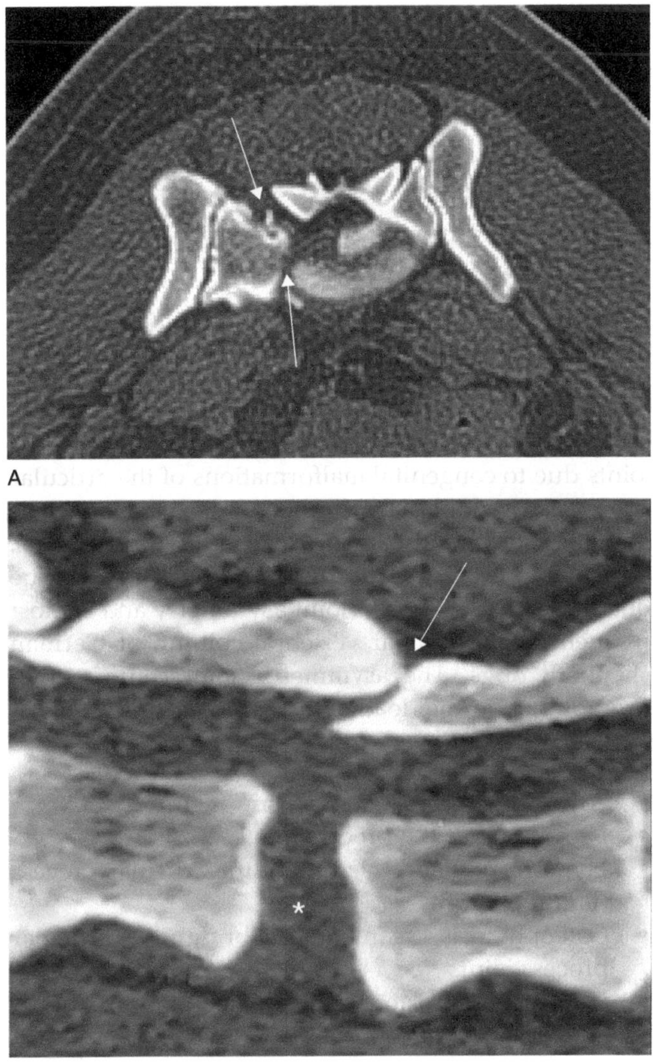

Figure 22.13 (A) Transverse CT image (lumbosacral junction) of a dog that was hit by a car. There is a sagittal fracture through the cranial aspect of the sacrum (arrows) with right sacroiliac luxation and narrowing of the vertebral canal. Soft tissue-dense material compressing the epidural fat and the cauda equina likely represents hemorrhage and/or herniated disk material. (B) Adult dog with T13–L1 subluxation. Sagittally reconstructed CT image shows malarticulation between the articular processes (arrow), increased intervertebral space (asterisk) and a step between the vertebral bodies of T13 and L1.

canis. A fungal cause is also possible, particularly in the German shepherd dog. Hematogeneous dissemination from the bladder or other foci is common. Foreign bodies or iatrogenic cases are other etiologies.

CT features (Figure 22.14)

- Severe irregular bone destruction involving the vertebral end plates and adjacent vertebral body.
- Associated bone deposition, primarily on the ventral aspect of the affected spinal unit.

Meningomyelitis

Inflammation of the meninges and spinal cord can occur with a number of infectious and idiopathic processes. Granulomatous meningoencephalitis may involve the spinal cord as well as the brain. Several systemic infectious processes can cause intramedullary cord lesions. Feline infectious peritonitis is the most common cause of cord inflammation in the cat, while cryptococcus lesions are seen in both species. Other viral, fungal, protozoal and bacterial etiologies are possible, and aberrant intramedullary parasite migration has been reported.

CT features

- Post-contrast (IV):
  - difficult to diagnose confidently with CT
  - contrast enhancement of the spinal cord, often patchy
  - contrast enhancement of the meninges
  - may have cord swelling.

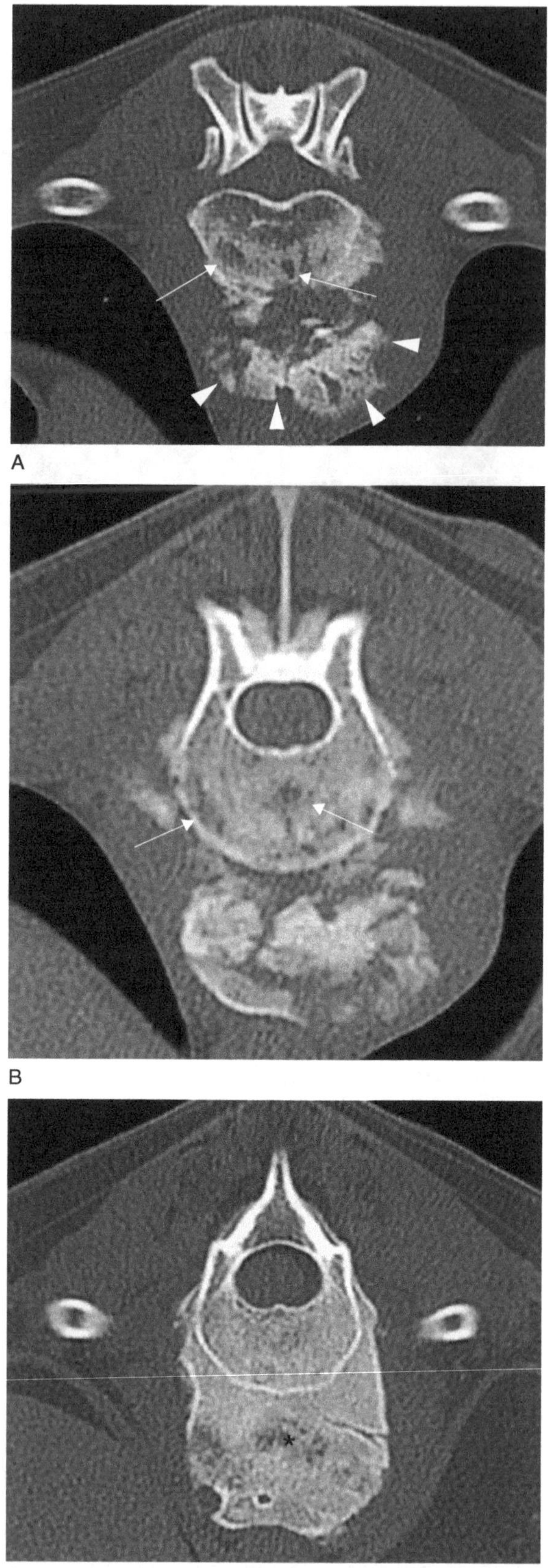

Figure 22.14 Adult dog with discospondylitis. Transverse CT images show (A) areas of bone lysis at the caudal end plate of the vertebral body of T9 (arrows) and irregular new bone proliferation ventrally (arrowheads), (B) T10 with similar areas of lysis in the middle part of the vertebral body (arrows), and (C) an organized, smooth bone proliferation ventral to T11 (asterisk).

Degeneration

Articular process joint arthrosis and articular process joint tropism

Osteoarthritis of the articular process joint develops secondary to abnormal loading of the articular process joints due to congenital malformations of the articular processes (hypoplasia) or other underlying developmental (osteochondrosis) or degenerative conditions. Articular process joint tropism is a term to describe bilateral articular process joint asymmetry and is most frequent in the lumbar vertebral column of German shepherd dogs. The asymmetric joint conformation promotes abnormal loading and osteoarthritis.

CT features

- Articular process joint tropism (Figure 22.15A).
- Narrowing of the process joints.
- Hypertrophy and sclerosis of the articular process (Figure 22.15B).
- Osteophytosis, sometimes bridging, articular process joints.
- Subarticular erosions and/or subchondral cysts.

Intraspinal articular cysts

Intraspinal articular cysts may be subdivided in ganglion cysts, synovial cysts and cysts arising from ligaments and intervertebral disks. Synovial cysts arise from synovial outpouching through weakened capsular tissue of the articular processes, while ganglion cysts arise from the periarticular connective tissue of intervertebral joints. Both are thought to develop secondary to degenerative joint disease. The differentiation is done by histological examination as synovial cysts are lined with synovium-like epithelial cells whereas ganglion cysts are not.

CT features (Figure 22.16)

- Soft tissue-dense cystic formation located immediately adjacent to a degenerated articular process.

Dural mineralization

Plaque-like dural mineralization commonly occurs in isolation as an incidental finding, even in relatively

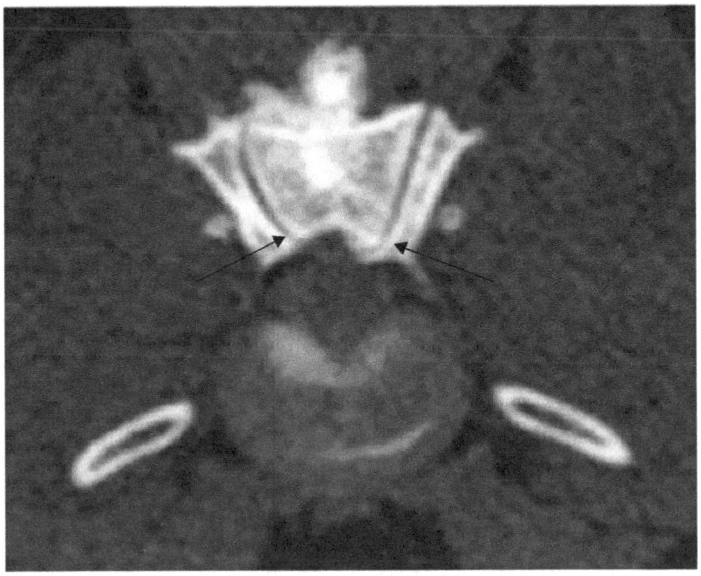

A

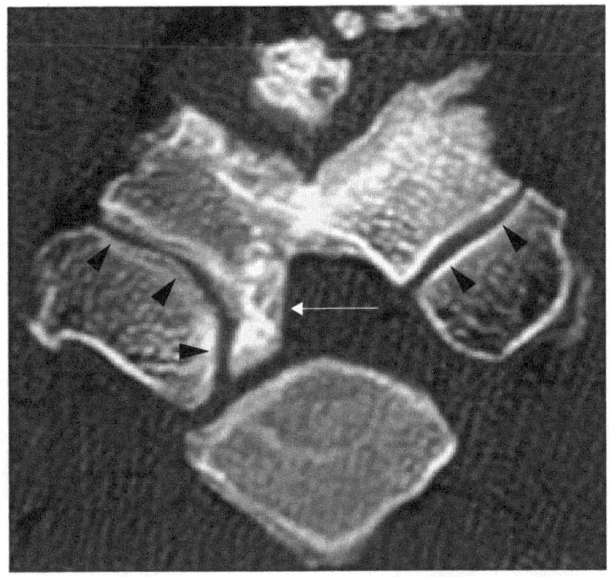

B

Figure 22.15 Two adult dogs with articular process joint arthrosis. (A) Transverse CT image shows asymmetry between the articular process joints (arrows). (B) Transverse CT image shows severe hypertrophy of the left articular process joint (arrow). Both joint spaces are narrowed (arrowheads), slightly irregular and the subchondral bone is sclerotic.

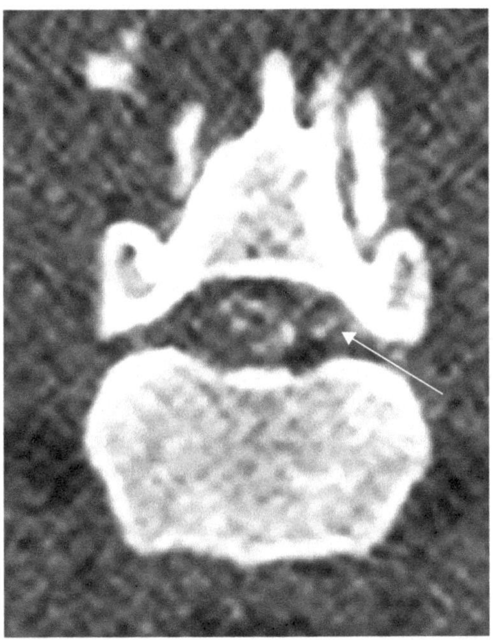

Figure 22.16 Adult dog with a ganglion cyst. Transverse CT image shows a soft tissue-dense cystic formation (arrow) located immediately adjacent to an articular process.

young dogs. The etiology is unknown. It can also occur in association with neoplasia, but other features of disease are then present.

CT features (Figure 22.17)

- Mineral-dense foci around the spinal cord.
- CT myelography: hard to see due to adjacent subarachnoid contrast.

Degenerative disk disease

Hansen type I disk disease is common in chondrodystrophic long-backed small breeds such as the Dachshund, often starting at a very young age. It consists of a metaplasia of the gelatinous nucleus pulposus into dehydrated and mineralized material. These changes per se do not cause clinical signs. However, minimal stress on the hardened central disk may then lead to complete rupture of the annulus fibrosus and extrusion of disk material into the vertebral canal at the disk space and adjacent vertebrae, leading to extradural spinal cord compression, extradural or intradural hemorrhage and intramedullary spinal cord swelling causing acute onset para- or tetraparesis.

Hansen type II disk disease can be seen in all dogs and in cats, usually at an advanced age. Mineralization of the nucleus pulposus is common but not always present. There is only partial fiber rupture of the annulus fibrosus with bulging of the disk into the vertebral canal. This protrusion causes a more localized and chronic form of spinal cord compression and chronic onset of clinical signs often starting with pain.

Vacuum phenomenon, gas collections within the intervertebral space, is sometimes seen in degenerative disk disease. It is due to the liberation of gas,

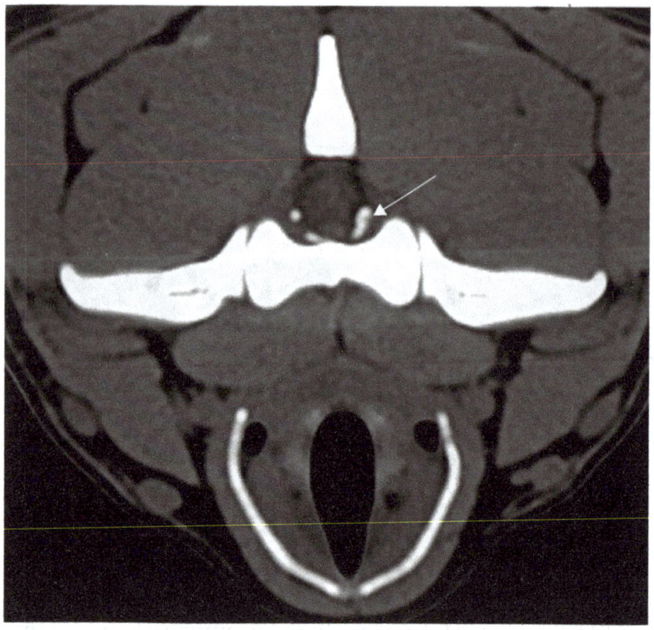

Figure 22.17 Transverse CT image of a dural mineralization (arrow) at C1 in a neurologically normal dog.

principally nitrogen, from surrounding tissues and accumulation within disk fissures. The vacuum sign indicates diskal degeneration but not spinal cord compression.

CT protocol

Mineralized extruded material can be seen on non-contrast images, but CT myelography is generally recommended for better delineation of the spinal cord and identification of non-mineralized compressive disk material. Multiplanar reconstructions are very helpful in delineating the extent and site of a lesion.

CT features (Figures 22.18–22.20)

- Disk degeneration is often present at multiple sites including that of the compression – stippled mineral-dense material present at the disk space.
- Linear or circular gas within the intervertebral space (vacuum phenomenon).
- CT myelography
  - compression and displacement of the spinal cord
  - compression of the epidural space
  - soft tissue-dense material at the site of compression.
- Post-contrast (IV):
  - hyperdense material (hemorrhage) often extending cranially or caudally from the site of compression
  - variable cord changes including hypodensity (edema), contrast filling (myelomalacia)
  - cord swelling.

Degenerative lumbosacral stenosis

Degenerative lumbosacral stenosis is characterized by intervertebral disk degeneration, ligamentous hypertrophy, bone proliferations and degenerative changes of the dorsal articular facet joints, all of which can contribute to compression of the cauda equina.

CT features (Figures 22.21, 22.22)

- Dorsal protrusion of the lumbosacral disk.
- Dorsal displacement of the nerve roots and loss of surrounding fat.
- Bone proliferation on the vertebral bodies and dorsal articular process joints.
- Foraminal stenosis is evidenced by a narrowing of the intervertebral foramen and loss of foraminal fat.
- Swelling of the nerve roots of the cauda equina may be present.
- Acquiring image series in flexion and extension will allow assessment of a dynamic component of the cauda equina compression, with the compression being more severe in extension unless a lumbosacral instability is present (severe also in flexion).

Degenerative myelopathy

Degenerative myelopathy is a neurodegenerative disease process. German shepherd dogs are most commonly affected, although it has been described in other breeds. CT is most useful in ruling out other causes of progressive neuropathy, but certain non-specific features have been associated with the disease in affected animals.

CT features

- Spinal cord small and deformed.
- Spinal stenosis.
- Paraspinal muscle atrophy.

Neoplasia

CT protocol

Intravenous contrast medium application is recommended in any case where neoplasia is suspected. Contrast enhancement of the lesion will help in differentiation neoplastic lesions from hyperplastic lesions of the paravertebral ligaments and spinal cord

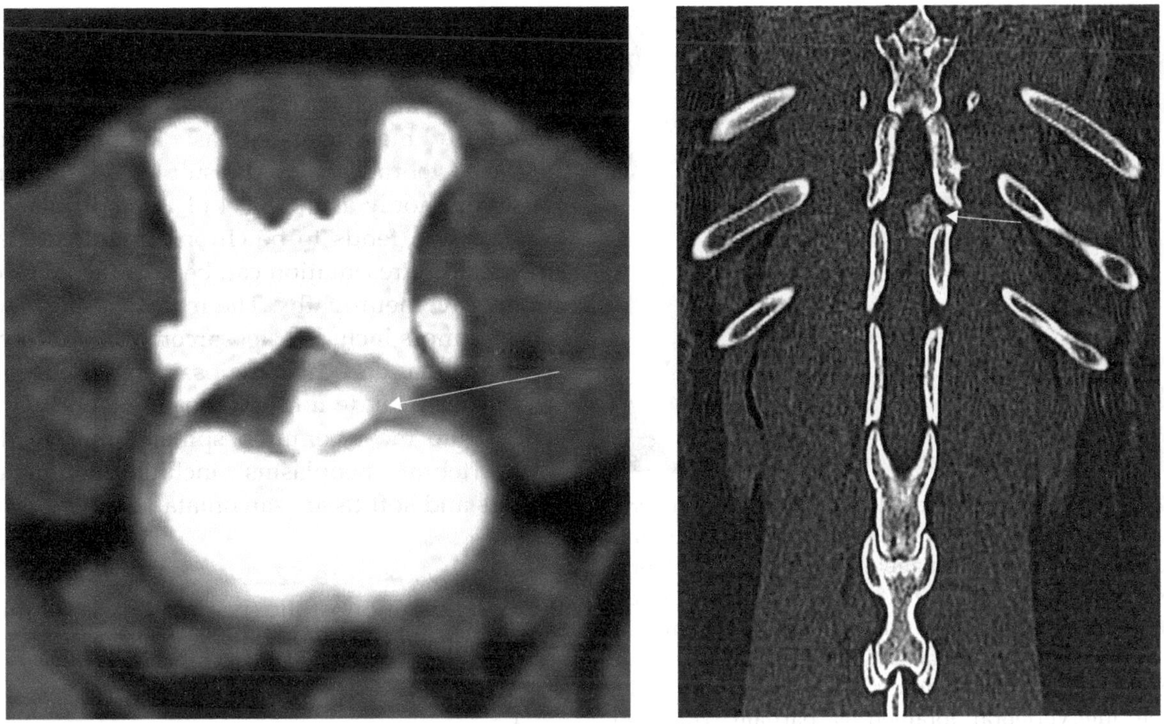

A B

Figure 22.18 Adult Dachshund with a discus hernia. (A) Transverse CT image shows severe lateralized extradural compression by an extruded mineralized disk (arrow). (B) Dorsally reconstructed CT image of the same dog, allowing accurate lesion localization (arrow).

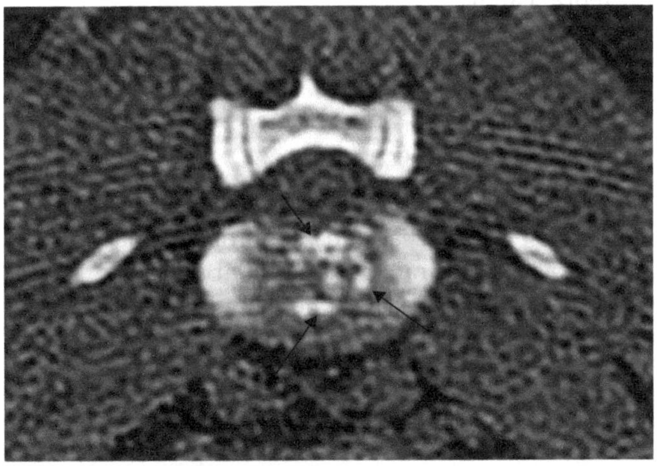

Figure 22.19 Adult dog with an in situ mineralized degenerative disk. Transverse CT image shows stippled mineral-dense material at the disk center (arrows).

adnexa, although non-neoplastic mass lesions may also contrast enhance. CT myelography is also helpful in delineating the spinal cord from any adjacent soft tissue lesion, and in differentiation of extradural, intradural and intramedullary lesions.

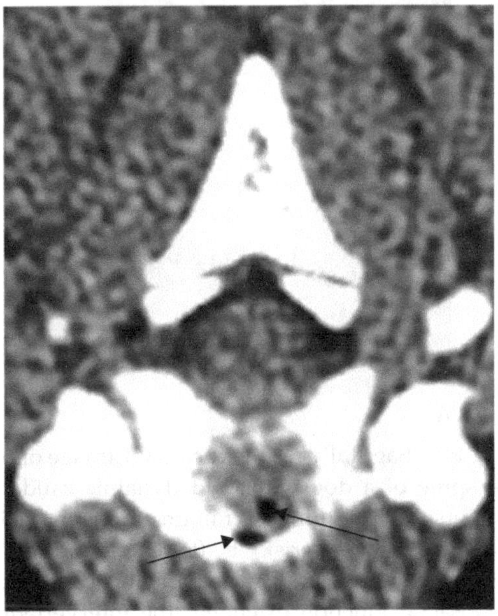

Figure 22.20 Adult Dachshund with discus hernia. Transverse CT images show a gas bubble (vacuum phenomenon) within intervertebral space (arrows).

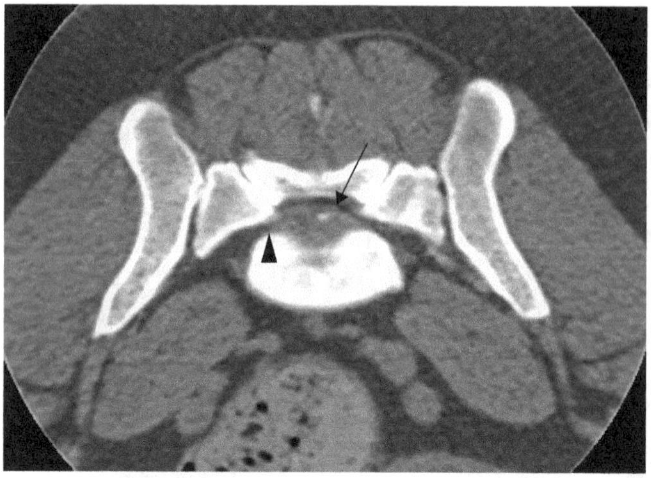

Figure 22.21 Adult dog with degenerative lumbosacral stenosis, compression of the cauda equina and right foraminal stenosis. Transverse CT image shows the intervertebral disk protruding dorsally, leaving only a thin sliver of epidural fat in the vertebral canal (arrowhead). The herniated material contains a focal mineralization seen as a hyperdense dot. The disk protrusion is more severe on the right side, where the intervertebral foramen is partially occluded (arrow). The nerve roots of the cauda equina are not visible separate from the herniated disk material (compressed).

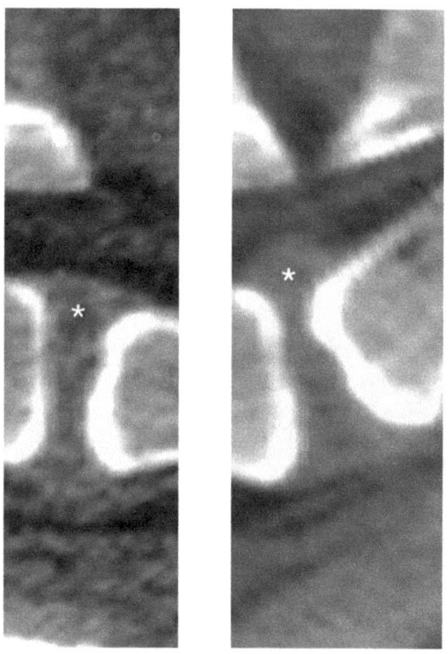

A B

Figure 22.22 Sagittally reconstructed CT image of the lumbosacral spine of a dog with mild dynamic cauda equina compression. (A) The lumbosacral junction is in flexion, the intervertebral disk (asterisk) is flattened and the cauda equina is not compressed. (B) The patient is positioned with the lumbosacral junction extended, the intervertebral disk (asterisk) protrudes much further dorsally, narrowing the vertebral canal and attenuating the epidural fat around the cauda equina.

Extradural

Extradural tumors are the most common category of neoplasms affecting the spinal cord. Primary bone tumors and metastatic neoplasia to bone can encroach on the vertebral canal and result in cord compression, most commonly at the level of the thoracic spine. As compression tends to be chronic, focal cord atrophy may result. Presentation can be of an acute or chronic progressive neuropathy. The most common focal vertebral tumors include osteosarcoma, chondrosarcoma, fibrosarcoma and hemangiosarcoma, while diffuse neoplasms include multiple myeloma and lymphosarcoma (the most common spinal tumor in the cat). Paravertebral neoplasms include neuroendocrine tumors and soft tissue sarcomata.

CT features (Figure 22.23)

- Location: monostotic (primary) or randomly polyostotic (secondary).
- Usually very subtle osteolysis with or without periosteal reaction.
- Occasionally osteosclerotic appearance.
- Pathologic compression fracture common.
- Perivertebral soft tissue mass extension into thorax possible.
- Small circular lesions within the body.
- Soft tissue- or mineral-dense mass within the vertebral canal.
- Displacement of the spinal cord.
- Post-contrast (IV): enhancement of the lesion.

Intradural extramedullary

Meningioma, neurofibrosarcoma, lymphosarcoma, nerve root neoplasia and nephroblastoma can all appear as intradural extramedullary lesions. Nerve root neoplasia, such as peripheral nerve sheath tumors, may have intramedullary and intradural components. Most affect older dogs and cats, but nephroblastomas are typical in young dogs and occur specifically between T10 and L2.

CT features (Figure 22.24)

- CT myelography is necessary to define location as intradural.
- Widened subarachnoid space
  - a 'golf tee' is apparent in the contrast column on sagittal and dorsal reconstructions
  - the tumor may extend into the spinal cord and can appear more intramedullary
  - with nerve root tumors there is often widening of the intervertebral foramen and presence of a

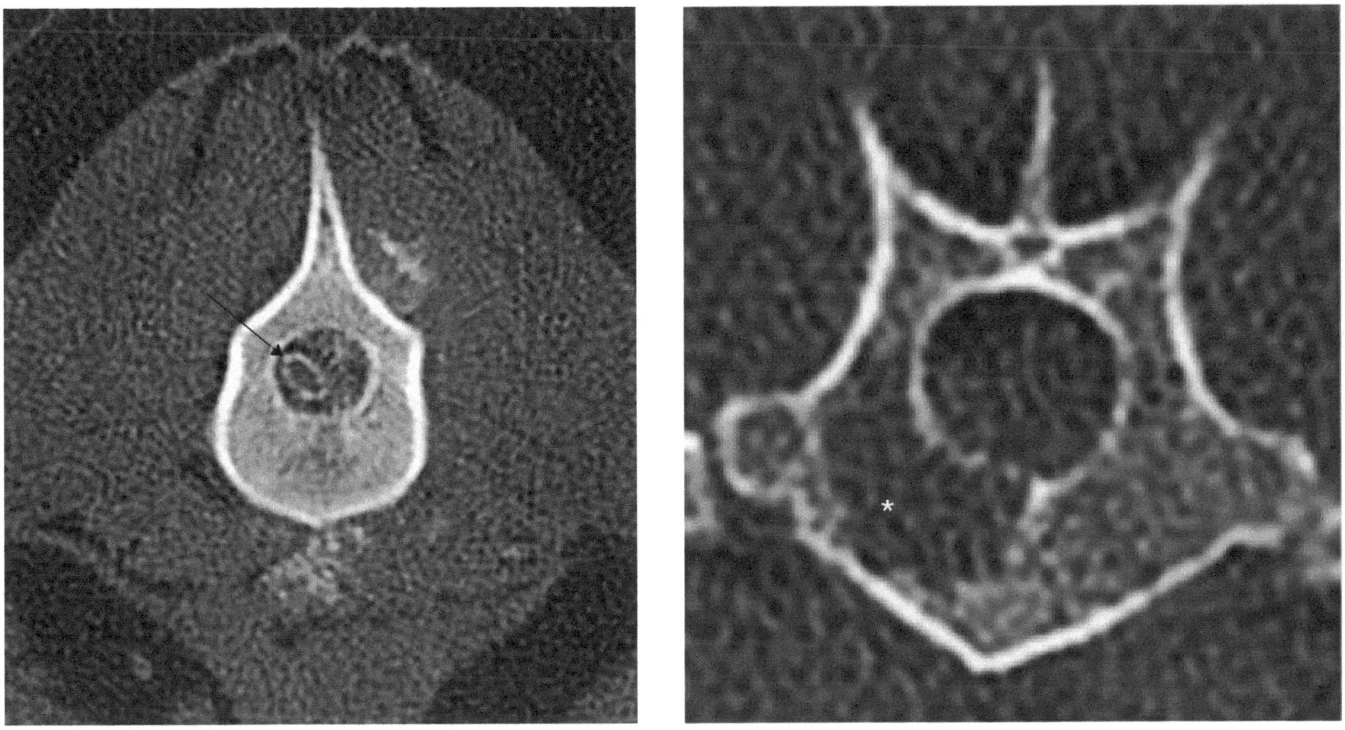

A B

Figure 22.23 (A) Adult dog with metastatic osteosarcoma. Transverse CT myelogram shows marked spinal cord compression (arrow) (image courtesy of N. Nelson, Ohio State University). (B) Adult dog with multiple myeloma. Transverse CT image shows decreased density on the right half of the vertebral body (asterisk).

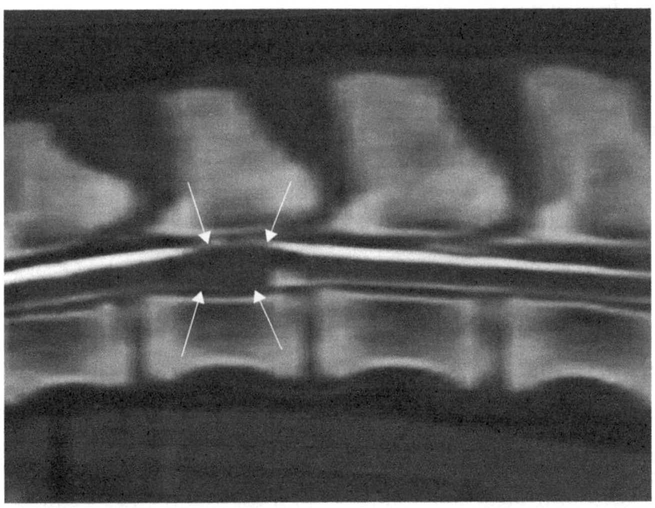

Figure 22.24 Young dog with a nephroblastoma. Sagittally reconstructed CT myelogram shows an intradural extramedullary lesion (arrows) (image courtesy of N. Nelson, Ohio State University).

contrast-enhanced tubular structure consistent with nerve root enlargement.

Intramedullary

Glial cell tumors are the most common intramedullary tumors in dogs, while lymphosarcoma is most common in cats. Intramedullary metastases are rare.

CT features

- CT myelography: focal spinal cord swelling.
- Post-contrast (IV): enhancement of the spinal cord.

Vascular disorders

Fibrocartilaginous embolism

Fibrocartilaginous embolism is acute infarction of the spinal cord that results from vascular occlusion by fibrocartilage from the nucleus pulposus. Large dogs are most commonly affected, but spinal cord infarction has also been described in the cat. A typical presentation is acute-onset asymmetric neuropathy that is non-painful and non-progressive after the first 24h. CT diagnosis is by exclusion of other causes of spinal cord disease.

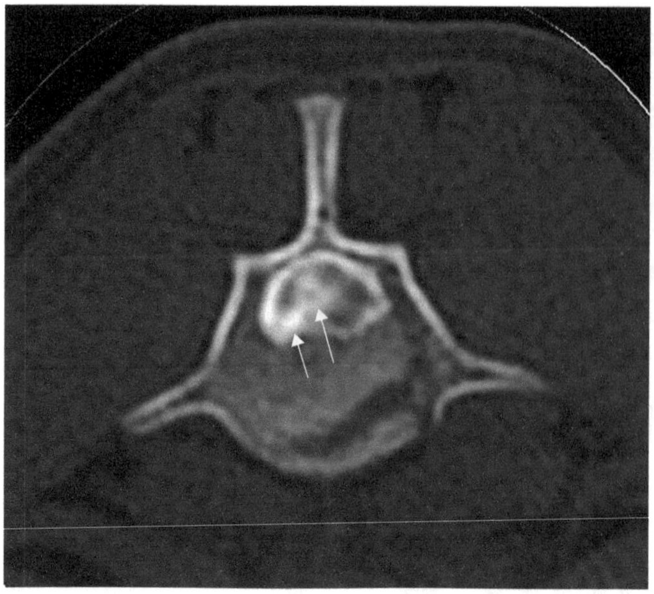

Figure 22.25 Adult dog that was hit by a car and developed myelomalacia at the site of a lumbar fracture. Transverse CT myelogram shows swelling of the spinal cord that contains multiple hyperdense areas (contrast medium) (arrows).

CT features

- Post-contrast (IV): focal spinal cord swelling may be present.

Myelomalacia

Myelomalacia is hemorrhagic infarction of the spinal cord. It can occur secondary to any acute spinal cord injury and may be focal or extend cranially. Ascending myelomalacia is usually fatal.

CT features (Figure 22.25)

- Most often seen in association with other lesions (trauma, disk extrusion).
- Hyperdense area within the spinal cord.
- CT-myelography
  - contrast medium within the cord parenchyma
  - spinal cord swelling.

Idiopathic/Nutritional

Hypervitaminosis A

Hypervitaminosis A is a nutritional disorder of cats due to excessive feeding with vitamin A. It is characterized by severe exostosis of the joints and vertebrae, particularly the cervical vertebrae. This disorder may lead to pain and rigidity and in severe cases it may cause nerve root and spinal nerve compression.

Calcinosis circumscripta

Calcinosis circumscripta has been described as a rare cause of compressive spinal cord dysfunction in young dogs, mostly between C1 and C2.

Disseminated skeletal hyperostosis

Disseminated skeletal hyperostosis results in extensive ventral vertebral new bone formation, including endplates and body, often spanning more than three vertebrae.

Further reading

Axlund TW and Hudson JA (2003) Computed tomography of the normal lumbosacral intervertebral disc in 22 dogs. *Vet Radiol Ultrasound* **44**: 630–4.

Dennison SE, Drees R, Rylander H, Yandell BS, Milovancev M, Pettigrew R and Schwarz T (2010) Evaluation of different computed tomography techniques and myelography for the diagnosis of acute canine myelopathy. *Vet Radiol Ultrasound* **51**: 254–8.

Drees R, Dennison SE, Keuler NS and Schwarz T (2009) Computed tomographic imaging protocol for the canine cervical and lumbar spine. *Vet Radiol Ultrasound* **50**: 74–9.

Gnirs K, Ruel Y, Blot S *et al.* (2003) Spinal subarachnoid cysts in 13 dogs. *Vet Rad Ultrasound* **44**: 402–8.

Jones JC and Inzana KD (2000) Subclinical CT abnormalities in the lumbosacral spine of older large-breed dogs. *Vet Radiol Ultrasound* **41**: 19–26.

Kinns J, Mai W, Seiler G *et al.* (2006) Radiographic sensitivity and negative predictive value for acute canine spinal trauma. *Vet Radiol Ultrasound* **47**: 563–70.

Ramirez III O and Thrall DE (1998) A review of imaging techniques for canine cauda equina syndrome. *Vet Radiol Ultrasound* **39**: 283–96.

Schwarz T, Owen MR, Long S and Sullivan M (2000) Vacuum disk and facet phenomenon in a dog with cauda equina syndrome. *J Am Vet Med Assoc* **15**: 862–4.

Sharp NJH, Cofone M, Robertson ID, DeCarlo A, Smith GK and Thrall DE (1995) Computed tomography in the evaluation of caudal cervical spondylomyelopathy of the Doberman pinscher. *Vet Radiol Ultrasound* **36**: 100–8.

CHAPTER TWENTY-THREE

Heart and Vessels

Marc-André d'Anjou and Tobias Schwarz

Imaging Protocol (Table 23.1)

The advent of multislice CT has expanded the capacity of CT to assess cardiovascular disorders. With single-slice CT, protocols must be adapted to favor the acquisition of high-resolution images along the Z-axis in the shortest possible time. Once the region of interest is identified after scanning the entire thorax, slice thickness may be further reduced to better highlight small structures. Test bolus injection should be used whenever possible to determine the peak enhancement, and to select the best acquisition start time after contrast medium injection start. This is essential for assessment of the more distant pools and lumens such as left ventricle and aorta that suffer from contrast dilution with peripheral vein injection. In case of soft tissue masses; a delayed acquisition should also be performed to assess tissue perfusion after the clearance of contrast medium from the great vessels. The complex anatomy of the heart and great vessels is best depicted with multiplanar reformation (MPR), maximum intensity projection (MIP), shaded surface display (SSD) or volume rendering.

CT: Anatomy

Heart and pericardium (Figure 23.1)

The heart is a complex muscular structure composed of four chambers that can readily be distinguished when filled with iodinated contrast medium. The atria are separated by a thin interatrial septum that may not be well defined with CT, whereas the ventricles are separated by a thicker interventricular septum and outlined by walls that can be consistently recognized. Atrioventricular valves are relatively perpendicular to the transverse plane and can be recognized in most cases, particularly if slice thickness is less than 3 mm. The pericardial cavity can be filled with hypodense fat, particularly in obese patients, in which case the fibrous pericardium (smooth, 1–2 mm thick) becomes distinct from the underlying myocardium. The cardiac apex is normally oriented to the left of the midline, although it may be central or right-sided in some animals.

Great vessels (Figure 23.1)

The pulmonic trunk and aortic root are similar in width. The pulmonic and aortic valves can be identified with thin-slice acquisitions, particularly with MPR. Contrast-enhanced CT allows evaluation of the ventricular outflow tracts, the lumen of the aortic arch and its branches, and of the pulmonary arteries. The pulmonic trunk and arteries fill rapidly and intensely with contrast medium after peripheral venous injection, while the aorta fills later (±10 s post-injection) after systemic hemodilution. Time and intensity of enhancement of the cranial and caudal vena cava depend on the site and rate of injection. Injection through a large catheter via the cranial vena cava allows rapid injection of large boluses but results in beam-hardening streak artifacts that can compromise the visibility of nearby structures. Injecting into a peripheral vein results in more uniform contrast filling and reduces the presence of artifacts. Reducing contrast medium concentration may also help, particularly with a central intravenous catheter. The use of a pressure injector is advised.

Anatomic and physiologic variants and incidental findings

Coronary artery branching (Figure 23.2)

Five different anatomical pattern of the right and left coronary artery branching have been identified in

Veterinary Computed Tomography, First Edition. Edited by Tobias Schwarz, Jimmy Saunders.

Table 23.1
CT imaging protocol for single-slice CT angiography of heart and great vessels.

Series	Pre-contrast	+/– Delayed post-contrast	Angiography
Decubitus	Ventral		
Scan margins	Caudal to cranial extent of lungs		
Voltage (kVp)	120		
Current (mAs)	200		
Tube rotation time (s)	0.5–1.0		
Slice width (mm)	3 (<10 kg), 5 (>10 kg)		3 (<10 kg), 5 (>10 kg)*
Pitch	1.5	1.5–2.0	
Helical image reconstruction interval	0.5 × slice width		
Kernel frequency	Medium		
Motion control	+/– manual ventilation		
Contrast medium application site	N/A	**Caudal vena cava:** cephalic or external jugular **Cranial vena cava:** saphenous vein **Heart, aorta or pulmonary arteries:** external jugular or cranial vena cava	
Contrast medium type	N/A	Iodinated	
Contrast medium dose	N/A	400–800 mg iodine/kg bw	
Contrast medium injection mode	N/A	Automated	
Scan delay post start contrast injection	N/A	Based on test bolus injection and peak enhancement of the region(s) of interest	
Window level (HU)	40	200–400	100–600 dependent on contrast medium concentration
Window width (HU)	200–2000 Dependent on contrast medium concentration		

dogs. An anomalous origin of the left coronary artery can lead to subvalvular pulmonic stenosis and has therapeutic consequences. Multislice helical CT angiography offers a minimally invasive, quick and efficient way of assessing the coronary artery branching pattern in dogs for diagnosis and treatment planning.

Adaptive cardiovascular changes (Figure 23.3)

The size and shape of the heart and great vessels depend on the phase of the cardiac and respiratory cycle and external pressure changes. To some degree this is visible on CT exams and should be taken into account when assessing cardiovascular structures.

Cardiovascular gas emboli (Figure 23.4)

Numerous gas bubbles can be seen in most dogs and cats undergoing a CT examination in the veins of the thorax, shoulder and vertebral system without any related clinical signs during or after the procedure. They are often present already before contrast medium application and are a normal phenomenon of vascular catheterization. Gas location depends on the venous catheter site and recumbency of the animal, as the gas accumulates in the highest location.

Aortic and cardiac mineralization

Mineralization of the aortic wall or other cardiac vessels can be recognized incidentally. It affects mainly

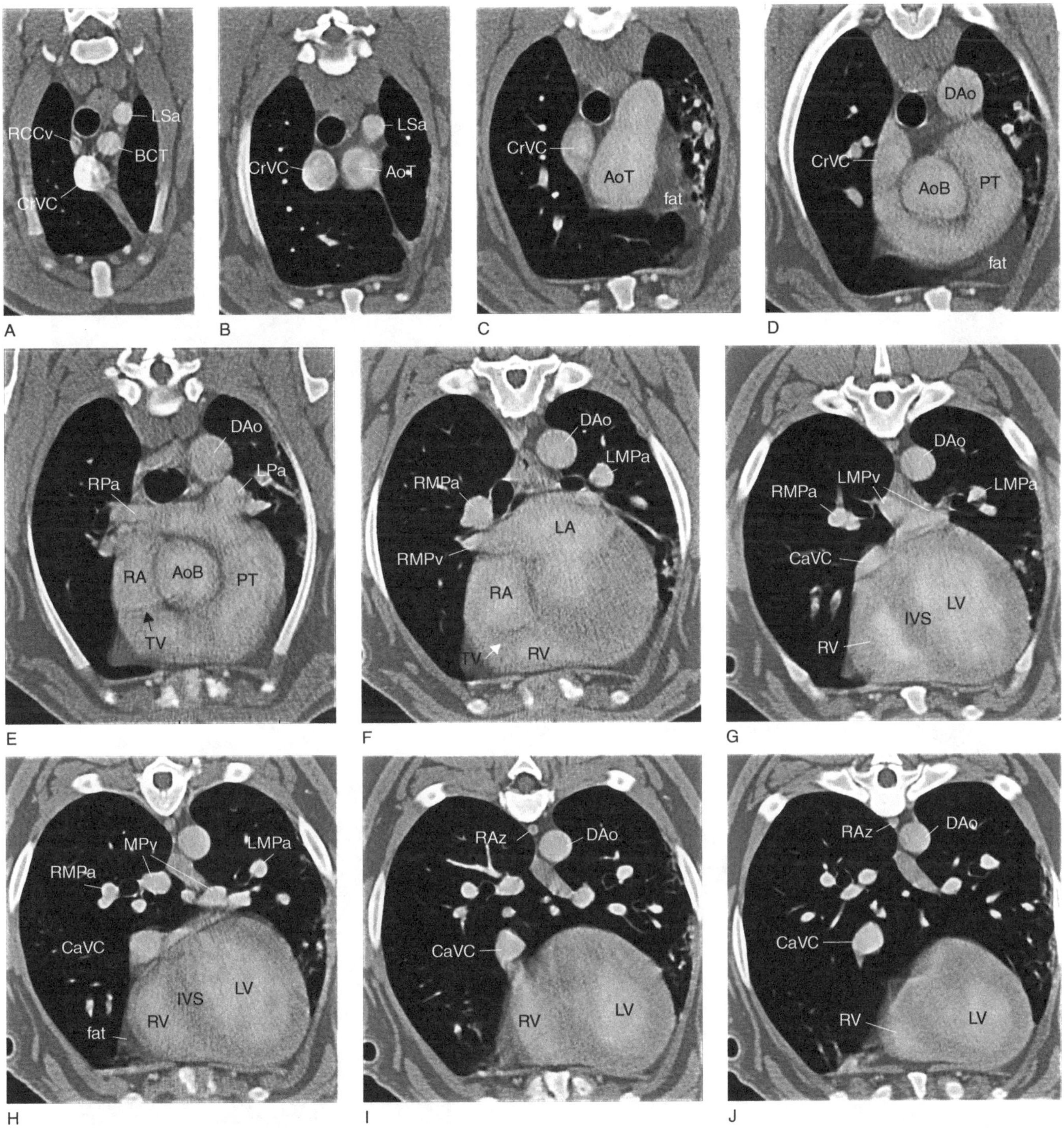

Figure 23.1 Normal CT angiographic anatomy of the heart and great vessels. Transverse images A–J represent successive, but not contiguous, images from cranial to caudal. AoB = aortic bulb; AoT = aortic trunk; BCT = brachiocephalic trunk; CaCV = caudal vena cava; CrCV = cranial vena cava; DAo = descending aorta; IVS = interventricular septum; LA = left atrium; LMPa = left main pulmonary artery; LPa = left pulmonary artery; LSa = left subclavian artery; LV = left ventricle; MPv = main pulmonary veins; PT = pulmonic trunk; RA = right atrium; RAz = right azygos vein; RCCv = right costocervical vein; RPa = right pulmonary artery; RMPa = right main pulmonary artery; RMPv = right middle pulmonary vein; RV = right ventricle; TV = tricuspid valve.

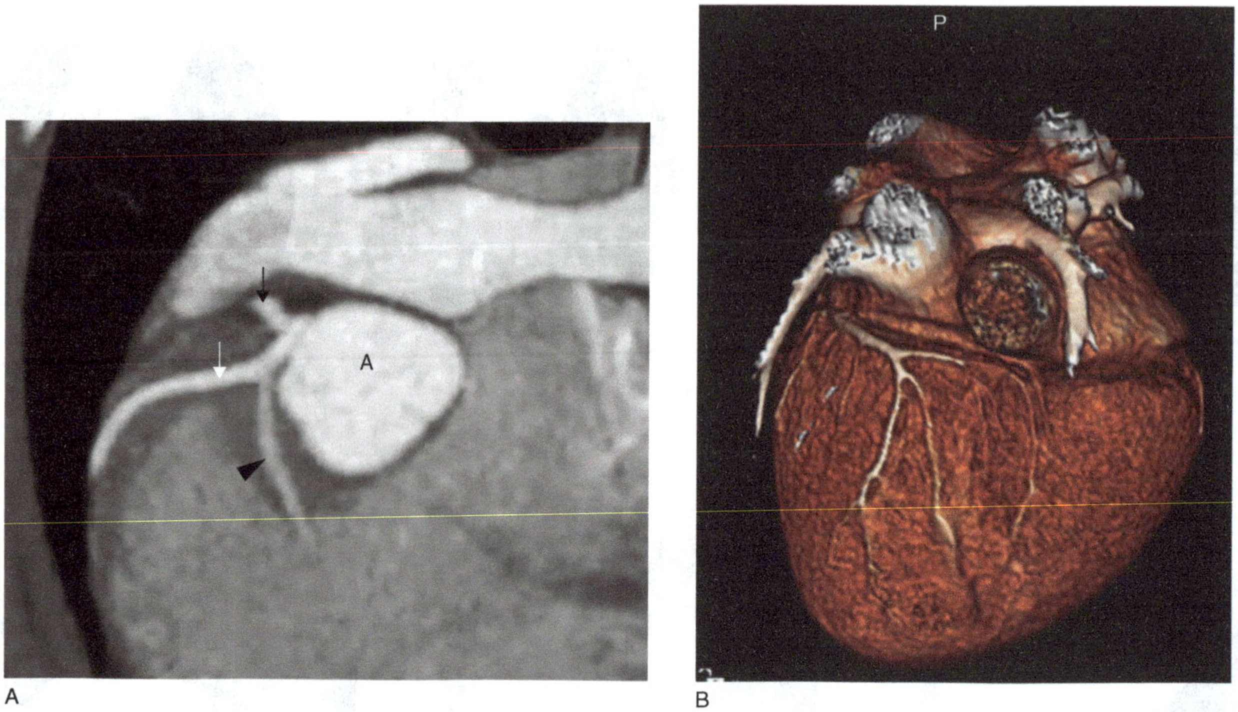

Figure 23.2 Coronary CT angiogram of a normal dog using 64-slice CT technology. (A) Transverse CT angiogram showing the aorta (A) and the following left coronary artery branches: the circumflex (black arrow), interventricular paraconal (white arrow) and septal branch (arrowhead). (B) Volume-rendered image of the heart viewed from a right caudal perspective demonstrating the left circumflex coronary artery (images courtesy of Randi Drees).

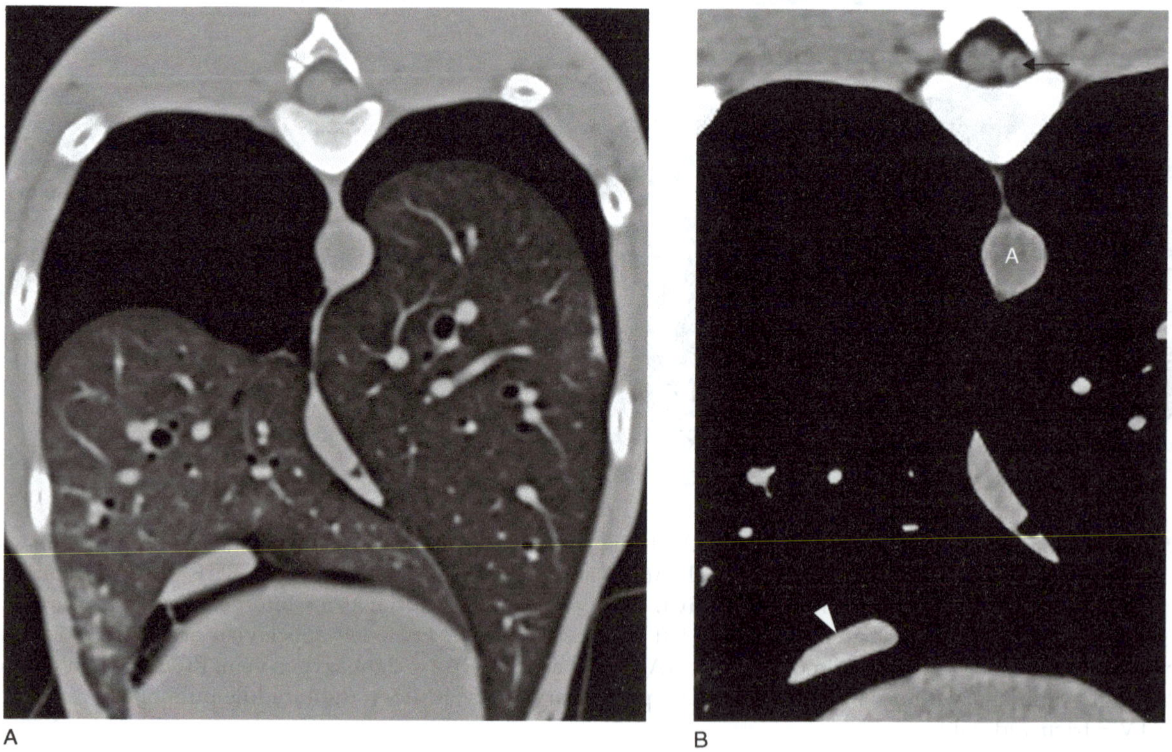

Figure 23.3 (A) Transverse CT image of a dog with marked pneumothorax. (B) Due to the raised extravascular pressure, the caudal vena cava (arrowhead) is partially collapsed whereas the left vertebral venous sinus (arrow) is enlarged as a means of alternative venous return. The size of the aorta (A) is not affected.

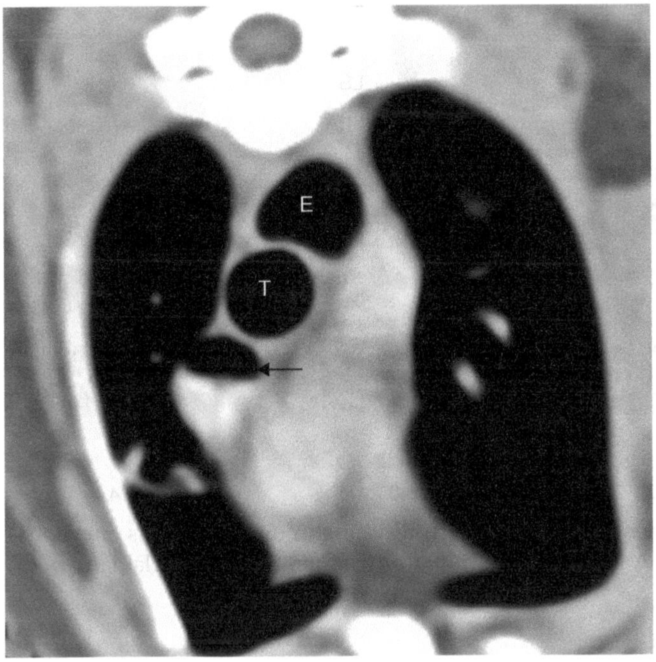

Figure 23.4 Transverse CT image of a cat with a small gas cap in the cranial vena cava (arrow), ventral to trachea (T) and esophagus (E). This is a normal phenomenon after vascular catheterization, often already present before contrast medium administration.

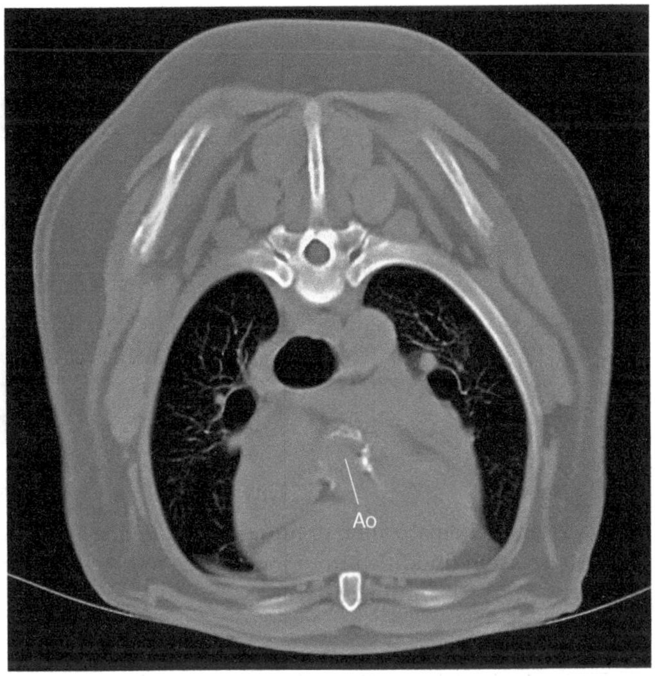

Figure 23.5 Transverse CT image of a dog with incidental mineralization of the aortic bulb. An irregular, hyperdense partial rim involves the wall of the aorta (Ao).

older, large-breed dogs (particularly Rottweiler and Irish wolfhound) and is usually degenerative in origin. Mineralization of the descending aorta can also be associated with atherosclerosis, spirocercosis or hyperadrenocorticism.

CT features (Figure 23.5)

- Curvilinear or amorphous hyperattenuation of mineral value involving the aortic wall, particularly in the bulb region, or other cardiac arteries such as coronaries.

Disease Features

Malformation/Developmental disorders

Malformations may appear during fetal development and represent incidental findings, such as a left-sided cranial vena cava. Conversely, cardiac and vascular anomalies may become clinically significant. Contrast-enhanced CT, especially with multislice units, can complement echocardiography in treatment planning of such malformations, particularly embolization or stenting. Because of its tomographic nature and higher contrast resolution, CT angiography is performed with peripheral venous injection, i.e. non-selectively, and has replaced conventional angiography.

Vascular ring anomalies (Figure 23.6)

Persistence of the right aortic arch accounts for ±90% of vascular ring anomalies in dogs and cats. The esophagus is most commonly affected and its compression varies in site and severity according to the specific type of malformation. Characterization of these anomalies is best performed with contrast-enhanced CT. Injection of air through a catheter placed in the esophagus may help in confirming the site and level of compression.

CT features (Figure 23.7)

- **Types 1–3**: dextra position of the aorta, associated with leftward displacement of the trachea.
- **Type 1** (most common): compression of the esophagus typically at the heart base by a non-enhancing left ligamentum arteriosum that extends dorsally between the pulmonic trunk and a right-sided aorta.
- **Type 2 or 3:** compression of the esophagus cranial to the heart base in cases of aberrant left subclavian artery that crosses craniodorsally over the esophagus (type 2). The presence of an aberrant right ligamentum arteriosum in this case prevents another site of compression at the heart base. If a left ligamentum arteriosum is present, two sites of compression may be found (type 3).

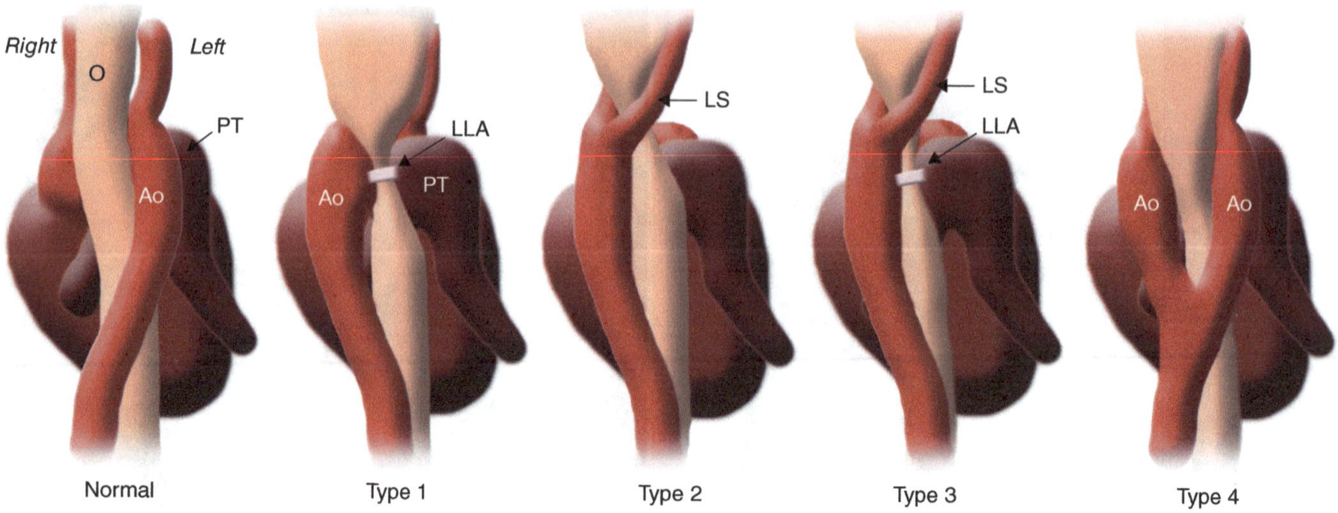

Figure 23.6 Schematization of normal and abnormal development of the aortic arch resulting in different levels of esophageal compression (modified from Joly *et al.* 2008). Ao = Aorta; LLA = left ligamentum arteriosum; LS = left subclavian artery; O = esophagus; PT = pulmonic trunk.

- **Type 4**: double aortic arch joining to form a ring around the esophagus caudal to the heart base.
- Other vascular malformations such as anomalous subclavian artery may also result in esophageal entrapment.

Patent ductus arteriosus

Patency of the ductus arteriosus connecting the fetal main pulmonary artery with the aorta is a common congenital malformation in dogs and, less frequently, cats. Persistent shunting can occur in a left-to-right or right-to-left direction of flow. Left-to-right shunts have a distinctive machinery murmur that is lacking in right-to-left shunts. CT can aid in the diagnosis of more difficult right-to-left patent ductus cases and can be used for shunt size assessment for therapy planning.

CT features (Figure 23.8)

- Distinct ductus diverticulum connecting proximal descending aorta with the main pulmonary artery. A tapered ductus diverticulum may be clinically silent.
- Distinct patterns of contrast enhancement in levo- and dextro-phase CT angiography depending on shunt type.

Aberrant bronchoesophageal artery

In dogs and cats the bronchoesophageal artery arises from several thoracic aortic branches and supplies the bronchi with systemic blood with venous drainage via the azygos system. As a rare anomaly in dogs, the artery can form a shunt with a pulmonary artery and clinical signs similar to a left-to-right patent ductus arteriosus can occur.

CT features

- Levo-phase angiogram demonstrating contrast enhancement of multiple small aortic branches converging into a single tortuous shunt vessel entering the right pulmonary artery and flow of contrast medium into the pulmonary arterial circulation.

Cardiac valvular stenoses and insufficiencies (Figure 23.9)

Although CT is currently not widely used for most cardiac conditions in small animals, the potential of multislice CT examination of the heart is encouraging. The typical vascular and chamber enlargements seen in canine and feline valvular heart diseases, such as aortic and pulmonic stenosis, mitral and tricuspid insufficiencies can be recognized on CT.

Vascular dissection, aneurysm and stenosis (Figure 23.10)

Aneurysms can affect veins such as the cranial vena cava, but are more commonly seen in the thoracic aorta in association with patent ductus arteriosus, aortic coarctation, aortic wall degeneration, *Spirocerca lupi* infection or systemic hypertension. Aneurysms of cardiac chambers have also been described and can be congenital or traumatic. Aortic dissection can also be

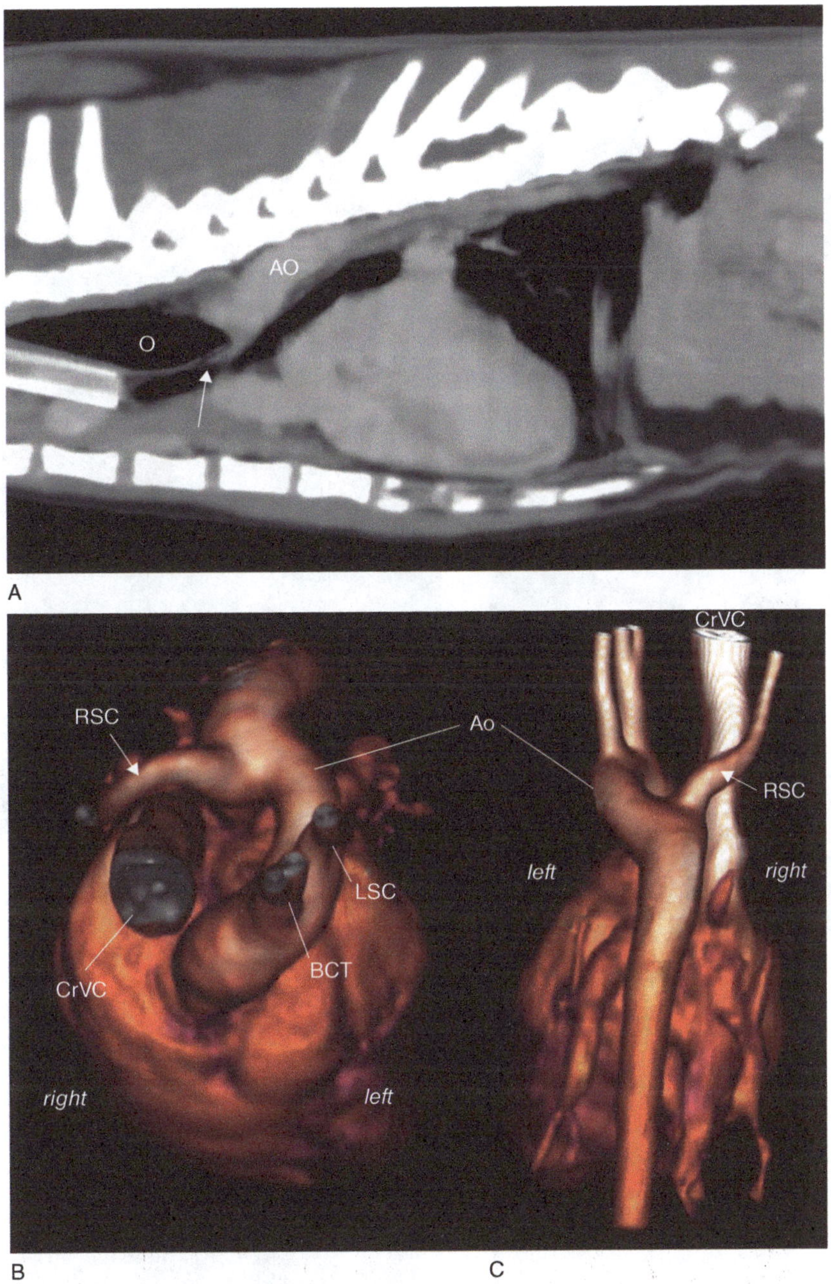

Figure 23.7 Five-month-old cat with an aberrant right subclavian artery. (A) Sagittally reconstructed CT image shows esophagus (O) dilatation in the cranial thorax and compression by an aberrant right subclavian artery (arrow) that originates directly from the aorta (Ao). (B) and (C) 3-D reconstructed CT images on which the anomaly can be clearly depicted from cranial (B) and dorsal (C) views. BCT = brachiocephalic trunk; CrVC = cranial vena cava; LSC = left subclavian artery; RSC = right subclavian artery (images courtesy of Franck Durieux).

encountered, with characteristic visualization of the intimal flap on CT. Trauma may result in false aneurysm, i.e. focal wall rupture with eccentric accumulation of blood limited by the adventitial layer, or complete rupture. Pulmonary artery stenosis has been reported in a dog. The use of a pressure injector is essential to adequately enhance the aortic lumen and to identify these anomalies, particularly in regard to the dissection flap. These linear defects must also be differentiated from streaks artifacts due to motion or beam hardening.

CT features (Figure 23.11)

- **Aneurysm**: focal, smooth dilatation of the vessel or chamber lumen.

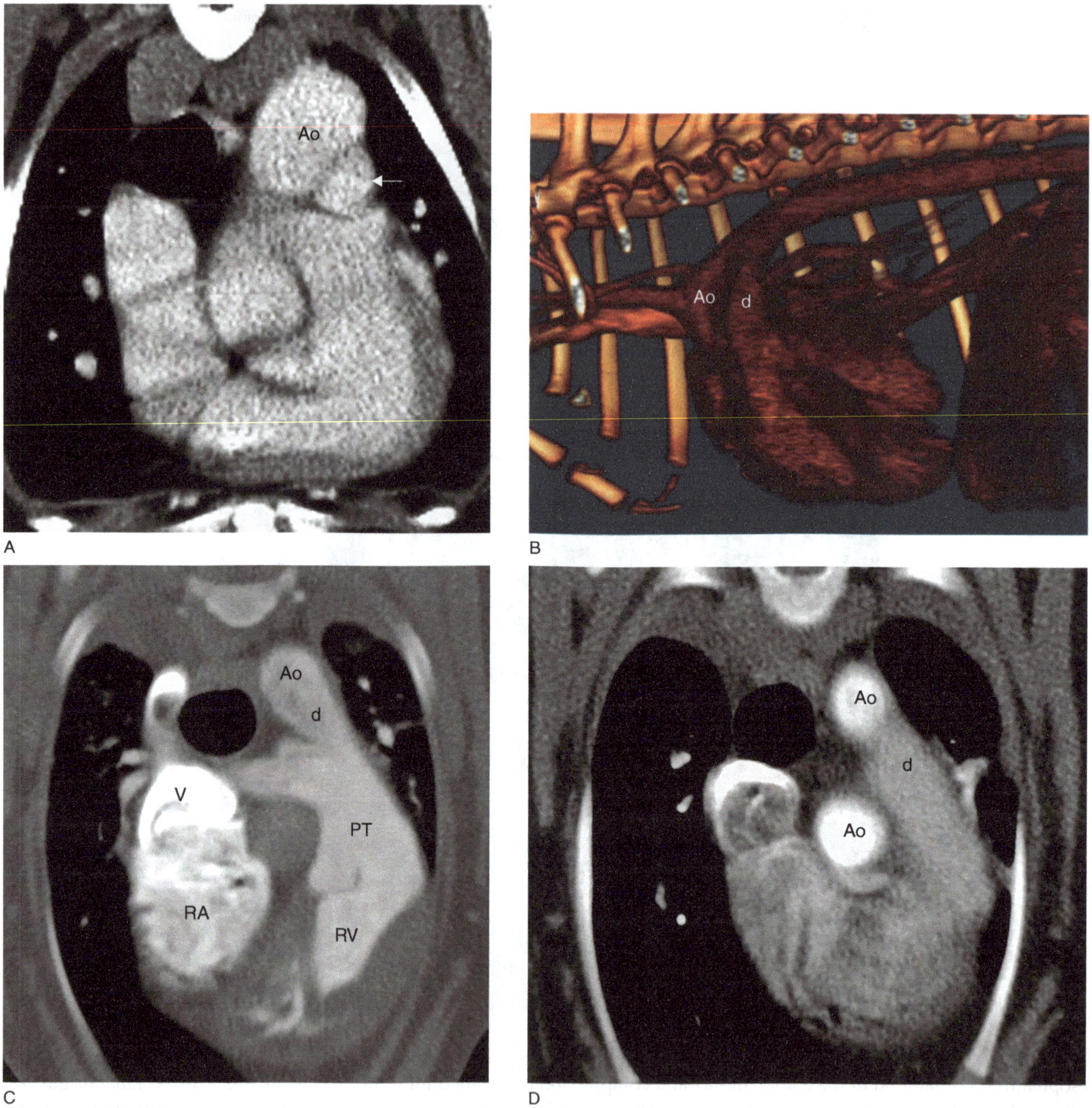

Figure 23.8 (A) Transverse CT image of a dog with a clinically silent patent ductus arteriosus diverticulum (arrow) ventral to the descending aorta (Ao). (B) Volume-rendered view at the right heart of a different, clinically affected dog with a large patent ductus arteriosus (d) joining the aorta (Ao). (C) Dextro-phase CT angiography demonstrates a contrast-enhanced cranial vena cava (V), right heart (RA, RV), pulmonic trunk (PT), patent ductus arteriosus (d), and descending aorta (Ao). (D) Levo-phase CT angiography shows the stronger contrast enhancement in the aortic arch (Ao) than in the patent ductus arteriosus (d). The combination of these features confirms a right-to-left shunt direction (B to D images courtesy of Björn Åblad).

- **Pseudoaneurysm**: focal outpouching of contrast medium through a defect in the wall.
- **Dissection**: curvilinear contrast-filling defects indicating intimal flap, with higher enhancement of the true lumen during the peak phase of aortic enhancement. The false lumen tends to be larger than the true lumen. The intimal flap may also be calcified on pre-contrast images.
- **Stenosis**: focal constriction of the lumen with post-stenotic enlargement.

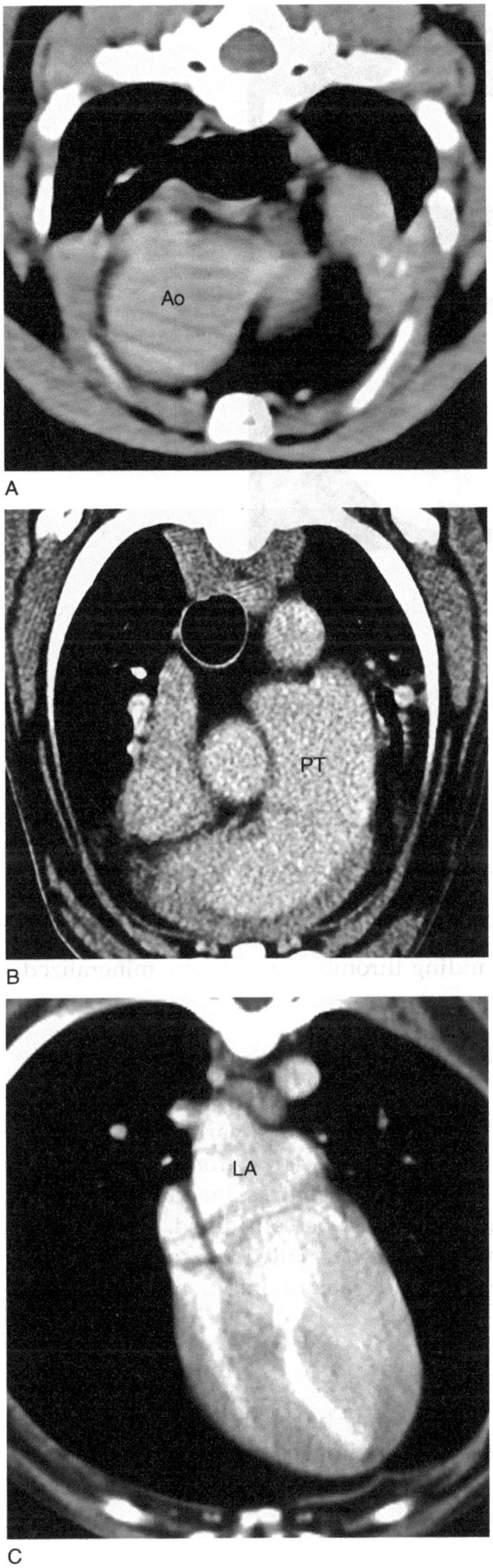

Figure 23.9 (A) Transverse CT image of a cat with bulbous dilatation of the aortic arch (Ao) in a cat with confirmed aortic stenosis. (B) Transverse CT image of a dog with confirmed pulmonary hypertension showing dilatation of the pulmonic trunk (PT). (C) Transverse CT image of a dog with confirmed mitral valve insufficiency showing marked left atrial (LA) dilatation and deviation of adjacent mediastinal structures.

Cardiac neoplasia

Hemangiosarcomas usually involve the right atrium or ventricle and may lead to pericardial effusion. Most heart base tumors are chemodectomas, but thyroid carcinomas and invasive tumors involving the lung base or bronchial lymph nodes must also be considered. Other neoplasia that can involve the heart of dogs and cats include mesothelioma and lymphoma.

CT features (Figure 23.12)

- Mass of soft tissue attenuation showing variable contrast enhancement, with borders that can be ill defined or well defined, smooth or irregular, infiltrating the myocardium or pericardium, often protruding into a vascular lumen, into a cardiac chamber (right atrium typically), or into the pericardium.
- Pericardial effusion and thromboembolism may be present.

Other disorders

Pericardial effusions

Pericardial effusion may be idiopathic, neoplastic, cardiogenic, inflammatory, infectious or hemorrhagic in origin. Cardiac tamponade develops when the pericardial pressure is equal to or above the right heart-filling pressure and characterized by a smaller right ventricle. With marked effusion, heart swinging motion may lead to motion artifacts.

CT features (Figure 23.13)

- Accumulation of fluid into the pericardium with an HU value that depends on the presence of hemorrhage. Hyperdense clots may also form in the pericardial sac.
- May be associated with the presence of a soft tissue mass attached to the myocardium or pericardium that can usually be better outlined after contrast enhancement.

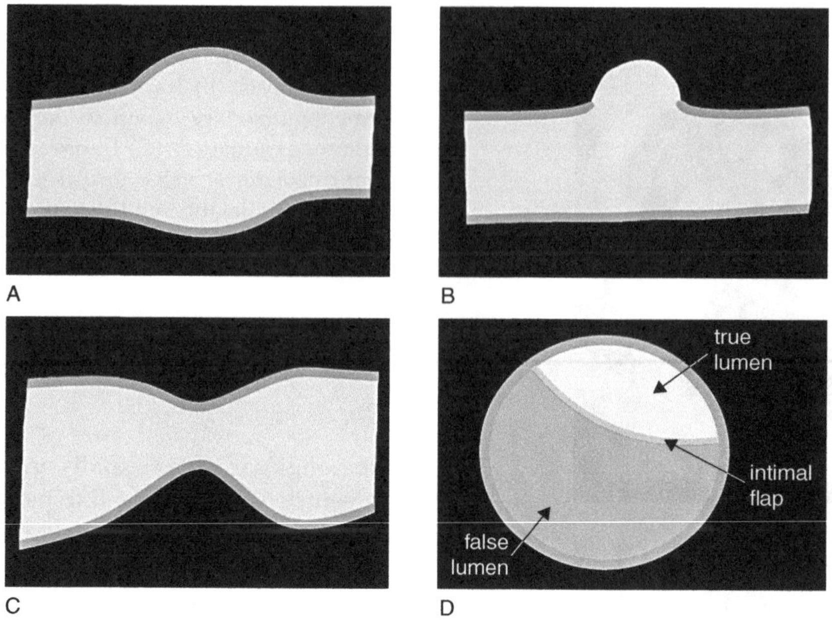

Figure 23.10 Schematization of vascular wall anomalies. (A) Aneurysm, (B) pseudoaneurysm, (C) stenosis, (D) dissection.

Vena cava thrombosis

Thrombosis of the cranial or caudal vena cava may be spontaneous or be secondary to vascular compression or invasion by thoracic or abdominal malignancy. The detection of thrombosis requires complete and uniform filling of the venous lumen with contrast medium. Injection through a cephalic or external jugular vein is recommended for the caudal vena cava while the saphenous vein is recommended for the cranial vena cava. Non-uniform mixing of contrast medium with blood or streaming of opacified blood following rapid injection represents a major pitfall that can lead to a false positive diagnosis. By using a venous access where contrast medium homogeneously mixes with blood in a capillary system (pulmonary or systemic) before entering the vessel of interest, this artifact can be minimized. Serial CT acquisitions pre- and post-contrast are recommended to confirm the persistence of the filling defect consistent with venous thrombosis. The distinction between soft tissue infiltration of the vessel lumen and thrombosis may be difficult to achieve, particularly if the invasive process is poorly vascularized and does not enhance on delayed acquisitions after contrast medium injection.

CT features (Figure 23.14)

- Well-defined, longitudinal filling defect that is usually fusiform or oblong, and partially or completely surrounded with contrast medium.
- Long-standing thrombi may become mineralized.

Pulmonary thromboembolism

Pulmonary embolism represents a life-threatening condition that can result from a variety of causes. As for the detection of vena cava thrombosis, technical aspects in the delivery of contrast medium and timing of CT acquisitions must be considered. Opacification of pulmonary arteries is usually more uniform regardless of the site and rate of injection, which helps prevent misdiagnoses.

CT features (Figure 27.18)

Pulmonary arteries may be enlarged and tortuous on pre- and post-contrast images, proximal to the site of embolism, with poor visibility of smaller peripheral arteries.

- Well-defined, longitudinal filling defect that may be surrounded with contrast medium, or abrupt

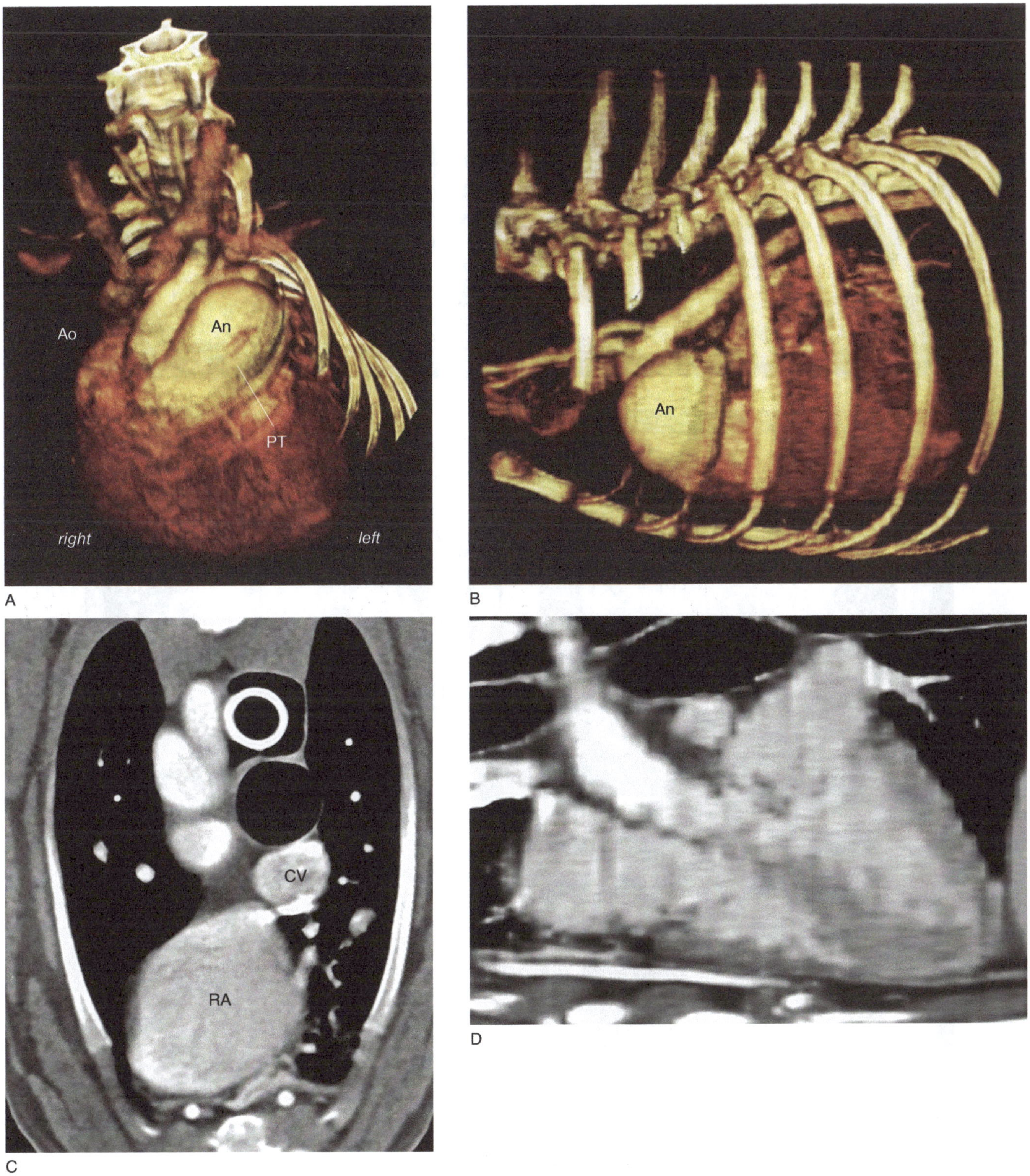

Figure 23.11 (A) Cranial and (B) left lateral volume rendering views of an incidental pulmonic trunk aneurysm in a dog. The lumen of the pulmonic trunk (PT) is markedly focally enlarged (An). Ao = aorta (images courtesy of Franck Durieux). (C) Aneurysmal right atrium (RA) ventral to the cranial vena cava (CV) in the cranial mediastinum of a dog. (D) The sagittal reconstruction shows the cranial extent of the aneurismal right atrium (images courtesy of Anu Lappalainen).

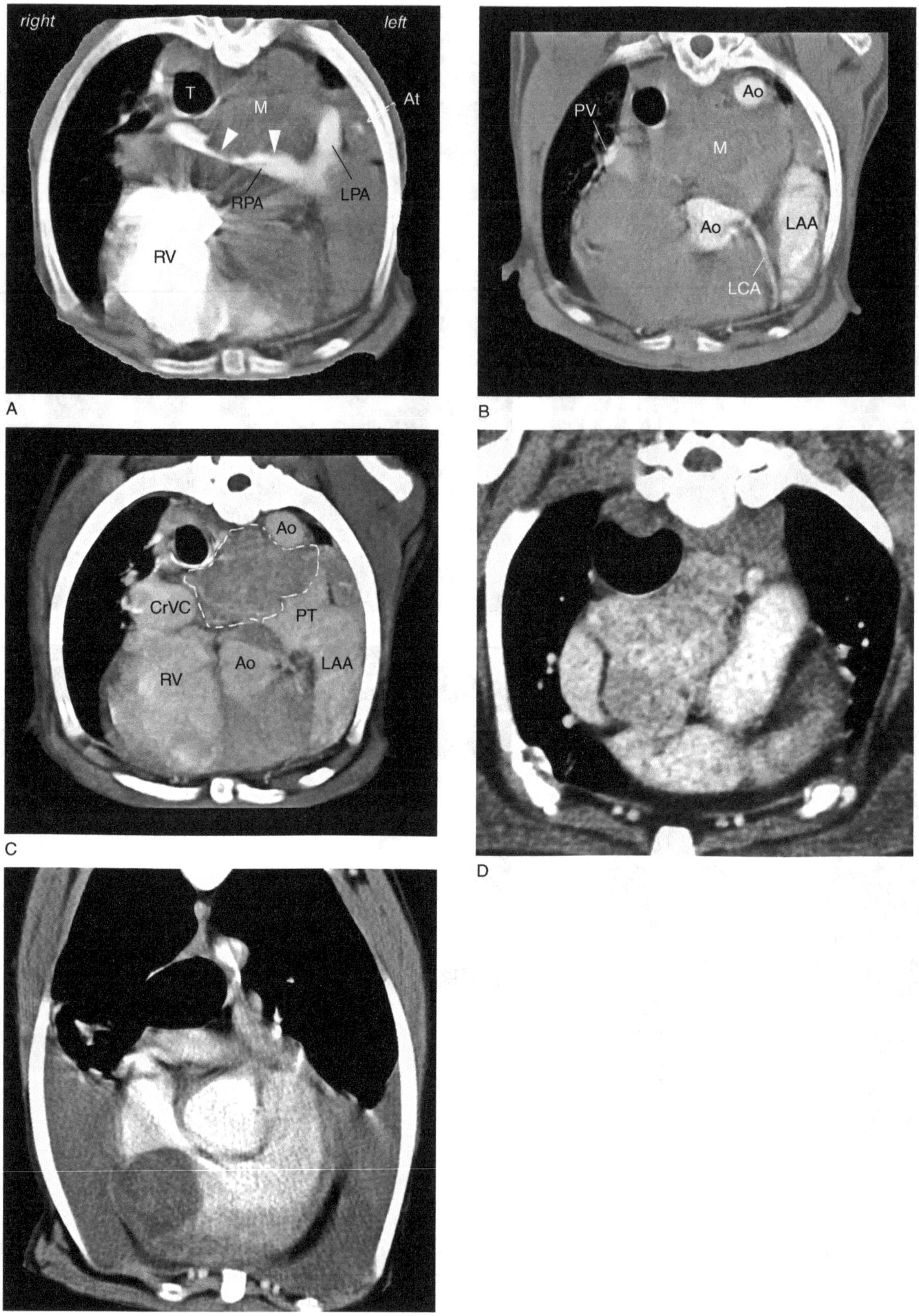

A B C D E

Figure 23.12 Transverse CT angiograms of canine cardiac neoplasia. (A–C) Heart base mass in a dog. (A) During the initial pulmonary arterial phase, the soft tissue mass (M) is seen to invade (arrowheads) the right pulmonary artery (RPA) and displace the left pulmonary artery (LPA) and trachea (T). Streak artifacts radiate from the contrast enhanced right ventricle (RV). There is focal lung atelectasis. (B) 10 s later, the contrast bolus reaches the left heart. The mass (M) displaces the descending aorta (Ao) and is associated with mild, heterogeneous enhancement. (C) 2 min post-injection, all compartments are filled with diluted contrast medium and the mass (interrupted line) shows mild enhancement but remains poorly defined. CrVC = cranial vena cava; LAA = left atrial appendage; LCA = left coronary artery; PT = pulmonic trunk; PV = pulmonary vein. (D) Incidentally diagnosed chemodectoma in a dog causing deviation of great vessels and other mediastinal structures. (E) Right atrial hemangiosarcoma, ruptured pericard and hemothorax in a dog. The non-enhancing nature of the mass probably relates to hematoma formation.

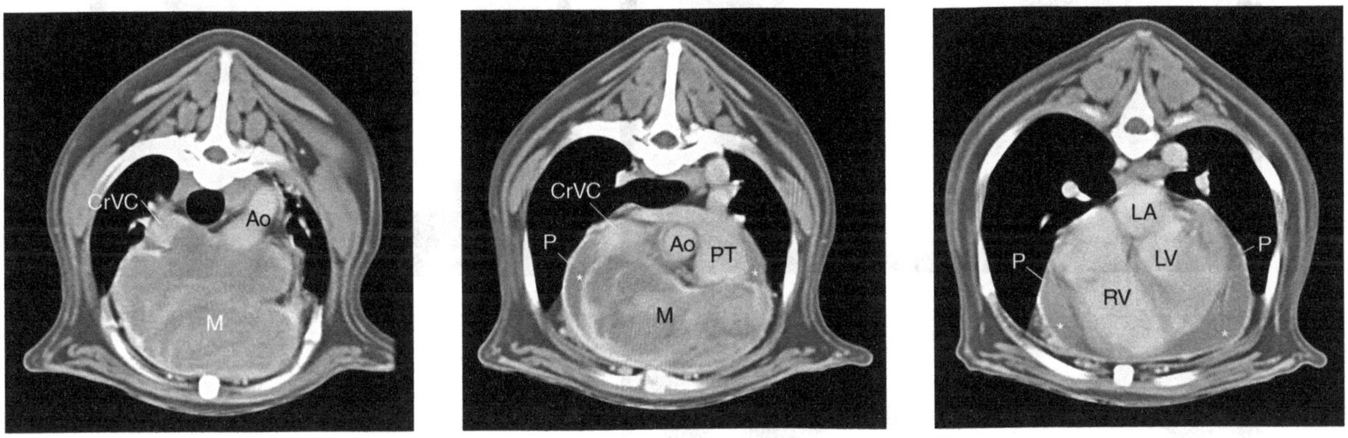

A B C

Figure 23.13 Transverse CT images of ectopic thyroid carcinoma in a dog. (A) Immediately and (B) 2 min post-injection, a large, lobulated mass (M) is visible at the cranial aspect of the heart, protruding into the pericardial sac (P) and is (C) associated with pericardial effusion (asterisk). CrVC = cranial vena cava; Ao = aorta; PT = pulmonic trunk; LA = left atrium; LV = left ventricle.

interruption in the opacification of arteries in case of complete obstruction.

- Secondary pulmonary hyperattenuation as the result of hemorrhage, edema and/or necrosis, sometimes with pleural effusion.

Further reading

De Rycke LM, Gielen IM, Simoens PJ and van Bree H (2005) Computed tomography and cross-sectional anatomy of the thorax in clinically normal dogs. *Am J Vet Res* **66**: 512–24.

Davidson BL, Rozanski E, Tidwell AS and Hoffman AM (2006) Pulmonary thrombo-embolism in a heartworm-positive cat. *J Vet Intern Med* **20**: 1037–41.

Joly H, d'Anjou MA and Huneault L (2008) Imaging diagnosis-CT angiography of a rare vascular ring anomaly in a dog. *Vet Radiol Ultrasound* **49**: 42–6.

Kirberger RM and Zambelli A (2007) Imaging diagnosis – aortic thromboembolism associated with spirocercosis in a dog. *Vet Radiol Ultrasound* **48**: 418–20.

MacGregor JM, Winter MD, Keating J, Tidwell AS and Brown DJ (2006) Peripheral pulmonary artery stenosis in a 4-month-old West Highland White Terrier. *Vet Radiol Ultrasound* **47**: 345–50.

Schwarz T, Sullivan M, Störk CK, Willis R, Harley R and Mellor DJ (2002) Aortic and cardiac mineralization in the dog. *Vet Radiol Ultrasound* **43**: 419–27.

Schwarz T, Willis R, Summerfield NJ and Doust R (2005) Aneurysmal dilatation of the right auricle in two dogs. *J Am Vet Med Assoc* **226**: 1512–16.

Salvolini L, Renda P, Fiore D, Scaglione M, Piccoli G and Giovagnoni A (2008) Acute aortic syndromes: role of multi-detector row CT. *Eur J Radiol* **65**: 350–8.

Tidwell AS (2000) Uses of computed tomography in cardiopulmonary disease. In: Bonagura JD (ed.) *Kirk's current veterinary therapy XIII*, pp 709–10. Philadelphia, PA: WB Saunders.

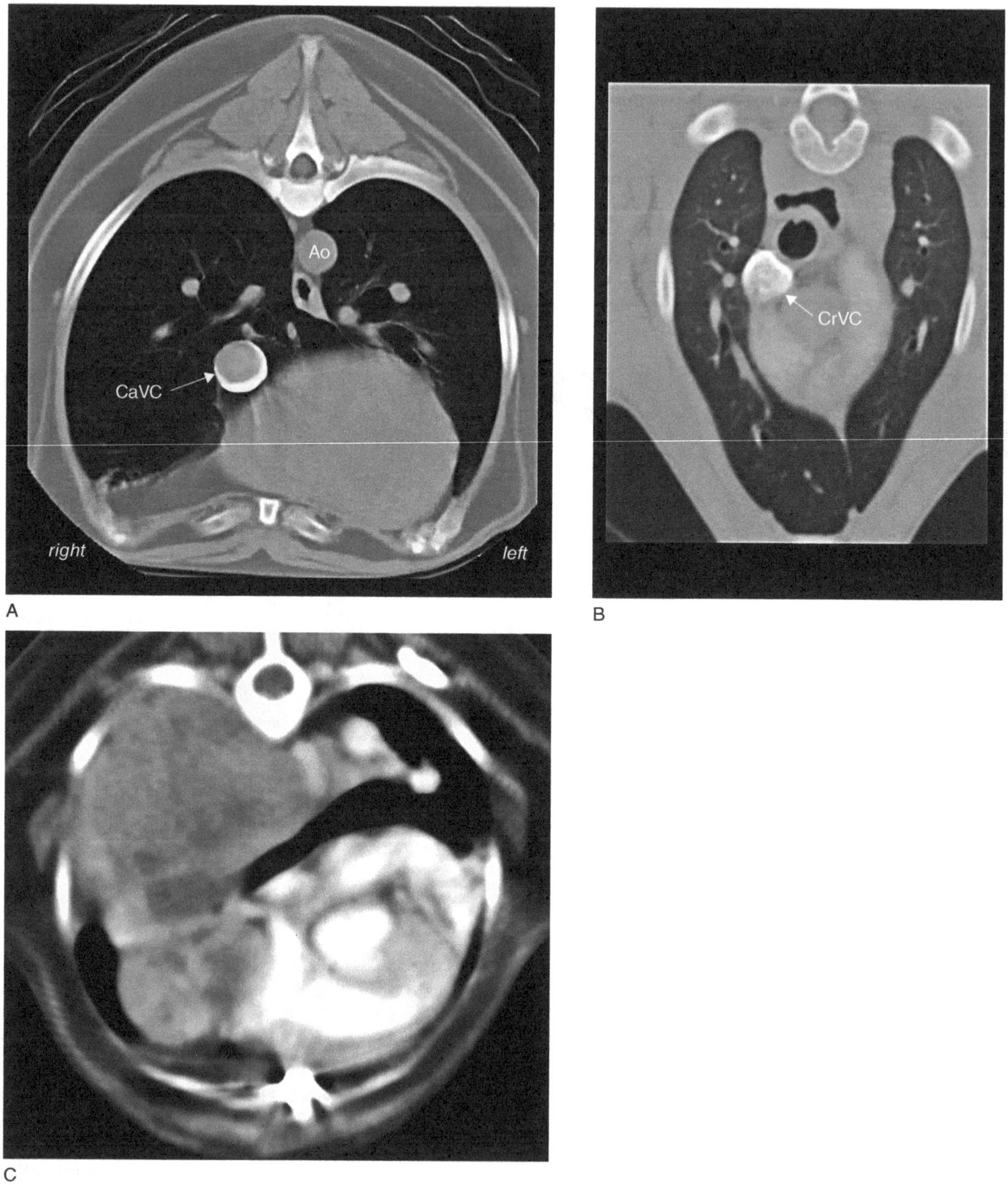

Figure 23.14 Transverse CT images of caval disorders. (A,B) Thrombosis of the caudal vena cava (CaVC; arrowed) in a dog caused by an adrenal tumor. (A) There is a marked filling defect in the dorsal caval lumen. (B) Streamlining resulting in pseudothrombosis of the cranial vena cava (CrVC; arrowed). A filling defect is present due to incomplete mixing of contrast medium and blood. (C) Cranial mediastinal mass (thymoma) in a cat causing cranial vena cava thrombosis.

CHAPTER TWENTY-FOUR

Trachea

Tobias Schwarz and Jimmy Saunders

Imaging Protocol (Table 24.1)

The cervical trachea cannot be assessed properly with a tracheal tube in place. Options are to remove the tube immediately prior to scanning or to use intubation-free anesthetic or sedation protocols. Respiratory motion is desirable for tracheal imaging and essential for assessment of collapse. Using a very small helical reconstruction interval minimizes the blurring artifact. To assess tracheal collapse, the patient should be sedated or better consciously restrained and a helical scan of the entire trachea is acquired first. Then three series of dynamic CT for 30 s periods are performed over the cervical and thoracic trachea and the mainstem bronchi. In conscious patients, it might be best not to obtain scout radiographs, but to start with the helical CT and quickly perform the dynamic CT series at locations determined on the first series.

CT: Anatomy and Normal Variants

The trachea is a semi-rigid tube that connects the larynx to the bronchial system. It ends at the level of the fourth to fifth intercostal space with a crest, the carina. The trachea consists of C-shaped cartilages opened dorsally and interconnecting tracheal ligaments and respiratory mucosa. The dorsal opening of the cartilages is connected by the tracheal muscle and connective tissue. The trachea is slightly wider than it is high.

The esophagus is adjacent to the trachea dorsally in the cranial cervical part, then left dorsolaterally towards the thoracic inlet and then again dorsally at the carina. Other adjacent structures include the thyroid glands, the carotid sheath and its content in the cervical part, the longus colli muscles, the cranial vena cava and aortic arch in the thoracic part (Figure 24.1).

CT allows real-time evaluation of the trachea during the respiratory cycle. Alterations in tracheal luminal pressure are responsible for the degree of tension on the dorsal tracheal membrane and thus for the shape of the trachea. With increased intratracheal pressure (cervical trachea in expiration, thoracic trachea in inspiration), the trachea appears rounded. If the intratracheal pressure is lower than in its surroundings (cervical trachea in inspiration, thoracic trachea in expiration) it can show a dorsal flattening or even a slight concavity of the dorsal membrane into the tracheal lumen (Figure 24.2). The mean percentage of change in tracheal cross-sectional area of healthy dogs (not breed specific) between inspiration and passive expiration has been reported to be ±6%, with observed changes up to 24%. This degree of change closely resembles that in humans.

A marked invagination of the dorsal tracheal muscle into the tracheal lumen is commonly observed on CT at the level of the caudal cervical trachea, reducing the height of the tracheal lumen. It is accompanied by a slight rotation of the tracheal height axis. This finding corresponds to the misnamed 'pseudocollapse' described on radiography, which in fact is a true, albeit partial, collapse but without contributable respiratory signs (Figure 24.3). The tracheal dynamics are also influenced by external conditions (pharyngeal, laryngeal, intrathoracic).

Disease Features

Congenital/Malformation

Tracheal hypoplasia

Tracheal hypoplasia corresponds to a reduction >50% of the cross-sectional lumen over all the tracheal length.

Veterinary Computed Tomography, First Edition. Edited by Tobias Schwarz, Jimmy Saunders.

Table 24.1
CT imaging protocol (intravenous contrast study: standard protocol; *see* Chapter 5).

Series	Pre- and post-contrast
Decubitus	Ventral or lateral
Scan margins	Larynx ←→ Carina
Voltage (kVp)	120
Current (mAs)	60–150
Tube rotation time (s)	0.5–1
Slice width (mm)	2–3
Kernel frequency	Medium
Collimator pitch	2
Helical image reconstruction interval (mm)	0.5 × slice width
Motion control	None, respiratory motion is desirable
Window level (HU)	−250
Window width (HU)	1500

The disorder is more common in English bulldogs and English mastiffs, although it has been described in other breeds. The condition is rarely seen in cats. Dogs and cats with mucopolysaccharidosis VII may show similar lesions.

CT features (Figure 24.4)

- Reduced diameter of the trachea.
- Tracheal wall thickening.
- Tracheal cartilages overlapping.
- Tracheal rings almost complete with negligible dorsal muscle.
- Common concurrent congenital abnormalities: megaesophagus, pulmonic or aortic stenosis.
- Mucopolysaccharidosis VII: reduced tracheal diameter with thickened, misshapen cartilages.

Inflammation/Infection

Tracheitis

Tracheitis may be due to an infectious agent (virus, bacteria, parasite – *Oslerus osleri*) or may have a non-infectious origin (prolonged barking, tracheal collapse, chronic cardiac disease, irritation by gas or dust).

CT features (Figure 24.5)

- Tracheal wall thickening.
- Narrowing of the trachea in cross-sectional area.
- *Oslerus osleri*: soft tissue-dense nodules in the trachea.
- CT examination may also be normal.

Trauma

Tracheal hemorrhage

Tracheal hemorrhage can be secondary to an external or an internal trauma (intubation accident) or more commonly due to generalized bleeding disorders (rodenticide intoxication).

CT features

- Tracheal wall thickening due to submucosal hemorrhagic infiltration.
- Other sites of hemorrhage are frequently found: mediastinum, lungs.

Tracheal laceration and avulsion

Tracheal laceration and avulsion are mostly associated with severe trauma such as road traffic accidents, bite injuries, post-surgery wound dehiscence or overzealous intubation (mainly in cats).

CT features

- Laceration in the tracheal wall.
- Irregular tracheal wall/lumen, misshapen trachea.
- Absence of tracheal rings in case of complete rupture.
- A pneumomediastinum is commonly identified, localized or generalized.

Tracheal stenosis

Segmental tracheal stenosis may be congenital or, more commonly, acquired as a consequence of laceration/avulsion. It may be asymptomatic despite a reduction in diameter of 80% in lumen size.

CT is very useful for planning, guidance and follow-up of stent placement procedures in dogs with tracheal stenosis. CT reconstructed images allows to determine accurately the extent and degree of stenosis allowing adequate selection of the size of tracheal stents.

CT features (Figure 24.6)

- Thickened tracheal wall.
- Reduced tracheal diameter.
- Dorsal and 3-D reconstructions allow exact location and extent of the stenosis to be determined.

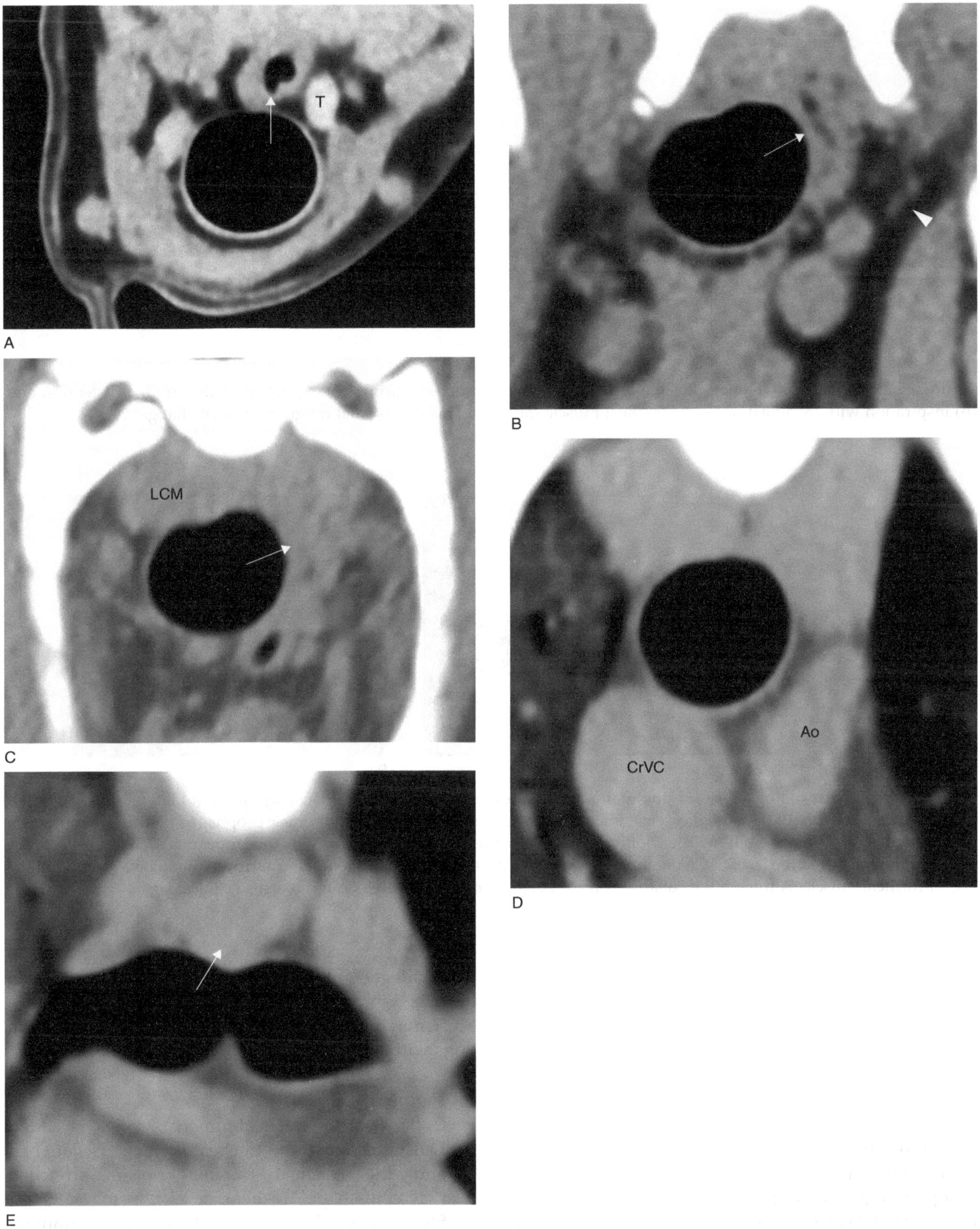

Figure 24.1 Transverse CT images of the trachea in the normal dog during the respiratory pause at the level of (A) C3, (B) C6, (C) T1, (D) T3 and (E) T5. Note the positional change of the esophagus (arrows) and adjacent thyroid glands (T), carotid sheath (arrowhead), longus colli muscle (LCM), cranial vena cava (CrVC) and aortic arch (Ao).

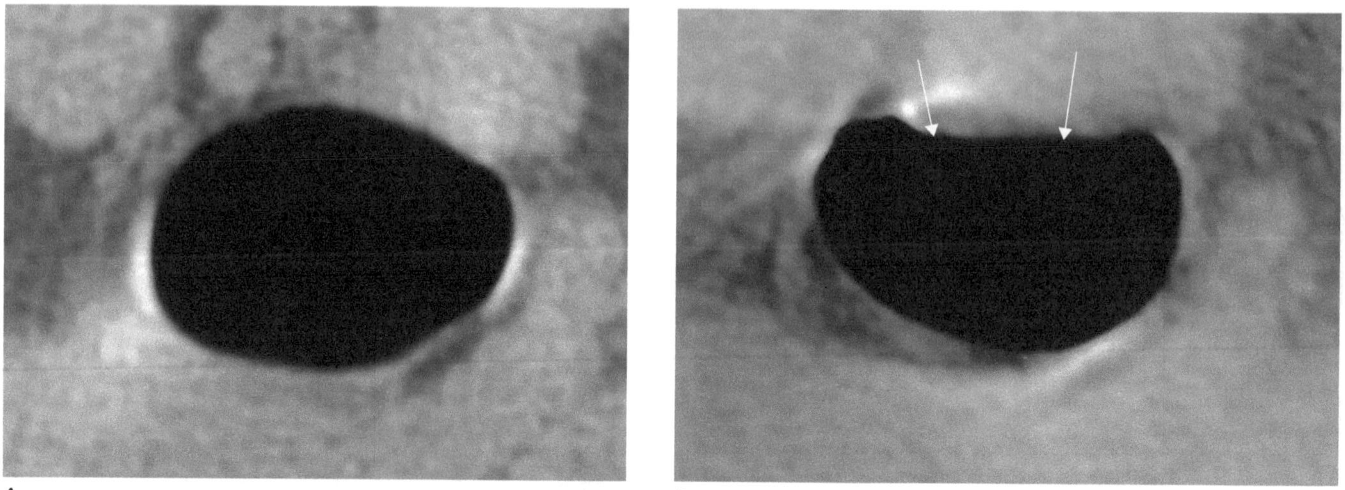

A B

Figure 24.2 Transverse CT images of the canine mid-cervical trachea during (A) expiration with rounded distention and (B) inspiration with invagination of the tracheal muscle (arrows). This is a normal range of luminal change.

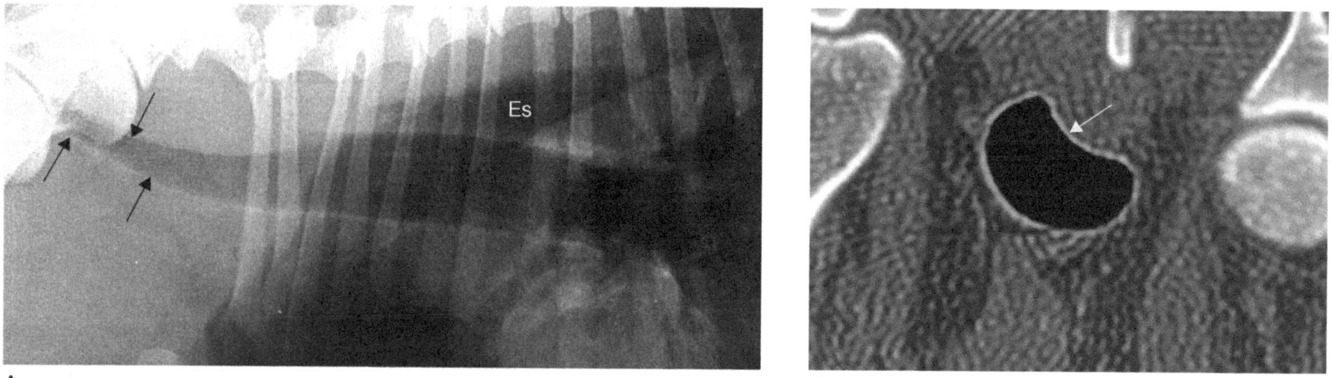

A B

Figure 24.3 11-year-old mixed-breed dog without respiratory signs. (A) Tracheal close-up of a right lateral thoracic radiograph shows a collapse of the caudal cervical trachea (arrows) and a gas-distended thoracic esophagus (Es). Superimposition of the esophagus or longus colli muscle is often erroneously referred to as the reason for this appearance. (B) Transverse CT image of the trachea at the level of C6 demonstrates the true partial collapse of the trachea (arrow) due to invagination of the dorsal tracheal muscle. Although the collapse is real, it is probably not severe enough to cause clinical signs.

Degenerative

Tracheal collapse

Tracheal collapse is a progressive, degenerative disease of the tracheal rings, predominantly affecting middle-aged to older small and toy-breed dogs. It may be inspiratory (cervical region), expiratory (thoracic region) or mixed.

Cervical collapse may also be the consequence of nasopharyngeal or laryngeal obstruction via the negative intratracheal pressure created by an inspiratory effort. This should particularly be considered in cats where degenerative ring disorders have only been described in mucopolysaccharidosis.

CT may be used for monitoring stent placement in dogs with tracheal collapse.

CT features (Figure 24.7)

- Collapse of the tracheal lumen.
- During collapse the tracheal cartilage is flattened and the tracheal muscle appears stretched ('crescent-shape' trachea).
- Stent-check CT can differentiate stenotic granulation from fluid accumulation.

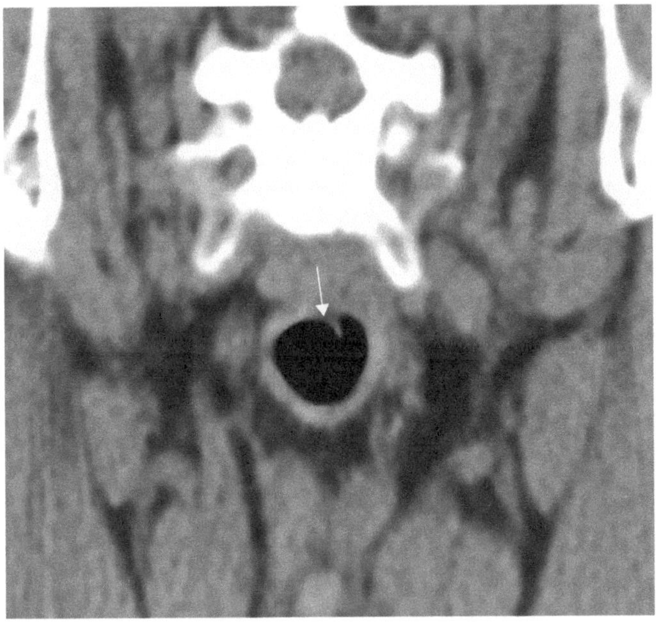

Figure 24.4 Adult dog with mucopolysaccharidosis VII. Transverse CT image of the cervical trachea shows marked hypoplasia and an abnormally overlapping tracheal cartilage (arrow).

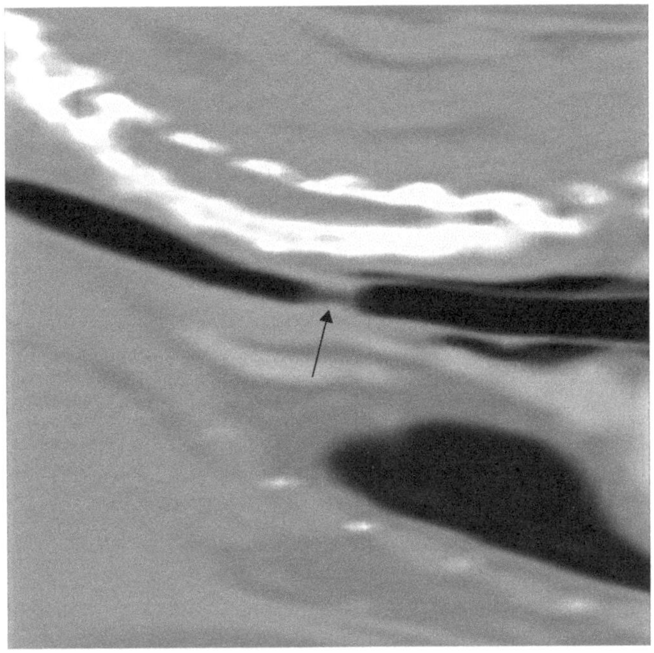

Figure 24.6 Sagittally reconstructed thoracic CT image of a cat with a stenosis of the cranial thoracic trachea (arrow).

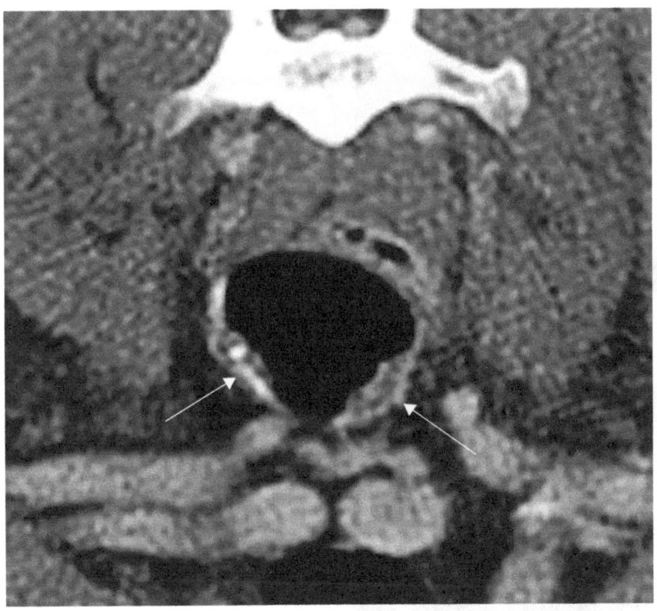

Figure 24.5 Adult dog with tracheitis. Transverse CT image of the caudal cervical trachea shows a bilateral ventrolateral proliferation of the tracheal mucosa (arrows).

Neoplasia

Tracheal neoplasia

Tracheal neoplasia is rare in dogs and cats. Tumors may affect primarily the trachea (osteochondroma, chondrosarcoma, carcinomas in dogs, lymphoma or carcinomas in cats) or invade it extramurally (thyroid carcinoma, lung neoplasia, aortic body tumor, esophageal tumor).

CT features (Figure 24.8)

- Soft tissue-dense mass arising from the tracheal wall.
- Post-contrast: moderate to severe enhancement.

Further reading

Kara ME, Turan E, Dabanoglu I and Ocal MK (2004) Computed tomographic assessment of the trachea in the German shepherd dog. *Ann Anat* **186**: 317–21.

Leonard CD, Johnson LR, Bonadio CM and Pollard RE (2009) Changes in tracheal dimensions during inspiration and expiration in healthy dogs as detected via computed tomography. *Am J Vet Res* **70**: 986–91.

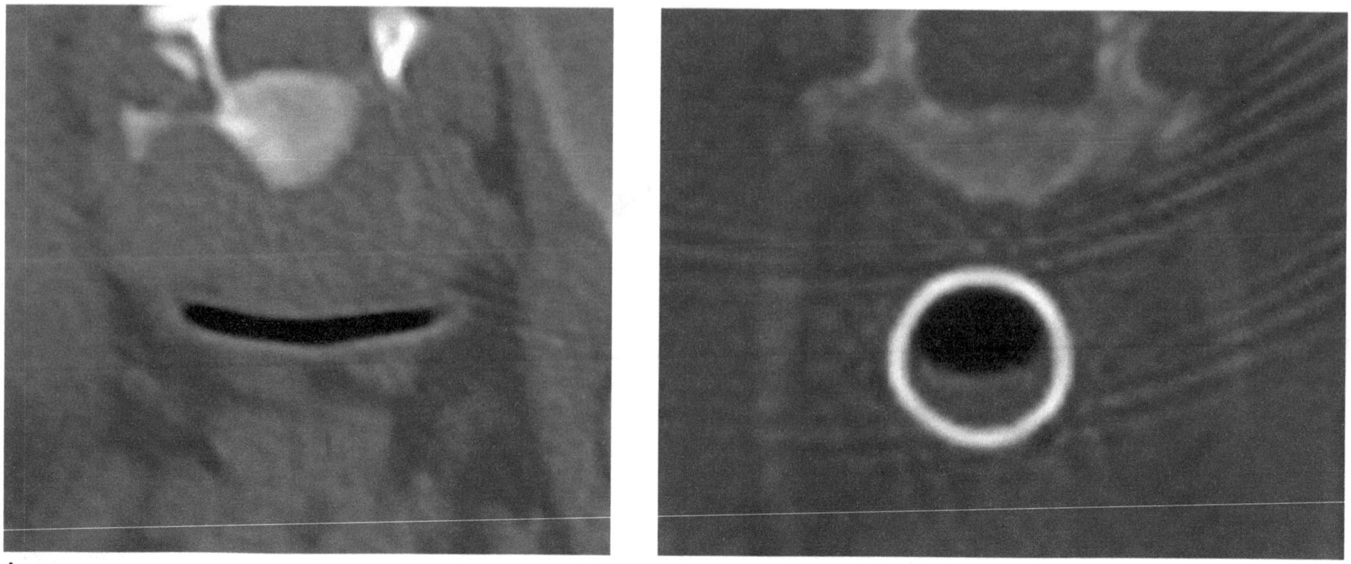

Figure 24.7 Tracheal CT study of two different dogs with tracheal collapse. (A) Transverse CT image shows an almost complete collapse of the caudal cervical trachea in a Papillon with severe attributable respiratory signs. The complete loss of C-shape of the tracheal cartilage indicates chondromalacia. (B) Transverse CT image of a Yorkshire terrier with respiratory distress several weeks after stent placement for tracheal collapse. The meniscus-shaped fluid–gas interface indicates intraluminal fluid accumulation consistent with airway infection, ruling out stenotic granulation.

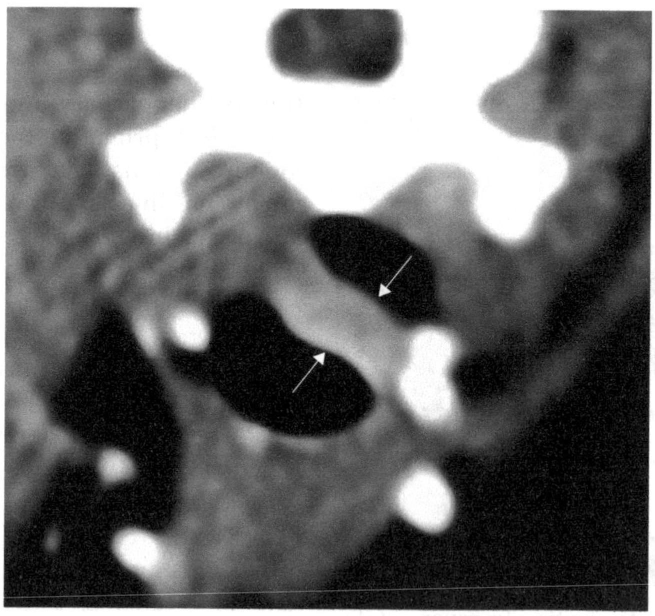

Figure 24.8 Adult cat with a lymphoma. Post-contrast transverse CT image of the cranial trachea shows a moderately contrast-enhancing mass arising from the dorsal tracheal wall (arrows).

CHAPTER TWENTY-FIVE

MEDIASTINUM

Audrey Petite and Robert Kirberger

IMAGING PROTOCOL (TABLE 25.1)

Images are also viewed in lung and bone windows allowing different aspects of a disease to be evaluated.

CT: ANATOMY AND NORMAL VARIANTS

The mediastinum is the thoracic midline space comprised between the left and right pleural cavities. The mediastinum is continuous with the soft tissues of the neck cranially through the thoracic inlet. It is continuous caudally with the retroperitoneum through the aortic hiatus. In dogs and cats, the mediastinum contains the thoracic trachea (*see* Chapter 24) and the esophagus, lymph nodes, the thymus, the thoracic duct, several important nerves, the heart and the great vessels (*see* Chapter 23). The mediastinum also contains a variable amount of fat deposits. Although in cats the width of the cranial mediastinum is fairly consistent (Box 25.1), brachycephalic and/or obese dogs accumulate a large amount of mediastinal fat, which is responsible for widening of the mediastinum (Figure 25.1). On CT, the fat present in the cranial mediastinum provides a natural contrast with the other mediastinal structures and may help their visualization.

The mediastinum has three anatomic reflections: cranioventral, caudoventral and the plica venae cavae (Figure 25.2A). For interpretation purposes, it is classically divided into three sections: cranial, middle and caudal (Figure 25.2B and Table 25.2).

Although the mediastinum represents the midline space of the thoracic cavity, it runs obliquely craniocaudally from right to left. The ventral cranial mediastinum lies slightly to the right due to the extension of the cranial left lung lobe across the midline. Caudally, the accessory lobe extends to the left across the midline, locating the caudal mediastinum to the left.

Mediastinal shift is an important radiographic interpretative concept that can be applied to CT imaging. It refers to a displacement of the mediastinum from its original location. It is usually due to a pathologic process inducing a change in volume of one hemithorax. An increased hemithoracic volume displaces the mediastinum away from the process, while a decreased volume displaces the mediastinum towards the process. Causes of mediastinal shift are numerous (Box 25.2).

Esophagus

The esophagus is a tubular structure that connects the oropharynx to the stomach at the level of the cardia. It is composed of four soft tissue layers: fibrous, muscular, submucous and mucous, which are not distinguishable on CT. The esophagus is divided into three portions: cervical, thoracic and abdominal. In its cervical portion, it runs dorsally and to the left of the trachea to finish laterally and to its left at the level of the thoracic inlet. In its thoracic portion, the esophagus crosses dorsally over the tracheal bifurcation with the aortic arch on its left. It then lies more or less midline, to the right of the descending aorta until it reaches the esophageal hiatus of the diaphragm. The abdominal portion is very short and wedge-shaped, merging with the cardia of the stomach.

In CT, the esophagus can be followed along its entire length. It adopts a rounded to ovoid shape of soft tissue density in the neck, cranial and middle mediastinum. In the caudal mediastinum, it often adopts a more triangular shape (Figure 25.2A). Its lumen may be highlighted by a variable amount of air, particularly

Veterinary Computed Tomography, First Edition. Edited by Tobias Schwarz, Jimmy Saunders.

Table 25.1
CT imaging protocol (intravenous contrast study: standard protocol; *see* Chapter 5).

Series	Pre- and post-contrast: mediastinal window
Decubitus	Ventral or dorsal
Special positioning	Placement of orogastric tube or air insufflation of the esophagus when necessary
Scan margins	Thoracic inlet ←→ Insertion of the diaphragm on L3
Voltage (kVp)	120
Current (mAs)	60–150
Tube rotation time (s)	1
Slice width (mm)	3–5
Kernel frequency	Medium smooth
Collimator pitch	1.75
Helical image reconstruction interval	0.5 × slice width
Motion control	Induced respiratory pause with manual hyperventilation
Window level (HU)	+40
Window width (HU)	400

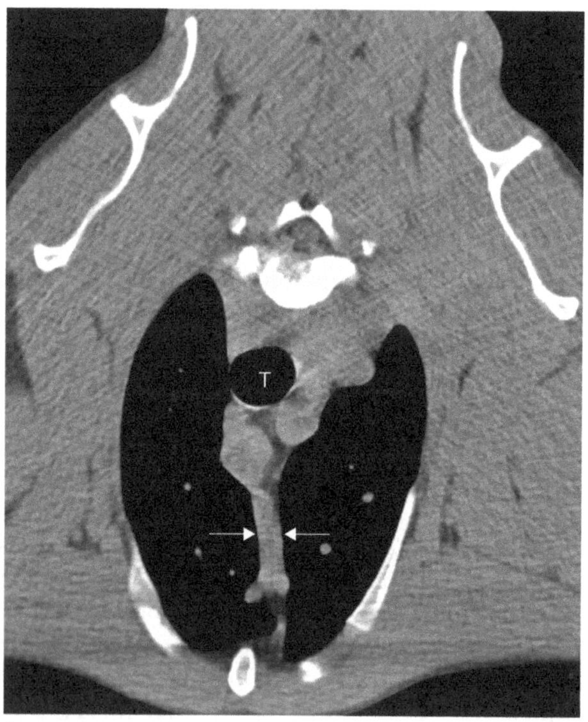

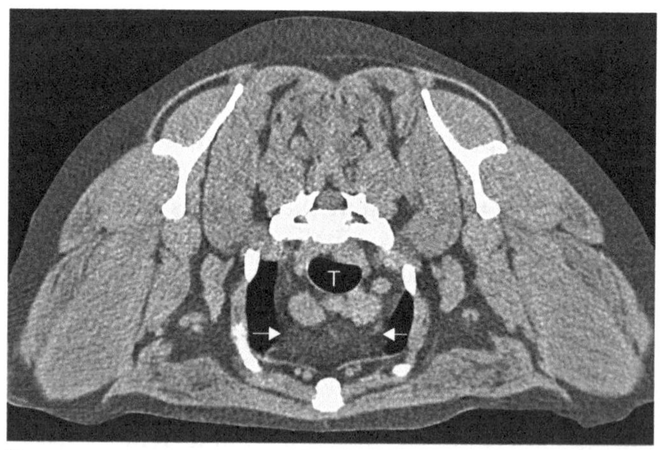

Figure 25.1 Post-contrast transverse CT image of the cranial mediastinum in (A) a greyhound and (B) an English bulldog. Both images are set with the same window (level 40 HU, width 400 HU). In addition to the difference in cranial mediastinal width (between arrows), note the better contrast provided by the mediastinal fat in the bulldog. T = trachea.

Box 25.1 Cranial mediastinal width
Dog: should be less than twice the width of the vertebral column
Cat: should have a similar width to the vertebral column

when animals are anesthetized. Occasionally, the caudal esophagus contains some fluid due to regurgitation, and a distinct horizontal fluid line can be seen. When visualization of the esophagus is hindered by surrounding structures or lesions, an orogastric tube can be placed. If an esophageal condition is suspected,

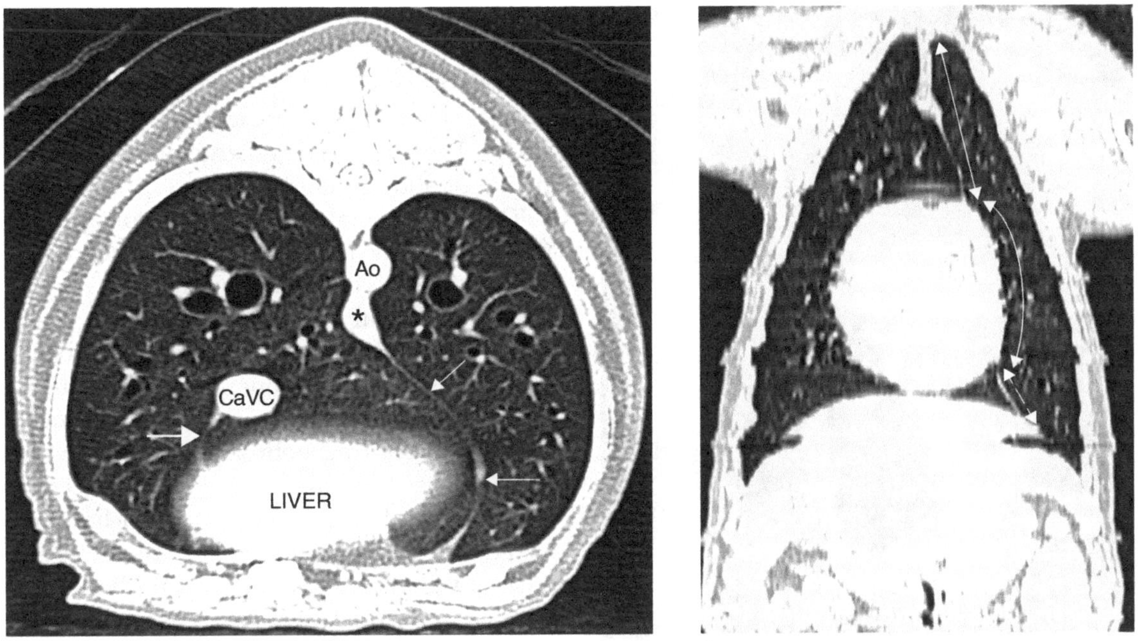

Figure 25.2 CT anatomy of the mediastinum. (A) Transverse CT image: caudoventral (small arrows) and plica venae cavae (large arrow). (B) Dorsally reconstructed CT image: cranial (continuous straight arrow), middle (curved arrow) and caudal (dashed arrow) mediastinum. Ao = aorta; CaVC = caudal vena cava; * = esophagus.

Table 25.2
The three mediastinal sections and their content.

Mediastinal area	Main structures present
Cranial	Trachea, esophagus, thymus, thoracic arteries, veins and lymphatics, brachiocephalic trunk and cranial vena cava
Middle	Heart, aortic arch, ascending aorta, esophagus, carina and bronchial lymph nodes
Caudal	Esophagus, caudal vena cava, descending aorta, azygos vein, thoracic duct and vagal nerves

Box 25.2 Common causes and direction of mediastinal shift

Away from the process
Unilateral pneumothorax
Unilateral pleural effusion
Unilateral lobar overinflation
Large pulmonary mass(es)
Unilateral diaphragmatic hernia or rupture

Towards the process
Unilateral lung collapse (Figure 25.3)
Pleural adhesions secondary to pleural disease

an additional endotracheal tube is passed into the esophagus to inflate the esophagus just prior to the scan. The distended air-filled esophagus allows better delineation of the intraluminal component of any mural mass. If the esophagus and stomach are distended with air, virtual endoscopy allows generation of images similar to a direct endoscopic examination (Figure 25.4). It is important to distend the esophagus adequately to avoid mistaking smaller nodules for esophageal folds. In cases where the mass totally occludes the esophagus precluding the passage of the endoscope, virtual endoscopy allows visualization of structures beyond the mass and/or retrograde viewing of the mass.

Lymph nodes

In the mediastinum, three groups of lymph nodes are present: the sternal, the mediastinal and the bronchial lymph nodes.

The sternal lymph nodes, also known as retrosternal or presternal, are located at the level of the second

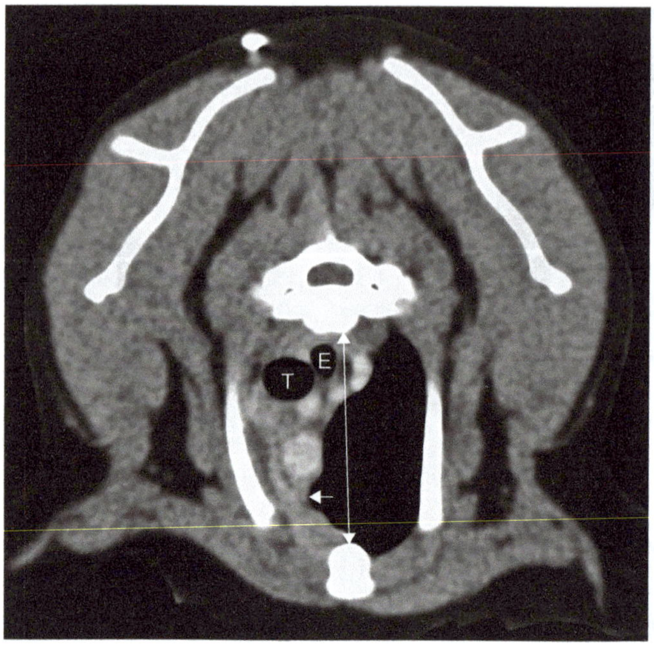

Figure 25.3 Transverse CT image of an adult cat with complete right lung lobe collapse and a mediastinal shift (arrow) towards the lesion (completely deviated to the right). The midline double arrow line represents the normal location of the mediastinum. E = esophagus; T = trachea.

sternebra. Although they are usually paired, a large individual variation exists, the left one being more consistently present than the right. They drain the lymphatics from the thoracic wall and the abdominal cavity. Therefore, their enlargement should raise a suspicion of abdominal disease.

The mediastinal lymph nodes consist of a chain of nodes along the large vessels of the heart in the cranial mediastinum. Their number and size vary.

The bronchial lymph nodes are divided into two groups, the pulmonary and the tracheobronchial lymph nodes. The pulmonary ones are most frequently absent, but when present are distributed along the main bronchi. Three tracheobronchial lymph nodes are normally present and are located at the level of the carina. The right and left tracheobronchial lymph nodes are ovoid structures found on their respective side of the base of the main bronchi. The middle or bifurcational tracheobronchial lymph node is more V-shaped and lies caudal to the angle created by the bifurcation of the trachea. It is the largest of the three nodes.

With CT, the normal lymph nodes are barely visible but a moderate enlargement can be demonstrated. CT assessment of mediastinal lymphadenopathy repre-

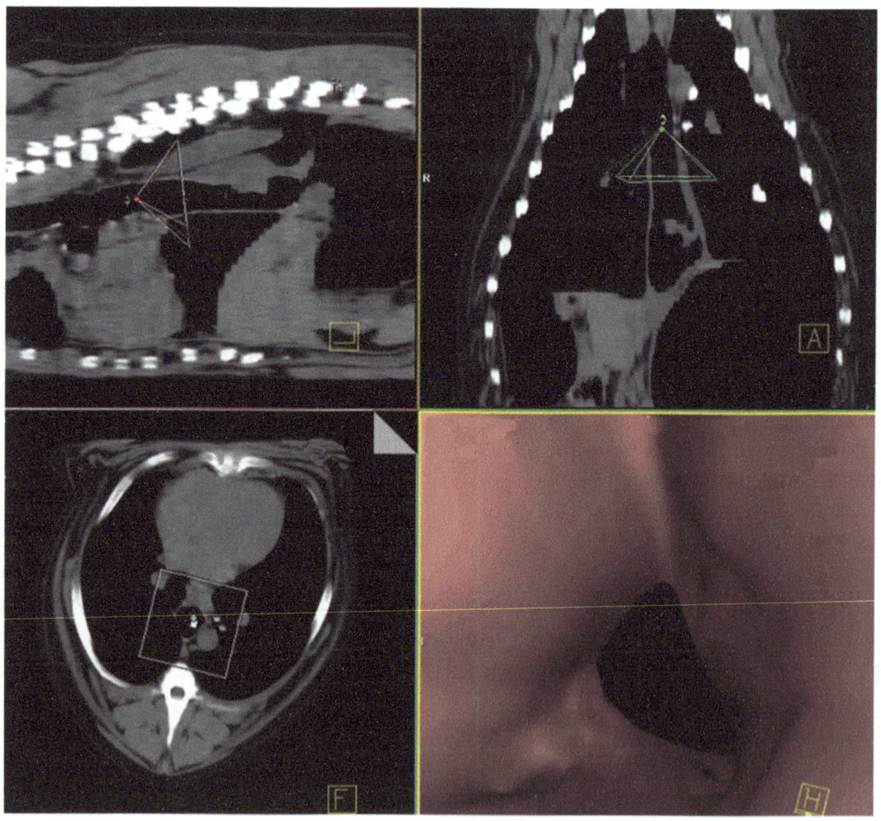

Figure 25.4 Screenshot from a virtual endoscopy of an air-insufflated esophagus generated from CT images of a dog with a caudal esophageal mass. The prism-shaped viewfinder is looking down the esophagus with the virtual endoscopic picture seen on the bottom right of the image. Small nodules can be seen on the left ventrolateral surface of the esophagus. The viewfinder can be moved backwards and forwards to give a real-time endoscopic appearance.

Table 25.3
CT features associated with mediastinal lymphadenopathy.

Group of lymph nodes	CT features associated to lymphadenopathy
Sternal	One or two soft tissue densities dorsal to second sternebra
Mediastinal	Soft tissue density associated with a widening of the cranial mediastinum, elevation of the thoracic trachea, if gross enlargement
Tracheobronchial	Soft tissue density in their respective location Right and left: caudal and ventral displacement of the ipsilateral main bronchus, associated to a variable degree of compression Middle: widening of the angle created by the mainstem bronchi, which can be slightly deviated ventrally

sents an important part of the routine oncologic staging and pre-surgical planning. Enlarged lymph nodes can be identified as rounded homogeneous soft tissue densities in their respective location. They are associated with a mass effect, which displaces or compresses the adjacent structures (Table 25.3).

Thymus

The thymus is mainly a lymphoid structure located in the cranial mediastinum, which has a role in the T-lymphocyte maturation. Its size varies with the animal's age. Already relatively large at birth, it grows until sexual maturity; thereafter it progressively involutes during the rest of the animal's life, the lymphoid tissue being replaced by fatty tissue.

Thoracic duct

The thoracic duct is formed by a single or multiple lymphatic ducts that coalesce in the cranial part of the thorax. It originates from the cisterna chyli, which is located ventrally to L4 and drains the pelvic and abdominal viscera as well as the pelvic limbs. It enters the thoracic cavity through the aortic hiatus and runs dorsally to the aorta and ventrally to the azygos vein. It crosses to the left of the aorta more or less at the level of T6. It may join any major cranial vein, including the left external jugular vein, the left subclavian vein, the left brachiocephalic vein, the azygos vein or the cranial vena cava. On a plain CT, the lymphatic ducts are usually not visible in the thorax and merge with the rest of the surrounding soft tissue structures. In the cranial abdomen the cisterna chyli can sometimes be seen as a hat-shaped structure draping dorsally over the aorta. The lymphatic visualization is not improved with intravenous contrast administration unless there is increased alternative lymphatic uptake in case of reduced renal clearance of vascular contrast medium. CT lymphangiography allows a better detection of the number and topography of the lymphatic ducts than radiography.

Nerves

In normal circumstances, the nerves crossing the mediastinum are not visible with CT.

Disease Features

Congenital

Esophageal diverticulum

Esophageal diverticulum refers to a sacculation of the esophageal wall, which can be congenital or acquired. Ingesta accumulate in the diverticulum and can cause significant esophagitis.

CT features

- Focal dilatation of the esophagus in the cranial mediastinum.
- Presence of mixed attenuating content corresponding to filling with ingesta.
- Possible signs of aspiration pneumonia.

Megaesophagus

Strictly speaking, a megaesophagus refers to the dilatation of a part of or the entire esophagus. It can be congenital or, more commonly, acquired secondary to neuromuscular or other diseases, esophageal obstruction or intoxication. General anesthesia induces in most dogs and cats a moderate esophageal distention, which is incidental.

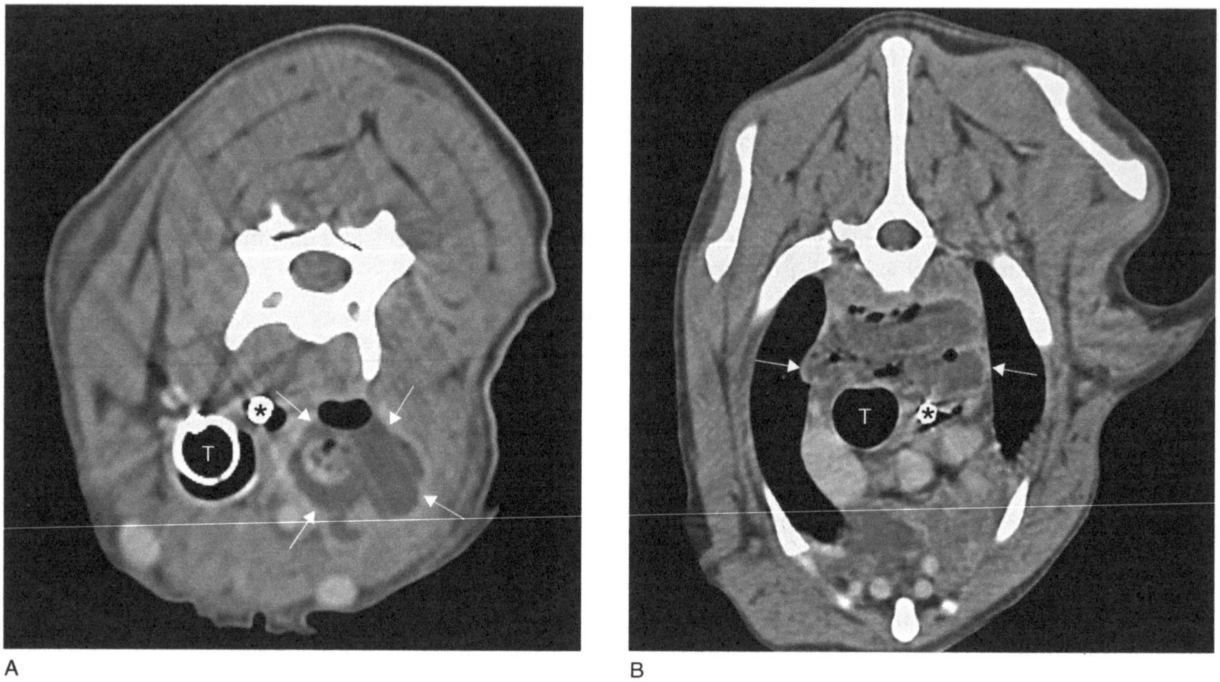

Figure 25.5 Transverse CT images of a dog with a perforating cervical esophageal foreign body leading to (A) paraesophageal abscess delineated with a contrast enhancing thin wall (arrows) and (B) moderate pneumomediastinum and mediastinitis (arrows). * = esophagus; T = trachea.

CT features

- Visualization of the esophageal walls over a variable length.
- Presence of non-attenuating gas within the esophageal lumen.
- Possible signs of aspiration pneumonia.

Trauma

Pneumomediastinum

Pneumomediastinum corresponds to the presence of free gas, usually air, in the mediastinum. It is most commonly the result of a traumatic event affecting any cervical or thoracic structure in direct contact with air (thoracic, tracheal, esophageal or cervical injury). Spontaneous pneumomediastinum can occur following severe respiratory disease. If all identifiable causes have been ruled out, idiopathic pneumomediastinum is diagnosed. Although a pneumomediastinum can lead to a pneumothorax, a pneumothorax is never the cause of pneumomediastinum. CT is particularly useful to investigate the cause of pneumomediastinum. Both the neck and the chest should be scanned, starting from the oropharynx. If esophageal or tracheal perforation is suspected, 5–10ml of non-ionic water-soluble iodinated contrast medium can be administered into the organ of concern. The CT scan should be repeated after enough time to allow contrast extravasation (5–10min).

CT features (Figure 25.5)

- Presence of non-attenuating gas tracking along the mediastinal structures, resulting in enhancement of their visualization.
- The full thickness of the trachea and esophagus are visible.
- Visualization of individual vessels is enhanced.
- Non-attenuating gas is often simultaneously found along the fascial planes of the neck, subcutaneously and in the retroperitoneum.
- If a perforating foreign body is present, a focal area of hypo- or hyperattenuation, depending on the attenuation properties of the foreign body, may be seen in the periphery of the perforated organ.
- Extravasation of contrast medium may be seen in the fascial planes surrounding the perforation site.

Esophageal stricture

Esophageal stricture usually develops as a consequence of a traumatic or inflammatory lesion of the esophageal mucosa. The clinical signs vary greatly with the degree of stenosis.

CT features

- Under normal circumstances, the stricture is not visible.
- Moderate esophageal gas distention proximal to the stenotic portion.
- Insufflation of gas in the esophagus may enhance visualization of the stricture.

Esophageal foreign body

Retained esophageal foreign bodies are common in dogs. They are most frequently found at the thoracic inlet, the heart base or the esophageal hiatus. Occasionally, perforation can occur and cause mediastinitis.

CT features

- Direct visualization of the foreign body depends on its density.
- Moderate esophageal gas distention proximal to the foreign body.
- Enhanced visualization achieved with gas insufflation in the esophagus.

Infection/Inflammation

Esophagitis

Inflammation or ulceration of the mucosal surface of the esophagus is usually secondary to gastroesophageal reflux, chronic vomiting or direct trauma to the mucosa. In extreme cases, perforation can cause mediastinitis.

CT features (Figure 25.6)

- No abnormalities are usually detected with CT.
- Occasionally, moderate focal esophageal dilatation ± presence of fluid/ingesta.

Mediastinitis

Mediastinitis is an inflammatory or infectious process affecting the mediastinum. A large number of etiologies may be responsible for mediastinitis (Box 25.3). Mediastinitis can be generalized or focal, depending on the cause.

CT features (Figure 25.5)

- Moderate widening of the affected part of the mediastinum, due to thickening of the mediastinal pleura and variable amount of effusion.
- Irregular outline of the mediastinum.

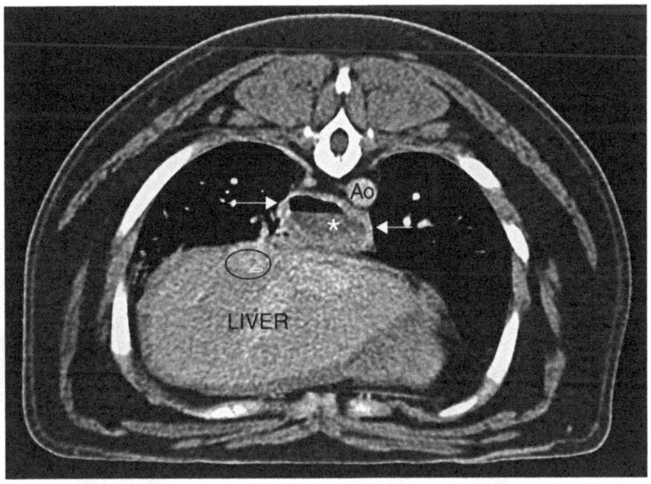

Figure 25.6 Post-contrast transverse CT image of an English bulldog with chronic vomiting and esophagitis. The thoracic esophagus (arrows) is moderately distended and partially fluid-filled (asterisk) due to esophageal reflux. Ao = aorta; black oval = caudal vena cava.

Box 25.3 Causes of mediastinitis

Primary
Fungal: *Histoplasma, Cryptococcus*
Bacterial: *Actinomyces, Nocardia*
Parasitic: *Spirocerca lupi*
Cats: mediastinal Feline Infectious Peritonitis

Secondary
Esophageal perforation
Tracheal perforation
Extension from pleural, pulmonary, pericardial or cervical disease

- Increased attenuation of the mediastinal content due to accumulation of exudate, chyle.
- Mediastinal lymph node enlargement may be present depending on the cause.
- In case of mediastinits secondary to tracheal or esophageal perforation, mediastinal air (pneumomediastinum) may be present.
- Mild contrast uptake may be seen in areas of active inflammation and in the thickened mediastinal pleura.

Spirocercosis

Spirocerca lupi is a nematode that is a common cause of mediastinal pathology in endemic areas. Following penetration of the gastric wall, the larvae migrate to

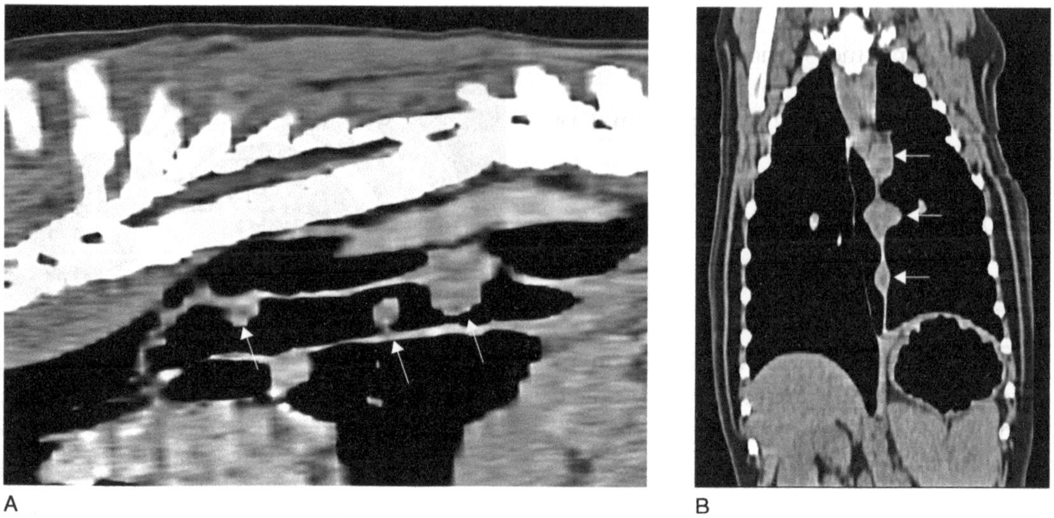

Figure 25.7 (A) Sagittally and (B) dorsally reconstructed CT images of a dog with three spirocercosis nodules (arrows) in an air-insufflated esophagus, two cranial luminal and a caudal mural nodule.

the aorta through the arteries, then to the esophageal wall. There, they transform into their adult form. The typical imaging appearance is that of a caudodorsal mediastinal mass as a result of a terminal esophageal mural nodule or nodules, which bulge into the esophageal lumen (Figure 25.7). Depending on the mass size, it may be readily seen on routine thoracic radiographs, particularly dorsoventral/ventrodorsal (DV/VD) projections. Nodules may also occur in the hilar region, where they are more difficult to detect radiographically. CT is the modality of choice to evaluate masses that are located on the esophageal serosal surface which cannot be fully evaluated endoscopically or when pleural or mediastinal fluid effaces structures on the radiograph. With time, the nodules may undergo neoplastic transformation or may lead to other complications. The latter and possible pathology from the primary migration route or aberrant migration are given in Table 25.4. CT is used for surgical planning and prognostication in spirocercosis patients. In endemic areas, all the potential pathological processes must be assessed on a thoracic CT, even if the dog has been presented for a different problem, because of the sensitivity of CT in detecting even small, clinically insignificant masses. An additional endotracheal tube is passed into the esophagus to inflate the esophagus just prior to the scan. The routine scan is usually followed by a CT angiogram to assess mass perfusion and to detect aortic aneurysms and thrombi (Figure 25.8). Images are viewed in mediastinal, bone and lung windows, allowing evaluation of different aspects of the disease.

CT features

Benign masses often have a more hypodense central region indicative of a fluid or necrotic component with a soft tissue density periphery that will enhance with the CT angiogram. Benign nodules that have undergone neoplastic transformation to osteosarcoma or fibrosarcoma have a more homogeneous soft tissue density with patchy enhancement after CT angiography.

Neoplasia

Mediastinal neoplasia can have numerous origins, but all result in the presence of a mediastinal mass. The location of the mass is the key point in the differential diagnosis and for interpretation purposes. The mediastinum can be divided into five areas: cranioventral, craniodorsal, perihilar, caudoventral and caudodorsal. Also, mediastinal masses can have a non-neoplastic etiology. Table 25.5 summarizes the differential diagnosis of mediastinal masses according to their location and the CT features potentially associated with the mass effect.

The internal CT features of mediastinal neoplasia largely depend on the origin of the tumor. Most commonly, the tumor has a homogeneous soft tissue density with a variable contrast enhancement according to its degree of perfusion. Hypoattenuating areas may be present in the core of the lesion corresponding to a necrotizing center.

Table 25.4
Pathology that may be seen on a thoracic CT examination in cases with spirocercosis. Pathology is given in order of most to least likely.

Possible forms and complications associated with spirocercosis	
Primary pathology	Caudal esophageal mass or masses (Figure 25.7) Large masses compress main stem bronchi and trachea depending on location Neoplastic masses tend to be large, occur in older dogs (6.4 ± 1.91 vs 4.93 ± 2.87 years in benign cases) and may show pulmonary metastasis or mass mineralization Hilar esophageal mass or masses Gastric mass in cardia region
Pathology secondary to normal or aberrant migration	Spondylitis (Figure 25.9) Aortic dystrophic mineralization (Figure 25.10) Aortic aneurysm Abnormally located mass Aortic rupture with periaortic streak-like hemorrhage or marked hemorrhage resulting in hemomediastinum or more commonly acute death due to hemothorax Focal thoracic hematoma, often associated with a blood vessel Thoracolumbar extradural cord compression Thoracolumbar intramedullary spinal cord swelling Aortic thrombus formation (Figure 25.8)
Complications	Hypertrophic osteopathy, primarily in malignant cases Esophageal perforation with mediastinitis and/or pyothorax Pleuritis Pneumomediastinum Aspiration pneumonia Pneumothorax Gastro-esophageal intussusception

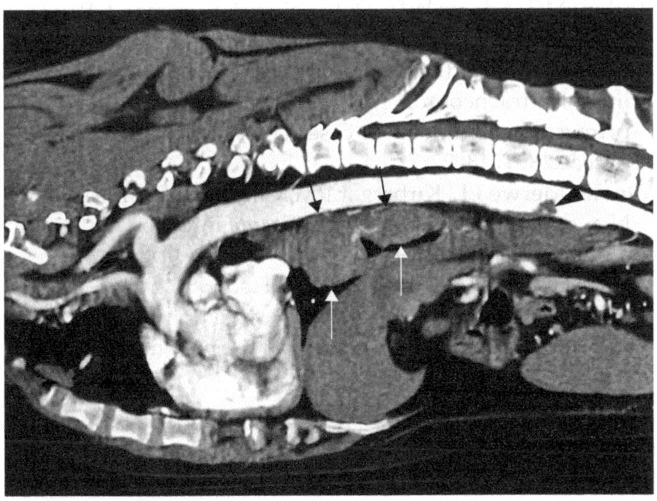

Figure 25.8 Sagittally reconstructed CT-angiogram of a dog with spirocercosis. There is a multilobulated irregular caudal esophageal mass (arrows) with mild aneurysmal dilatation of the aorta at the origin of a ventrally located aortic thrombus (arrowhead). The dog presented with iliac thromboembolism.

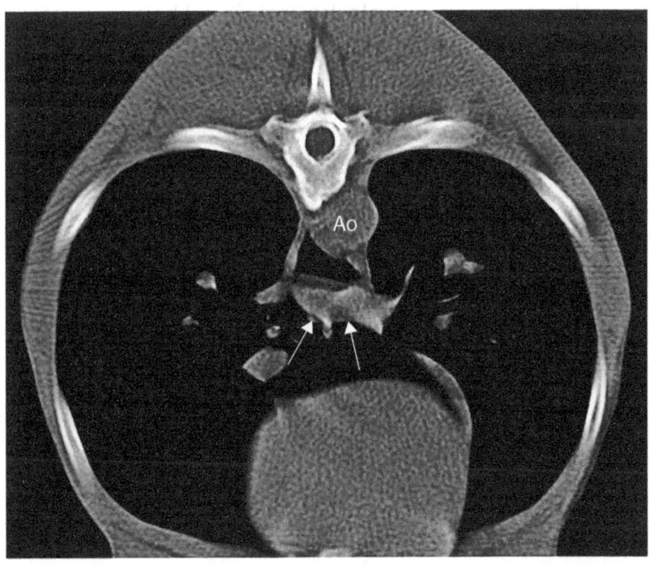

Figure 25.9 Transverse CT image in a dog with spondylitis secondary to aberrant *S. lupi* larval migration. Small nodules are visible in the ventral esophagus (arrows). Ao = aorta.

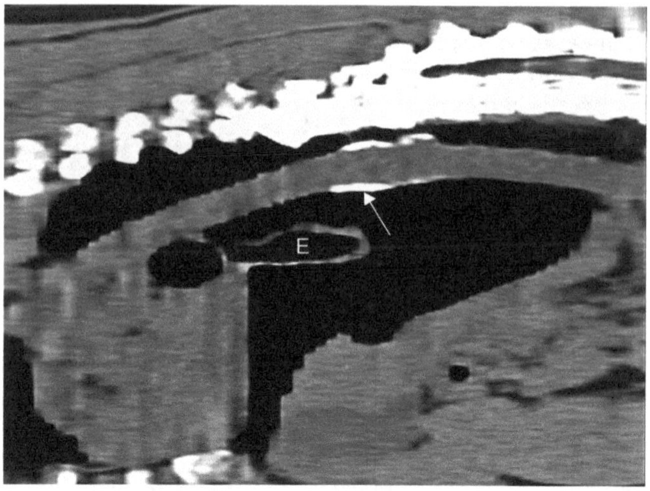

Figure 25.10 Sagittally reconstructed CT image of a dog with spirocercosis. There is dystrophic aortic calcification of the dorsal and ventral intima (arrow). E = air-filled esophagus.

Other masses

Cysts

Mediastinal cysts are usually benign, incidental findings that occur in both dogs and cats. They can go unnoticed until their size leads to compressive effects. Occasionally they rupture and can cause mediastinitis. They can have a pleural, branchial, thymic, lymphatic, bronchogenic or neoplastic origin. They are most commonly found in the cranioventral mediastinum, but can occasionally be located in the caudal mediastinum.

CT features (Figure 25.13)

Rounded mass lesion with variable mass effect on surrounding structures (cf. Table 25.5).

- Thin wall of soft tissue density.
- Fluid density filling the lesion.
- Mild contrast enhancement of the wall.

Granuloma/Abscess

An abscess or a granuloma can develop in the mediastinum secondary to an infectious or a traumatic process.

CT features (Figure 25.11)

- Rounded mass lesion with variable mass effect on surrounding structures (cf. Table 25.5).
- Thick, irregular wall of soft tissue density.
- Mixed soft tissue/fluid/gas density filling the lesion.
- Mild contrast enhancement of the wall.

Further reading

Ballegeer EA, Adams WM, Dubielzig RR, Paoloni MC, Klauer JM and Keuler NS (2010) Computed tomography characteristics of canine tracheobronchial lymph node metastasis. *Vet Radiol Ultrasound* **51**: 397–403.

Dvir E, Kirberger RM and Malleczek D (2001) Radiographic and computed tomographic changes and clinical presentation of spirocercosis in the dog. *Vet Radiol Ultrasound* **42**: 119–29.

Esterline ML, Radlinsky MAG, Biller DS, Mason DE, Roush JK and Cash WC (2005) Comparison of radiographic and computed tomography lymphangiography for identification of the canine thoracic duct. *Vet Radiol Ultrasound* **46**: 391–5.

Paoloni MC, Adams WM, Dubielzig RR, Kurzman I, Vail DM and Hardie RJ (2006) Comparison of results of computed tomography and radiography with histopathologic findings in tracheobronchial lymph nodes in dogs with primary lung tumors: 14 cases (1999–2002). *J Am Vet Med Assoc* **228**: 1718–22.

Van der Merwe LL, Kirberger RM, Clift S, Williams M, Keller N and Naidoo V (2008) *Spirocerca lupi* infection in the dog: a review. *Vet J* **176**: 294–309.

Yoon J, Feeney DA, Cronk DE, Anderson KL and Ziegler LE (2004) Computed tomographic evaluation of the canine and feline mediastinal masses in 14 patients. *Vet Radiol Ultrasound* **45**: 542–6.

Table 25.5
Differential diagnosis of mediastinal masses according to their location and associated CT features.

Mediastinal area	Differential diagnosis	CT features
Cranioventral (Figure 25.11)	Lymphoma Thymic diseases (thymoma, lymphosarcoma, cysts, hematoma, hyperplasia, amyloidosis)	• Soft tissue/mixed density mass • Widening of the cranioventral mediastinum • Elevation ± compression of the trachea • Caudal displacement of the heart and carina • Caudal displacement of the cranial lung lobes ± pulmonary atelectasis • Pooling of contrast in the veins of the neck and thoracic limbs
Craniodorsal (Figure 25.12)	Esophageal diseases Neural or neuroendocrine tumors Vertebral or paravertebral tumors (Aortic aneurysm, chemodectoma or thymoma reported)	• Soft tissue/mixed density mass, dorsal to the thoracic trachea • Ventral depression ± compression of the trachea • Ventral or lateral displacement of the esophagus if extra- or intra-mural esophageal mass • Variable amount of esophageal dilatation proximal to the lesion
Perihilar	Perihilar lymphadenopathy Heart-based tumors Esophageal diseases Bronchogenic cyst Vascular or cardiac enlargement	• Soft tissue/mixed density mass • Displacement ± compression/obstruction of the corresponding mainstem bronchus • If mass is caudal to the carina, widening of the angle created by the tracheal bifurcation ± possible compression of the carina
Caudoventral	Diaphragmatic lesions Peritoneo-pericardial hernia	• Soft tissue/mixed density mass • Widening of the caudoventral mediastinum or plica venae cavae • Displacement of the caudal vena cava • Displacement ± atelectasis of the accessory lung lobe
Caudodorsal (Figure 25.13)	Esophageal diseases Neural tumors Hiatal hernia Diaphragmatic mass	• Soft tissue/mixed density mass • Widening of the caudodorsal mediastinum • Ventral or lateral displacement of the esophagus if extra- or intra-mural esophageal mass • Variable amount of esophageal dilation proximal to the lesion
Any location	Primary mediastinal tumors (hemangiosarcoma, lipoma/sarcoma, histiocytic sarcoma) Abscess/granuloma Hematoma	• According to the location (cf. above)

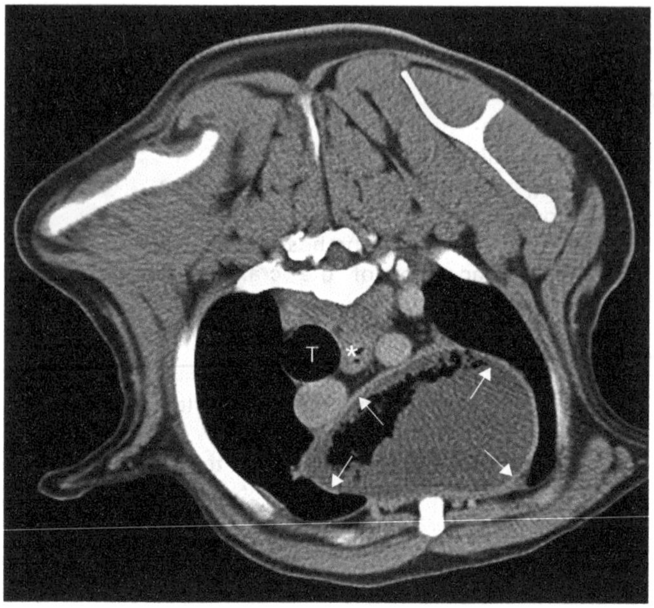

Figure 25.11 Post-contrast transverse CT image of a dog with a cranioventral mediastinal abscess. It is delineated with a contrast-enhancing wall (arrows) and has a mixed fluid and gas content. * = esophagus; T = trachea.

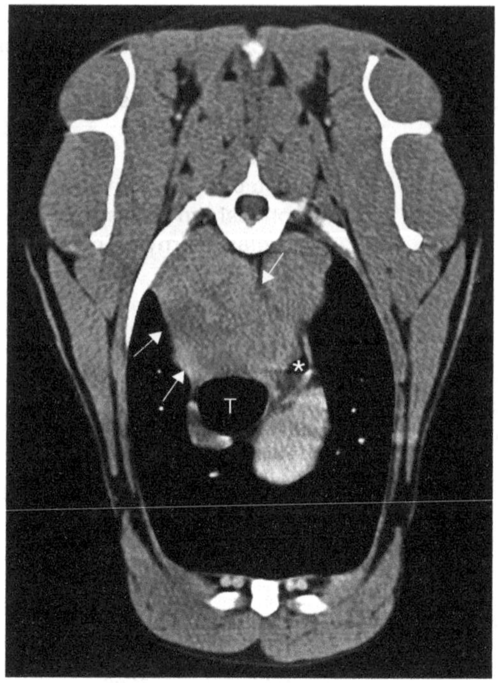

Figure 25.12 Post-contrast transverse CT image of a dog with a craniodorsal mediastinal paravertebral leiomyosarcoma (arrows). The trachea (T) is ventrally displaced and the esophagus is displaced to the left (asterisk).

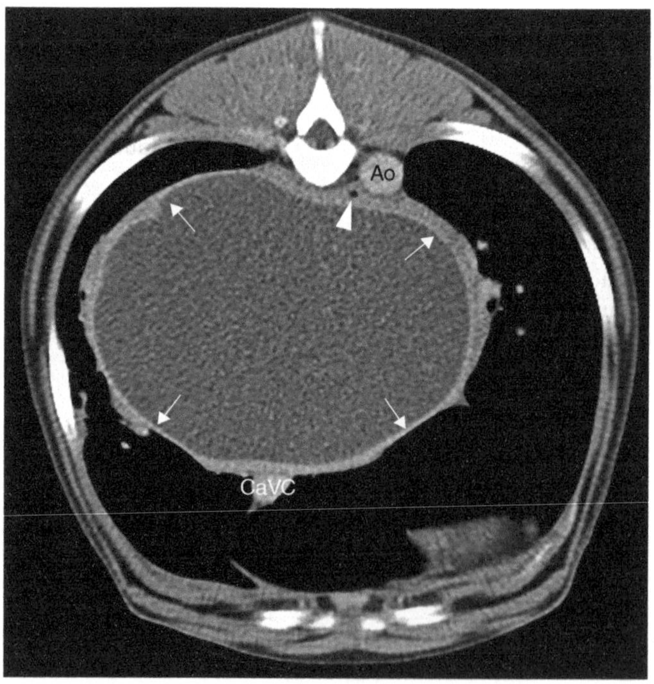

Figure 25.13 10-month-old dog with a paraesophageal cyst. Post-contrast transverse CT image shows a caudodorsal mediastinal mass delineated with a contrast-enhancing thin wall (arrows) and is fully fluid filled. It produces a significant mass effect on the aorta (Ao), caudal vena cava (CaVC) and esophagus (arrowhead).

CHAPTER TWENTY-SIX

Lungs and Bronchi

Tobias Schwarz and Victoria Johnson

Imaging Protocol

See Table 26.1.

CT: Anatomy and Normal Variants

The bronchi (Figures 26.1 and 26.2)

The bronchi are air-conducting tubes with bands of smooth muscle and flattened overlapping cartilage rings for support. The bronchial tree consists of a left and right principal bronchus, each of which subdivides into lobar bronchi and then further arborizes into segmental bronchi within each lobe. The segmental bronchi ventilate a small area of lung within a lobe and continue to branch into smaller and smaller tubes down to the respiratory bronchioles.

The bronchi are clearly visualized on high-frequency reconstruction images with lung window settings as round, air-filled tubes with hyperdense walls tapering towards the periphery. The walls may be mineralized centrally in dogs; this is most marked and most peripheral in chondrodystrophic breeds. In cats, normal bronchial walls should not be mineralized. Bronchioles are usually not visualized within 10 mm of the peripheral surface of the lung. Virtual bronchoscopy of normal bronchi reveals smooth-walled tubular structures which taper gradually and are round in cross-section. Smaller bronchioles cannot be assessed with this technique.

Normal bronchial wall thickness can be assessed by measuring the internal and external cross-sectional areas (CSA) of the bronchus, generating the bronchial wall CSA by subtraction of the internal from the external CSA, and dividing the bronchial wall CSA by the external bronchial CSA. This ratio should not exceed 0.5. A bronchoarterial diameter ratio can be used to assess overall bronchial size for bronchiectasis with a normal range of 0.8 to 2. A bronchial diameter that exceeds twice the diameter of the adjacent pulmonary artery indicates bronchiectasis.

In dogs the pulmonary artery CSA should be between 0.4 and 0.6 of the external CSA of the adjacent bronchus. Both measurements should be obtained at the level of the T8 vertebra.

The lung parenchyma (Figures 26.1 and 26.3–26.6)

The lung parenchyma consists of a vast and thin-walled alveolar airspace, interstitium with feeding bronchovascular and lymphatic structures. Like humans, dogs and cats have a bronchoarterial lung type, in which a centrilobular artery accompanies the bronchus and pulmonary veins separate from the bronchus at segmental level. Unlike humans (type II lung), dogs and cats do not have distinctive septa between lung lobules (type III lung). The pulmonary interstitium is not very prominent in dogs and cats.

High-resolution CT settings with a lung window are best to visualize details of aerated lung anatomy. High-resolution CT is not a specific preset on most CT units, but is achieved with a combination of optimized settings for maximal image detail which includes a high-frequency reconstruction algorithm, minimal slice width, no or low pitch, high mAs settings, a small field of view and the largest available image matrix. The lung parenchyma should be reasonably homogeneous with a tolerable noise level, with density levels in the negative range. Mean density levels that are applicable for all lobes and different CT settings have been established in dogs as −713 HU in expiration and −846 HU in inflated inspiratory CT. The soft tissue-dense pulmonary vessels can be followed to the fourth-degree

Veterinary Computed Tomography, First Edition. Edited by Tobias Schwarz, Jimmy Saunders.

Table 26.1
CT imaging protocol (intravenous contrast study: standard protocol; *see* Chapter 5).

Series	Pre- and post-contrast	High resolution lung
Decubitus	Ventral	
Scan margins	Caudal extent of lung → Thoracic inlet	
Voltage (kVp)	120	
Current (mAs)	160	200 to 300
Tube rotation time (s)	0.5 to 1	
Slice width (mm)	3–5	1
Kernel frequency	High	
Collimator pitch	1.5	0–1
Helical image reconstruction interval (mm)	1.5 to 2.5	
Motion control	Required	
Window level (HU)	−100	
Window width (HU)	2000	

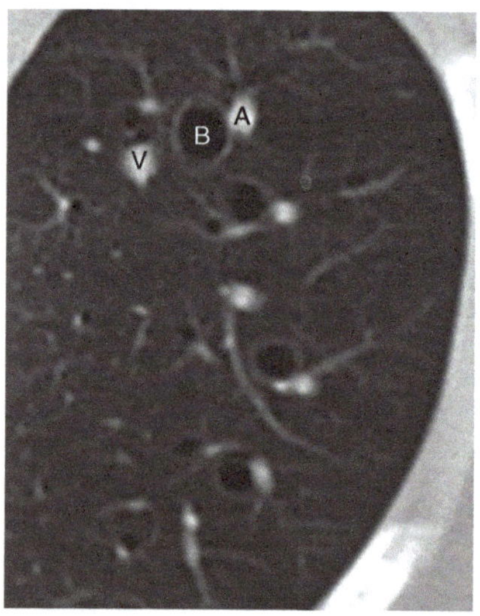

Figure 26.1 Close-up of a transverse high-resolution CT image of normal canine lung. The bronchi (B) have thin, dense walls. The pulmonary arteries (A) are directly adjacent to the bronchi, whereas the veins (V) travel in a distance. Small lung vessels are visible in the lung periphery but not interlobar septa.

branch as tubular soft tissue structures. Arteries and veins can be distinguished by their relationship to the bronchus. The pleural lining of the lung is usually a very faint hyperdense line, and consequently it can be difficult to define the exact lung lobe borders on CT. Orthogonal reconstructions as well as lower and narrower window settings are helpful in this respect. The branching of the bronchial tree is also helpful to determine the lung lobe anatomy, in particular for the right middle lobe, which can easily be identified by its unique dorsoventral bronchial orientation. Finally the lack of visible vasculature in the lung periphery can aid the identification of lung borders.

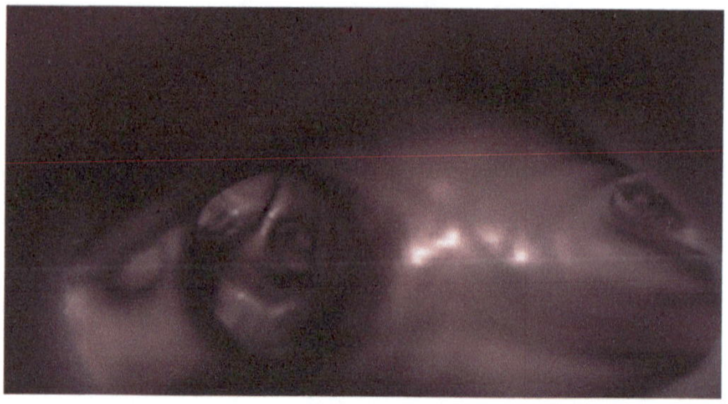

Figure 26.2 Normal virtual bronchoscopy image with a view from the distal trachea into the right mainstem bronchus. Note the smooth, rounded appearance of the bronchus and its divisions.

Heterotopic pulmonary bone formation (pulmonary osteoma) frequently occurs in large breed dogs, particularly collie breeds, and manifests on CT images as 1–3 mm dense nodules throughout the parenchyma and subpleurally. Although these nodules consist of bone, measured density values are frequently still in the negative HU range, due to volume averaging with the air-dense lung.

A degree of peripheral atelectasis (synonym *collapse*) is ubiquitous in lung CT examinations of dogs and cats. Only a fraction of the normal lung capacity is needed at rest and prolonged recumbency and general anesthesia with oxygen instead of air lead to collapse of lung space. Atelectasis (Box 26.1) occurs in the most dependent part of the lung and is most marked with compression by other organs. There are many causes of lung collapse that should be differentiated. Even if atelectasis is physiologic, it can mask pathologic lung lesions such as soft tissue nodules. It may be necessary to repeat the CT exam with the patient positioned with the atelectatic lung in the non-dependent position and hyperventilated prior to scanning.

Intravenous contrast medium application is rarely helpful to assess aerated lungs, but it is very useful for all soft tissue structures of the thorax, including non-aerated lung. Collapsed or consolidated lung and the pleural lining show a strong contrast enhancement. Therefore the contrast uptake is helpful to differentiate pleural fluid from lung tissue, as well as vascularized lung tissue from necrotic, infarcted, abscessed or cystic

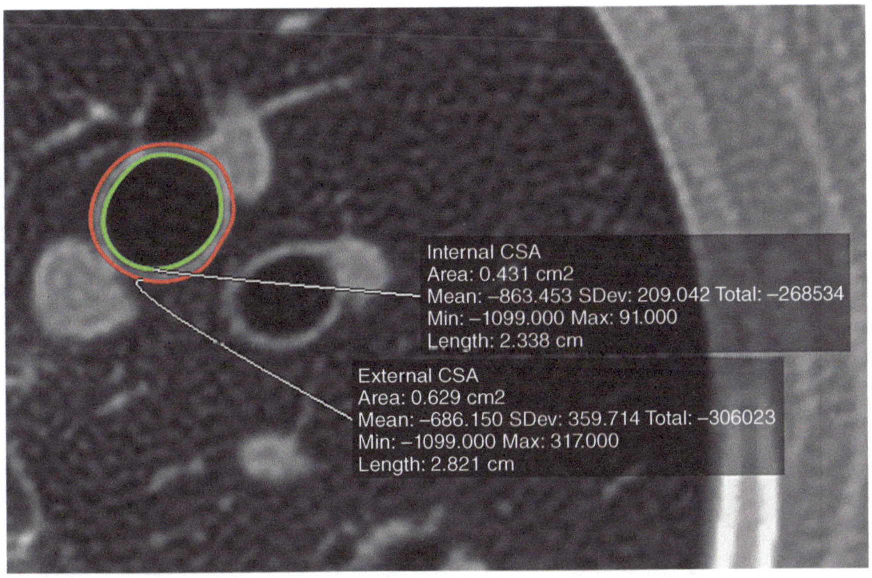

Figure 26.3 Close-up transverse CT image of a normal left canine caudal lobar bronchus with regions of interest drawn to measure the external (red circle, 0.6 cm^2) and internal (green circle, 0.4 cm^2) bronchial cross-sectional areas (CSA). The resulting bronchial wall CSA is 0.2 cm^2 and the ratio between it and the external bronchial CSA is 0.33 (normal range ≤ 0.5).

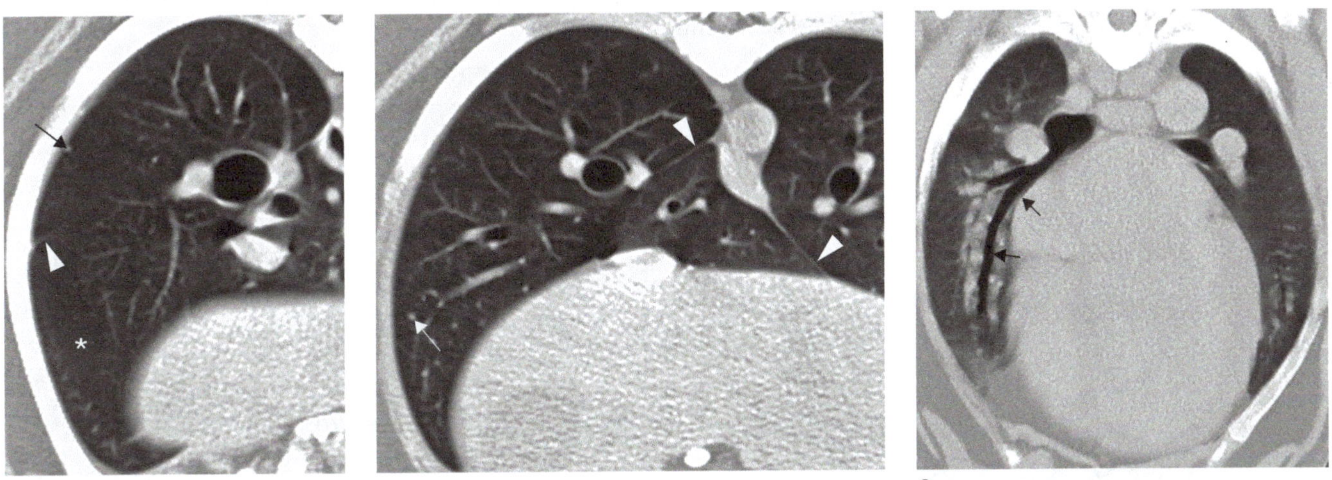

Figure 26.4 Transverse CT images with features for canine lung lobe identification. Faintly hyperdense pleural lines are seen between (A) the right middle and caudal lobe (arrowheads) and (B) around the accessory lobe (arrowheads). There is an absence of pulmonary vessels in the periphery of the right middle lobe (asterisk) and there are numerous small, dense pulmonary osteomas (arrows). (C) The right middle lobar bronchus (arrows) is the only bronchus with a dorsoventral orientation, helping to identify this lobe.

lung. The contrast uptake in inflammatory or infiltrative lung (consolidation) cannot be differentiated from atelectatic lung.

CT Disease Features

Malformations/Developmental

Bronchial collapse

Bronchial collapse is commonly seen in small or toy breed dogs and is often found in conjunction with tracheal collapse (*see* Chapter 24). The underlying cause is a progressive degeneration of the bronchial cartilage leading to an unstable bronchial wall. The disease is often accompanied by other complicating factors such as obesity and chronic bronchitis.

CT features (Figure 26.7)

- Flattened or narrow bronchi (appreciated best in transverse section).
- Collapse occurs during expiration so best to acquire images during this phase of respiratory cycle.

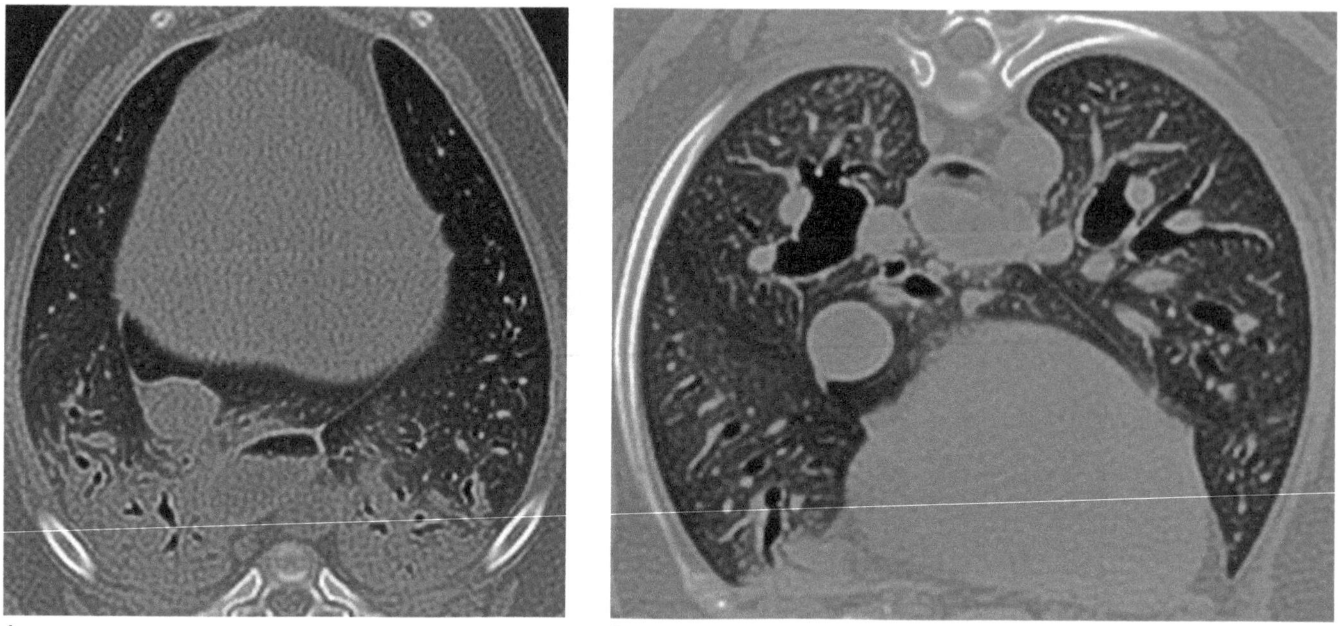

A B

Figure 26.5 (A) Transverse CT image with pronounced atelectasis in dependent dorsal lung areas in a dog. This is a physiologic feature but can mask pathology. (B) Repeat CT scan with the dog in ventral recumbency post hyperventilation shows the re-aerated dorsal lung and the beginning atelectasis ventrally.

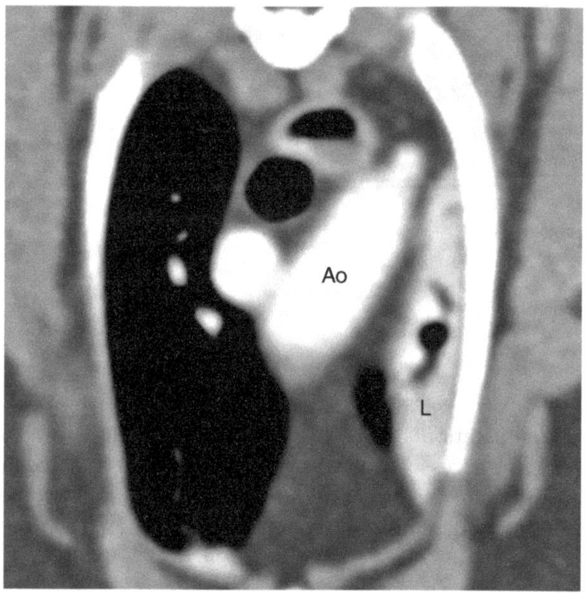

Figure 26.6 Transverse CT image with normal contrast enhancement of a collapsed left cranial lung lobe (L). Ao = aorta.

Box 26.1 Forms of lung atelectasis

- ***Passive atelectasis***
  - hypostatic lung collapse (physiologic)
  - mild pneumothorax or pleural effusion
  - small compressive mass lesion
- ***Compression atelectasis***
  - tension pneumothorax
  - marked pleural effusion
  - large compressive mass lesion
- ***Resorption atelectasis***
  - oxygen supplementation (physiologic)
  - airway obstruction
- ***Adhesive atelectasis***
  - congenital lack of surfactant
  - acute respiratory distress syndrome
- ***Cicatrization atelectasis***
  - lung fibrosis
  - adhesive pleuritis

- May see dynamic changes if a static CT series is acquired while the patient breathes normally (see tracheal collapse).
- Possible additional pathology such as pneumonia and right-sided heart enlargement (cor pulmonale).

Trauma

Blunt external forces or internal trauma (barotrauma) can lead to rupture of pulmonary capillaries, causing hemorrhage and inflammatory reaction with lung lobe swelling (contusion) and bronchial or airspace rupture, leading to bulla formation, pneumomediastinum and pneumothorax. A bronchial tear may occur secondarily to iatrogenic barotrauma (positive pressure ventilation, bronchoscopy), lung lobe torsion or parasitic infestation. The rupture results in gas tracking into the mediastinum, fascial planes and subcutis.

CT features (Figure 26.8)

- Swollen soft tissue-dense lung lobe in consolidation.
- Bulla formation.

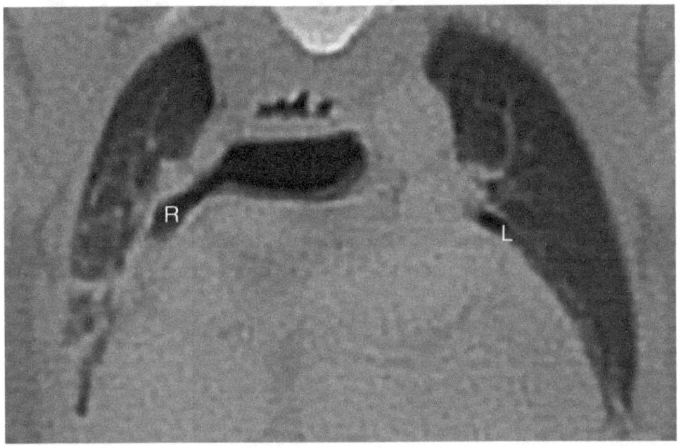

Figure 26.7 Transverse CT image of the tracheal bifurcation in a Yorkshire terrier. The right stem bronchus (R) is partially collapsed and the left one (L) is completely collapsed.

- Pneumomediastinum.
- Pneumothorax.

Infection/Inflammation

Bronchitis

Chronic canine bronchitis typically affects middle-aged and older dogs with chronic airway inflammation, smooth muscle hypertrophy and mucous gland hyperplasia. Potential causes of canine bronchitis include infectious, inflammatory or allergic disease, dynamic airway collapse and bronchiectasis.

Feline bronchial disease is a term used to include a multitude of small airway diseases in the cat. The condition results from airway inflammation, reversible obstructive disease, bronchial wall edema and hypersecretion of mucus. Respiratory tract parasites (*Aelurostrongylus, Capillaria, Paragonimus* spp.) can also create or contribute to the condition and should be excluded. Hyperinflation may result from air trapping distal to the obstructed airways. Right middle lung lobe collapse is a common sequel and on occasion chronic rib fractures may be seen.

CT features (Figure 26.9)

- Thickened bronchial walls and peribronchial cuffing.
- Intraluminal soft tissue-dense material.

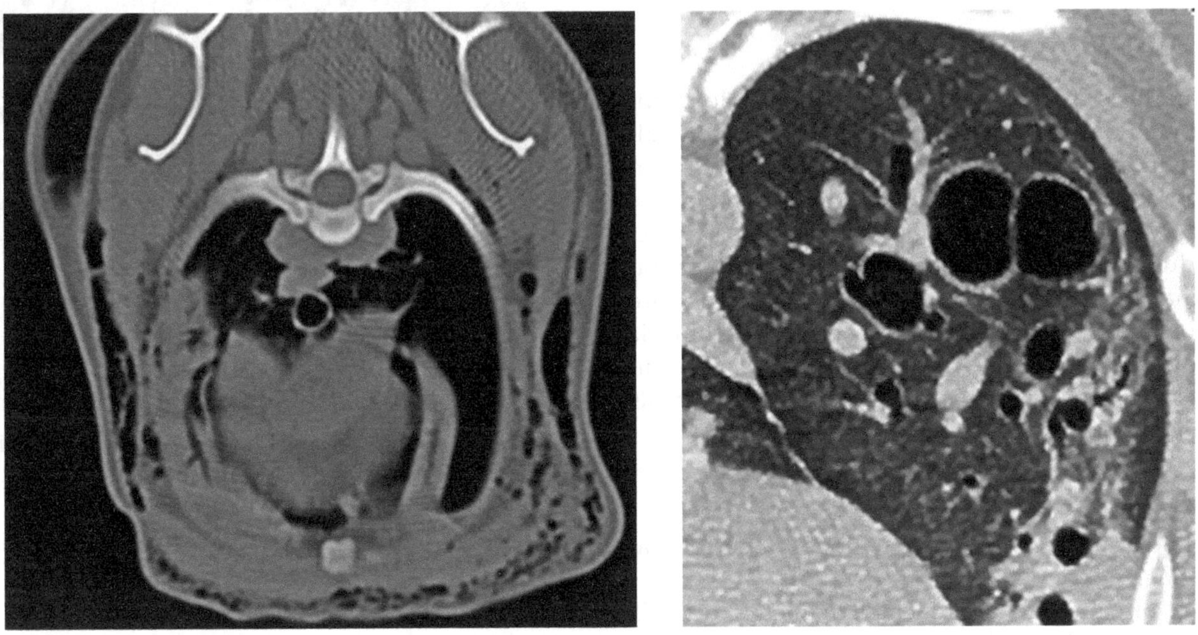

A B

Figure 26.8 Transverse CT images in two different dogs. (A) Thorax trauma with marked subcutaneous emphysema, pneumomediastinum, pneumothorax and right cranial and left cranial lung lobe consolidation, consistent with a contusion. (B) Traumatic bullae formation in the left caudal lung lobe.

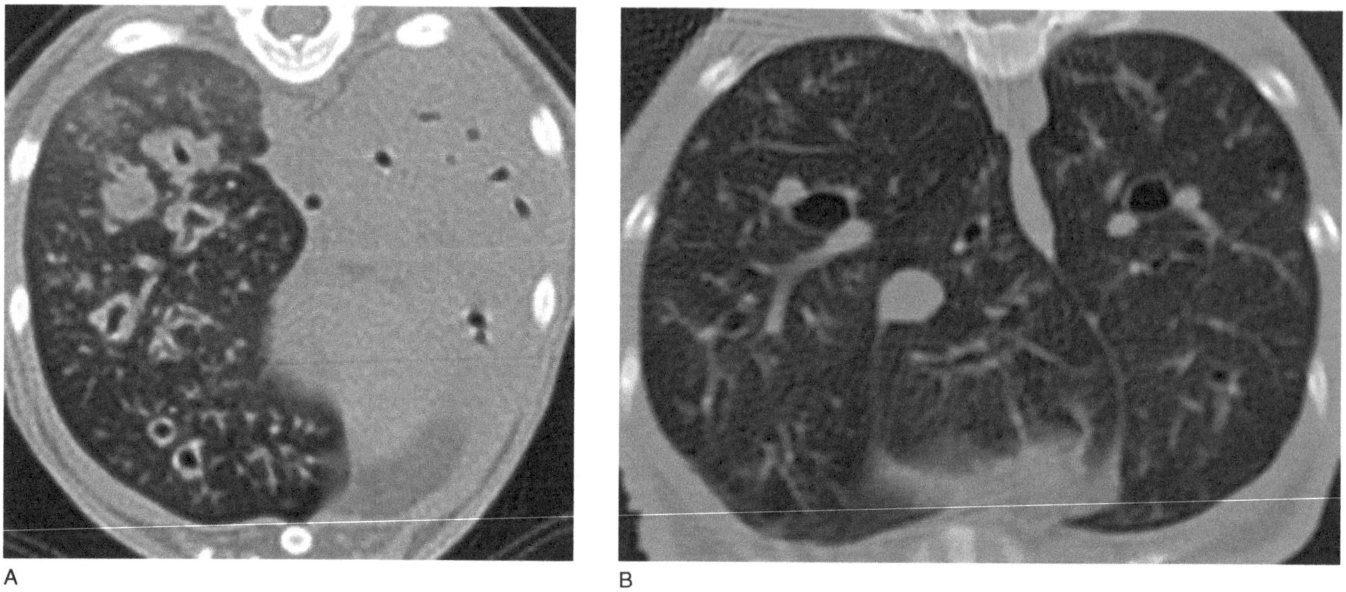

Figure 26.9 Transverse CT images. (A) Canine bronchopneumonia with complete left caudal lung lobe consolidation and irregular thickening of the right caudal bronchial walls. (B) Feline bronchitis with increased wall thickening of peripheral bronchi.

- Right middle lung lobe collapse in cats (mucus plug).
- Rib fractures (more commonly seen in cats).
- Hyperlucency and peripheral bronchiectasis with air trapping in cats.
- Co-existing features of pneumonia, bronchiectasis or bronchial collapse.

Bronchiectasis

Bronchiectasis is characterized by irreversible bronchial dilatation. The changes may be focal or generalized, cylindrical or saccular shaped. The disease can occur in association with primary ciliary dyskinesia, secondary to long-standing or severe respiratory infections, due to airway obstruction or as a complication of radiation treatment. Secondary infections are common and difficult to completely resolve. In fibrotic lung diseases in dogs, traction bronchiectasis can occur. The distorted, fibrosed lung architecture pulls the bronchi into irregular dilated shapes.

CT features (Figure 26.10)

- Cylindrical or saccular distentions of peripheral bronchi.
- Lack of tapering of bronchial diameter towards periphery, visible bronchi within 1 cm of lung margin.
- Bronchoarterial ratio exceeds 2.0.
- Co-existing features of pneumonia or fibrosis.

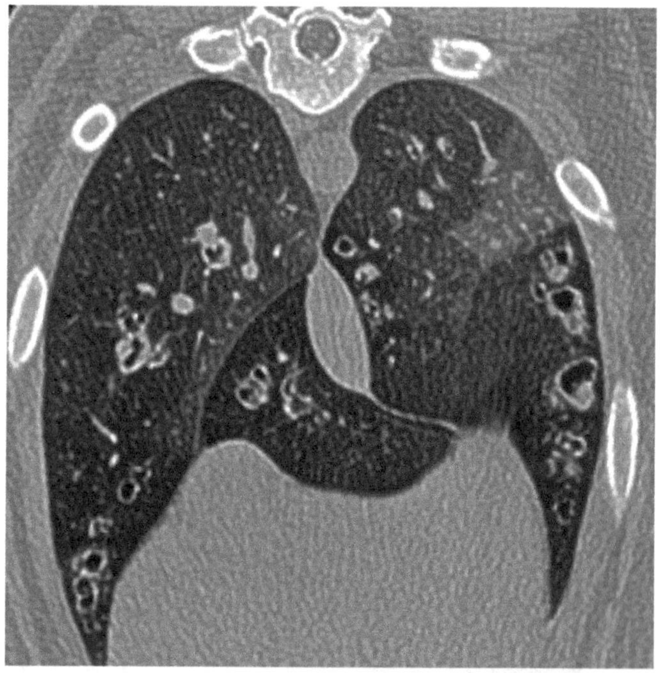

Figure 26.10 Transverse CT image with severe bronchiectasis with thick-walled, cylindrically and saccularly distended peripheral bronchi in a dog with immotile cilia syndrome.

Bronchial foreign body

Inhaled bronchial foreign bodies may cause obstruction, irritation, inflammation and laceration. The size of the foreign body dictates the level at which it will cease movement. The caudal lobes are more commonly

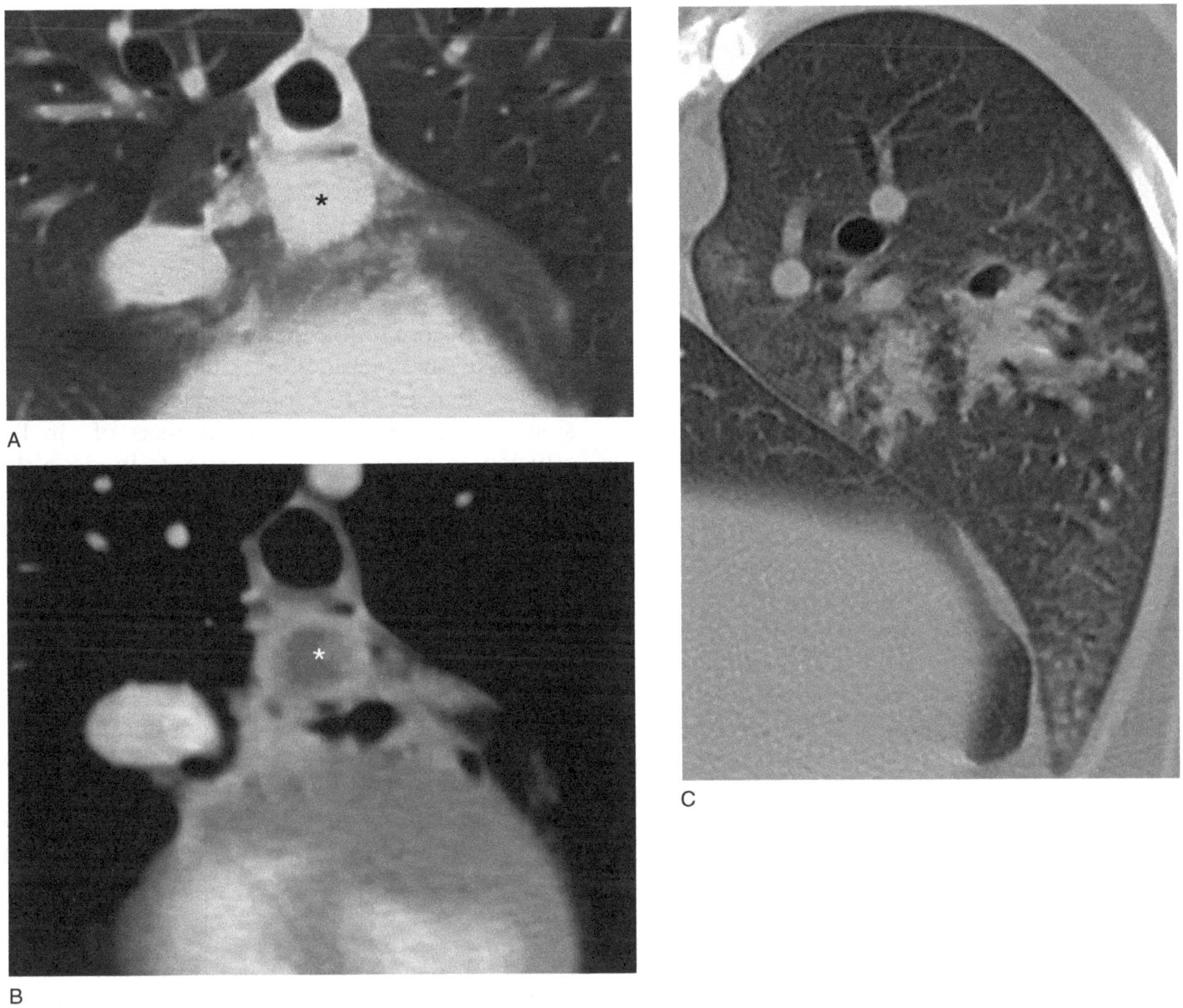

Figure 26.11 (A) Transverse CT image with round, soft tissue lesion in (asterisk) the center of the accessory lobe in a dog with a migrating grass awn. (B) The post-contrast image shows rim enhancement with non-enhancing content (abscess) (asterisk). (C) Occlusion and exudate formation in the bronchial tree of a dog that inhaled pine needles.

affected. Chronic foreign bodies result in pneumonia and even abscessation.

CT features (Figure 26.11)

- Presence of foreign material within a bronchus (not always seen):
  - high density (bone, stone, tooth, metal fragment, dental calculus etc.)
  - soft tissue density (grass awn, toys, food fragments, etc.)
  - neither type will show any enhancement with intravenous contrast administration.
- Focal pneumonia or abscess formation. The abscess typically shows peripheral enhancement with a non-enhancing fluid-dense core surrounding the foreign material.
- Lobar atelectasis due to obstructive resorption atelectasis.
- Hyperlucency and increased lobar volume if a check-valve effect is created by an incompletely obstructing foreign body.

Lung infection and inflammation

Bacterial, viral, fungal and parasitic pneumonia and bronchopneumonia as well as allergic and idiopathic inflammatory changes of the lung manifest with often marked density changes and different distribution patterns of the alveolar space. The specific CT patterns of different inflammatory lung diseases have not been established yet in dogs and cats but some general rules can be applied.

CT features (Figure 26.12)

- Propensity towards soft tissue opacification (similar to radiographic alveolar pattern).
- Propensity towards ventral airspace filling in hematogeneous bacterial pneumonia.
- Peribronchial thickening in allergic and parasitic airway conditions.
- Perivascular thickening in parasitic vascular infection.
- Associated perihilar lymphadenopathy, most marked in fungal pneumonia.
- Nodule and mass formation (abscess, granuloma) is less common.

Granulomatous lung diseases and abscess formation

Pulmonary abscess formation can be a sequel to pneumonia, inhaled, penetrated or migrating foreign body infection, or severe pleural infection. Granuloma formation can be seen in fungal disease, canine eosinophilic pneumonia, mycobacterial disease and lymphomatoid granulomatosis. Contrast-enhanced CT is essential to differentiate these lesions from other inflammatory or neoplastic conditions, although there remains some overlap.

CT features (Figures 26.13 and 26.14)

- Pulmonary soft tissue nodule or mass.
- Abscess characterized by non-enhancing material or gas and a regular contrast-enhancing wall.
- Abscess may contain opaque foreign body.
- Granulomas often have irregularly shaped large mass formation, often with central necrosis and are usually not cavitated.
- Multifocal small nodular granulomas can be difficult to differentiate from metastatic lung lesions.
- Granulomatous disease often has very marked associated perihilar lymphadenopathy, more so than with abscess and neoplasia.

Lung fibrosis

Interstitial fibrosis can be the end stage of various chronic pulmonary conditions. *Idiopathic pulmonary fibrosis* is a chronic progressive condition of unknown etiology seen in older terrier breed dogs with progressive exercise intolerance and inspiratory crackles on auscultation. It has also been reported in cats.

CT features (Figure 26.15)

- Diffuse ground-glass opacity (similar to radiographic interstitial pattern).
- Bands of dense lung tissue perpendicular to the pleural surface.
- Peribronchial and subpleural soft tissue opacities.
- Mild traction bronchiectasis.

Lung lobe torsion

Torsion of a lung lobe is a rare condition in dogs (extremely rare in cats) with twisting and occlusion of the perihilar lobar bronchus, lobar pulmonary vein and later artery with progressive swelling. Resorption atelectasis and venous congestion lead to a soft tissue-dense, often enlarged, maloriented lung lobe, occasionally with residual small pockets of air. Pleural effusion is almost always present. In deep-chested dogs the right middle lobe, and in small breed dogs with barrel-chest formation the left cranial lobe, are most commonly affected. Multiplanar and paddle-wheel reconstruction as well as virtual bronchoscopy generated from thin-sliced images are helpful to follow the bronchial tree and check for patency. Contrast-enhanced CT can assist differentiating vascularized collapsed lung from a necrotic torsed lung lobe. Equally, positional changes on a repeat CT examination should reveal reinflation of collapsed lung in a non-dependent position but consistent atelectasis of a torsed lobe. With pleural effusion aerated lung lobes often float and become folded and this should not be confused with torsion.

CT features (Figure 26.16)

- Collapsed or swollen lung lobe with lung apex pointing in abnormal direction and maloriented bronchovascular structures.
- Accumulation of small air pockets (vesicular pattern).
- Abruptly interrupted patency of a bronchus, blunted appearance, fish-mouth like appearance in virtual bronchoscopy.
- Lack of contrast enhancement with arterial occlusion and necrosis.

Pulmonary edema

Cardiogenic pulmonary edema is a common sequel of heart disease in dogs and cats, less commonly seen is non-cardiogenic permeability edema formation. CT should be an excellent imaging modality to assess edema formation, but it has not been extensively used yet in veterinary cardiology.

CT features (Figure 26.17)

- Patchy areas of soft tissue infiltrate in lungs.
- Enlarged pulmonary veins in cardiogenic edema.

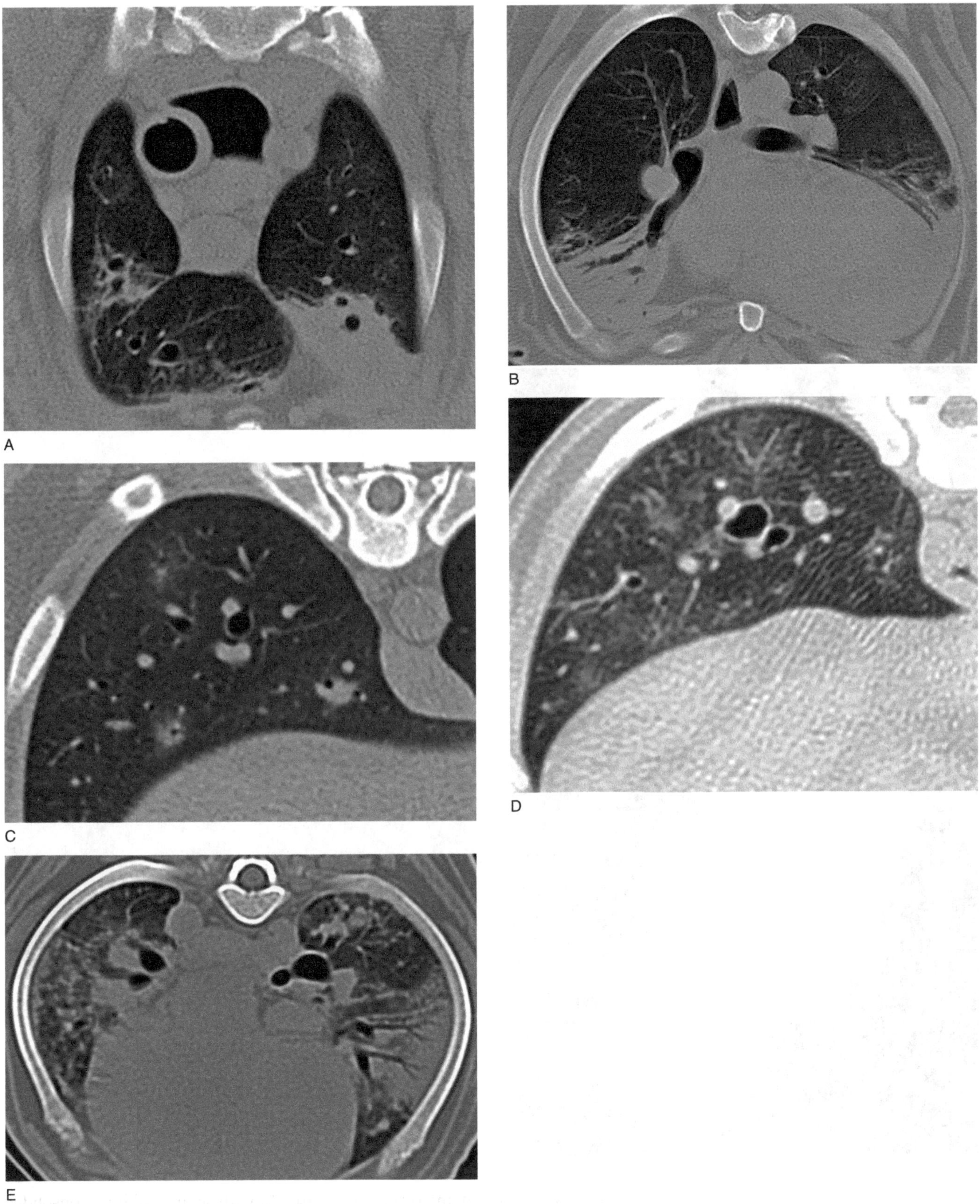

Figure 26.12 Transverse CT image with canine bacterial pneumonia with ventral consolidation of (A) left cranial and (B) right middle lung lobe. (C) Septic peribronchial foci in right caudal and accessory lung lobe in a pyrexic dog. (D) Patchy areas of ground-glass opacity in a histologically confirmed case of interstitial pneumonia. (E) Patchy alveolar infiltrate and vascular enlargement in a dog with angiostrongylosis (image courtesy of Lars Knudsen Granly).

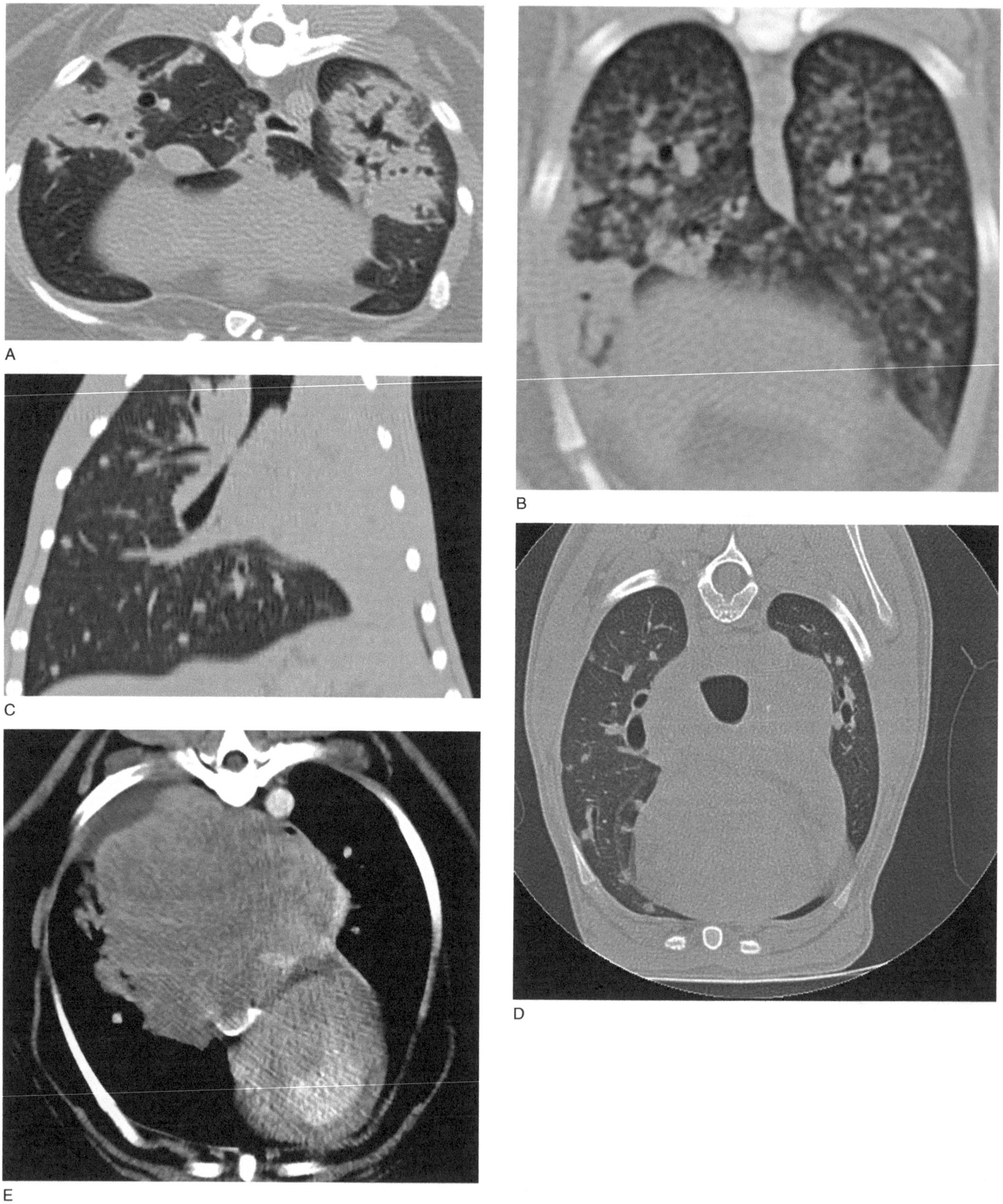

Figure 26.13 Transverse CT images of confirmed cases of granulomatous lung disease (A) with segmental lung consolidation (cause unknown) and (B) miliary nodular changes and lung consolidation in tuberculosis in two cats. (C) Dorsally reconstructed CT images with numerous soft tissue nodules, left lung consolidation and perihilar lymphadenopathy (cause unknown) and (D) massive perihilar lymph node granuloma and nodules throughout the lungs (cause unknown) in two dogs. (E) Large mass formation in the right caudal lung lobe in a dog with an eosinophilic granuloma.

Pulmonary vascular embolic events and infarction

Pulmonary arterial embolism can occur as a consequence of thromboembolic disease, iatrogenically dislodged intravascular material, fat and bone marrow embolism due to trauma or bone-marrow compressive surgery, septic, neoplastic or parasitic embolism.

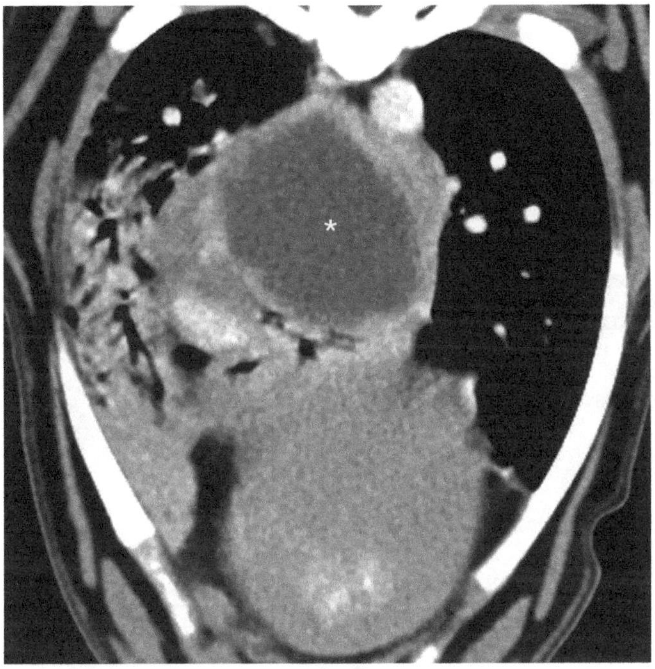

Figure 26.14 Transverse CT image with pneumonia in the right lung with abscess formation in the accessory lobe with a markedly contrast-enhancing rim and non-enhancing content (asterisk).

In pulmonary thromboembolism the bronchoarterial ratio can exceed 2.0 in the thrombosed vessel segment and be diminished in the post-occluded vascular bed. Peripheral wedge-shaped areas of lung consolidation are consistent with infarcted lung. Pulmonary CT angiography can reveal filling defects in thrombosed vessels.

Diffuse metastatic neoplasia of the lungs (synonym *pulmonary carcinosis*) has been documented in dogs with hematogeneous tumor emboli in the lung capillaries, leading to obstruction of blood flow, ischemia and infarction.

CT features (Figure 26.18)

- Iatrogenically dislodged material in pulmonary artery.
- Enlarged thrombus containing arterial segment.
- Collapsed post-thrombotic arterial segment and pulmonary vein.
- Pleural-based, wedge-shaped lung consolidation.
- Filling defect of pulmonary artery segment in CT angiography.
- Wedge-shaped and froth-like bands of subpleural infiltrate, general ground-glass opacity, scattered small nodules and areas of ground-glass opacity in pulmonary carcinosis.

Neoplasia

Primary pulmonary and bronchial and infiltrative tumors

Pulmonary, bronchial and bronchoalveolar carcinomas are relatively common, usually slowly growing single

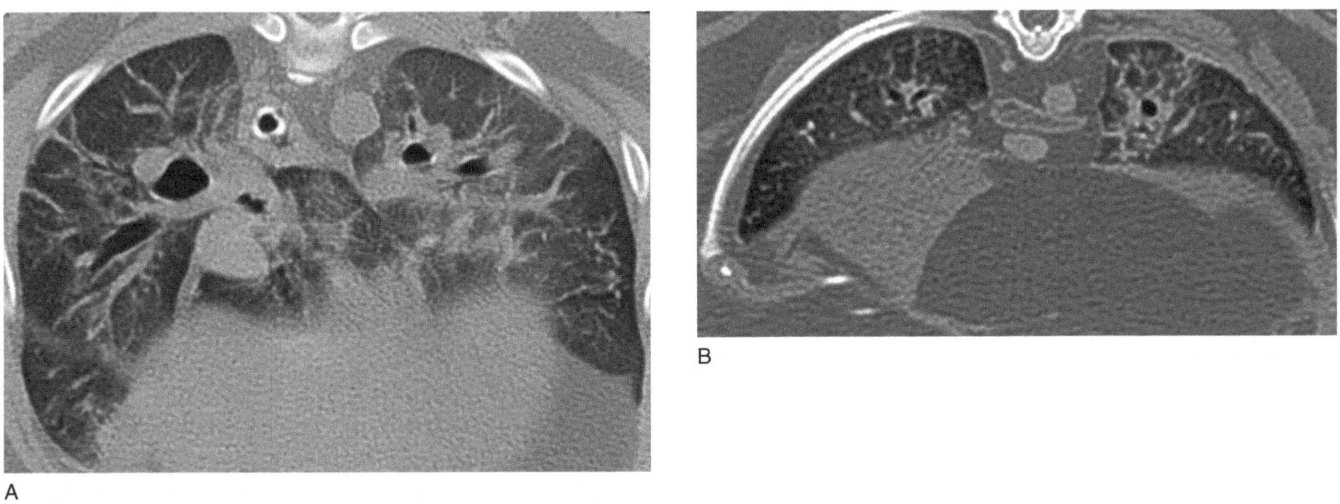

Figure 26.15 Transverse CT image with generalized ground-glass opacity and parenchymal fibrous band in (A) a West Highland white terrier with idiopathic pulmonary fibrosis and (B) a domestic shorthair cat with suspected fibrotic changes.

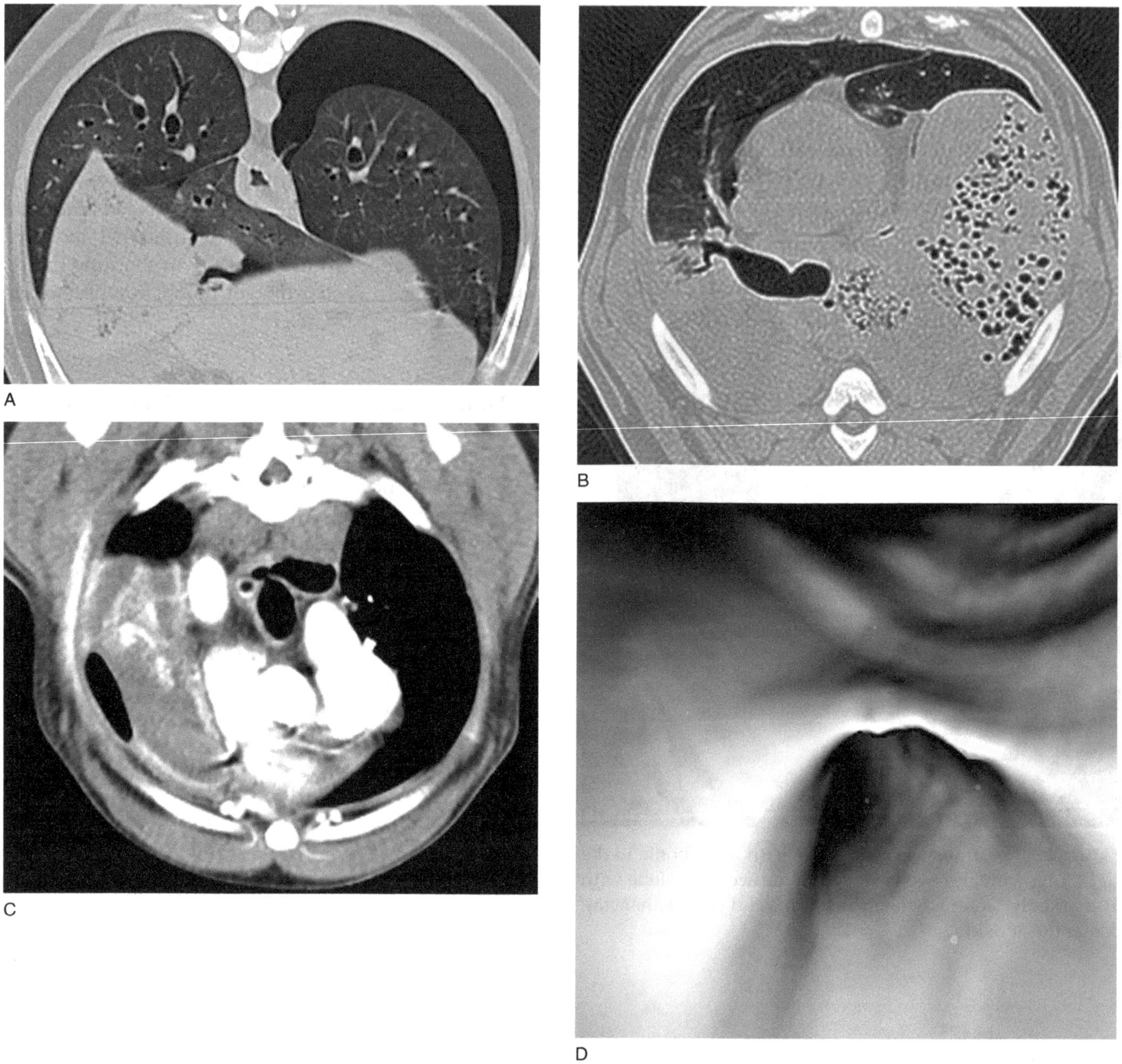

Figure 26.16 (A) Torsed consolidated right middle lung lobe of which the apex points dorsally, compressing the right caudal lobe. Marked left pneumothorax. (B) Torsed consolidated left caudal lung lobe with a vesicular gas pattern and pleural effusion in the dorsally dependent part. (C) Lack of uniform contrast enhancement of a torsed right cranial lobe and mild pleural effusion in a pug. (A–C = transverse CT images.) (D) Virtual bronchoscopy image with a view into the torsed right middle lobar bronchus with an ovoid fish-mouth appearance.

masses in dogs and cats that will eventually cavitate (gas or fluid filled) and seed metastases to the lungs and other organs. CT is very valuable in assessment of these lesions for possible surgical resection and the presence of pulmonary, pleural or lymph node metastases. Solitary pulmonary neoplasia often only deviates bronchial structures and thus remains clinically silent longer than bronchial neoplasia that occludes airways immediately. Canine multicentric neoplasia such as lymphoma typically leads to diffuse interstitial lung infiltrate, whereas it only very rarely affects the lungs in cats. Other locally infiltrative canine neoplasias such as histiocytic sarcoma and lymphomatoid granulomatosis present with large poorly marginated areas of soft tissue infiltrate of the lungs and perihilar lymph nodes. There are cystic lung tumors that can

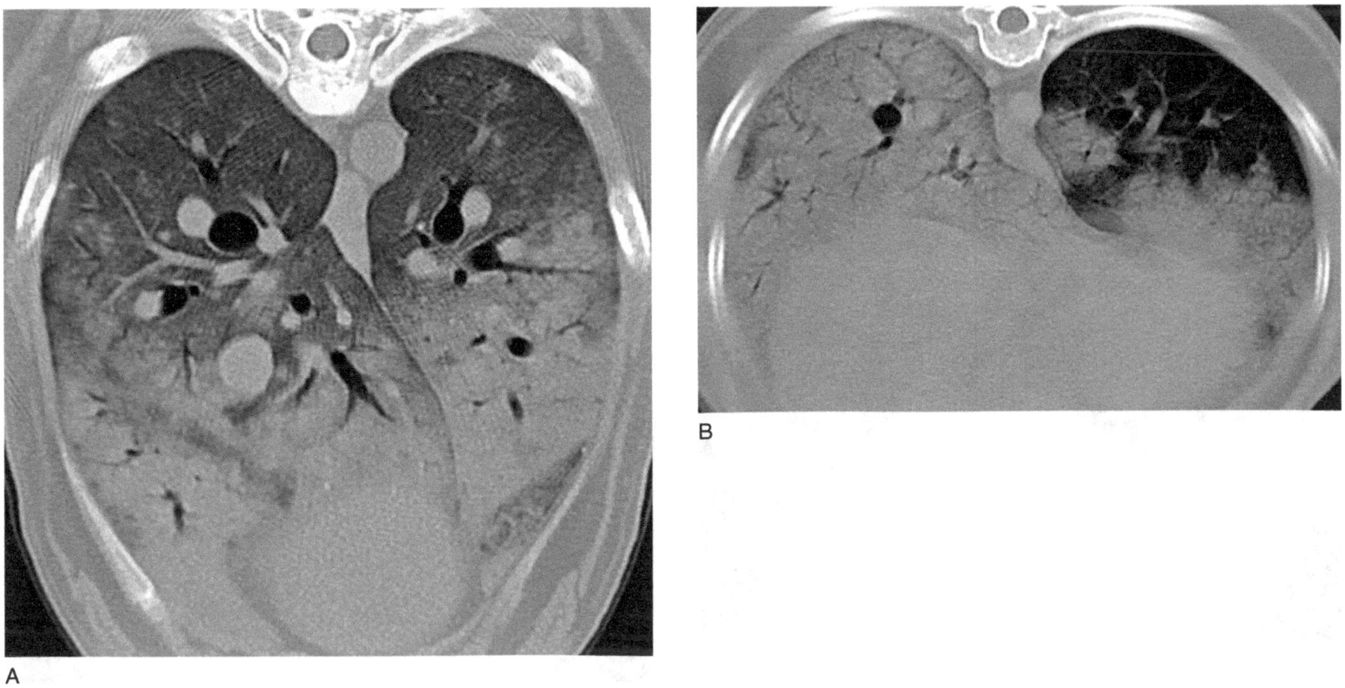

Figure 26.17 (A) Transverse CT image with non-cardiogenic pulmonary edema in a dog with suspected paraquat intoxication. There is marked diffuse alveolar airspace filling, particularly in caudoventral lung areas. (B) Marked edematous and inflammatory infiltrate in ventral lung areas in a dog with acute respiratory distress syndrome.

mimic pulmonary and mediastinal abscessation and cysts. Primary lung neoplasia has many features similar to granulomatous lung disease and both should be considered in the differential diagnosis.

CT features (Figures 26.18 and 26.19)

- Soft tissue mass, central mineralization more common in cats than in dogs.
- Gas and/or non-enhancing fluid content in larger masses.
- Multilobulated fluid-filled cysts in cystic adenocarcinoma.
- Deviation and compression of bronchovascular structures with pulmonary neoplasia.
- Bronchial wall and lumen invasion with bronchial neoplasia.
- Usually show strong enhancement and central necrotic non-enhancing regions.
- May have enlarged perihilar tracheobronchial lymph nodes.
- May have evidence of pulmonary or pleural metastatic disease.
- Feline bronchial neoplasia may be diffuse with areas of alveolar consolidation, bronchial thickening, interstitial infiltrates and mineralization.

Metastatic lung neoplasia

The lungs are the most common site for distant metastases in dogs and cats. Most metastases develop as soft tissue nodules in the pulmonary interstitium. Lymphangitic spread is less common and can lead to diffuse or alveolar septal metastases. Hemangiosarcoma metastases are often hemorrhagic and have less well-defined margins. In general, pulmonary metastases are less well-defined in cats than in dogs. Local metastatic spread can develop along bronchovascular structures. Both granulomatous disease and neoplasia can cause nodules that may be difficult to differentiate without further clinical information (*see* Box 26.2).

CT features (Figures 26.18 and 26.20)

- Soft tissue nodules within parenchyma.
- Distinct from vessels, which are tubular and therefore continuous on continuous slice images.
- May have feeding vessel.
- More indistinct margins in cats and with hemangiosarcoma.
- Variety of sizes with advanced primary neoplasia.
- Very rarely mineralize.

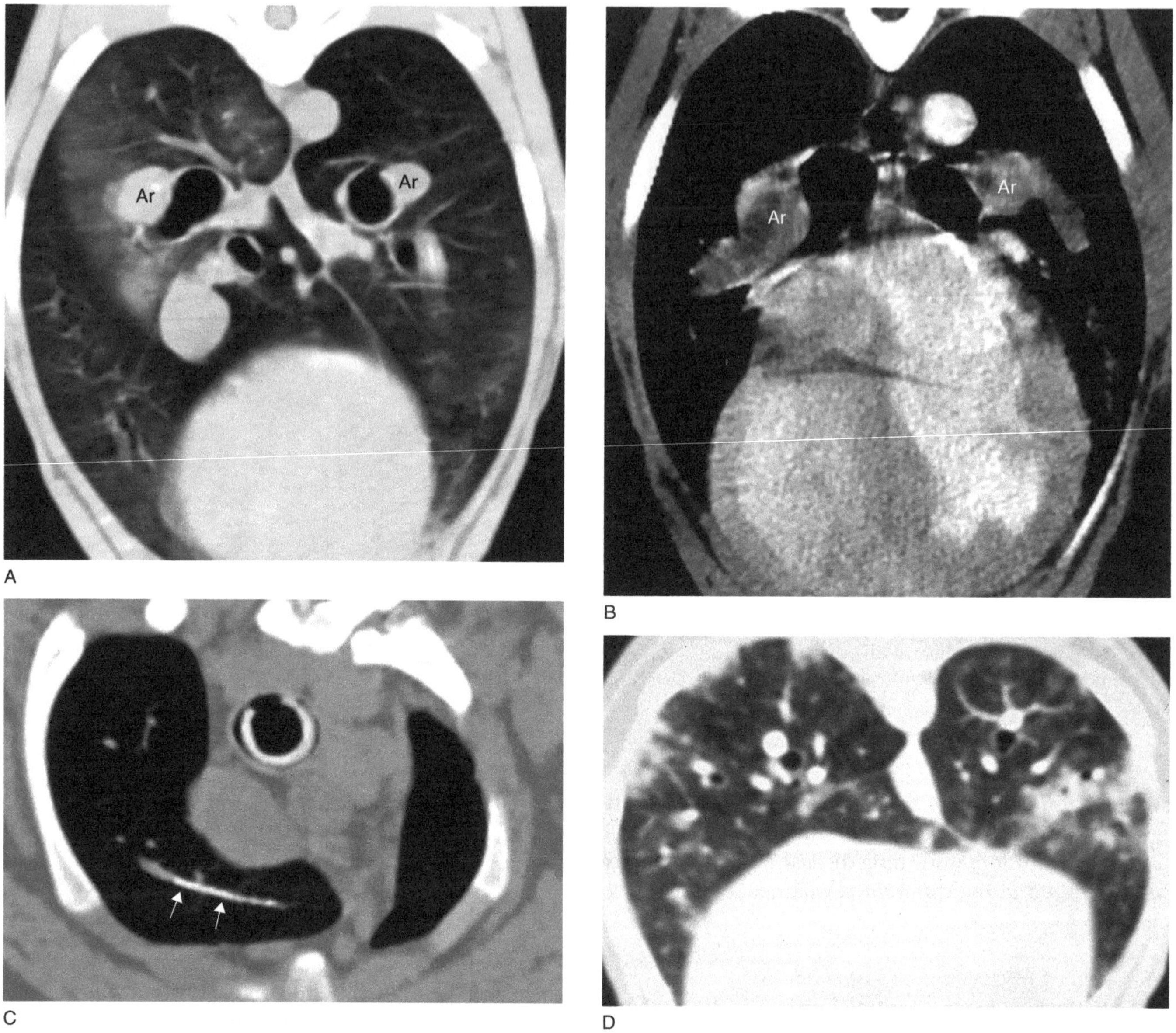

Figure 26.18 Transverse CT image with (A) enlarged pulmonary arteries (Ar), pleural-based lung opacification on survey CT and (B) luminal arterial filling defects (Ar) in pulmonary angiography CT in canine pulmonary thromboembolism. (C) Clinically silent dislodged catheter fragment (arrows) in the right cranial lung lobe artery of a dog (image courtesy of Tiziana Liuti). (D) Pulmonary carcinosis causing numerous small tumor emboli and subpleural lung infarcts.

Figure 26.19 Transverse CT images of primary lung tumors. (A) Large cavitated soft tissue mass (M) involving bronchi and lung tissue of the accessory lung lobe in feline bronchoalveolar carcinoma. (B) Right caudal lung lobe tumor (asterisk) in a cat with typical central gas and mineralization. (C) A slow-growing pulmonary carcinoma (asterisk) causing bronchial deviation (image courtesy of L. Jarrett). (D) Pulmonary adenocarcinoma in a dog (asterisk) with heterogeneous contrast enhancement indicative of necrosis. (E) Cystic bilobed adenocarcinoma of the accessory lobe in a dog mimicking a mediastinal cyst (asterisks). (F) Diffuse ground-glass opacity with canine lymphoma.

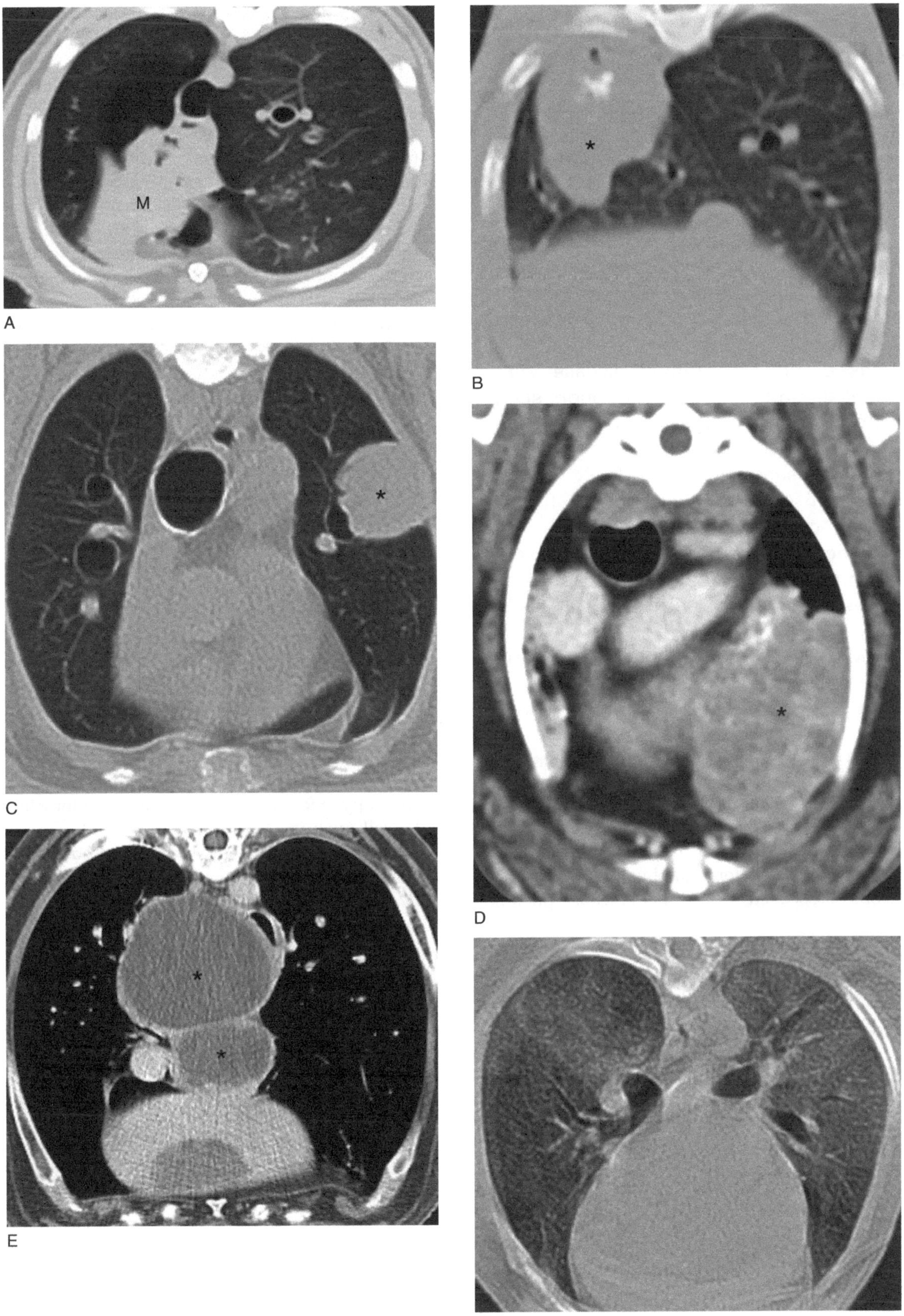
M
A
B
C
D
E
F

Box 26.2 Ditzels

This is a medical term to describe small lung nodules with unknown potential for malignancy in humans. Due to the high sensitivity of CT, very small nodules are also visible in dogs and cats, and not all of them are neoplastic. The following rules can be applied.

- 1–2 mm in size, very dense lesions throughout the lungs in dogs are most likely incidental pulmonary osteomas. Due to partial volume effect, densitometry is not reliable to confirm mineralization.
- In areas of endemic fungal disease with known likelihood for nodule formation, such as histoplasmosis, fungal origin should be considered more likely.
- Metastatic disease is more likely to be present with an identified primary tumor with high metastatic potential. The more chronic the primary tumor is, the more likely it is the patient would have advanced metastatic disease, with nodules of a range of sizes.
- A follow-up CT scan in 4–6 weeks should be considered.

Further reading

Au JJ, Weisman DL, Stefanacci JD and Palmisano MP (2006) Use of computed tomography for evaluation of lung lesions associated with spontaneous pneumothorax in dogs: 12 cases (1992–2002). *J Am Vet Assoc* **228**: 733–7.

Cannon MS, Wisner ER, Johnson LR and Kass PH (2009) Computed tomography bronchial lumen to pulmonary artery diameter ratio in dogs without clinical pulmonary disease. *Vet Radiol Ultrasound* **50**: 622–4.

Henninger W (2003) Use of computed tomography in the diseased feline thorax. *J Small Anim Pract* **44**: 56–64.

Nemanic S, London C and Wisner ER (2006) Comparison of thoracic radiographs and single breath-hold helical CT for detection of pulmonary nodules in dogs with metastatic neoplasia. *J Vet Intern Med* **20**: 508–15.

Johnson VS, Corcoran BM, Wotton PR, Schwarz T and Sullivan M (2005) Thoracic high-resolution computed tomography findings in dogs with canine idiopathic pulmonary fibrosis. *J Small Anim Pract* **46**: 381–8.

Johnson VS, Ramsey IK, Thompson H *et al.* (2004) Thoracic high-resolution computed tomography in the diagnosis of metastatic carcinosis. *J Small Anim Pract* **45**: 134–43.

Joly H, D'Anjou M, Alexander K and Beauchamp G (2009) Comparison of single-slice computed tomography protocols for detection of pulmonary nodules in dogs. *Vet Radiol Ultrasound* **50**: 279–84.

Morandi F, Mattoon JS, Lakritz J, Turk JR and Wisner ER (2003) Correlation of helical and incremental high-resolution thin-section computed tomographic imaging with histomorphometric quantitative evaluation of lungs in dogs. *Am J Vet Res* **64**: 935–44.

Schultz RM, Peters J and Zwingenberger A (2009) Radiography, computed tomography and virtual bronchoscopy in four dogs and two cats with lung lobe torsion. *J Small Anim Pract* **50**: 360–3.

Seiler G, Schwarz T, Vignoli M and Rodriguez D (2008) Computed tomographic features of lung lobe torsion. *Vet Radiol Ultrasound* **49**: 504–8.

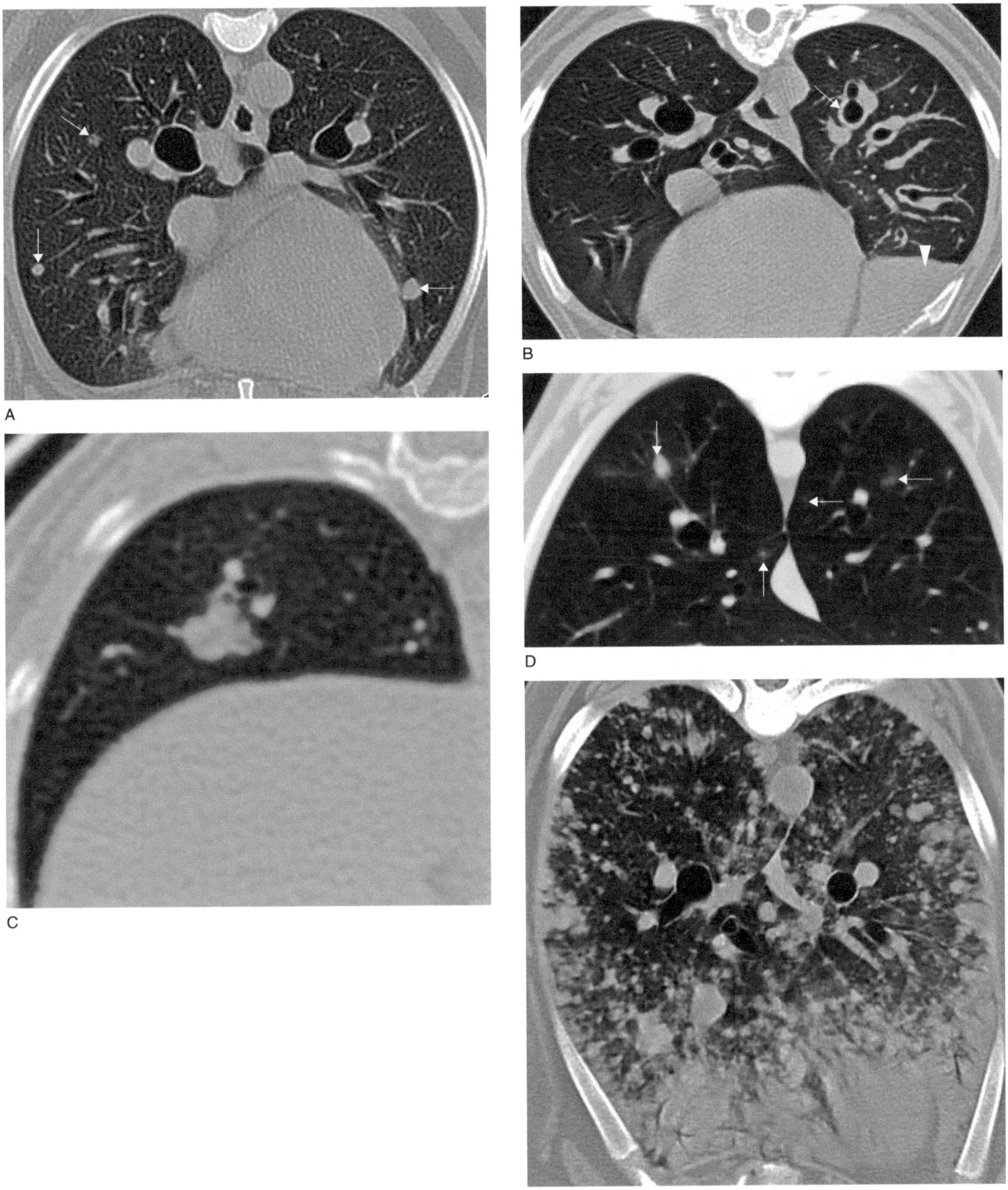

Figure 26.20 Transverse CT images of metastatic lung neoplasia. (A) Regularly shaped nodular metastases (arrows) in a range of sizes in a dog with anal gland carcinoma. The faint opacity of the dorsal node is due to volume averaging with aerated lung. Nodules can be differentiated from vessels that are tubulous and taper towards the lung periphery. (B) Direct metastases along bronchial walls (arrow) in the left caudal lobe in a dog with left cranial lobar consolidation (arrowhead) due to perihilar bronchial carcinoma. (C) Irregularly marginated lung metastasis typically seen in cats. (D) Poorly marginated lung metastases (arrows) in a canine anaplastic carcinoma. (E) Poorly marginated coalescing pulmonary metastases of a canine hemangiosarcoma due to hemorrhage and infarction.

CHAPTER TWENTY-SEVEN

Pleura

Wilfried Mai

Imaging Protocol

See Table 27.1.

CT: Anatomy

The pleural membrane is composed of a single layer of mesothelial cells that overlie a connective tissue layer containing blood vessels and lymphatics. There is a parietal pleura that covers the inner surface of the wall of the thorax (costal wall, diaphragm and mediastinum) and a visceral pleura that lines the lung surface and forms the interlobar fissures. The two layers of pleura (parietal and visceral) cannot be distinguished normally on CT. Because they are thin and oblique relative to the plane of the scan, the normal major fissures are also not usually visible on CT. In some patients though, just as on radiographs, normal fissures perpendicularly aligned to the scanning plane can be seen as thin lines of soft tissue attenuation.

There is a thin space between the two pleural layers called the pleural cavity. This cavity is a potential space that contains 2–3 ml of serous fluid, which acts a lubricant to minimize friction during respiration.

In planning for the CT, one must remember that the diaphragmatic pleura, the costodiaphragmatic and lumbodiaphragmatic pleural recesses extend well caudal to the lung bases and that scans caudal to the diaphragmatic dome must be obtained to evaluate these parts of the pleura completely.

In normal patients, a 1–1.5 mm thick opaque line is commonly seen at the periphery of the lung especially between adjacent rib segments: this stripe primarily represents the innermost intercostal muscle when present, combined with the two pleural layers and some extrapleural fat (Figure 27.1).

No significantly enhanced visibility of the pleura should be seen after contrast medium injection. If this is the case, then thickening of the pleura and primary or reactive pleural disease should be suspected.

The kernel frequency for pleural imaging should be in the medium range, and without additional edge enhancement to avoid rebound artifacts that can mimic pneumothorax and pleural thickening (see Figure 4.19D).

Disease Features

Pneumothorax

CT is usually not used to diagnose pneumothorax. However, it is frequently used in patients with spontaneous pneumothorax to rule out ruptured cavitary pulmonary lesions such as blebs or bullae as a cause of the pneumothorax (*see* Chapter 26).

CT features

- Free pleural air is easily recognized using lung window/level settings as a non-attenuating space between the parietal and visceral pleura accumulating in the highest (non-dependent) area of the pleural cavity (Figure 27.2).
- Non-ruptured pulmonary blebs or bullae appear as rounded regions of low pulmonary parenchymal density, with focal changes to the vascular pattern (disruption by pruning or distortion around the low-density region).
- Ruptured pulmonary bullae are very difficult to identify as their appearance is non-specific (focal area of alveolar consolidation).
- Imaging should be performed after thoracic drains have been placed to drain the pneumothorax and imaging should be performed under mild positive pressure ventilation to prevent pulmonary atelectasis. Even if a lesion has been localized previously and an assessment of the entire thorax is not needed, the scanning area should always include

Veterinary Computed Tomography, First Edition. Edited by Tobias Schwarz, Jimmy Saunders.

Table 27.1
CT imaging protocol (intravenous contrast study: standard protocol; *see* Chapter 5).

Series	Pre- and post-contrast
Decubitus	Ventral
Special positioning	Thoracic limbs extended cranially to avoid inclusion in field of view
Scan margins	Last pair of ribs ←→ Manubrium
Voltage (kVp)	120
Current (mAs)	Small/medium thorax:160; large thorax: 200*
Tube rotation time (s)	1
Slice width (mm)	Small thorax: 2; medium thorax: 3; large thorax: 5
Sequential slice interval (mm)	Small thorax: 4; medium thorax: 5; large thorax: 7
Kernel frequency	Medium
Collimator pitch	Small thorax: 2.0; medium thorax: 1.7; Large thorax: 1.4
Helical image reconstruction interval	Small thorax: 2; medium size thorax: 3; Large thorax: 5
Motion control	• Hyperventilate immediately prior to scan – apnea during scan • Alternatively use paralytic agent – constant infusion of 3 µg/kg/min of cisatricurium** Mechanical ventilation is required after CT scan for several minutes
Window level (HU)	Mediastinal: +40; lung: +700
Window width (HU)	Mediastinal: 400; lung: 1500

*Thorax: small <15 kg; medium 16–30 kg; large >30 kg body weight.
**Nimbex, cisatracurium bensylate 2 mg/ml, Abbott Laboratories, North Chicago, IL.

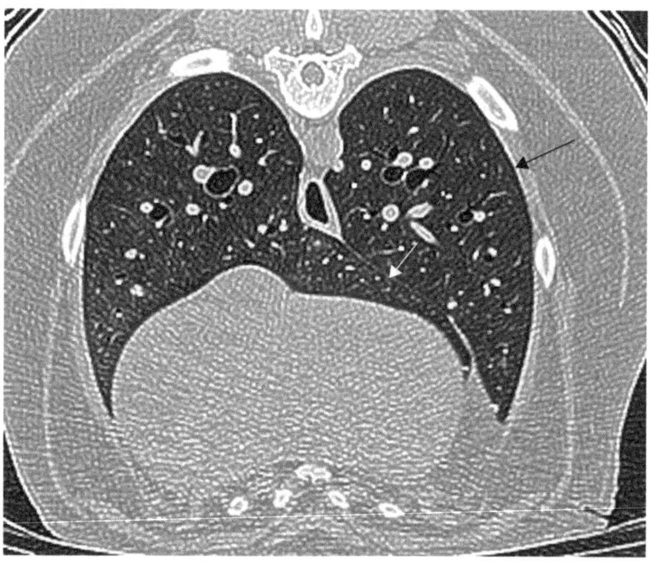

Figure 27.1 Transverse CT image of the thorax in a normal dog, high-resolution CT. A thin opaque line is seen at the periphery of the lung representing the summation of the innermost intercostal muscle combined with the two pleural layers and some extra-pleural fat (black arrow). The mediastinal pleura between the accessory and the left caudal lung lobe is also visible (white arrow).

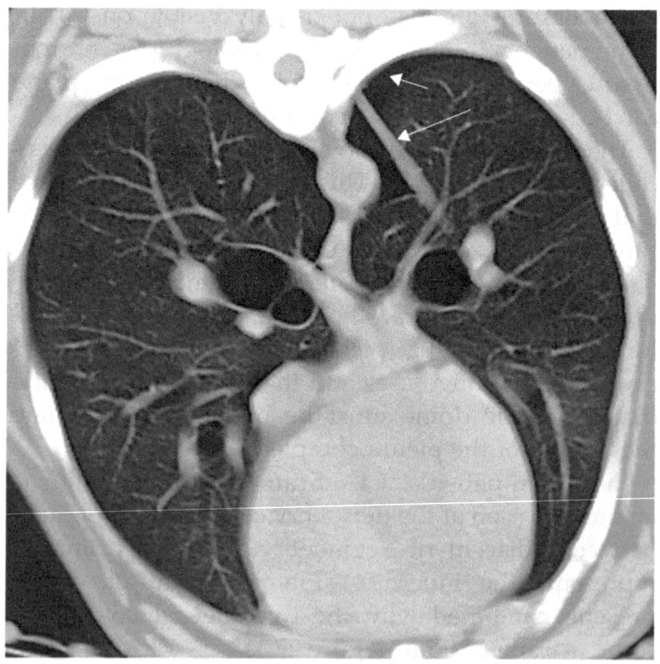

Figure 27.2 Migrating foreign body (long arrow) and spontaneous pneumothorax (short arrow) in a dog with chronic cough (image courtesy Dr Schultz and Dr Zwingenberger, University of California, Davis).

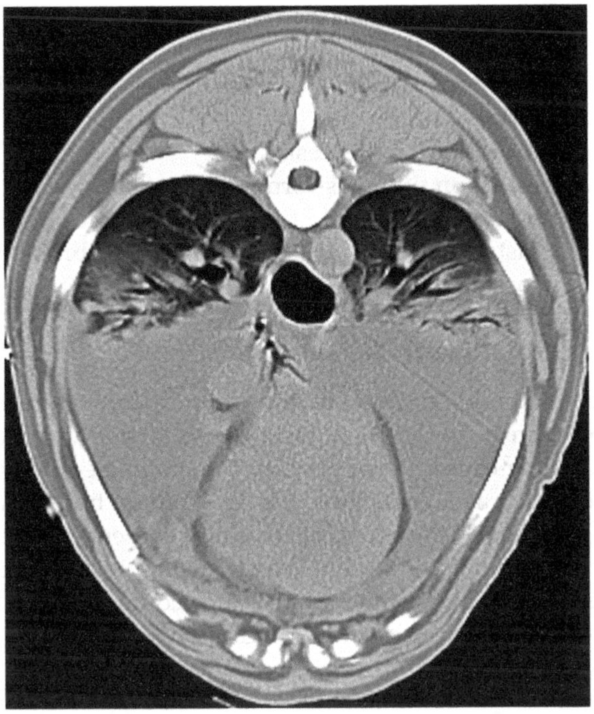

Figure 27.3 Free pleural effusion appearing crescentic and demonstrating gravitational shift in a dog.

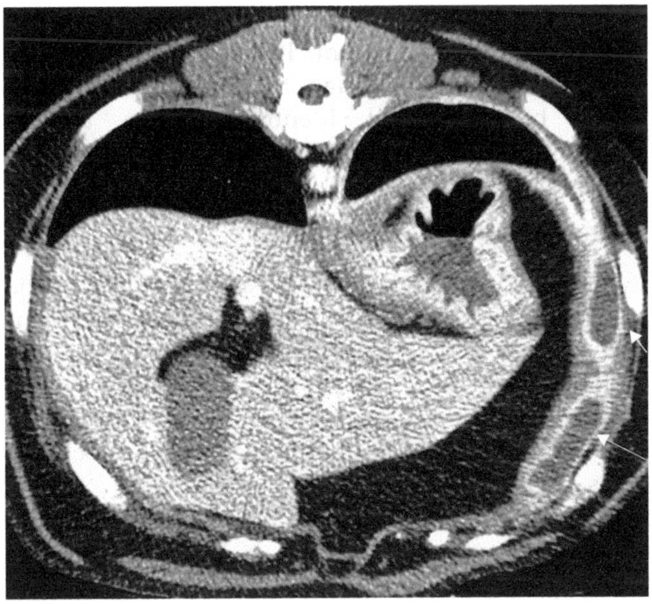

Figure 27.4 Post-contrast transverse CT in a dog with a pyothorax. Elliptic and lenticular effusion with pleural enhancement is seen (arrows) consistent with loculated effusion.

the highest point of the pleural cavity to identify the magnitude of the pneumothorax.
- Sensitivity of CT to identify ruptured bullae or small-sized intact bullae is relatively low.

Pleural effusion

General considerations

Pleural fluid can easily be recognized on thoracic CT, with most effusions having a density close to that of water.

CT numbers cannot be used to predict the nature of pleural effusion with the exception of hemothorax (see below). In addition, the presence of pleural thickening is suggestive of an exudate rather than a transudate.

On cross-sectional images, effusions can be crescentic, elliptical or lenticular in shape:

- Crescentic and dependent effusions are usually free fluid although in theory one should demonstrate that the effusion moves with patient movement to confirm this (unlikely to be done in practice) (Figure 27.3).
- Elliptical and lenticular effusions are more likely to represent loculated fluid (Figure 27.4).

Hemothorax

Hemothorax can result from trauma, or is the consequence of coagulation disorders or associated with an intrathoracic neoplasm.

CT features

- Hemorrhagic effusion on CT is usually dense (>50 HU) and may appear inhomogeneous, especially with the dependent regions having CT numbers higher than that of water.
- In some cases a 'fluid–fluid' interface may be seen ('hematocrit effect', due to the linear separation of cellular and liquid components of blood).

Chylothorax

Chylothorax is the accumulation of chyle within the pleural space, which leads to dyspnea. This manifests as a pleural disease, although it results from changes associated with the thoracic duct or its tributaries located within the mediastinum.

CT features

- CT lymphangiography can be performed after pre-surgical direct catheterization of a mesenteric lymphatic vessel or ultrasonographically guided injection of a mesenteric lymph node, using iodinated contrast medium. It has proven to be an efficient way to image the thoracic duct and its branches and identify leakage and/or lymphangiectasia-type changes.

Pyothorax (pleural empyema)

Pyothorax or pleural empyema is a purulent septic pleural effusion. CT can be useful in the management of pyothorax to determine the extent and distribution of lesions and look for possible causes. CT is also useful in patients refractory to traditional treatment with thoracic drains to identify loculated or pocketed areas of effusion.

CT features

- Pyogenic effusions are commonly unilateral or asymmetrical.
- Pleural thickening (especially parietal, less often visceral) is commonly seen on post-contrast series (Figure 27.5).
- A 'split-pleura' sign can be observed, when the thickened visceral and parietal pleural layers are split apart by and surround the empyema. This can also be seen in the costodiaphragmatic recesses of the pleural space due to fluid entrapment in the costophrenic reflection of the parietal pleura (Figure 27.4).
- Pockets of loculated effusion appear lenticular or elliptical in shape.
- Presence of air in the effusion is usually the result of:
  - recent thoracocentesis
  - infection with gas-forming bacteria
  - a bronchopleural fistula, which could for instance result from a migrating bronchial foreign body (see below).

Pleural foreign bodies

Pleural foreign bodies are not common and can result from direct penetration from external thoracic wall trauma or from chronic migration of an inhaled foreign body such as a grass awn. Inhaled foreign bodies can migrate along the bronchial tree and can end-up penetrating the visceral pleura to enter the pleural space. Lesions of pleuropneumonia and complications of pyothorax and/or pneumothorax can result from this migration.

CT features

- CT allows better characterization and localization of lesions induced by pulmonary migrating foreign body than radiographs.
- Common findings include:
  - focal interstitial to alveolar pulmonary opacities most commonly seen in one caudal lung lobe or the accessory lung lobe

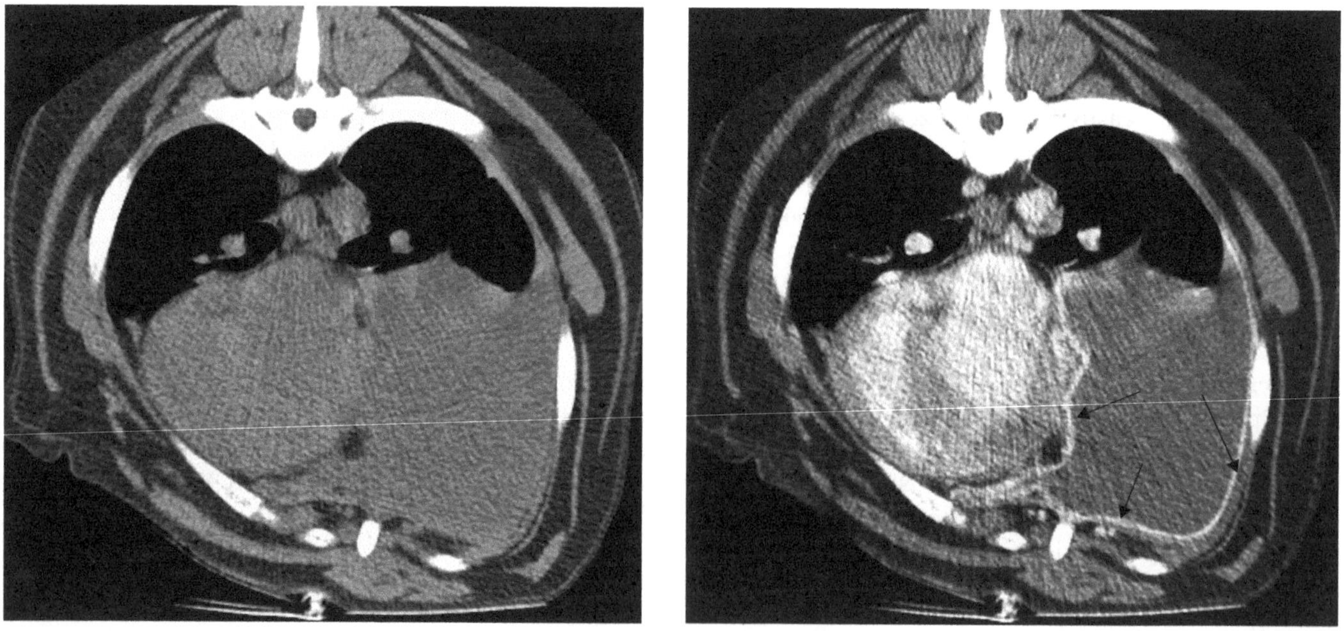

Figure 27.5 Pre- (left) and post- (right) transverse contrast CT in a dog with a pyothorax showing severe left-sided effusion causing mediastinal shift to the right as well as parietal pleural enhancement and thickening seen on the post-contrast image (arrows).

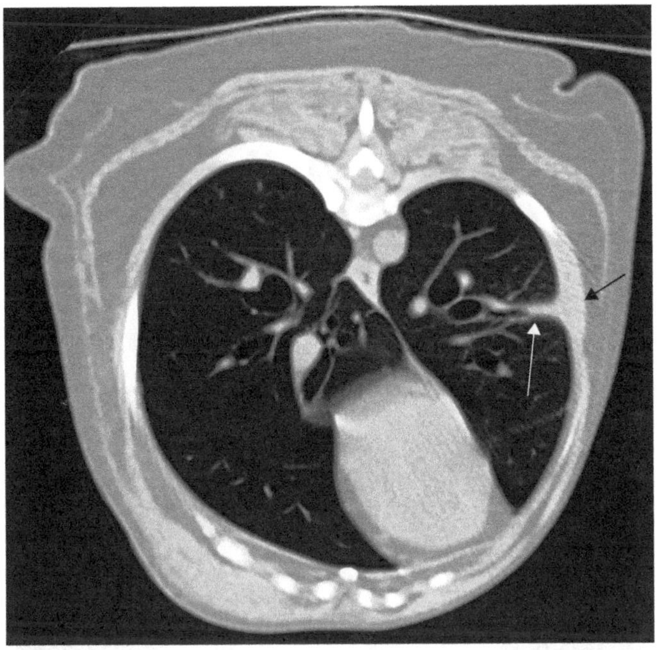

Figure 27.6 Post-contrast transverse CT in a poodle with a migrating grass awn. An enhancing fistula tract (white arrow) is seen in the left caudal lung lobe and there is focal thickening of the pleural at that level (black arrow) (image courtesy Dr Schultz and Dr Zwingenberger, University of California, Davis).

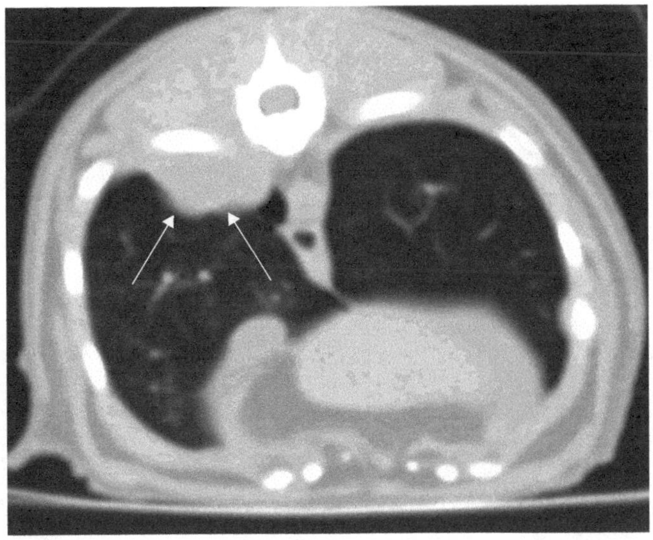

Figure 27.7 Siamese cat with a history of infiltrative thymoma that had been debulked surgically some months prior to this CT. A pleural mass is seen in the right caudal thorax appearing as a soft tissue-attenuating lesion that is broad-based towards the parietal pleura and displaces the lung ventrally. This was a pleural metastasis of the thymoma.

- pleural effusion
- focal pleural thickening and enhancement (Figure 27.6)
- pneumothorax (Figure 27.2)
- foreign body contrast enhancing tract (Figure 27.6)
- visualization of the foreign body itself (Figure 27.2).

Pleural masses

Pleural masses can be present as a manifestation of pleural spread of cancerous lesions (pleural carcinomatosis) or as a manifestation of primary neoplastic infiltrate, in particular mesothelioma. The differential diagnosis will rely on the history (prior knowledge of a primary distant neoplasm) and/or on CT findings (e.g. concomitant finding of pleural lesions and a mass lesion in the lung).

Mesothelioma is a highly aggressive neoplasm with an extremely poor prognosis. It is characterized morphologically by gross pleural thickening which can be 'en plaque', nodular or create mass lesions. The tumor usually spreads by local infiltration of the pleural.

CT features

- CT is very useful in confirming the presence and extent of pleural masses: irregular or nodular thickening of the pleura is identified (Figure 27.7).
- Post-contrast series are useful to distinguish the neoplastic tissue from associated fluid collections or strands of fibrin and hemorrhage (Figure 27.8).
- In cases of mesothelioma, pleural effusion might be the only recognizable finding. All portions of the pleura can be affected, including mediastinal pleural masses. Concurrent pericardial masses or pericardial effusion is common.

Further reading

Au JJ, Weisman DL, Stefanacci JD and Palmisano MP (2006) Use of computed tomography for evaluation of lung lesions associated with spontaneous pneumothorax in dogs: 12 cases (1999–2002). *J Am Vet Med Assoc* **228**: 733–7.

Burk RL (2009) Computed tomography of thoracic disease in dogs. *J Am Vet Med Assoc* **199**: 617–21.

De Rycke LM, Gielen IM, Simoens PJ and van Bree H. Computed tomography and cross-sectional anatomy of

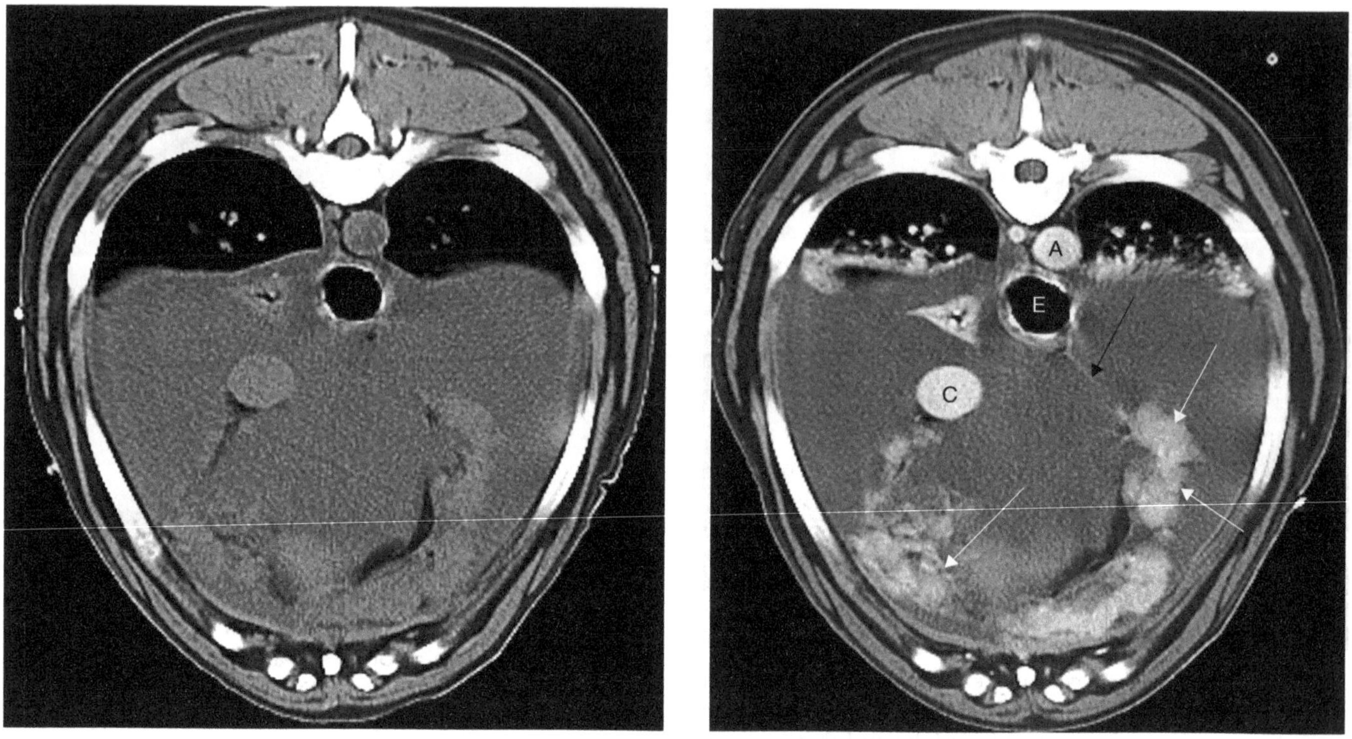

Figure 27.8 Pre- (left) and post- (right) contrast enhanced transverse CT image in a dog with a confirmed pleural mesothelioma. Irregularly marginated and strongly enhancing pleural lesions (white arrows) are identified attached to the caudoventral mediastinal reflection (black arrow) and the diaphragmatic parietal pleura. A = aorta, C = caudal vena cava, E = esophagus (image courtesy Dr Valdes-Martinez, Colorado State University).

the thorax in clinically normal dogs. *Am J Vet Res* **66**: 512–24.

Esterline ML, Radlinsky MG, Biller DS, Mason DE, Roush JK and Cash WC (2005) Comparison of radiographic and computed tomography lymphangiography for identification of the canine thoracic duct. *Vet Radiol Ultrasound* **46**: 391–5.

Henninger W (2003) Use of computed tomography in the diseased feline thorax. *J Small Anim Pract* **44**: 56-64.

Swinbourne F, Baines EA, Baines SJ and Halfacree ZJ (2011) Computed tomographic findings in canine pyothorax and correlation with findings at exploratory thoracotomy. *J Small Anim Pract* **5**: 203–8.

Zwingenberger A and Schultz RM (2008) Radiographic, computed tomographic, and ultrasonographic findings with migrating intrathoracic grass awns in dogs and cats. *Vet Radiol Ultrasound* **49**: 249–55.

CHAPTER TWENTY-EIGHT

Thoracic Boundaries

Jimmy Saunders, Massimo Vignoli and Ingrid Gielen

Imaging Protocol

Similar to pleura; *see* Chapter 27.

CT: Anatomy and Normal Variants

The boundaries of the thoracic cavity consist of the thoracic skeleton (vertebral column, ribs, sternum), the cranial and caudal thoracic apertures, and the covering soft tissue structures (thoracic, pectoral, spinal and other musculature, subcutaneous fat and skin).

The thoracic skeleton consists of 13 thoracic vertebrae, which articulate cranially with a corresponding rib pair and eight sternebrae. The first sternebra is called the manubrium and the last one the xiphoid process (Figure 28.1). The first nine ribs articulate with the sternum through the costal cartilages. The cranial thoracic aperture, also called thoracic inlet (Figures 28.2 and 28.3), is a small passage for the trachea, esophagus, muscles, vessels and nerves. The deep fascia as well as pectoral, scalenius and longus colli muscles enclose it. The diaphragm is a dome-shaped musculotendinous organ that attaches to the costal arch and covers the caudal thoracic aperture (Figure 28.4). It develops from six embryogenic segments into two muscular masses, the crura diaphragmatica and a central collagenous tendon. The normal adult diaphragm has three openings: the dorsal aortic hiatus (for the aorta, azygos vein and thoracic duct), the central esophageal hiatus (for the esophagus) and the dextroventral caval foramen (for the caudal vena cava). The soft tissue mantle of the rib cage should normally be thin and even.

Feline anatomical specificities

Dogs have a curved sternum, which is square in cross-section, while cats have a cylindrical straight sternum with a flat xiphoid process. Malposition of xiphoid process in cats is usually not traumatic. Vertebral body shape in cats is more cylindrical than in dogs. Vertebral arrangement is physiologically more flexible in cats (allowing bending of back).

Disease Features

Malformation/Developmental

Congenital abnormalities of the thoracic skeleton are relatively common, particularly in dogs, and are most often incidental. Vertebral, costal and sternal abnormalities are often combined and should be assessed in conjunction.

Spinal abnormalities

See Chapter 22.

Rib cage abnormalities: chondrodysplasias

Abnormal cartilage development may cause proportionate (all bones affected) or disproportionate dwarfism (affecting primarily facial bones and/or appendicular skeleton). These features are often inherited and selectively bred, such as disproportionate dwarfism in dachshunds and basset hounds (unusual 'cottage loaf' thorax conformation).

Veterinary Computed Tomography, First Edition. Edited by Tobias Schwarz, Jimmy Saunders.

Congenital hypothyroidism is a disproportionate dwarfism caused by arrested thyroid activity.

Mucopolysaccharidosis is a group of rare genetic connective tissue disorders in dogs and cats with generalized skeletal deformities.

CT features

- Chondrodystrophic breed chest conformation: inward deviation of ventral rib component (Figure 28.5A).
- Congenital hypothyroidism: delayed physeal closure, shortened, often kyphotic vertebrae.

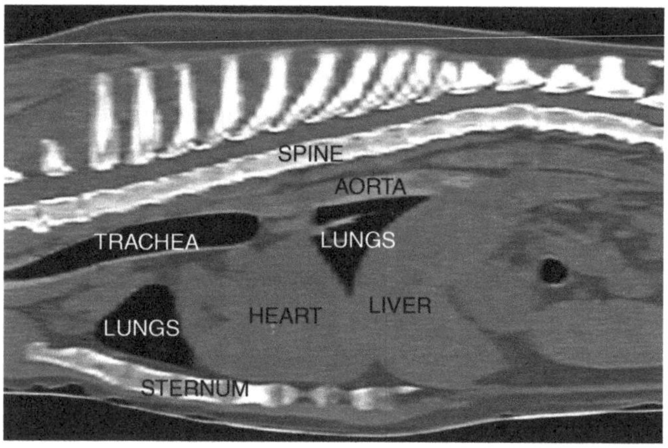

Figure 28.1 Sagittally reconstructed CT image shows the main thoracic structures.

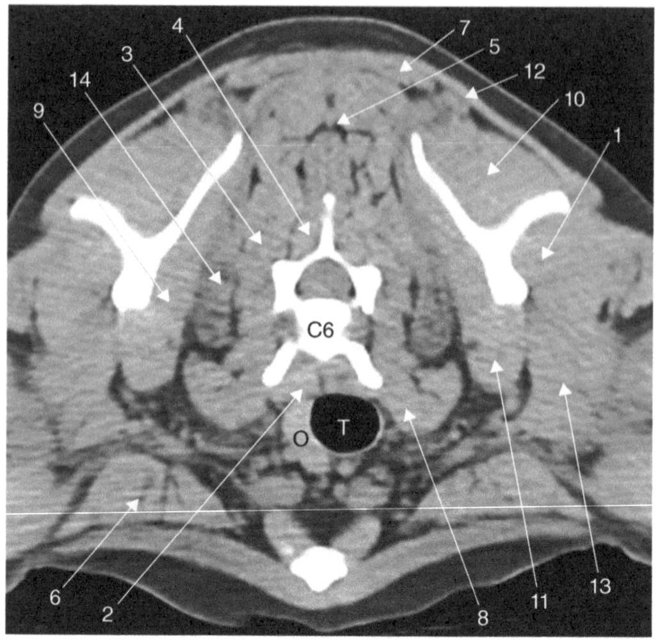

Figure 28.2 Transverse CT image at the thoracic inlet. 1 = infraspinatus m.; 2 = long m. of the neck; 3 = longissimus m.; 4 = multifidus m.; 5 = nuchal ligament; 6 = pectoralis m.; 7 = rhomboid m.; 8 = scalenus m.; 9 = subscapular m.; 10 = supraspinatus m.; 11 = teres major m.; 12 = trapezius m.; 13 = triceps (long head) brachii m.; 14 = ventral serrate m.; C6 = sixth cervical vertebra; O = esophagus; T = trachea.

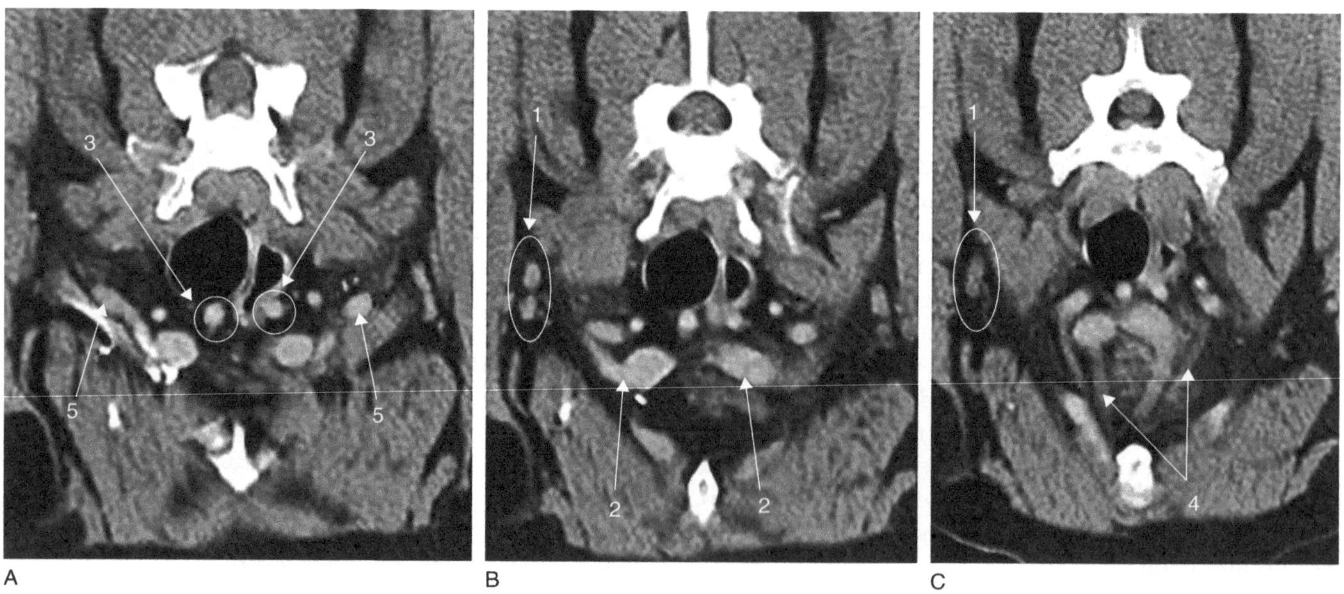

Figure 28.3 Transverse CT image of the vascular structures and lymph nodes at the thoracic inlet. 1 = axillary lymph node (fat); 2 = confluence of the axillary veins into the brachiocephalic veins; 3 = common carotid arteries; 4 = internal thoracic vein and artery; 5 = origin of the axillary arteries.

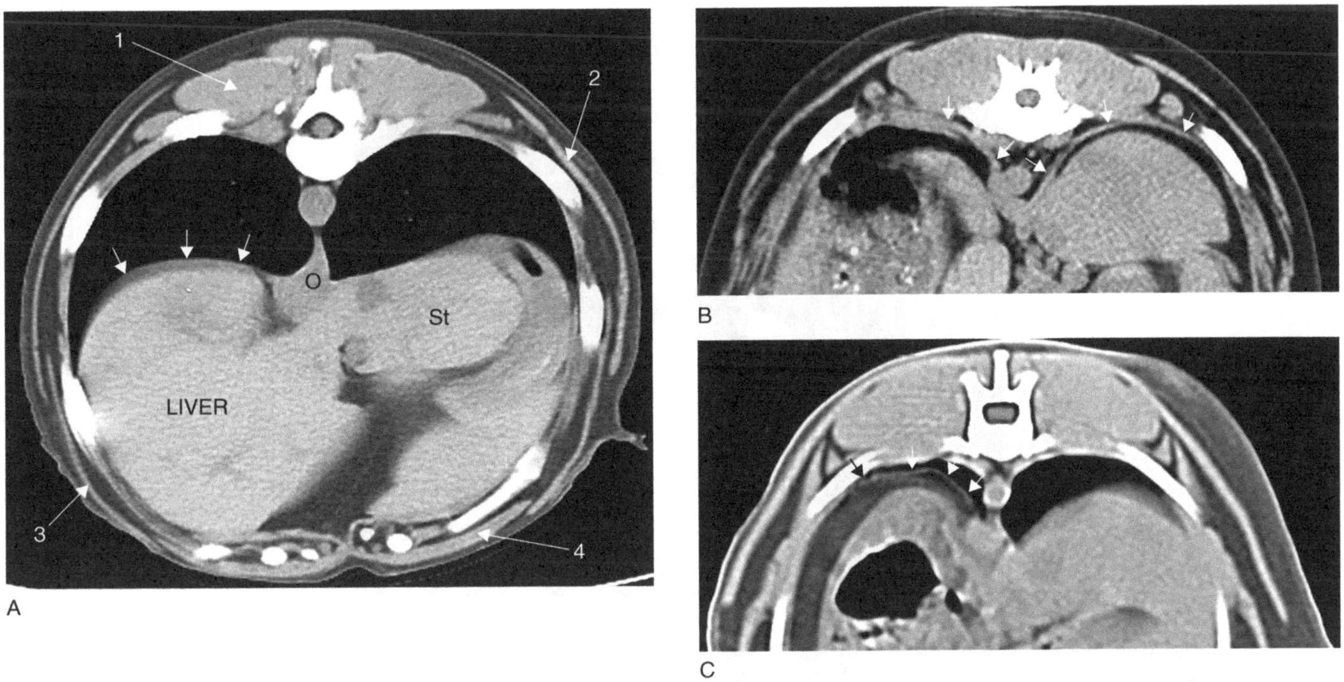

Figure 28.4 (A) Transverse CT image at the level of the caudal thorax (diaphragm – arrows). 1 = juxta-vertebral m.; 2 = latissimus dorsi m.; 3 = oblique m.; 4 = rectus abdominis m. O = esophagus; St = stomach. (B,C) Transverse CT image shows the diaphragm (arrows).

- Mucopolysaccharidosis: oar-shaped ribs, endplate sclerosis, widened and fused vertebrae, degenerative joint disease and spondylosis, often *Pectus excavatum* (see below) (Figures 28.5B and 28.5C).

Sternal abnormalities

A variation in the size and number of sternebrae, and in the shape of the manubrium and xiphoid process is commonly seen and is usually incidental. Sternal dysraphism is the failure of the left and right cartilaginous sternal precursors to fuse. It leads to a ventral defect that is closed by the thoracic fascia and pleura only. In the absence of diaphragmatic defects, sternal dysraphism has no adverse respiratory or circulatory consequences. Pectus excavatum (funnel chest) is a congenital or developmental abnormality with variable decrease in the thoracic dorsoventral diameter due to inward deviation of the sternum. It can affect normal respiratory physiology in severe cases.

CT features

- Abnormal number and shape of sternebrae is easily recognizable.
- Ventrally deviated xiphoid process in cats.
- Sternal dysraphism: split sternum or xiphoid process (Figure 28.6A).
- Pectus excavatum (Figure 28.6B):
  - inward deviation of the sternum into the thoracic cavity
  - decrease in thoracic dorsoventral diameter.

Diaphragmatic abnormalities

Diaphragmatic hernia

Diaphragmatic hernias are congenital anomalies due to agenesis of a portion of the diaphragm or lack of fusion between the parts of the primitive diaphragm. They are usually found in young animals with no history of trauma. In contrast to diaphragmatic ruptures, the prolapsed abdominal organs are contained within a pleural (pleuroperitoneal hernia) or pericardial (peritoneopericardial hernia) hernial sac.

A hiatal hernia corresponds to herniation of any abdominal organ through the esophageal hiatus. It is most often congenital in origin, but can be acquired following repair of chronic diaphragmatic rupture, traumatic event, esophageal/upper respiratory tract pathologies or neuromuscular disorders. Three main

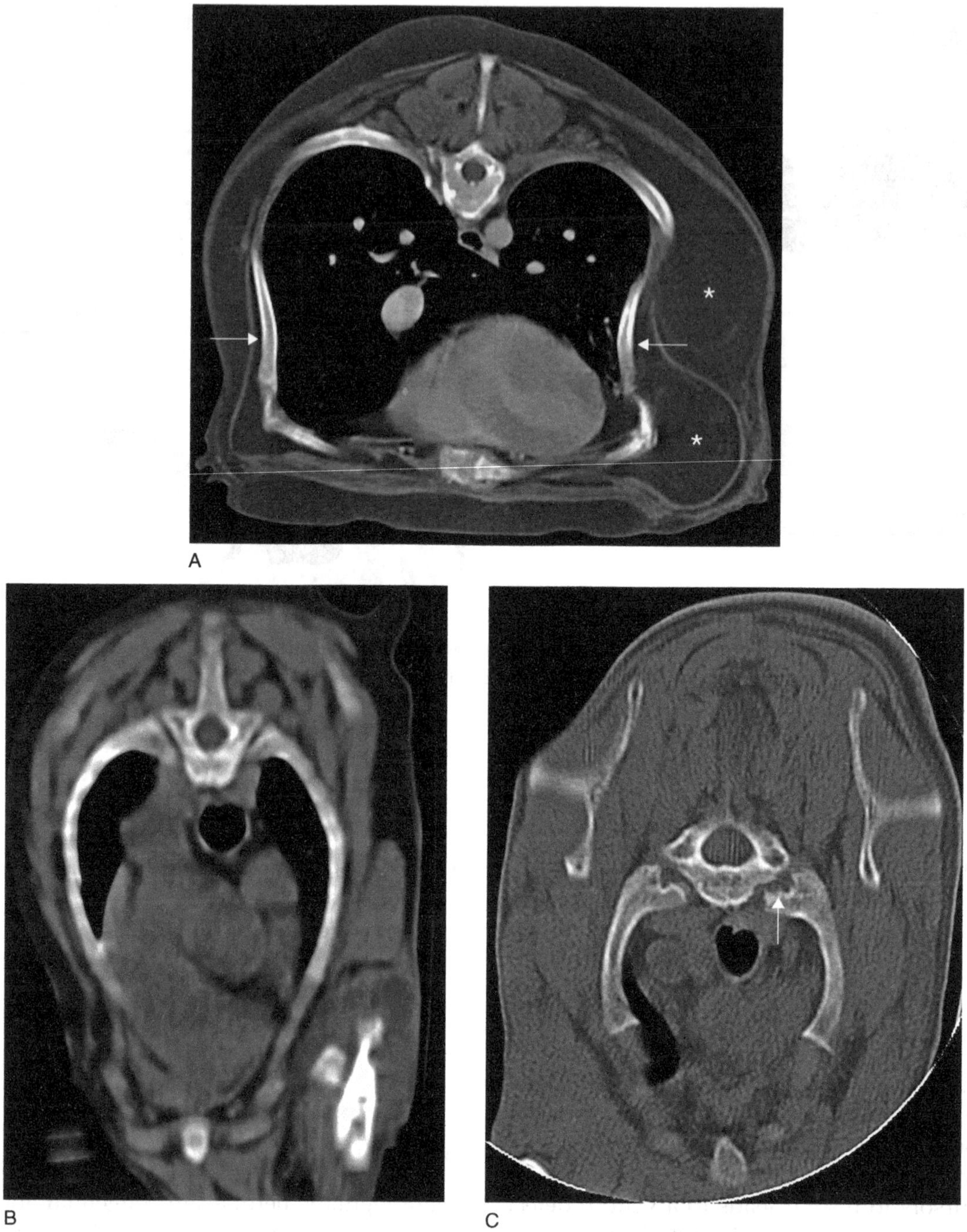

Figure 28.5 Two dogs with rib cage abnormalities. (A) Transverse CT image of a normal basset hound shows inward rib deviation (arrows). A lipoma is also visible (asterisks). (B,C) Transverse CT images of dogs with mucopolysaccharidosis show deformation of the rib cage ('oar-shaped' ribs) and small degenerative changes (arrow).

types of hiatal hernia are recognized in animals: short-esophagus hiatal hernia, sliding hiatal hernia and paraesophageal hiatal hernia. Chinese Shar-Pei dogs are predisposed for hiatal hernias.

CT features

- Hiatal hernia (Figure 28.7):
  - stomach visible within the thoracal esophagus
  - thickened wall of the esophagus, mainly dorsal
  - gas may be present in the esophagus and surround the stomach.

Trauma

Spinal fractures

See Chapter 22.

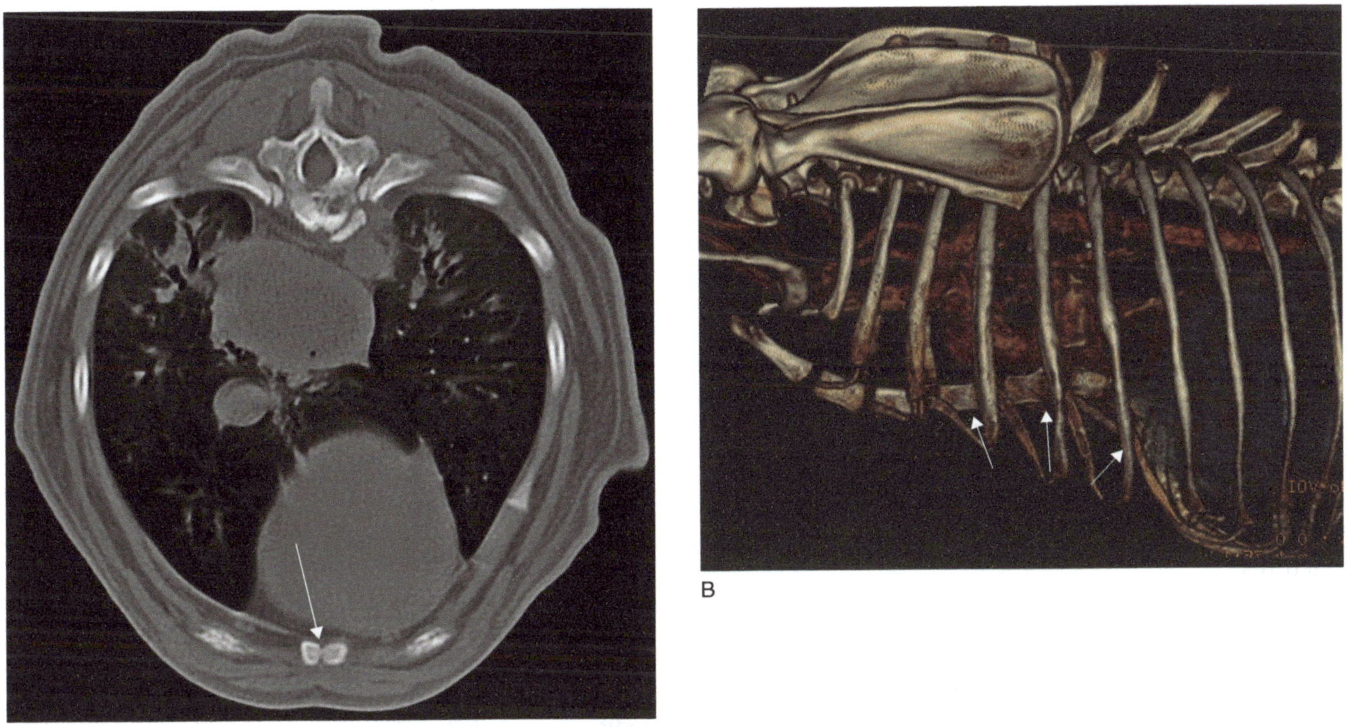

A B

Figure 28.6 CT of congenital abnormalities. (A) Transverse CT image of a dog with spinal dysraphism shows a split xiphoid process (arrow). Additional findings are a fluid-dilated esophagus, dorsal lung hypostasis and vertebral bone reaction. (B) Volume rendering three-dimensionally reconstructed CT image viewed from the left side of a dog with pectus excavatum showing inward deviation of the sternum into the thoracic cavity with a decreased dorsoventral thoracic diameter (arrows).

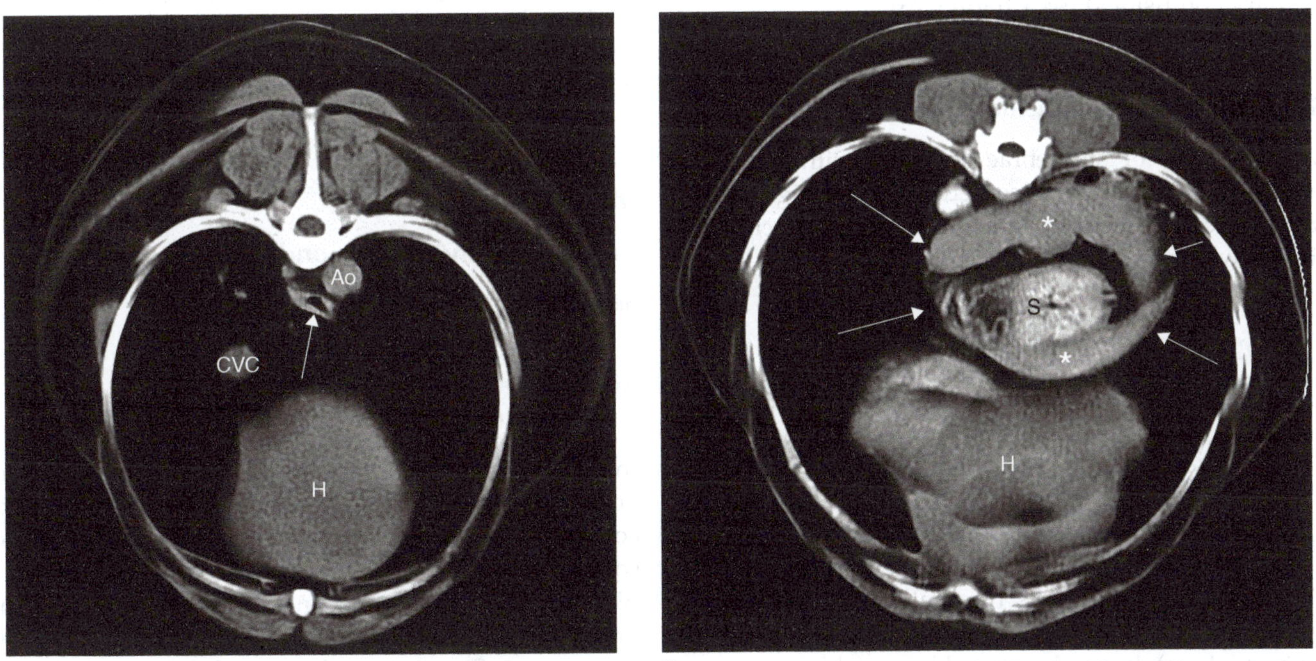

A B

Figure 28.7 Adult dog with a hiatal hernia. (A) Transverse CT image shows the esophagus being slightly dilated by gas (arrow). (B) Post-contrast transverse CT image shows the hyperdense stomach (S) within a dilated esophagus (arrows). The wall of the esophagus is thickened (asterisks) and some gas is visible between the stomach and the dorsal wall of the esophagus. Ao = aorta; CVC = caudal vena cava; H = heart.

Rib fractures

Most rib fractures are traumatic in origin, although pathologic or stress fractures are not uncommon. Traumatic rib fractures may be transverse, oblique or segmental, and are often multiple and sequential. They are currently associated with displaced fragments that can cause lung trauma and penetrating injuries, open or closed pneumothorax. Possible underlying diseases of pathologic or stress fractures are osteopenic (chronic feline renal disease or other causes of hyperparathyroidism), osteolytic (rib neoplasia) or respiratory conditions inducing repeated stress on costal muscle attachments (feline asthma, chronic canine bronchial disease or lobar emphysema). Due to the anatomical orientation of the ribs, CT is not the most appropriate modality for demonstration of rib fractures.

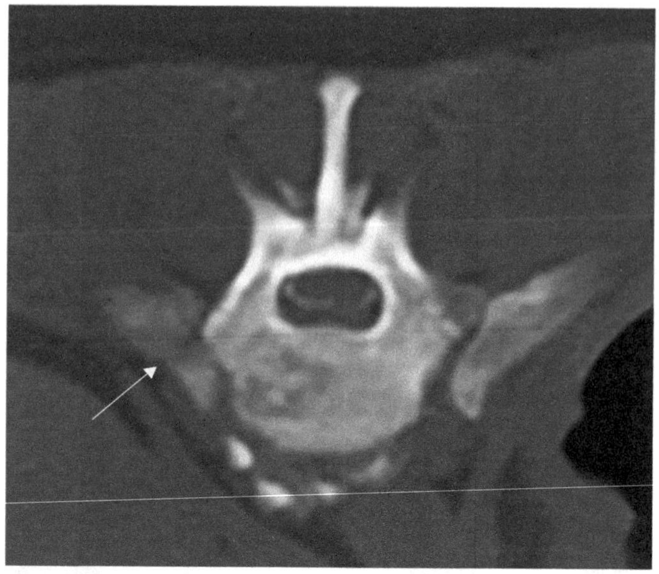

Figure 28.8 Transverse CT image of an adult dog with a rib fracture involving the proximal insertion of the rib (arrow). New bone formation associated with spondylosis deformans is visible at the ventral aspect of the vertebral body.

CT features (Figure 28.8)

- Malalignment altered direction, abnormal spacing) of the fractured rib(s), usually obvious.
- Bone fragments:
  - sharp fracture margins with recent trauma
  - unsharp fracture margins suggest a pathological fracture.
- Adjacent soft tissue swelling.
- Associated lung lesions (pneumothorax, pulmonary contusions) (*see* Chapter 26).

Sternal fracture and dislocation

Malalignment of sternebrae, with or without prior trauma, is frequently observed and is insignificant unless accompanied by intra- and extrathoracic soft tissue swelling or clinical signs.

CT features

- Usually obvious dislocation.
- Malposition of xiphoid process in cats is usually not traumatic.

Diaphragmatic rupture

Diaphragmatic rupture is traumatic in origin (often misnamed 'acquired diaphragmatic hernia' as there is no hernial sac). It may be caused by a sudden increase in intra-abdominal pressure while the glottis is open. The side, size and shape of the rupture are variable. The liver, stomach, small intestines and omentum are the organs that most frequently prolapse.

CT features (Figure 29.9)

- Presence of a diaphragmatic defect.
- Discontinuity of the (hemi)diaphragm with intrathoracic abdominal organs and/or peritoneal fat – best seen on multiplanar reconstructions.
- Displacement of normal thoracic structures.
- Pleural fluid.

Infection

Spondylitis and discospondylitis

See Chapter 22.

Ribs, thoracic wall, sternal osteomyelitis and abscessation

Infections of the thoracic wall result from foreign bodies, lacerations, bite wounds or surgical wound contamination. They are often very painful, even more so than neoplasia. Migrating foreign bodies such as plant material (grass awns) may penetrate via the skin, or wooden skewers via the gastrointestinal tract. They can cause inflammatory disease, abscess/granuloma, fistulous tract in the thoracic wall region or even lead to pleural effusion. Fungal or parasitic (hepatozoonosis) osteomyelitis and cellulitis may occur in endemic areas.

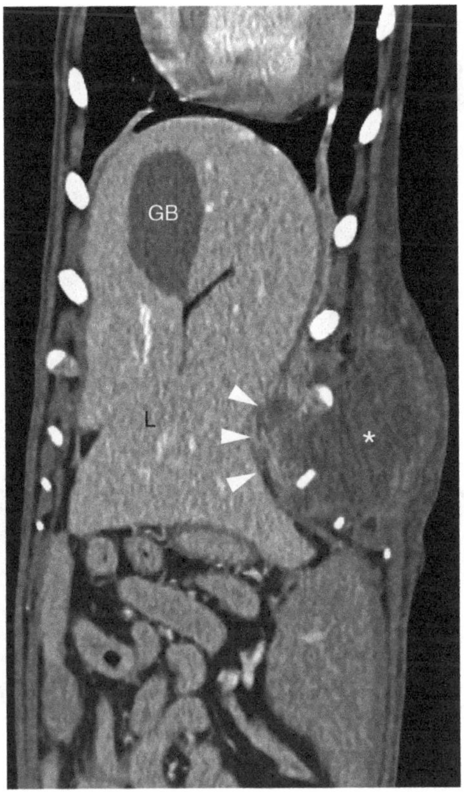

Figure 28.9 Adult dog with a chest wall abscessation secondary to a grass awn penetration. Post-contrast dorsally reconstructed CT image shows a left-sided mass (asterisk) displacing the ribs medially. The tenth rib is malaligned and the space between the tenth and eleventh ribs is increased. The mass comes in close contact with the liver and there is loss of detail of the liver margin (arrowheads). GB = gallbladder; L = liver.

Chest wall abscessation is uncommon, but may be a sequel to trauma (bites, penetrating foreign body) or a complication of midline thoracotomy (sternotomy). An intermittently discharging sinus may be present.

CT features (Figure 28.9)

- Periosteal reaction around affected rib/sternebra.
- Osteolysis or sclerosis.
- Soft tissue swelling – lucent gas tracts may be seen with a discharging sinus.
- Pleural thickening and effusion.
- Displacement, even invasion, of adjacent thoracic or abdominal organs.

Neoplasia

Spinal neoplasia

See Chapter 22.

Rib tumors

Primary rib tumors are uncommon, with osteosarcoma and chondrosarcoma most frequently seen, whereas fibrosarcoma, hemangiosarcoma and benign neoplasms (osteoma, chondroma, osteochondromatosis) are only rarely seen. Pleural neoplasia (mesothelioma) can metastasize by contiguity to the ribs locally and be difficult to differentiate from other types of neoplasia. Multiple myeloma frequently affects ribs along with vertebrae and other bones. Primary bone lymphoma or bone involvement in multicentric lymphoma is rare but may affect young animals.

CT features (Figures 28.10–28.12)

- Osteolysis, mostly extended but can be subtle.
- Irregular to sunburst periosteal reaction and amorphous new bone.
- Soft tissue component may induce inwards displacement or involve pleural and pulmonary structures and involve the thoracic wall.
- Displacement or involvement of adjacent ribs.
- Fractures with unsharp margins (pathologic fracture).
- *Primary rib tumors*: monostotic, preferentially distal third of rib, displaced adjacent ribs which are otherwise normal, often very large intrathoracic component.
- *Metastatic rib tumors*: often polyostotic, but randomly oriented, preferentially middle and proximal third of rib, often small at time of detection.
- *Soft tissue tumor invading ribs*: soft tissue mass with variable external component, osteolysis, periosteal reaction, fractures at multiple adjacent ribs; any part of rib can be affected.
- *Mesothelioma*: abundant pleural effusion, no external chest wall mass, periosteal reaction on several ribs possible.
- *Multiple myeloma*: multiple punctate lucencies without periosteal reaction or sclerosis.
- *Lymphoma*: irregular periosteal reaction and punctate or diffuse lysis, metaphyseal area in bone lymphoma.
- Osteochondromatosis (Figure 28.13); *see* Chapter 22.
- Aneurysmal bone cyst: blow-out appearance, marked cortical thinning with minimal bone formation. May affect the diaphysis or the metaphysis.

Thoracic wall tumors

The most common soft tissue mass of the thoracic wall is fibrosarcoma, which is particularly common in cats.

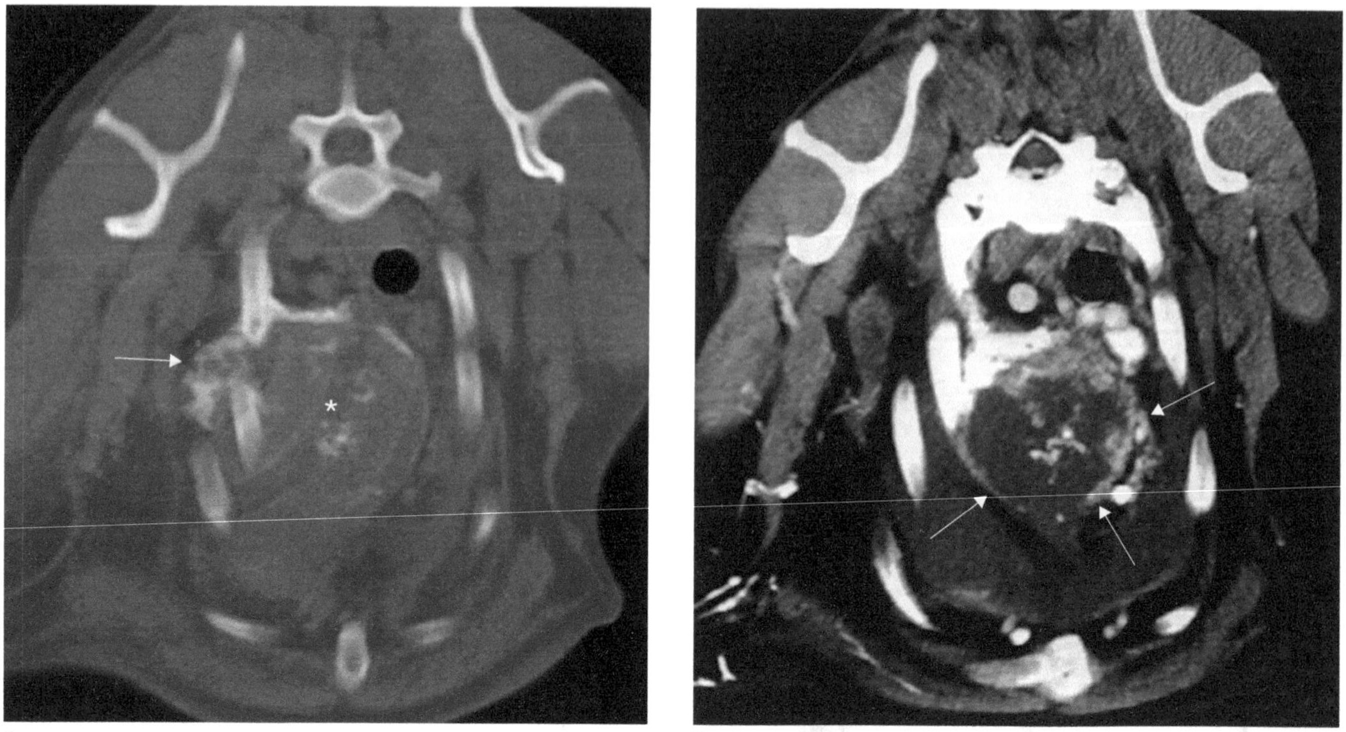

A B

Figure 28.10 Adult dog with first rib chondroma. (A) Transverse CT image shows a round, well-delineated calcified mass (asterisk) in continuity with the first left rib (arrow). There is osteolysis of the first rib which is in close contact with the second rib (arrow). (B) Post-contrast transverse CT image shows peripheral contrast enhancement of the mass (arrows) which invades the thoracic cavity compressing and displacing the cranial mediastinal structures to the right side.

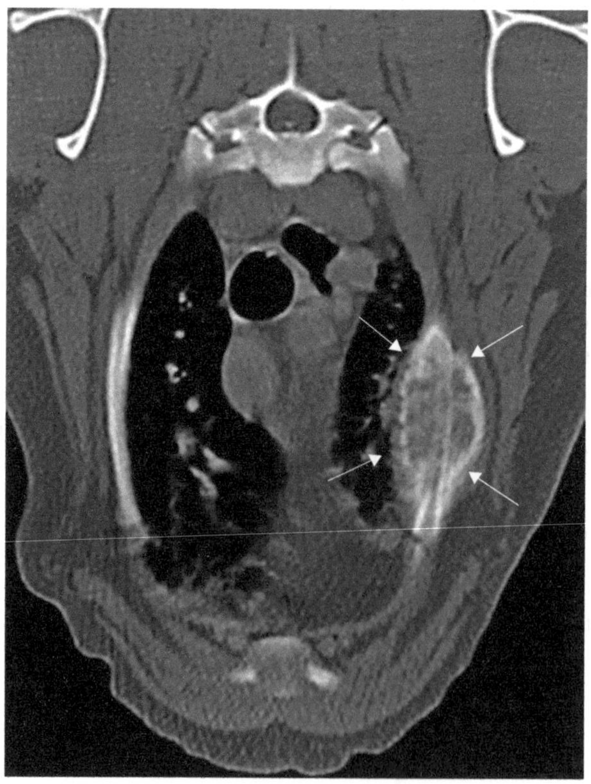

Figure 28.11 Adult dog with a primary rib tumor (osteoblastic chondrosarcoma). Transverse CT image shows an expansile bone mass centered on the mid-diaphysis of a rib (arrows). In the middle of the mass the outline of the affected rib is still visible, showing zones of lysis.

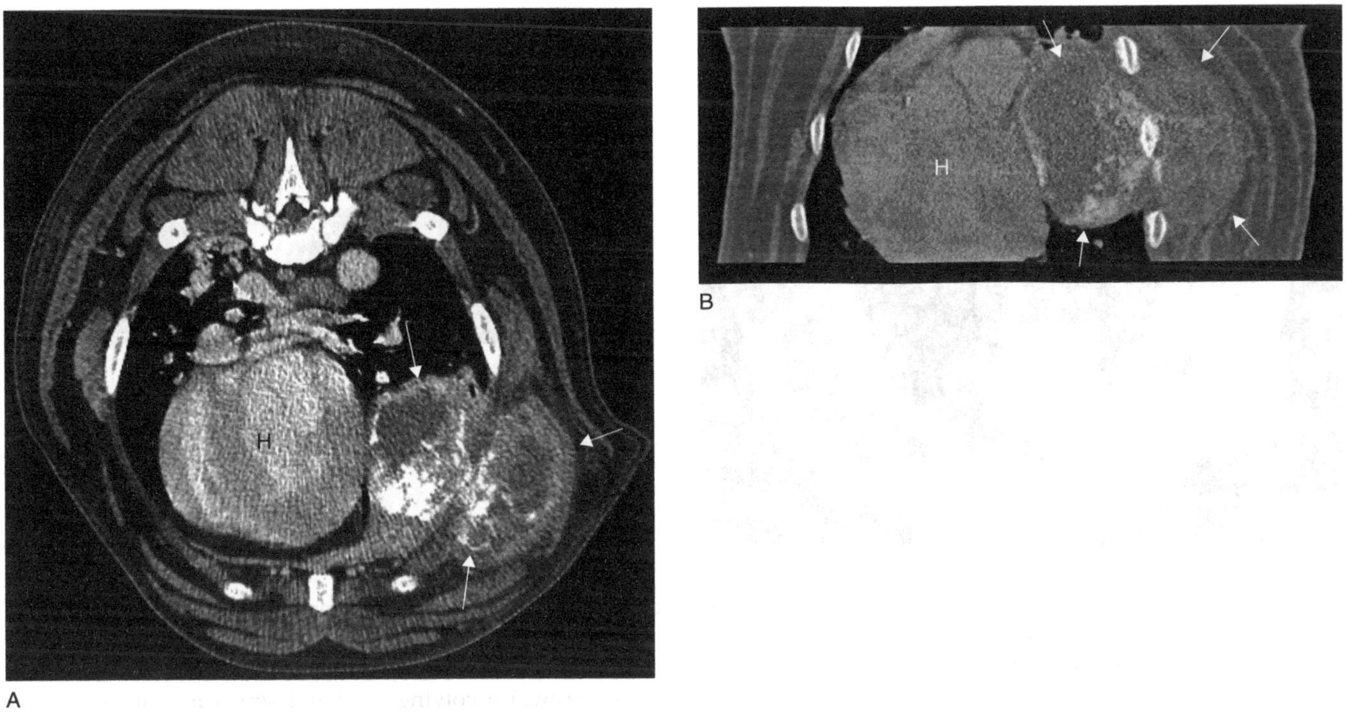

Figure 28.12 Adult dog with chondrosarcoma. (A) Post-contrast transverse CT image shows a round soft tissue-density mass, with central calcified tissue (arrows), centered on the rib cage. The mass extends into the thorax on one side and into the subcutaneous tissues on the other side. (B) Dorsally reconstructed CT image shows the calcified mass (arrows) involving the thoracic wall musculature and extending into the thorax. The heart is displaced to the right. H = heart.

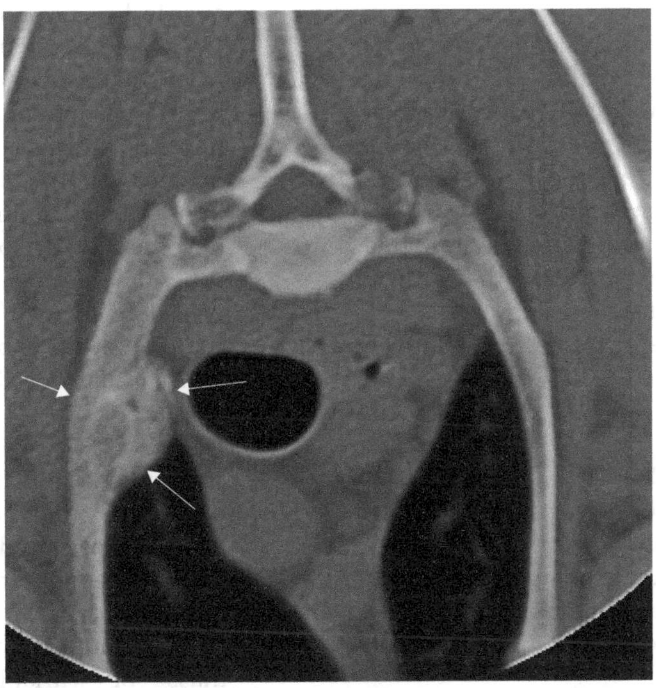

Figure 28.13 Cartilaginous exostosis in a dog. Transverse CT image shows a slightly irregular lesion (arrows) originating at the medial aspect of proximal diaphysis of the rib. This new bone formation has a density equivalent to the normal rib.

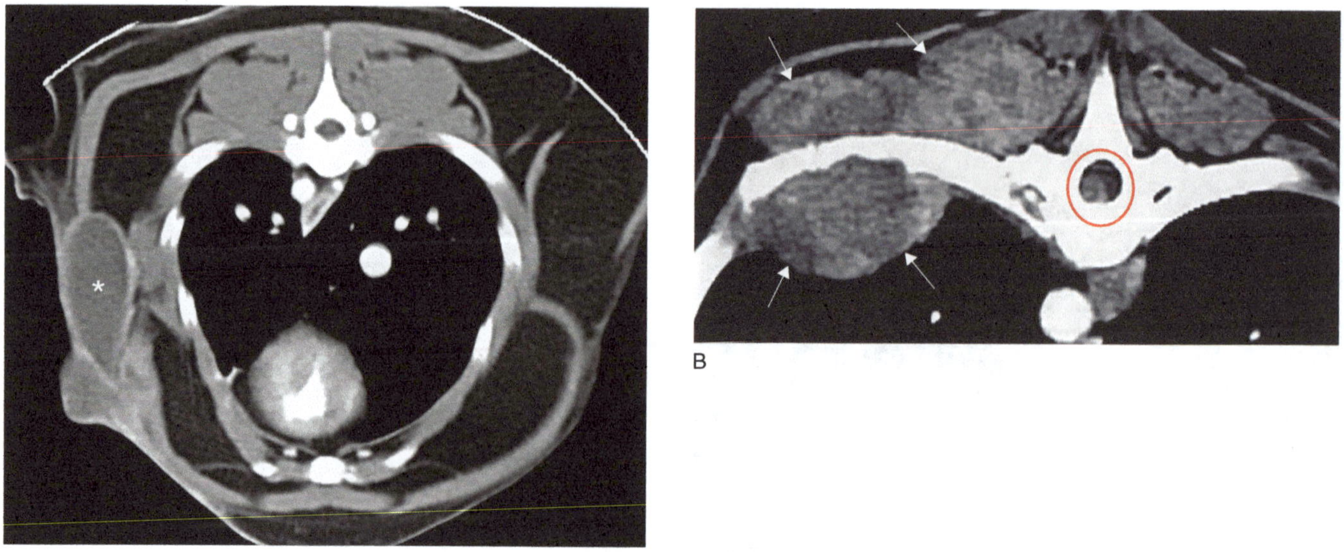

A B

Figure 28.14 Injection site associated fibrosarcoma may show different levels of tissue invasion in the cat. (A) Post-contrast transverse CT image shows a subcutaneous poorly delineated mass, hyperdense compared to the surrounding muscles. In addition a well-delineated oval cystic component with ring enhancement is visible (asterisk). (B) Post-contrast transverse CT image shows a large inhomogeneous, moderately enhancing mass (arrows) involving the longissimus muscle. The mass induces rib erosion and extends into the thorax. Within the vertebral canal (red ring) there is also a contrast-enhancing extradural mass (extension of fibrosarcoma) compressing the spinal cord.

It can usually be distinguished from diffuse processes, such as cellulitis or hemorrhage, by its focal distribution and its propensity to grow towards the thoracic cavity. It can be difficult to differentiate from primary rib tumors.

Lipoma is common in the subcutaneous layers of the thoracic wall. It is characterized as soft moveable masses that, occasionally, slowly grow to cause a mass effect on internal thoracic organs. Infiltrative lipoma and liposarcoma can also infiltrate the inter- and intramuscular layers of the thoracic wall.

Peripheral nerve sheath tumors are slow-growing, locally invasive tumors that extend along the pathway of nerve roots and rarely metastasize.

Metastatic tumors in the soft tissues are relatively common.

CT features

- Fibrosarcoma (Figure 28.14):
  - subcutaneous mass located at the lateral or dorsal aspect of the thoracic wall
  - aspect variable from single homogeneous, well-delineated mass to large inhomogeneous mass invading the surrounding soft tissues, mainly muscles
  - post-contrast: enhanced mildly to moderately, ring enhancement common.
- Lipoma (Figure 28.15):
  - can be difficult to differentiate from obesity-related fat deposition
  - no or mild enhancement on post-contrast
  - simple lipoma: homogeneous fat-dense lesion (HU = –40 to –150), which distinguishes them from soft tissue masses, capsule
  - infiltrative lipoma: locally aggressive, infiltration of muscles and fibrous tissue, no metastases
  - liposarcoma: infiltrative, inhomogeneous may have fat and/or soft tissue density.
- Peripheral nerve sheath tumor (Figure 28.16):
  - well-defined oval, spherical or fusiform mass centered at the expected location of a nerve
  - periscapular muscle atrophy
  - displacement of adjacent muscles and vessels
  - sometimes regional invasion into thoracic cavity or dorsally into vertebral canal
  - post-contrast: mild to severe, homogeneous or heterogeneous, rim enhancement in about half of the cases.
- Metastatic tumor in soft tissues (Figure 28.17):
  - mass of variable density, mineralization possible
  - post-contrast: marked contrast enhancement.

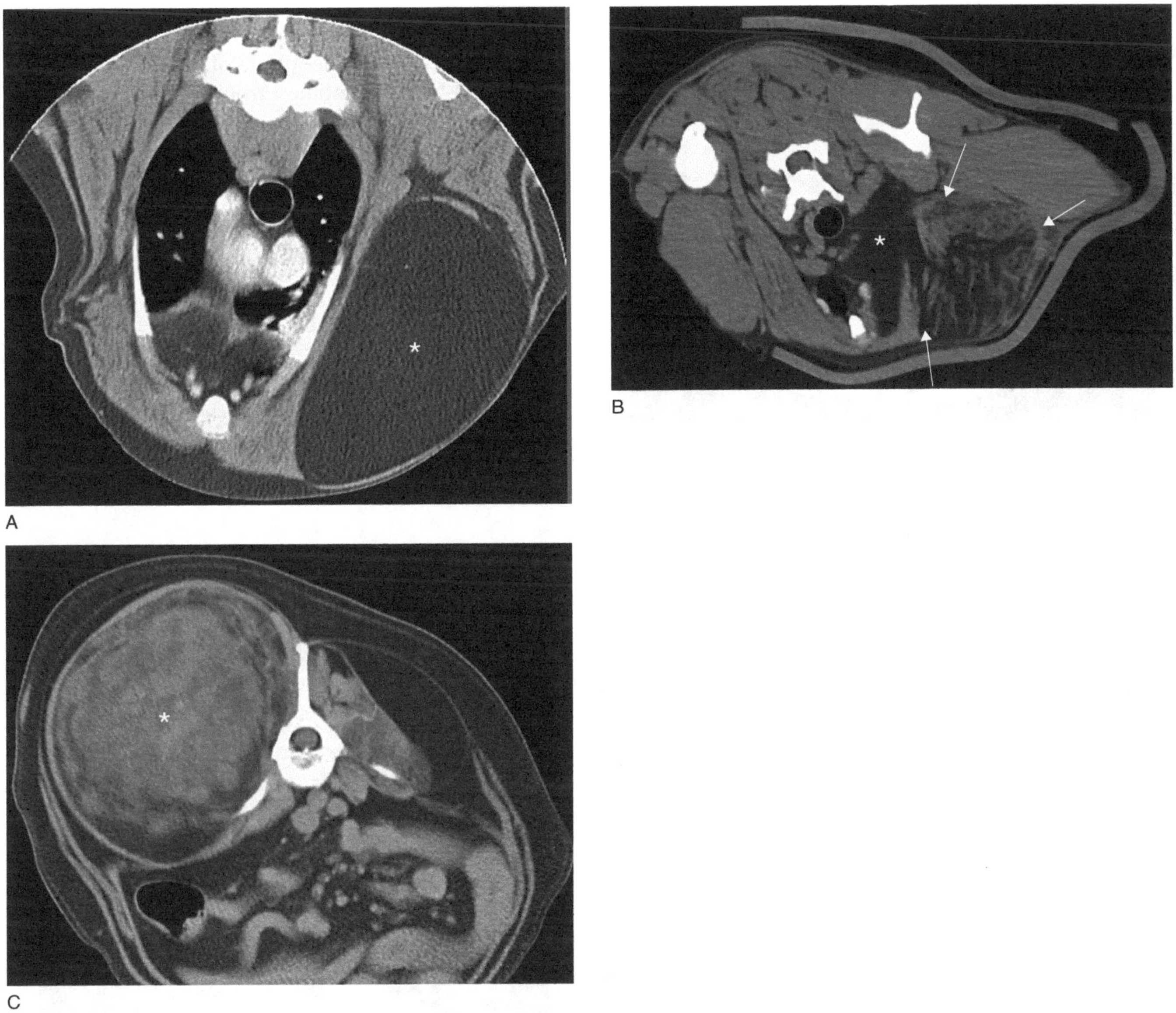

Figure 28.15 Three adult dogs with lipomatous masses. (A) Adult dog with simple lipoma. Transverse CT image shows a well-delineated, homogeneous fat density mass (asterisk) in the thoracic wall. (B) Adult dog with infiltrative lipoma. Transverse CT image (level thoracic vertebra) shows a mass located between the trachea, the vertebral column, the triceps brachialis muscle and the ventral skin. The mass is partly homogeneous with a fat density (asterisk) and partly inhomogeneous (fat/soft tissue density). The mass is locally aggressive and infiltrates the surrounding muscles (arrows). (C) Adult dog with liposarcoma. Transverse CT image shows an inhomogeneous mass (asterisk) at the location of the juxtavertebral muscles.

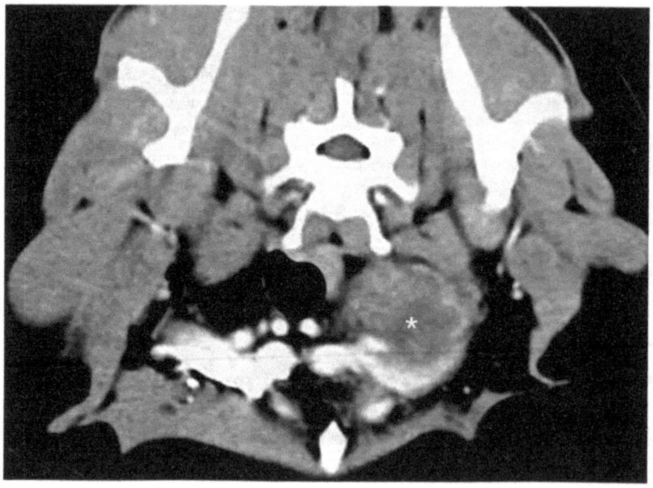

Figure 28.16 Adult dog with malignant peripheral nerve sheath tumor. Post-contrast transverse CT image shows a round mass with mild rim enhancement (asterisk) located at the thoracic inlet.

Sternal neoplasia

Primary or secondary neoplasia of the sternum is rare and should be differentiated from osteomyelitis.

Radiographic findings

- Combination of osteolytic and irregular osteoproductive lesions.
- May grow into the thorax and reach a large size.

Further reading

Watine S, Hamaide A, Peeters D *et al.* (2003) Resolution of chylothorax after resection of rib chondroma in a dog. *J Small Anim Pract* **44**: 546–9.

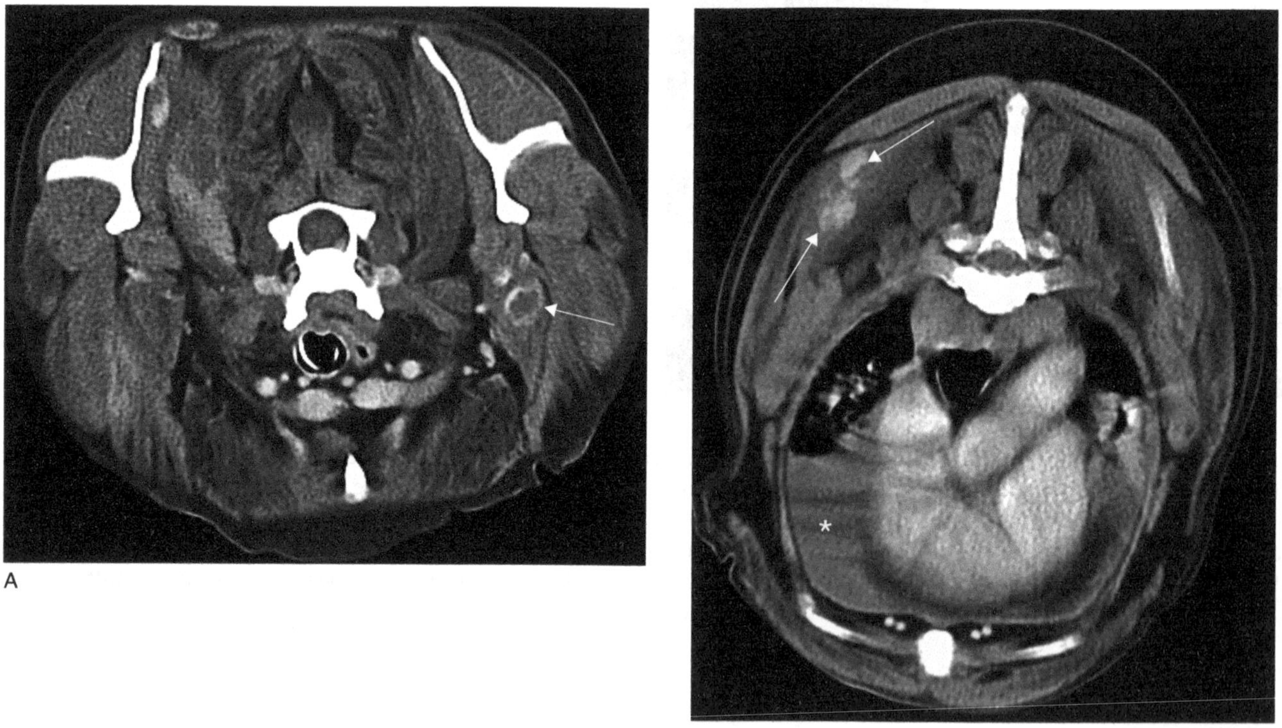

A

B

Figure 28.17 Adult dog with chest wall (muscles) metastases of a splenic hemangiosarcoma. (A) Post-contrast transverse CT image at the level of the thoracic inlet shows a round mass with ring enhancement (arrow) in the teres major muscle. (B) Post-contrast transverse CT image at the level of the T6 shows two heterogeneously enhancing hyperdense masses in the muscle in the distal aspect of a swollen infraspinatus muscle (arrows). Pleural effusion is also present (asterisk).

CHAPTER TWENTY-NINE

Liver, Gallbladder and Spleen

Federica Rossi, Federica Morandi and Tobias Schwarz

General Imaging Protocol

See Table 29.1.

Contrast Imaging Protocols

Biliary contrast medium excretion (Figure 29.1)

Specific biliary contrast media have not been applied to veterinary patients in CT yet. However, all commercially available iodine- and gadolinium-based contrast media have a small biliary excretion fraction. This is sufficient to see a late hepatic enhancement approximately 10 min post application of intravenous iodinated contrast medium. This late hepatic enhancement is useful to delineate the neighboring organs of equal density from the liver, such as the diaphragm and the pancreas.

Approximately 30–60 min post intravenous contrast medium application the hepatic and extrahepatic biliary ducts and gallbladder accumulate contrast-enhanced bile. This can be used to assess the patency of the bile ducts in clinical cases and is promising for further clinical applications.

Transsplenic CT Portography (Table 29.2)

The injection of iodinated non-ionic contrast medium into the splenic parenchyma has been described in transsplenic CT portography (TSCTP) in dogs, a procedure analogue to ultrasound-guided percutaneous spleonoportography, as an alternative to dual-phase CT angiography (DPCTA) for evaluation of the portal vasculature. This technique is not suitable for cats due to their smaller and thinner spleen.

CT: Anatomy and Normal Variants

Liver

The liver is located in the cranial abdomen, cranially it is in direct contact with the diaphragm and caudally with the stomach, pancreas, duodenum and right kidney. The diaphragm and the liver parenchyma are seen as one continuous structure in CT, except with late-phase post-contrast CT. Variable amounts of hypodense peritoneal fat surround the ventral and caudal surfaces of the liver, helping to identify the hepatic margins, lobes and hilar vessels.

Liver size can be subjectively evaluated by assessing the distance between the diaphragm and the stomach, the portion of the liver covered by the costal arch, and the caudal extension and shape of the hepatic margins. Moreover, quantitative CT can be used to calculate liver size. In a study comparing dogs with portosystemic shunts and control dogs, normal liver volume normalized to body weight has been reported to be $24.5 \pm 5.6\,cm^3/kg$.

The liver is divided into four main lobes (left, right, quadrate and caudate lobes), four sublobes (medial and lateral left and right sublobes) and two processes (caudate and papillary processes of caudate lobe). If two lobes are in direct contact, the interlobar fissures are not consistently identified in CT. Single lobes can be more easily recognized ventrally where some peritoneal fat is present. However, the enhancement of

Veterinary Computed Tomography, First Edition. Edited by Tobias Schwarz, Jimmy Saunders.

Table 29.1
Imaging protocol.

Series	Pre-contrast	Post-contrast
Decubitus	Ventral	
Scan margins	Liver and gallbladder: diaphragm to cranial pole of the right kidney Spleen: left lateral liver lobe to middle or caudal abdomen	
Scan mirection	***Dual-phase CT angiography*** – Arterial phase: cranial to caudal – Venous phase: caudal to cranial	
Voltage (kVp)	120–140	
Current (mAs)	100–160	
Tube rotation time (s)	0.5–1	
Slice width (mm)	2–5	
Kernel frequency	Low to medium	
Collimator pitch	1–2	
Helical image reconstruction interval	½ of the slice width	
Motion control	Hyperventilation to achieve expiratory apnea	
Contrast medium application site	N/A	Cephalic or jugular vein
Contrast medium type	N/A	Iodinated
Contrast medium dose	N/A	800 mg iodine/kg bw
Contrast medium injection mode	N/A	Automatic injection is preferred
Scan delay post start contrast injection	N/A	***Standard post-contrast*** – No delay for the liver – Delayed scan for splenic diseases. **Dual-phase *CT angiography*** – Arterial phase: 9–16 s – Venous phase: 10–35 s
Window level (HU)	+40	
Window width (HU)	300	

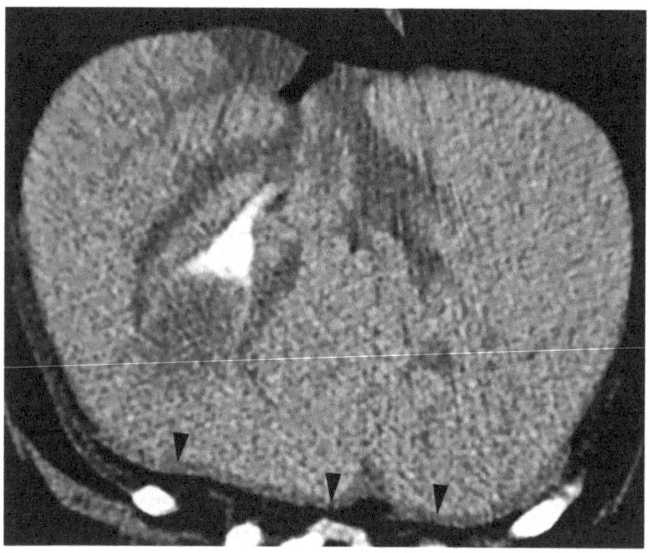

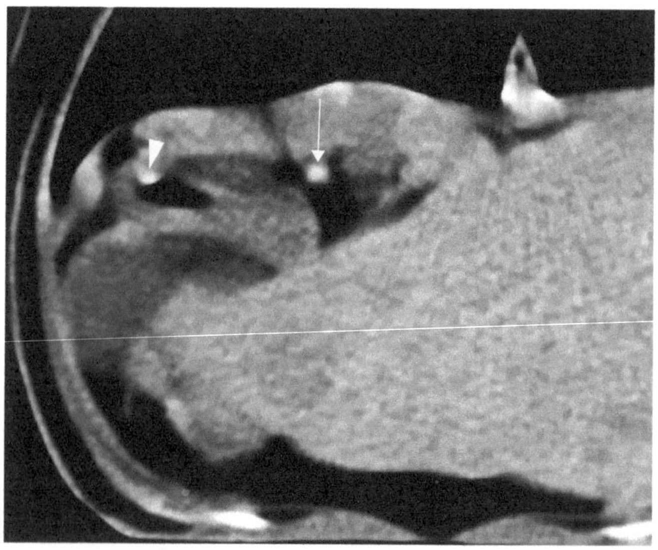

A B

Figure 29.1 (A) Transverse CT image showing biliary excretion of gadolinium based contrast media 50 min post MRI scan. The hepatic parenchyma is enhanced, differentiating it from the non-enhancing diaphragm (arrowheads), and contrast-enhanced bile accumulates in the gall bladder and cystic duct. (B) Contrast-enhanced bile in the extrahepatic common bile duct (arrow) and its duodenal papilla (arrowhead) in a dog 50 min post intravenous administration of iodinated contrast medium.

Table 29.2
Transsplenic CT portography

Access site	Spleen (preferentially under CT guidance)*
Route of administration	Non-selective injection in the splenic parenchyma
Needle size	20 or 22 ga, 1½" length, attached to a preloaded extension set
Injection method	Manual under CT guidance*
Contrast agent	Iodinated (water-soluble)
Type	Tri-iodinated, non-ionic, low-osmolar
Generic name	Omnipaque
Concentration	175 mg iodine/ml or lower to minimize high-density streak artifacts
Volume	Ranging from 3 ml for a small dog (Yorkshire terrier) to 15 ml for a large dog (adult Golden retriever)
Rate of injection	1–3 ml as a bolus, followed by steady injection of the remaining volume at about 0.4 ml/s
Duration of injection	5–30 s depending on animal size
Scan trigger	Beginning of contrast injection
Side effects and risks	Subcapsular (Figure 29.2) or intraperitoneal leakage of contrast medium, if severe, can lead to non-diagnostic studies. Potentially splenic hemorrhage
Undesired effects	*Streaks*: because of the targeted delivery of contrast medium, vascular opacification is usually higher and less homogeneous (incomplete mixing with blood) in TSCTP than in DPCTA, resulting in streamlining and high-density streak artifacts (Figures 29.3 and 29.4). This may limit the ability to identify shunts, particularly in the the right and central divisional branches of the portal vein (left hepatic contrast medium propensity)

*To perform a transsplenic injection, the operator must stay in the room during image acquisition and needs to be protected from radiation with a permanent shield, protective lead clothing or other means to comply with the relevant radiation protection legislation. An extension set, in addition to avoiding needle motion during injection, allows the operator to maintain a greater distance to the gantry, thereby minimizing exposure.

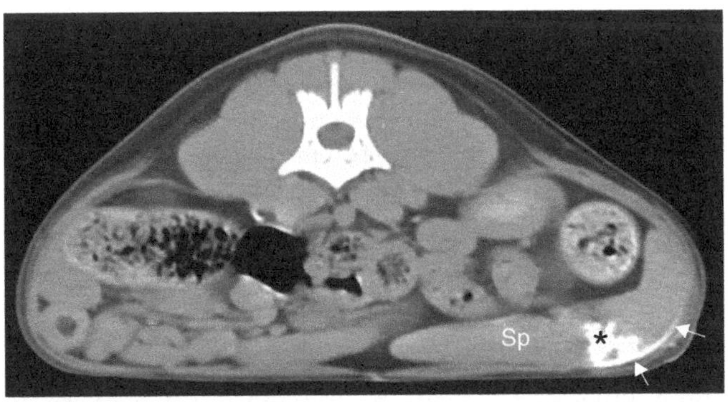

Figure 29.2 Transverse 3 mm helical image taken during transsplenic CT portography. Notice the focal area of contrast medium accumulation (asterisk) in the parenchyma of the spleen (Sp). There is also a small subcapsular accumulation of contrast medium (arrows).

the liver parenchyma and of the vasculature in the post-contrast scan and the presence of the gallbladder enable the recognition of different anatomical regions and structures (Tables 29.3–29.5, Figure 29.5).

The liver parenchyma shows a homogeneous density in the range of about 60–70 HU in dogs and 42–65 HU in cats, values depending on technical settings (kVp, mA, slice width). After contrast medium administration, the enhancement is intense and homogeneous.

The intrahepatic vasculature includes an arterial supply and a double venous system (hepatic and portal veins). In dual-phase CT angiography, arterial and venous vessels can be identified. The hepatic artery arises from the celiac artery, it runs cranially and after giving off the gastroduodenal artery it enters the liver with a a variable number of branches ventral to the portal vein at the porta hepatis. Intrahepatic arteries are seen in the arterial phase as small vessels running in association with the portal vein wall (Figure 29.5E). The largest hepatic veins are often visible already before contrast administration as hypodense tubular structures (Figure 29.5F); they become more evident in the arterial phase as filling defects surrounded by enhancing hepatic parenchyma. During the venous phase, they contrast enhance and are then easily recognizable (Figure 29.5G). The largest hepatic

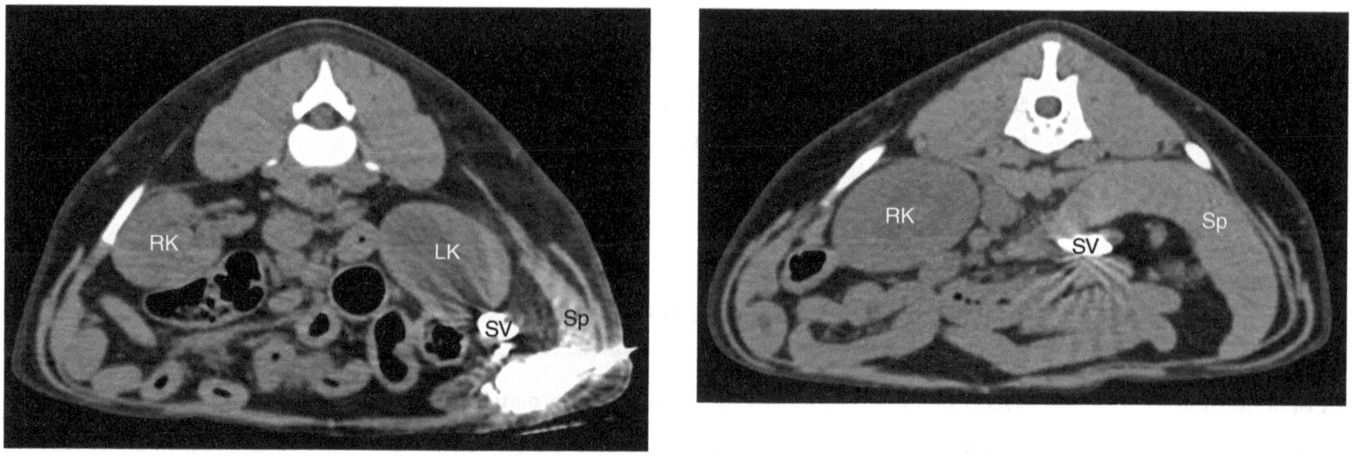

Figure 29.3 Transverse 2 mm helical images taken during transsplenic CT-portography. Notice the streak artifact arising from the high density contrast medium within the spleen (Sp) and splenic vein (SV). LK = left kidney; RK = right kidney.

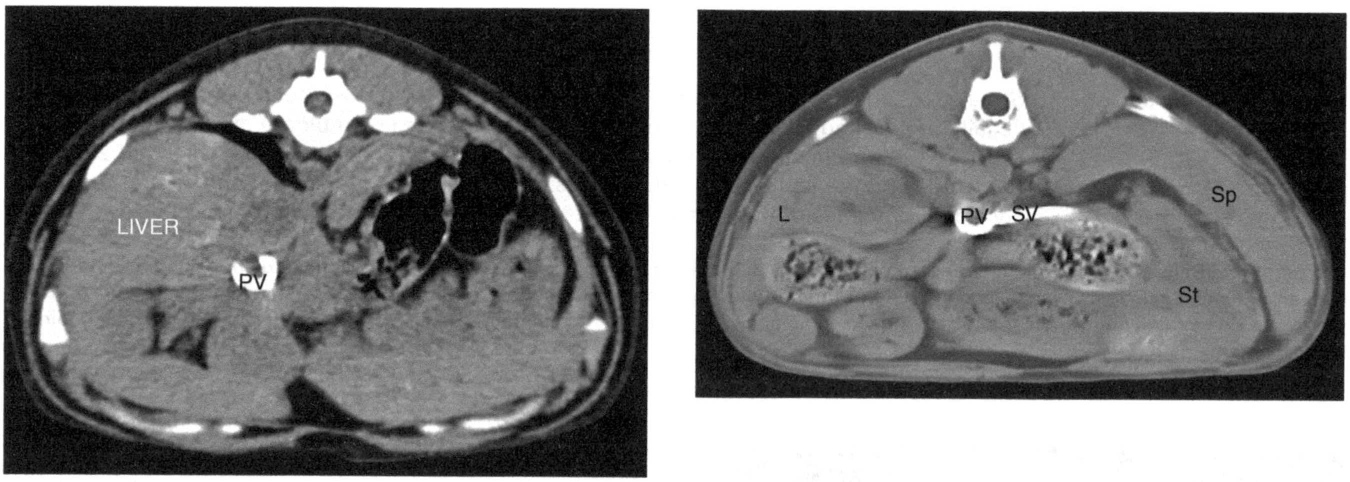

Figure 29.4 Streamlining in two different dogs after transsplenic contrast medium injection, shown at different windows; both images were acquired at 3 mm collimation helically. Notice the peripheral distribution of contrast medium in the portal vein (PV), predominantly ventral and left-sided, where the splenic vein enters the portal vein. L = liver; Sp = spleen; SV = splenic vein; St = stomach.

veins are the branches draining the left medial and lateral lobe; they can be followed entering the caudal vena cava as a common vessel, the hepatic ampulla, in the cranial liver. The right medial and quadrate hepatic veins converge dorsally to the gallbladder. Smaller hepatic veins drain from the caudate and right lateral lobe. Intrahepatic portal vasculature can be distinguished in CT during the venous phase following the division of the main portal vein into the two main right and left branches which supply the different liver lobes. Maximum intensity projection and 3-D reconstructions are useful for better spatial representation of the hepatic vessels.

Gallbladder and biliary system

The gallbladder is easily recognized in CT because of its location between the right medial and quadrate hepatic lobes in the dog (between two parts of the right medial lobe in the cat), its pear shape and typical density. Depending on the amount of bile, the size and position of the gallbladder can vary. When distended, it extends more cranially making contact with the diaphragm. The gallbladder wall is not normally seen as a separate structure. On post-contrast CT, some thin enhancement along the wall is seen mainly where the gallbladder is adjacent to peritoneal fat. The bile is

Table 29.3
Anatomic details of the cranial liver, at the level of the CVC and esophageal hiatus (Figure 29.5A) scan plane 1

CT region visible	Location, shape, density	Relationship with surrounding structures
Liver parenchyma/ lobes	Liver parenchyma occupies the entire cranioventral abdomen, homogeneous pre- and post-contrast	Diaphragm (dorsally and laterally), CVC (dorsally and to the right), esophagus (dorsally in the mid-plane), falciform fat (ventrally), apex of the gallbladder (ventrally and to the right)
CVC	Oval flattened, enhancing in the post-contrast scan	Liver parenchyma (ventrally)

CVC = caudal vena cava.

Table 29.4
Anatomic details of the middle liver (Figure 29.5B and C) scan plane 2 and 3.

CT region visible	Location, shape, density	Relationship with surrounding structures
Liver parenchyma/ lobes	Fissures between liver lobes sometimes visible ventrally, QL and RML separated by the GB. Homogeneous parenchyma divided by hepatic veins	Diaphragm (dorsally and laterally), cardia and stomach fundus (dorsally to the left), falciform fat (ventrally), gallbladder (ventrally, to the right)
CVC and hepatic veins	CVC: oval, located dorsally on the right. HVs confluence toward the CVC visible dorsally to the right, HVs are hypodense to liver in pre-contrast study and in arterial phase, high density in venous phase	Vessels are surrounded by homogeneous hepatic parenchyma
Portal vein and collaterals	PV: round, located ventrally and slightly to the right of the CVC Portal veins visible running toward the periphery, low density in pre-contrast study and in arterial phase, highly attenuating in venous phase	Vessels are surrounded by homogeneous hepatic parenchyma
GB and CBD	GB: pear-shaped, hypodense structure, variable size, located ventral and on the right, the wall is partially enhancing in post-contrast scan. CBD sometimes seen ventral to PV running towards duodenum	GB: between RML and QL

CBD = common bile duct; CVC = caudal vena cava; GB = gallbladder; HV = hepatic vein; PV = portal vein; QL = quadrate lobe; RML = right medial lobe.

hypodense to the hepatic parenchyma both in pre- and post-contrast images; HU values are variable depending on the density of the biliary content. High-density material is sometimes visible in CT, collecting in the dependent part of the gallbladder. On delayed post-contrast studies biliary accumulation of contrast medium is a normal phenomenon. The biliary system is not consistently identified in CT. Only part of the common bile duct can sometimes be recognized as a round hypodense structure located ventral to the portal vein. Intrahepatic ducts are not normally seen.

Spleen

The long tongue-shaped spleen is a mobile organ located in the left hypogastric region. It is only fixed by its dorsal extremity to the stomach. If the stomach is empty, it can be in direct contact with the left lateral lobe of the liver, while in the case of gastric distention its position is more caudal (Figure 29.6A). Since animals are under general anesthesia for CT, splenomegaly is a common finding. The abundant hypodense fat contained in the gastrolienal ligament at the splenic hilus

Table 29.5
Anatomic details of the caudal liver (Figure 29.5D) scan plane 4.

CT region visible	Location, shape, density	Relationship with surrounding structures
Liver parenchyma/ lobes	Caudal part of the LLL and RLL visible ventrally. RLL visible dorsally and to the right, it covers the CP of the CDL extending toward the right kidney. The PP is visible in the midplane, triangular shape	LLL and RLL: laterally in contact with abdominal wall, medially with peritoneal fat RLL: in contact dorsally with right diaphragmatic crus, medially with PV and CVC, ventrally with CP. CP in contact ventrally with duodenum, pancreas, colon, caudally with right kidney PP: between aorta (dorsally), CVC and PV (to the right), branches of hepatic arteries. Variable contact with head of the spleen, stomach, pancreas and colon. Surrounded by fat
Ao, CVC, PV	In the dorsal-mid abdomen (Ao), more ventrally and slightly to the right (CVC and PV), round shape, of similar size	Ao surrounded by caudal attachments of diaphragmatic crura, CVC and PV by liver parenchyma and peritoneal fat. Portal lymph nodes sometimes visible to the left and right of the PV

Ao = aorta; CDL = caudate lobe; CP = caudate process; CVC = caudal vena cava; LLL = left lateral lobe; PP = papillary process; PV = portal vein; RLL = right lateral lobe; RML = right medial lobe.

is helpful to visualize the converging splenic vessels and tributaries lymph nodes.

In pre-contrast images, the spleen shows a homogeneous density. In the arterial phase, the enhancement of the splenic parenchyma is very heterogeneous as a consequence of the irregular distribution of the contrast medium in the red and white pulp (Figure 29.6B and C). This phenomenon should not be interpreted as pathological; however, it may mask a splenic lesion. Therefore, a complete evaluation of this organ requires a delayed CT scan in the venous phase.

Disease Features

Malformation/Developmental

CT enables the recognition of some anatomical variants and malformation of the liver, biliary system and spleen (Table 29.6). These conditions are sometimes discovered as an incidental finding.

Trauma

In trauma patients, CT can be used to establish the extent of a lesion and the involvement of abdominal organs. Subcapsular hematomas of the spleen and liver are lenticular bloody collections adjacent to the organ's margins. Diffuse hemorrhage or fractures of the parenchyma can be detected in the post-contrast sequences as non-enhancing foci or bands. Traumatic herniation of liver or spleen into the thorax can be easily diagnosed with CT. The post-contrast study can be useful to detect hypovascular areas due to direct trauma, torsion or stretching of vessels.

CT features (Figure 29.9)

- Deformation of splenic or hepatic margins (subcapsular hematoma).
- Abnormal position (herniation) of the liver or spleen.
- Post-contrast: hypodense irregular areas (diffuse hemorrhage) or more defined regions (hematomas, parenchymal fractures, vascular infarcts).

Splenic and hepatic infarcts and torsion

Infarcts of the spleen and liver can be due to thrombosis and embolism or can be secondary to torsion. CT findings of isolated splenic torsion have been described. The post-contrast study enables evaluation of the entire vascular bed and parenchyma. The area supplied by the occluded vessel is visible as peripheral, low-density, non-enhancing band with well-defined margins.

CT features (Figure 29.10)

- Free peritoneal fluid.
- Enlarged and abnormally positioned spleen/liver lobe.

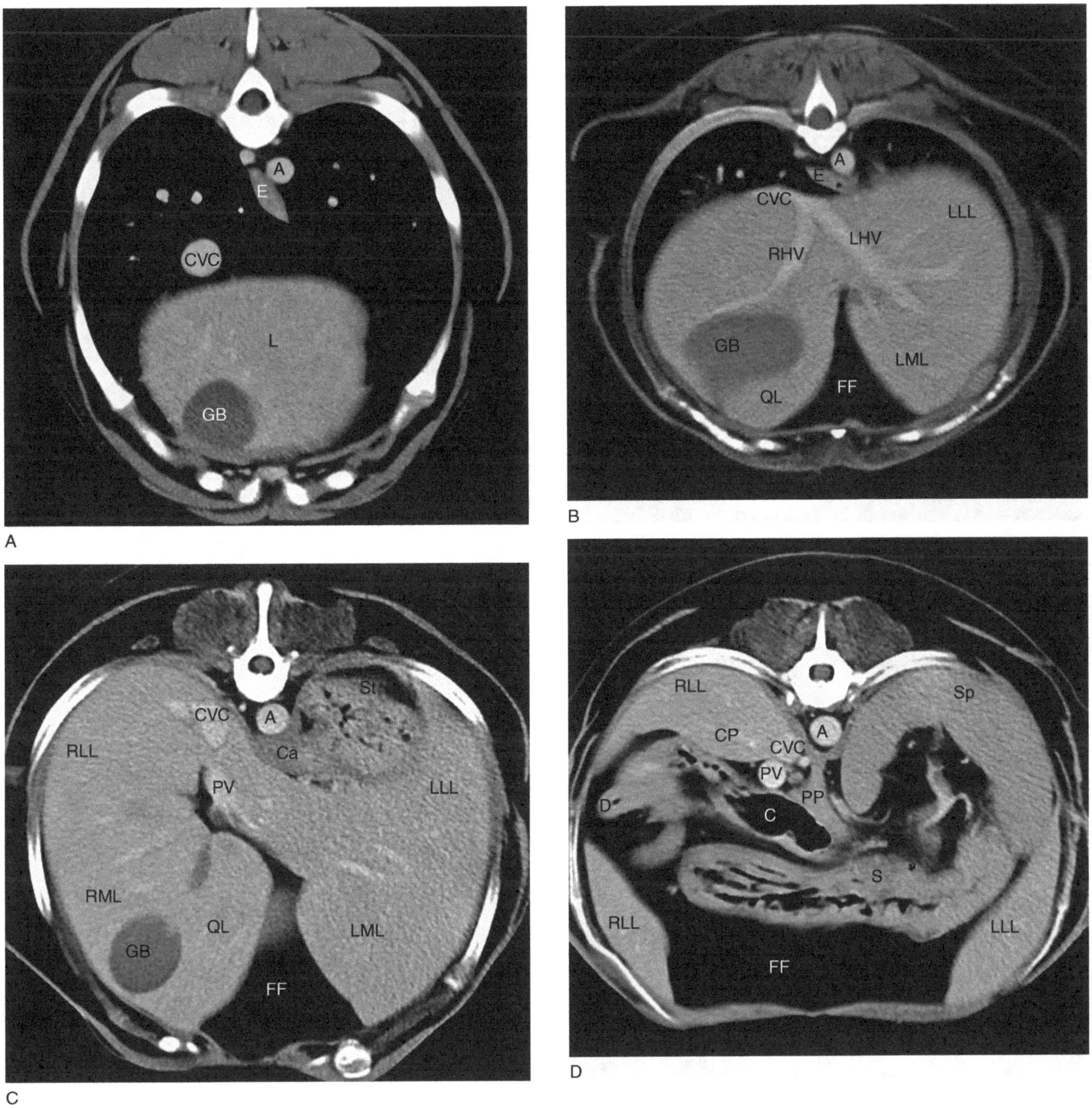

Figure 29.5 Post-contrast CT images of a normal dog representing the anatomy of the liver and biliary system: (A) cranial, (B,C) middle and (D) caudal aspect of the liver. (E) Hepatic arteries (arrows) are small tortuous vessels running parallel with the portal veins, (F) hepatic veins are hypodense in the pre-contrast study and, (G) enhancing structure in the venous phase of the contrast study. A = aorta; CP = caudate process; C = colon; Ca = cardia; CVC = caudal vena cava; D = duodenum; E = esophagus; FF = falciform fat; GB = gallbladder; LHV = left hepatic vein; L = liver; LLL = left lateral lobe; LML = left medial lobe; PP = papillary process; PV = portal vein; RHV = right hepatic vein; RLL = right lateral lobe; RML = right medial lobe; QL = quadrate lobe; St = stomach; Sp = spleen.

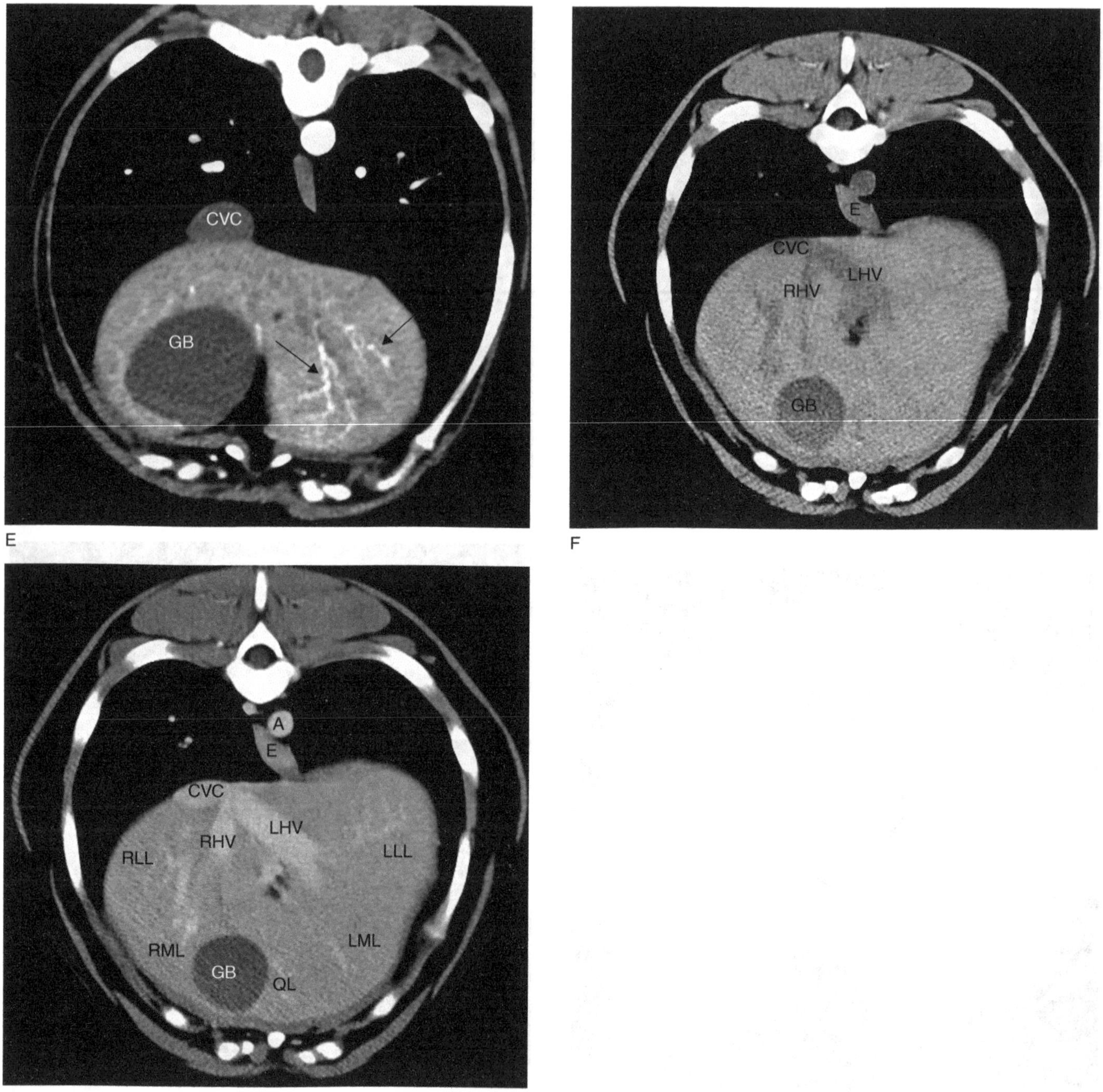

Figure 29.5 (*Continued*)

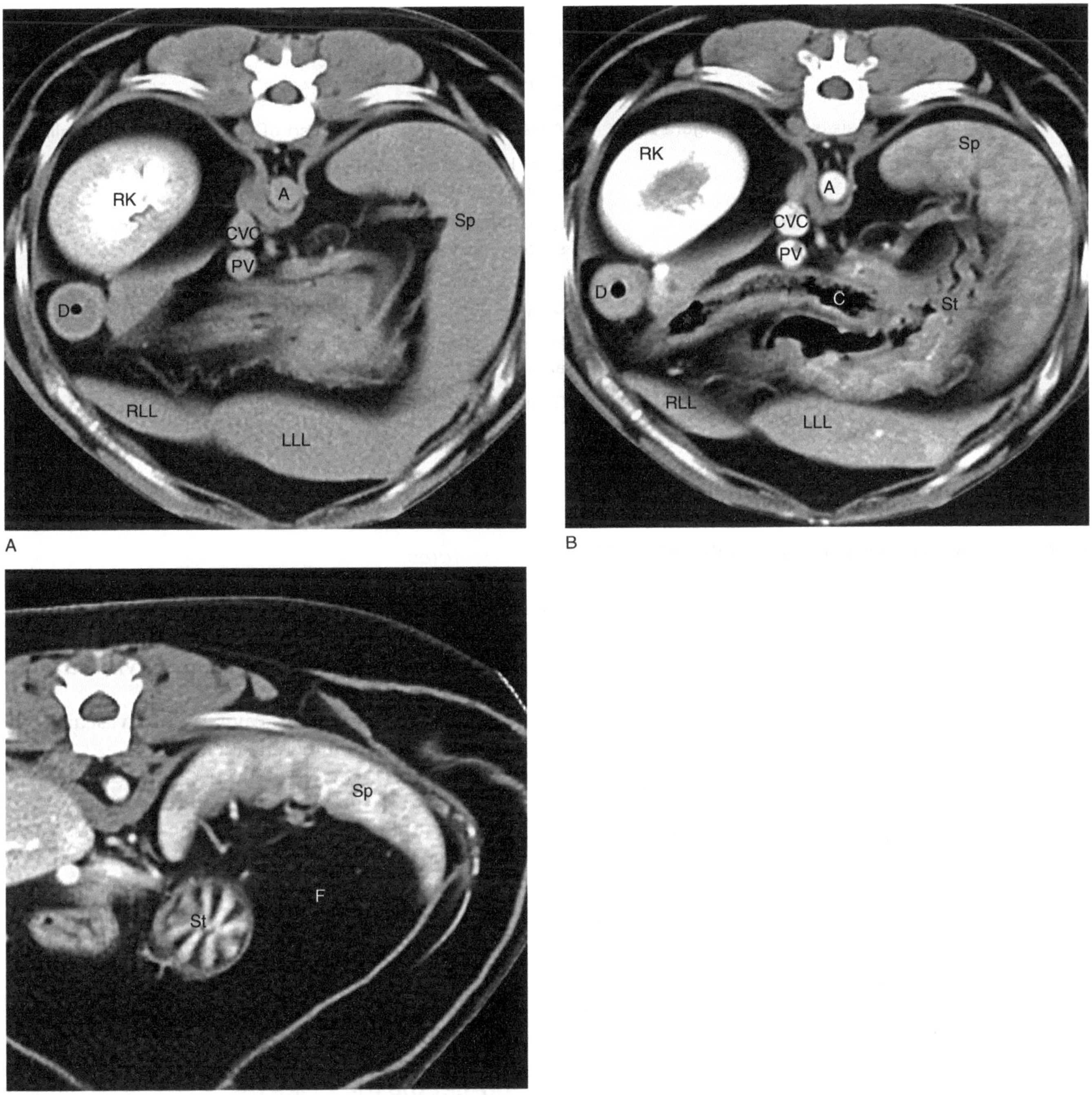

A
B
C

Figure 29.6 Normal canine (A,B) and feline (C) spleen during the venous (A) and the arterial (B,C) phase. The dorsal extremity of the spleen is located under the rib cage surrounded by the fat of the gastrolienal ligament. (B,C) In the arterial phase, the parenchyma is heterogeneous because of the irregular distribution of the contrast medium in the red and white pulp. (A) The same spleen becomes more homogeneous in the venous phase. A = aorta; C = colon; CVC = caudal vena cava; D = duodenum; F = fat; LLL = left lateral liver lobe; PV = portal vein; RK = right kidney; RLL = right lateral liver lobe; Sp = spleen; St = stomach.

Table 29.6
Malformation of the liver, biliary system and spleen.

Condition	CT findings
Liver lobes or GB agenesis/hypoplasia (Figure 29.7)	Absence of reduced size of part of the liver, GB not visualized
Congenital diaphragmatic hernia	Liver lobes and/or GB localized in the thorax into the pericardium, diaphragm discontinuous
Bilobed GB or GB duplication (cats)	GB separated in two parts by a septum or presence of two separated GBs
Vascular malformations of the liver	Decreased liver volume, presence of abnormal vessels (*see* Chapter 36)
Accessory spleen	Island of ectopic splenic tissue localized in the peri-splenic area
Hepatic cysts (polycystic disease, cats) (Figure 29.8)	Round, low-density, non-enhancing structures

GB = gallbladder.

- Corkscrew-like soft tissue mass at the splenic hilus (pedicle) – splenic torsion.
- Post-contrast: lack of enhancement in the affected areas.

Diffuse non-neoplastic parenchymal diseases

Acute inflammation, congestion and storage diseases often produce hepatomegaly or splenomegaly. Wheras parenchymal CT density changes associated with diffuse liver diseases are well documented in humans, there is very little information available about animals. Lower attenuation values of the liver have been reported in cats and tortoises with hepatic lipidosis. Calcification is seen in patients with metabolic conditions such as Cushing's disease and in association with chronic hepatitis.

CT features

- Hepato-, splenomegaly: increased size and rounded margins.
- Metabolic conditions, chronic hepatitis: calcified areas that appear as hyperdense foci of variable size and location may be present.

Focal non-neoplastic parenchymal diseases

Differential diagnosis includes many types of benign condition and focal neoplasia.

CT features

- Focal hepatic and splenic lesions:
  - often seen as hypo- to hyperdense foci to the normal surrounding parenchyma
  - post-contrast: normally improved visualization.
- Alveolar echinoccocosis:
  - multiple cystic or cavitary non-vascularized lesions with mineralization.
- Hepatic abscesses, hepatic necrosis secondary to neoplasia or immune-mediated diseases:
  - multiple non-enhancing lesions can be seen.
- Splenic focal lesions:
  - malignant lesions (hemangiosarcoma) show lower attenuation values than benign conditions (hematomas and focal nodular neoplasia) (Figure 29.11).

Gallbladder and biliary system – non-neoplastic diseases

CT features

- Biliary calculi in the gallbladder or common bile duct lumen:
  - foci of mineral density are seen with calcium-containing concretions
  - the dilated common bile duct can be recognized ventral to the portal vein.
- Intrahepatic biliary ducts distention due to complete long-term biliary obstruction:
  - tortuous tubular structure, non-enhancing and hypodense to the surrounding parenchyma.

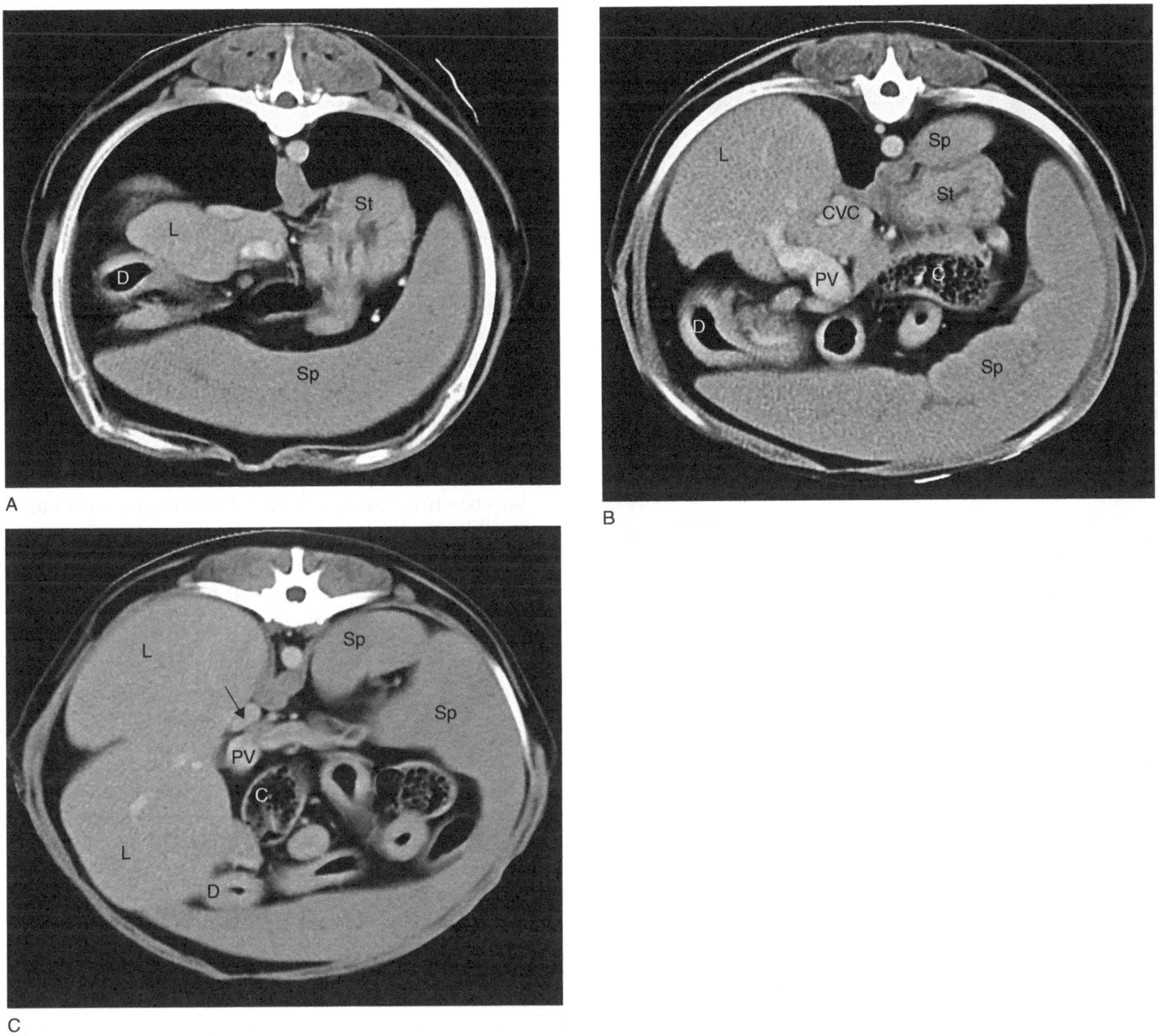

Figure 29.7 Post-contrast images of the cranial (A), middle (B) and caudal (C) aspect of the liver in a dog with congenital liver malformation. The liver extends only to the cranial right abdomen; the stomach and the spleen are in direct contact with the left diaphragm. The right liver consists of two lobes with rounded margins. The gallbladder is not visualized. C = colon; CVC = caudal vena cava; D = duodenum; L = liver; PV = portal vein; St = stomach; Sp = spleen.

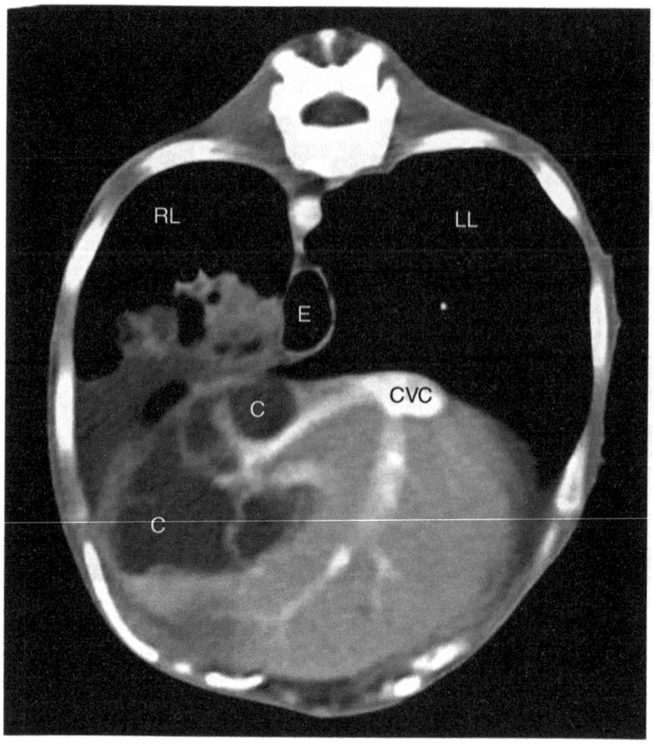

Figure 29.8 Persian cat with a carcinoma of the right caudal lung lobe and polycystic disease (incidental finding). Post-contrast CT image shows an irregular cystic structure (C) in the right middle and dorsal liver. This hypodense, multilobulated cyst is divided by enhancing septa. C = hepatic cyst; CVC = caudal vena cava; E = esophagus; LL = left lung lobe; RL = right lung lobe.

- Emphysematous cholangitis (Figure 29.12):
  - accumulation of gas in the gallbladder wall and/or lumen
  - presence of gas around the gallbladder and loss of continuity of the wall suggest gallbladder rupture secondary to necrosis
  - peritoneal effusion is normally present due to biliary peritonitis.

Neoplasia

Primary or metastatic neoplasia can have variable size and CT appearance. Dual-phase CT can be useful to detect small liver lesions, because lesions may only enhance in the arterial phase or appear as low-density lesions in the venous phase.

CT features

- Primary tumors tend to be large irregular masses associated with anarchic vascularization. Cystic component is present with hepatic cystadenoma or cystadenocarcinoma, frequently seen in the cat.
- Splenic and hepatic hemangiosarcomas: large non-vascularized areas.
- Metastases: frequently seen as multiple round hypodense nodules.

Advantages of pre-treatment CT in patients with hepatic or splenic neoplasia

- Evaluation of the exact size and extension of a mass (useful mainly in the case of big masses), differentiation between peripheral hepatic or splenic lesions from masses arising from adjacent organs (sometimes difficult to assess with ultrasound) (Figure 29.13).
- Assessment of the involvement of the main vascular structures such as caudal vena cava, aorta and portal vein (Figure 29.14).
- Staging of diseases (evaluation of tributaries, lymph nodes, detection of possible metastases in the thorax or abdomen) (Figures 29.14C and D, 29.15).

Further reading

Echandi RL, Morandi F, Daniel WT, Paquette JL and Daniel GB (2007) Comparison of transplenic multidetector CT portography to multidetecetor CT angiography in normal dogs. *Vet Radiol Ultrasound* **48**: 38–44.

Fife WD, Samii VF, Drost WT, Mattoon JS and Hoshaw-Woodard S (2004) Comparison between malignant and nonmalignant splenic masses in dogs using contrast-enhanced computed tomography. *Vet Radiol Ultrasound* **45**: 289–97.

Irausquin RA, Scavelli TD, Corti L *et al.* (2008) Comparative evaluation of the liver in dogs with a splenic mass by using ultrasonography and contrast-enhanced computed tomography. *Can Vet J* **49**: 46–52.

Nakamura M, Chen HM, Momoi Y and Iwasaki T (2005) Clinical application of computed tomography for the diagnosis of feline hepatic lipidosis. *J Vet Med Sci* **67**: 1163–5.

Patsikas MN, Rallis T, Kladakis SE and Dessiris AK (2001) Computed tomography of isolated splenic torsion in a dog. *Vet Radiol Ultrasound* **42**: 235–7.

Stieger SM, Zwingenberger AL, Pollard RE, Kyles AE and Wisner R (2007) Hepatic volume estimation using quantitative Computer Tomography in dogs with portosystemic shunts. *Vet Radiol Ultrasound* **48**: 409–13.

Zwingenberger AL and Schwarz T (2004) Dual-phase CT angiography of the normal canine portal and hepatic vasculature. *Vet Radiol Ultrasound* **45**: 117–24.

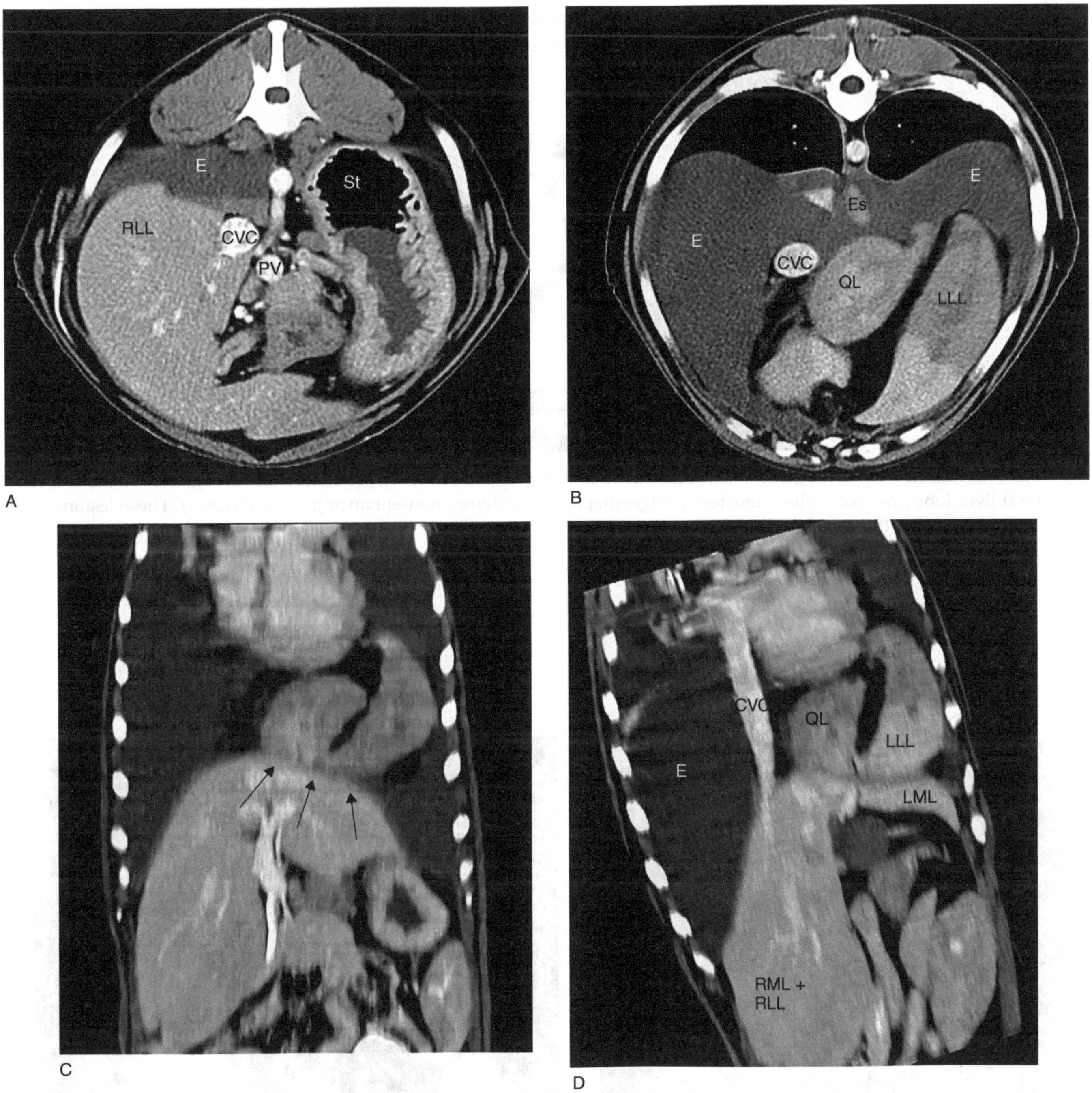

Figure 29.9 Thorax and cranial abdomen of an adult Border collie that was hit by a car and is suffering from diaphragmatic rupture. (A,B) Post-contrast and (C,D) 2-D maximum intensity projection reconstructions. In the thorax, pleural effusion is visible. The quadrate and left lateral liver lobes are herniated into the left caudal hemithorax between the caudal vena cava and the cardiac apex. The two lobes are oriented cranially, the parenchyma shows extended hypoperfused areas due to vascular stretching and torsion. The diaphragmatic tear is demonstrated by the maximum intensity projection reconstructions (arrows). CVC = caudal vena cava; E = effusion; Es = esophagus; LLL = left lateral liver lobe; LML = left medial liver lobe; PV = portal vein; QL = quadrate lobe; RLL = right lateral liver lobe; RML = right medial liver lobe; St = stomach.

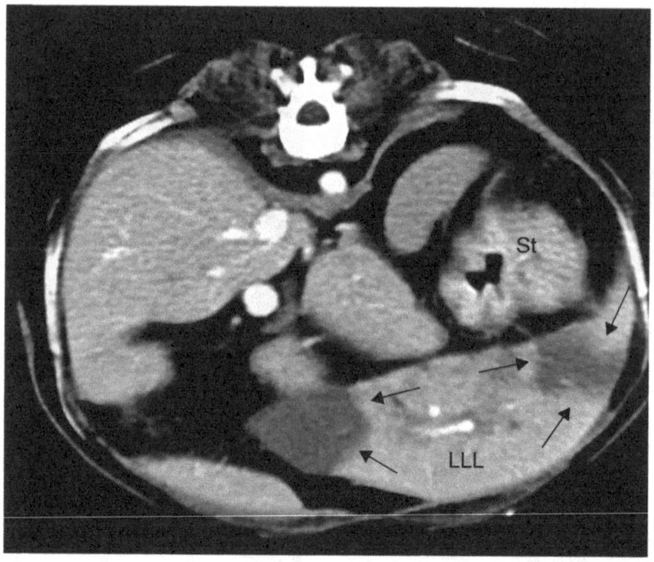

Figure 29.10 Adult Maltese dog with vasculitis due to *Ehrlichia* spp. infection. Post-contrast CT image shows the enlarged left lateral liver lobe and two well-delineated, wedge-shaped, hypodense, non-enhancing areas (arrows). These lesions were not demonstrated by ultrasound. LLL = left lateral liver lobe; St = stomach.

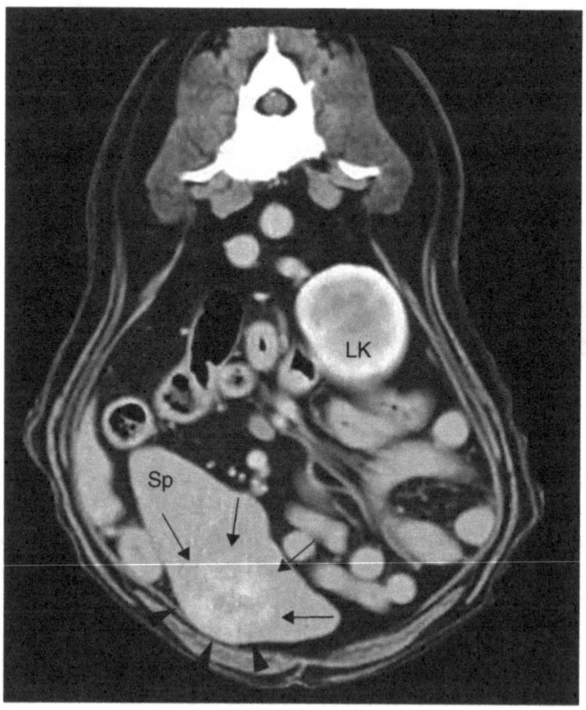

A

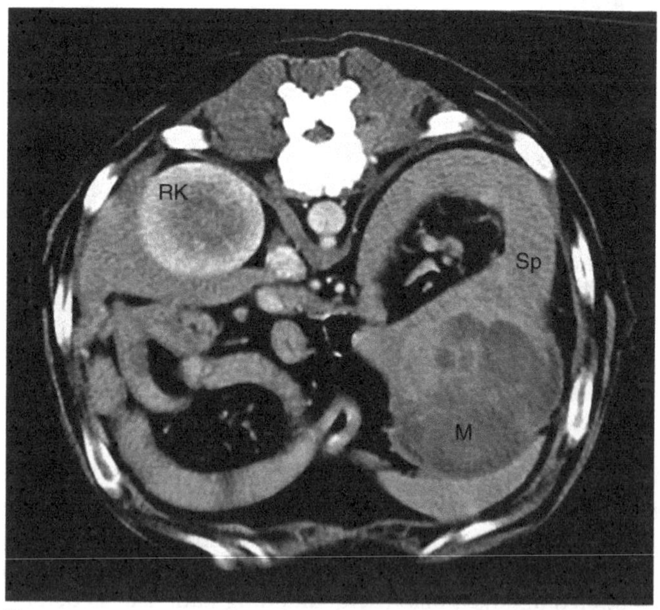

B

Figure 29.11 Splenic focal lesions in two different dogs. (A) Adult dog with benign hyperplasia: post-contrast CT image shows a 4 cm round, slightly protruding nodule, with some irregular enhancement in the venous phase (arrows). (B) Adult dog with hemangiosarcoma: post-contrast CT image shows a 6 cm round mass with large irregular hypodense areas. LK = left kidney; M = mass; RK = right kidney; Sp = spleen.

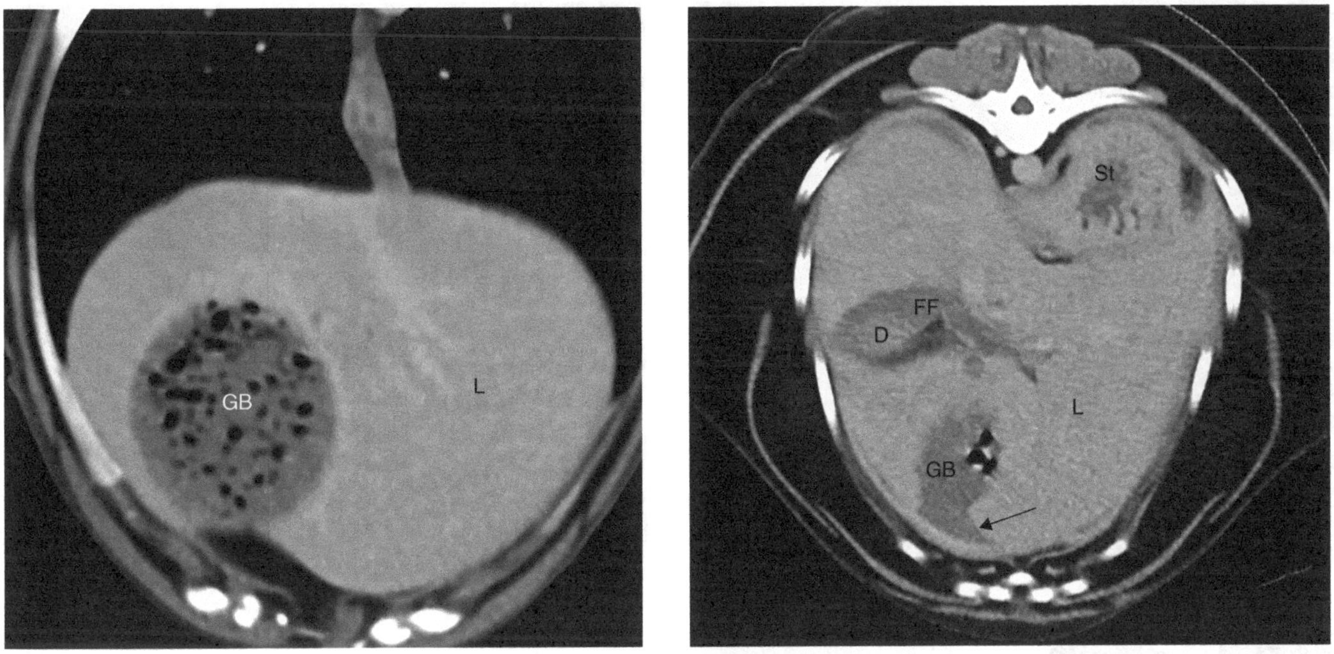

A B

Figure 29.12 Emphysematous cholecystitis in two different dogs. (A) Post-contrast CT image shows multiple oval gas bubbles in the lumen of the gallbladder. The gallbladder has a normal round shape. (B) Post-contrast CT image shows a loss of the normal contour of the cranial aspect of the gallbladder. There are some small air bubbles in the lumen and a small quantity of free fluid accumulated around its apex (arrow) and the duodenum. In this dog, rupture of the gallbladder and biliary peritonitis was found in surgery. D = duodenum; FF = free fluid; GB = gallbladder; L = liver; St = stomach.

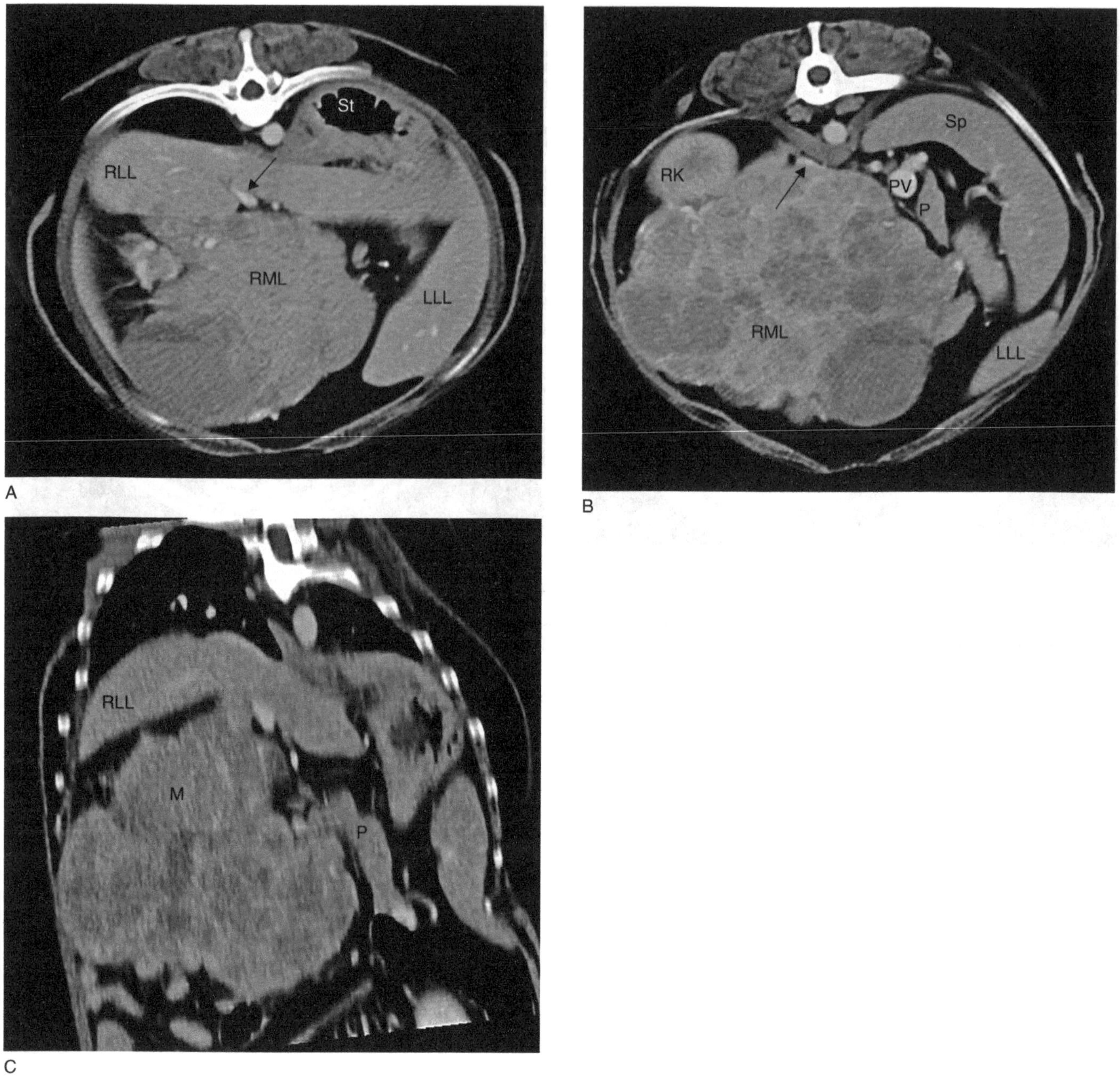

Figure 29.13 Adult dog with hepatoma. (A,B) Post-contrast and (C) 2-D reconstructed CT image show that the lesion is a large pedunculated liver mass arising from the right medial lobe and extending caudally between the pancreas, the right kidney and small intestine. The caudal vena cava is severely compressed (arrow). LLL = left lateral liver lobe; M = mass; P = pancreas; PV = portal vein; RK = right kidney; RLL = right lateral liver lobe; RML = right medial liver lobe; Sp = spleen; St = stomach.

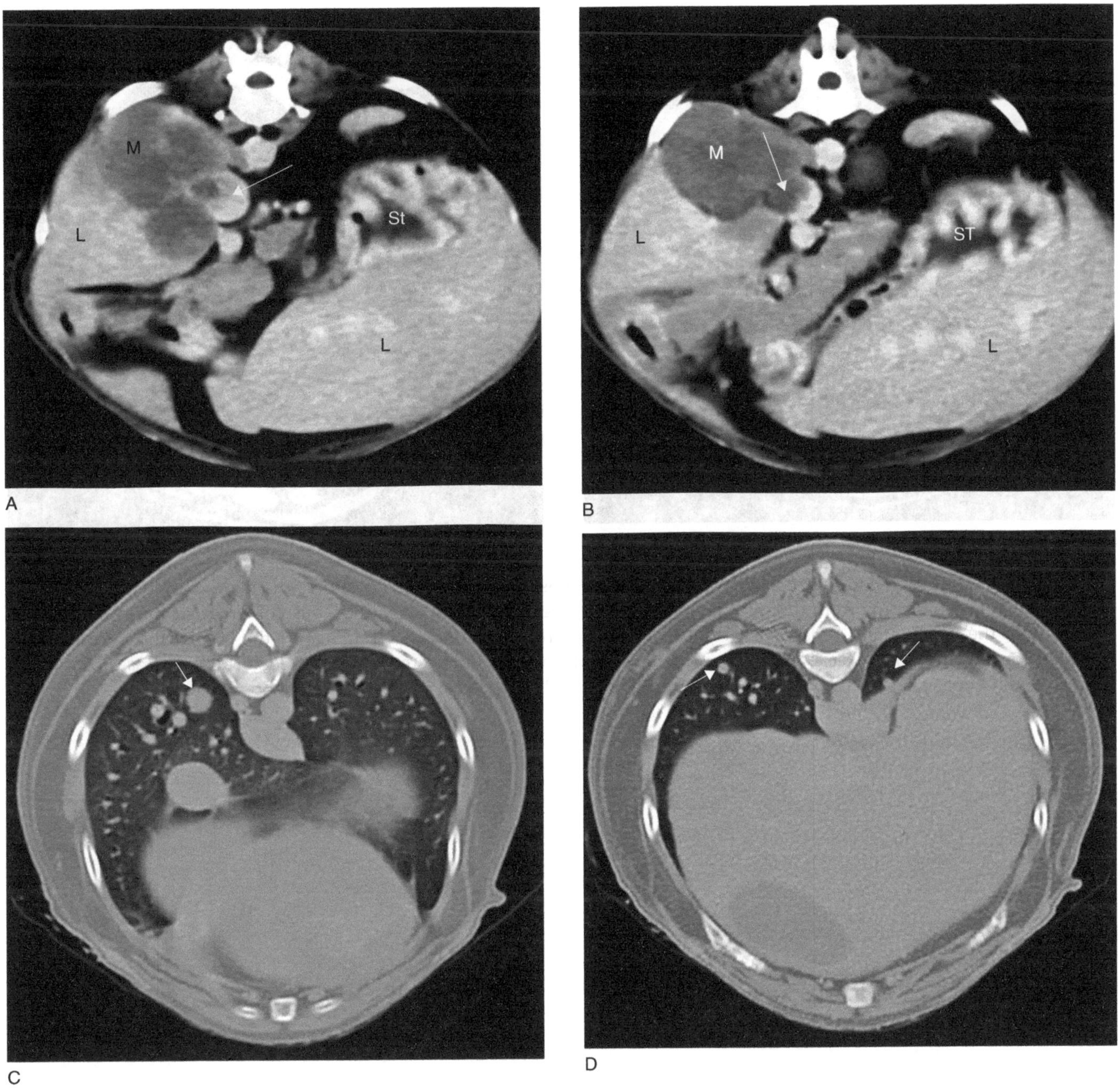

Figure 29.14 Adult dog with hepatic adenocarcinoma. (A,B) CT images of the abdomen show a hypodense liver mass located dorsal and on the right, adjacent to the caudal vena cava. The lesion extends into the lumen of the vessel producing a round filling defect (arrow). (C,D) CT images of the caudal lung show small round nodules in the caudal right lobe representing lung metastases (arrows). L = liver; M = mass; ST = stomach.

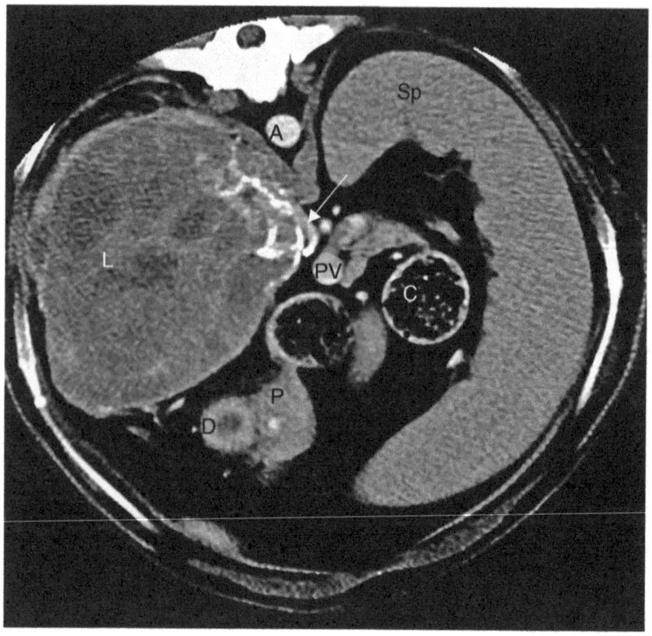

A

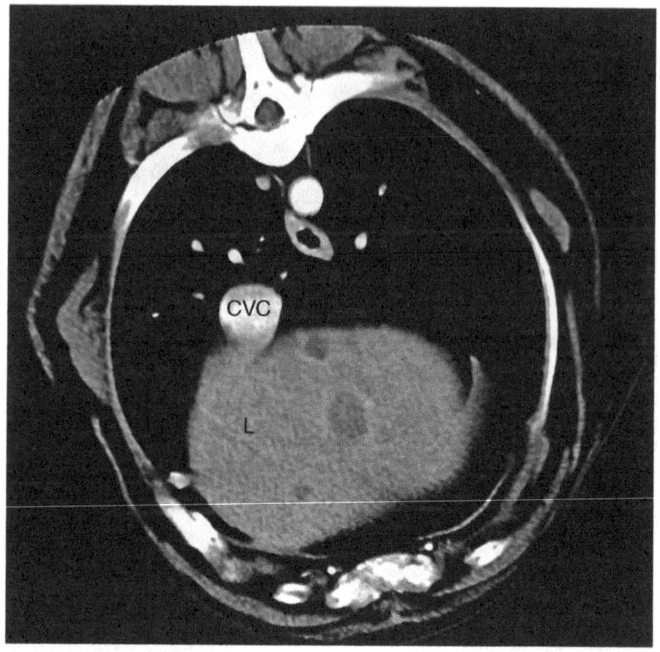

B

Figure 29.15 Adult dog with hepatic adenocarcinoma. (A) Post-contrast CT image shows the main mass which is a 10 cm diameter oval lesion, arising from the right lateral lobe, with heterogeneous density because of irregular mineralization, in contact with the right caudal vena cava (CVC) wall (arrow). (B) Post-contrast CT image of the cranial liver shows three hypodense round nodules. These lesions were detected only by CT and were demonstrated to be metastases. A = aorta; CVC = caudal vena cava; C = colon; D = duodenum; L = liver; P = pancreas; PV = portal vein; Sp = spleen.

CHAPTER THIRTY

PANCREAS

Ana V. Cáceres

IMAGING PROTOCOL

See Tables 30.1, 30.2.

CT: ANATOMY AND NORMAL VARIANTS

The pancreas is a U-shaped organ located caudal to the liver and stomach. It consists of three segments: the body, the right lobe and the left lobe. There is no clear demarcation between each segment but certain landmarks can been used. The body of the pancreas is dorsoventrally flattened and is located adjacent to the *porta hepatica* ventral to the portal vein, medial to the gastroduodenal angle, between the pylorus and the transverse colon. The right lobe is located adjacent to the right abdominal wall, dorsal, dorsolateral or dorsomedial to the descending duodenum. The caudal extremity of the right lobe terminates in an abrupt medial angulation at the caudal duodenal flexure. The left pancreatic lobe is adjacent to the body of the stomach and extends caudally adjacent to the splenic vein, transverse and descending colon (Figure 30.1). CT dimensions of the pancreas are shown in Table 30.3. The right lobe follows the duodenum and the left lobe parallels the greater curvature of the stomach (Figure 30.2).

Feline anatomical specificities

The feline pancreas consists of two lobes; it is ±12 cm long and ±1–2 cm wide. Unlike in dogs there is an acute angle between the two lobes, probably because there is no pancreatic body. In cats, the pancreas appears homogeneous during the venous phase. The mean HU of the pre-contrast pancreas was found to be 37.45 ± 7.19. The pancreas is hypodense to the liver and spleen and enhances immediately after IV contrast administration, peaking immediately and then gradually clearing but remaining hypodense compared to the spleen.

Pancreatic angiography and contrast enhancement

The normal pancreatic angiography has been described in dogs. Vascular and pancreatic enhancements are shown in Tables 30.4 and 30.5. On dual-phase there is heterogeneous arterial and homogeneous venous pancreatic enhancement.

Veterinary Computed Tomography, First Edition. Edited by Tobias Schwarz, Jimmy Saunders.

Table 30.1
CT imaging protocol.

Series	Pre-contrast	Dynamic	Dual phase			Delayed post-contrast
Decubitus	Ventral					
Scan margins	Diaphragm → L5	Pancreatic body → Area of interest (no motion)	Body Rt lobe Lt lobe	Arterial Cd Body → Cr body Cr pancreas → Cd Rt lobe Cr pancreas → Cd Lt lobe	Portal Diaphragm → Cd pancreas Cd Rt lobe → Diaphragm Cd Rt lobe → Diaphragm	Diaphragm → L5
Voltage (kvp)	120					
Current (mAs)	130					
Tube rotation time (s)	1					
Slice width (mm)	Dogs: <20 kg 3 mm; >20 kg 5 mm					
Kernel frequency	Soft tissue algorithm					
Collimator pitch	Dogs: <20 kg 1.7; >20 kg 1.4					
Helical image recon interval	2 mm					
Motion control	Hyperventilation or ventilator					
Contrast medium application site and type	None	Cephalic/Iohexol 240 mg I/ml				None
Contrast medium dose		0.5 ml/kg	2.2 ml/kg			None
Contrast medium injection mode		Automatic – 5 ml/s				None
Scan delay post start contrast injection		No delay	Dependent on the Dynamic scan Arterial ≈ 7 s		Portal ≈ 12.2 s	5–10 min
Window level (HU)	+350					
Window width (HU)	50					

Cd = caudal, Cr = cranial, Le = left, Rt = right.

Table 30.2
CT protocols.

Condition	Pre-contrast	Dynamic	Dual-Phase	Post-contrast	Delay
Pancreatitis	✓			✓	✓
Pancreatic cysts and pseudocyst	✓			✓	✓
Exocrine pancreatic tumor	✓			✓	✓
Endocrine pancreatic tumors	✓	✓	✓		✓

Disease Features

Malformation/Developmental

Pancreatic cyst, pseudobladder

Pancreatic cyst is a collection of fluid lined with cuboidal epithelium that lacks communication with the pancreatic duct. Pancreatic cysts and pseudobladder are believed to be congenital. In humans, pancreatic cysts can be unilocular or multilocular and can be from microscopic to several centimeters large. Pancreatic cysts have been described in cats, more commonly in the Persian or Persian crossbred with polycystic kidney and liver disease.

CT features
- Cystic structure(s) with thin and smooth wall.
- Post-contrast: no contrast enhancement of the cyst or the wall (macrocystic pancreatic lesions).

Infection/Inflammation

Pancreatitis and pancreatic necrosis

Pancreatitis in small animals is divided into acute or chronic types on the basis of clinical findings and pathologic criteria. Acute pancreatitis is more common in dogs and chronic pancreatitis affects mainly cats. CT can be useful for evaluation and diagnosis of pancreatic necrosis, abscess and thrombosis. In human medicine the diagnosis of pancreatic necrosis plays an important role in determining prognosis, due to its higher mortality rate, especially with concurrent infection. Pancreatic necrosis is defined as focal or diffuse areas of non-viable pancreatic parenchyma involving more than 30% of the gland.

CT features of acute pancreatitis (Figure 30.3)
- Pancreatic mass effect or enlargement.
- Hypodense central or peripheral areas.
- Peritoneal effusion.
- Post-contrast:
  - lack of contrast enhancement
  - lazy or ill-defined peripancreatic mesentery
  - in severe cases peripancreatic vasculature thrombosis.

CT features of chronic pancreatitis in dogs and cats
- Post-contrast: patchy and heterogeneous contrast enhancement.

Pancreatic pseudocyst

Pancreatic pseudocysts are believed to represent dilatation of the pancreatic duct. Pancreatic pseudocysts are a sequela of pancreatitis or pancreatic trauma, they have been defined as a collection of pancreatic fluid enclosed by a wall of fibrous or granulation tissue. Pseudocysts may regress spontaneously, or persist with or without clinical implications, and can be of various sizes. The pathogenesis for the formation follows pancreatic inflammation, accumulation of enzyme-rich fluid, lack of absorption and pancreatic duct communication, therefore the pseudocyst is usually rich in pancreatic enzymes and sterile.

CT features (Figure 30.4)
- Round or oval fluid collection with a thin, ill-defined capsule or thick wall.
- Small mineralizations have also been reported in rare cases.
- Post-contrast: capsule/wall enhances after contrast administration.

Pancreatic abscess

Pancreatic abscesses are mainly the result of acute pancreatitis and pancreatic necrosis can develop as a complication from pancreatic pseudocyst. Although pancreatic abscesses are infrequently reported, mortality rates have been reported to range between 50 and 86%. Most pancreatic abscesses in dogs yield negative bacterial culture results and are thought to be sterile. Pancreatic abscesses seem to occur more frequently in

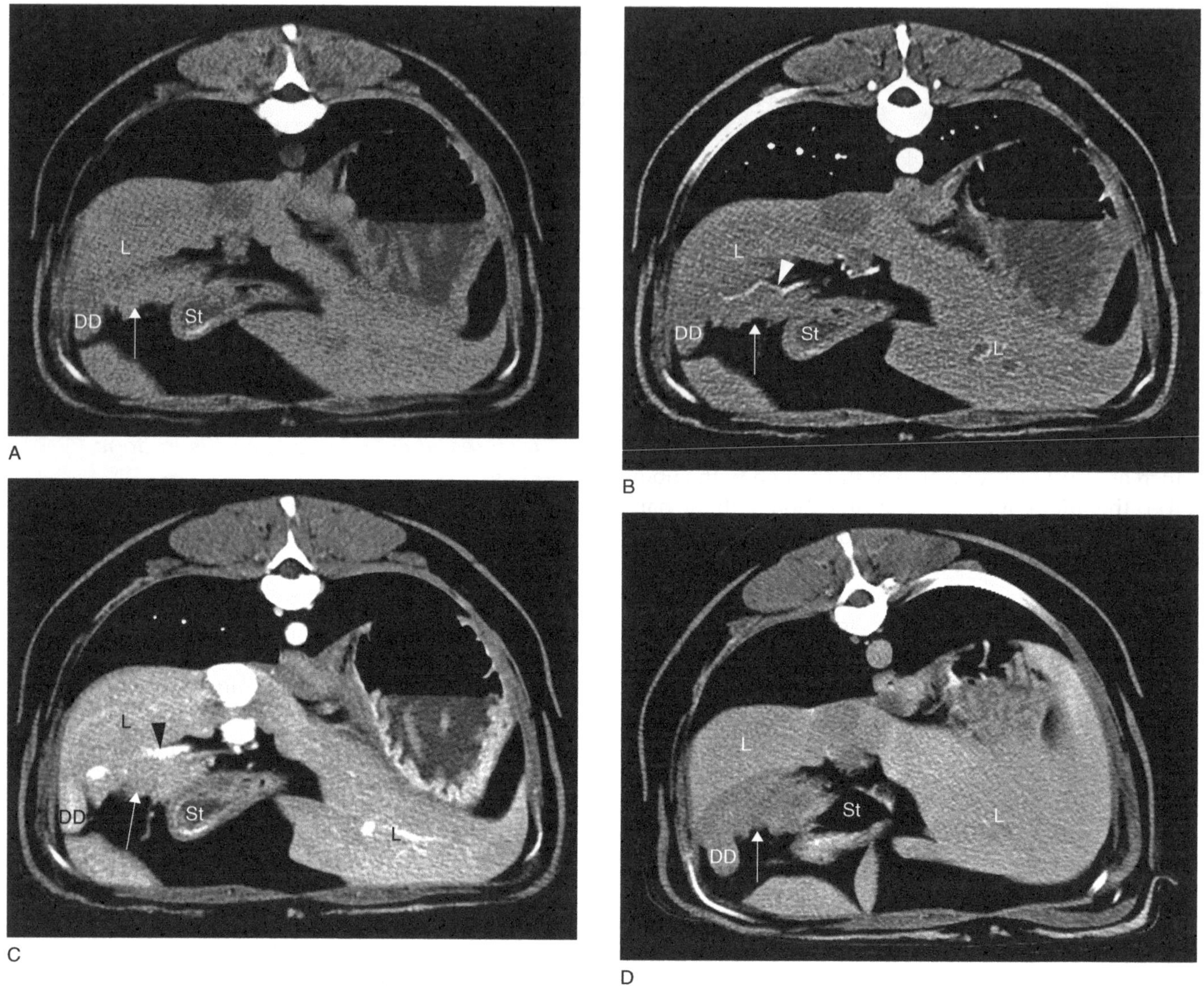

Figure 30.1 (A–D) CT images at the level of the pancreatic body (arrow) of a normal dog. (A) Pre-contrast phase: the pancreas is isodense to the liver and gastrointestinal tract. (B) Arterial phase: the gastroduodenal artery (arrowhead) is seen dorsal to the pancreatic body and shows early inhomogeneous enhancement. (C) Portal phase: the gastroduodenal vein dorsal to the body (arrowhead) and homogeneous contrast enhancement. (D) Delay phase: the pancreas is hypodense compared with the liver due to faster clearance. L = liver; DD = descending duodenum; St = stomach antrum. (E, F) Illustration of the pancreatic blood supply in dogs and cats (adapted from Caceres *et al.* 2006, with permission). (E) Arterial blood supply. Ao = aorta; CdPDA = caudal pancreaticoduodenal artery; CeA = celiac artery; CrMA = cranial mesenteric artery; CrPDA = cranial pancreaticoduodenal artery; GDA = gastroduodenal artery; HA = hepatic artery; HBr = hepatic branches of the hepatic artery; LGA = left gastric artery; LGEA = left gastroepiploic artery; RGA = right gastric artery; RGEA = right gastroepiploic artery; SpA = splenic artery. (F) Venous drainage. CdMV = caudal mesenteric vein; CdPDV = caudal pancreaticoduodenal vein; CrMV = cranial mesenteric vein; CrPDV = cranial pancreaticoduodenal vein; GDV = gastroduodenal vein; LGEV = left gastroepiploic vein; LGV = left gastric vein; PV = portal vein; RGEV = right gastroepiploic vein; RGV = right gastric vein; SpV = splenic vein.

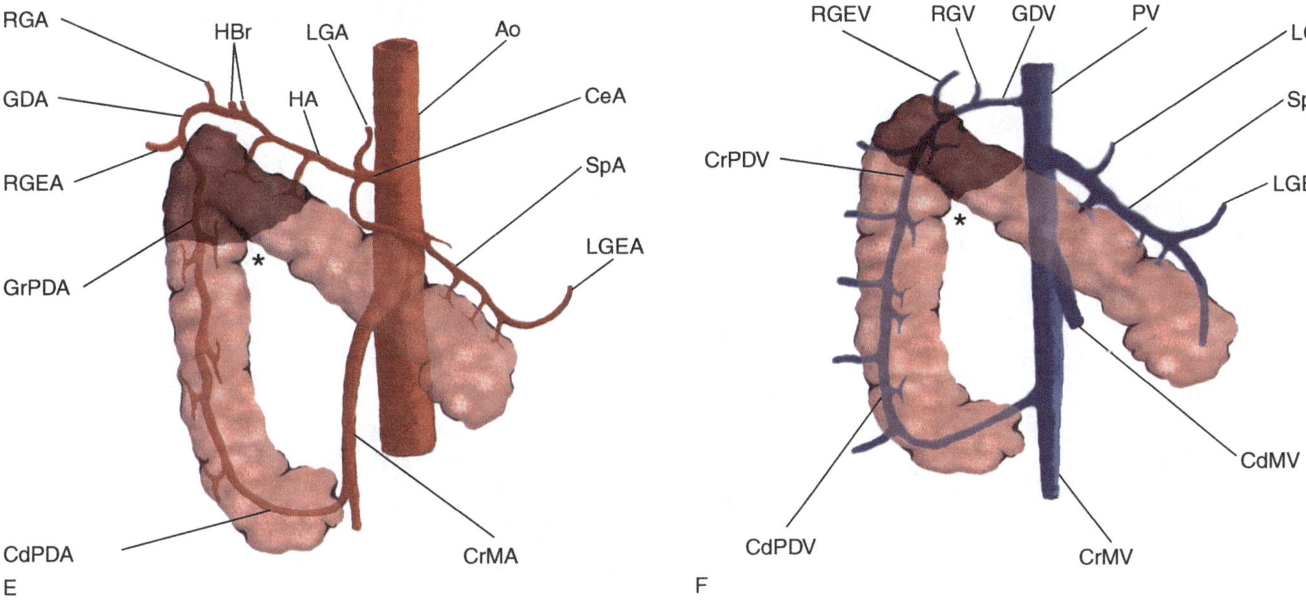

Figure 30.1 *(Continued)*

Table 30.3
Pancreatic dimensions of nine beagle mix dogs.

Pancreatic region	Median height (cm)	Median width (cm)	Median length (cm)
Right lobe	1.6 (1.2–2.1)	1.9 (1.4–2.4)	9.9 (8.3–12.0)
Left lobe	1.2 (0.8–1.9)	1.6 (0.7–2.8)	6.4 (3.6–6.7)
Body	1.4 (0.8–2.5)	4.8 (3.5–7.7)	Not measured

the right lobe, while pancreatitis and pancreatic necrosis seem to have no association to any lobe. In humans pancreatic abscess are thought to develop from translocation of bacterial from the adjacent inflamed colon.

CT features

- Cystic structure with ill-defined or irregular thick capsule.
- Low dense material in the center with gas bubbles.
- Post-contrast:
  - absence of central contrast enhancement
  - variable peripheral enhancement.

Neoplasia

Exocrine pancreatic tumor (adenoma, carcinoma)

Exocrine pancreatic tumors are rare in dogs and cats. There is no sex predilection but the Airedale terrier, boxer, Labrador retriever and cocker spaniels are at increased risk. Pancreatic neoplasia is very aggressive and has often metastasized to the liver and local lymph nodes or less common lungs at the time of diagnosis. Paraneoplastic alopecia and superficial necrolytic dermatitis have been described in a cat with pancreatic carcinoma.

Pancreatic hyperplasia may mimic neoplasia when it develops into a large mass, but the former is a benign focal enlargement that typically has similar pre- and post-contrast density characteristics of the normal gland (Figure 30.5).

CT features

- Hypodense pancreatic mass compared to the normal enhancing pancreas in all phases.
- In pancreatic tumor there is a 'cuff' of soft tissue encasing the peripancreatic vessels, while in pancreatitis there are perivascular striations.

Endocrine pancreatic tumor (insulinoma, gastrinoma, glucagonoma, somatostatinoma)

Insulinoma is the most common endocrine pancreatic neoplasm in dogs, ferrets and humans, but is rare in cats. They are typically functional secreting tumors that arise from the islet cells. More than 95% of insulinomas in dogs are malignant and about 40–50% of the tumor have visibly metastasized at the time of surgery. Large breed dogs are over represented.

Gastrinomas (Zollinger–Ellison syndrome) are rare gastrin-producing, non-β islet cell pancreatic tumors that result in gastric acid hypersecretion and gastrointestinal ulceration. The disease usually develops in middle-aged dogs and there in no breed predilection reported.

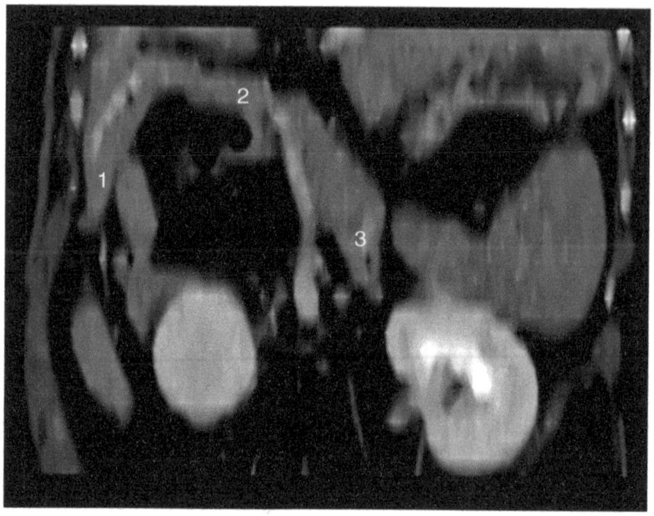

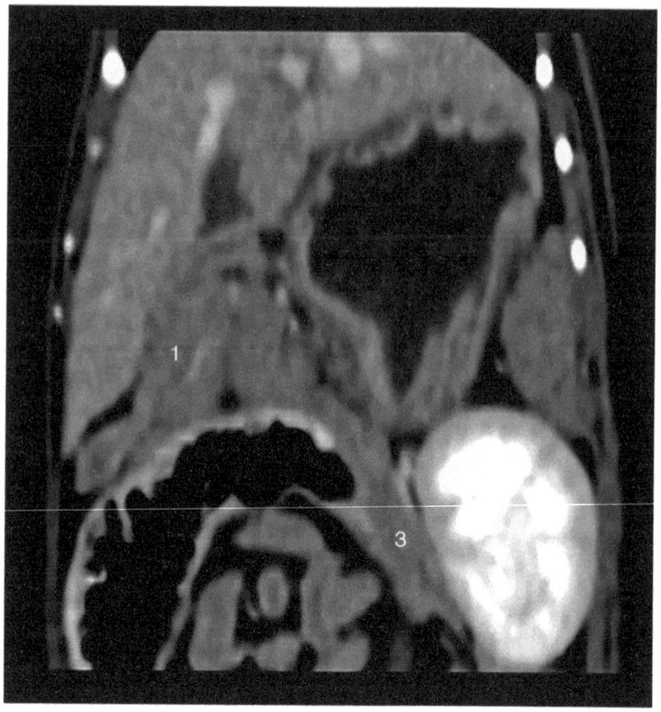

Figure 30.2 Dorsally reconstructed CT image of the normal pancreas (A) in a dog and (B) in a cat. In the cat, the angle of the pancreas is more acute than in the dog and the left pancreatic lobe extends to the caudal aspect of the left kidney. 1 = right lobe; 2 = body; 3 = left lobe.

Table 30.4
Vascular enhancement of nine beagle mix dogs at the level of the ***porta hepatis***.

Abdominal vessel	Median TA* (s)	Median TP† (s)
Aorta	6.3 (5.0–8.9)	10.5 (6.0–13.6)
Gastroduodenal artery	7.0 (5.2–9.2)	12.0 (9.7–14.0)
Gastroduodenal vein	12.0 (10.9–16.0)	23.0 (17.0–27.0)
Portal vein	12.2 (10.7–15.1)	32.0 (24.9–42.4)

*Time of appearance: time at 15% of peak contrast enhancement post start contrast medium injection.
†Time to peak: time between start of contrast medium injection and peak contrast enhancement.

Table 30.5
Pancreatic parenchymal enhancement of nine beagle mix dogs.

CT phase	Pancreas mean density (HU)	Liver mean density (HU)
Pre-contrast	61 (56–68)	65 (60–70)
Arterial	130 (96–164)	94 (84–108)
Venous	129 (110–155)	151 (132–168)
Delayed†	91 (78–110)	110 (84–136)

†Performed in five dogs.

Glucagonoma (alpha cell) and somatostatinoma (delta islet cell) are rare pancreatic neoplasia.

CT features (Figure 30.6)

- Dual-phase preferred.
- Small pancreatic mass that may or may not deform the surface. In the diffuse form only increase in thickness may be seen.
- Iso- to hypodense on pre-contrast.
- Post-contrast:
  - markedly contrast-enhancing (hyperdense) mass in the arterial phase, less commonly isodense
  - iso- to hyperdense in the portal phase
  - may see invasion to peripancreatic vasculature
  - contrast-enhancing, normal to mildly enlarged regional lymph nodes.

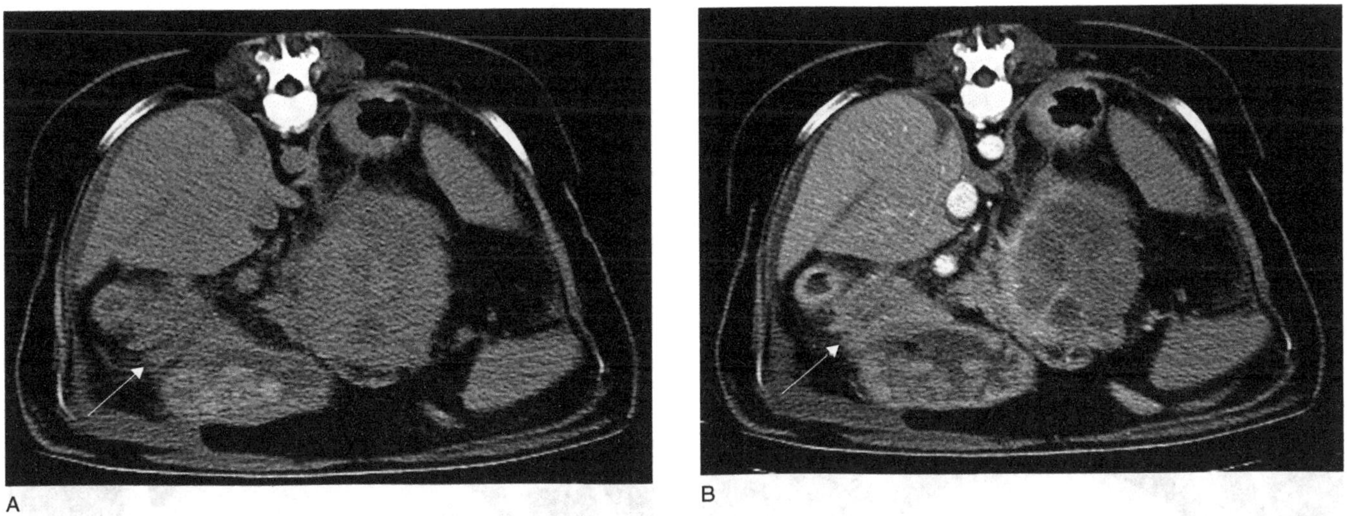

Figure 30.3 Adult dog with pancreatitis. (A) Pre-contrast CT image shows an enlarged, rounded pancreatic body (arrow) with inhomogeneous density (hyperdense center and hypodense peripancreatic mesentery). The duodenum is seen dorsolaterally and contains a mild amount of gas. (B) Post-contrast CT image at the same location shows heterogeneous contrast enhancement of the pancreas (arrow) with a less dense center, a mild enhancement of the peripancreatic mesentery, focal effusion ventrolateral to the pancreas. There is also focal enhancement and increased thickness of the medial wall of the stomach adjacent to the left lobe of the pancreas.

Further reading

Caceres AV, Zwingenberger AL, Hardam E, Lucena JM and Schwarz T (2006) Helical computed tomographic angiography of the normal canine pancreas. *Vet Radiol Ultrasound* **47**: 270–8.

Forman MA, Marks SL, De Cock HE *et al.* (2004) Evaluation of serum feline pancreatic lipase immunoreactivity and helical computed tomography versus conventional testing for the diagnosis of feline pancreatitis. *J Vet Intern Med* **18**: 807–15.

Head LL, Daniel GB, Tobias K, Morandi F, DeNovo RC and Donnell R (2003) Evaluation of the feline pancreas using computed tomography and radiolabeled leukocytes. *Vet Radiol Ultrasound* **44**: 420–8.

Iseri T, Yamada K, Chijiwa K *et al.* (2007) Dynamic computed tomography of the pancreas in normal dogs and in a dog with pancreatic insulinoma. *Vet Radiol Ultrasound* **48**: 328–31.

Jaeger JQ, Mattoon JS, Bateman SW and Morandi F (2003) Combined use of ultrasonography and contrast enhanced computed tomography to evaluate acute necrotizing pancreatitis in two dogs. *Vet Radiol Ultrasound* **44**: 72–9.

Robben JH, Pollak YW, Kirpensteijn J *et al.* (2005) Comparison of ultrasonography, computed tomography, and single-photon emission computed tomography for the detection and localization of canine insulinoma. *J Vet Intern Med* **19**: 15–22.

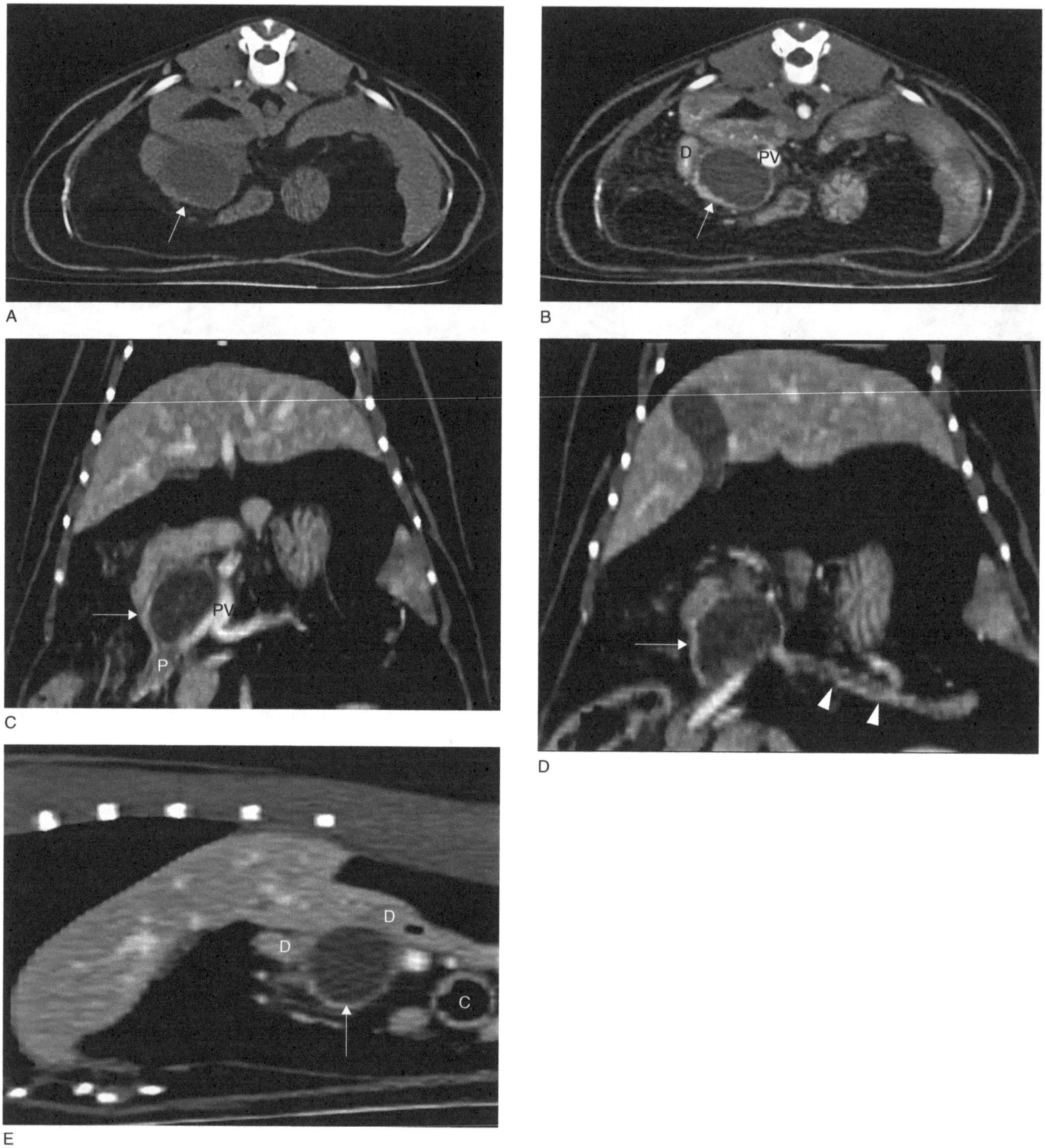

Figure 30.4 Adult cat with pancreatic pseudocyst (based on fluid analysis) in the cranial aspect of the pancreas. (A) Pre-contrast CT image shows an oval, hypodense cystic structure within the pancreas (arrow). (B) Post-contrast CT image shows the rim-enhancing cystic structure (arrow) and peripancreatic mesenteric inflammation. The cyst shows a slightly thickened and irregular portion on the ventrolateral aspect of the wall, representing portion of the right pancreatic lobe. D = duodenum; PV = portal vein. (C) Dorsally reconstructed CT image shows the pancreatic pseudocyst (arrow) to the right of the portal vein (PV). It is adjacent to the proximal aspect of the right pancreatic lobe (P). (D) Dorsally reconstructed CT image shows the pseudocyst (arrow) and the left pancreatic lobe (arrowheads). The left lobe is small sized and irregularly marginated. (E) Sagittally reconstructed CT image shows the relationship between the pseudocyst (arrow), duodenum (D) and transverse colon (C).

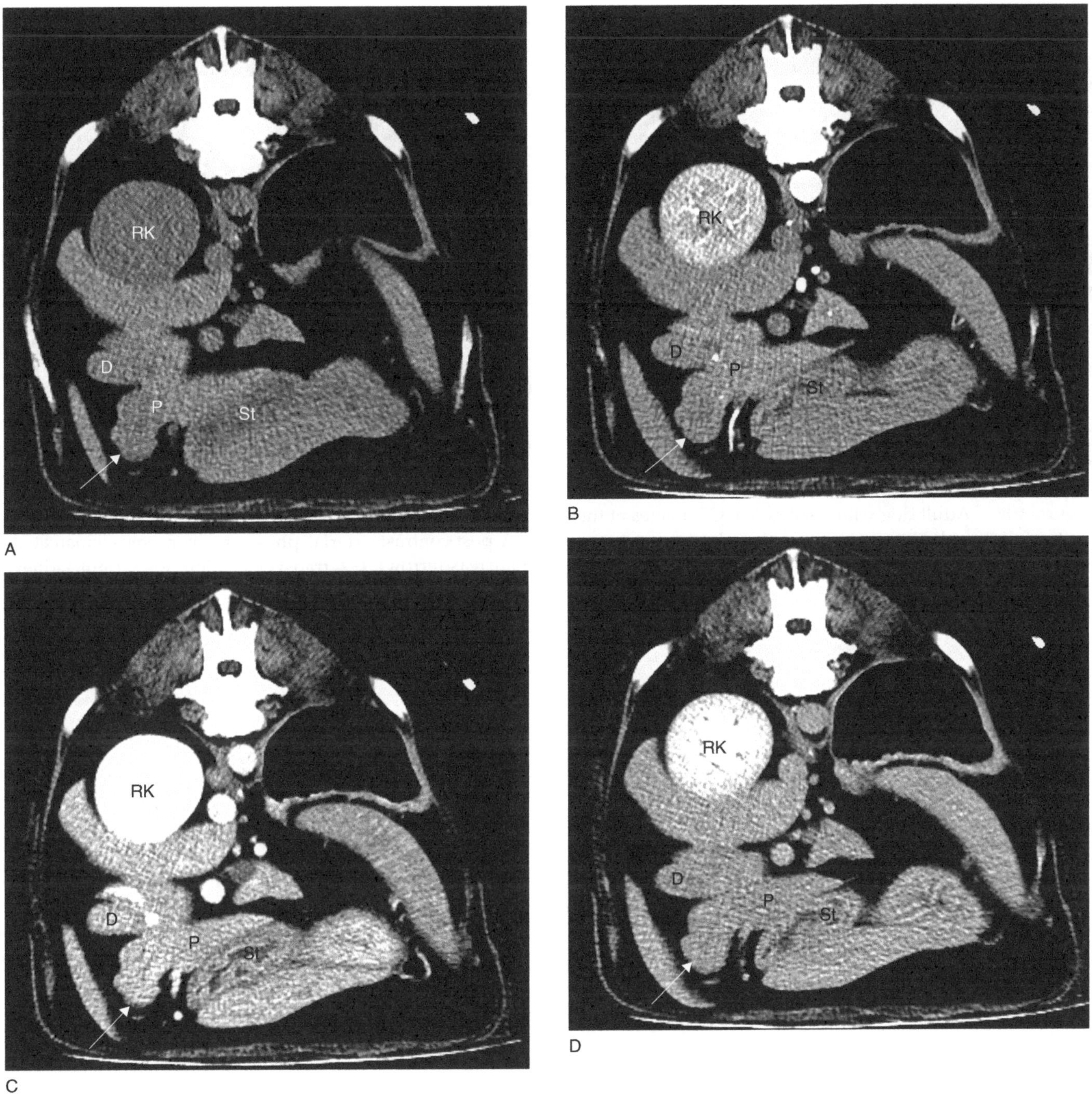

Figure 30.5 Adult dog with pancreatic hyperplasia. CT images at the level of the pancreatic body. (A) Pre-contrast phase, (B) arterial phase, (C) portal phase, (D) delay phase. There is a pedunculated slightly irregular, mildly hypodense mass extending ventrally from the body of the pancreas (arrow). There is no differential arterial enhancement from the rest of the pancreas which is isodense in the portal and delay phases. D = duodenum; P = pancreas; RK = right kidney; St = stomach.

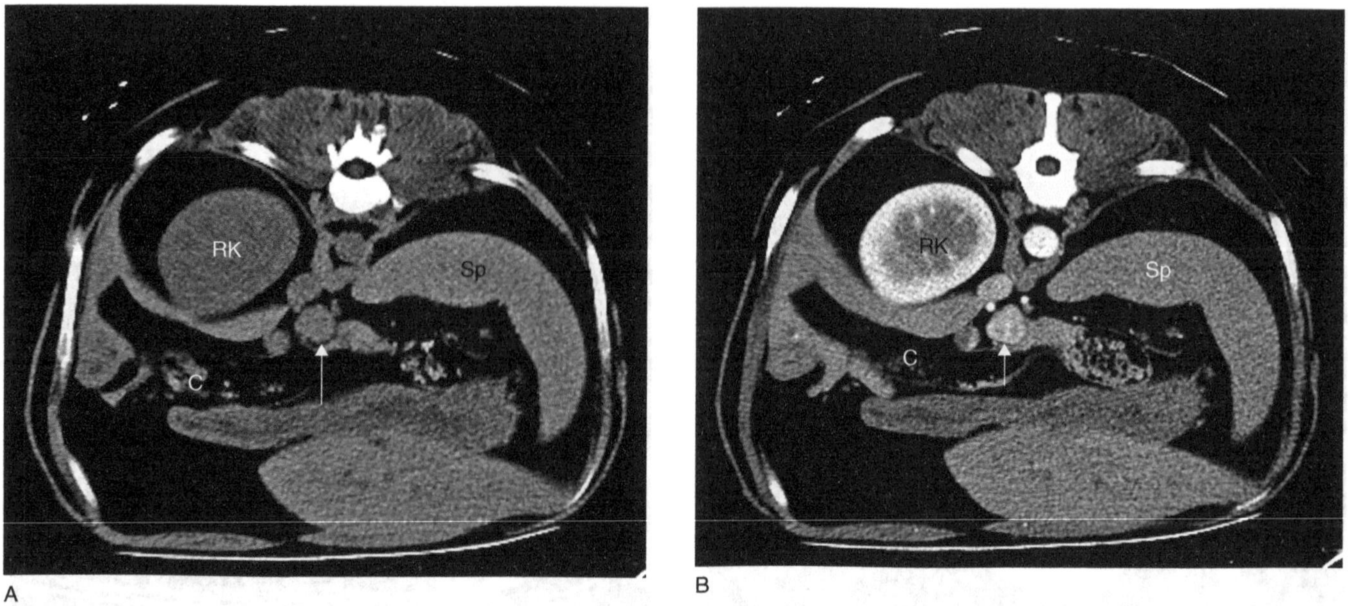

Figure 30.6 Adult dog with insulinoma. CT images at the level of the proximal aspect of the left pancreatic lobe. (A) A pre-contrast image shows focal pancreatic enlargement (arrow). (B) A post-contrast arterial phase shows a well-demarcated, markedly contrast enhancing mass deforming the shape of the pancreas (arrow). C = transverse colon; RK = right kidney; Sp = spleen.

CHAPTER THIRTY-ONE

Gastrointestinal Tract

Massimo Vignoli and Jimmy Saunders

Imaging Protocol

See Table 31.1. CT gastroenterography allows optimal visualization of the gastric and proximal intestinal wall. Fluid (Table 31.2) can be put into the stomach via a gastric tube and manual injection of 30 ml/kg bw. Scanning can start immediately after injection of contrast. Oral administration of water completed by intravenous injection of contrast medium is the most appropriate combination for visualization of the stomach and proximal intestine.

CT: Anatomy and Normal Variants

Stomach

The stomach is a hollow organ located caudal to the liver. From left to right, it is divided into a cardiac sphincter, a fundus, a body, a pyloric antrum and a pyloric sphincter. The stomach has a musculoglandular wall designed to store large volumes of food and continue the digestive process. Its inner lining secretes acids and enzymes to break down food. Additionally, the gastric mucosa has folds that help grind and digest food. Once the initial gastric phase of the digestive process is completed, the partially digested food exits the stomach through the pyloric sphincter into the duodenum. Liquids are emptied in an exponential pattern without evidence of a lag phase. In contrast to this, solid food is emptied with a lag phase of varying length, depending on the composition and temperature of the ingesta, and follows a more linear pattern afterwards.

The size and shape of the stomach vary depending of the size of the animal, the gastric content and the degree of distention (Figure 31.1). For CT imaging of the stomach, adequate distention is essential (Figures 31.1B,C). If the stomach is not well distended, diseases may be overlooked or, conversely, the collapsed gastric wall may mimic disease.

Small intestine

The small intestine follows the stomach. It is a tube-like structure of about 2.5 times the animal's total body length and consists of three parts: duodenum, jejunum and ileum. The duodenum is quite short and receives enzymes and other secretions from the pancreas and liver via the pancreatic and common bile ducts (Figure 31.2). The jejunum is the middle and longest portion (±90% of the length). It is rich in villi, which are small, finger-like structures that protrude inwards into the food contents and increase the absorption surface for the nutrients. Villi are not visible on CT. The short ileum connects to the large intestine. On post-contrast CT, the normal bowel wall shows marked contrast enhancement allowing detection of hypoperfused areas.

Large intestine

The large intestine connects the small intestine to the anus. It has several distinct parts: the cecum (near the junction with the small intestine, the colon (longest portion) and the rectum (final portion). The primary function of the large intestine is to absorb water from feces as needed, thus keeping the hydration level of the body constant.

Veterinary Computed Tomography, First Edition. Edited by Tobias Schwarz, Jimmy Saunders.

Feline anatomical specificities (Figure 31.3)
The stomach is left-sided with the pylorus mostly located at the level of the vertebral column. The gastric folds are less numerous and thinner than those in the dog. On CT, an intramural lucent band and hypodense layer corresponds to fat in the gastric submucosa. This band is a normal anatomic feature. The normal small intestine contains less gas in cats than in dogs. The feline cecum is very short.

Disease Features

Gastrointestinal foreign body

It is very common for dogs and cats, especially young ones, to ingest objects other than food. Most of this foreign material, such as small pieces of bone, passes through the gastrointestinal tract without, or with minimal, clinical incidence. Sometimes larger objects become partially or completely lodged. Most common obstructive foreign bodies are latex teat, plastic objects, string/rope/fishing lines, stones or balls, but many others have been reported. In dogs, the jejunum is the most common location of discrete foreign objects, while in cats the distribution is more uniform. Linear foreign bodies are most commonly anchored at the pylorus in dogs and around the tongue in cats. Foreign bodies may cause bowel perforation.

Table 31.1
CT imaging protocol (intravenous contrast study: standard protocol; *see* Chapter 5).

Series	Pre- and post-contrast gastroenterography
Decubitus	Ventral
Scan margins	Cranial abdomen ⟷ Caudal pelvis
Voltage (kVp)	120–140
Current (mAs)	100 (cats and small dogs); 250 (big dogs)
Tube rotation time (s)	0.8–1
Slice width (mm)	1.25–5
Kernel frequency	Low to medium
Collimator pitch	1–2
Helical image reconstruction interval	½ of the slice width
Motion control	Hyperventilation to achieve expiratory apnea
Window level (HU)	+40
Window width (HU)	300–400

Table 31.2
Contrast procedures for the gastrointestinal tract

Study	Agent	Features
Gastroenterography	Positive contrast agents	– do not mix uniformly with gastric contents, and pseudotumors can be created – may mask subtle lesions, particularly when combined with IV contrast – can complicate 3-D reconstructions – optimal distention of the small intestine (barium)
	Water	– inexpensive, well-tolerated – allows good visualization of the enhancing wall – improved visualization of the gastric wall – better detection of subtle disease – does not interfere with 3-D reconstructions – suboptimal distention of the small intestine (because of rapid transit)
	Positive contrast agent followed by water	– positive contrast material will fill the distal small bowel loops, and the water will distend the stomach and proximal small bowel
Intravenous contrast		– used in addition of oral agents – improved visualization of disease processes

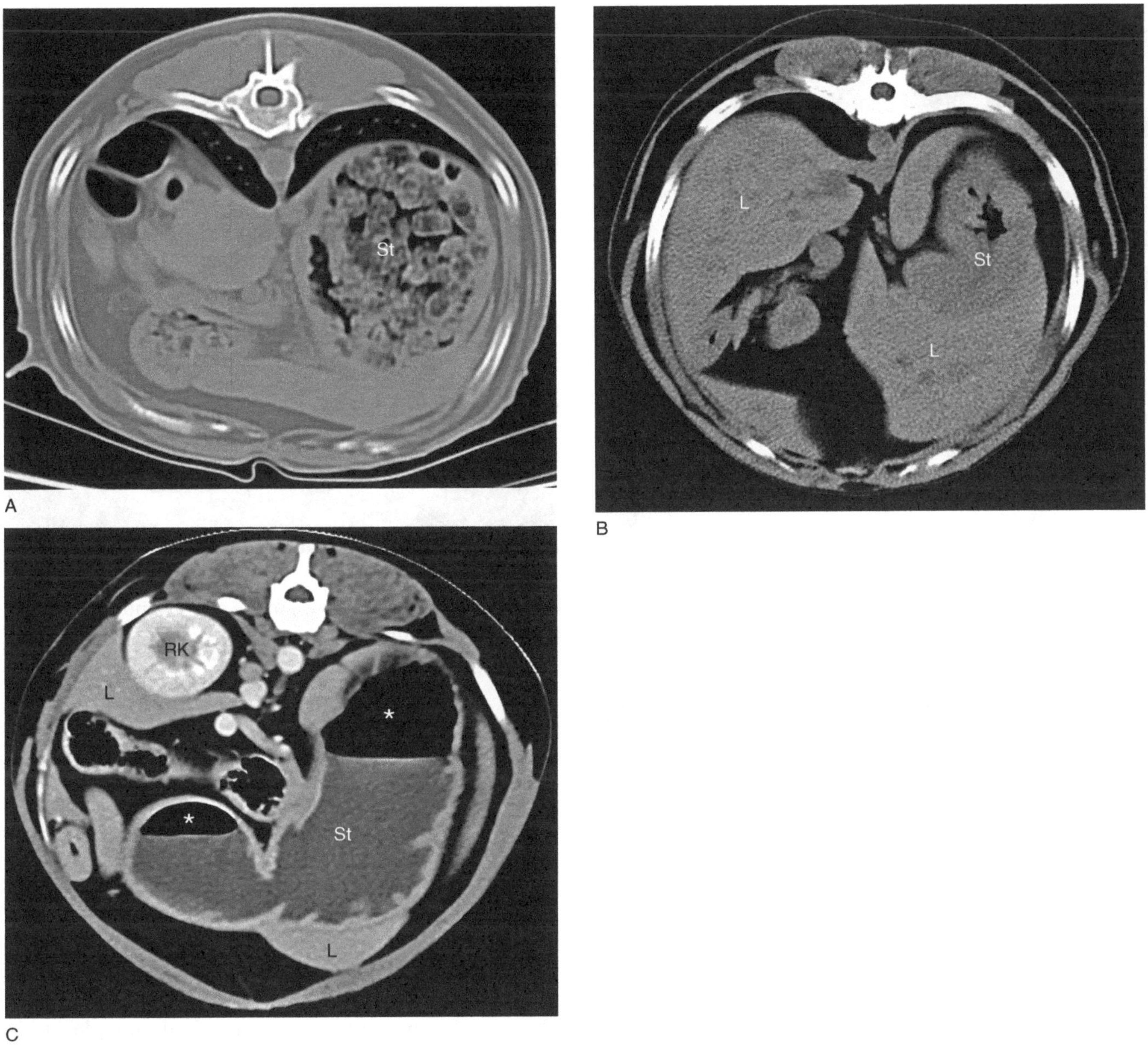

Figure 31.1 Transverse CT images at the level of the stomach. (A) Stomach filled with solid food. (B,C) Normal stomach in a medium-sized dog, (B) before and (C) after administration of water (30 ml/kg) in the stomach. CT gastrography using water greatly improves the visualization of the stomach wall. A small amount of gas is present in the dilated stomach (asterisks). L = liver; RK = right kidney; St = stomach.

CT features (Figure 31.4)

- Have not been reported.
- Anticipated features on CT:
  - foreign material may show different densities
  - fluid surrounds the foreign bodies
  - if secondary obstruction: intestinal wall thickening due to inflammation.

Gastrointestinal perforation

Possible causes of gastrointestinal perforation include ruptured ulceration following steroid and/or NSAID therapy, dehiscence after surgery, chronic non-neoplastic bowel disease, localized granuloma or neoplasia leading to necrosis, foreign body or, mainly for the large intestine, fractured bone fragments.

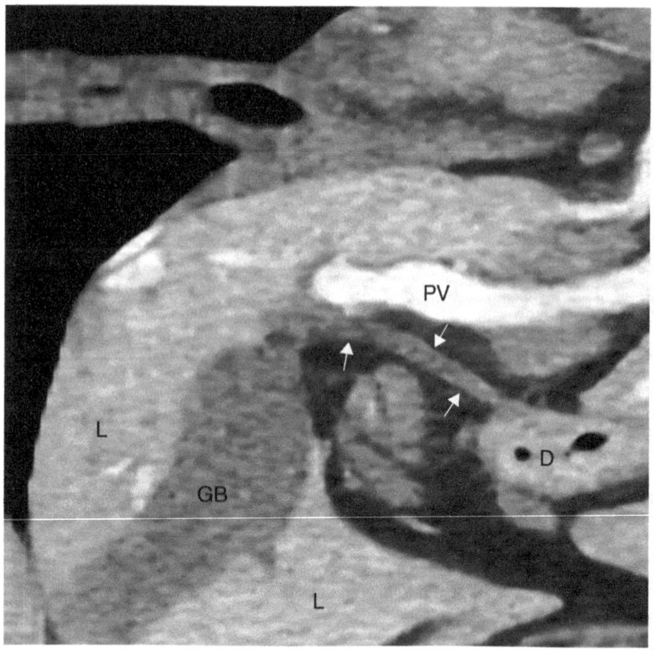

Figure 31.2 Sagittally reconstructed CT image shows the biliary duct (arrows) originating in the gallbladder (GB) and entering the duodenum (D). L = liver; PV = portal vein.

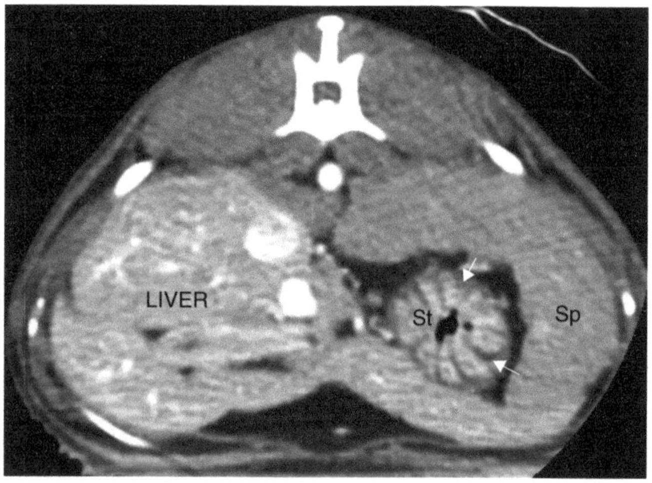

Figure 31.3 Post-contrast transverse CT image shows hypodense layers (arrows) in the gastric wall of an adult cat corresponding to normal fat. Sp = spleen; St = stomach.

CT features (Figure 31.5)

- Small pockets of extraluminal gas.
- Small amount of peritoneal free fluid.
- Intestinal wall thickening.
- Post-contrast (IV): enhancement of the surrounding inflamed tissue.
- CT gastroenterography: contrast visible outside the intestinal lumen.

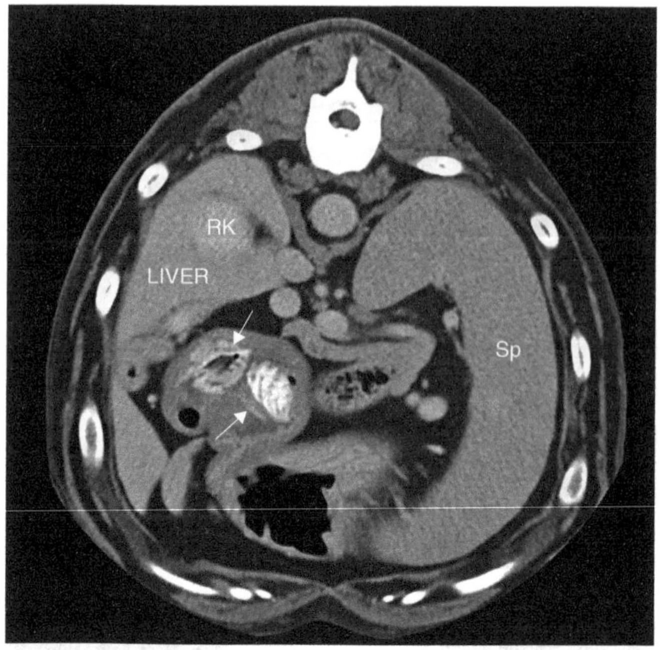

Figure 31.4 Transverse CT image of an adult dog with two foreign bodies (peach stones) in the pyloric antrum (arrows) surrounded by fluid. RK = right kidney; Sp = spleen.

- Depending on the cause, a neoplastic or granulomatous mass, foreign body or bone fragment may be seen.

Gastrointestinal neoplasia

The most common gastrointestinal neoplasia is malignant lymphoma in the cat, and adenocarcinoma in the dog followed by smooth muscle tumors. A strong breed predisposition for gastric tumors is present in rough collies, Staffordshire terriers and Belgian shepherd dogs.

CT features (Figures 31.6–31.8)

- Have not been reported.
- Anticipated features on CT:
  - inhomogeneous, soft tissue mass of variable size (mostly large at presentation) in the gastric/intestinal wall
  - lymphoma: symmetric or asymmetric thickening of the gastric/intestinal wall over a variable distance
  - contrast (IV) enhancement.

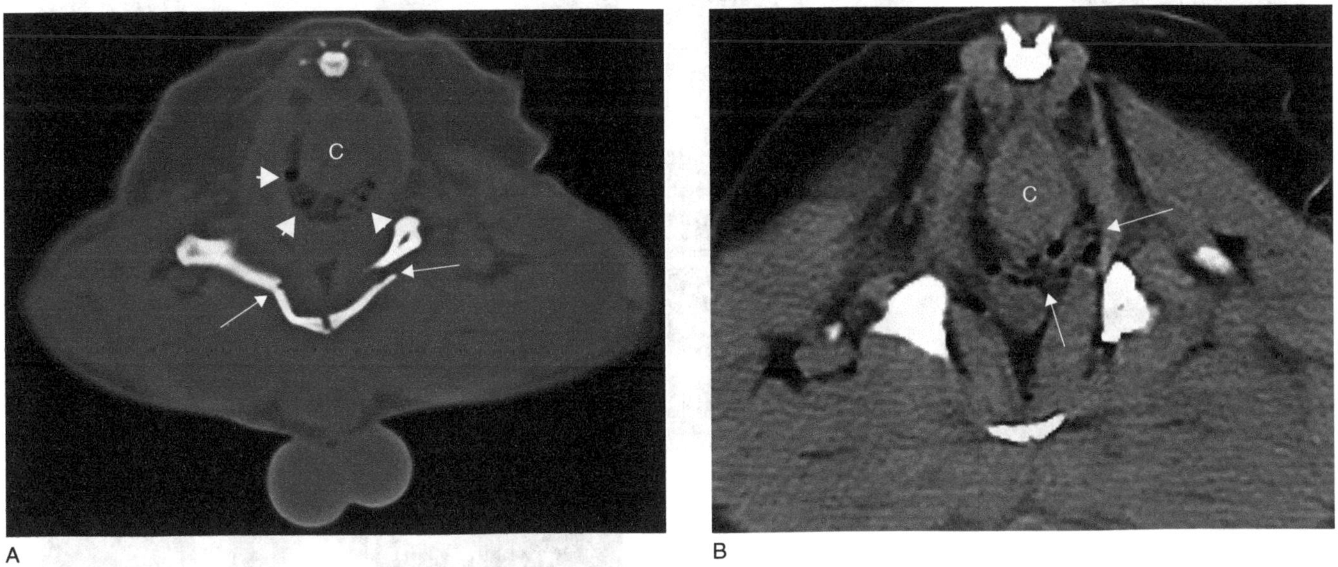

Figure 31.5 Miniature poodle with colonic laceration. It was in a car accident 6h prior to CT. (A) Transverse CT image shows gas bubbles outside the colon (short arrows). Pelvic fractures are visible (long arrows) with sharply delineated fracture ends. (B) Transverse CT image shows colonic laceration with gas bubbles exiting the colon (arrows). C = colon.

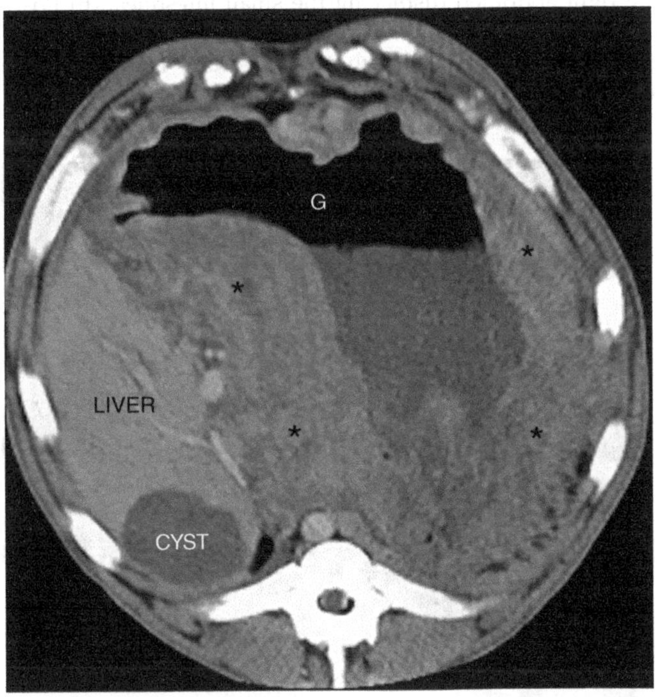

Figure 31.6 Adult dog with gastric adenocarcinoma. Transverse CT image (dog in dorsal decubitus) shows a soft tissue density mass involving almost the complete stomach wall (asterisks). The stomach is moderately filled with fluid and also contains gas (G). A cyst is present in the liver.

Further Reading

Fant P, Caldin M, Furlanello T *et al.* (2004) Primary gastric histiocytic sarcoma in a dog–a case report. *J Vet Med A Physiol Pathol Clin Med* **51**: 358–62.

Hylands R (2005) Veterinary diagnostic imaging. Longitudinal intestinal perforation at the level of the proximal duodenum near the pylorus resulting in a septic peritonitis. *Can Vet J* **46**: 748–50.

Terragni R, Rossi F, Laganga P *et al.* (2010) Evaluation of the stomach wall by helical hydro-CT: normal technique and clinical cases. *Proc Annual ESVONC Meeting*, p. 45. Turin, Italy.

Yamada K, Morimoto M, Kishimoto M and Wisner ER (2007) Virtual endoscopy of dogs using multi-detector row CT. *Vet Radiol Ultrasound* **48**: 318–22.

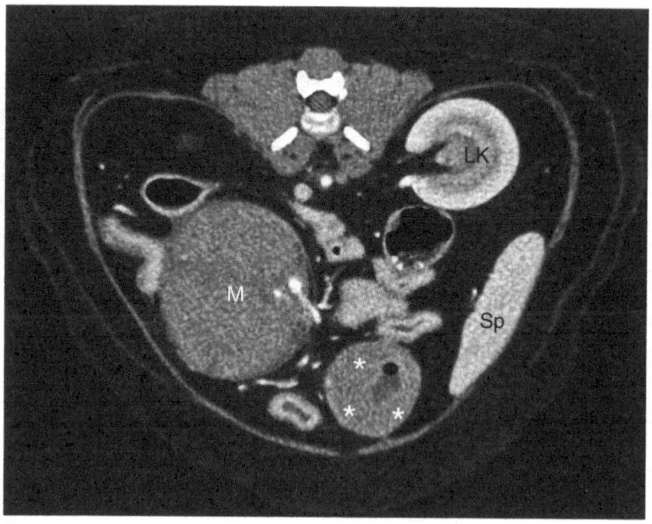

A

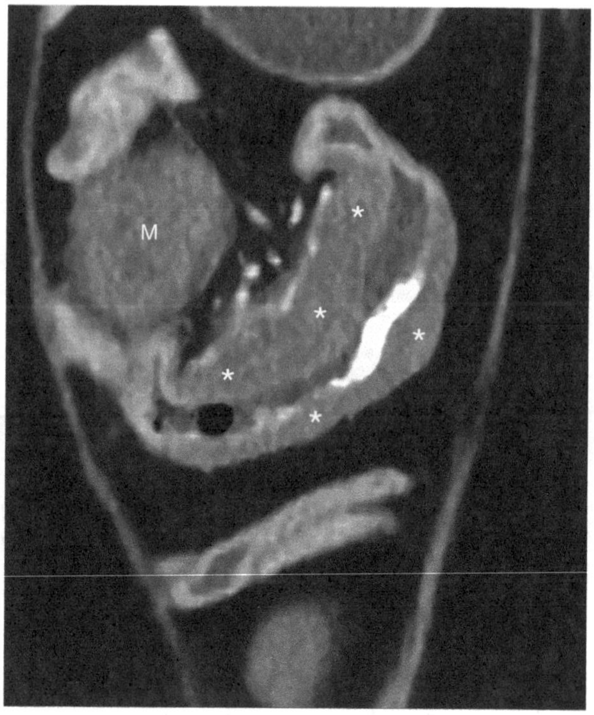

B

Figure 31.7 Adult cat with intestinal lymphoma. (A) Post-contrast transverse CT image shows a transverse slice of the small intestine filled with mucus and gas with a severely thickened and asymmetric wall (asterisks). A large circular mass (M), diagnosed as a tumoral lymph node after biopsy, is visible in the right abdomen displacing the small intestines. (B) Post-contrast dorsally reconstructed CT image shows an asymmetric thickening of the small intestinal wall over a few centimeters (asterisks). The intestinal lumen is filled with mucus, a small gas bubble and a trace of contrast medium. The previously described lymph node is visible (M). LK = left kidney; SP = spleen.

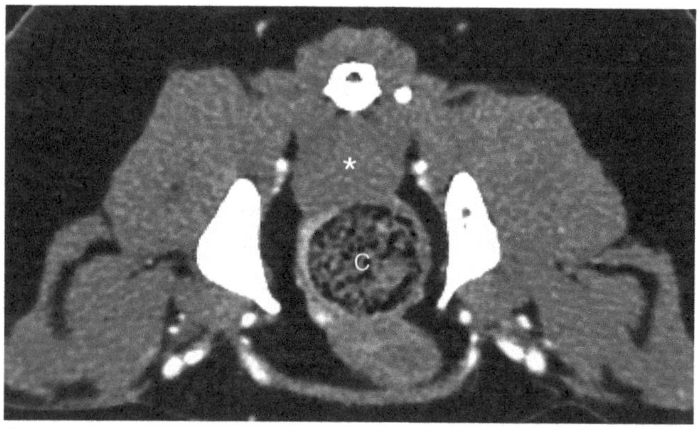

A

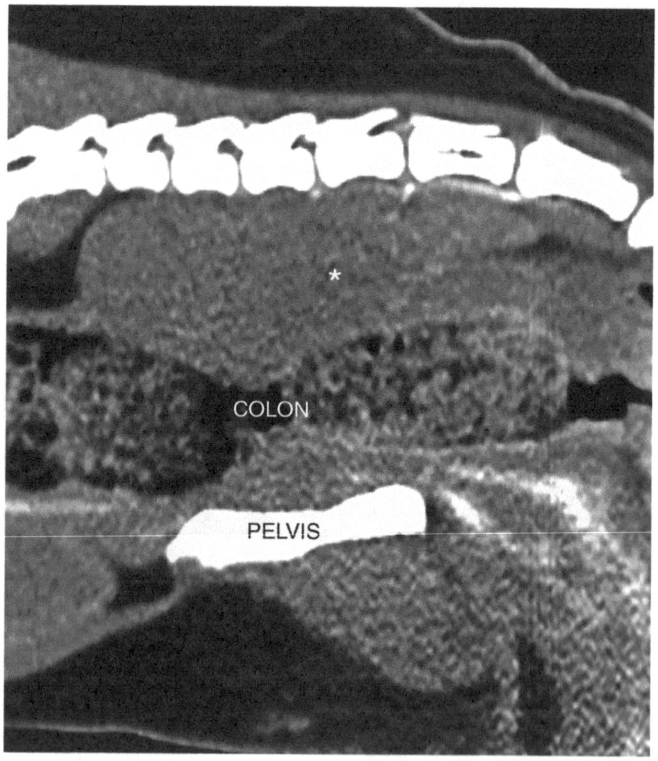

B

Figure 31.8 Adult dog with a leiomyoma of the large intestine. (A) Transverse CT image shows a circular isodense mass (asterisk) located between the tail and the dorsal wall of the large intestine (C). (B) Sagittally reconstructed CT image shows the mass (asterisk) extending from the level of the sacrum to at least the seventh coccygeal vertebra.

CHAPTER THIRTY-TWO

Urinary System

Tobias Schwarz

Imaging Technique

See Table 32.1.

CT: Anatomy and Normal Variants (Figures 4.24C, 32.1–32.3)

The kidneys can be well visualized on CT and their size, shape, density, location and number can be assessed. Parenchymal-phase post-contrast images show cortical and later medullary contrast medium uptake which can be inhomogeneous. On excretory phase images there is a hyperlucent halo around the contrast-enhanced renal pelvis, due to beam hardening (*see also* Chapter 4, beam hardening).

The ureters, urinary bladder and urethra should be followed on the pre-contrast series first to rule out ureterolithiasis that would be obliterated on excretory phase images by contrast-enhanced urine. The distal ureters are closely located to the descending colon. A large fecal-filled colon can make the ureteral identification more difficult.

Parenchymal phase images are helpful to visualize the contrast-enhancing mucosa of the ureters, urinary bladder and urethra.

Excretory phase images should be performed with an elevated pelvis, so that the gravitationally dependent contrast-enhanced urine pools in the cranioventral bladder, away from the clinically relevant trigone area and vesicourethral junction.

The female urethra can be outlined with a retrograde vaginogram study; however, urethral filling is not consistently achieved with this technique (see also Chapter 33, Vagina).

Urological Abnormalities

Renal abnormalities

Abnormal renal shape, size, density and contrast enhancement can be well visualized with CT. Glomerular filtration rate can be estimated with applied software; however, this is still not widely available in veterinary practice. Secondary effects of renal insufficiency and failure can also be evident on CT images, such as gastric wall mineralization, increased excretion via alternative pathways (biliary, intestinal mucosa) or increased lymphatic uptake and bone demineralization.

CT features (Figures 32.4 and 32.5)

- Irregular small kidneys with chronic renal disease.
- Non-enhancing wedge-shaped areas with infarcts.
- Pelvis distention with pyelonephritis and hydronephrosis.
- Mineralized concretions with urolithiasis.
- Irregular contrast-enhancing or non-enhancing masses with neoplasia.
- Gastric or aortic wall mineralization, osteopenia, marked excretion of contrast medium into gallbladder and intestinal lumen in case of renal insufficiency and failure.

Ureteral abnormalities

Pre-contrast CT is a quick and efficient imaging modality to screen for ureterolithiasis in dogs and cats. Ureteral distention and lack of peristalsis can be assessed on serial examinations or dynamic CT. The parenchymal and excretory phases can be helpful to

Veterinary Computed Tomography, First Edition. Edited by Tobias Schwarz, Jimmy Saunders.

Table 32.1
CT imaging protocol.

Series	Pre-contrast	Post-contrast parenchymal phase	Post-contrast excretory phase	Post-contrast excretory phase ureterovesical junction dynamic CT
Decubitus	Ventral with pelvis elevated			
Scan margins	Cranial pole right kidney to anus			Stationary at caudal bladder neck
Voltage (kVp)	120			
Current (mAs)	120–200			
Tube rotation time (s)	1			
Slice width (mm)	3–5			5 using maximum number of image channels (e.g. 4 × in 4-slice CT)
Pitch/Temporal slice interval and duration	1.5–2			1 s slice interval for 30 s
Helical image reconstruction interval	Half of slice width			Equal to tube rotation time
Kernel frequency	Medium			
Motion control	Not required			
Contrast medium application site	N/A	Cephalic or external jugular vein		
Contrast medium type	N/A	Iodinated		
Contrast medium dose	N/A	400 mg I/kg bw		
Contrast medium injection mode	N/A	Manual		
Scan delay post start contrast injection	N/A	None	2–4 min	5–10 min
Window level (HU)	100–200		300–500	
Window width (HU)	300–500		1000–1600	

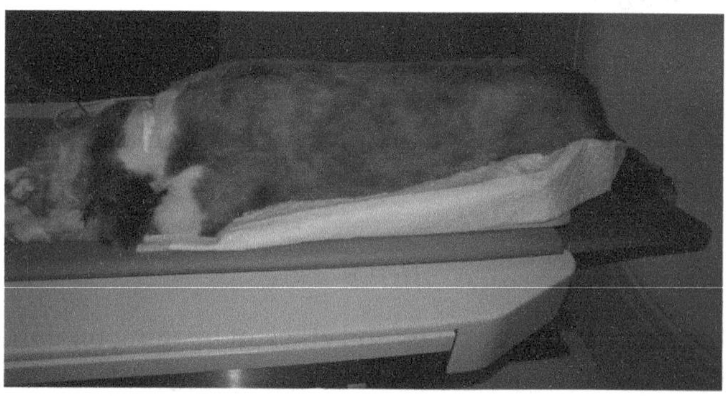

Figure 32.1 For a urologic CT examination the patient should be positioned in ventral recumbence with the pelvis elevated on a wedge with a 5° to 10° angle.

assess luminal distention if a pre-contrast series was performed.

CT is the modality of choice to assess the normo- or ectopic ureteral ending, since it requires no colonic enema preparation and is quick and easy to perform. Due to the higher specific gravity, contrast-enhanced urine sinks to the bottom of the urinary bladder. To demonstrate the entrance point of a ureter, the jet of contrast-enhanced urine drizzling through the non-enhanced higher urine layers needs to be visualized. If the contrast-enhanced ureter continues caudal from this point, a partially ectopic ureter is present. If the ureter is completely ectopic and only connects to the urethra, the urethral lumen is contrast enhanced and contrast-enhanced urine runs back to the urinary bladder. Ectopic ureters can also connect to the vagina. If the patient is not properly positioned in ventral

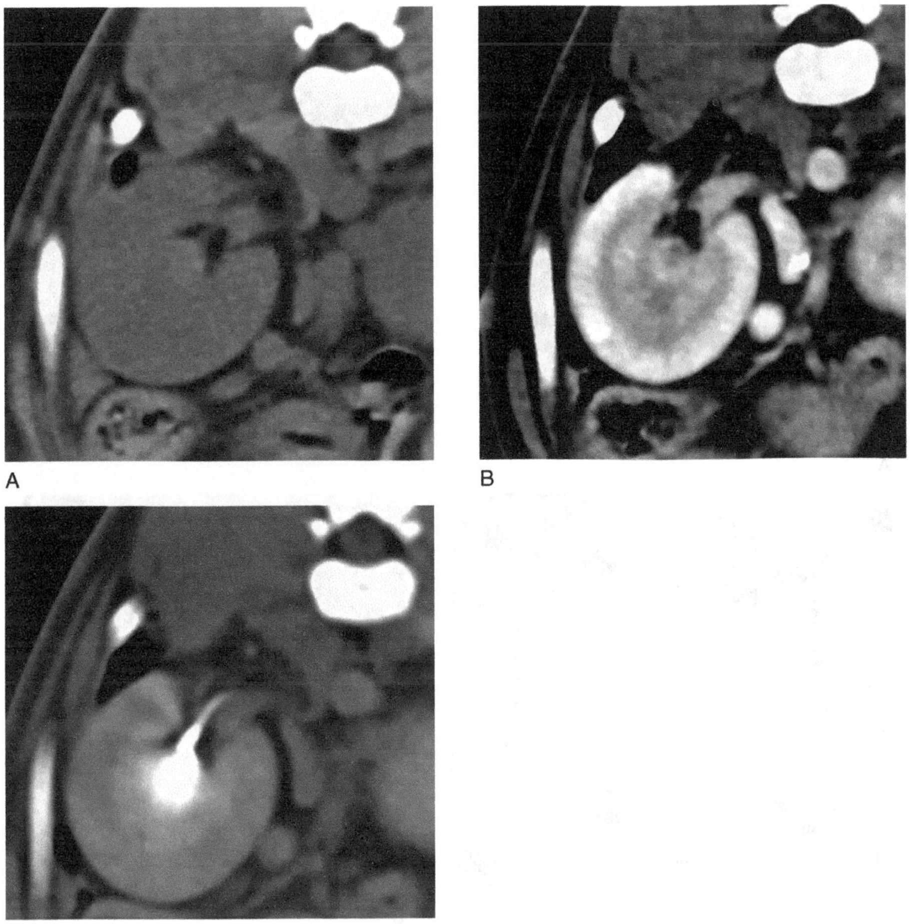

A B C

Figure 32.2 Normal CT features of a right canine kidney, transverse images. (A) On the pre-contrast image the renal parenchyma is homogeneously soft tissue dense. The renal pelvis lining is often slightly hyperdense and is surrounded by hilar fat. The ureter can be identified. (B) In the parenchymal contrast enhancement phase, the renal cortex is most markedly contrast enhancing. (C) In the excretory phase, the renal pelvis and ureter are strongly contrast enhancing. Beam hardening creates a dark halo around the renal pelvis.

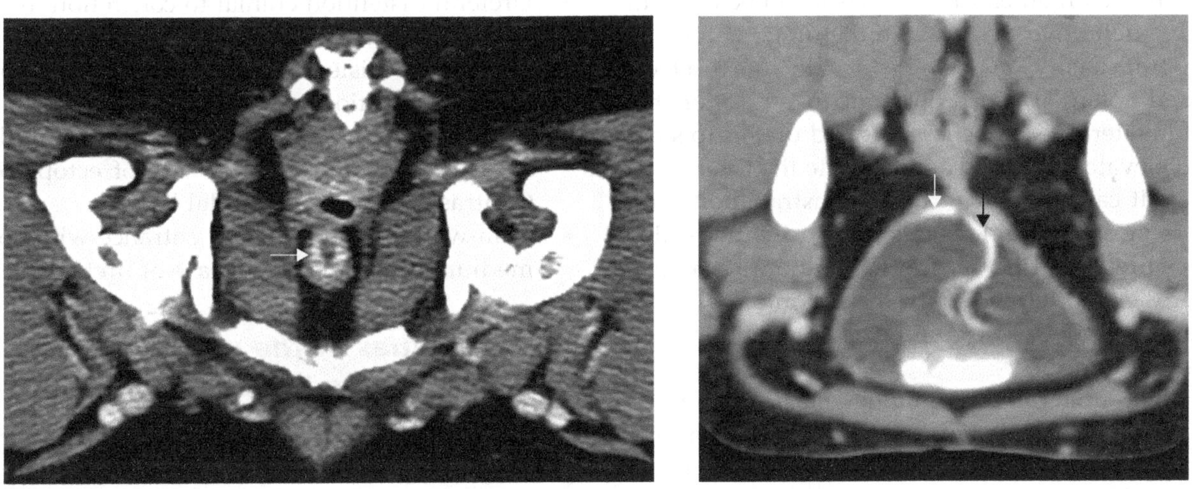

A B

Figure 32.3 Transverse CT images. (A) Normal mucosal enhancement of the pelvic urethra (arrow) in a male dog after intravenous contrast medium application. (B) Normal location of both ureterovesical junctions (arrows) in a dog. A left urine jet (black arrow) drizzles through the non-enhanced urine towards the bottom of the urinary bladder.

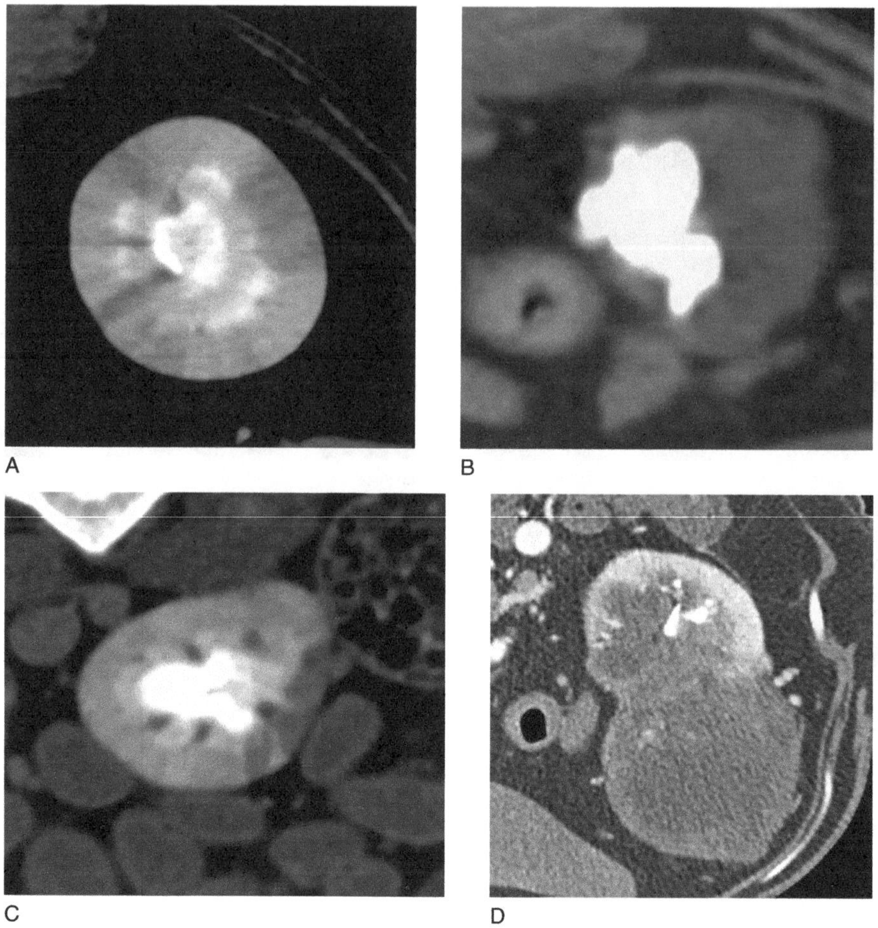

Figure 32.4 Transverse CT images of the kidney. (A) Small, irregular feline kidney with a wedge-shaped non-enhancing cortical area consistent with chronic nephritis and infarction. (B) Large nephrolith in a feline renal pelvis. (C) Distended, contrast enhanced renal pelvis and wedge-shaped non-enhancing cortical area in a dog with pyelonephritis and renal infarction. (D) Non-contrast-enhancing renal carcinoma mass in a dog.

recumbency with an elevated pelvis it can be difficult to reach a definitive diagnosis. If the ureter enters the bladder from a very lateral angle (usually due to a fecal distended colon) it can be helpful to reposition the patient in lateral recumbency (affected ureter up side) with an elevated pelvis to demonstrate the ureteral jet this way. It can be difficult to demonstrate both ureteral jets in one imaging series due to the peristaltic nature of ureteral urine transport. Therefore a dynamic CT over the bladder neck with the maximum number of image channels is recommend to monitor both ureters over time.

For other ureteral abnormalities such as a ureterocele or ureteritis it is important to scan during the parenchymal and excretory phases to be able to assess the mucosal lining and peristalsis.

CT features (Figures 32.5–32.9)

- Mineralized intraluminal concretions in ureterolithiasis.
- Ureteral distention cranial to concretion in case of obstructive ureterolithiasis.
- Uniformly distended ureter with hydroureter (ectopic, infection).
- Contrast-enhanced ureter entering caudal bladder neck, urethra or vagina in case of ectopic ureter. Contrast jet in too far caudal location.
- Thin-walled cystic ureteral entrance with contrast medium accumulation in case of ureterocele.

Abnormalities of the urinary bladder and urethra (Figures 32.9, 32.10 and 33.11)

Although CT is not the modality of choice to investigate these organs, it can be useful to assess them to provide a complete urologic work-up or in cases of suspected secondary changes due to other diseases, such as urolithiasis and cystitis secondary to portosystemic shunts. Wall thickening, mass formation and urolithiasis can be documented using CT. An intrapel-

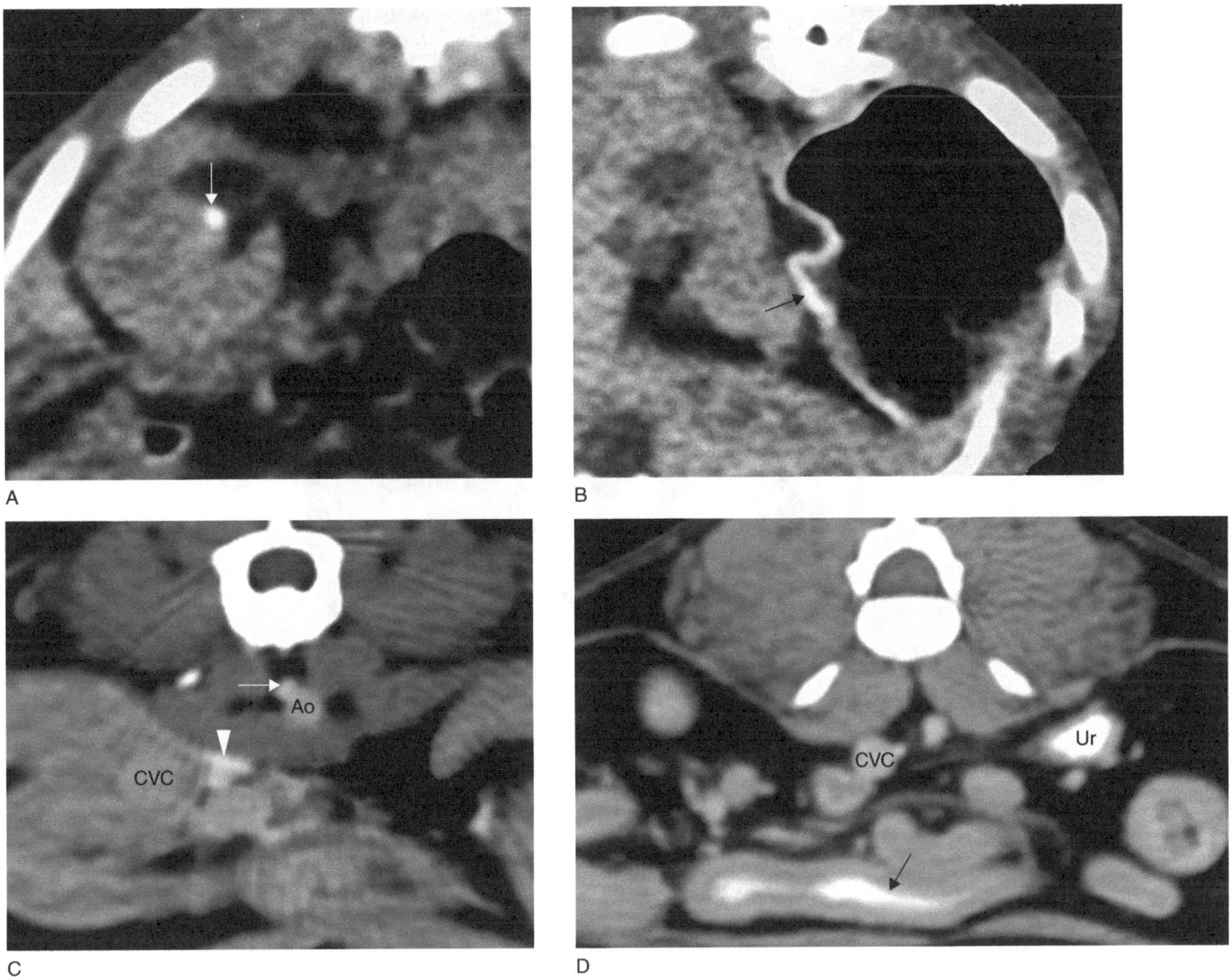

Figure 32.5 Transverse CT images showing secondary features of renal failure. (A,B) Chronic renal failure in a guinea pig with (A) obstructive renolithiasis (white arrow) and (B) a mineralized gastric wall (black arrow) due to secondary uremic gastritis. (C,D) Chronic renal failure in a cat with obstructive urolithiasis. (C) Increased contrast medium uptake in afferent abdominal lymph vessels (arrowhead) and the cisterna chyli (white arrow), located dorsolaterally to the aorta (Ao). (D) Intestinal mucosal contrast medium excretion (black arrow). CVC = caudal vena cava. Ur = obstructive ureterolith.

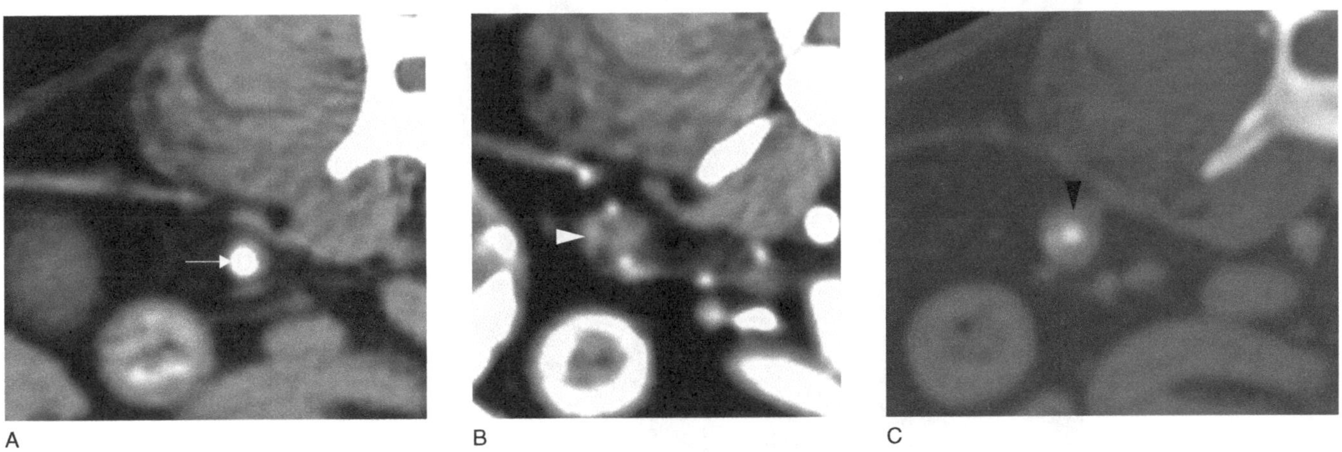

Figure 32.6 Diagnosis of obstructive urolithiasis in a cat with the help of different CT techniques, transverse images. (A) Mineral-dense concretion (arrow) in the right ureter on pre-contrast CT. (B) Parenchymal-phase contrast CT proximal to the concretion demonstrates mucosal enhancement (arrowhead) and luminal distention. (C) Excretory CT at the same location demonstrates ureteral wall thickening and luminal distention (arrowhead), indicative of obstruction.

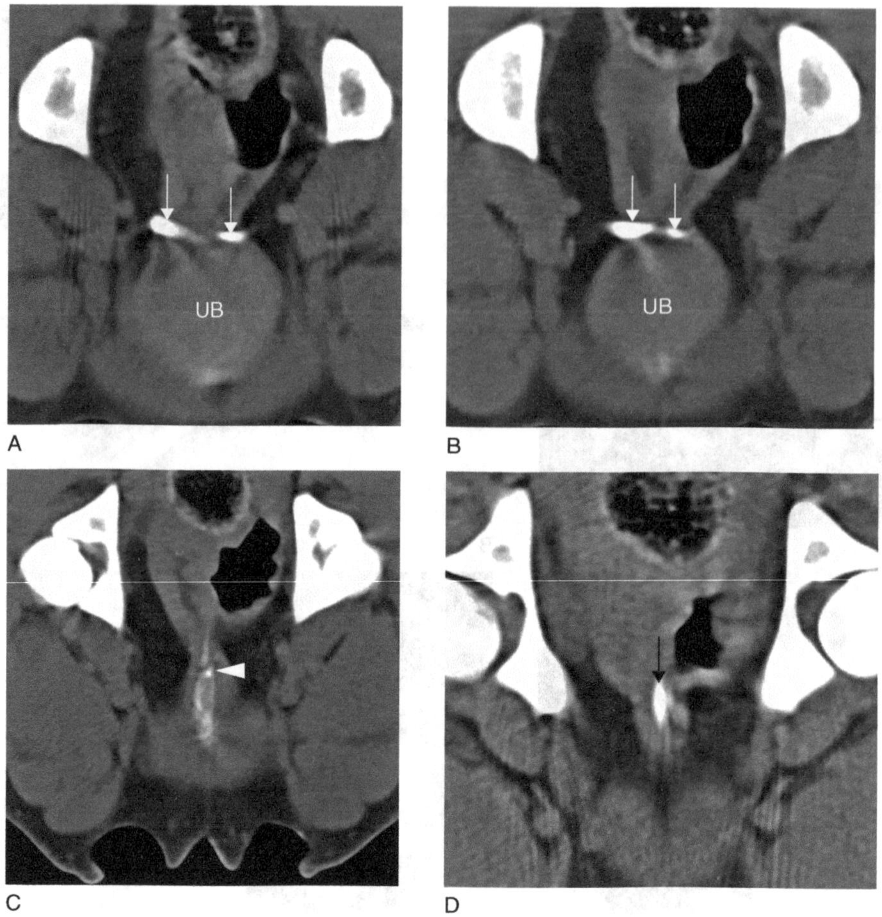

Figure 32.7 Transverse CT images showing bilateral ectopic ureters in a bitch. (A,B) Both ureters (arrows) travel caudally beyond the normal trigone area of the urinary bladder (UB). The right ureter is distended. (C) The smaller left ureter (arrowhead) enters the urinary bladder lumen at the vesicourethral junction and creates a drizzling urine jet, proving its entrance. (D) The distended right ureter joins further caudally the pelvic urethra and releases contrast-enhanced urine into it (arrow).

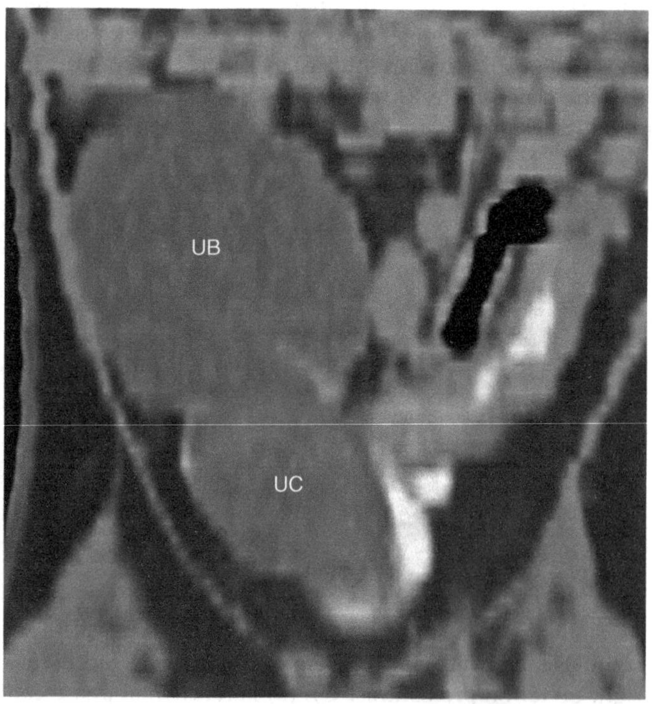

Figure 32.8 Dorsal plane image of an ureterocele (UC) in a cat forming a thin-walled cyst within the lumen of the urinary bladder (UB).

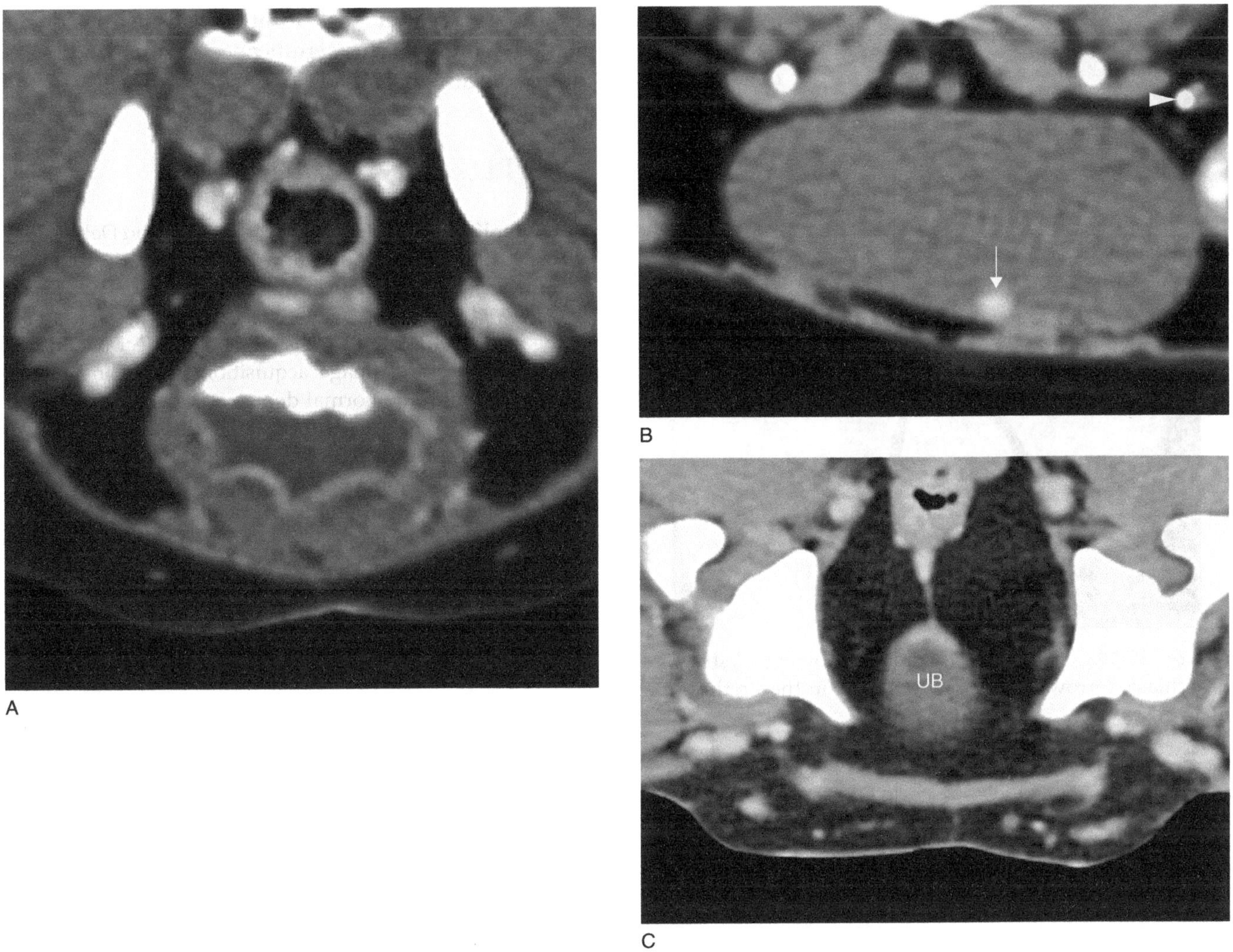

Figure 32.9 Transverse CT images of urinary bladder disorders. (A) Chronic cystitis in a dog with a portosystemic shunt with a thickened urinary bladder wall and pronounced mucosal enhancement. Dorsal contrast medium pooling due to dorsal recumbency. (B) Cystic (arrow) and ureteral (arrowhead) urolithiasis in a cat. (C) The urinary bladder (UB) extends caudally to the level of the hip joints, consistent with an intrapelvic bladder neck. However, this is a male dog with no signs of incontinence.

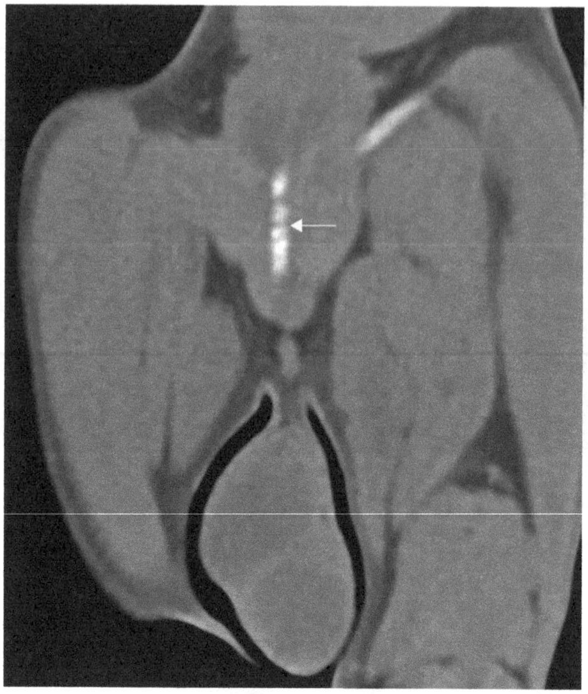

Figure 32.10 Transverse CT image showing obstructive urolithiasis (arrow) in the pelvic flexure in the urethra of a male dog.

vic urinary bladder neck location can also be documented with CT. The significance of this finding is controversially discussed.

Further Reading

Alexander K, Dunn M, Carmel EN, Lavoie JP and Del Castillo JRE (2010) Clinical application of Patlak plot CT-GFR in animals with upper urinary tract disease. *Vet Radiol Ultrasound* **51**: 421–7.

Barthez PY, Begon D and Delisle F (1998) Effect of contrast medium dose and image acquisition timing on ureteral opacification in the normal dog as assessed by computed tomography. *Vet Radiol Ultrasound* **39**: 524–7.

Rozear L and Tidwell AS (2003) Evaluation of ureter and ureterovesicular junction using helical computed tomographic excretory urography in healthy dogs. *Vet Radiol Ultrasound* **44**: 155–64.

Samii VF, McLoughlin MA, Mattoon JS *et al.* (2004) Digital fluoroscopic excretory urography, digital fluoroscopic urethrography, helical computed tomography, and cystography in 24 dogs with suspected ureteral ectopia. *J Vet Int Med* **18**: 271–81.

CHAPTER THIRTY-THREE

Genital Tract

Jimmy Saunders, Federica Rossi and Tobias Schwarz

Imaging Protocol

See Table 33.1.

CT: Anatomy and Normal Variants

The female genital tract

The ovaries are found close to the caudal poles of the kidneys and are generally ovoid in shape (Figure 33.1). They are continued by the uterine horns, cervix and vagina. The appearance of the female tract varies according to the different phases of the normal cyclus.

Retrograde CT vaginography allows assessment of the cervix, vagina propria, vestibulovaginal junction, vestibule and clitoral groove (Figure 33.2). Filling of the urethra is inconsistent with this method.

The male genital tract

The testes are situated in the scrotum from the age of 8–12 weeks. The prostate is a bilobed, ovoid-shaped retroperitoneal gland encircling the neck of the urinary bladder and the proximal urethra (Figure 33.3). It enlarges from birth to maturity and hyperplasia begins around middle age. The size of the gland varies between individuals and depends on the hormonal status. Scottish terriers have a prostate gland up to four times the size of other similarly sized and aged dogs.

On CT, a normal prostate gland appears homogeneous. The capsule and parenchyma cannot be differentiated. The median septum becomes prominent on post-contrast images. The normal prostate gland has a density between 40 and 70 HU on pre-contrast CT, and between 90 and 150 HU on post-contrast studies.

Disease Features

Malformation/Intersexuality

Intersexuality can be defined as the presence of both male and female sexual characteristics in the same individual. There are multiple medical conditions that can lead to intersexuality (Table 33.2) and variations within categories are common, leading sometimes to complex combinations.

CT features (Figure 33.4)

- Presence of male and female genital structures in the same individual.
- The genital structures may be normal or abnormal (incomplete, aberrant, underdeveloped).

The gonads

Retained testis and testis neoplasia

Cryptorchidism has a prevalence of 0.8–10% in male dogs and is due a sex-linked autosomal recessive trait that affects most commonly small breeds. Retained testes are usually small and atrophied and are located between the kidney and the inguinal ring. Castration is recommended because retained testes are 13 times more likely to develop neoplasia, especially sertoli cell tumors, than normal testes and are at increased risk for torsion. These tumors are functional and often metastasize to the regional lymph nodes, liver and lungs.

CT features (Figure 33.5A)

- Non-tumoral retained testis:
  - presence of an oval, well-delineated soft tissue density mass along the expected course of testicular descent (abdominal, inguinal, prescrotal).

Veterinary Computed Tomography, First Edition. Edited by Tobias Schwarz, Jimmy Saunders.

Table 33.1

CT imaging protocol (intravenous contrast study: standard protocol; *see* Chapter 5).

Series	Pre- and post-contrast	Retrograde CT vagino(urethro)graphy (Figure 33.2)
Decubitus	Ventral	Lateral or ventral
Scan margins	Cranial abdomen ⟷ Anus	L4 ⟷ Anus
Voltage (kVp)	120–140	
Current (mAs)	100 (cats and small dogs); 250 (big dogs)	
Tube rotation time (s)	0.8	
Slice width (mm)	1.25–5	
Kernel frequency	Low to medium	
Collimator pitch	1– 2	
Helical image reconstruction interval	½ of the slice width	
Motion control	Hyperventilation to achieve expiratory apnea	General anesthesia
Contrast medium application site	N/A	Vagina (balloon tip catheter)
Contrast medium type	N/A	Iodinated
Contrast medium dose	N/A	– Adequate distention on the scout pilot – Guidelines: 10 mg iodine/ml, 1 ml/kg bw or 20–120 ml (spayed dogs < intact dogs)
Contrast medium injection mode	N/A	Manual
Scan delay post start contrast injection	N/A	Immediately
Window level (HU)	+40	
Window width (HU)	300–400	

- Tumoral retained testis:
  - large, sometimes heterogeneous, soft tissue density mass with moderate contrast enhancement located in the central abdomen, mostly ventral
  - calcifications may be present
  - liver, lungs or regional lymph node metastases.

Ovarian neoplasia

Ovarian neoplasia accounts for 1% of all tumors in both the dog and cat. Tumor types are variable and include epithelial cell tumors, germ cell tumors, sex cord stromal tumors and metastatic disease.

CT features (Figure 33.5B)

- Large, sometimes heterogeneous, soft tissue density mass with moderate contrast enhancement located in the central abdomen, mostly ventral.
- Teratoma: large, irregular solid component containing coarse calcifications.

The prostate gland

Prostate gland disorders include squamous metaplasia, benign hyperplasia, inflammation, neoplasia and cysts. Concurrent disease conditions frequently coexist in the same prostate gland of older dogs. The neoplastic gland frequently contains foci of benign hyperplasia, cystic glandular dilatation and significant inflammation making imaging diagnosis challenging.

The CT features of prostatic disorders have not been reported. Anticipated CT features based on a limited number of cases and ultrasonographic features are suggested.

Benign prostatic hyperplasia

Benign prostatic hyperplasia is a diffuse disorder dependent on age-related alterations in testosterone

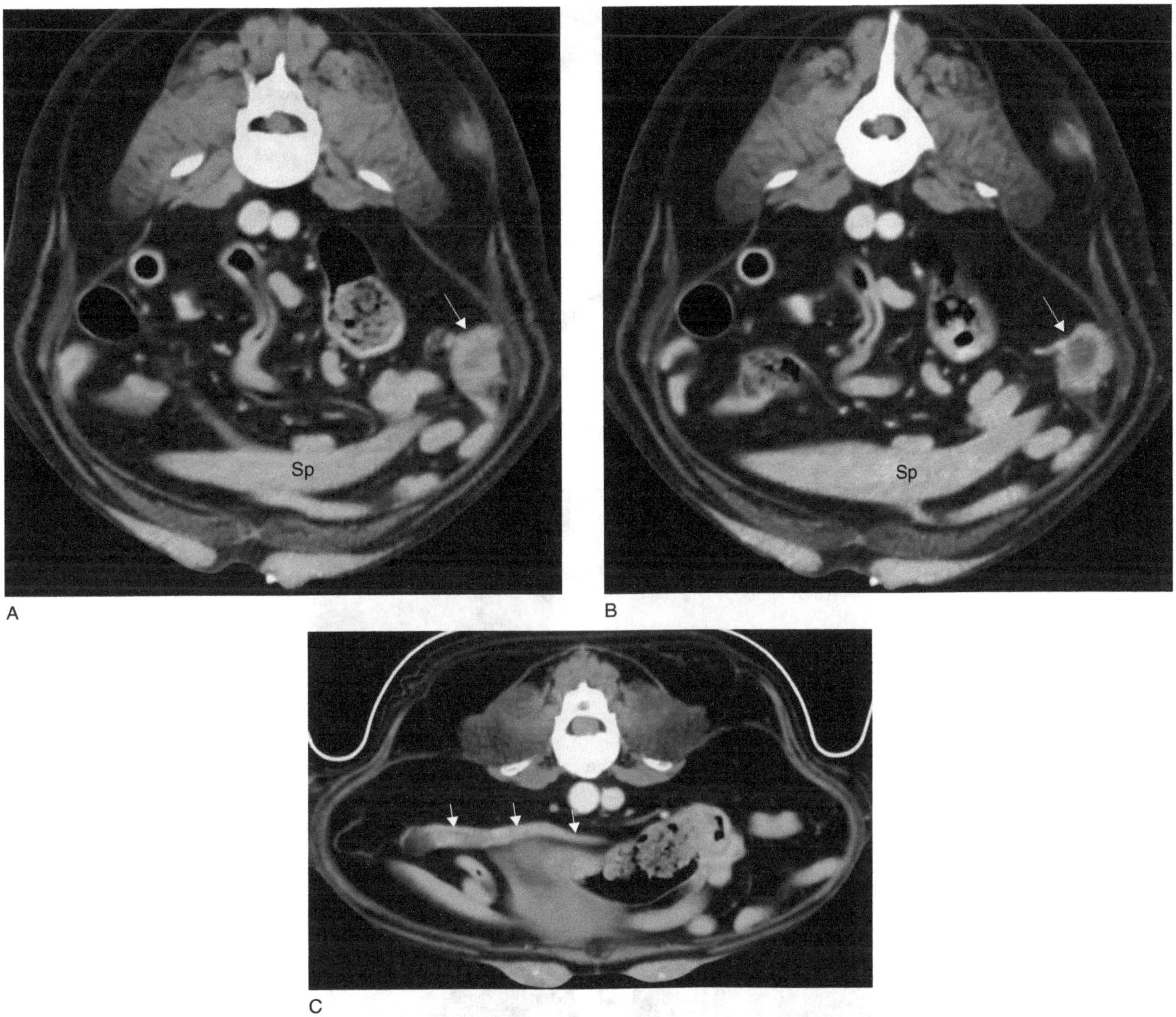

Figure 33.1 Transverse CT images of the female genital tract in a normal female dog. (A) The left ovarium and its ovarian bursa (arrow) are visible along the left abdominal wall. Sp = spleen. (B) The left ovarium during the estrus is visible at the same location (arrow) and shows a hypodense center (fluid content). (C) The uterus is visible is the center of the abdomen (arrows).

and estrogen ratios. It initiates with sexual maturity and affects almost all intact male dogs older than 7 years of age. Glandular hyperplasia mostly seen in young dogs (intra-alveolar increase in papillary proliferations of prostatic secretory epithelium along with an increased stromal component) is believed to progress to complex hyperplasia in older dogs (cystic and/or atrophied glands along with significant periglandular chronic inflammation).

CT features

- Symmetrical or asymmetrical prostatomegaly.
- Heterogeneity of the parenchyma.
- Hyperdense foci: fibrosis or vascular changes, mineralizations less likely.
- Cystic hyperplasia (cysts of different size and numbers).
- Capsule intact.
- No evidence of lymphadenopathy.

Prostatic neoplasia

Prostatic neoplasia is an uncommon disorder that affects both sexually intact and castrated dogs equally. Overall, these tumors are aggressive malignant epithelial neoplasms, mostly adenocarcinomas. At

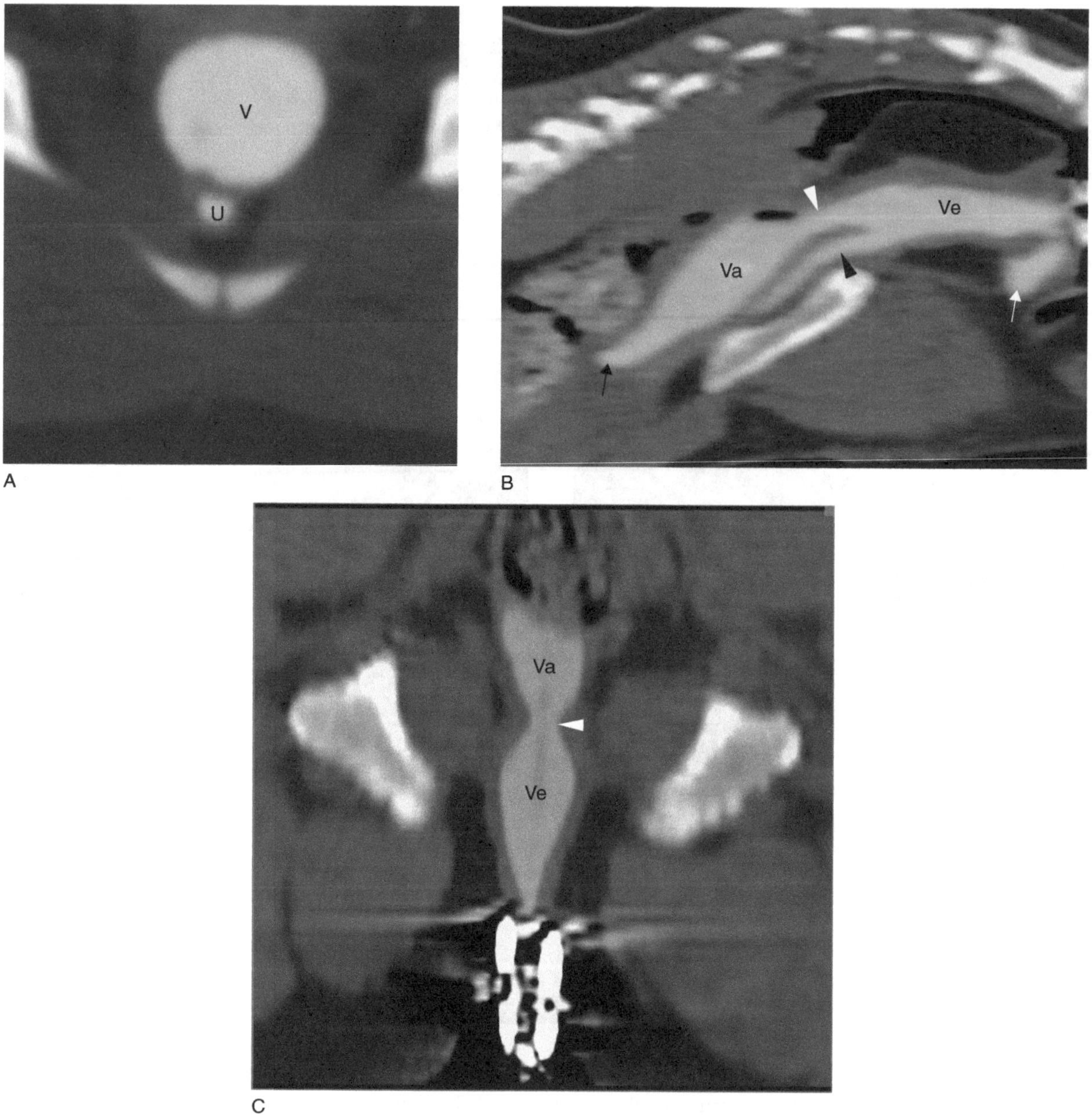

Figure 33.2 CT retrograde vaginourethrogram in the normal bitch. (A) Transverse CT image shows the dilated vagina (V) and ventral to it, the urethra (U). (B) Sagittally reconstructed CT image shows the cervix (black arrow), vagina propria (Va), vestibulovaginal junction (white arrowhead), vestibule (Ve), urethra (black arrowhead) and clitoral fossa (white arrow), all are well outlined. (C) Dorsally reconstructed CT image shows the vagina (Va), vestibule (Ve) and vestibulovaginal junction (arrowhead).

presentation, 80% of the affected dogs have regional lymph node and/or lung metastases.

CT features (Figure 33.6)

- Symmetrical or asymmetrical prostatomegaly.
- Focal or multifocal poorly defined hypodense areas.
- Cyst or cyst-like structures.
- Mineralization may be present.
- Post-contrast (IV): moderate (e.g. leiomyoma) to marked (e.g. adenocarcinoma) heterogeneous enhancement.
- Metastases:
  - lymph nodes: enlarged, sometimes irregularly delineated and heterogeneous lymph nodes

Table 33.2
Classification of the intersexual conditions.

Intersexuality	Genotype	Gonadal sex	Phenotype
Hermaphrodism	XX > XY	Mixed	
Sex reversal	XX	Male	Male
	XY (gene translocation)	Female	Female
Pseudo-hermaphrodism	Male (XY)	Male	Female
	Female (XX)	Female	Male

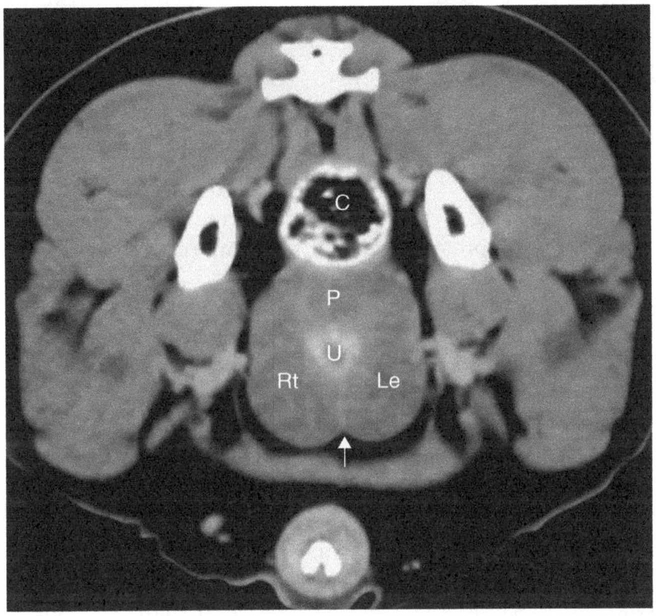

Figure 33.3 Transverse CT image of the prostate gland in a normal male dog. The gland is divided into two lobes by a median septum (arrow). C = colon; Le = left lobe (prostate); P = prostate; Rt = right lobe (prostate); U = urethra.

- bone: mainly proliferative: smooth, palisading new bone, with possibly small osteolytic lesions
- metastases in the lungs, abdominal organs, brain, long bones and pelvic musculature are not infrequent.

Prostatitis/Prostatic abscess

Prostatitis may be acute or chronic and is mainly the result of a urinary tract infection or the extension of a testicular or epididymal disease. Regional lymphadenopathy may be present. A prostatic abscess is a complication of a prostatitis or an infection of benign cyst.

CT features (Figure 33.7)

- Symmetrical or asymmetrical prostatomegaly.
- Focal or multifocal poorly defined hypodense areas.
- Cyst or cyst-like structures.
- Small foci of mineralization are possible.
- Focal fluid accumulation in caudal abdomen.
- Regional lymphadenopathy, less severe than for neoplasia.
- Abscess: one or more large cavities with irregular, thickened walls and hyperdense content.
- Post-contrast (IV): heterogeneous enhancement.

The caudal genital tract

The caudal part of the genital tract includes the vagina and vestibule in the bitch and the urethra and penis in the male dog. Computed tomography can be used to determine the extent of disease process of this part of the genital tract in the female (Figures 33.8–33.10) or in the male (Figure 33.11) dog.

The cat

Male genital tract disorders are extremely rare in the cat. Female genital tract disorders are more frequent but do are not indications for CT.

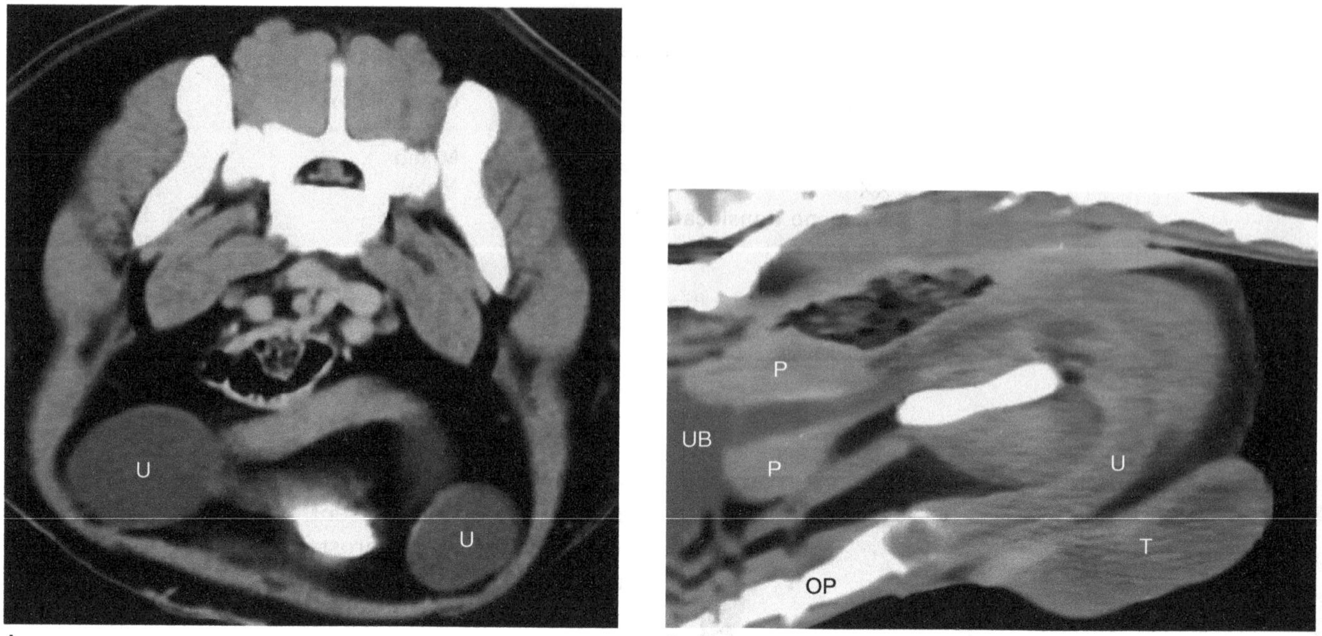

A

B

Figure 33.4 Two-year-old (female) hermaphrodite dog. (A) Transverse CT image with two round uterine horns filled with fluid (U). (B) Sagittally reconstructed CT image shows the urinary bladder (UB), prostate gland (P), urethra (U), os penis (OP) and testis (T).

FURTHER READING

Ragetly GR, Bennett A, Chow EP and Naughton JF (2009) What's your diagnosis? *J Am Vet Med Assoc* **234**: 1127–8.

Smith J (2008) Canine prostatic disease: a review of anatomy, pathology, diagnosis, and treatment. *Theriogenology* **70**: 375–83.

Vegter AR, Kooistra HS, van Sluijs FJ *et al.* (2010) Persistent Mullerian duct syndrome in a miniature Schnauzer dog with signs of feminization and a sertoli cell tumour. *Reprod Dom Anim* **45**: 447–52.

Wang KY, Samii VF, Chew DJ *et al.* (2006) Vestibular, vaginal and urethral relationships in spayed and intact normal dogs. *Theriogenology* **66**: 726–35.

Wang KY, Samii VF, Chew DJ *et al.* (2006) Vestibular, vaginal, and urethral relations in spayed dogs with and without lower urinary tract signs. *J Vet Intern Med* **20**: 1065–73.

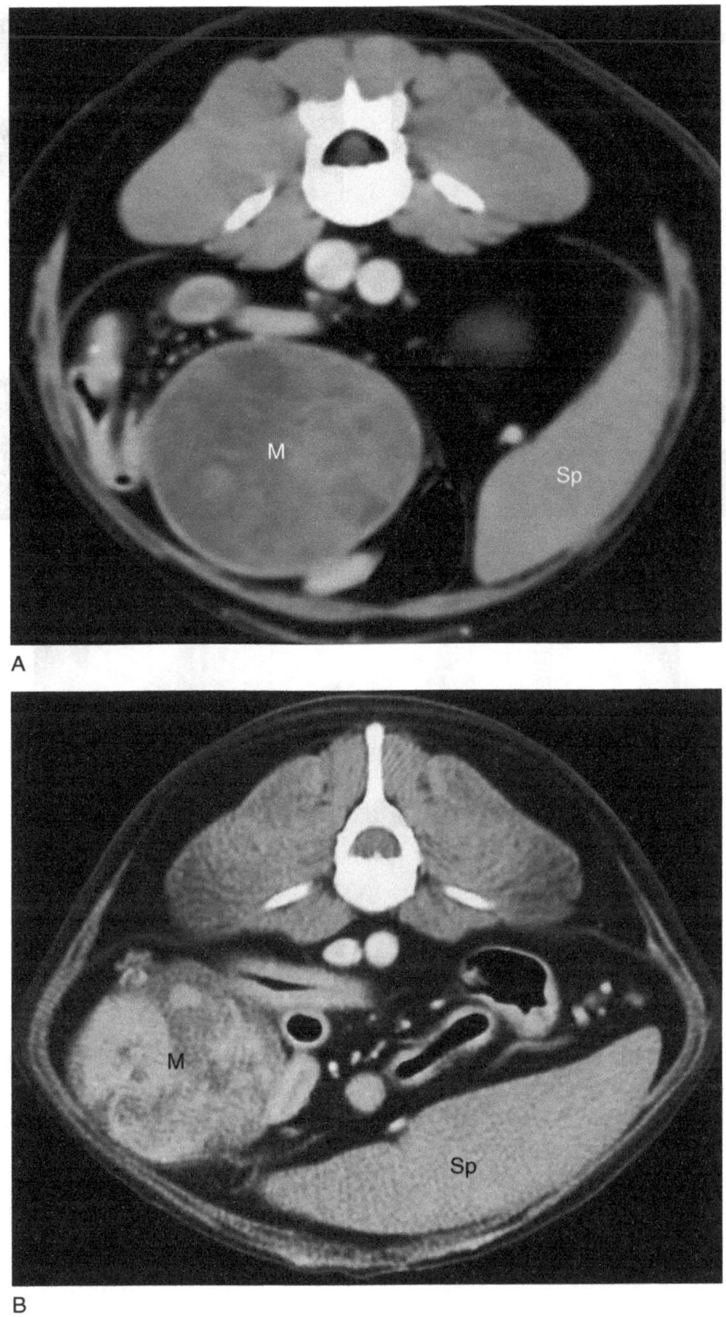

Figure 33.5 Adult dogs with gonadal tumors. (A) Post-contrast transverse CT image of a male dog with testicular neoplasia. A large, round, soft tissue density mass (M) is present in the right ventral abdomen. This mass is slightly heterogeneous and shows mild contrast enhancement. It displaces the small intestines dorsally and to the right. (B) Post-contrast transverse CT image of an adult female dog with ovarian adenocarcinoma shows an irregularly delineated, heterogeneously enhanced large mass (M) displacing the intestines dorsally and medially. Sp = spleen.

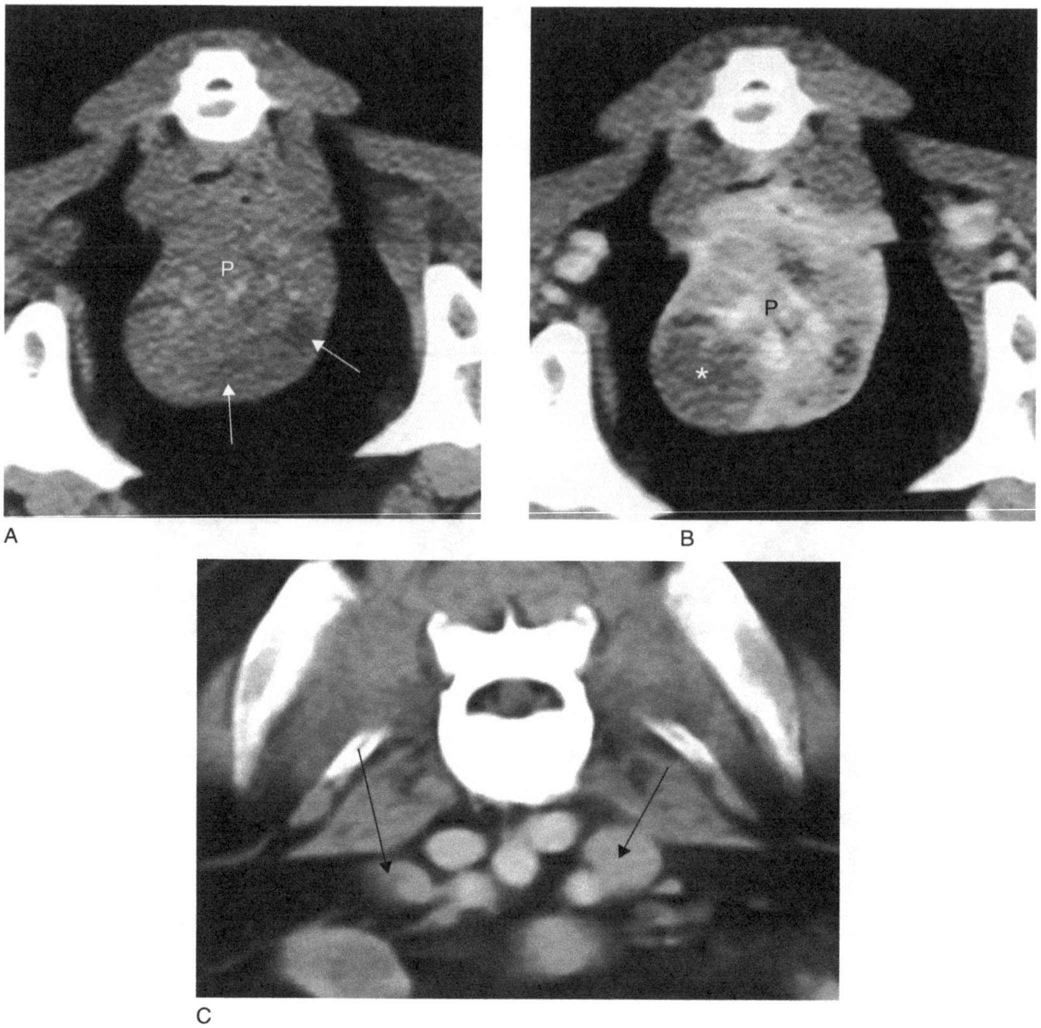

Figure 33.6 Adult dog with prostatic adenocarcinoma. (A) On the transverse CT image, the prostate gland (P) shows multiple small hyperdense foci and some hypodense areas (arrows). (B) Post-contrast transverse CT image shows marked heterogeneous contrast enhancement. One large (asterisk) and multiple smaller hypodense areas are visible. (C) Transverse CT image shows enlarged medial iliac lymph nodes (arrows).

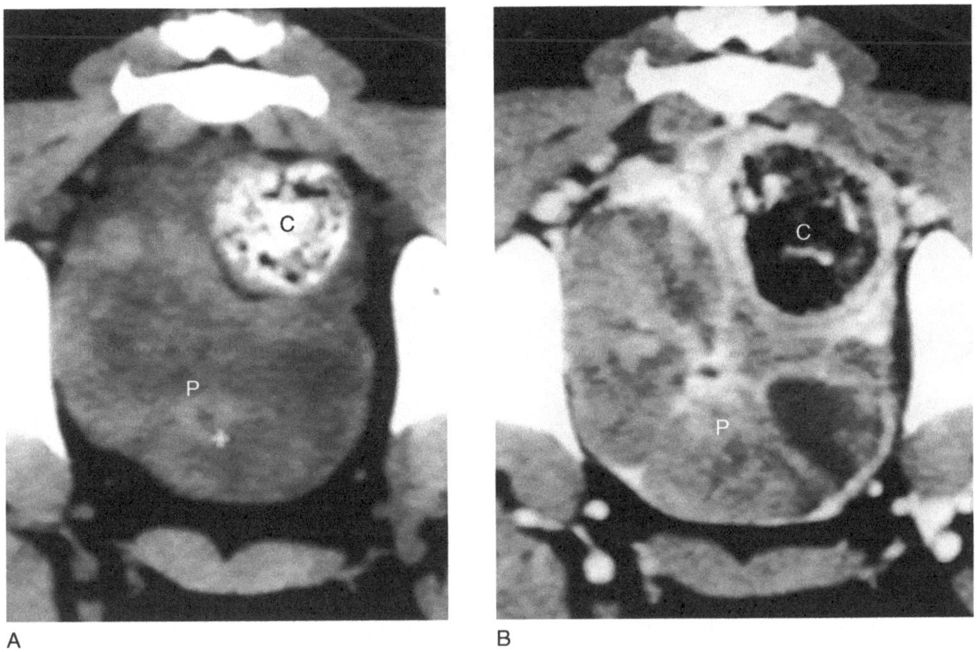

Figure 33.7 Adult dog with prostatic abscess. (A) Transverse CT image shows an enlarged, mildly heterogeneous prostate gland. (B) Post-contrast transverse CT image shows peripheral enhancement and multiple large hypodense areas. C = colon; P = prostate gland.

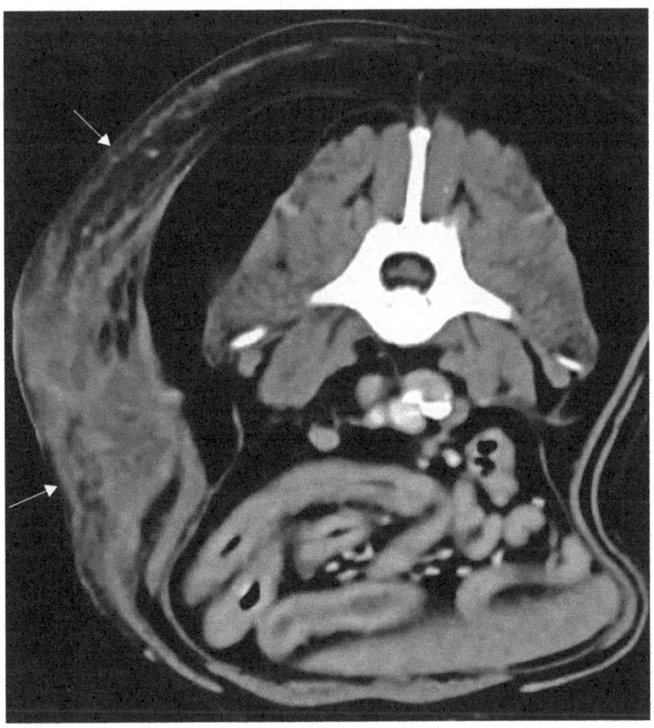

Figure 33.8 Adult dog with a fistula secondary to an ovarian stump abscess. Post-contrast transverse CT image shows edematous swelling of the right abdominal body wall (arrows). Areas of mild contrast enhancement alternate with hypodense zones.

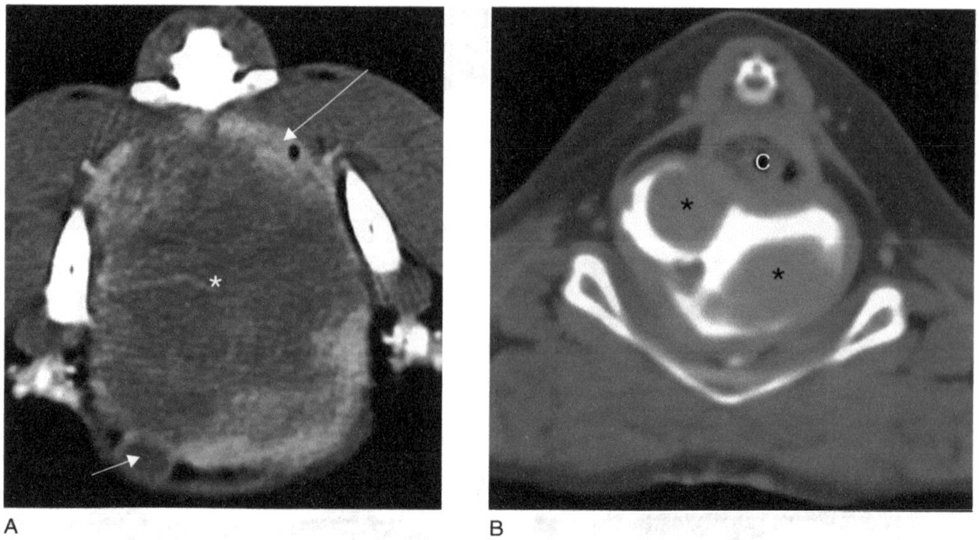

Figure 33.9 CT studies of two patients with vaginal neoplasia. (A) Post-contrast transverse CT image of an adult bitch with vaginal fibroma. A large, mildly contrast enhancing vaginal mass (asterisk) is visible within the pelvis. The colon is displaced dorsally and to the left (long arrow) and the urethra ventrally and to the right (short arrow). (B) Transverse CT vaginogram of an adult bitch with neoplasia of the urethra extending into the vagina. The vagina shows two large filling defects (asterisks). C = colon.

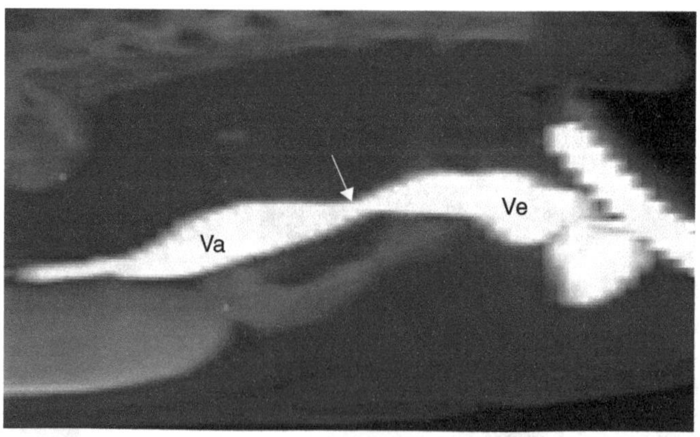

Figure 33.10 Sagittally reconstructed CT retrograde vaginogram shows congenital stenosis of the vestibulovaginal junction (arrow). Va = vagina; Ve = vestibule.

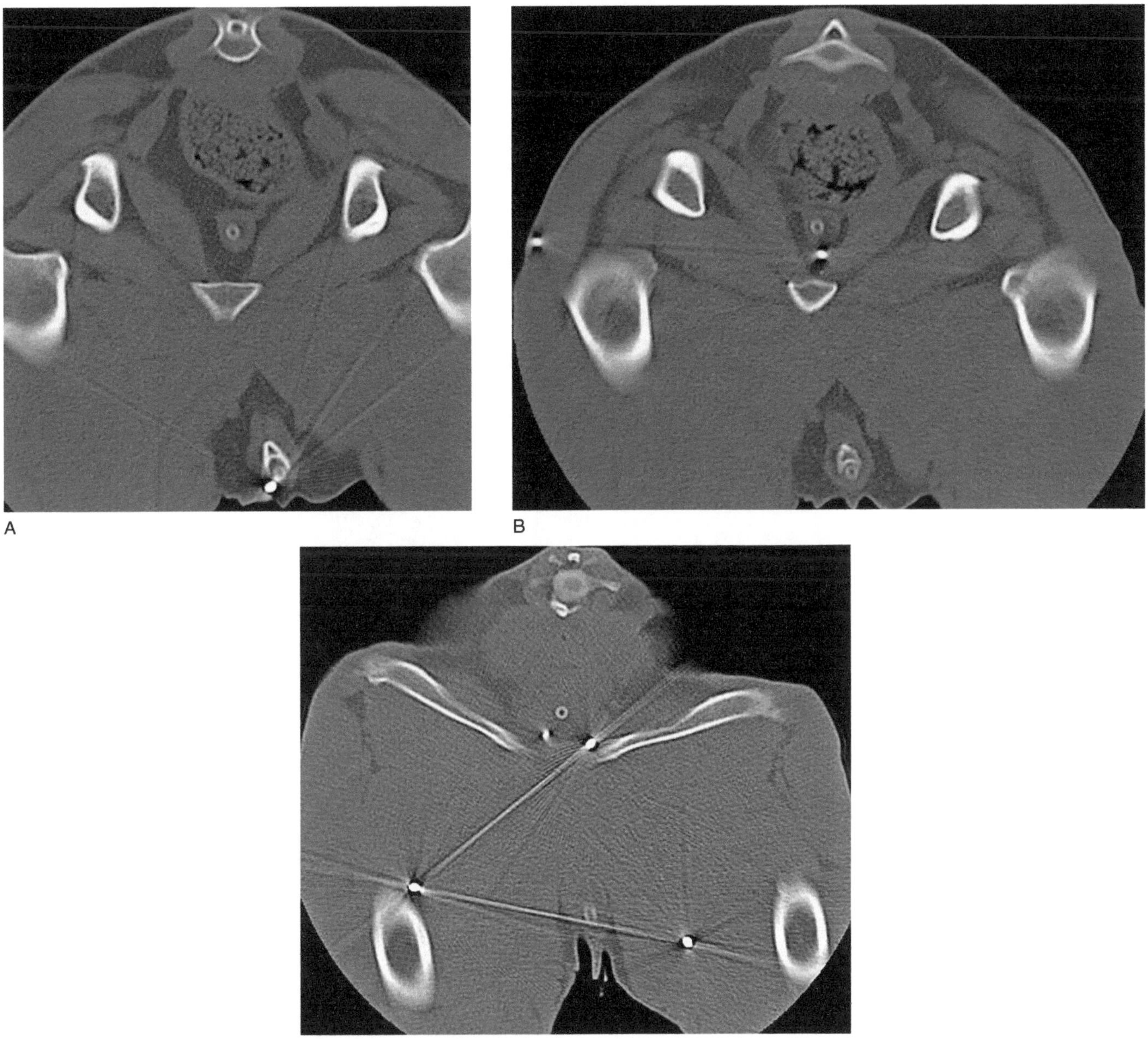

A B C

Figure 33.11 Adult male dog with gun shot injury. Transverse CT images show bullets close to (A) the catheterized penile and (B) pelvic urethra (C) as well as in the thigh musculature.

CHAPTER THIRTY-FOUR

ADRENAL GLANDS

Federica Morandi

IMAGING PROTOCOL

See Table 34.1.

CT: ANATOMY AND NORMAL VARIANTS

The adrenal glands are located medial to the cranial aspect of the kidneys. The left adrenal is the largest, with a peanut shape, and the right is smaller and more rounded. The left adrenal gland lies ventrolateral to the aorta, between the origin of the cranial mesenteric and left renal arteries. The right adrenal gland is lateral to, and in close association with, the caudal vena cava, cranial to the right renal artery and vein. Normal adrenal glands have homogeneous density, approximately equal to that of the kidneys. On transverse CT images, the shape and size of the adrenal glands can vary due to slightly variable orientation of each gland within the abdomen. There is no correlation between a dog's body weight and adrenal measurements (Table 34.2).

CT DISEASE FEATURES

Malformation/Developmental

Congenital hypoadrenocorticism

In dogs, hereditary hypoadrenocorticism due to single autosomal recessive gene has been documented in standard poodles, Portuguese water dogs and Duck Tolling retrievers. Other breeds with reported increased risk of hypoadrenocorticism include Great Danes, Rottweilers, West Highland White terriers, soft-coated Wheaten terriers, bearded collies and Leonbergers.

CT features

- Have not been reported.
- Anticipated features on CT:
  - because hypoadrenocorticism is most commonly due to complete loss of adrenal gland cortical function, small, atrophic adrenal glands should be visible on CT.

Infection/Inflammation

Granulomatous infection/inflammation of the adrenal glands have been occasionally reported in cases of systemic mycoses (aspergillosis, blastomycosis, cryptococcosis, coccidioidomycosis and histoplasmosis), angiostrongylosis, neosporosis and peliosis hepatis. There are no published data on the specific CT appearance of these diseases.

Endocrine

Hyperadrenocorticism

Adrenal hyperplasia in hyperadrenocorticism (Cushing's syndrome) may be due to a primary pituitary neoplasm (up to 85% of the cases) or primary adrenal neoplasm. Symmetric or asymmetric enlargement of the adrenal glands has been reported with pituitary-dependent hyperadrenocorticism; however, in up to 23% of dogs with pituitary-dependent hyperadrenocorticism, the adrenal glands can be normal in size and morphology. In dogs in which the disease is due to a secreting adrenocortical tumor, the contralateral adrenal gland should become atrophied at long term. CT may be particularly useful in the evaluation of individual cases, such as large breed dogs (especially those with deep-chested conformation or obesity) in which the adrenal glands (particularly the right) may not be visible on ultrasound. In cases of marked enlargement of the adrenal glands, CT may be useful in ruling out vascular invasion (Figure 34.1).

Veterinary Computed Tomography, First Edition. Edited by Tobias Schwarz, Jimmy Saunders.

Table 34.1
Imaging protocol.

Series	Survey abdomen pre-contrast	Targeted pre-contrast	Targeted angiogram phase
Decubitus	Ventral		
Scan margins	Diaphragm ⟷ L7	T12-13 ⟷ Caudal aspect of the left kidney	
Voltage (kVp)	120	130	
Current (mAs)	150	175	
Tube rotation time (s)	1		
Slice width (collimated or binned, mm)	5	2	
Sequential slice interval (mm)	5	2	
Kernel frequency	Standard (medium)		
Collimator pitch	1.25	1	
Contrast medium application site	N/A		Peripheral vein (cephalic)
Contrast medium type	N/A		Iodinated, non-ionic
Contrast medium dose	N/A		770 mg I/kg bw
Contrast medium injection mode	N/A		Manual or automatic (3 ml/s)
Scan delay post start contrast injection	N/A		– **Targeted angiogram phase**: simultaneous to injection – **Targeted post-contrast**: 5 min
Window level (HU)	+40		Between +35 and +50
Window width (HU)	350		Between 350 and 600

Table 34.2
Hounsfield units and mean volume of the adrenal glands using multidetector CT.

	Right adrenal	Left adrenal
Attenuation values (HU)		
– pre-contrast	34.3 ± 7.0	36.0 ± 5.3
– post-contrast	97.4 ± 12.4	101.5 ± 10.6
Mean volume (cm³)	0.55 ± 0.19	0.60 ± 0.17

Feline anatomical specificities
In the cat, both adrenal glands have a similar, ovoid shape. In older cats, adrenal glands can incidentally mineralize while retaining normal morphology.

CT features

- No difference in adrenal attenuation values has been found between dogs with pituitary-dependent hyperadrenocorticism and normal dogs.
- Increased adrenal volume has been documented in dogs with pituitary-dependent hyperadrenocorticism compared with normal dogs:
  - $1.60 \pm 1.25\,cm^3$ in dogs with microadenoma
  - $2.88 \pm 1.60\,cm^3$ in dogs with macroadenoma.
- Small mineralizations have also been reported in rare cases.
- Hypodense, rounded or ovoid nodular lesions of variable size.
- Post-contrast: minimal to no contrast enhancement can be seen in affected adrenal glands.

Neoplasia

Adrenal tumors can arise from the adrenal cortex (adenoma, carcinoma) or medulla (pheochromocytomas, ganglioneuroma), and they may be functional (secreting excessive amounts of one or more hormones) or non-functional. Other non-functional adrenal tumors include myelolipomas and teratomas. Metastases to the adrenals have been reported in up to 20% of canine and 15% of feline neoplasias, with pulmonary, mammary, prostatic, gastric and pancreatic

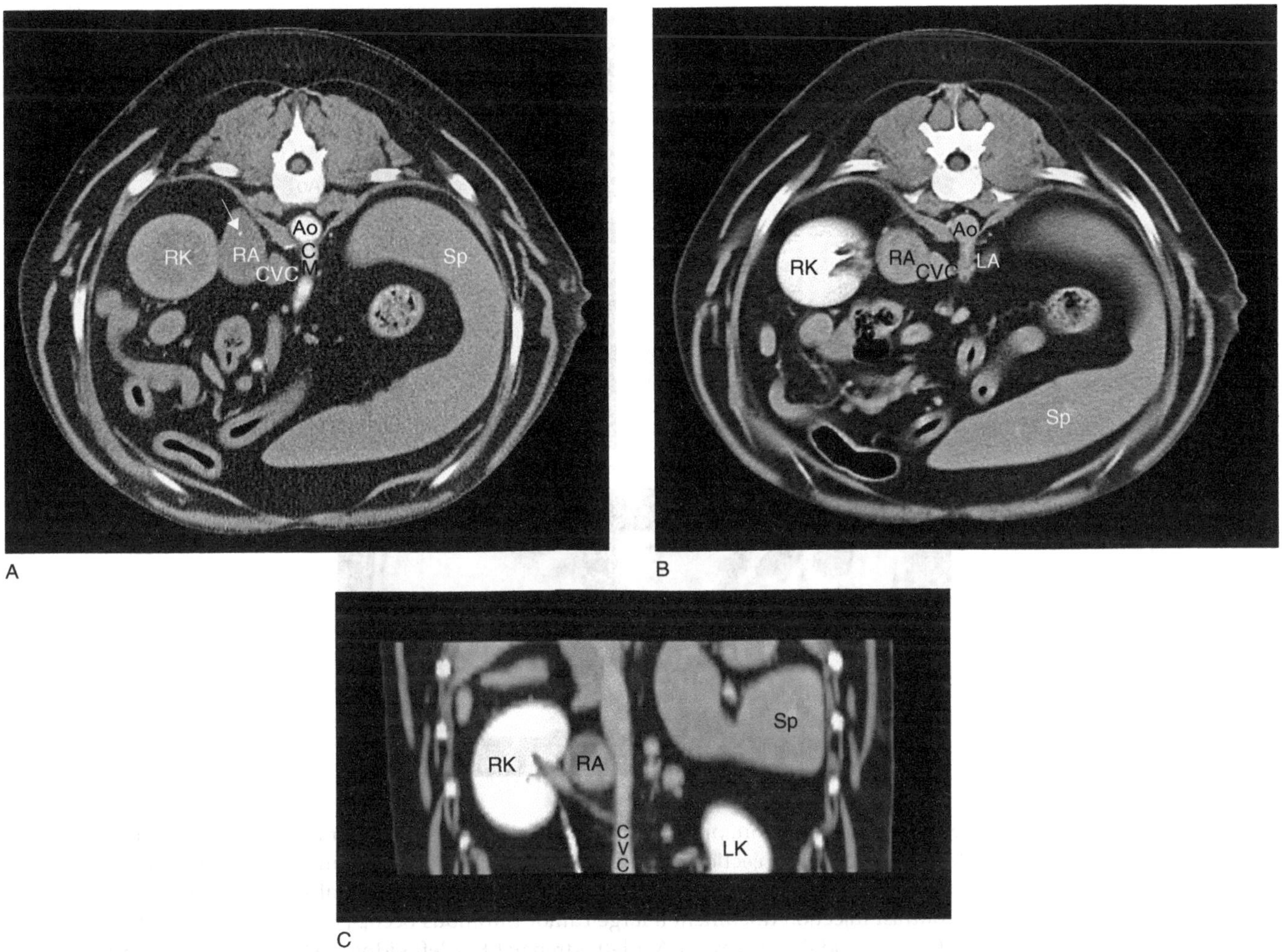

Figure 34.1 Adult dog with pituitary-dependent hyperadrenocorticism. Transverse CT images taken (A) during contrast injection, (B) 5 min after contrast injection and (C) post-contrast dorsal reformatted CT image. There is a markedly enlarged, slightly heterogeneously enhancing right adrenal gland (RA) containing a small speckle of mineralization (arrow) and deforming, but not invading, the caudal vena cava. Only a small portion of the left adrenal gland (LA) is visible on Figure 34.1B and is normal in size. Ao = aorta; CM = cranial mesenteric artery; CVC = caudal vena cava; LK = left kidney; RK = right kidney; Sp = spleen.

carcinomas, and melanoma having the highest rates of adrenal metastasis in dogs.

CT protocol

- When evaluating adrenal masses with suspect vascular invasion, an acquisition during the angiogram phase (timed synchronously with contrast injection) can be very useful in confirming thrombus formation (Figure 34.2); the thrombus appears as a filling defect within the otherwise contrast-filled vessel.
- A post-contrast acquisition (5–10 min after contrast injection) provides information regarding pattern of enhancement of the adrenal mass and thrombus: a tumor thrombus (neoplastic tissue invading a vessel) will show contrast enhancement similar to the adrenal mass, while a clot will not.

CT features

- To date, no specific data correlating CT characteristics and histopathologic diagnosis exist in canine and feline patients, unlike in human medicine.
- Evaluation of adrenal masses is limited to their size, morphology, location and regional vascular invasion (Figures 34.3 and 34.4).
- Fine needle aspirate or biopsy is needed for a conclusive diagnosis.
- Adrenal tumors can have homogeneous or heterogeneous parenchyma.
- Post-contrast: variable contrast enhancement.

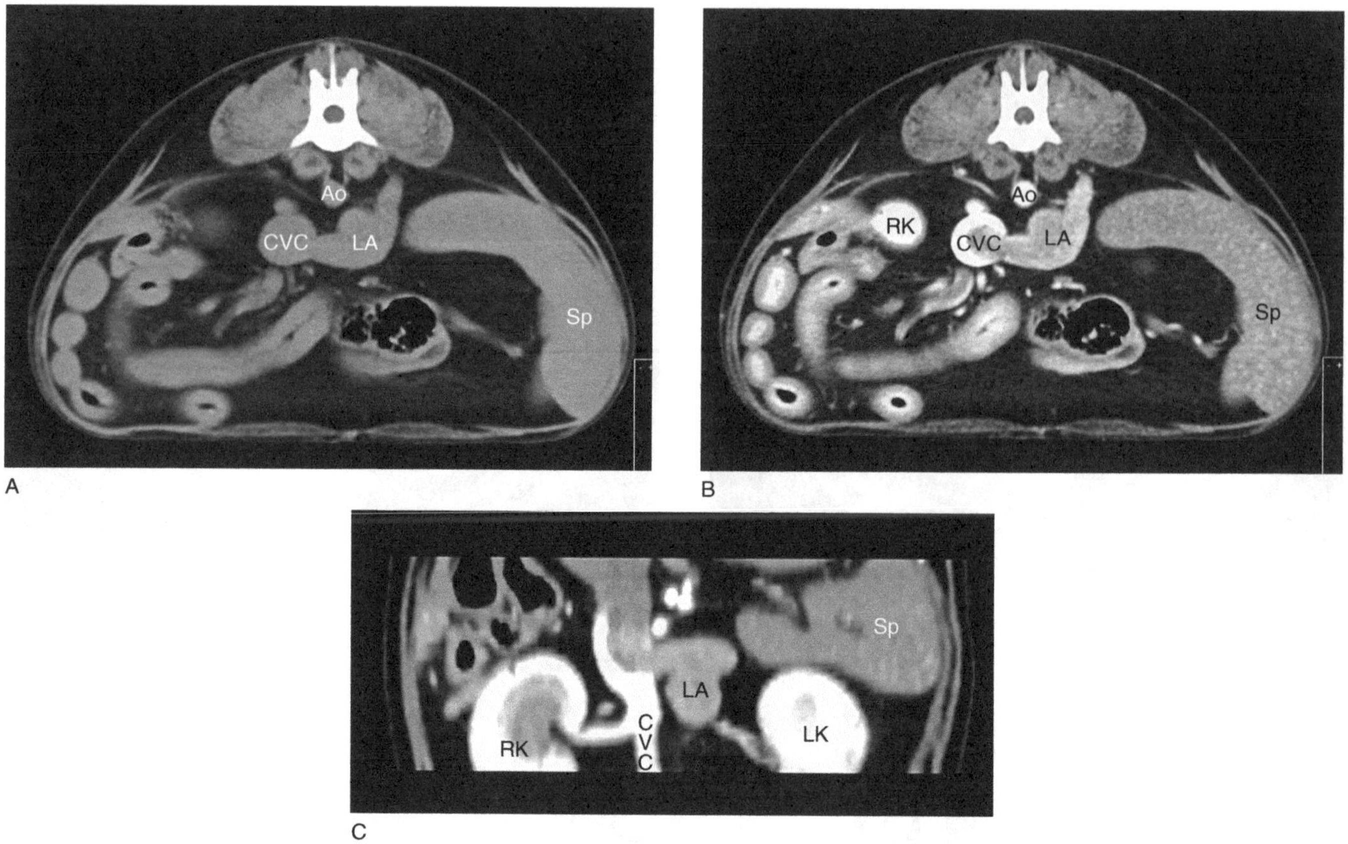

Figure 34.2 Adult dog with persistent hypertension, presumably due to a pheochromocytoma. Transverse CT images taken (A) before contrast injection, (B) during contrast injection and (C) dorsally reformatted CT image during contrast injection. There is a large, lobulated left adrenal (LA) mass, which extends to silhouette with the caudal vena cava on the pre-contrast image. Images obtained during contrast injection document a large tumor thrombus occupying the majority of the lumen on the caudal vena cava. Ao = aorta; CVC = caudal vena cava; LA = left adrenal; LK = left kidney; RK = right kidney; Sp = spleen.

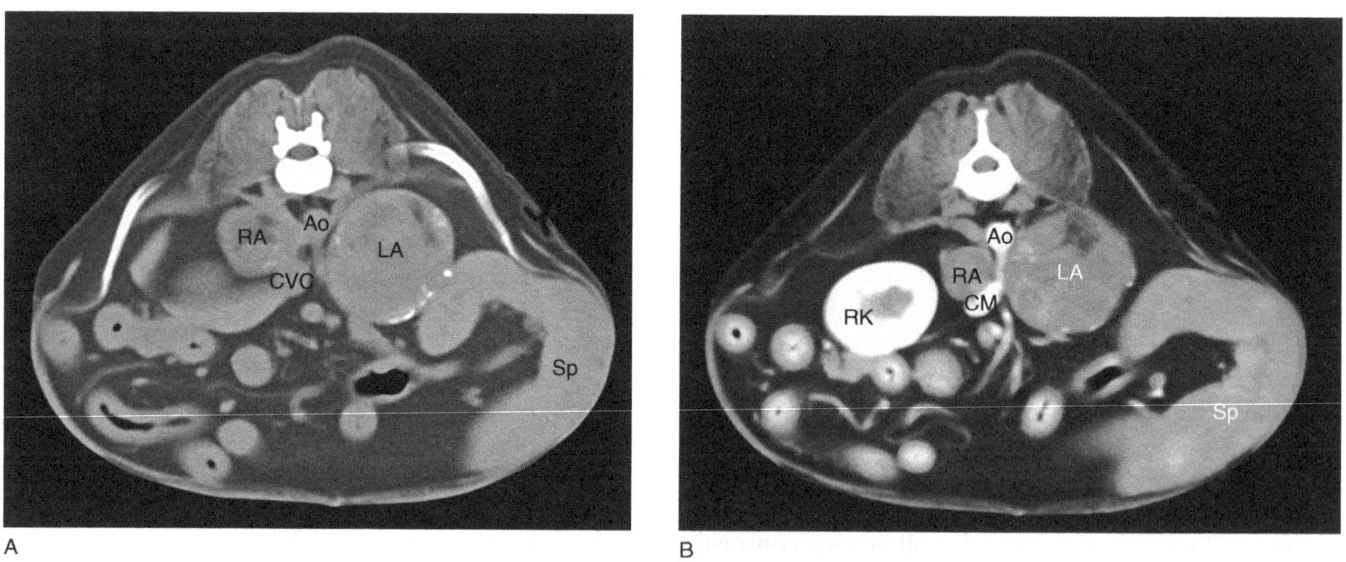

Figure 34.3 (A) Transverse CT image of an adult dog showing both the right (RA) and left (LA) adrenal glands markedly enlarged. Both glands have heterogeneous density with the left adrenal containing mineral densities at the periphery. (B) Post-contrast transverse CT image of the same dog showing attenuation of contrast flow within the cranial mesenteric artery (CM) due to compression by the adjacent adrenal glands. Ao = aorta; CM = cranial mesenteric artery; CVC = caudal vena cava; RK = right kidney; Sp = spleen.

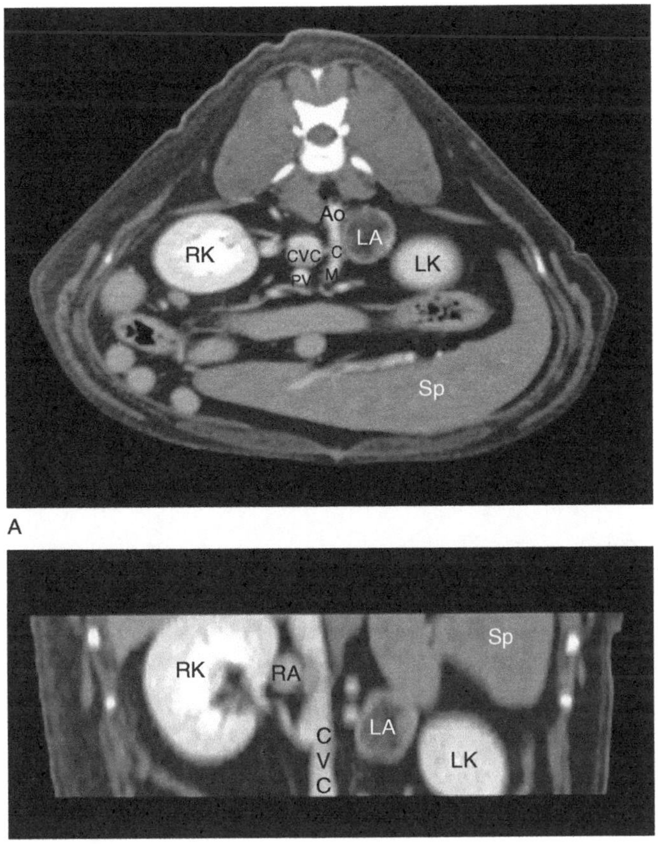

Figure 34.4 Adult dog with adrenal myelolipoma and adenoma. (A) Post-contrast CT image showing a markedly enlarged, smoothly marginated and heterogeneous left adrenal gland (LA). The gland shows a predominantly fat density and minimal, predominantly peripheral, contrast enhancement. (B) Post-contrast dorsally reconstructed CT image of both glands, with the right adrenal (RA) showing homogeneous contrast enhancement. The right adrenal gland is only mildly enlarged and deviates the caudal vena cava to the left. Ao = aorta; CM = cranial mesenteric artery; CVC = caudal vena cava; LK = left kidney; PV = portal vein; RK = right kidney; Sp = spleen.

- Mineralizations are most common with adrenocortical tumors, but have also been reported with pheochromocytomas.

Further Reading

Bertolini G, Furlanello T, De Lorenzi D and Caldin M (2006) Computed tomography of canine adrenal gland volume and attenuation. *Vet Radiol Ultrasound* **47**: 444–8.

Bertolini G, Furlanello T, Drigo M and Caldin M (2008) Computed tomographic adrenal gland quantification in canine adrenocorticotroph hormone-dependent hyperadrenocorticism. *Vet Radiol Ultrasound* **49**: 449–53.

Caoili EM, Korobkin M, Francis IR *et al.* (2002) Adrenal masses: characterization with combined unenhanced and delayed enhanced CT. *Radiology* **222**: 629–33.

Morandi F, Mays JL, Newman SJ and Adams WH (2007) Imaging diagnosis – bilateral adrenal adenomas and myelolipomas in a dog. *Vet Radiol Ultrasound* **48**: 246–9.

CHAPTER THIRTY-FIVE

Systemic and Portal Abdominal Vasculature

Tobias Schwarz

Imaging Technique

Imaging protocol

See Table 35.1.

Imaging principles (Figure 35.1)

CT allows identification of a wide range of attenuation values permitting visualization of vascular contrast enhancement even after passage through and hemodilution in the pulmonary and systemic capillary bed during the first vascular cycle. Helical CT allows scanning of long body parts in a short time span. Therefore helical CT angiography enables visualization of contrast-enhanced abdominal vessels using only a peripheral venous injection of iodinated contrast medium. Thus more invasive, costly, labor- and time-intensive selective angiographic procedures can be replaced by CT. Multislice CT improves the image quality further and allows better timing of vascular phases.

During an abdominal CT angiography, contrast medium is injected into the cephalic or external jugular vein as a bolus. Use of a power injector is essential for most vascular studies and preferential for all. The bolus passes the heart and pulmonary circulation and then enters the abdominal aorta and arterial system. Very soon after this, the renal veins and the pre-renal segment of the caudal vena cava contrast enhance with streamlining of pre- and post-caval blood. Several seconds later the portal vein tributaries, portal vein and branches as well as the post-renal cava and peritoneal organs contrast enhance.

A pure arterial vascular phase lasts only for 5–15 s in the canine and feline abdomen (shorter in smaller animals). The peak enhancement times also vary considerably (5–15 s post start injection), depending on the size of the animal (earlier in smaller animals), cardiovascular conditions, injection speed and pressure. The portal and caval phases last longer (25–60 s) but their peak enhancement times also vary. A CT angiography cannot be easily repeated within a short time span due to the abundance of contrast-enhanced structures and patient safety considerations. Correct timing of vascular phase imaging is therefore essential and three different options are available:

- Educated guessing with the help of published values (Frank *et al.* 2003). There is a moderate chance of missing the peak enhancement by guessing.
- Performing a test bolus dynamic CT scan at the organ level of interest to determine the peak enhancement times of vascular phases.
- Use of automated bolus tracking software. This is a very convenient method; however, there are some serious drawbacks using this technology with currently available software options (see Chapter 6).

All methods of planning only assess the start and peak enhancement times, not the end times. The end of the vascular phases can be estimated by the duration of the bolus injection and study of published values (Zwingenberger *et al.* 2004). In practice, however, this is usually not relevant. The limiting factor for pure arterial phase imaging is the onset of the venous phase, which can be measured by test bolus. The venous phase is usually long enough that if the scan started early on during this phase, it can be successfully imaged and even repeated, if restarted within 1 min.

Suppression of respiratory motion artifacts in the cranial abdomen is essential for all abdominal vascular studies, particularly because the study cannot easily be repeated. Rigorous hyperventilation immediately prior to scanning is most commonly performed; inspiratory bag holding or drug-induced apnea can also be considered. Further details on motion artifact control

Veterinary Computed Tomography, First Edition. Edited by Tobias Schwarz, Jimmy Saunders.

Table 35.1
CT imaging protocol.

Series	Pre-contrast	Test bolus	Arterial phase	Venous phase
Decubitus	Ventral			
Scan margins	Left atrium to hip joint	Stationary at porta hepatis or organ of interest	Caudal abdomen to cranial liver margin	Thoracic inlet to hip joint
Voltage (kVp)	120			
Current (mAs)	80–120		120–200	
Tube rotation time (s)	1	2	0.5–1.0	
Slice width (mm)	5		2–5	
Pitch/Temporal slice interval	Pitch of 2	2s slice interval	Pitch of 1–1.5	
Helical image reconstruction interval	Equal to slice width	Equal to tube rotation time	Half of slice width	
Kernel frequency	Medium			
Motion control	Required			
Contrast application site	N/A	Cephalic or external jugular vein		
Contrast medium type	N/A	Iodinated		
Contrast medium dose	N/A	200 mg I/kg bw	800 mg I/kg bw	
Contrast medium injection mode	N/A	Automated, 3–5 ml/s, maximum pressure: 300 psi (2000 kPa) Injection line needs to be screwed into catheter		
Scan delay post start contrast injection (s)	N/A	0–4	Based on test bolus	
Window level (HU)	100–200			
Window lidth (HU)	300–500			

can be found in Chapter 4. The scanning direction should always be selected with the examination finishing in the caudal abdomen, furthest away from the artifact-prone diaphragm when the patient eventually starts breathing again. This means a caudal scan direction for a single-phase scan and successive cranial and then caudal direction for a dual-phase scan technique, despite the fact that this is against the flow direction of the vascular phases.

It is not absolutely necessary to perform a dual-phase study for all abdominal vascular indications. Particularly with a limited X-ray tube heat capacity or patients with poor respiration control it might be advisable to concentrate on the vascular system of primary interest. However, if there are no such restrictions it is very helpful to assess both the arterial and venous contrast enhancement of the abdomen for:

- confident identification of arteries and veins, particularly in case of multiple extrahepatic shunts
- identification of arteriovenous fistulae, venous thrombosis and other abnormalities of the non-selected vascular system
- identification of hepatic veins, which are best seen during the arterial phase scan as negatively contrasted against the hepatic parenchyma
- identification of tortuous enlarged hepatic arteries as a secondary sign of portosystemic shunts.

Vascular Anatomy and Normal Variations

Abdominal aorta and branches (Figures 35.2–35.4)

The abdominal aorta runs in the left dorsal retroperitoneal space and gives off in caudal succession the celiac, right and left phrenicoabdominal, cranial mesenteric, right and left renal, right and left testicular/ovarian, caudal mesenteric, right and left deep circumflex iliac, left and right external iliac arteries before dividing into right and left internal iliac arteries. These branches are all visible on arterial-phased, low-pitched CT angiography studies.

Common incidental anatomic variations in dogs and cats include multiple left and right renal arteries, as

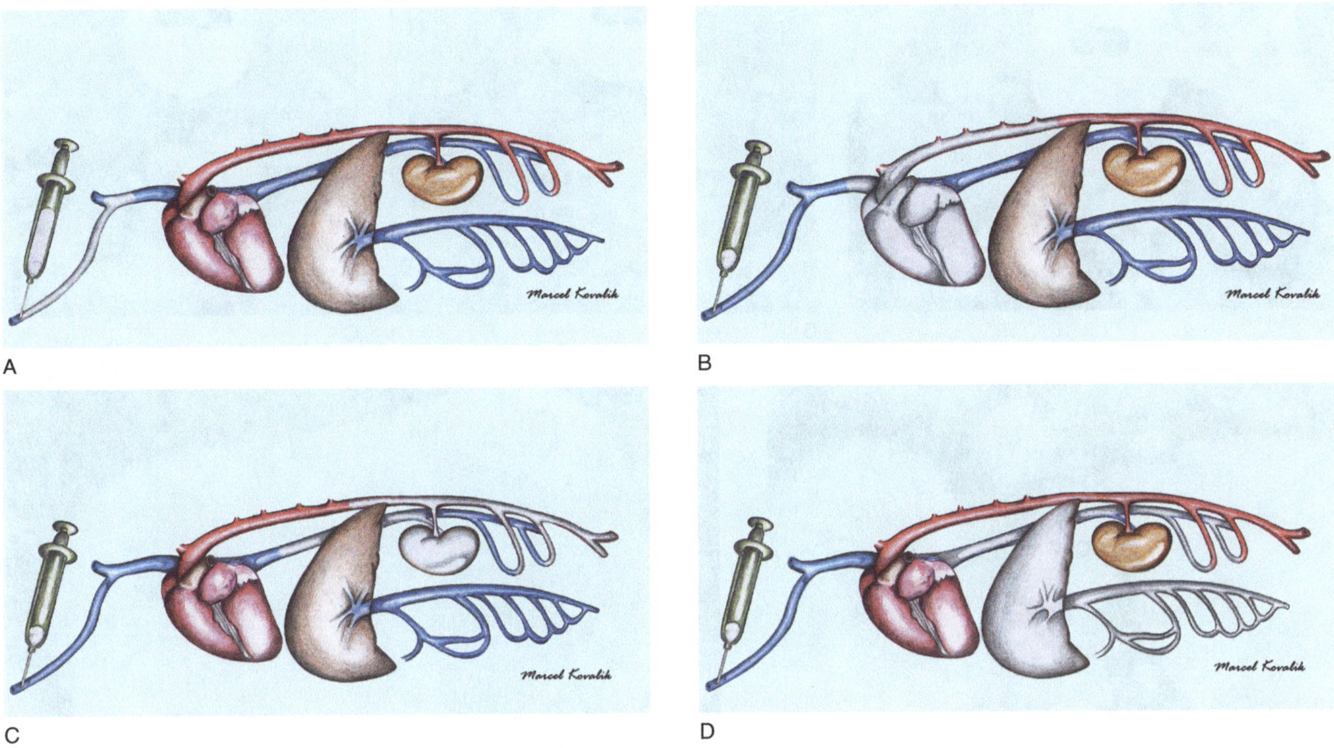

Figure 35.1 The contrast bolus during a contrast medium injection can be seen as a train that runs in vessels instead of on rails. The aim of a CT angiography is to catch the train in the abdomen and ride it along its journey. (A) Contrast medium is injected as a tight bolus into the cephalic vein and travels through the cranial vena cava towards the heart. (B) The bolus train passes through the heart and pulmonary circulation and enters the abdominal aorta. For arterial phase imaging it is now time to catch the train. (C) The bolus train soon passes the kidneys and enters the pre-renal caudal vena cava. For caval imaging it is best to wait for the next bolus train that will carry homogeneously contrast-enhanced pre- and post-renal caval blood. (D) After passage through the systemic capillary system, two bolus trains run in parallel through the caval and portal venous systems, leading to parenchymal hepatic and other abdominal organ enhancement. The CT angiography has now arrived at its final destination.

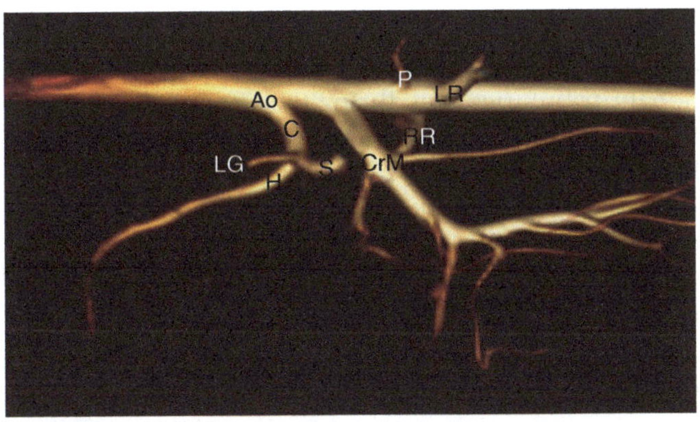

Figure 35.2 Volume rendering 3-D reconstruction image of the canine cranial abdominal aorta (Ao), viewed from the left, with celiac (C), cranial mesenteric (CrM), left phrenicoabdominal (P), right (RR) and left renal (LR) artery branches. The celiac artery trifurcates into left gastric (LG), hepatic (H) and splenic (S) artery, whereas the cranial mesenteric artery divides into ileocolic, caudal pancreaticoduodenal and many jejunal branches.

well as different branching patterns of the hepatic arteries.

Caudal vena cava and tributaries (Figures 35.3, 35.4 and 35.18)

The caudal vena cava (CVC) runs in the right dorsal abdomen from the right dorsal aspect of the liver towards the right ventral margin of the aorta in the caudal abdomen. Further caudally the CVC moves right and then dorsal to the aortic bifurcation. The CVC is formed by the confluence of the common iliac veins. In cranial succession the deep circumflex iliac, right testicular/ovarian, left and right renal, left and right phrenicoabdominal, and hepatic veins join the CVC. There are usually two right hepatic veins entering the CVC separately, and the majority of left hepatic veins form a large vessel; the hepatic ampulla then joins the CVC from the left. These tributaries are

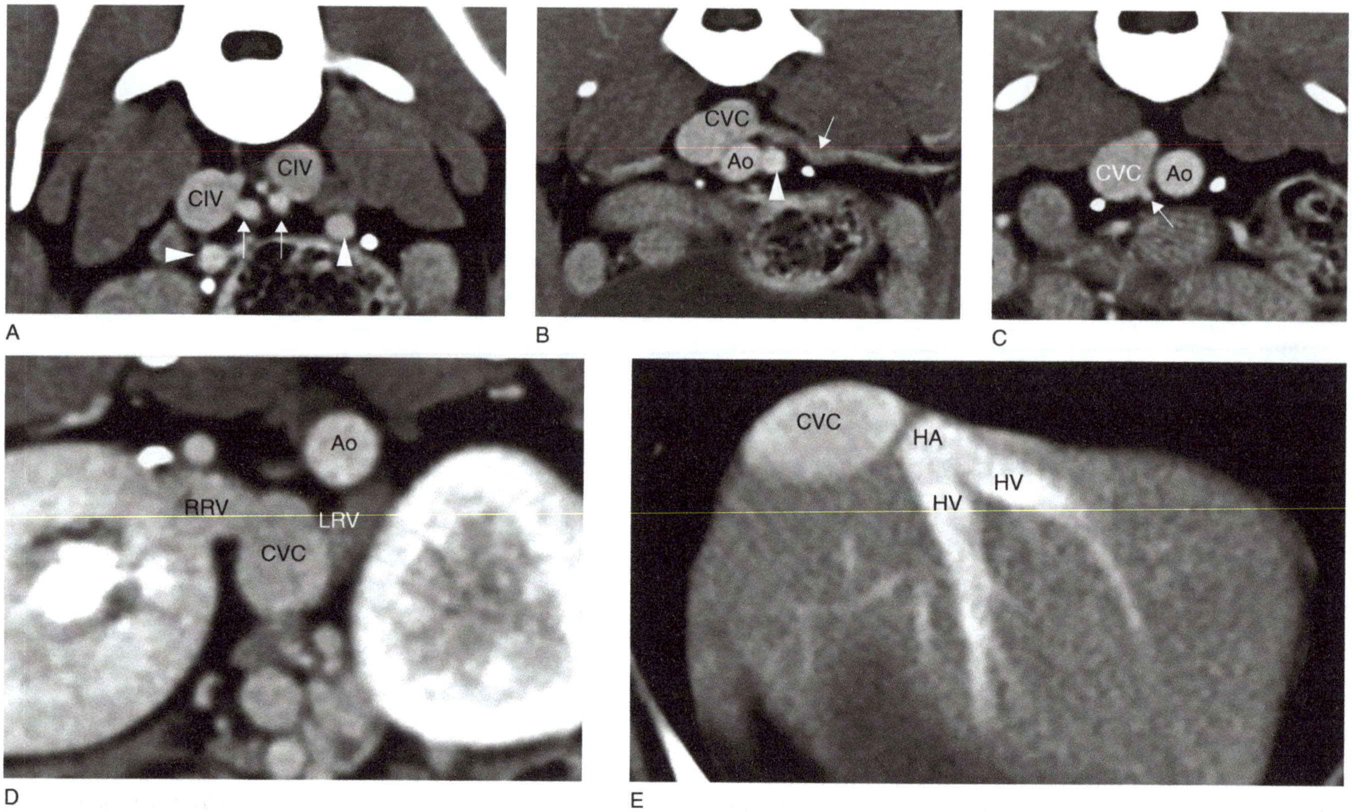

Figure 35.3 Canine caval and aortic anatomy. (A) The common iliac veins at the level of L7 (CIV) form the caudal vena cava, whereas the internal iliac arteries (arrows) form the aorta. The external iliac arteries (arrowheads) are the last branches of the aorta. (B) Caudal vena cava (CVC) with tributary deep circumflex iliac vein (arrow) at the level of L6. The aorta (Ao) receives the left external iliac artery (arrowhead). (C) The CVC receives the right ovarian vein (arrow) at the level of L5. (D) Right (RRV) and left (LRV) renal veins join the CVC. Multiple extrahepatic shunt vessels ventrally. (E) Left hepatic veins (HV) form the ampulla (HA) that joins the CVC just cranial to this level.

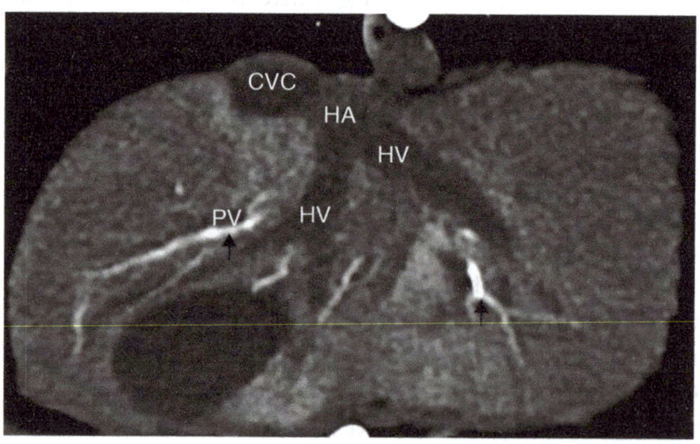

Figure 35.4 Arterial phase image of a normal canine liver showing the moderately contrast-enhancing parenchyma, enhanced hepatic arteries (arrows) that run parallel to non-enhancing portal veins (PV). The hepatic veins (HV), ampulla (HA) and CVC stand out as non-enhanced vessels.

all visible on low-pitched CT angiography studies, the hepatic tributaries best during the arterial phase where they are negatively contrasted against the enhancing hepatic parenchyma.

Common incidental anatomic variations in dogs and cats include a split CVC (usually in the post-renal caval segment) and multiple left and right renal veins. The left testicular/ovarian vein normally drains into the left renal vein, but can occasionally drain directly into the CVC.

Portal vein, tributaries and branches (Figures 35.4–35.6 and 35.9A)

The jejunal and ileal veins form the cranial mesenteric vein, which makes an S-shaped dorsal and then cranial turn to receive the much smaller caudal mesenteric vein (usually from dorsal) at which point they form

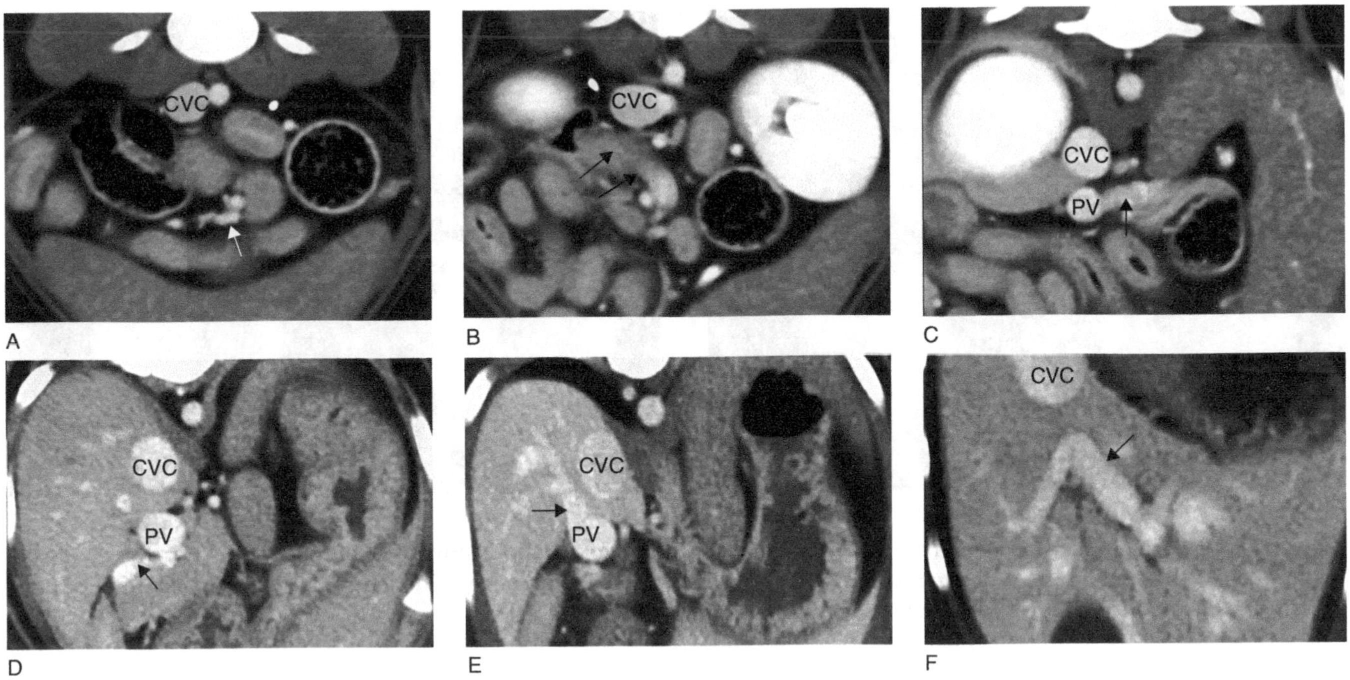

Figure 35.5 Normal canine portal vein anatomy. (A) The jejunal veins (arrow) in the mid-abdomen form the cranial mesenteric vein. (B) The cranial mesenteric vein (arrows) makes an S-shaped turn towards dorsal and then cranial and receives the caudal mesenteric vein (not pictured) to form the portal vein (PV). (C) The portal vein receives the large tributary splenic vein (arrow) from the left side in the cranial abdomen and increases in diameter. (D) The last tributary of the portal vein is the small gastroduodenal vein (arrow), which it receives just caudal to the porta hepatis, from right ventral. (E) Upon entrance into the liver the portal vein immediately gives off its short right branch (arrow). (F) The remainder is the left portal branch (arrow). CVC: caudal vena cava.

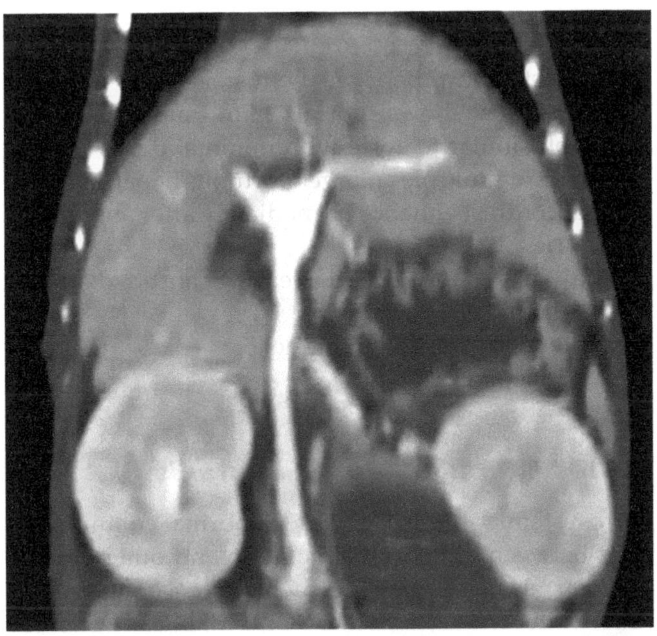

Figure 35.6 Dorsal view of the portal vein in a cat with a bulbous distention at the porta hepatis without associated clinical signs.

the portal vein. The portal vein then receives the large splenic vein from the left and, just caudal to the porta hepatis, the small gastroduodenal vein from right ventral. With each tributary the portal vein enlarges in diameter. Directly cranial to the gastroduodenal vein entrance the portal vein enters the liver and immediately gives off the short smaller right branch that supplies the right lateral and caudate lobe, and continues as the larger left branch supplying the remaining lobes of the liver. The hepatic arteries run parallel to the portal veins in the caudal aspect of the liver. The hepatic veins run separately in the cranial aspect of the liver.

There is great variation in the feeding pattern of the caudal mesenteric vein. In cats, the portal vein can have a bulbous distention prior to the liver entrance. The hepatic portal branches can already be seen during the arterial phase, where they run adjacent to the contrast enhancing arteries, as non-enhanced vessels.

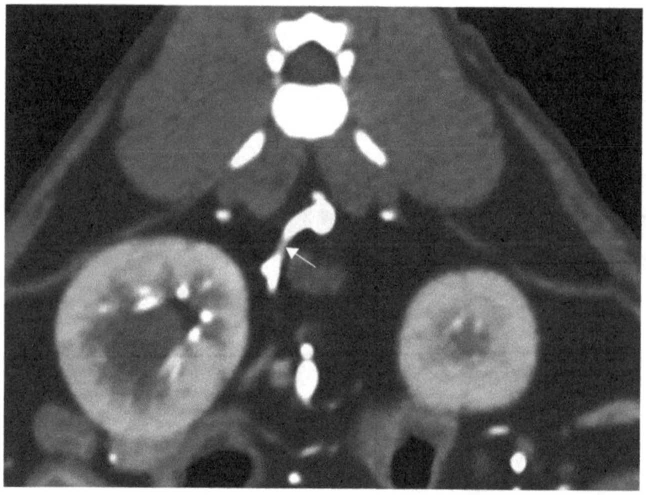

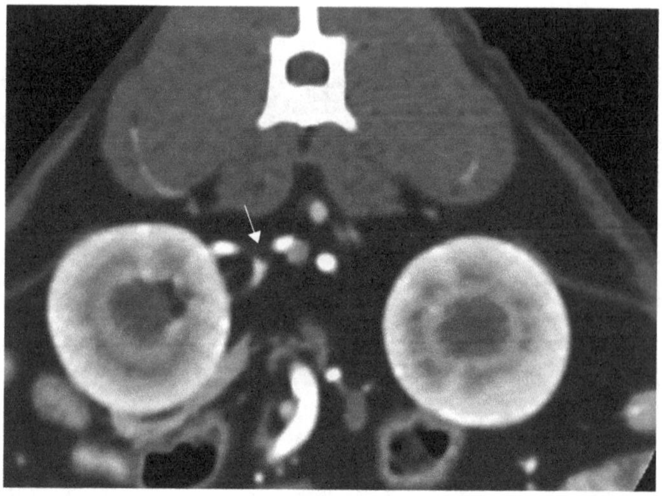

Figure 35.7 Normal renal vascular anatomy assessment in a renal donor cat. (A) Single right renal artery (arrow) giving off two branches. (B) Single right renal vein (arrow) receiving two tributary branches. The length of the common stem of both vessels is measured for surgical planning (images courtesy of Ana V. Cáceres).

Assessment of Normal Vascular Structures (Figure 35.7)

CT can be used to identify individual anatomic patterns for specific surgical procedures such as determination of stem length of renal arteries and veins for renal transplant surgery, or hepatic artery distribution patterns for interventional vascular procedures. A dual-phase, low-pitched imaging protocol with good respiration control is essential for diagnosis. A test bolus is highly recommended, particularly in cats with very short arterial peak enhancement times.

Vascular Diseases

Aortic thrombosis

Thromboembolic disease of the abdominal aorta results in the formation of a saddle thrombus at the aortic bifurcation. Abdominal ultrasound is usually quick and efficient in diagnosing this condition; however, CT angiography might be indicated if intravascular thrombolytic therapy is planned and complete assessment of the thrombus extent is needed.

CT features

- Filling defect in aorta and branching arteries on contrast-enhanced CT.

Arterioportal hepatic fistula

This is a are rare congenital abnormality in dogs in which the hepatic arteries feed into the portal vein with a single vessel or multiple (synonym *arteriovenous malformation*) tortuous shunt vessels, resulting in portal hypertension, hepatic encephalopathy and ascites. They are often combined with portosystemic shunts, complicating diagnosis.

CT features (Figure 35.8)

- Almost always peritoneal effusion.
- Test bolus shows portal vein time–attenuation graph similar to aorta with minimal delay.
- Single or multiple enlarged tortuous hepatic vessels that contrast enhance immediately after abdominal arteries.
- May have abruptly decreasing aortic diameter caudal to celiac artery.
- Distended portal vein branches.
- Microhepatia.

Portosystemic shunts (Figure 35.9)

Portosystemic shunts (PSS) are abnormal communications between the portal circulation and other venous vascular systems causing hepatic encephalopathy, raised bile acids and other abnormalities. Portosystemic shunts can be classified according to different criteria.

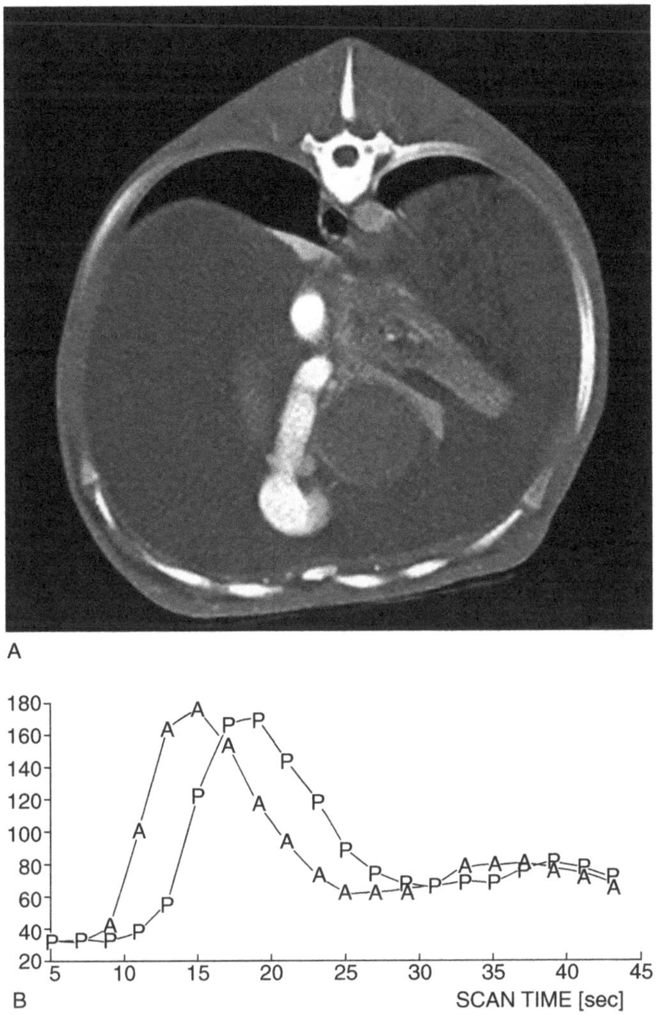

Figure 35.8 (A) Arterial phase image of the cranial abdomen of a dog with an arterioportal fistula. There is marked peritoneal effusion, marked microhepatia and a large tortuous vessel that contrast enhances shortly after the aorta. (B) The time-density graph (time on X-axis, HU values on Y-axis) derived from density measurements of a dynamic CT scan (test bolus). The aortic enhancement curve (A) is has a sharp rise and decline, typical for arterial vessels. The portal curve (P) is only minimally delayed and similar. This is indicative of an arterioportal fistula (courtesy of Allison Zwingenberger).

- Connected vascular systems (each with further subtypes for exact branch):
  - porto-caval shunts
  - porto-azygos shunts
  - porto-internal-thoracic-vein shunts
  - porto-esophageal varices.
- Relation to the liver:
  - left-divisional intrahepatic
  - central-divisional intrahepatic
  - right-divisional intrahepatic
  - extrahepatic
  - intra- and extrahepatic components.
- Number of shunt vessels:
  - single
  - multiple
  - multiple entrances, single exit
  - single entrance, multiple exits.
- Shunt fraction:
  - incomplete shunting
  - complete shunting with no remaining anatomic portal vein.
- Assumed etiology:
  - congenital
  - acquired.

The classification of PSS is an evolving process, as more and more shunt types and combinations according to the different criteria are being identified with advanced imaging modalities. PSS are relatively common in dogs, and the most common shunt types are single extrahepatic in small breed dogs and single intrahepatic in large breeds. The left-divisional intrahepatic shunt is synonymous with a patent ductus venosus Arantii. PSS are rare in cats, the most common type here is an extrahepatic portoazygos shunt. Intrahepatic PSS are usually of assumed congenital origin, whereas extrahepatic shunts can be congenital or secondary to some form of portal hypertension. The assumption that multiple extrahepatic shunts are always acquired is not correct.

Microvascular portal vein dysplasia is a condition where shunting only occurs at microscopic level, requiring a liver biopsy for confirmation. CT is used to rule out a macroscopic shunt. Dynamic CT has potential to aid in further diagnostic by calculation of the hepatic perfusion index (see Chapter 2).

CT features

General features (Figure 35.10)

- Microhepatia.
- Renomegaly (inconsistent).
- Urolithiasis.
- Cachexia.
- Enlarged tortuous hepatic arteries.
- Periportal edema (unknown significance).
- Gastric foreign bodies (allotriophagia).
- Reduced portal vein diameter cranial to shunting portal tributary vein (extrahepatic shunt).
- Cessation or reduction of portal enhancement distal to intrahepatic shunt origin.

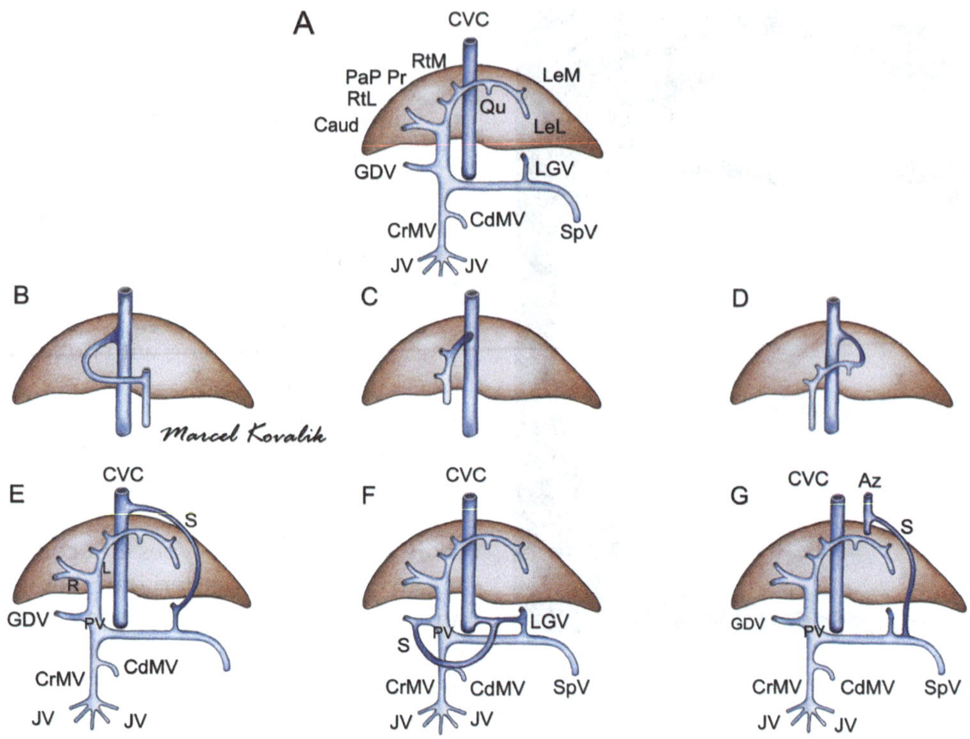

Figure 35.9 (A) Normal portal vein anatomy (light blue) with confluence of cranial (CrMV) and caudal (CdMV) mesenteric veins, splenic (SpV) and gastroduodenal (GDV) vein tributaries. The portal vein grows in diameter after each tributary. Upon liver entrance the portal vein branches into a short right branch, supplying the caudate (Caud) and right lateral lobes (RtL). The remaining left branch supplies the papillary process (Pap Pr), right medial (RtM), quadrate (Qu), left medial (LeM) and left lateral (LeL) lobes of the liver. CVC = caudal vena cava. (B) Right-divisional intrahepatic shunt originating from the right portal branch. (C) Short bulbous central-divisional intrahepatic shunt, originating from an early left portal branch. (D) Left-divisional intrahepatic shunt (patent ductus venosus), originating from the left portal branch and connecting to the hepatic ampulla. (E) Extrahepatic shunt (S) originating from the left gastric vein (LGV) connecting to the CVC directly cranial to the liver. JV = jejunal veins; L = left branch; PV = portal vein; R = right branch. (F) Extrahepatic shunt originating from gastroduodenal and left gastric veins connecting directly to the CVC. (G) Extrahepatic shunt originating from the splenic vein and connecting to the azygos vein (Az).

Single right-divisional intrahepatic portosystemic shunt (Figures 35.9B and 35.11)

- Wide tortuous intrahepatic shunt vessels in right lateral lobe.
- Originates from right portal branch directly at liver entrance.
- Connects to CVC from right with one or multiple connections.

Single central-divisional intrahepatic portosystemic shunt (Figures 35.9C and 35.12)

- Short bulbous intrahepatic shunt vessel in central part of liver.
- Connects left branch with CVC.
- Usually narrowed lumen at either shunt end.

Single left-divisional intrahepatic portosystemic shunt (Figures 35.9D and 35.13)

- Wide tortuous intrahepatic shunt vessel in left liver half.
- Originates from left portal branch, curves lateral, then dorsal, to connect to the hepatic ampulla.

Common single extrahepatic shunt types (Figures 35.9E–G and 35.14)

- Originating from the left gastric vein, curving along the minor curvature of the stomach, continuing over the dorsal liver margin to connect to the CVC between liver and diaphragm.
- Originating from the gastroduodenal and left gastric veins, merging to feed into the CVC from the left, cranial to the kidneys.

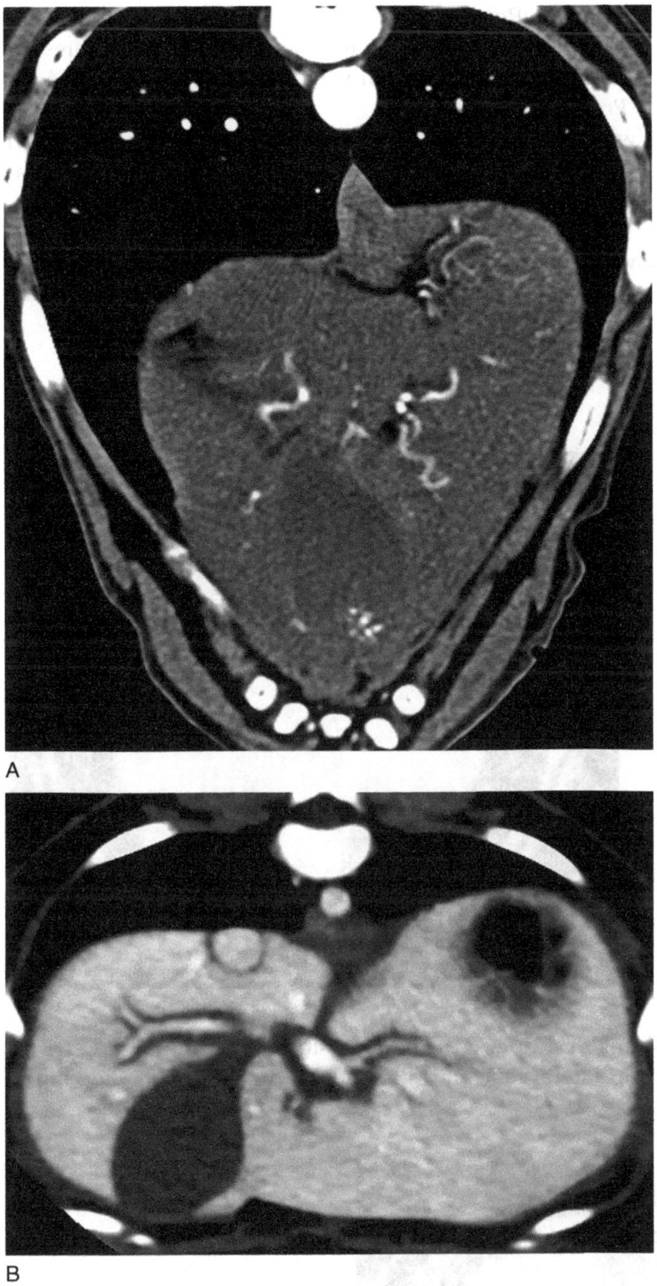

Figure 35.10 General features of canine portosystemic shunts. (A) Microhepatia with enlarged tortuous hepatic arteries. (B) Periportal hypodense halo consistent with portal wall edema, a non-specific sign of unknown significance.

- Originating from the splenic vein and connecting to the azygos vein.

Common multiple extrahepatic shunt types (Figure 35.15)

- Multiple small chaotic vessels between great vessels and left kidney and around left kidney, less commonly right kidney.
- Esophageal vascular enlargement with varix formation.

Portal vein thrombosis (Figure 35.16)

Portal vein thrombosis is a rare consequence of systemic disease occasionally seen in dogs with primary or secondary coagulopathies, resulting in portal hypertension and ascites. CT is an excellent modality to confirm or rule out a portal vein thrombosis by demonstration of a filling defect in venous phase CT. It is very important to inject contrast medium via the cephalic or jugular vein and to scan not too early during the venous phase. Preferentially two scans should be performed during the venous phase to rule out any pseudothrombosis caused by streamlining of native and contrast-enhanced blood.

Segmental caudal vena cava aplasia (Figures 35.17 and 35.18)

This is an increasingly frequently reported congenital anomaly in dogs in which the pre-renal CVC segment between the kidneys and the liver has not been formed. Post-renal caval blood is shunted to a right or anomalous left azygos vein. The condition can be incidental as the cavo-azygos shunt is a functional conduit, but it is associated with significant morbidity in about 25% of cases, due to either thrombosis in the aneurismal cavo-azygos shunt vessel or associated portosystemic shunts. In some cases the portal vein completely connects to the azygos vein, making it inoperable. CT angiography is therefore an excellent modality to assess the need for and possibility of surgical intervention.

Vascular neoplasia and tumor invasion (Figure 35.19)

CT angiography is an excellent modality to assess tumor vascularity, vascular invasion and tumor thrombosis of abdominal neoplasia. Most commonly, screening of caval invasion of adrenal neoplasia is performed.

References

Frank P, Mahaffey M, Egger C and Cornell KK (2003) Helical computed tomography in 10 normal dogs and 10 dogs with a portosystemic shunt. *Vet Radiol Ultrasound* **44**: 392–400.

Zwingenberger AL and Schwarz T (2004) Dual-phase CT angiography of the normal canine portal and hepatic vasculature. *Vet Radiol Ultrasound* **45**: 117–24.

Further Reading

Cáceres AV, Zwingenberger AL, Aronson LR and Mai W (2008) Characterization of normal feline renal vascular anatomy with dual-phase CT angiography. *Vet Radiol Ultrasound* **49**: 350–6.

Cáceres AV, Zwingenberger AL, Hardam E, Lucena J and Schwarz T (2006) Helical computed tomographic angiography of the normal canine pancreas. *Vet Radiol Ultrasound* **47**: 270–8.

D'Anjou MA and Huneault L (2008) Imaging diagnosis – complex intrahepatic portosystemic shunt in a dog. *Vet Radiol Ultrasound* **49**: 51–5.

Schwarz T, Rossi F, Wray JD *et al.* (2009) Computed tomographic and magnetic resonance imaging features of canine segmental caudal vena cava aplasia. *J Small Anim Pract* **50**: 341–9.

Zwingenberger AL, McLear RC and Weisse C (2005) Diagnosis of arterioportal fistulae in four dogs using computed tomographic angiography. *Vet Radiol Ultrasound* **46**: 472–7.

Zwingenberger AL, Schwarz T and Saunders HM (2005) Helical CT angiography of canine portosystemic shunts. *Vet Radiol Ultrasound* **46**: 27–37.

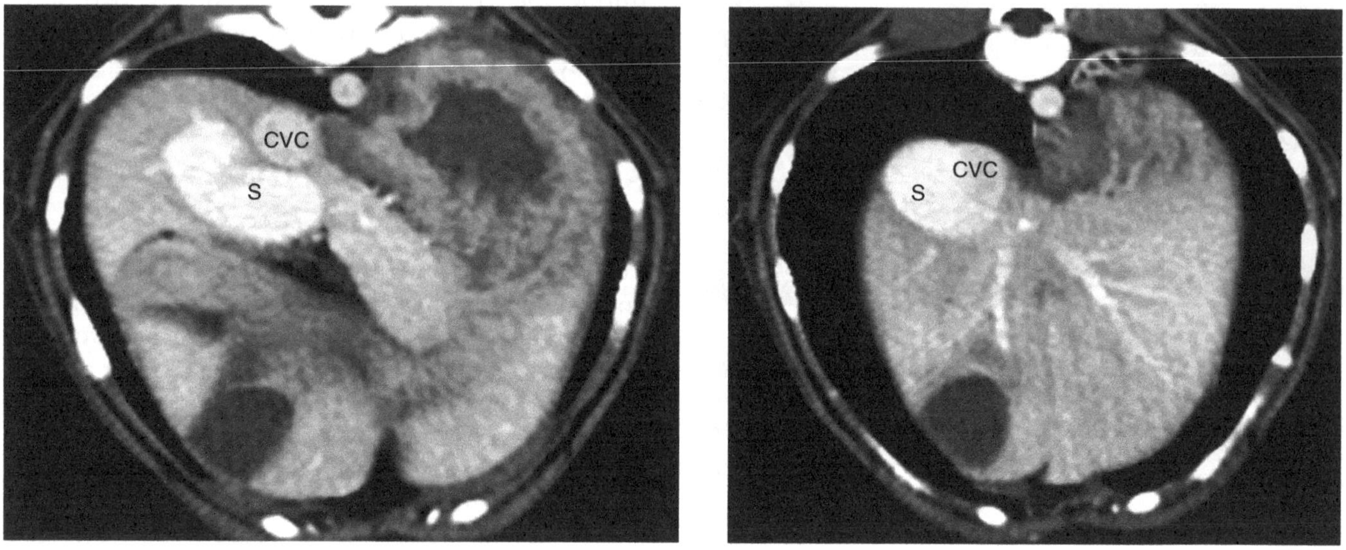

B

Figure 35.11 Single right-divisional intrahepatic portocaval shunt in a dog. (A) The large tortuous shunting vessel (S) emerges from the right portal vein branch, travels through the right lateral lobe and (B) connects from the right side to the caudal vena cava (CVC) close to its hepatic exit point.

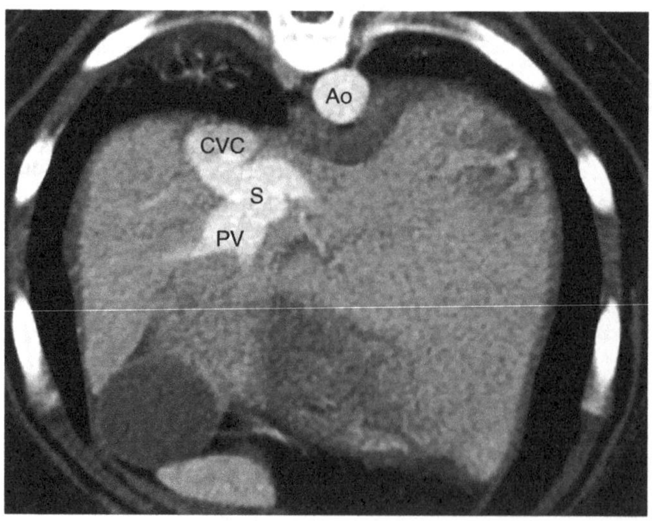

Figure 35.12 Single central-divisional intrahepatic portocaval shunt in a dog with a short bulbous shunting vessel (S) connecting the caudal part of the left portal vein branch (PV) through a small orifice from ventral to the caudal vena cava (CVC). Ao = Aorta.

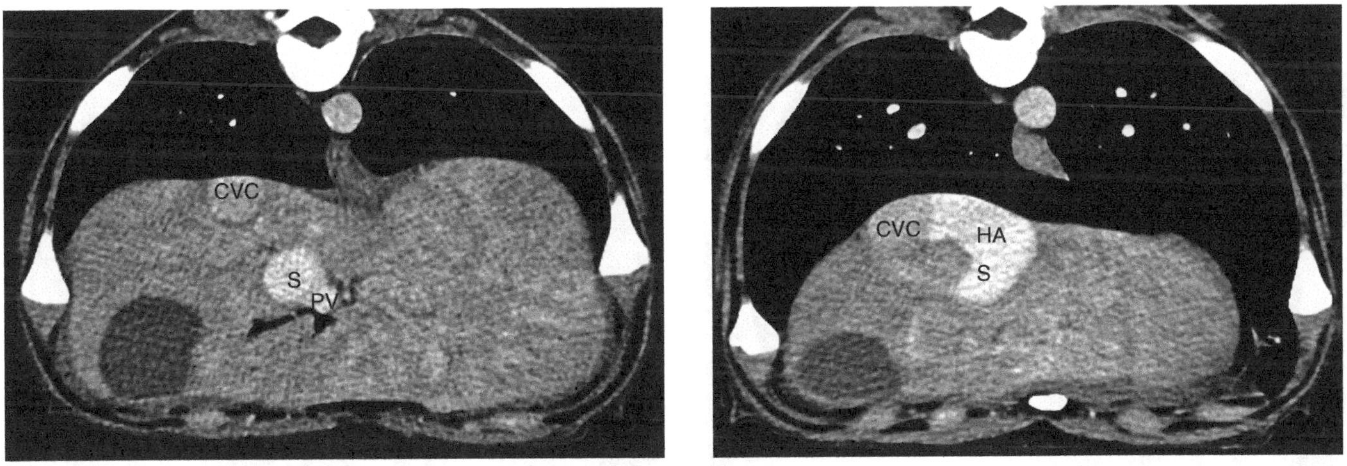

A B

Figure 35.13 Single left-divisional intrahepatic portocaval shunt in a dog with (A) a large tortuous shunting vessel (S) emanating from the lateral part of the left portal vein branch (PV) and (B) performing a leftward turn to connect to the hepatic ampulla (HA) which flows into the caudal vena cava (CVC).

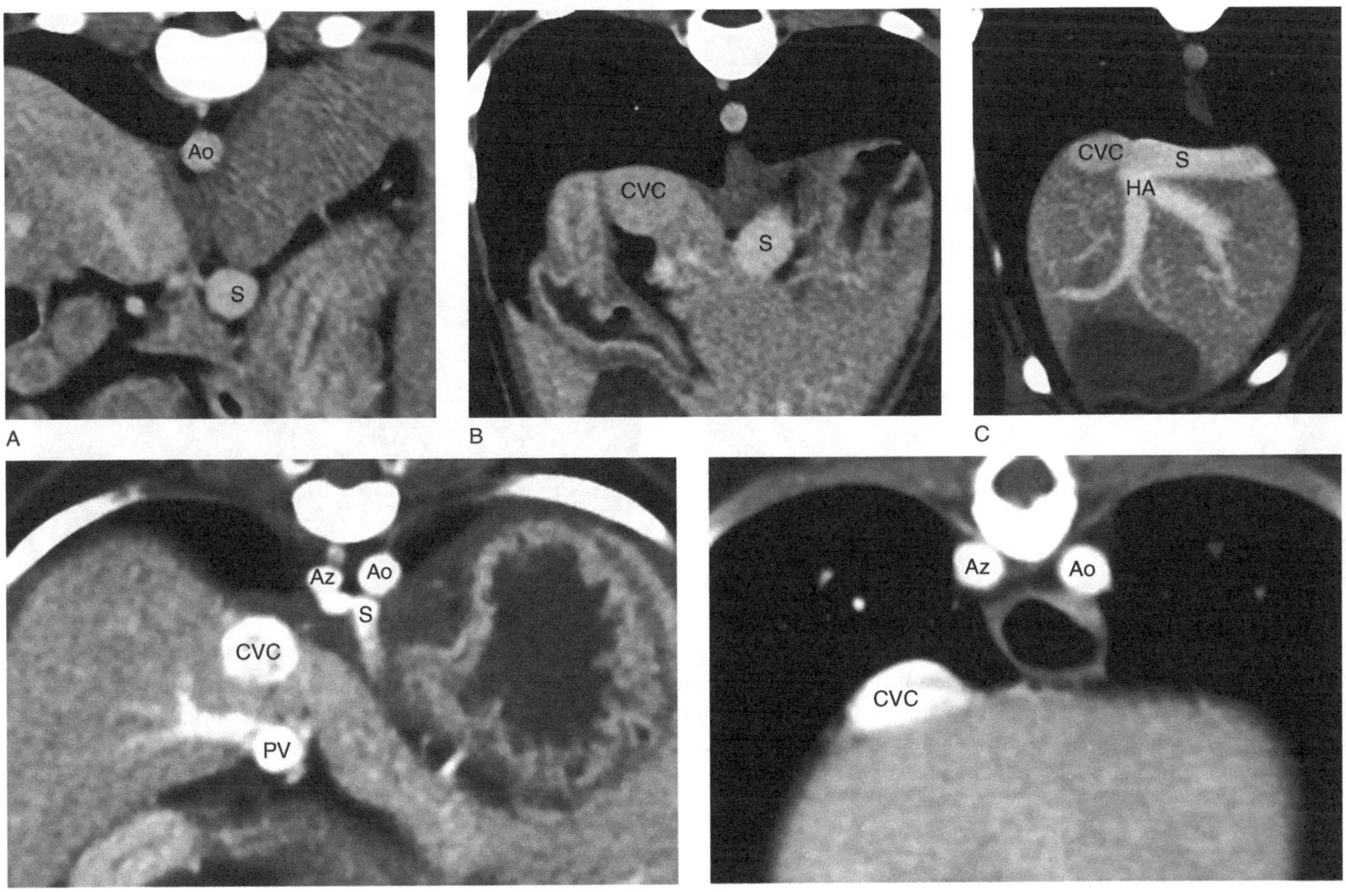

A B C D E

Figure 35.14 (A–C) Single extrahepatic shunt (S) in a dog (A) emanating from the left gastric vein, traveling along the minor curvature of the stomach and (B) then dorsal to the left liver margin to (C) connect to the caudal vena cava (CVC) directly cranial to its liver exit at which point the CVC also receives the hepatic ampulla (HA). (D,E) Single extrahepatic portoazygos shunt in a dog where (D) the shunt vessel (S) can be seen entering the right azygos vein (Az) which (E) further cranially is enlarged. Ao = aorta; PV = portal vein.

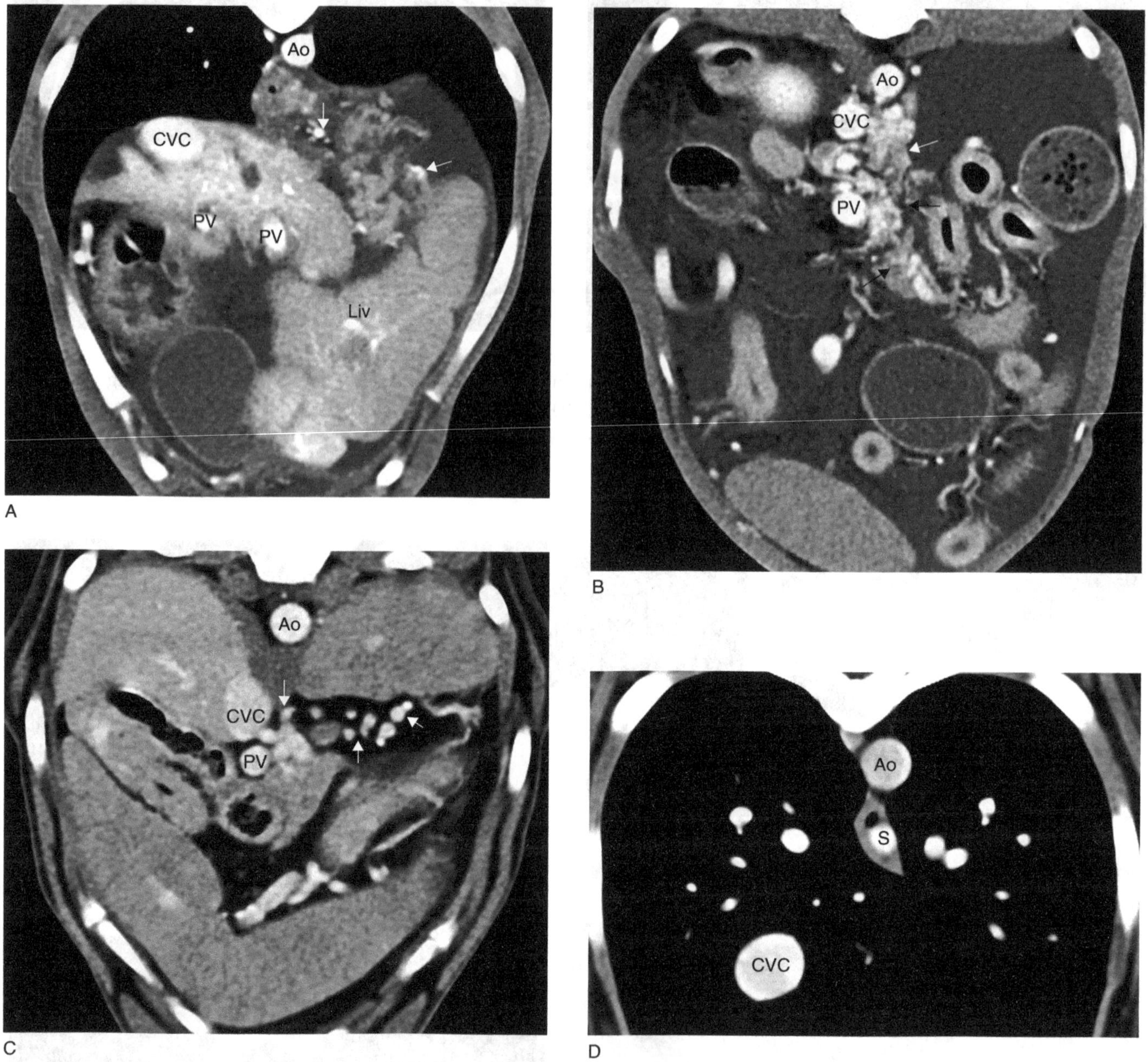

Figure 35.15 (A,B) Multiple extrahepatic shunts in a dog. The chronically diseased liver (Liv) is abnormally small and irregular causing marked ascites and multiple extrahepatic portocaval shunts (arrows). Ao = aorta; CVC = caudal vena cava; PV = portal vein. (C,D) Multiple extrahepatic shunts and esophageal varix in a dog. (C) Multiple small shunt vessels (arrows) emanating from the portal vein (PV) and connecting to the CVC. (D) In the caudal thorax a distended shunt vessel (S) can be seen in the esophageal wall, indicating a varix formation.

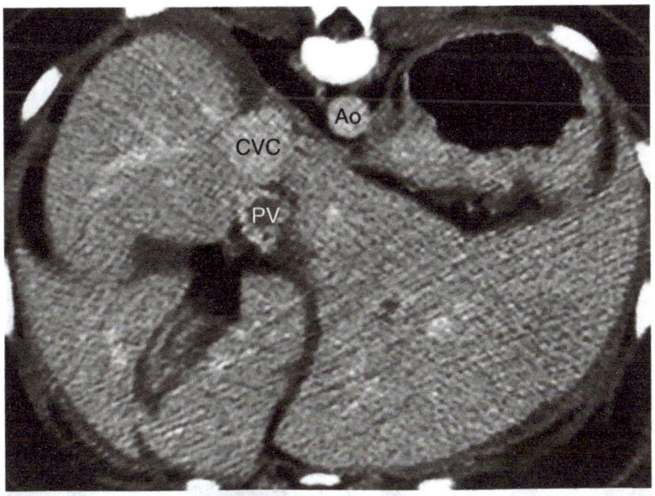

Figure 35.16 Portal vein thrombosis in a dog following an accidental steroid medication overdose. The portal vein (PV) contains a hypodense filling defect, compared to the contrast enhancement in caudal vena cava (CVC) and aorta (Ao). The liver lobes are separated by a hypodense rim, indicating ascites.

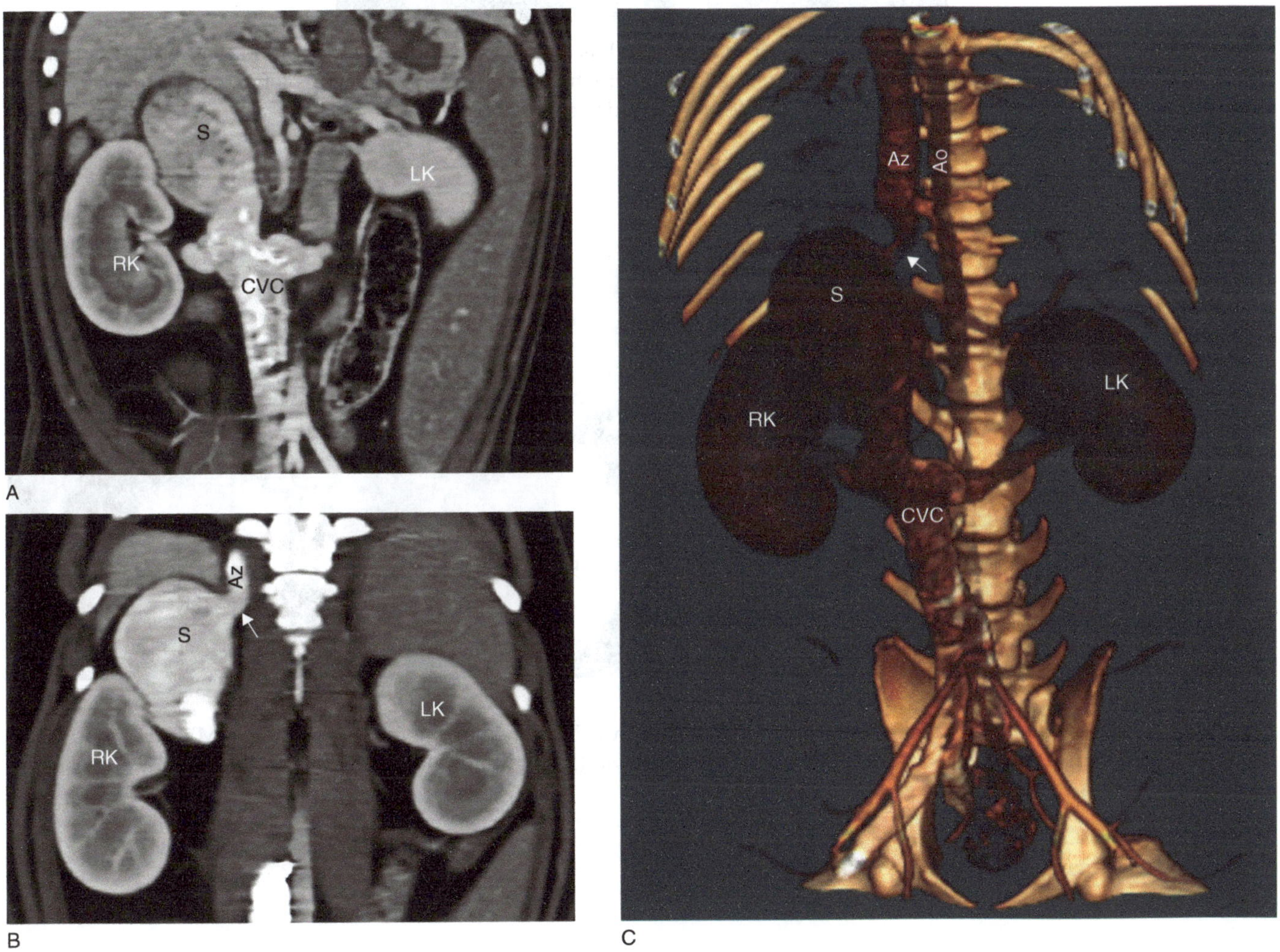

Figure 35.17 Segmental caudal vena cava aplasia in a dog. (A) The post-renal segment of the caudal vena cava (CVC) is entering a large bulbous shunting vessel (S), located right and dorsal to the right kidney (RK) with mixed contrast medium uptake, suggestive of turbulent flow. LK = left kidney. (B) The shunting vessel feeds via an isthmian conduit (arrow) into the right azygos vein (Az). (C) Volume-rendered 3-D image of the abdomen, viewed from ventral (cranial on top), displaying the cavo-azygos shunt vessel (arrow) and its relation to the kidneys and aorta (images courtesy of Fraser McConnell). Ao = aorta.

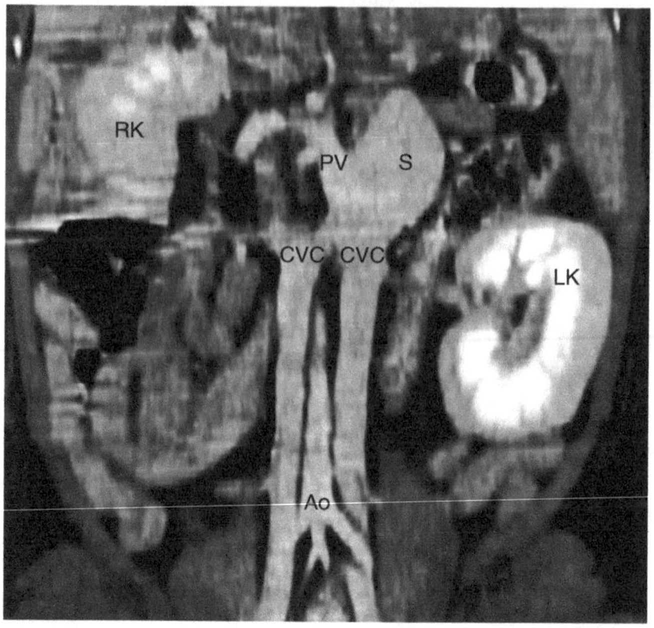

Figure 35.18 Split caudal vena cava (CVC) in a dog that also has segmental caudal vena cava aplasia. A right and a left CVC can be seen entering a large bulbous shunting vessel (S), which connects to an anomalous left azygos vein. The portal vein (PV) also feeds into the shunt vessel. Ao = aorta; LK = left kidney; RK = right kidney.

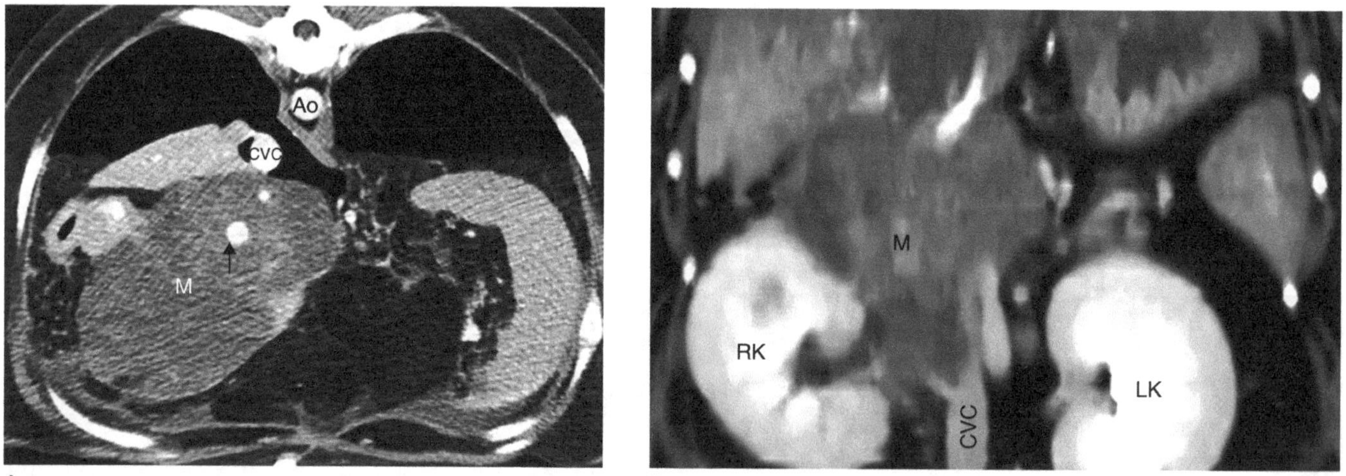

Figure 35.19 (A) Mesenteric hemangiosarcoma in a dog with a large hemorrhagic omental mass (M) surrounding the irregular portal vein (arrow). Ao = aorta, CVC = caudal vena cava. (B) Right adrenal adenocarcinoma (M) in a dog causing invasion of the CVC. LK = left kidney; RK = right kidney.

CHAPTER THIRTY-SIX

Abdominal Lymph Nodes and Lymphatic Collecting System

Federica Rossi, Michail Patsikas and Erik R. Wisner

Imaging Protocol

See Table 36.1.

CT: Anatomy and Normal Variants

Abdominal lymph nodes

Several abdominal lymph nodes can be routinely identified in CT. In the authors' experience, left hepatic, splenic, jejunal, medial iliac and superficial inguinal lymph nodes are usually recognized in normal dogs. Less consistently seen are the gastric, pancreaticoduodenal, colic, hypogastric, sacral, aortic and renal lymph nodes, which are easily visualized if enlarged (Figure 36.1).

In the cat, there are no significant differences in the presence and location of abdominal lymph nodes; the abundance of abdominal fat increases the conspicuity of these very small structures.

In CT, normal lymph nodes appear as small, round to elongated structures, with a density in the range of soft tissues and surrounded by low attenuating fat. The dimensions of the lymph nodes vary; in the authors' experience, the ratio of the longitudinal to the transverse diameter is normally ≥ 2. To identify the lymph nodes, the best way is to follow the abdominal vessels in the post-contrast study and look for small enhancing structures adjacent to the associated artery or vein. The long axis of lymph nodes is usually parallel to that of adjacent vessels. Because lymph nodes are highly vascularized structures, normal nodes intensely enhance but to a lesser extent than adjacent vessels. No differentiation between the cortex and medulla is possible in a standard CT examination but the fat filled hilus appears as a low density region located eccentrically in the node.

Collecting system – lymphatic vessels, cisterna chyli and thoracic duct

The peripheral system of lymphatic vessels and the lymph collecting ducts (cisterna chyli and thoracic duct) are difficult to detect on CT unless contrast enhanced.

To perform a CT lymphography, two techniques are possible.

- Interstitial or indirect lymphography, for the visualization of the lymphatic vessels and lymph nodes directly draining from the injected area. The contrast medium is injected into tissues within the lymphatic drainage volume.
- Direct lymphography, for the visualization of the cisterna chyli and thoracic duct. The injection is made directly into a lymph vessel or lymph node (*see* Table 36.1).

Indirect lymphography

Normally, contrast medium injected interstitially enters into the draining lymphatic vessels almost immediately following injection. The draining lymphatic vessels and the sentinel lymph node are often well-visualized 1 minute after the injection. The sentinel lymph node is the first lymph node that receives lymph flow from the injected area and appears as an oval-shaped structure with a greater diameter than the lymphatic vessels. Contrast medium is homogene-

Veterinary Computed Tomography, First Edition. Edited by Tobias Schwarz, Jimmy Saunders.

Table 36.1
CT imaging protocol.

Series	Pre-contrast	Post-contrast	Indirect CT lymphography*	Direct CT lymphography**
Decubitus	Ventral		Ventral or dorsal (injected area opposite to the table top)	A. Ventral B. Dorsal
Scan Margins	13th thoracic vertebra > Sacral bone		13th thoracic vertebra or more cranially if draining lymphatic vessels enter in the thorax > Sacral bone	Thoracic inlet > Popliteal lymph node
Voltage (kVp)	120–140			
Current (mAs)	100–160			
Tube rotation time (s)	1 or 2			
Slice width (mm)	2–5***			
Kernel frequency	Medium			
Collimator pitch	1–2			
Helical image reconstruction interval	½ of the slice width			
Motion control	Hyperventilation to get expiratory apnea			
Contrast medium application site	N/A	Peripheral vein	Intratissue (subcutaneous, intraparenchymal, intralesional) by means of a 27-gauge needle Gentle massage of the anatomic location	A. Popliteal lymph node (25 ga butterfly needle). Gentle massage of the injected area B. Mesenteric lymph node(s) 27-ga 1¼" needle
Contrast medium type	N/A	Iodinated	Iodinated, non-ionic, water-soluble 300 to 370 mg iodine/ml, absorbed by the initial lymphatic vessels	Iodinated, non-ionic, water-soluble 300–370 mg iodine/ml
Contrast medium dose	N/A	800 mg iodine/kg bw	0.5 to 1 ml depending on the size of the injected area	A. 1 ml/kg B. 1.5–2 ml/lymph node
Contrast medium injection mode	N/A	Manual or automated (preferably)	Manual, slow injection. The total dose can be divided in many sites.	A. Manual, 2 ml/min B. Manual in 90–120 s
Scan delay post start contrast injection	N/A	First scan: immediately Delayed scan: 3–5 min	First scan 1 min after injection Delayed scan: 5–10 min	A. First scan: immediately Delayed scan: 5–10 min B. 5 min
Window level (HU)	+40			
Window width (HU)	300			

*To localize the draining lymphatic vessels and sentinel lymph node.
**To visualize the cisterna chyli and thoracic duct.
***In some patients, additional thinly collimated images may be required to fully characterize the thoracic duct and its branches, particularly near its convergence with the cranial vena cava.

ously distributed into the normal lymph node and lymphatic vessels, which are easily recognized by their high density. Five minutes after the injection, lymphatic vessels coursing from the sentinel lymph node to more proximal nodes are usually visualized. The 3-D reconstructed post-contrast CT images provide a comprehensive anatomy of the lymphatic vasculature and the location of the sentinel lymph node(s) (Figure 36.2).

Direct lymphography

The topographic anatomy of the cisterna chyli and of the thoracic duct can be easily identified with percuta-

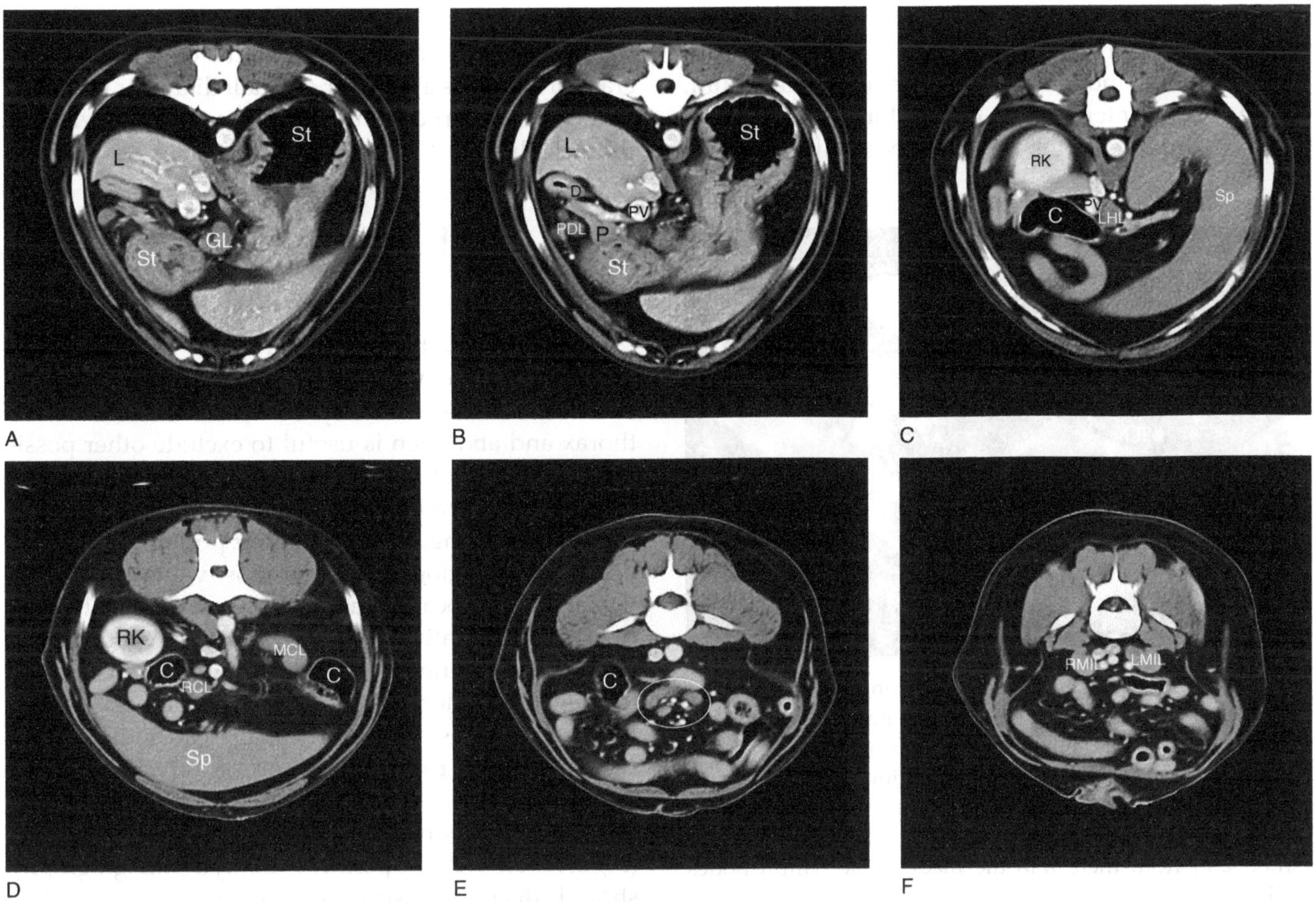

Figure 36.1 Adult dog with multicentric lymphoma. (A–F) Transverse CT images show moderate enlargement and rounding of all abdominal lymphocenters increasing their visibility. The following lymph nodes are visible: gastric (A), pancreatico-duodenal (B), left hepatic (C), right and middle colic (D), jejunal (E) and medial iliac (F) lymph nodes. C = colon; D = duodenum; GL = gastric lymph nodes; L = liver; LHL = left hepatic lymph node; LMIL = left medial iliac lymph node; MCL = medial colic lymph nodes; P = pancreas; PDL = pancreatico-duodenal lymph nodes; PV = portal vein; RCL = right colic lymph nodes; RK = right kidney; RMIL = right medial iliac lymph node; Sp = spleen; St = stomach. The circle encloses jejunal lymph nodes.

neous injection of contrast medium into the popliteal lymph node. The proper dose and administration rate of contrast medium are essential for successful visualization (Table 36.1).

CT lymphangiography following ultrasound-guided percutaneous injection of contrast medium into mesenteric lymph nodes has been recently proposed as a less invasive alternative to conventional mesenteric lymphangiography which requires cannulation of a surgically exposed mesenteric lymphatic vessel. Following the initial unenhanced CT scan, one or two mesenteric lymph nodes are localized and injected. An echogenic 'bloom' can sometimes be detected as contrast medium accumulates in the node and a slow delivery rate is important to maximize retention of contrast medium within the node and associated afferent lymphatic vessels. In the authors' experience, this injection technique is much more successful in dogs than in cats and the imaging study may have to be aborted if contrast medium delivery is unsuccessful.

CT imaging findings

The efferent lymphatic vessels of the popliteal lymph node, the lymph nodes of the iliosacral lymphocenter, the cisterna chyli and the thoracic duct are best visualized on CT images acquired immediately after the injection of the contrast medium. Normally, there is no leakage of the contrast medium into the abdominal and thoracic cavity. The cisterna chyli, a lymphatic reservoir, is located ventral to the first four lumbar vertebrae, it is bordered ventrally by the aorta and dorsally by the azygous vein and becomes the thoracic duct as it passes cranially through the aortic hiatus. In the dog, the thoracic duct crosses to the left, dorsal to the aorta, at approximately the level of the sixth thoracic vertebra and enters the cranial mediastinum, where it may enter the left external jugular vein, the left subclavian vein, the left brachiocephalic vein, the azygos vein, the cranial vena cava or other veins. As the thoracic duct arises from cisterna chyli and travels cranially, it gives a number of small diameter branches that travel a short distance and re-anastomose with the thoracic duct.

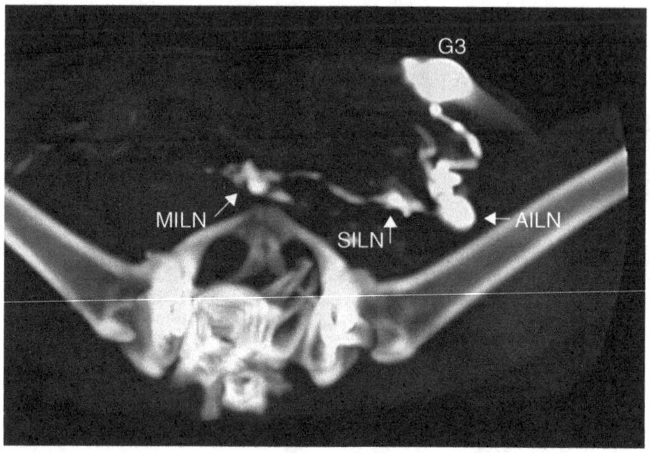

Figure 36.2 3-D reconstructed CT lymphogram 5 min after injection of contrast medium into the parenchyma of the third mammary gland (G3) in a normal cat (dorsal decubitus) shows mammary lymphatic vessels draining into the accessory inguinal lymph node (AILN). Efferent lymphatic vessels from AILN drain into the superficial inguinal lymph nodes (SILN) and from there into the medial iliac lymph nodes (MILN).

Disease Features

Trauma

Chylothorax due to traumatic rupture of the thoracic duct is common while chyloabdomen secondary to lesions of the cisterna chyli is quite rare. CT of the thorax and abdomen is useful to exclude other possible underlying causes of chylous effusion (neoplasia, caudal vena cava thrombosis, lung lobe torsion, pericardial thickening, other pleural or peritoneal lesions).

CT lymphangiography is of most value in defining the anatomic location and character of the thoracic duct in preparation for surgery (Figure 36.3). The abnormal appearance of the duct and its branches may explain the underlying cause of chylothorax. Overt, localized contrast medium leakage can indicate thoracic duct wall rupture (Figures 36.4, 36.5), whereas distention and multiplication of small terminal branches may suggest obstructive lymphangectasia (Figure 36.6). Post-operative CT lymphangiography should document successful ligation by complete

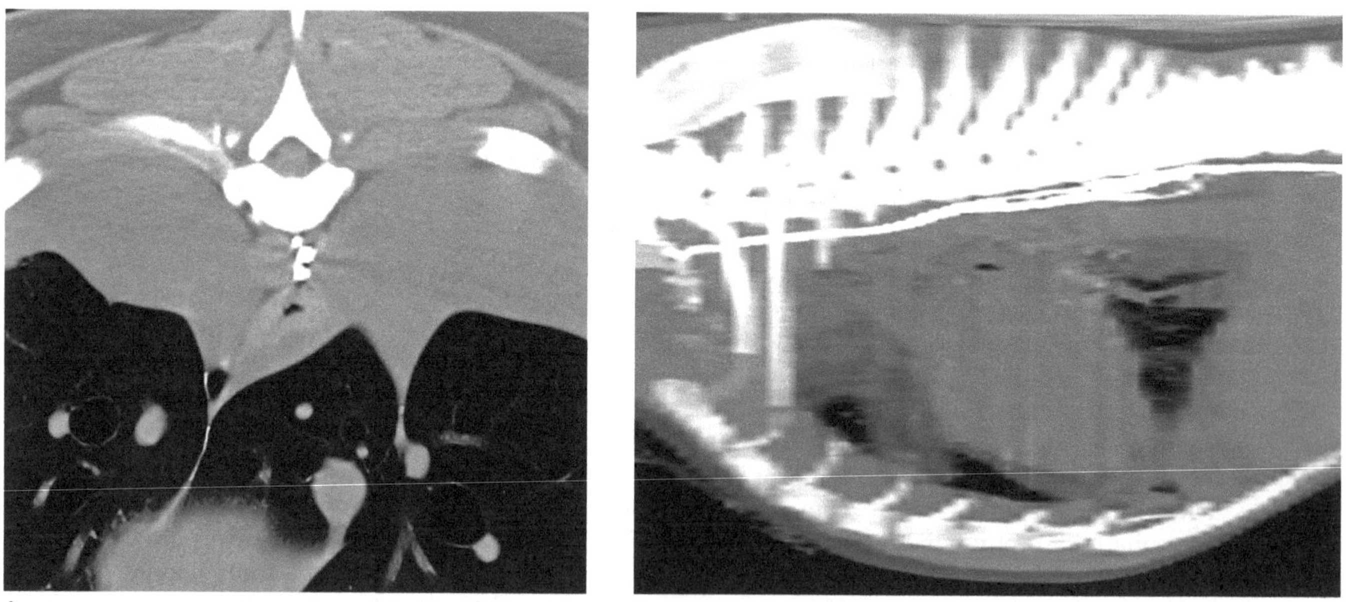

A B

Figure 36.3 Dog with chylothorax. (A) Transverse CT image acquired at the level of the caudal thorax with the dog in dorsal recumbency and following iodinated contrast medium administration into a mesenteric lymph node. At least three parallel thoracic duct branches are identified in cross-section adjacent to the descending aorta. **(B)** Sagittally oriented maximum intensity projection (MIP) of the same dog documents the path of the redundant thoracic duct and its termination near the thoracic inlet.

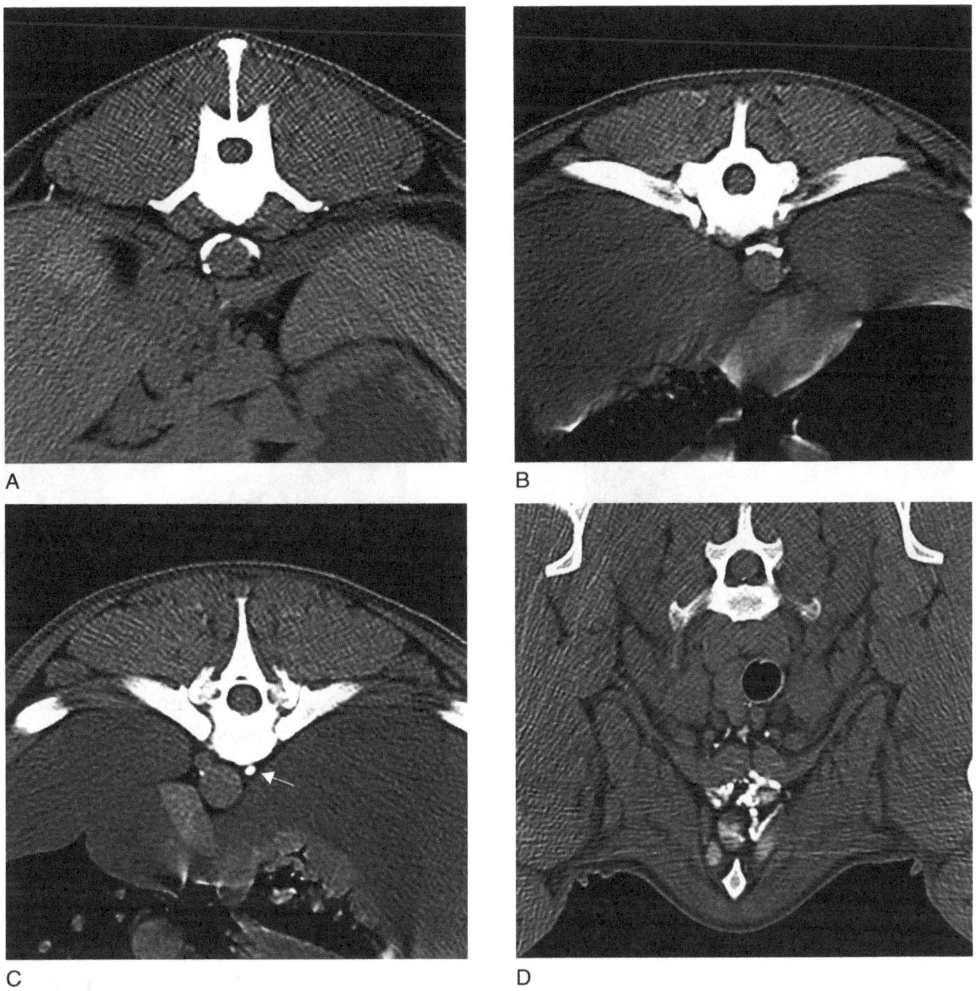

Figure 36.4 Adult dog with idiopathic chylothorax. Direct CT lymphogram images at the level of L2 (A), T12 (B), T11 (C) level and through the cranial mediastinum (D). The cisterna chyli (A) and the thoracic duct with its branches (B,C) filled with contrast medium are clearly visualized. The thoracic duct is localized on the left side of the aorta (C, arrow). Another small collateral vessel lies on the right between the aorta and azygos vein. An anastomotic vessel is visible at the level of T12 (B). In the cranial mediastimum, multiple dilated lymphatic vessels are visualized (D).

truncation of the thoracic duct contrast column and its parallel branches, if any, cranial to the ligation site.

In patients in whom the thoracic duct is ligated, CT lymphography is also performed preoperatively for surgical planning and immediately postoperatively to verify duct ligation. Postoperative studies are of particular importance in patients with multiple duct branches coursing in parallel, since thoracic duct duplication may make complete ligation more challenging.

Visceral lymph nodes can be enlarged if chronic cavitary effusion is present. Abdominal trauma can produce lymphadenomegaly because of edema or hemorrage due to direct injury or secondary to inflammation of the peritoneum or other abdominal viscera.

CT features

- Pleural and/or abdominal effusion.
- Direct CT lymphography:
  - loss of visualization or interruption of the thoracic duct or its branches
  - extravasation of contrast medium into the pleural space.
- Associated lymphadenomegaly (with chronic effusion or direct trauma).

Lymphadenitis

Abdominal lymphadenitis due to inflammation or infection of peritoneal organs is often recognized. Reactive lymph nodes are enlarged and therefore easily identified. They tend to be rounded and homogeneous; however, sometimes there is a change in

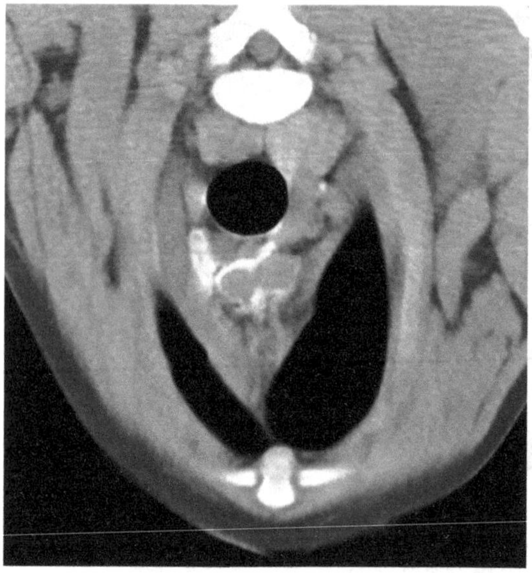

Figure 36.5 Dog with chylothorax. Transverse CT image acquired near the thoracic inlet with the dog in dorsal decubitus and following iodinated contrast medium administration into a mesenteric lymph node. Contrast medium surrounds the confluence of the two external jugular veins. A similar pattern of uncontained contrast medium was also present further caudally. The imaging diagnosis was thoracic duct rupture near its termination at the cranial vena cava with resultant lymphatic fluid leakage.

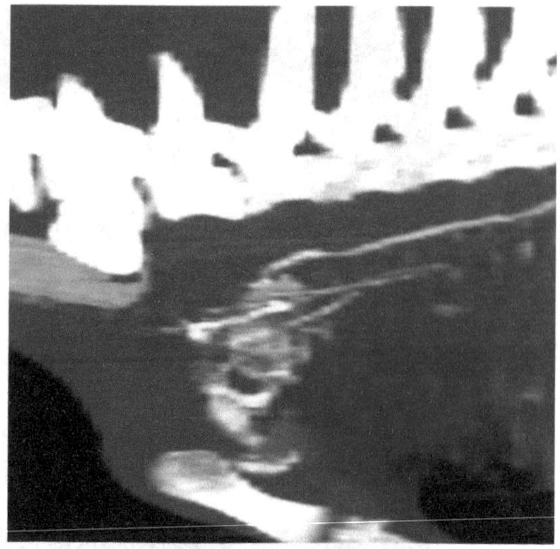

Figure 36.6 Dog with chylothorax. Sagittally oriented maximum intensity projection from a thoracic CT study following iodinated contrast medium administration into a mesenteric lymph node. The thoracic duct courses cranially and terminates in a complex of markedly distended terminal lymphatic vessels. The imaging diagnosis in this patient was obstructive lymphangectasia.

shape and density due to abscess or cyst formation within an affected node.

CT features

- Lymphadenomegaly.
- Acute cases:
  - often rounded lymph nodes with regular shape and margins.
- Chronic cases:
  - lymph nodes more irregular in shape and heterogeneous
  - hypodense areas with abscessation, necrosis or cysts formation (Figure 36.7)
  - hyperdense foci in case of calcification.

Neoplasia

Abdominal lymphadenomegaly is often seen in oncologic patients. Because of the exquisite anatomical detail provided by CT, it can be used to differentiate enlarged lymph nodes from masses arising from other abdominal viscera. CT enables precise evaluation of all lymphocenters and identification of possible site of metastases in animals having primary neoplasia. Following peritumoral contrast medium administration, indirect CT lymphography may be used to characterize the anatomic distribution and morphological features of sentinel and more distant lymph nodes. In general, lymph nodes containing macroscopic metastases have heterogeneous contrast medium uptake with metastatic deposits typically appearing as contrast filling defects. In patients with multicentric lymphoma, several and more distant lymph centers may be involved (Figure 36.1). Typically, lymphomatous lymph nodes are more uniformly enlarged and have a mildly heterogeneous "foamy" appearance following contrast medium administration. CT features can be overlapping with inflammatory conditions.

CT features

- Lymphadenomegaly.
- Often irregular shape.
- Post-contrast: heterogeneous density (Figure 36.8) because of hyper- or hypodense foci due to hemorrhage, necrosis, cysts formation or mineralization.
- Indirect CT lymphography: often heterogeneous or lack of opacification in indirect CT lymphography (Figure 36.9).
- Invasion of surrounding fat, vessels, other soft tissue or bony structures (Figure 36.10).

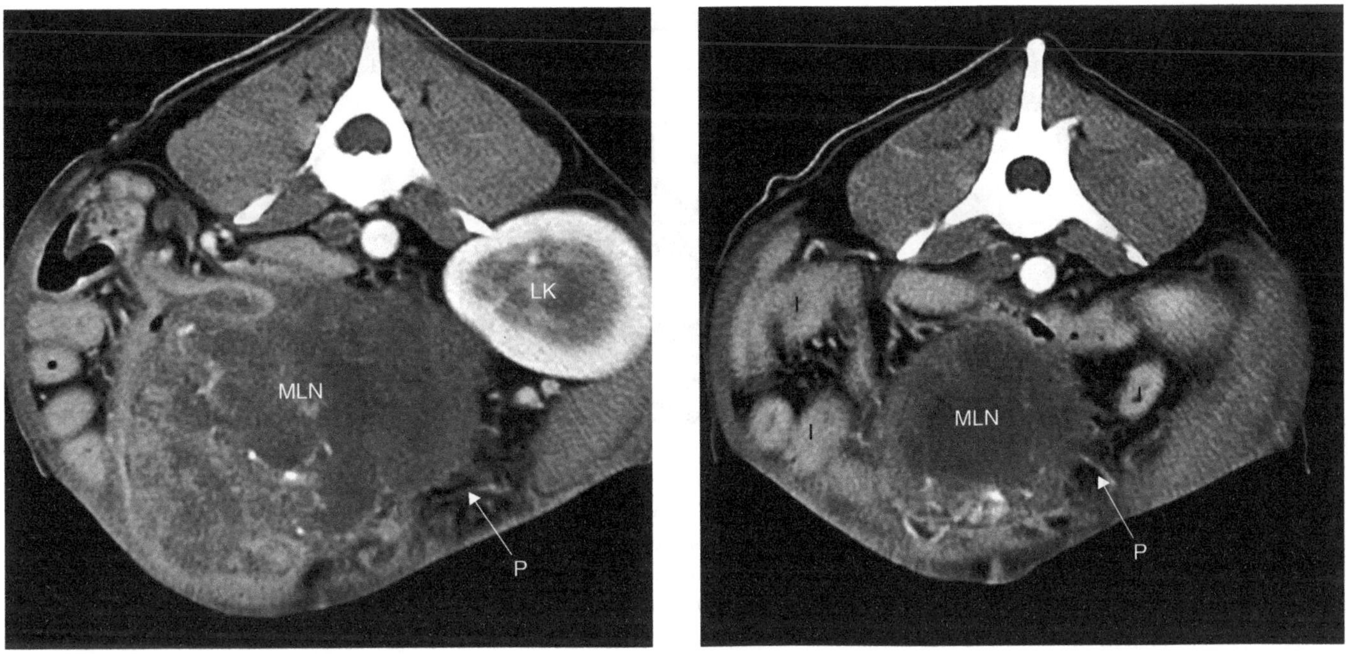

A B

Figure 36.7 Adult dog with a peritoneal abscess originating from a mesenteric lymph node. Post-contrast transverse CT images of the (A) mid- and (B) caudal abdomen show a severely enlarged mesenteric lymph node (MLN) that is also heterogeneous because of variable contrast medium uptake and multifocal mineralization. The abscessed lymph node is surrounded by thickened peritoneum (P) and small intestinal loops (I). LK = left kidney.

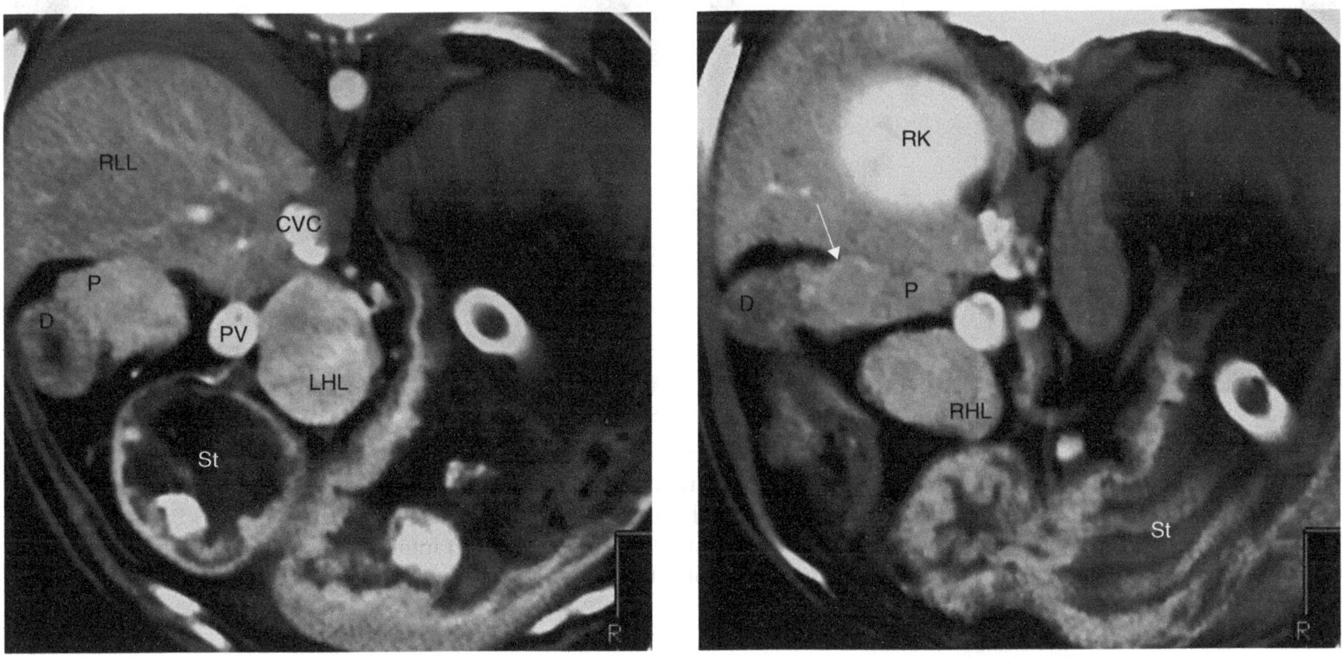

A B

Figure 36.8 Adult dog with primary pancreatic neoplasia (gastrinoma). (A,B) Post-contrast 3-D volume rendering reconstructed CT images of the hepatic hilus region. The left and right hepatic lymph nodes (LHL and RHL), confirmed to be metastatic, are increased in diameter with irregular shape and heterogeneous density. The pancreas (P) is enlarged, and a high-density nodule is visible (B, arrow). CVC = caudal vena cava; D = duodenum; PV = portal vein; RK = right kidney; RLL = right lateral liver lobe; St = stomach;.

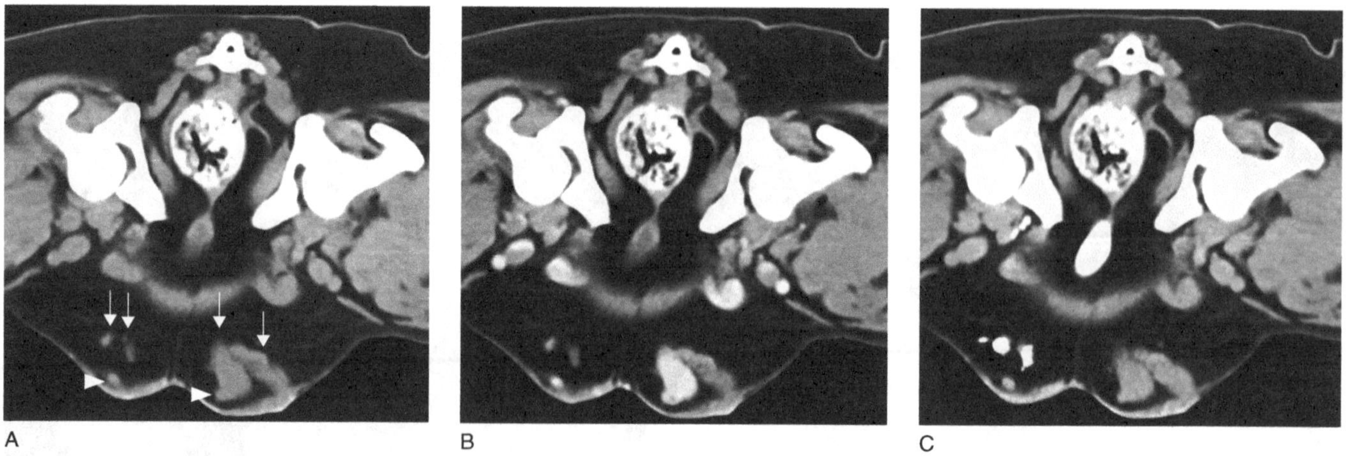

Figure 36.9 Adult dog with neoplasia of the fourth left mammary gland. (A) Transverse CT image shows two metastatic left and two normal right superficial inguinal lymph nodes (arrows). The left-sided lymph nodes are enlarged with irregular shape and heterogeneous density (arrowheads demonstrate superficial vessels). (B) Post-contrast transverse CT image shows heterogeneous enhancement of the left-sided lymph nodes immediately after intravenous injection of the contrast medium. (C) Indirect CT lymphogram 1 min after injection of the contrast medium into the neoplastic and collateral normal mammary glands failed to opacify left sided lymph nodes.

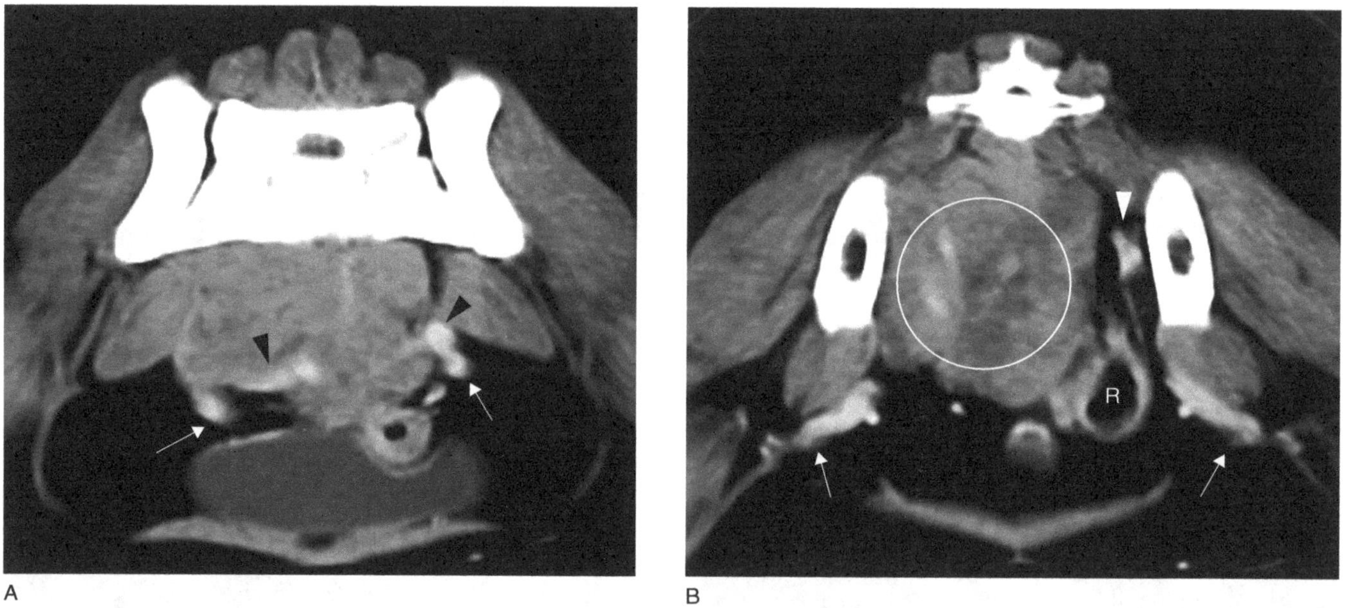

Figure 36.10 Metastatic hypogastric lymph nodes in an adult dog with primary anal sac carcinoma. (A) Post-contrast CT image shows infiltration of the sublumbar fat and musculature. The external iliac arteries (arrows) and common iliac veins (arrowheads) are visible. The veins on the right are ventrally displaced and compressed by the mass. (B) Post-contrast CT image shows the right and left femoral veins are clearly identified (arrows). The left internal iliac vein is visible (arrowhead), while the right left internal iliac vein and their branches enter the mass (circle). The rectum (R) is displaced ventrally and towards the left.

Further reading

Esterline ML, Radlinsky MG, Biller DS, Mason DE, Roush JK and Cash WC (2005) Comparison of radiographic and computed tomography lymphangiography for identification of the canine thoracic duct. *Vet Radiol Ultrasound* **46**: 391–5.

Fossum TW, Mertens MM, Miller MW *et al.* (2004) Thoracic duct ligation and pericardectomy for treatement of idiopathic chylothorax. *J Vet Intern Med* **18**: 307–10.

Johnson EG, Wisner ER, Kyles A, Koehler C and Marks SL (2009) Computed tomographic lymphography of the thoracic duct by mesenteric lymph node injection. *Vet Surg* **38**: 361–7.

Naganobu K, Ohigashi Y, Akiyoshi T, Hagio M, Miyamoto T and Yamaguchi R (2006) Lymphography of the thoracic duct by percutaneous injection of iohexol into the popliteal lymph node of dogs: experimental study and clinical application. *Vet Surg* **35**: 377–81.

Papadopoulou PL, Patsikas MN, Charitanti A *et al.* (2009) The lymph drainage of the mammary glands in the cat: a lymphographic and computerized tomography lymphographic study. *Anat Histol Embryol* **38**: 292–9.

Patsikas MN, Papadopoulou PL, Charitanti A *et al.* (2010) Computed tomography and radiographic indirect lymphography for visualization of the mammary lymphatic vessels and the sentinel lymph node in normal cats. *Vet Radiol Ultrasound* **51**: 299–304.

Suga K, Ogasawara N, Yuan Y, Okada M, Matsunaga N and Tangoku A (2003) Visualization of breast lymphatic pathways with an indirect computed tomography lymphography using a nonionic monomeric contrast medium iopamidol: preliminary results. *Invest Radiol* **38**: 73–84.

CHAPTER THIRTY-SEVEN

LONG BONES

Ryan M. Schultz and Erik R. Wisner

CT: ANATOMY AND NORMAL VARIANTS

The CT appearance of long bones is similar to that seen on conventional radiographs. However, due to a lack of anatomic superimposition, there may be better definition of medullary bone architectural detail and better delineation of endosteal cortical margins.

Long bone physeal closure times are age dependent in dogs and cats and are well-documented in other sources. Physes appear as lucencies of variable width and definition depending on anatomic location and patient age. The appearance of physes can be somewhat confusing when viewed in-plane and are often better evaluated on images reformatted along the long axis of the bone (Figure 37.1).

Table 37.1 shows the anatomic differences between canine and feline long bones.

DISEASE FEATURES

Malformation/Developmental

Angular limb deformities

Angular limb deformities such as radius curvus, tibial torsion and femoral varus or torsion can result from trauma or developmental orthopedic disease. These types of deformities in dogs have been associated with a variety of clinical disorders including lameness, gait alteration, joint incongruity, patellar instability, Osgood–Schlatter-like syndrome and osteoarthrosis. Radiographs may cause a false appearance of tibial torsion due to image distortion from beam angle and magnification artifacts whereas CT does not.

CT features (Figure 37.2)

CT can be used in dogs with angular limb deformities for preoperative corrective osteotomy planning as the torsional or angular deformity of the bone can be accurately and quantitatively characterized by CT.

Panosteitis

Panosteitis is a self-limiting disorder of unknown cause primarily affecting the appendicular skeleton of immature large breed dogs with male and German shepherd dogs overrepresented. Onset of the disorder is typically at 5 to 12 months of age, but panosteitis has been reported to occur in dogs as young as 2 months and as old as 7 years. Lesions in a particular location may resolve as others develop and imaging findings do not always correlate with clinical signs. This pattern leads to the typical history of shifting leg lameness.

CT features (Figure 37.3)

- Lesions may be monostotic or polyostotic.
- Ill-defined intramedullary bone opacities may be surrounded by intramedullary fat or extend to the endosteal surface of the cortex.
- Regional periosteal or endosteal production may be evident and the lesions often arise near a nutrient foramen. The lesions eventually resolve leaving a residual coarse to normal appearing trabecular bone architecture.

Incomplete ossification of the humeral condyle

Incomplete ossification of the humeral condyle most often occurs in Spaniel breeds and may lead to pathologic humeral condylar fractures following normal physical activities. Two separate humeral condylar ossification centers appear radiographically at approximately 22 days of age and fuse by 84 days. In dogs with incomplete ossification, the two ossification centers remain separated by a thin fibrous fissure. Pathologic fractures are often Y- or T- fractures of the humeral condyle and epicondyle, but fractures limited

Veterinary Computed Tomography, First Edition. Edited by Tobias Schwarz, Jimmy Saunders.

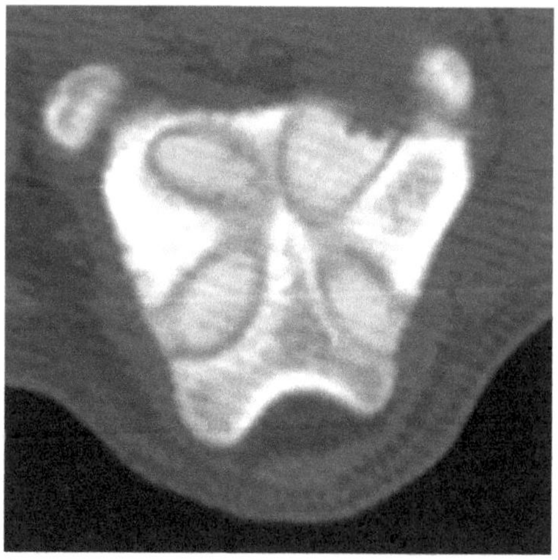

A

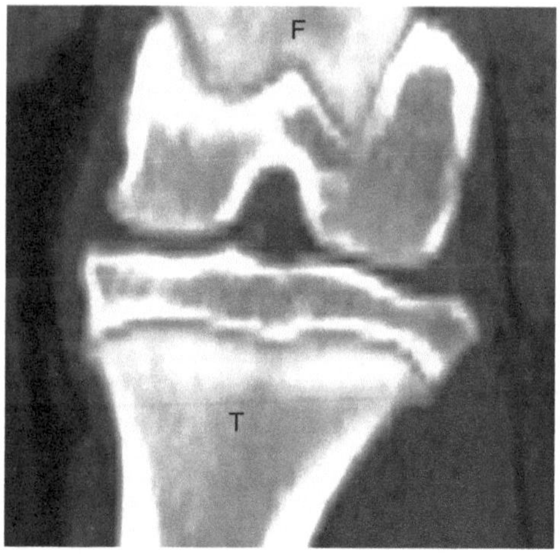

B

Figure 37.1 Six-month-old Labrador retriever with apparent open physes. (A) Transverse CT image shows the complex anatomy of a portion of the distal femoral physis, the metaphysis and the epiphysis. (B) Frontally reformatted maximum intensity projection image of the distal femoral and proximal tibial physes. The anatomy of the physes is easier to evaluate on images reformatted along the long axis of the bone. F = femur; T = tibia.

Table 37.1
Anatomic differences between canine and feline long bones.

Structure	Canine	Feline
Supratrochlear foramen of humerus	Present	Absent
Supracondylar foramen of humerus	Absent	Present – the brachial artery and median nerve traverse this structure
Coronoid fossa of the humerus	Absent	Present
Clavicle	Remnant	Well developed and ossified
Coracoid process of the scapula	Rudimentary	Well developed
Hamate and suprahamate processes of the acromion of the scapula	Absent	Present

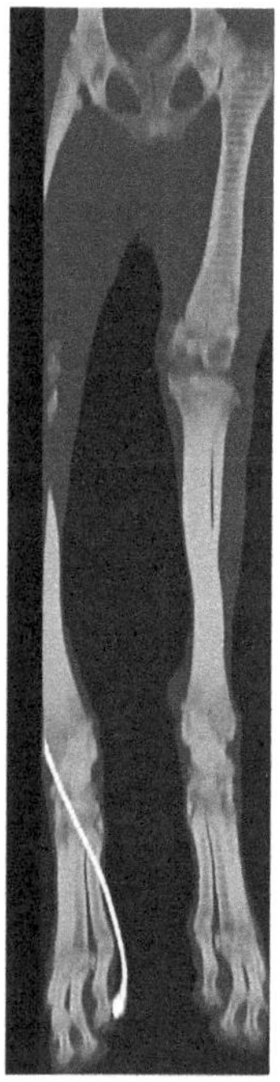

Figure 37.2 Maximum intensity projection CT image centered on the left pelvic limb of a dog with an angular limb deformity. There is an S-shaped deformity of the tibia, rotational deviation of the tarsus relative to the tibia, and the stifle and tarsal joints malalign. This study was performed for preoperative planning to calculate osteotomy angles for a corrective osteotomy of the tibia.

only to the lateral or medial aspects of the condyle also occur. This disorder is often bilateral and evaluation of the contralateral humerus is indicated in young dogs that are presented with spontaneous unilateral humeral condylar fractures.

CT features (Figure 37.4)

- Thin lucent vertical fissure centrally in the humeral condyle that may extend from the elbow joint to the supratrochlear foramen. This fissure is usually surrounded by sclerotic bone.

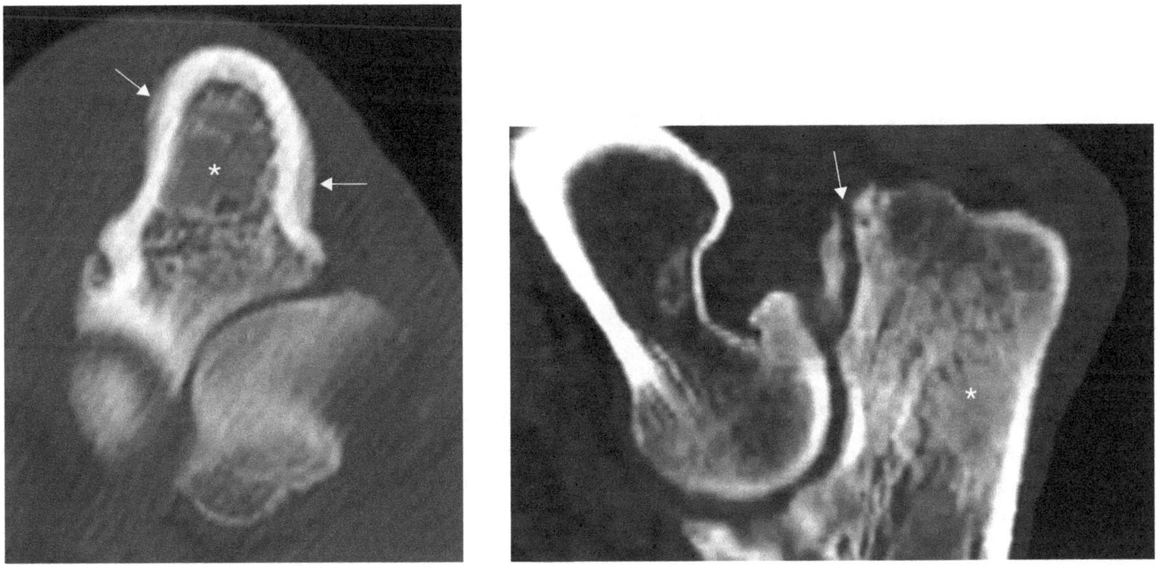

A B

Figure 37.3 Young German shepherd dog with panosteitis and an ununited anconeal process. (A) Transverse CT image shows an intramedullary bone density (250 HU) in the proximal ulna (asterisk) associated with a mild surrounding periosteal productive response (arrows). (B) Sagittally reformatted CT image again reveals the proximal intramedullary density (asterisk). A vertical linear fissure is also visible in this image documenting the presence of an ununited anconeal process (arrow).

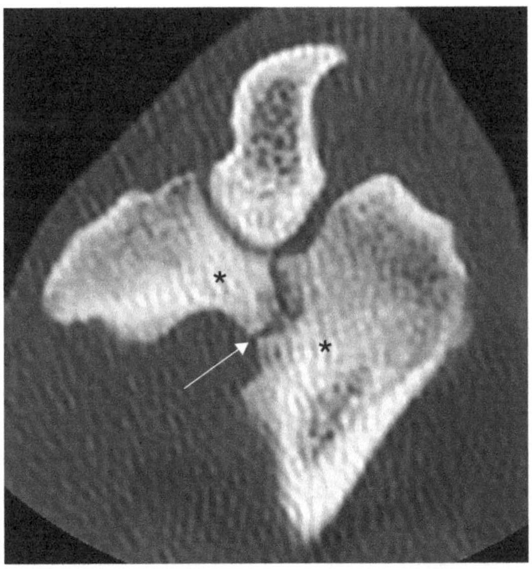

Figure 37.4 Distal humeral condyle from a young Spaniel with incomplete ossification of the humeral condyle. Transverse CT image shows a soft tissue dense vertical fissure (arrow) with surrounding sclerosis (asterisks) in the middle of the humeral condyle. There is no displacement or fracture.

- Periosteal reaction is frequently present on the lateral aspect of the distal humeral metaphysis which is likely secondary to chronic instability.

Miscellaneous developmental disorders

Other developmental disorders such as cartilaginous exostosis, hypertrophic osteodystrophy, retained cartilage core, mucopolysaccharidosis, osteogenesis imperfecta, congenital hypothyroidism, and metaphyseal and epiphyseal dysplasia are initially diagnosed and adequately monitored using radiography.

Metaphyseal osteopathy (synonym: Hypertrophic osteodystrophy)

Initial findings are soft tissue swelling in the region of the metaphysis of the distal radius and ulna, the tibia and the metacarpal/metatarsal bones, and the occurrence of a radiolucent zone parallel to the physis within the metaphysis. Later on periosteal bone proliferation occurs and an extraperiosteal cuff of mineralization develops along the metaphysis. In mature dogs remnants of periosteal and extraperiosteal changes can be detected.

Trauma (Figure 37.5)

Currently CT is not routinely used for trauma or initial assessment of diaphyseal and metaphyseal long bone fractures in dogs and cats. Articular fractures and other complex fractures may be difficult to adequately characterize on radiographs and CT may be indicated for confirmation and preoperative planning for surgical fixation.

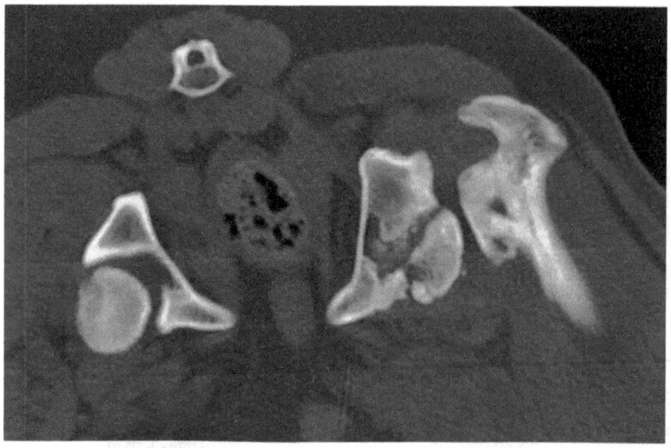

Figure 37.5 Young dog with a chronic fracture of the left femoral head. Transverse CT image shows a chronic fracture of the femoral head and a large amount of surrounding periarticular and periosteal production.

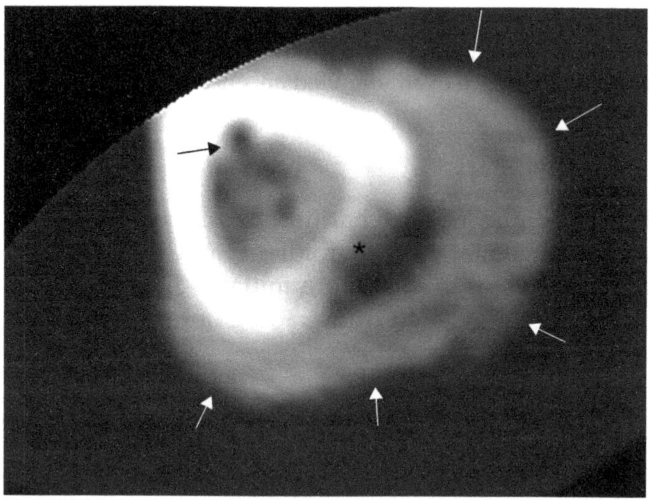

Figure 37.6 Adult dog with coccidioidomycosis osteomyelitis. Transverse CT image of the left tibia shows focal cortical destruction (asterisk) with a prominent adjacent periosteal and endosteal productive response (white arrows). This lesion surrounds the nutrient artery (black arrow) suggesting a hematogeneous etiology.

Infection/Inflammation

Osteomyelitis

Osteomyelitis typically occurs as the result of bacterial or fungal infection. Bacterial osteomyelitis is usually due to direct extension from a penetrating wound or adjacent soft tissue infection, surgical contamination or, in young dogs, from hematogeneous spread to the physis, metaphysis or epiphysis.

Mycotic osteomyelitis is spread hematogeneously and is therefore usually polyostotic. In the US, mycotic osteomyelitis typically occurs in young large breed sporting dogs located in specific geographic locations, including the southwest (coccidioidomycosis) and the southeast and Mississippi river valley regions (blastomycosis). Aspergillus is a less common cause of mycotic osteomyelitis, often as part of a multiorgan, systemic infection. Young female German shepherd dogs are predisposed. Bone infections cannot always be distinguished from bone neoplasms based on imaging appearance only.

CT features (Figure 37.6)

- Bacterial osteomyelitis:
  - variable depending on the initial cause and chronicity of the lesion
  - significant bone destruction and variable reactive periosteal production
  - bone fragments of increased density with sharply delineated cortical margins may be seen when devitalized (sequestered bone).
- Fungal osteomyelitis:
  - pronounced productive unstructured periosteal response with significant underlying bone destruction.

Aseptic necrosis of the femoral head

Aseptic necrosis of the femoral head, also termed Legg–Calve–Perthes disease, typically occurs in growing toy and small breed dogs. Necrosis of the subchondral bone of the femoral head results from a compromised blood supply and the disorder may be bilateral.

CT features

- Initially there is resorption of the subchondral bone of the femoral head followed by femoral head remodeling with surrounding periosteal and periarticular production during the chronic phase of the disease.
- Pathologic fracture of the femoral head may also occur.

Hypertrophic osteopathy (synonyms: Hyperthrophic pulmonary osteopathy, Marie's disease)

Hypertrophic osteopathy is a specific periosteal reaction, usually described as pallisading or columnar, that starts on the metacarpal and metatarsal bones and can progress proximally. The occurrence of this process is usually secondary to a mass in the thorax or abdomen and there are several current theories for the pathophysiology, including vascular, neurogenic or endocrine disturbances. The joints usually are not involved. Conventional radiography is currently adequate for accurate diagnosis of hypertrophic osteopathy.

Metabolic

Secondary hyperparathyroidism

Secondary hyperparathyroidism can cause bone resorption. Renal secondary hyperparathyroidsism primarily affects the mandible and skull. In young animals with nutritional secondary hyperparathyroidism the long bones may be affected. Radiographs are typically used to diagnose these diseases, although CT may be used to quantitatively assess bone density.

CT features

- Thinning or double cortices.
- Decreased bone density.
- Pathologic folding fractures.

Neoplasia

Primary and metastatic bone tumors

Primary long bone tumors typically occur at a single metaphyseal location. The more common sites include the proximal humerus, distal radius, distal femur and proximal tibia. The age distribution in dogs is bimodal with peaks at 2 years of age and a much larger peak in old age. The value of CT for accurate measurement of tumor length is controversial. Regardless, accurate determination of the size of a primary bone tumor is generally only important if a limb-sparing procedure is to be considered as a therapeutic option.

Metastatic tumors of the long bones occur most often from primary transitional cell, mammary, pulmonary and thyroid carcinomas. Metastatic lesions from sarcomas such as primary bone tumors and hemangiosarcomas also occur. Histiocytic sarcomas arising from, or metastasizing to, bone have also been reported.

CT features (Figures 37.7–37.9 and 38.13)

- Cortical bone destruction.
- Amorphous periosteal productive response.
- Long, ill-defined transition zone and a rapid rate of change.

Bone infarcts secondary to a primary bone tumor

Bone infarcts in the long bones are reported to occur secondary to bone sarcomas and occur most frequently in smaller dogs, especially miniature schnauzers and collie-type dogs. These infarcts have not been documented to be caused by actual neoplastic tissue and their pathophysiology is unknown.

CT features (Figure 37.10)

- Focal regions of hyperdensity within the medullary cavity of the long bones.
- Bone infarcts are most frequently distributed in the radius, ulna, tibia and distal third of the femur.

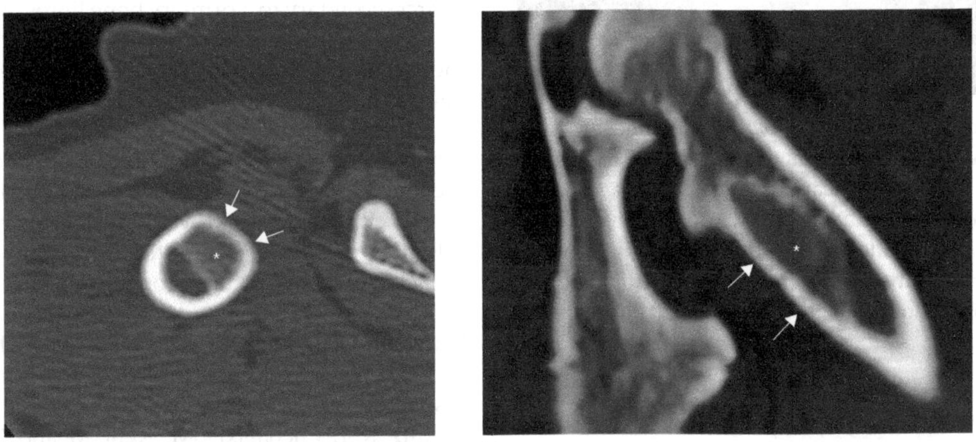

A B

Figure 37.7 Adult dog with a femoral osteoma. (A) Transverse CT image of the proximal aspect of the left femur shows a well-defined soft tissue mass (asterisk) with mild adjacent cortical thinning (arrows). No aggressive destruction or significant production is identified. (B) Frontally reformatted CT image shows the length of the well-defined intramedullary soft tissue mass (asterisk) with adjacent cortical thinning (arrows).

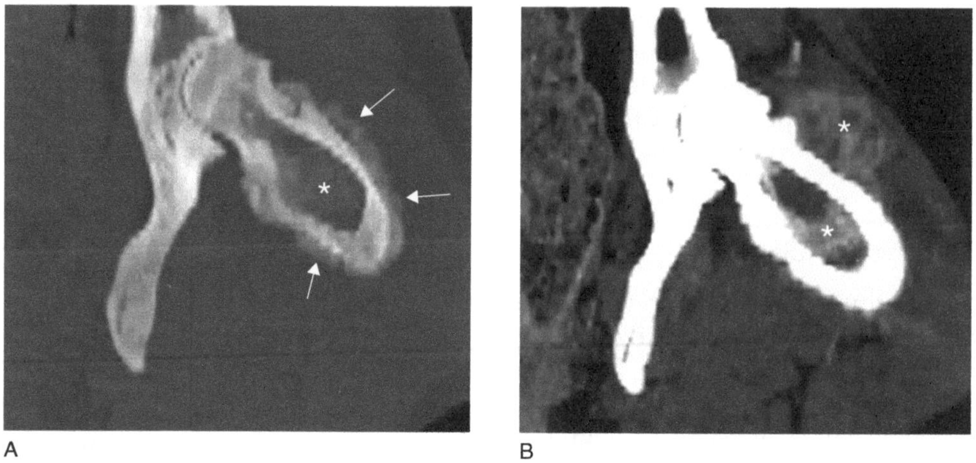

Figure 37.8 Frontally reformatted CT images from an adult dog with a femoral osteosarcoma. (A) There is a mixed productive and destructive soft tissue dense mass (asterisk) with periosteal proliferation (arrows) in the medullary cavity of the proximal left femur. (B) Contrast enhancement of the soft tissue mass extends beyond the femur into the surrounding musculature (asterisks).

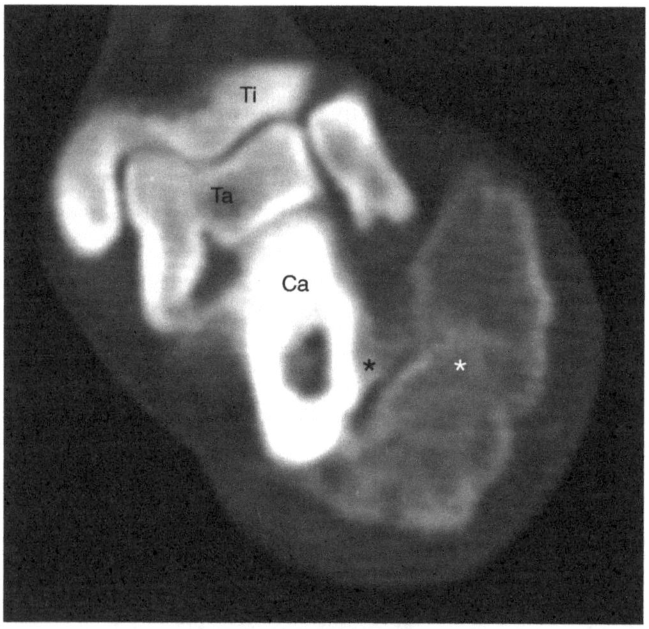

Figure 37.9 Adult dog with a parosteal osteosarcoma. Transverse CT image (right tarsus at the level of the distal tibia (Ti), talus (Ta) and calcaneus (Ca)) shows a large smoothly marginated mineralization (white asterisk) in the soft tissues lateral to the calcaneus. In addition, there is irregular periosteal proliferation (black asterisk) surrounding the calcaneus, which is connected to this mineralization in the soft tissue.

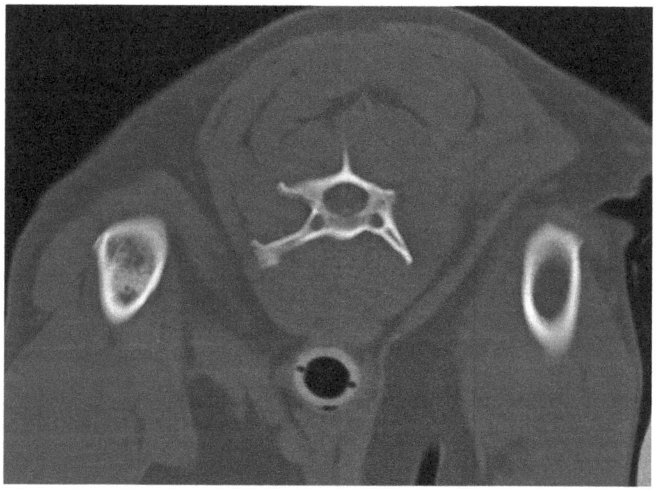

Figure 37.10 Adult small-breed dog with a suspected infarct secondary to a primary bone fibrosarcoma. Transverse CT image (proximal humerus and fourth cervical vertebra) shows intramedullary bone density in the right proximal humerus.

Further reading

Aper R, Kowaleski MP, Apelt D, Drost WT and Dyce J (2005) Computed tomographic determination of tibial torsion in the dog. *Vet Radiol Ultrasound* **46**:187–91.

Davis GJ, Kapatkin AS, Craig LE *et al.* (2002) Comparison of radiography, computed tomography, and magnetic resonance imaging for evaluation of appendicular osteosarcoma in dogs. *J Am Vet Med Assoc* **220**: 1171–6.

Dudley RM, Kowaleski MP, Drost WT and Dyce J (2006) Radiographic and computed tomographic determination of femoral varus and torsion in the dog. *Vet Radiol Ultrasound* **47**: 546–52.

Marcellin-Little DJ, DeYoung DF, Ferris KK and Berry CM (1994) Incomplete ossification of the humeral condyle in spaniels. *Vet Surg* **23**: 475–87.

Schultz RM, Puchalski SM, Kent M and Moore PF (2007) Skeletal lesions of histiocytic sarcoma in nineteen dogs. *Vet Radiol Ultrasound* **48**: 539–43.

Schultz RM, Johnson EG, Wisner ER, Brown NA, Byrne BA and Sykes JE (2008) Clinicopathologic and diagnostic imaging characteristics of systemic aspergillosis in 30 dogs. *J Vet Intern Med* **22**: 851–9.

CHAPTER THIRTY-EIGHT

Joints

Valerie Samii (stifle), Ingrid Gielen (shoulder, elbow, tarsus), Eberhard Ludewig (carpus), William M. Adams (hip), Ingmar Kiefer (carpus), Henri van Bree (shoulder, elbow, tarsus) and Jimmy Saunders

Imaging Protocols

General imaging protocol (Table 38.1)

Specific imaging protocols

The coxofemoral joint (Table 38.2)

CT arthrography (Table 38.3)

Imaging tips

- Use bone as well as soft tissue windows to detect bone involvement.
- Thin slice collimation, preferably sub-millimeter, is preferred for the assessment of intra-articular ligamentous structures both pre-contrast and post-arthrography. Post-intravenous contrast studies are typically performed only if neoplasia of the stifle joint or surrounding tissues is suspected.

CT: Anatomy and Normal Variants

The shoulder joint (Figure 38.1, Table 38.4)

The shoulder is a ball-and-socket joint, which allows movement in essentially every direction. However, most of the motion takes place in a cranial-to-caudal plane, resulting in mainly joint extension and flexion.

Bones contributing to the formation of the shoulder are the scapula (by the glenoid cavity) and the humerus (by its head). The joint consists of a single cavity that extends between the scapula and humerus. A subdivision of the joint capsule surrounds the tendon of origin of the biceps, and travels with it through the intertubercular groove as the tendon's synovial sheath. A thick band of ligamentous tissue, the transverse humeral ligament, bridges the groove from greater to lesser tubercle retaining the biceps tendon. The medial and lateral glenohumeral ligaments are thickenings of the respective surfaces of the joint capsule and not real ligaments. They are rather weak.

The strength of the heavy musculature surrounding the shoulder maintains its integrity. Because of this musculature, shoulder luxations/subluxations are rare.

Feline anatomical specificities

A clavicle is present in cats (a rudimentary clavicle may be present in large dogs). The shape of the scapula and the trabecular bone structure differs between dog and cat. The cat also has a caudally oriented proliferation on the acromion.

The elbow joint (Figure 38.2, Table 38.5)

The elbow is a hinge joint. Its main motion is flexion–extension, together with a small gliding component. A small amount of rotation is also possible allowing supination and pronation of the paw.

Three bones form the elbow: humerus, radius and ulna. Three separate compartments are identified, each of which plays an essential role in the normal function of the joint. The humeroulnar joint is formed proximally by the humeral trochlea and distally by the trochlear notch of the ulna. This compartment affords the main flexion–extension motion of the elbow. The

Veterinary Computed Tomography, First Edition. Edited by Tobias Schwarz, Jimmy Saunders.

Table 38.1
CT imaging protocol (intravenous contrast study: standard protocol; *see* Chapter 5).

Series	Pre-contrast	Bone
Decubitus	**All joints:** ventral recumbency (elbow, stifle also reported in lateral recumbency*; carpus, digits in dorsal recumbency)	
Special positioning	**Front limb:** full extension of the front limbs cranially, dog's head pulled back to the lateral side **Hind limb:** full extension of the hind limbs caudally	
Scan margins	**Shoulder:** from acromion (parallel to the humeroscapular joint space) distal part humeral head **Elbow:** from top olecranon ±3 cm distal to radial head **Carpus/digits:** from distal radius top of digits **Stifle:** from 1 cm proximal to patella 2 cm distal to tibial plateau **Tarsus:** from top calcaneus proximal metatarsal bones	
Voltage (kVp)	100–140	
Current (mAs)	100 (carpus)–240 (large hips)	
Tube rotation time (s)	0.5–2	
Slice width (mm)	0.5–2	
Sequential slice interval (mm)	Equal to slice width	
Helical image reconstruction interval	<1 mm	
Kernel frequency	Medium (stifle: high)	High
Window level (HU)	+50–60	+200–500
Window width (HU)	360–400 (280–500)	2500–3000

*Tibial plateau parallel to long axis of CT couch from cranial to caudal.

Table 38.2
CT imaging protocol for the hip joint.

Hips	Cancer suspicion	Post-trauma	Hip dysplasia
Decubitus	Affected side up	Dorsal	Ventral
Special positioning	Hips/stifles extended	Hips/stifles flexed	Hip/stifle flexed, abducted Foam wedge at pelvic inlet
Scan margins	From L6 → caudal perineum		
Voltage (kVp)	100–140		
Current (mAs)	140 (small hips)–240 (large hips)		
Tube rotation time (s)	0.5–2		
Slice width (mm)	5	1–3	
Axial slice interval (mm)	5	1–3	
Kernel frequency	Medium	High	
Windowing bone (HU)	L: +250 W: 1500		
Windowing post contrast (HU)	WL: +40 WW: 350		N/A
MPR/3-D	No/No	Yes/Yes	No/No

Table 38.3
CT arthrography.

Access site	Standard site for joint centesis
Route of administration	Intra-articular surgical preparation mandatory
Catheter size	22 ga
Injection method	– Aspirate joint to confirm needle position and for synovial fluid sampling – Manual injection
Contrast agent	Iodinated
Contrast medium type	Non-ionic, dimeric
Generic name	Omnipaque
Contrast medium concentration	30 mg/ml* (1/10 dilution of Omnipaque 300 mg with saline)
Osmolality	336 mOsm/kg H_2O (±232 mOsm/l)
Volume (ml/kg)	To palpable distention
Rate of injection (ml/s)	0.5 ml/s
Scan delay	Immediately after 2 min of repeated flexion and extension of joint to insure adequate contrast medium distribution within joint
Side effects	Mild synovitis
Undesired effects	– Extra-articular injection of contrast medium – Iatrogenic joint infection secondary to failure to perform surgical preparation prior to joint centesis and arthrography

*In general the contrast medium concentration needs to be very low to avoid artifacts.

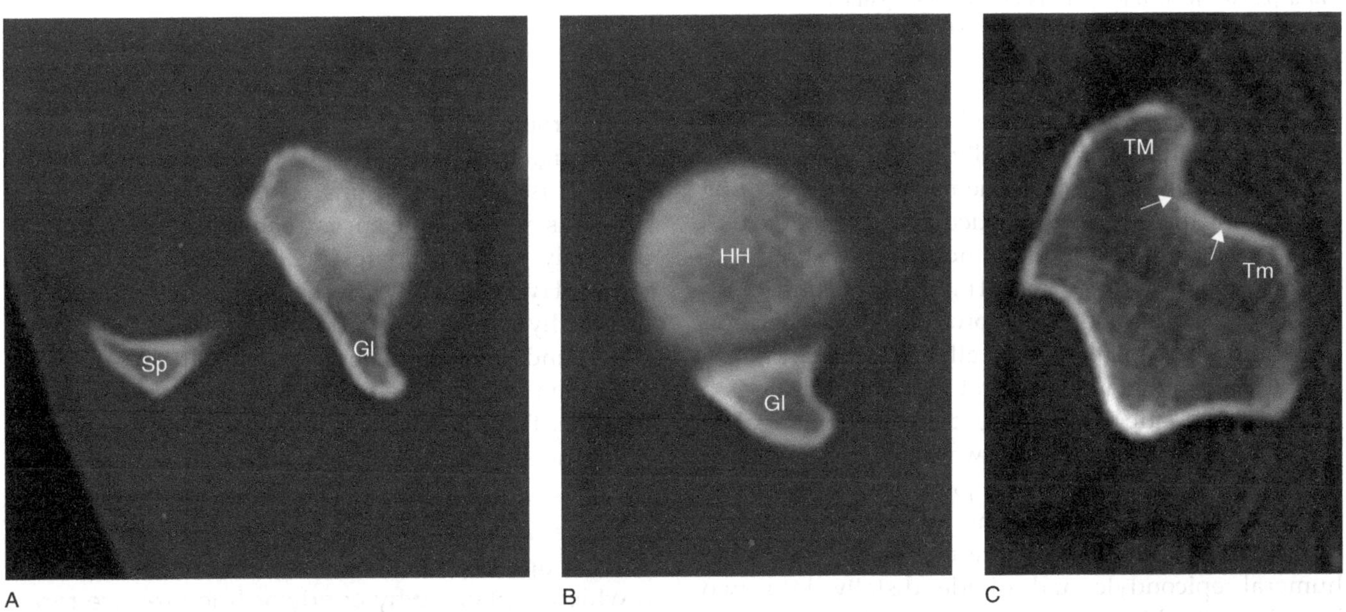

Figure 38.1 Reference transverse CT images of a normal right canine shoulder (shoulder joint musculature; *see* Figure 28.2). (A) Scapula at the level of the glenoid cavity (Gl): the caudal aspect of the glenoid cavity is well delineated; the distal part of the spine of the scapula (Sp) can be picked up at the lateral side. (B) Humerus at the level of the humeral head (HH): the normal delineation and subchondral density of the humeral head are illustrated; a part of the glenoid cavity (Gl) is visible. (C) Humerus at the level of intertubercular sulcus (arrows) of the biceps tendon: the sulcus is rounded and smoothly delineated, it is surrounded by the major tubercle (TM) laterally and by the minor tubercle (Tm) medially.

Table 38.4
Shoulder joint muscles.

Muscle name	Function	Origin	Insertion	Innervation
Biceps brachii	Extensor	Scapula: supraglenoid tubercle	Ulna: medial coronoid process Radial tuberosity	Musculocutaneous n.
Coracobrachialis[A]	Rotator (M) Adductor	Scapula: coracoid process	Humerus: lesser tubercle	Musculocutaneous n.
Deltoid	Abductor Flexor[B]	Scapula: acromion and spina	Humerus: deltoid tuberosity	Axillary n.
Infraspinatus[A,D]	Abductor[C]	Scapula: infraspinous fossa	Humerus: greater tubercle	Suprascapular n.
Subscapularis[A,E]	Adductor	Scapula: subscapularis fossa	Humerus: lesser tubercle	Subscapular n.
Supraspinatus[A]	Extensor	Scapula: supraspinous fossa	Humerus: greater tubercle	Suprascapular n.
Teres major	Adductor Rotator (M) Flexor[B]	Scapula: caudal border	Humerus: teres major tuberosity	Axillary n.
Teres minor	Abductor[C] Flexor	Scapula: infraglenoid tubercle	Humerus: teres minor tuberosity	Axillary n.
Triceps brachii (only long head)	Flexor	Scapula: caudal border	Ulna: olecranon	Radial n.

[A]All stabilizers of the shoulder joint;
[B]flexor when acting together;
[C]Teres minor helps Infraspinatus;
[D]Infraspinatus functions as a lateral collateral ligament;
[E]Subscapularis functions as a medial collateral ligament.

humeroradial joint is formed proximally by the humeral capitulum and distally by the radial head. This compartment provides the major weight-bearing function of the elbow. The articular circumference of the radial head and the radial notch of the ulna form the proximal radioulnar joint. This subjoint contributes to the rotary motion of the elbow. A single cavity comprises the joint capsule serving all three compartments. The medial and lateral collateral ligaments, located on the respective sides of the joint, steady the joint against excessive transverse motion towards the opposite side of the limb. They steady the joint against excessive transverse motion towards the opposite side of the limb. Both collateral ligaments attach proximally to the humeral epicondyle and divide distally into two branches, attaching separately to both the radius and the ulna. The annular ligament of the radius is a thin ligamentous band that passes transversally around the articular circumference of the radius (deep to the collateral ligaments), essentially surrounding the bone and maintaining its position against the ulna when the radius rotates. The oblique ligament is a relatively minor ligament on the cranial (flexor) surface of the joint. This ligament begins on the lateral side of the humerus dorsal to the supratrochlear foramen, crosses obliquely and terminates on the medial side of the radius. Hypothetically, this ligament assists in prevention of hyperextension. The olecranon ligament is a short band that extends between the lateral side of the olecranon and the medial side of the lateral humeral condyle. This ligament assists in retaining the proximity of the olecranon and the humerus.

Feline anatomical specificities
The supratrochlear foramen is absent in cats, which explains why condylar fractures are rare in this species. Instead, the feline humerus contains a supracondylar foramen through which the brachial artery and median nerve pass. The cat has greater rotation of the elbow and supination ability of the paw.

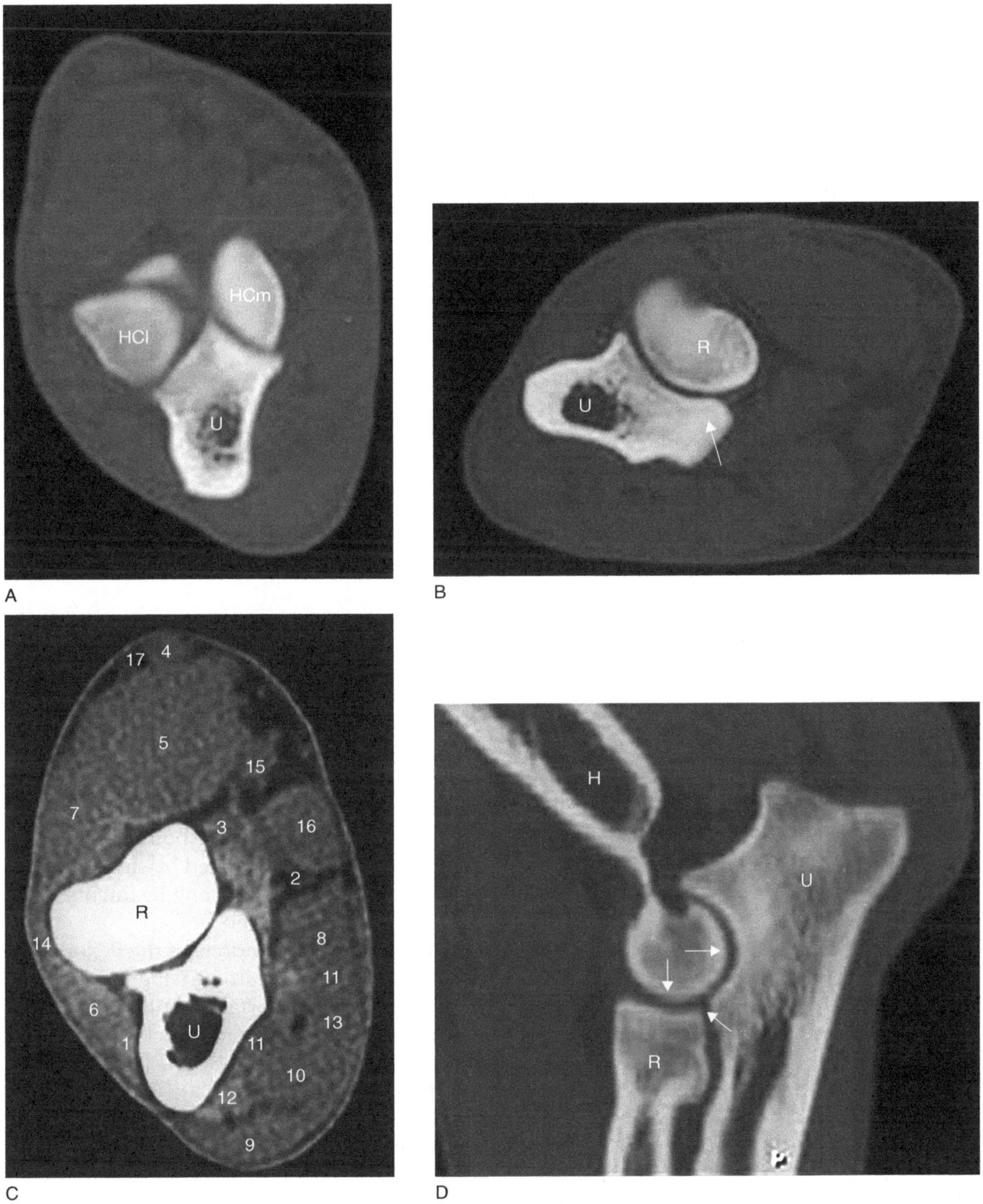

Figure 38.2 Reference CT images of the normal right canine elbow. (A) Transverse CT image at the level of the joint space: the normal aspect and density of the medial part of the humeral condyle (HCm) can be appreciated. HCl = lateral part of the humeral condyle. U = ulna. (B) Transverse CT image at the proximal level of the radius shows the normal delineation and subchondral density of the medial coronoid process (arrow). R = radius; U = ulna. (C) Transverse CT image at the level of the joint space (soft tissue window). 1 = anconeus m.; 2 = brachial a.; 3 = brachialis m.; 4 = cephalic v.; 5 = extensor carpi radialis m.; 6 = extensor carpi ulnaris m.; 7 = extensor digitorum communis m.; 8 = flexor carpi radialis m.; 9 = flexor carpi ulnaris m. (caput ulnare); 10 = flexor carpi ulnaris m. (caput humerale); 11 = flexor digitorum profundus m. (caput humerale); 12 = flexor digitorum profundus m. (caput ulnare); 13 = flexor digitorum superficialis m.; 14 = lateral collateral ligament; 15 = median v.; 16 = pronator teres m.; 17 = radial n. (lateral superficial branch). R = radius; U = ulna. (D) Sagittally reformatted CT image shows of a normal congruent elbow joint. The joint represent a parallel and narrow joint space (arrows) between humerus (H), radius (R) and ulna (U).

Table 38.5
Functional elbow musculature.

Muscle name	Function	Origin	Insertion	Innervation
Anconeus	Extensor[A]	Humerus: lateral and medial epicondyles	Ulna: olecranon	Radial n.
Biceps brachii	Flexor[B]	Scapula: supraglenoid tubercle	Ulna: medial coronoid process Radial tuberosity	Musculocutaneous n.
Brachialis	Flexor[B]	Humerus: proximocaudal	Ulnar and radial tuberosities	Musculocutaneous n.
Triceps brachii	Extensor[A]	Long head: infraglenoid tubercle – scapula Lateral, medial, accessory head: shaft – humerus	Ulna: olecranon	Radial n.
Pronator teres	Pronator forearm	Humerus: medial epicondyle	Radius: medial border	Median n.
Supinator[C]	Supinator forearm	Humerus: lateral epicondyle	Radius: proximal third, dorso-lateral	Radial n.

[A]Anconeus helps the Triceps brachii;
[B]Brachialis helps the Biceps brachii;
[C]An ossified sesamoid bone is present in the origin of the supinator muscle in large breed dogs and some cats.

The carpal joint and the digits (Figure 38.3, Table 38.6)

The seven bones of the carpus form a complex set of joints. A sesamoid bone medial to the middle carpal joint accompanies the abductor pollicis longus muscle. On the dorsal aspect of the second to the fifth digit, a single sesamoid bone can be seen. Adjacent to each of the metacarpophalangeal joints, paired sesamoid bones located palmar within tendons of insertion of the interosseous muscles are found in the second to the fifth digit. A single bone can be seen palmar to the first digit. These bony structures can be reliably identified with CT.

The joints of the carpus and of the distal limb are diarthrodial joints. The carpus has three major joints: the antebrachiocarpal joint, the middle carpal joint and the carpometacarpal joint. These joints are responsible for ±80%, ±15% and ±5% of carpal motion respectively. Intercarpal joints (joints between bones within the rows) are of minor importance with respect to the range of motion. The joint capsule of the carpus is composed of two non-communicating compartments. The proximal part covers the antebrachiocarpal joint, the distal radioulnar joint, and the joint of the accessory carpal bone. The distal part covers the joints of the middle carpal, the carpometacarpal and the intermetacarpal junctions.

The metacarpophalangeal joints are modified hinge joints. The proximal and distal interphalangeal joints represent saddle joints. Due to narrow joint spaces in some locations the bone interfaces cannot be visualized on CT.

Ligamentous support consists of medial and lateral collateral ligaments. In the carpus, additional intra-articular ligaments hold the bones in place. The accessory carpal bone is stabilized by short ligaments to the ulnar carpal bone and by long ligaments to the base of metacarpal bones IV and V.

The muscles and tendons of the flexor and extensor muscles are located around the carpus and on the dorsal and palmar surfaces of the joints of the feet. A number of these soft tissue structures can be differentiated in CT. However, due to the lack of fat, delineation is often difficult. Soft tissue structures with small dimensions (tendon sheaths, bursae, fasciae, nerves) hardly can be identified.

Feline anatomical specificities
Dorsal elastic ligaments retract the claw. In the retracted position, the distal phalanx is lateral to the middle phalanx.

The hip joint, pelvic bones and proximal femur (Figure 38.4, Table 38.7)

Patient positioning for pelvic CT depends on the purpose of the study. If it is for trauma assessment,

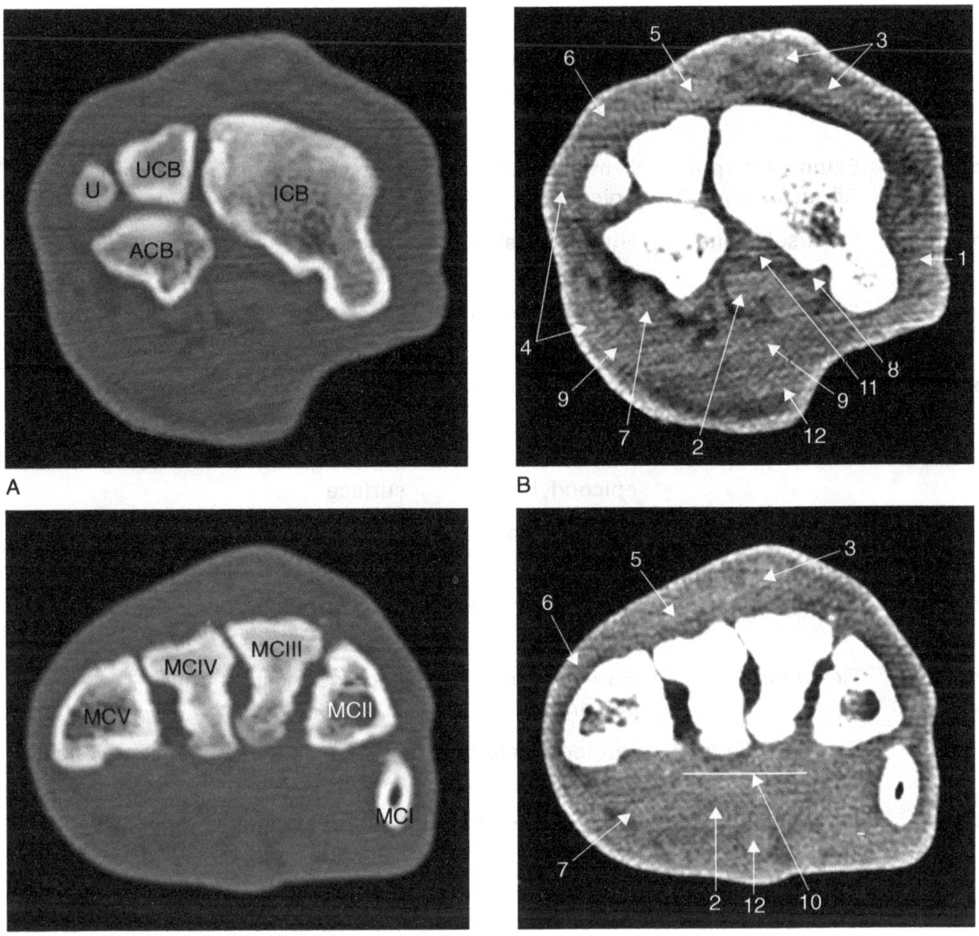

Figure 38.3 Reference transverse CT images of the normal right carpus at the level of (A,B) the carpal joint and (C,D) the proximal metacarpi. U = ulna; ACB = accessory carpal bone; ICB = intermediate carpal bone; UCB = ulnar carpal bone; MCI = first metacarpal bone; MCII = second metacarpal bone; MCIII = third metacarpal bone; MCIV = fourth metacarpal bone; MCV = fifth metacarpal bone. 1 = abductor pollicis longus m.; 2 = deep digital flexor tendon; 3 = extensor carpi radialis m.; 4 = extensor carpi ulnaris m.; 5 = extensor digitalis communis m.; 6 = extensor digitalis longus m.; 7 = fifth digit muscles; 8 = flexor carpi radialis m.; 9 = flexor retinaculum; 10 = palmar carpometacarpal fibrocartilage; 11 = palmar radiocarpal ligament; 12 = superficial digital flexor tendon.

symmetry with minimal stress is sought. For radiotherapy planning, the patient may be placed in a custom mattress to assure continuity of specific positioning for treatment planning. In large dogs, image quality of the hips will be compromised if the femurs are positioned perpendicular to the pelvis (Figure 38.4A). This is easily rectified using a high kV technique and either flexing or extending the hips (Figures 38.4B and 38.4C).

Assessment of the hips can be standardized by placing a wedge-shaped foam pad or rolled towel under the caudal abdomen with hips and stifles flexed, femurs abducted and tarsi extended, with the dog in ventral recumbency. The goal with this positioning is to measure the maximum acetabular depth for hip dysplasia evaluation. This depth is found on one of the three slices just cranial to the level of the obturator foramen. In dogs with poor acetabular conformation, the dorsal rim of the acetabulum may be abbreviated, resulting in a low acetabular angle (shallow acetabulum) (Figure 38.4D). In dogs with normal conformation, and those having had pubic symphysiodesis at a young age, the dorsal acetabular rim will extend ventrolaterally over the femoral head (deep acetabulum), yielding a high acetabular angle and low dorsal acetabular rim angle (Figure 38.4E).

Proximal to the greater trochanter of the femur a small nidus of bone is occasionally seen in the gluteal tendon; it is thought to be ossification of chronic avulsion injury to the tendons of insertion of the gluteal muscles. Likewise, a small focus of bone may be

Table 38.6
Functional carpal and digital musculature (small digital muscles are not included).

Muscle name	Function	Origin	Insertion	Innervation
Abductor pollicis longus	Extensor carpus Abductor (digit I)	Humerus: lateral epicondyle	Metacarpus I: proximal part	Radial n.
Extensor digitorum communis	Extensor digits	Humerus: lateral epicondyle	Distal phalanges digits II–V: processus extensorius	Radial n.
Flexor digitorum profundus	Flexor digits	Humerus: medial epicondyle	Third phalanges digits I–V: flexor tubercle	Ulnar n.
Extensor digitorum (I,II)	Extensor digits	Ulna: dorsolateral aspect	Metacarpi I: distal part common digital extensor	Radial n.
Extensor carpi radialis	Extensor carpus	Humerus: lateral epicondyle	Metacarpi II and III: dorsal–proximal surface	Radial n.
Extensor carpi ulnaris	Extensor carpus	Humerus: lateral epicondyle	Metacarpi V: proximo-lateral surface	Radial n.
Flexor carpi radialis	Flexor carpus	Humerus: medial epicondyle	Metacarpi II and III: proximal part	Median n.
Flexor carpi ulnaris	Flexor carpus	Humerus: medial epicondyle	Accessory carpal bone	Ulnar n.
Lateral digital extensor	Extensor digits	Humerus: lateral epicondyle	First phalanges digits III–V: dorsal aspect	Radial n.
Superficial digital flexor	Flexor digits	Humerus: medial epicondyle	Second phalanges digits II–V	Ulnar n.

present just proximal to the lesser trochanter, at the site of insertion of the iliopsoas muscle. These are usually incidental findings.

It is common for the pubic symphysis to be unfused at 2 years of age and 15% of large breed dogs still have an unfused pelvic symphysis at 7 years. It is this physis that is intentionally fused in immature dogs (juvenile pubic symphysiodesis) to improve hip conformation in those with excessive hip joint laxity. The iliac crest is also inconsistently fused with the body of the ilium in adult dogs, though in many it is fused by 2 years of age. The sacroiliac joint is made up of a large fibrocartilagenous synchondrosis, dorsocranial to a much smaller synovial portion of the joint. The ventral aspect of the sacroiliac joint may be fused in older dogs.

The stifle joint (Figure 38.5, Table 38.8)

The stifle joint is comprised of seven bones: femur, tibia, fibula, patella, medial and lateral fabellae, and the popliteal sesamoid bone.

The stifle is a complex joint with three compartments: the condyloid femorotibial, femoropatellar and proximal tibiofibular. The movement of the joint is primarily flexion and extension. However, the femoral condyles both roll and slide along the articular surface of the tibial plateau, enabling some degree of cranial and caudal displacement, distraction and compression, and internal and external rotation. The medial and lateral femorotibial and femoropatellar joint pouches all communicate. An infrapatellar fat pad is present caudal to the patellar tendon and cranial to the intra-articular ligaments and fibrocartilage of the femorotibial joint.

There are 15 intra- and extra-articular ligaments/tendons associated with the stifle joint. The most important are the cranial and caudal cruciate ligaments, and the medial and lateral collateral ligaments. The cranial cruciate ligament provides the primary check against internal rotation of the tibia during flexion. It originates from the caudomedial intercondyloid fossa of the femur and inserts on the cranial intercondyloid area of the tibia. The caudal cruciate ligament originates from the craniolateral aspect of the intercondyloid fossa of the femur. It crosses the cranial cruciate ligament medially and inserts on the lateral edge of the popliteal notch of the tibia. The collateral ligaments provide the primary check against external rotation of the tibia during extension and flexion. The lateral and medial meniscofibrocartilage are

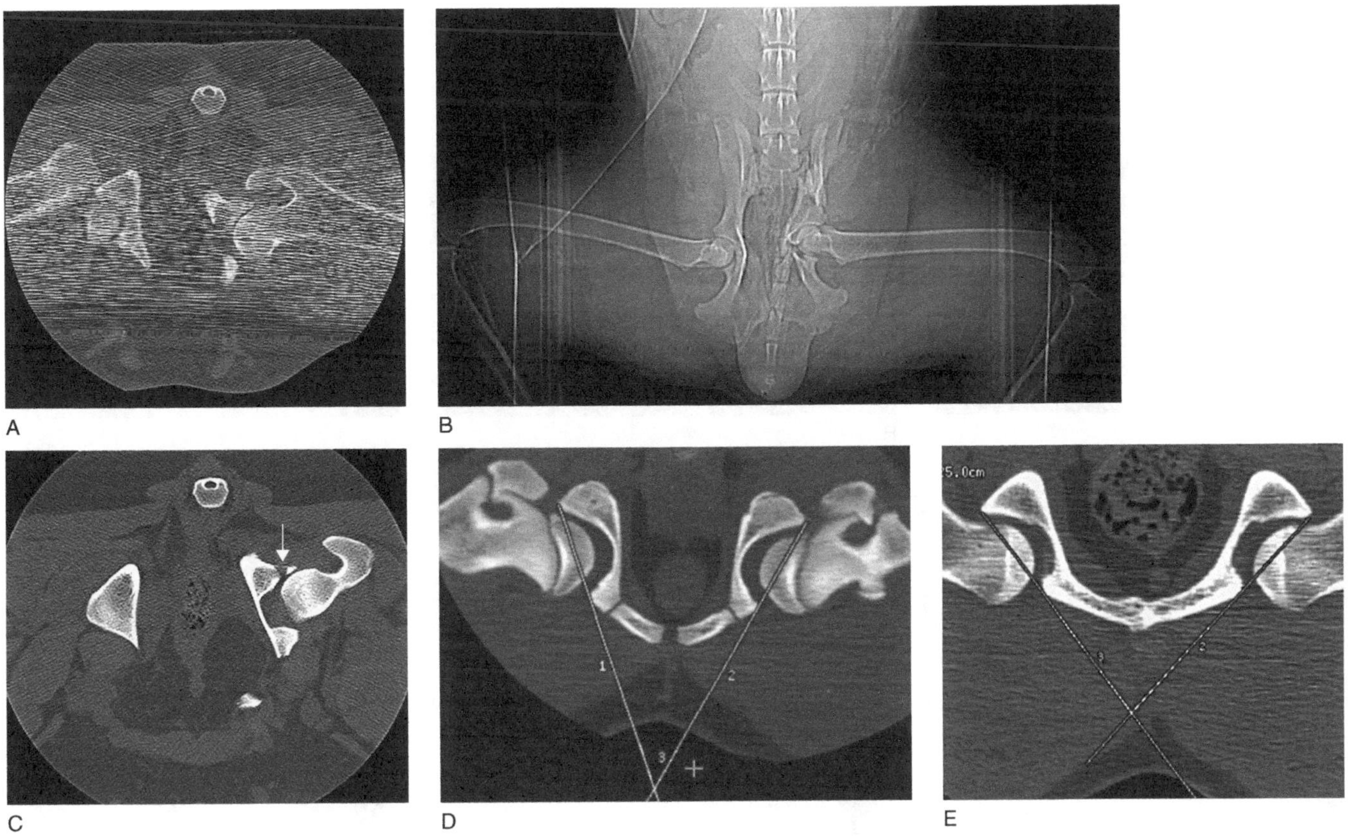

Figure 38.4 CT imaging of the hip joints. (A) Photon starvation artifact on a pelvic CT of an adult dog pelvis. (B) Scout image showing positioning of the femurs for the series containing image (A). (C) Similar acetabular location as (A) after the legs were extended, revealing an occult dorsal acetabular fracture (arrow) in this same dog. (D) Positioning and appropriate craniocaudal location for acetabular depth assessment by acetabular angle in a 16-week-old puppy with shallow acetabula. (E) Positioning and appropriate craniocaudal location for acetabular depth assessment by dorsal acetabular rim angle in the same dog at 2 years. This dog had pubic symphysiodesis at 16 weeks of age. Note the ventrolateral growth of the dorsal acetabular rims.

Table 38.7
Functional pelvic musculature (adapted by J. Saunders).

Muscle name	Function	Origin	Insertion	Innervation
Adductors/Gracilis/ Pectineus/Sartorius	Adductors	Pelvis	Medial femur, stifle, tibia	Obturator n.
Biceps femoris	Extensor	Pelvis: ischial tuberosity	Tibia	Sciatic n.
Gemelli/Obturator/Quadratus	Supinators	Pelvis: ischium and pubis	Femur: trochanteric fossa	Sciatic n.
Gluteus group	Extensor	Pelvis: iliac wing	Femur: greater trochanter	Gluteal n.
Iliopsoas	Flexor	Lumbar vertebrae: L2–L7	Femur: lesser trochanter	Lumbar spinal n.
Quadriceps (rectus femoris)	Flexor	Pelvis: ilium	Tibial tuberosity	Femoral n.
Semitendinosus Semimembranosus	Extensors	Pelvis: ischial tuberosity	Tibia and distal femur	Sciatic n.

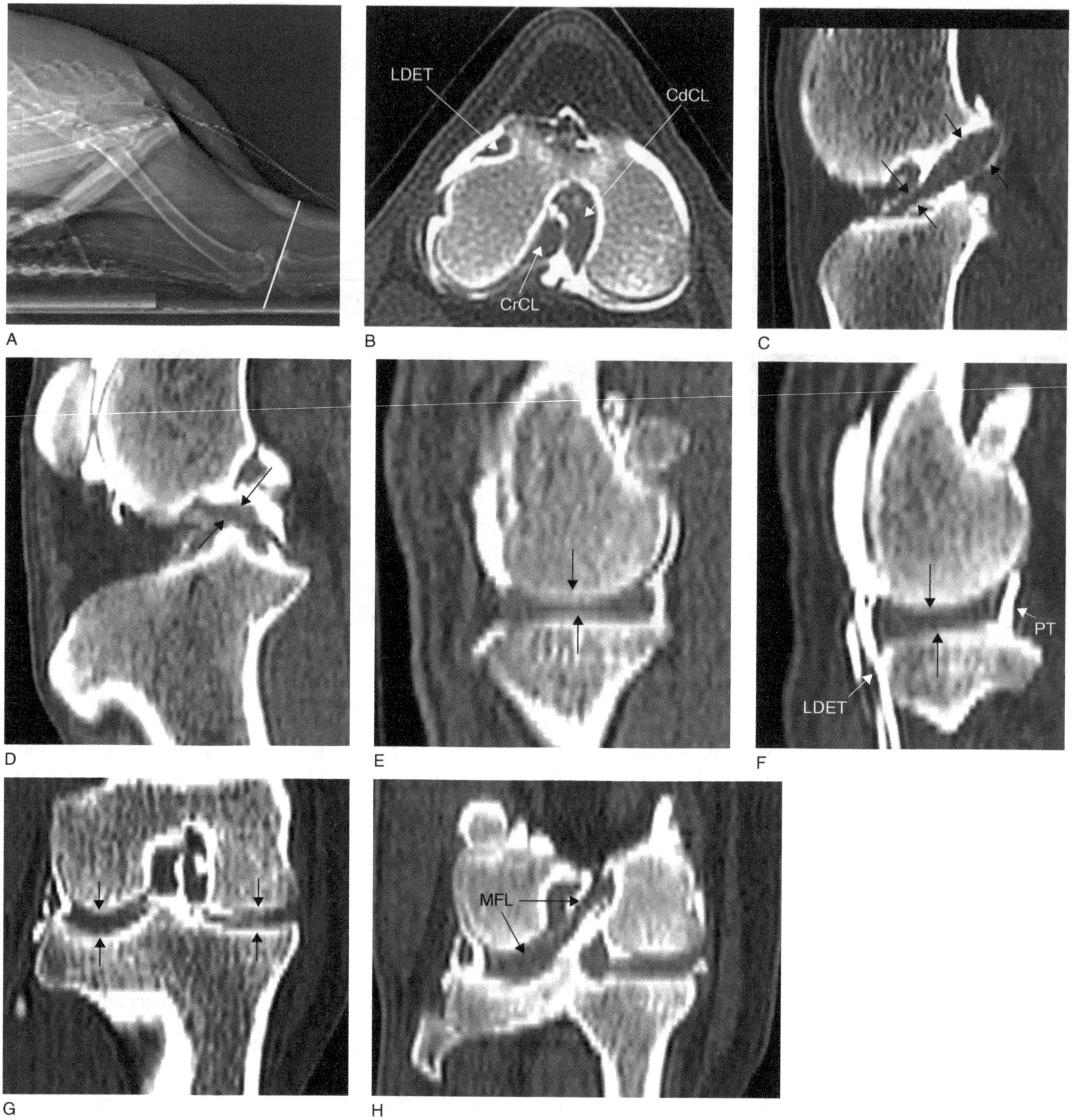

Figure 38.5 Reference CT images of the normal right canine stifle. (A) CT pilot image in ventral recumbency with the limb extended caudally. The white line designates the appropriate angle of transverse imaging through the joint (parallel to the tibial condyle). (B) Transverse CT arthrogram (1 mm transverse) shows the cranial cruciate (CrCL) and caudal cruciate (CdCL) ligaments and the long digital extensor tendon (LDET) at the level of the intercondyloid fossa of the femur. (C) Sagittally reconstructed CT image shows the cranial cruciate ligament (arrows). (D) Sagittally reconstructed CT image of the caudal cruciate ligament (arrows). (E) Sagittally reconstructed CT image of the medial meniscus (arrows). (F) Sagittally reconstructed CT image of the lateral meniscus (black arrows), long digital extensor tendon (LDET) and popliteal tendon sheath (PT). (G) Frontally reconstructed CT image of the medial and lateral menisci (arrows). (H) Normal frontally reconstructed CT image of the meniscofemoral ligament (MFL).

Table 38.8
Stifle joint musculature.

Muscle name	Function stifle	Origin	Insertion	Innervation
Biceps femoris	Extensor/Flexor	Pelvis: ischial tuberosity	Tibia	Sciatic n.
Popliteus	Flexor	Femur: popliteal fossa	Tibia: caudomedial	Sciatic n.
Quadriceps femoris	Extensor	– Vastus intermedius, medialis, lateralis: femur – Rectus femoris: ilium	Tibial tuberosity via patella	Femoral n.
Tensor fasciae latae	Extensor	Pelvis: Iliac crest	Patella	Gluteal n.

semi-lunar shaped disks between the femoral and tibial condyles. They increase stifle joint stability and congruency and serve as the shock absorbers of the stifle. The patellar tendon originates from the quadriceps femoris muscle and inserts on the tibial tuberosity. The patella, the largest of the sesamoid bones of the stifle joint, is imbedded in the patellar tendon. The tendon of origin of the long digital extensor is partially encased in an extension of the lateral femorotibial joint capsule. The medial and lateral fabellae are embedded in the tendons of the gastrocnemius muscles that originate on the supercondylar tuberosities of the caudodistal femur. The tendon of origin of the popliteus muscle contains a sesamoid bone as well. It originates caudally to the extensor fossa and just cranial and deep to the lateral collateral ligament. The tendon of origin is partially encased in an extension of the lateral femorotibial joint capsule.

In CT, the osseous structures and infrapatellar fat pad are clearly identifiable. Intra-articular contrast medium is necessary to clearly see the intra-articular soft tissue structures. Reformation of the acquired transverse or frontal planar images is necessary to fully assess the cruciate and meniscal structures (Figure 38.5).

Feline anatomical specificities
Cats have a more elongated patellar apex than dogs. Cats may also have meniscal ossicles as an incidental finding.

The tarsal joint (Figure 38.6, Table 38.9)

The tarsus is a hinge joint. Its main motion is flexion–extension, together with a small gliding component at the proximal intertarsal joint.

Seven bones compose the tarsus: the talus, calcaneus, central tarsal bone and the tarsal bones I–IV. They compose a proximal and a distal group. The talus (medially) and the calcaneus (laterally) surround the central tarsal bone in the proximal group. The tarsal bones I–III are relatively small in comparison with tarsal bone IV and are restricted to the medial half of the tarsus.

There are three main joints: the talocrural joint (providing the greatest range of motion), the intertarsal joints with two compartments (proximal and distal intertarsal compartments) and the tarsometatarsal joints. The tarsal joint capsule envelops the entire area of these joints like a sheath. It has seven subdivisions, four medial and three lateral. The largest component surrounds the tarsocrural joint. The main ligaments are the medial and lateral collateral ligaments, the extensor retinaculum, the flexor retinaculum, the plantar tarsal fibrocartilage and the special ligaments of which the long plantar ligament is the most clinically significant. Strain of this ligament is mostly associated with lameness.

The stifle joint muscles are responsible for movement in the tarsus. Because the flexor surface for the tarsus is positioned opposite to the flexor surface of the digits, the muscles that extend the tarsus flex the digits.

Feline anatomical specificities
The metatarsal bones are much longer than the metacarpal bones.

General Joint Disease Features

Developmental: osteochondrosis

Osteochondrosis is a common disorder in rapidly growing, large and giant breed dogs between 4 and 12 months of age. It is a disturbance in the process of endochondral ossification in a focal area of a

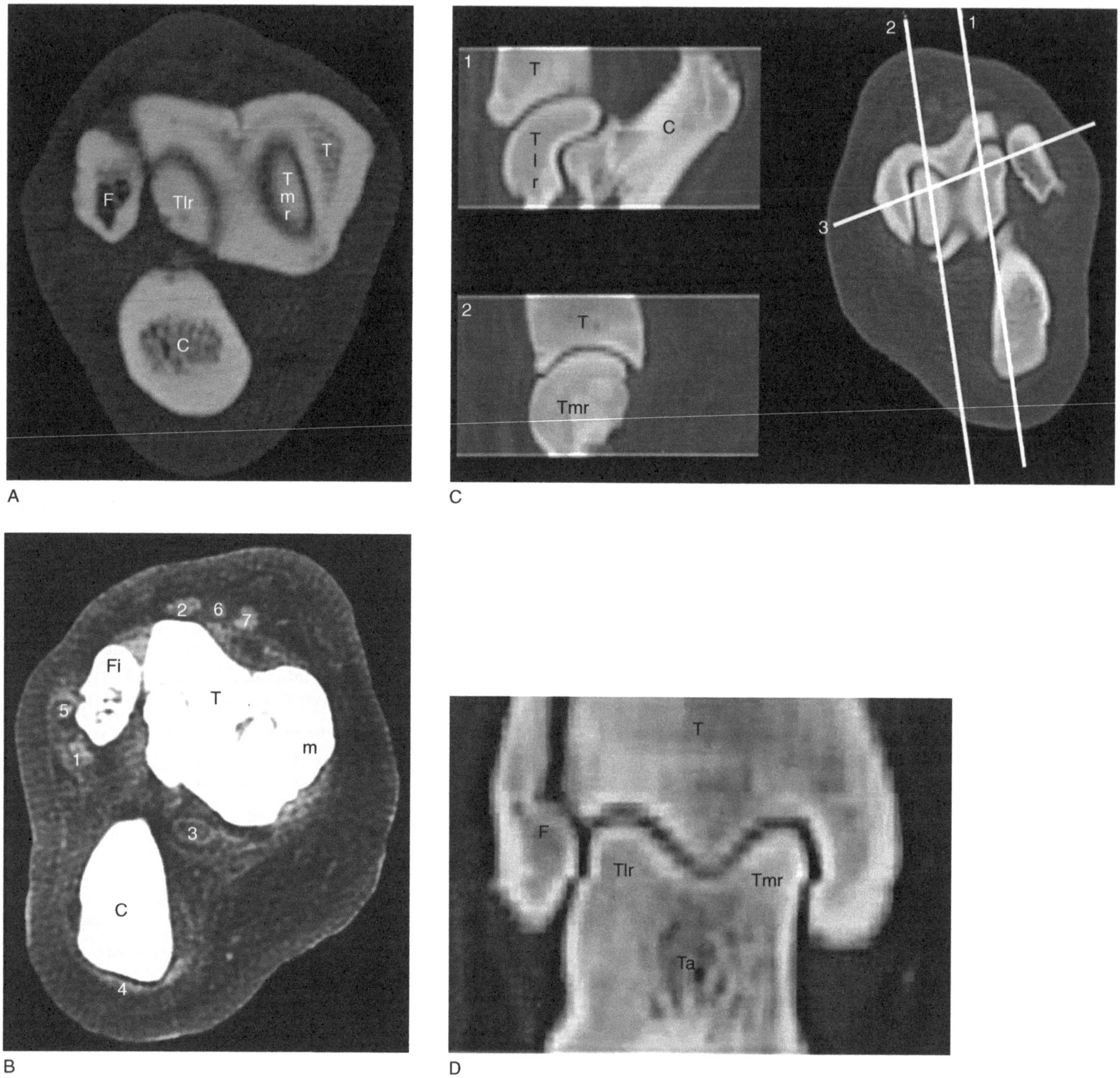

Figure 38.6 Reference CT images of the right normal canine tarsus. (A) Transverse CT image at the level of the proximal surface of the talar ridges: the oval shape and homogeneous density of the ridges can be noticed. (B) Transverse CT image (soft tissue window) at the level of the proximal surface of the talar ridges. 1 = extensor digitorum lateralis m.; 2 = extensor digitorum longus m.; 3 = flexor digitorum lateralis m.; 4 = flexor digitorum superficialis m.; 5=peroneus (fibularis) longus m.; 6 = tibialis cranialis a.; 7 = tibialis cranialis m. (C) Two sagittally reconstructed CT images (1, 2) and one in the frontal plane (3, *see* C) are presented. Image 1 (level lateral talar ridge) shows the joint space in the lateral sagittal plane. Image 2 (level medial talar ridge) shows the intact shape of the medial talar ridge. (D) Dorsal reconstructed CT image (white line 3 of B) shows both talar ridges and the curved congruent joint space (arrows). C = calcaneus; F and Fi = fibula; m = medial malleolus; T = tibia; Ta = talus; Tlr = lateral ridge of the talus; Tmr = medial ridge of the talus.

developing articular surface centered at the osteochondral junction. Local ischemia seems to be the key factor leading to failure of joint cartilage to undergo physiological calcification with consecutive cartilage necrosis, fragmentation and rupture. The subchondral bone becomes exposed to the synovial fluid (osteochondritis dissecans) causing synovitis, effusion, joint pain and lameness.

The common sites of osteochondrosis in the dog are reported in Table 38.10. Less common or controversial

Table 38.9
Tarsal joint musculature.

Name	Function	Origin	Insertion	Innervation
Tibialis cranialis	Flexor tarsus	Tibia: extensor sulcus	Metatarsus I or tarsal bone I and II	Deep fibular n.
Deep digital flexor	Flexor digits	Tibia, fibula: proximolateral and caudomedial	Third phalanges digits II–V: plantar surface	Tibial n.
Gastrocnemius	Extensor tarsus	Femur: lateral and medial supracondylar tuberosities (with two sesamoid bones)	Tuber calcanei	Tibial n.
Lateral digital extensor	Extensor digits	Lateral collateral ligament	First phalanx digit V: dorsolateral aspect	Peroneus n.
Long digital extensor	Extensor digits	Femur: extensor fossa of lateral condyle	Third phalanx digits I–V: extensor process	Peroneus n.
Peroneus brevis	Flexor tarsus	Tibia, fibula: distal part	Base metatarsal bone V	Superficial fibular n.
Peroneus longus	Flexor tarsus	Proximal fibula Tibia: lateral epicondyle, Stifle: lateral collateral ligament	Plantar surface tarsal bone IV, metatarsal bones I–IV	Deep fibular n.
Superficial digital flexor	Extensor tarsus Flexor digits	Femur: lateral supracondylar tuberosity	Plantar surface proximal and middle phalanges digits II–V	Tibial n.

Table 38.10
Common sites of osteochondrosis in the dog.

Joint	Location	Breeds predisposed
Vertebral	Sacrum >> seventh lumbar vertebra	German shepherd dog > boxer, Rottweiler
Shoulder	Caudal humeral head	Large and giant breeds (Great Dane, rottweiler, Labrador retriever, golden retriever, Bernese mountain dog, German shepherd dog) >> medium breeds (border collie)
Elbow	Medial aspect humeral condyle	
Stifle	Lateral femoral condyle (medial aspect) > medial femoral condyle	
Tarsus	Talar ridge (medial > lateral) > medial malleolus	Rottweiler and Labrador retriever

sites are the cervical vertebrae (*see* Chapter 22), scapular glenoid cavity, dorsal rim of the acetabulum, dorsal aspect lateral trochlear ridge and head of the head of the femur, patella and distal metaphysis of the ulna. In cats, osteochondrosis is rare and has been described at the humeral head, lateral femoral condyle and patella.

CT features (Figure 38.7)

- Flat to concave defect(s) (hypodense areas) in articular surface surrounded by regional subchondral sclerosis.
- Intra-articular osteochondral fragments may be present.
- Increased soft tissue density within joint secondary to effusion and/or joint capsular thickening.
- Periarticular degenerative osseous changes often present.
- CT arthrogram may demonstrate loss of articular cartilage.
- Tarsus: *see* Specific joint disease features, the tarsal joint.

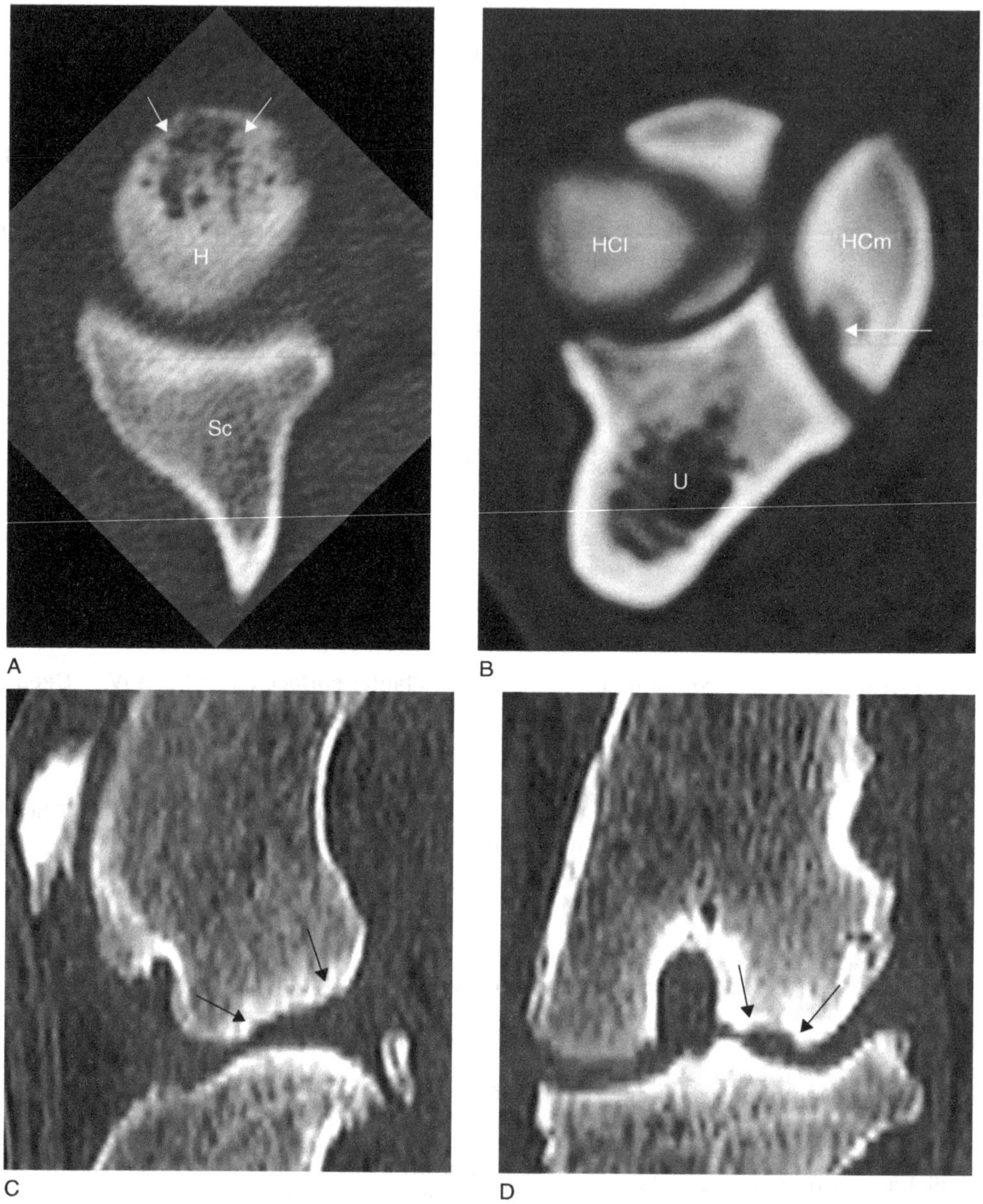

Figure 38.7 Osteochondrosis (OC)/osteochondritis dissecans (OCD). (A) OCD of the shoulder. CT image shows multiple hypodense focal areas (arrows) at the caudal head of the humerus (H). Sc = scapula. (B) OC of the elbow. CT image shows a hypodense area surrounded by a sclerotic rim (arrow) in the medial condyle of the humerus. HCl = lateral part of the humeral condyle; HCm = medial part of the humeral condyle; U = ulna. (C) Sagittally and (D) dorsally reconstructed CT images of the stifle. The medial femoral condyle appears flattened on the sagittal image (arrows) and on the frontal image, a lucency surrounded by a sclerotic rim is visible at the same location (arrows).

Trauma

Articular fracture

Articular (or intra-articular) fracture is a fracture within a joint or a fracture that involves the subchondral bone and articular cartilage.

The aims of CT studies are:

- To detect fractures: the identification of fractures in carpal or tarsal bones or detection of small (avulsed) fragments in all joints is challenging.
- To describe the extent of bone involvement: size and position of the fragments and the degree of involvement of articular surfaces.

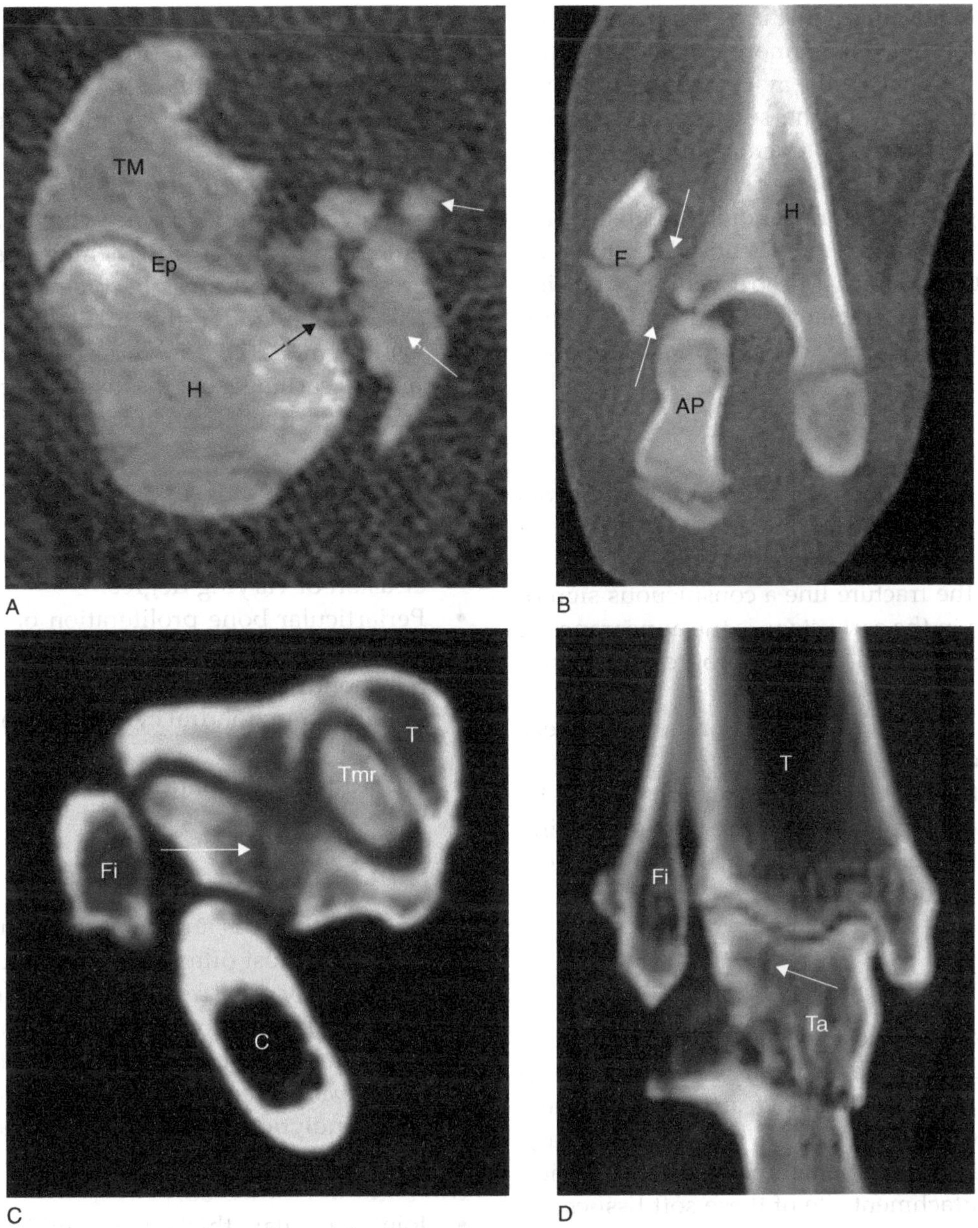

Figure 38.8 Intra-articular fractures. (A) Transverse CT image of the proximal humerus shows an epiphyseal fracture (black arrow). The trochanter minor is fractured and multiple fragments are present (white arrows). Ep = normal epiphysis; H = humerus; TM = trochanter major. (B) Frontally reconstructed CT image shows a fracture (F = distal fragments) of the lateral column of the humerus (H) in a young dog (arrows). AP = anconeal process. (C) Transverse and (D) frontally reconstructed CT images show an intra-articular fracture of the lateral talar ridge (arrow) of the talus. C = calcaneus; Fi = fibula; T = tibia; Ta = talus; Tmr = medial ridge of the talus.

- To map soft tissue changes: the location of the soft tissue damage and the identification of avulsed fragments can help to differentiate injury pattern (Figure 38.8).
- To identify and assess joint instability: functional (stress) CT investigations allows to localize and quantify a lack of ligamentous support.
- To control postoperative outcome: a complete reconstruction of bony surfaces reduces the risk of the development of degenerative changes. Inadequate forces on the joint cartilage (e.g. due to malpositioned fragments or limb deformities) result in subsequent degenerative joint disease. Despite artifacts due to metal implants (*see* Chapter 4) the integrity of surfaces often can be answered reliably. CT can also aid the decision to remove implants in cases of arthrodesis or osteosynthesis.

In immature animals, most fractures are periarticular Salter–Harris type I or II. Common articular fractures in the immature animal are the avulsion fracture of the supraglenoid tuberosity of the scapula, and for the elbow joint, Salter–Harris IV fractures of the humeral lateral condyle.

In adult dogs, the supraglenoid tuberosity, the humeral condyles (lateral > 'Y–T' condylar > medial), acetabular fractures, femoral head fractures, avulsion fractures of the cranial cruciate ligament and fractures of the small carpal and tarsal bones are common articular fractures.

CT features

- CT features of fractures depend on several factors (e.g. age and location of the fracture, degree of movability, size of the patient).
- Apart from the fracture line a conspicuous sign of organization in the early stage is the appearance of a resorptive zone, followed by progressive mineralization of the callus.
- Sagittal and frontal reconstructions can be very useful in these cases.
- Multiformat and 3-D reconstructions may be helpful in surgical planning – these post-processing methods require scan series using thin slices (<3 mm) for a good result.

Luxation/Subluxation

Joint luxation occurs most frequently as a result of trauma or, less commonly, secondary to poor joint conformation (*see* Specific disease features). Traumatic joint luxation is associated with soft issue damage (tendons, ligaments) and sometimes a small avulsion fracture at the attachment site of these soft tissues.

CT features (Figure 38.9)

- Joint capsular thickening and intracapsular effusion.
- Extracapsular swelling.
- Small osseous bodies (avulsion fragments) may be seen.
- Sagittal, frontal and 3-D reconstructions can be very useful.
- Stifle joint: cruciate +/– meniscal and collateral ligament tears probable.

Degenerative joint disease

Degenerative joint disease (osteoarthrosis, osteoarthritis) is a non-infectious progressive disorder of the weight-bearing joints affecting ±20% of dogs. It may be primary, due to aging (idiopathic). However, more frequently, it is the result of developmental (e.g. osteochondrosis, elbow or hip dysplasia) or acquired (e.g. trauma) disorders.

Early primary arthritis affects the cartilage that becomes yellow and opaque with localized areas of softening and surface roughening. As degeneration progresses, the soft areas become cracked and worn, exposing bone under the cartilage. The bone then begins to remodel and increases in density while any remaining cartilage begins to fray and osteophytes covered by cartilage form at the edge of the joint (Table 38.11).

CT features (Figure 38.10)

- Joint capsular thickening and/or intracapsular effusion of varying degree.
- Periarticular bone proliferation of varying degree depending on chronicity.
- Subchondral bone sclerosis.
- Possible perichondral cyst-like lesions in advanced cases.
- CT arthrogram: abnormal cartilage thickness.

Septic joint/Osteomyelitis

Infectious arthritis is an uncommon condition in dogs and cats. It is most often caused by bacterial contamination that may arise from direct penetration (surgical or traumatic), hematogenous dissemination or local spread from adjacent tissues. Several different bacteria, mostly *Staphylococcus intermedius*, *Staphylococcus aureus* and β-haemolytic streptococci, have been implicated.

CT features (Figure 38.11)

- Joint capsular thickening and/or intracapsular effusion of varying degree.
- Periarticular proliferation and subchondral bone lysis and sclerosis of varying degree depending on chronicity.
- Possible sequestra formation if chronic.
- Post-contrast (IV): enhancement of synovium may be seen.

Neoplasia

Synovial cell sarcoma

Synovial cell sarcoma is a rare, slow-growing neoplasm that arises from primitive mesenchymal precursor cells of the synovial membrane of joints and bursae. The elbow and stifle joints of middle-aged medium to

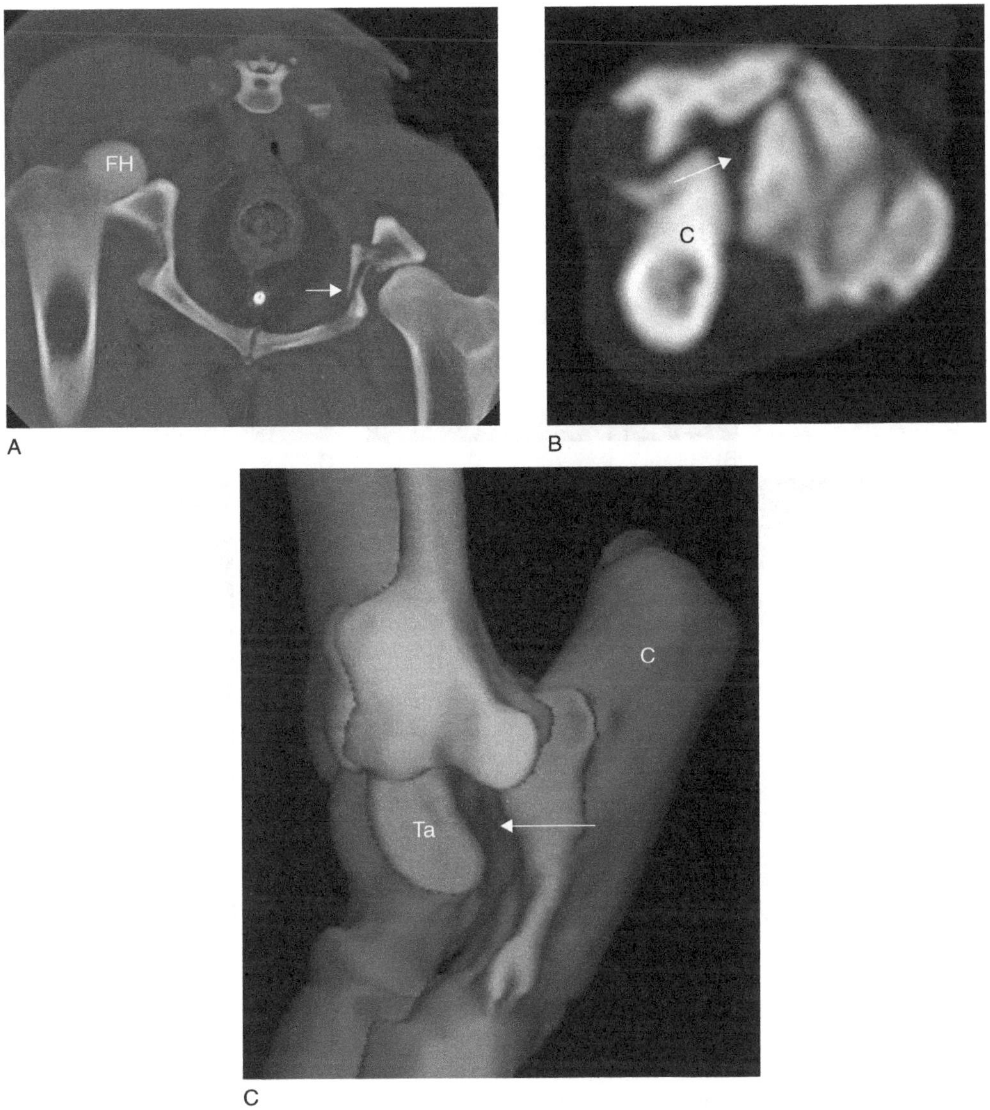

Figure 38.9 Joint luxations in two patients. (A) Young dog with right femoral head (FH) dorsal luxation and left medial acetabulum fracture (arrow). (B) Transverse and (C) 3-D reconstructed CT images of an adult cat showing a luxation (arrow) between talus (Ta) and calcaneus (C).

Table 38.11
Grading system for articular cartilage damage.

Grade	Description
0	Normal cartilage
I	Cartilage softening and swelling (chondromalacia)
II	Cartilage surface damage (fibrillation, wear lines, crack/fissure, fragmentation)
III	Deep cartilage damage (erosion) without bone exposure
IV	Deep cartilage damage with bone exposure
V	Bone damage (eburnation)

large breeds are more commonly affected. Tumor progression may occur by local invasion of surrounding bone and soft tissue, and metastasizes to regional lymph nodes and to the lungs.

Histiocytic sarcoma, synovial myxomas and other sarcomas are other less common joint tumors.

CT features (Figure 38.12)

- Joint capsular thickening and/or intra-articular mass effect and intracapsular effusion of varying degree.
- Subchondral lysis may or may not be seen depending on the aggressiveness and chronicity of the lesion.

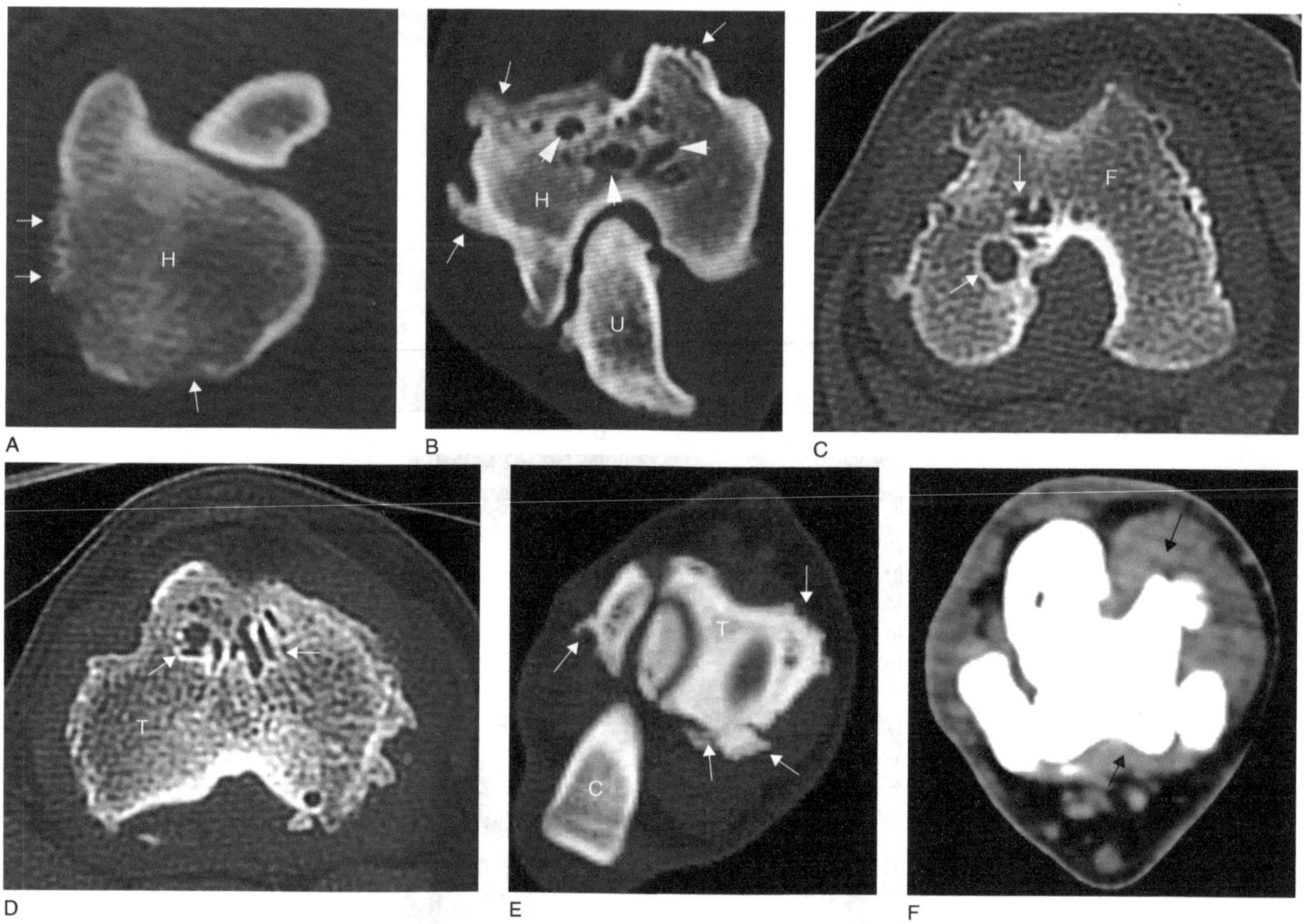

Figure 38.10 Degenerative joint disorders in different joints. (A) Shoulder: transverse CT image shows new bone formation at the level of the caudal humeral head (arrows). H = humerus. (B) Elbow: transverse CT image of the distal humerus shows new bone formation, multiple osteophytes (arrows) and subchondral cysts (arrowheads). H = humerus; U = ulna. (C,D) Stifle: transverse CT images show cyst-like lesions (arrows) lateral to the (C) intercondyloid area of the femur (F) and in the (D) subchondral bone of the cranial tibial (T) condyle. (E) Tarsus: transverse CT image shows new bone formation and multiple osteophytes at distal talus (T) and calcaneus (C) (arrows). (F) Tarsus: transverse CT image shows thickening of the tarsocrural joint capsule (arrows).

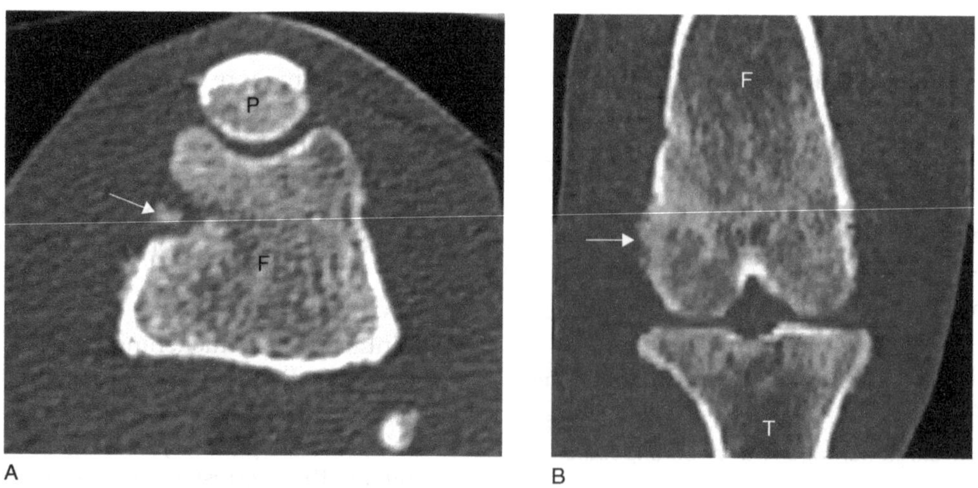

Figure 38.11 Adult dog with septic arthritis. (A) Transverse and (B) frontally reconstructed CT images show a sequestrum in the lateral femoral epicondyle (arrow). F = femur; P = patella; T = tibia.

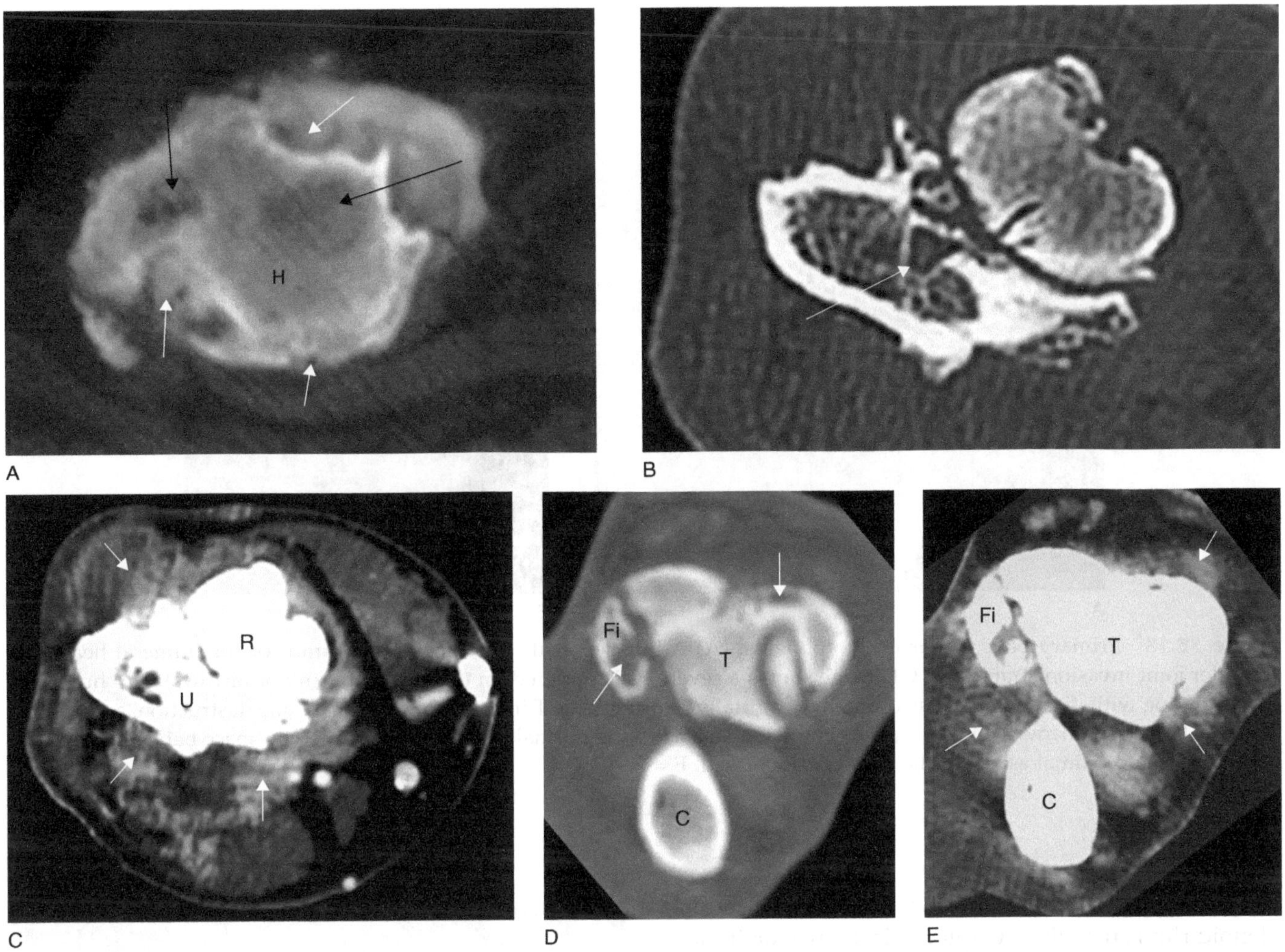

Figure 38.12 Adult dogs with synovial cell sarcoma (SCS). (A) Shoulder: CT arthrogram shows multiple lytic lesions within the humeral head (arrows). H = humerus. (B,C) Elbow: post-contrast transverse CT studies show (B) bone lysis (arrow) and (C) thickening of the neoplastic synovial membrane which is better seen after enhancement of the neoplastic process (arrows). R = radius; U = ulna. (D,E) Tarsus: transverse CT images show (D) bone destruction (arrows) of the fibula and dorsal aspect of the distal tibia and (E) the extent of the neoplastic synovium (arrows). C = calcaneus; Fi = fibula; T = tibia.

- Post-contrast (IV): enhancement of synovium and a mass may be seen.
- CT arthrogram: intra-articular filling defect created by a mass.

Primary or metastatic bone tumors

CT is used for staging surgical or radiotherapy planning and accurate aspirates or biopsy in patients with bone tumors. Osteosarcoma, the most common bone tumor, rarely invades the joint space, contrary to fibrosarcoma and hemangiosarcoma.

CT features (Figures 37.9 and 38.13)

- Osteolysis of the adjacent metaphysis with regional soft tissue swelling if cortical lysis or pathological fracture is present.
- Proliferative periosteal response.
- Joint capsular effusion may be an incidental finding.

Specific Joint Disease Features

The Shoulder Joint

Degenerative/Inflammatory

Incomplete ossification of the caudal glenoid rim

In immature dogs a separate ossification centre of the caudal rim of the glenoid has been suggested, although not proved. Some of these bone fragments are fused with the glenoid rim at maturity. If still present in the

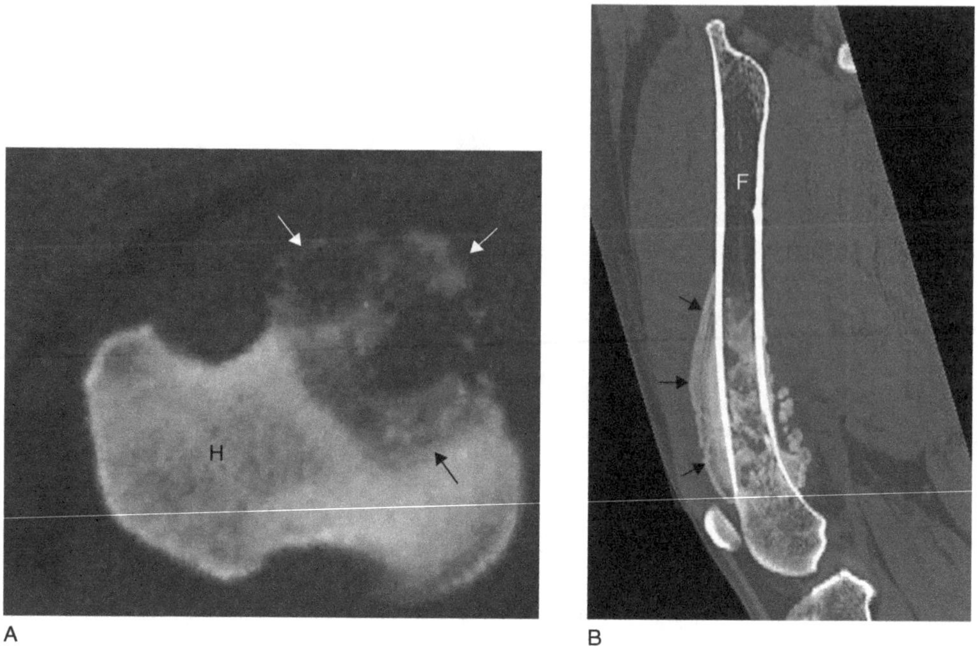

Figure 38.13 Primary bone tumor in two patients. (A) Adult dog with a primary bone tumor of the humeral head and shoulder joint invasion. Transverse CT image shows a severe lysis centered on the trochanter minor (arrows). H = humerus. (B) Adult dog with distal femoral osteosarcoma. Sagittally reformatted CT image shows cortical bone destruction, amorphous periosteal reaction (arrows) and a long transition zone between the normal and diseased bone. The space between the distal femur and the proximal aspect of the patella is increased. F = femur.

mature dog, incomplete ossification of the caudal glenoid rim is usually asymptomatic. However, it may result in pain if the fragment is unstable, and this can be demonstrated at arthroscopy.

CT features (Figure 38.14)

- Fragments causing clinical signs are mostly irregular or elongated instead of nicely rounded.
- Mild to moderate regional muscle atrophy.
- CT arthrogram: cartilage defect may be seen in front of the fragment.

Biceps lesions: tendinitis/tenosynovitis, rupture

The inflammation of the biceps tendon (bicipital tendinitis) and/or its tendon sheath (tenosynovitis) affects mostly large mature dogs causing a chronic, progressive lameness. The cause of the disorder is unclear, although a degenerative process and chronic repetitive trauma, such as an osteochondral fragment, are suggested etiologies. A tendinitis/tenosynovitis may result in tendon tear, partial or, rarely, complete tendon rupture and/or an avulsion fracture at the proximal insertion of the biceps. The disorder may be bilateral.

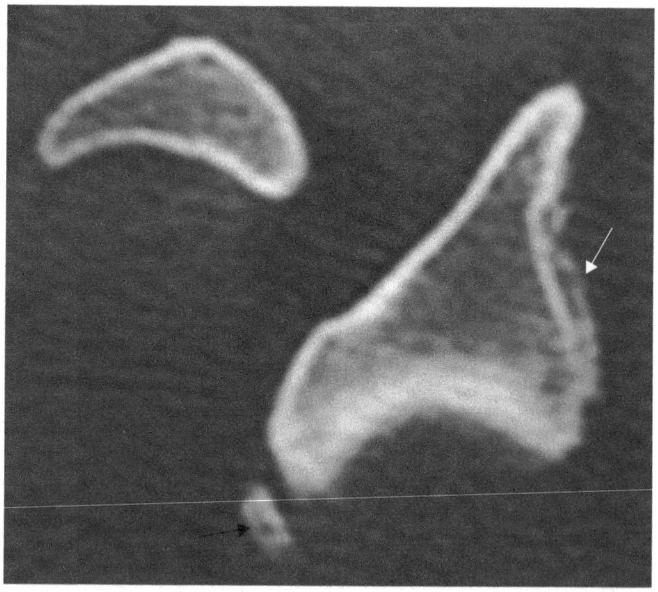

Figure 38.14 Young dog with a fragment in the caudal aspect of the glenoid rim. Transverse CT image shows an elongated bony fragment (black arrow) in the caudal aspect of the glenoid rim. Notice the new bone formation at the cranial part of the scapula (white arrow).

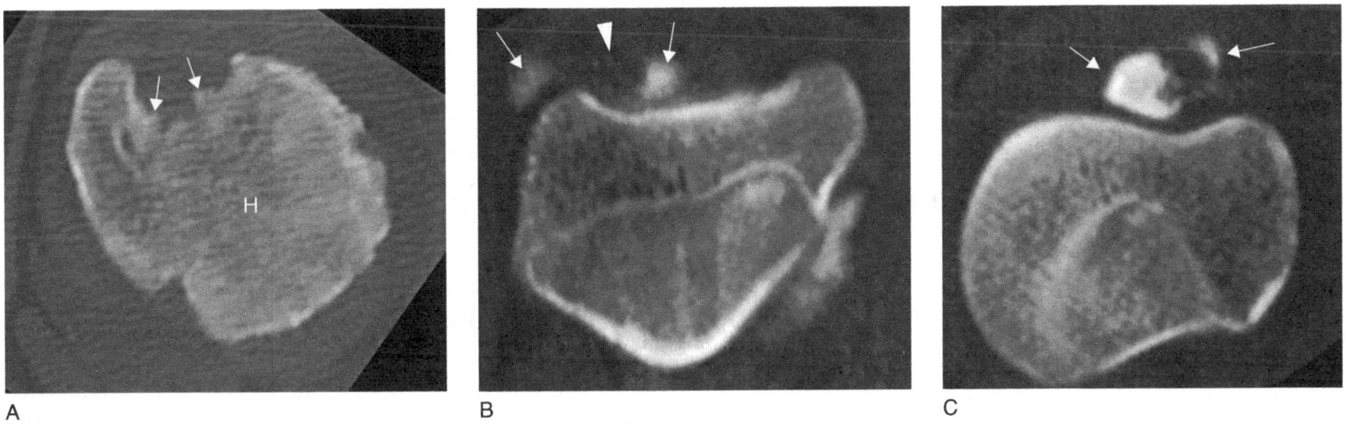

Figure 38.15 Transverse CT images of three patients with biceps tendon lesions. (A) Adult dog with inflammation of the biceps tendon. New bone formation is visible in the intertubercular sulcus of the biceps tendon (arrows). These bony spikes within the groove hinder the mechanical action and cause inflammation of the tendon. H = humerus. (B) Young dog with partial/complete rupture of the biceps tendon. CT arthrogram shows contrast material within the biceps tendon sheath (arrows). The biceps tendon is thickened and the normal integrity is absent (arrowhead). (C) Adult dog with avulsion fracture of the proximal insertion of the biceps tendon. Avulsed fragments are visible (arrows).

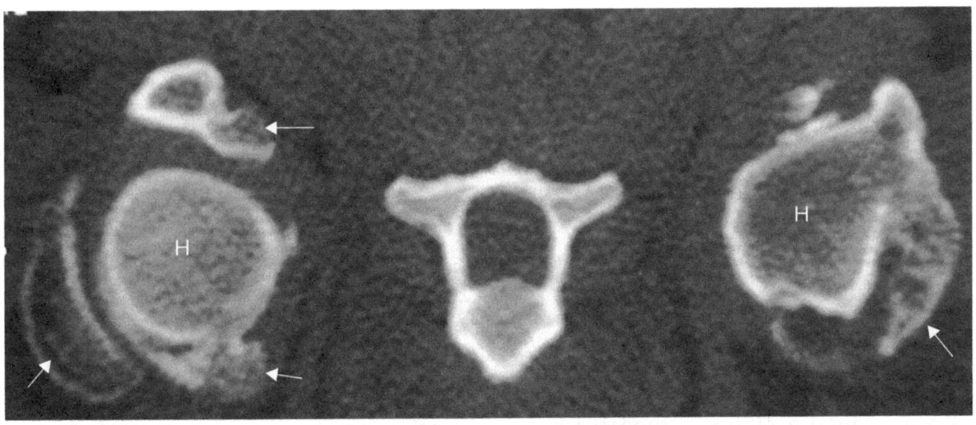

Figure 38.16 Adult dog with bilateral osteochondomatosis of the shoulder joints. Transverse CT image shows multiple calcified particles (arrows) within both joint cavities. H = humerus.

CT features (Figure 38.15)

- Fluid within the bicipital groove.
- Thickened bicipital tendon, possibly dystrophic calcification within it.
- Bony spikes present within the groove, hindering the mechanical action of the tendon.
- Mineralized fragments within the tendon sheath.
- Supraglenoid process: areas of hypodensity due to demineralization, bone proliferation, avulsed fragment.
- CT arthrogram: in case of tear/rupture, contrast material within the biceps tendon sheath (normal = biceps tendon identified as a well-delineated filling defect surrounded by contrast medium).

Neoplasia

Synovial osteochondromatosis of the shoulder joint

Shoulder synovial osteochondromatosis is a benign disorder in which the synovial lining of the joint or the bicipital tendon bursa undergoes a nodular cartilaginous, benign metaplasia producing multiple joint mice within the joint space causing chronic severe lameness. Synovial osteochondromatosis has rarely been described in the tarsal, stifle, elbow and carpal joints.

CT features (Figure 38.16)

- Multiple calcified particles with different densities can be defined within the joint cavity.

- CT arthrogram: presence of filling defects within the joint space.

The Elbow Joint

Malformation/Developmental

Elbow dysplasia

Elbow dysplasia can be separated into different pathologies, including fragmented medial coronoid process, ununited anconeal process, osteochondritis dissecans and incongruity(ies) of the elbow joint.

Chondromalacia

Chondromalacia refers to swelling, softening and degeneration of the articular hyaline cartilage. It may be observed at the level of the medial coronoid process as the only abnormality in dogs with elbow pain. Chondromalacia as observed in this case does not necessarily evolve to more severe forms of cartilage degeneration.

CT features (Figure 38.17)

- Transverse slices are the most appropriate for diagnosis.
- A mixture of hypo- and hyperdense bone is present at the medial coronoid process.
- There is no fragmentation of the coronoid process.

Fragmented medial coronoid process (FCP)

Fragmented medial coronoid process is the most common clinical entity causing elbow osteoarthrosis.

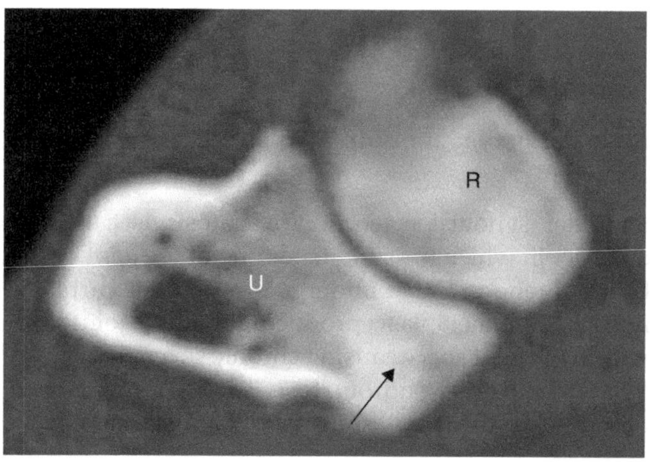

Figure 38.17 Adult dog with chondromalacia. Transverse CT image shows a mixture of hypo- and hyperdense bone at the medial coronoid process (arrow). R = radius; U = ulna.

In the normal dog, the medial coronoid process is first cartilaginous and ossifies at around 20 weeks of age. A disparate growth between radius and ulna or an incongruent trochlear notch may result in increased/abnormal pressure on the medial coronoid process causing fissuring or even fragmentation. The fragmentation may result in one or more fragment(s) that may or may not be displaced.

Kissing lesions are the result of erosion in articular cartilage and subchondral bone of the medial humeral condyle by a fragmented medial coronoid process. They have the same aspect as an osteochondritis dissecans lesion on radiography but a completely different CT aspect.

CT features (Figure 38.18)

- One or multiple fragments.
- The structures have to be examined on an appropriate bone window to accurately evaluate the subchondral bony structures, especially to visualize fissures, the appearance of which can be very discrete.
- Kissing lesions have a stripe-like form and are associated with a lot of new bone formation.

Ununited anconeal process (UAP)

In large breed dogs, the anconeal process of the ulna is a separate center of ossification that fuses at latest at 20–22 weeks of age. If the physis remains radiographically visible beyond this time, it is considered ununited. CT gives essential information for the surgeon to determine the surgical strategy. In cases of UAP, a check for an FCP is also indicated, as an association of both disorders is often present.

CT features (Figure 38.19)

- Irregular gap at the level of the humeral condyles and anconeal process.
- The position of the fragment in relation to the rest of the olecranon can best be evaluated on the sagittal reconstructions.

Elbow incongruity

Elbow incongruity is defined as a poor alignment of the joint surfaces of the elbow joint. Two features illustrate this disorder: an abnormal shape of the ulnar trochlear notch and a step between the radius and ulna. The radiographic evaluation of elbow incongruity provides low sensitivity, especially in discrete cases. CT improves the sensitivity.

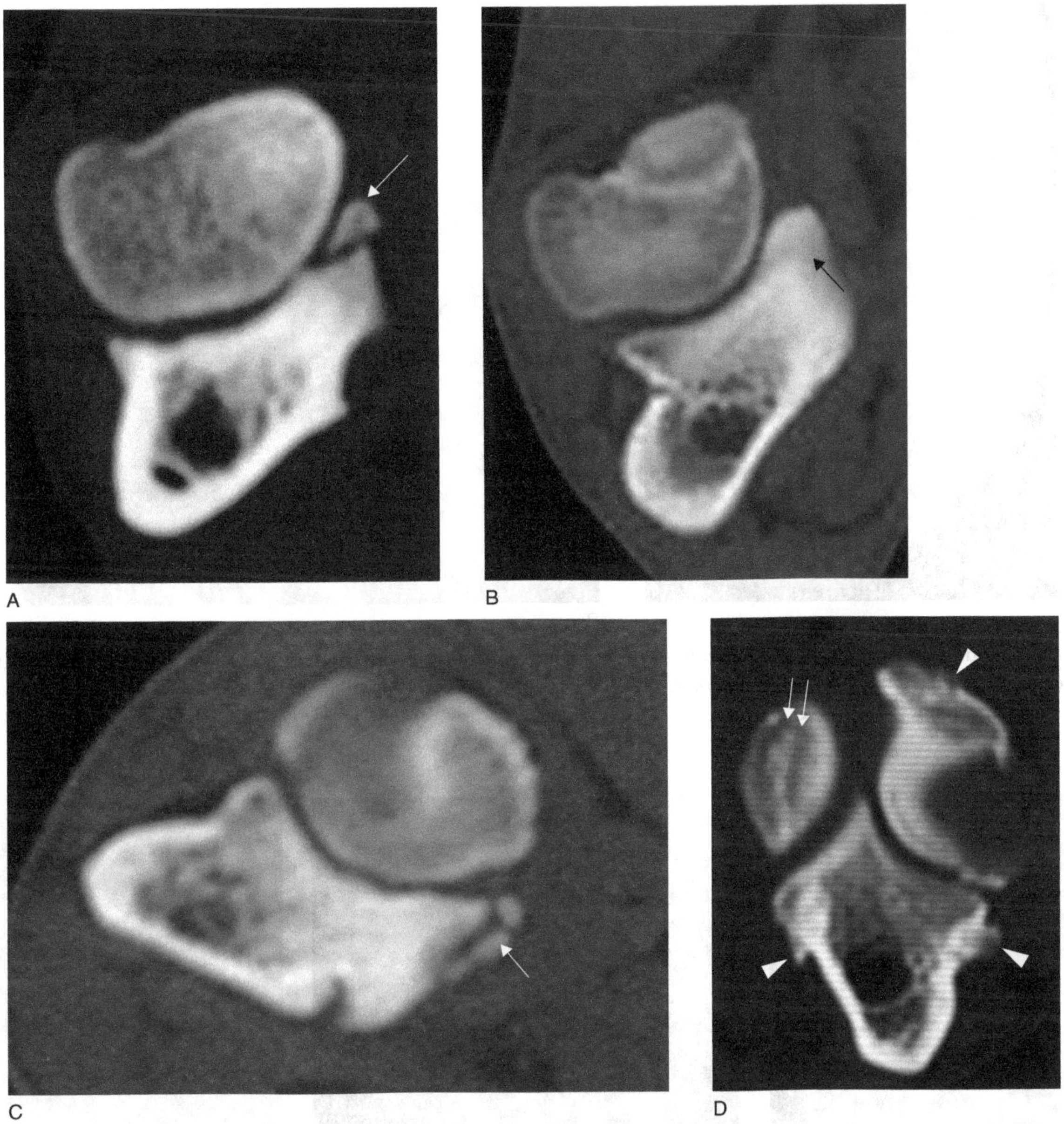

Figure 38.18 Transverse CT images of medial coronoid process fragmentation and associated disorder in four adult dogs. (A) A separate bone fragment is visible (arrow). (B) The process is thickened and sclerotic (arrow). (C) Fragmentation is present (arrow). (D) A mixed pattern of hyper- and hypodense stripes (white arrows) is present at the medial humeral condyle. New bone formation (arrowheads) of all bone structures can be appreciated. These findings represent kissing lesions.

CT features (Figure 38.20)

- Widened and diverging joint space at the level of the trochlear notch and anconeus. In normal elbows, this joint space appears narrow and parallel.
- On the sagittal and frontal reconstructions, a step between the radius and ulna can be appreciated.

Incomplete ossification of the humeral condyle

The humeral condyle consists of two parts (capitulum and trochlea) that develop as separate ossification centers. They appear ossified radiographically 14 ± 8 days after birth and fuse at 70 ± 14 days. An absence of bony fusion is sometimes observed, resulting in a mechanically weak midline composed of a thin cartilaginous plate predisposing it to humeral condylar fracture. This condition, also called intracondylar fissure, is commonly seen in spaniel breeds, where a genetic basis with recessive mode of inheritance is suspected. However, other dog breeds can also be affected.

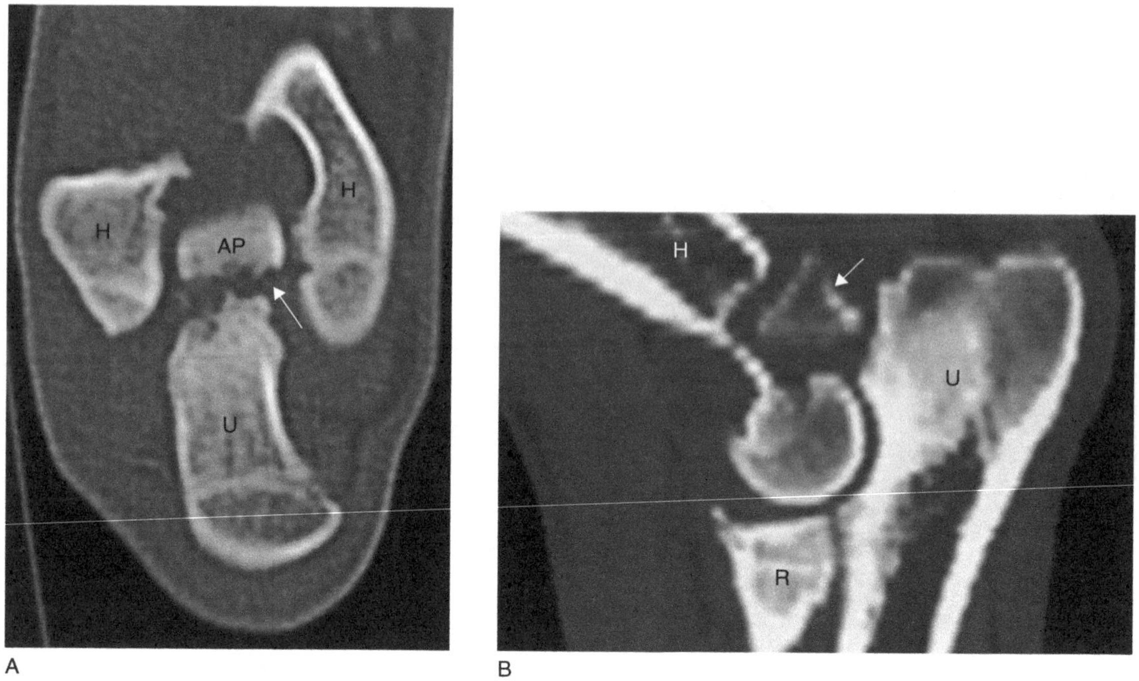

Figure 38.19 Young dog with ununited anconeal process. (A) Frontally reconstructed CT image shows a gap (white arrow) at the anconeal process (AP). (B) Sagittally reconstructed CT image shows the displaced and rotated ununited anconeal process (arrow). H = humerus; R = radius; U = ulna.

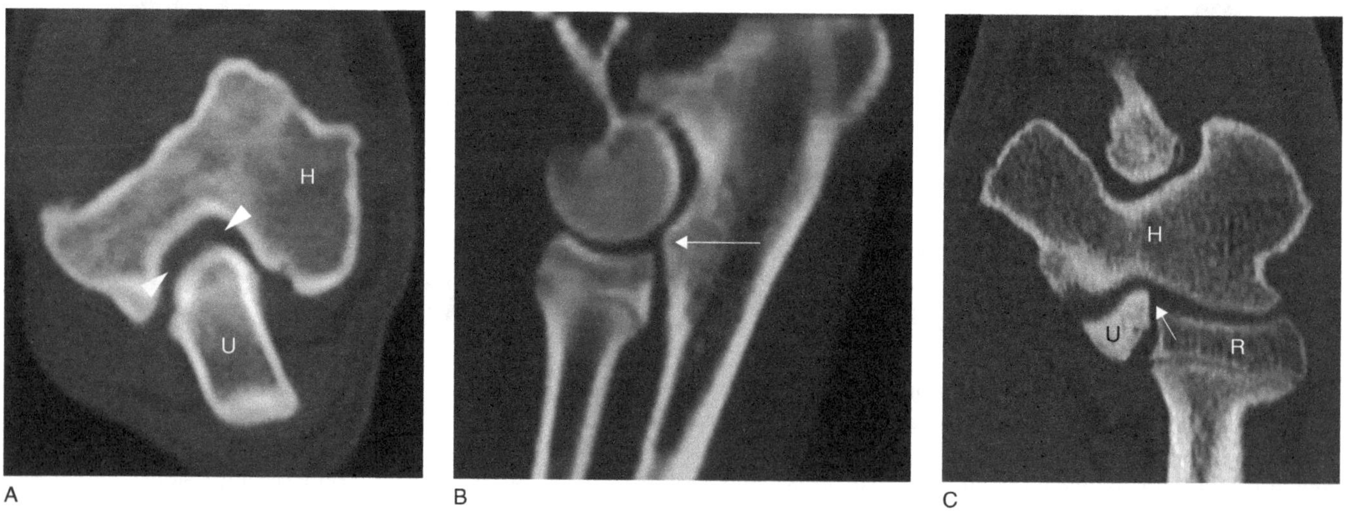

Figure 38.20 Young dog with elbow incongruency. (A) Transverse, (B) sagittally reconstructed and (C) frontally reconstructed CT images show the widened and diverging joint space (arrowheads). There is a step present, between radius and ulna (arrow). H = humerus; R = radius; U = ulna.

CT features (Figure 38.21)

- Saw-toothed intercondylar complete or incomplete hypodense defect with adjacent hyperdense margins and sclerosis.
- May be associated with degenerative changes or an atraumatic humeral condylar fracture, or even fragmented medial coronoid process.
- In dogs with a fractured humerus with underlying incomplete condylar ossification, a contralateral humeral condyle fissure, sclerosis and degenerative joint disease is seen in about 90% of the dogs.

Degenerative/Inflammatory

Mineralization of the insertion of the antebrachial flexor tendons

CT features (Figure 38.22)

- Calcifications within the soft tissues in the area of the medial humeral epicondyle.
- Avulsed fragments.
- Post-contrast: enhancement around these calcified bodies.

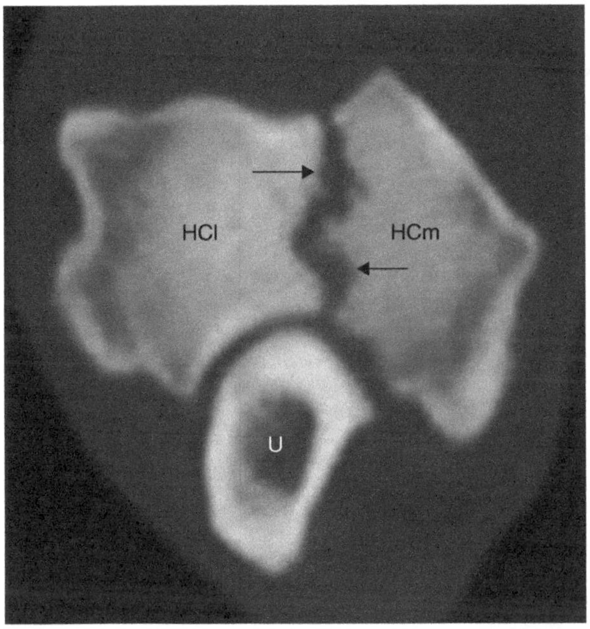

Figure 38.21 Adult dog with incomplete ossification of the humeral condyle. Transverse CT image shows a radiolucent area (arrows) surrounded by a sclerotic rim representing an intracondylar fissure. HCl = lateral part of the humeral condyle; HCm = medial part of the humeral condyle; U = ulna.

The Carpal Joint

Malformation/Developmental

Diverging number of bones

Aplasia and supernumerary bones can be seen in dogs and cats. Polydactyly is reported to be more common in cats than in dogs. In ectrodactyly the distal front limb is split. A part of the phalanges, the metacarpal and carpal bones are associated with the radius or the ulna.

CT features (Figure 38.23)

- Abnormal number of bones/phalanges.

Degenerative

Stenosing tenosynovitis of the abductor pollicis longus muscle

Overuse of the carpal joint may cause chronic inflammation, with proliferation of connective tissue of the synovial sheath, causing stenosis of the abductor pollicis longus muscle.

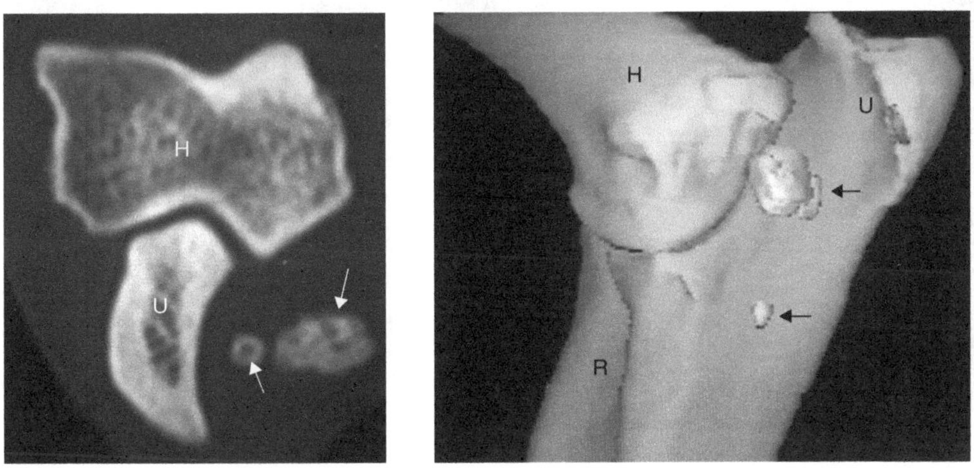

A B

Figure 38.22 Young dog with avulsion at the origin of the antebrachial flexor tendons. (A) Transverse and (B) 3-D reconstructed CT images show the avulsed fragments on the medial aspect of the ulna (arrows). H = humerus; R = radius; U = ulna.

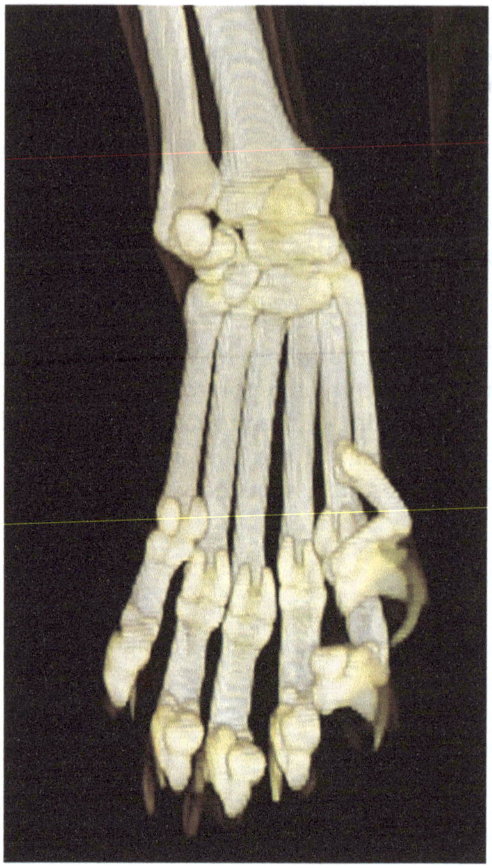

Figure 38.23 3D reconstructed CT image in an adult cat with polydactyly in the right front limb. The cat had six digits on each foot.

CT features

- Acute cases: soft tissue swelling.
- Advanced cases: proliferative bone reactions in the region of the fibro-osseous canal of the muscle (Figure 38.24).

Enthesiopathy of the short radial collateral ligament

In racing greyhounds, sprain of the short radial collateral ligament is described, causing an incomplete ligamentous tear and enthesiopathy at the site of the attachment of the ligament on the medial aspect of the distal radius.

CT features

- Soft tissue swelling.
- Periosteal reaction.
- Dystrophic calcification.
- Avulsion of parts of the origin of the ligament is also reported.

Specific Disease Features of the Digits

Neoplasia/Infection/Inflammation

Soft tissue swelling of one or more digits is a common cause of presentation for dogs and cats. Differential

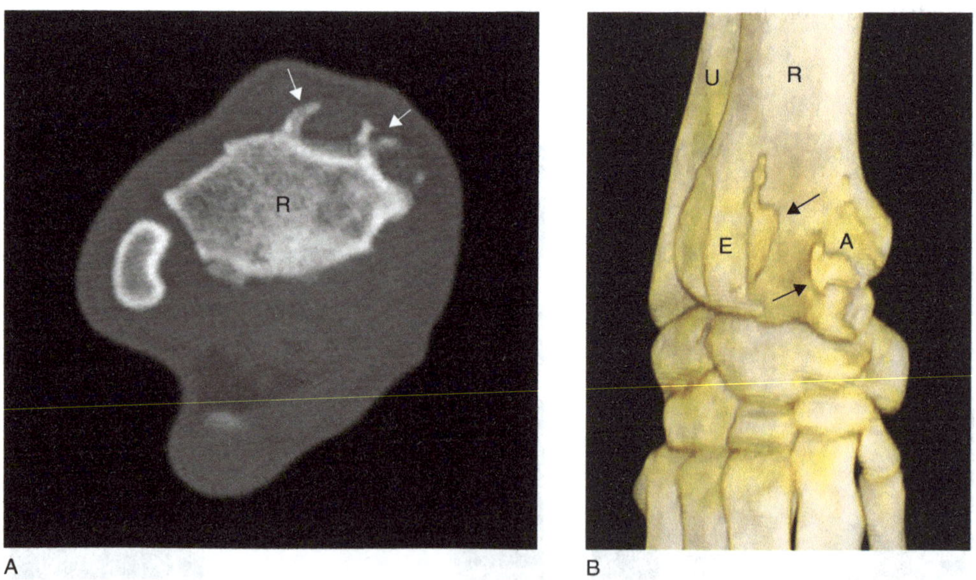

Figure 38.24 Adult dog with stenosing tenosynovitis of digital tendons. (A) CT image (just proximal to the antebrachiocarpal joint) shows barnacle-like proliferative bone reactions located in the craniomedial aspect of the radius (arrows). (B) 3-D reconstructions show the reactions (arrows) belonging to bony canals for the extensor carpi radialis muscle (E) and the abductor pollicis longus muscle (A). R = radius; U = ulna.

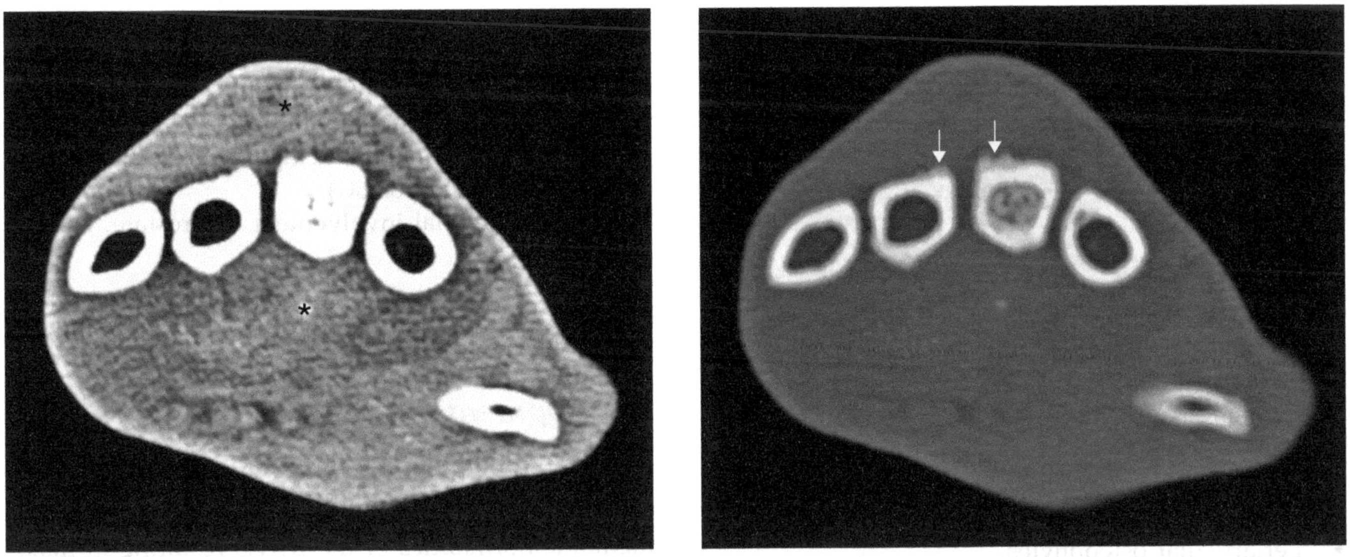

Figure 38.25 Adult dog with chronic infectious process, probably secondary to a foreign body. Transverse CT images (distal raw metacarpal bones) show (A) a dorsal and palmar soft tissue swelling adjacent to the third metacarpal bone (asterisks). In the palmar region the changes are accompanied with loss of definition of normal soft tissue structures. The lesion contains stippled mineralizations and (B) bony reaction on the dorsal aspect of the third and fourth metacarpal bone (arrows). The cortex of the third metacarpal bone is thickened and the medulla has an increased density.

diagnosis includes inflammation (paronychia – nail bed), neoplasia (subungual squamous cell carcinoma or others), infection (osteomyelitis, septic arthritis/pododermatitis, phlegmonia/abscess) and other rare disorders (synovial cyst).

Infection is caused by hematogeneous or local (penetrating wound/trauma) spread of bacteria. *Corynebacterium pyogenes*, *Clostridium* species, *Streptococcus* and *Staphylococcus* may be responsible for distinctive bony destruction and in the case of arthritis of severe cartilage damage.

A wide variety of tumor entities can affect the distal limb (primary and metastatic bone tumor, soft tissue tumors, primary joint neoplasm). Subungular squamous cell carcinoma is the most common type of digital tumor. Lung-digit syndrome is peculiar to the cat and can result in digital metastasis of primary pulmonary neoplasm.

CT features (Figure 38.25)

Etiological differentiation of these disorders based on soft tissue changes fails with CT. The growth behavior of the lesion and the distribution of bony changes are more valuable diagnostic means. Nevertheless, a definitive diagnosis is mostly only possible with histology.

- Soft tissue swelling.
- Signs of a foreign body inoculation (detection of foreign material, evidence of a tract).
- Degree of bone destruction: mostly severe lytic destruction of the involved bones, sometimes mixed pattern lysis-proliferation. Dependent on the stage/duration and the character (type of bacteria/tumor type) of the disease.
- Post-contrast (IV): homogeneous versus heterogeneous (central necrosis, foreign material).
- Phlegmon: inflammation is spread through tissue spaces over a large area and without definite margins.
- Mature abscess: exhibits a border.

The Coxofemoral Joint

Developmental

Canine hip dysplasia

Hip dysplasia is a complex inherited disease with a polygenic and multifactorial etiology. Almost all, breeds of dogs are affected, with predominance in large and giant breeds. The affected dog shows normal hips at birth but then develops joint laxity during adolescence and in most cases secondary osteoarthrosis.

CT features (Figure 38.26)

- Acetabular angle low – dorsal acetabular rim angle high.
- Fragmentation of the dorsal acetabular margin.

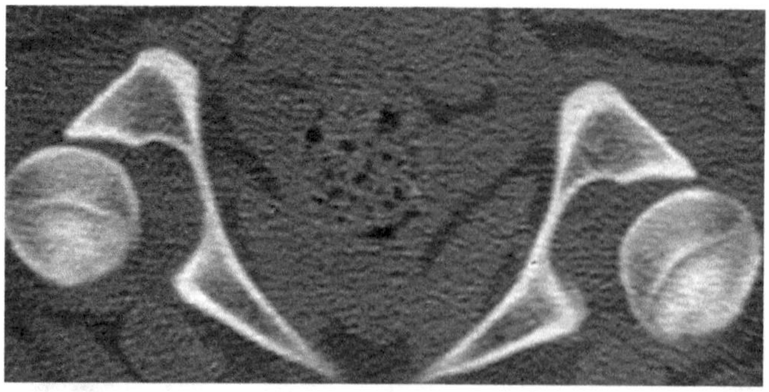

Figure 38.26 CT image of a dog with hip dysplasia shows the increased distance between the femoral head and acetabulum (subluxation).

- Enthesophytes at the femoral joint capsule attachment.
- Periarticular osteophytes.
- Subchondral sclerosis and cystic degeneration.

Trauma: luxation/subluxation

Luxation or subluxation occurs in both the hip joint and the sacroiliac joint. If there is excessive hip laxity secondary to trauma, an avulsion fracture fragment from the acetabulum may remain attached to the round ligament of the femur. If only one sacroiliac joint is luxated, look for a pelvic bone fracture.

Intrapelvic soft tissue injury is much more accurately assessed on CT than on radiographs, including sites and extent of hemorrhage, muscle tears and muscle attachment avulsion. Iliopsoas muscle and concomitant femoral nerve injuries have been reported, both with and without bone lesions. Muscle trauma is best assessed from images made immediately after contrast injection.

CT features (Figures 38.9A and 38.27)

- Fracture/luxation:
  - if pelvic fracture with displacement is identified, a second fracture or a sacroiliac luxation must also be present.
- Intrapelvic soft-tissue injury:
  - post-contrast (IV): hypodense regions indicating inflammation and/or hemorrhage.
- 3-D reconstructions may aid in surgical planning.

Neoplasia

CT is used for staging, surgical or radiotherapy planning and CT-guided aspirates or biopsy.

CT features

- Lack of contrast enhancement: necrotic, cystic or lipoma (Figure 38.28).
- Contrast enhancement: rim, heterogeneous or diffuse.
- Evaluate medial iliac and sacral lymph nodes: enlarged may only be reactive, but if also irregular or rim enhancing then metastases are probable (Figure 33.6C).
- Assess potential involvement of prostate, urethra or rectum.

The Stifle Joint

Developmental

Congenital patellar subluxation/luxation

Congenital patellar luxation is likely due to developmental abnormalities of the pelvis resulting in malalignment of the quadriceps complex (quadriceps tendon, patella, patellar ligament). The disorder can be seen as a medial luxation in small or toy-breed dogs (Shi Tzu, Llhassa, mini poodle) or as a lateral luxation in medium to large-breed dogs.

CT features (Figure 38.29)

- Patella laterally or medially displaced from trochlear groove of femur.
- Trochlear groove often shallow.
- Periarticular degenerative osseous changes often present.

Trauma

Cruciate ligament and meniscal cartilage avulsions/tears

The cranial cruciate ligament is by far the most commonly injured part of the stifle. Lameness associated with tearing or complete avulsion of the cranial cruciate ligament is regularly seen in clinical practice. Other or additional injuries may involve the caudal cruciate ligament and lateral or medial menisco-fibrocartilage.

CT features (Figures 38.30–38.32)

- Joint capsular thickening and intracapsular effusion always seen.
- Periarticular degenerative osseous changes often present.
- Small osseous bodies (osteochondromas or avulsion fragments) may be seen.
- CT arthrogram:
  - partial cruciate ligament tears: attenuation of the ligament +/− dissection of contrast medium within ligament

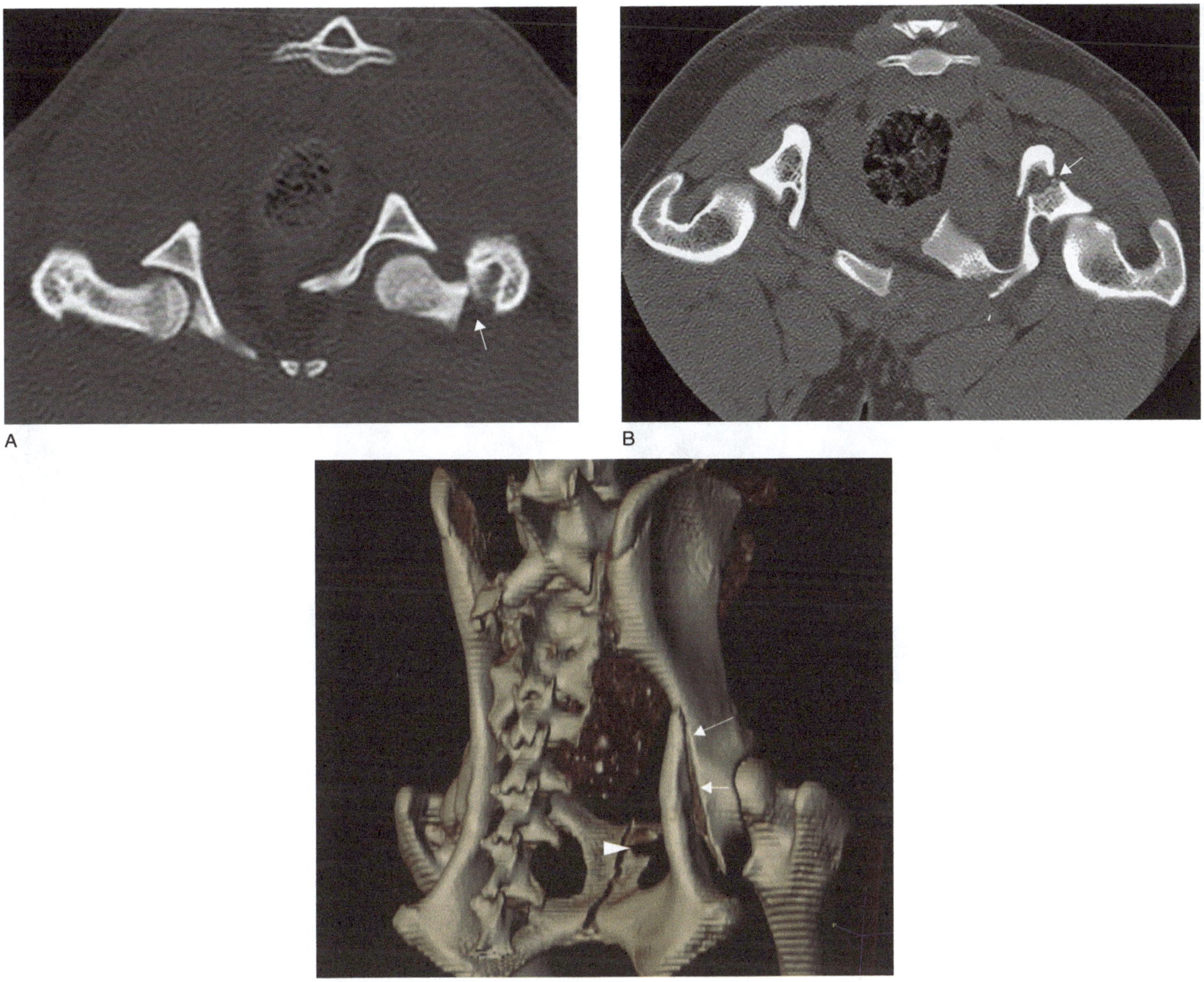

Figure 38.27 Pelvis fracture in two patients. (A) Right femoral neck fracture (arrow) in a 1-year-old peekapoo. (B) Left Ilial fracture (arrow), which mimicked acetabular fracture radiographically, and left pubic fractures in a dog. (C) Color 3-D reformatted pelvic CT of the same dog as (B), illustrating long oblique over-riding ilial fracture (arrows) and left pubic fracture (arrowhead). Right and left ilium wing fractures are also evident. Feces are in red.

- complete cruciate tears: inability to trace the ligament as a contiguous structure from the point of origin to the point of insertion
- meniscal fibrocartilage: dissection of contrast medium within the meniscus.

Long digital extensor tendonitis/tear/avulsion

Long digital extensor disorders occur mostly in immature, large-breed dogs as a result of long-standing trauma. The owners may overlook the initial trauma and the dogs are mostly presented with chronic lesions.

CT features (Figure 38.33)

- Joint capsular thickening and intracapsular effusion.
- Avulsion fragment may be seen.
- Sclerosis of the extensor fossa of the lateral femoral epicondyle may be seen.
- CT arthrogram:
  - tendonitis: thickening of the tendon and attenuation of intra-articular contrast distribution around the tendon
  - partial tendon tears: attenuation of the ligament +/− dissection of intra-articular contrast medium within the ligament.

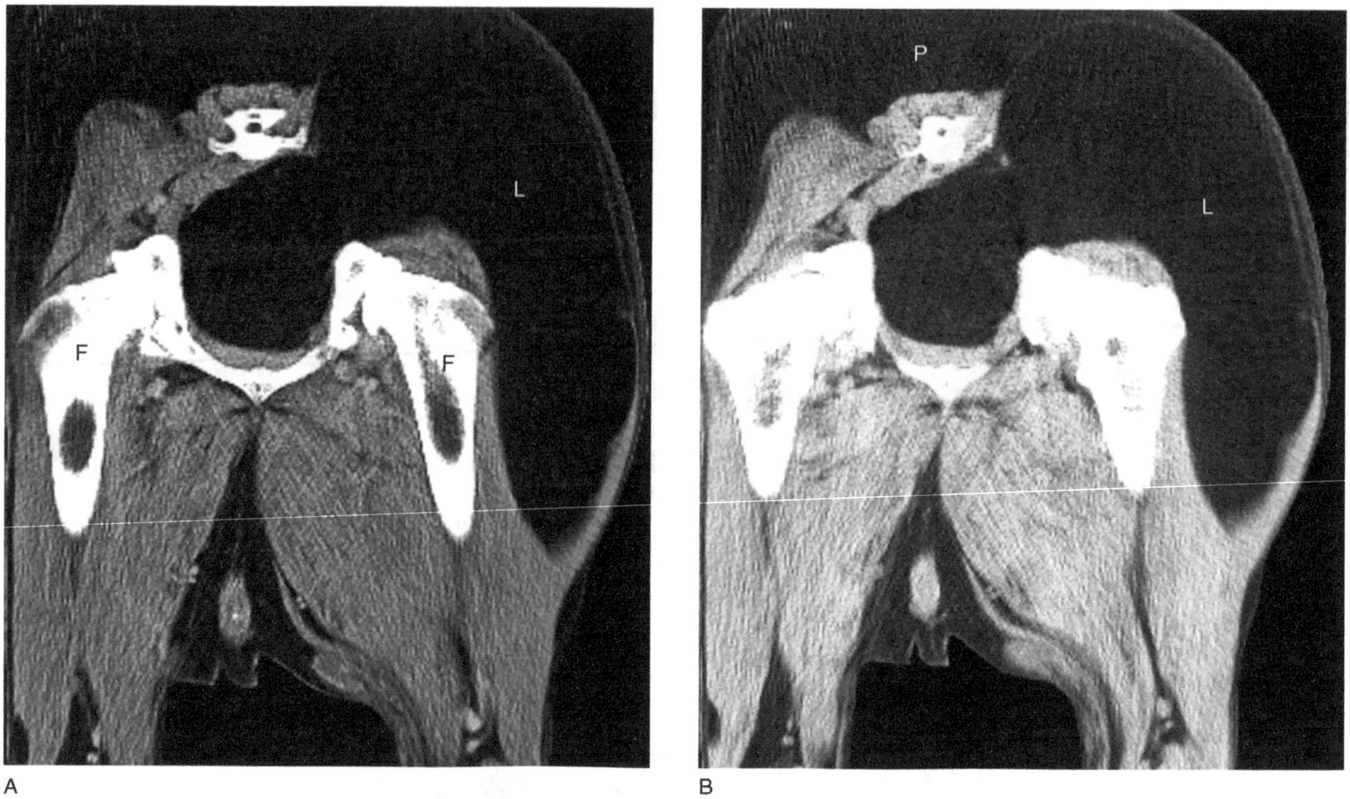

Figure 38.28 Adult dog with a lipoma. (A) Soft tissue window image of a large caudal thigh infiltrative lipoma (L) invading the pelvic canal and causing complete compression of the rectum. Advanced coxofemoral degenerative changes are evident but not well windowed. (B) Same image as (A), with a fat-enhancing window (320)/level (–70), shows the capsule between the lipoma (L) and perineal fat pad (P). F = femur.

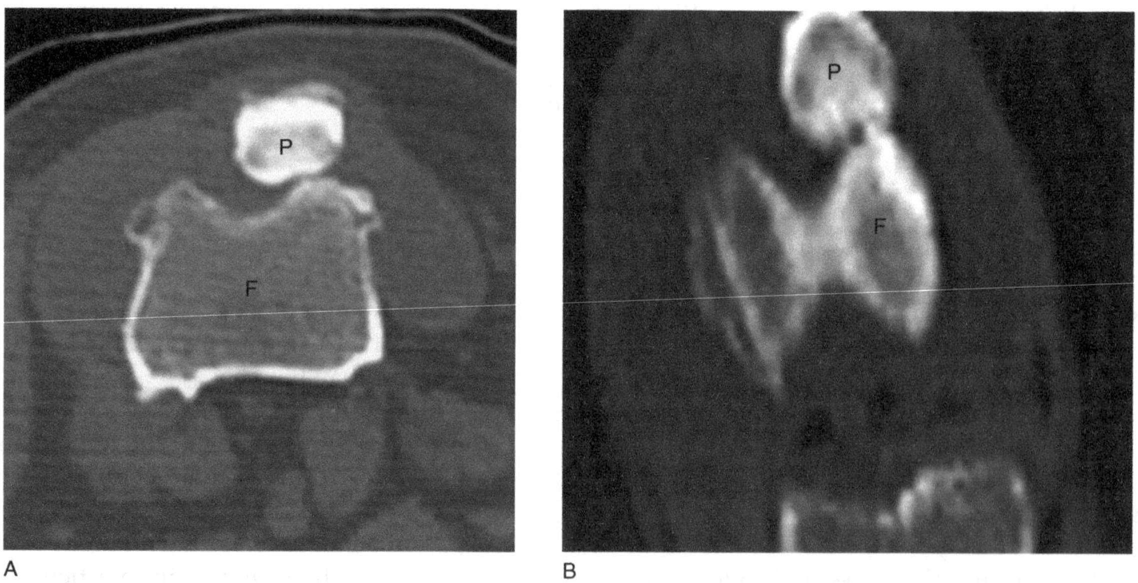

Figure 38.29 (A) Transverse and (B) frontally reformatted CT images of a patellar subluxation in a dog. F = femur; P = patella.

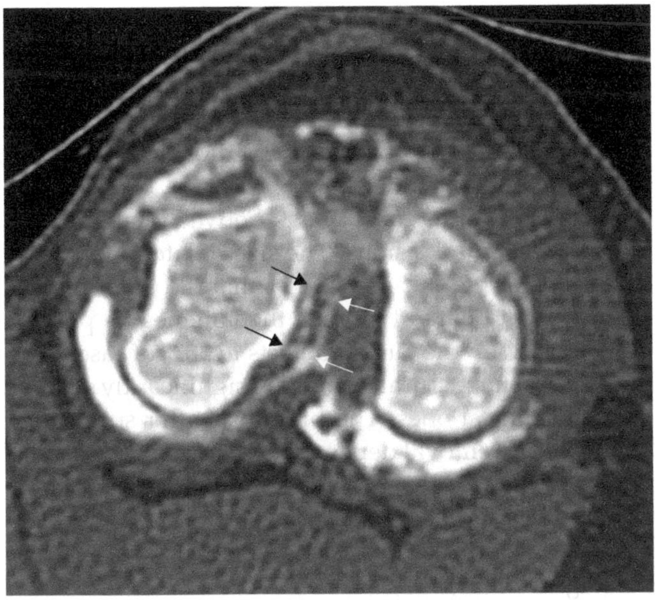

Figure 38.30 Transverse CT arthrogram of a partial cranial cruciate tear (arrows) in a dog.

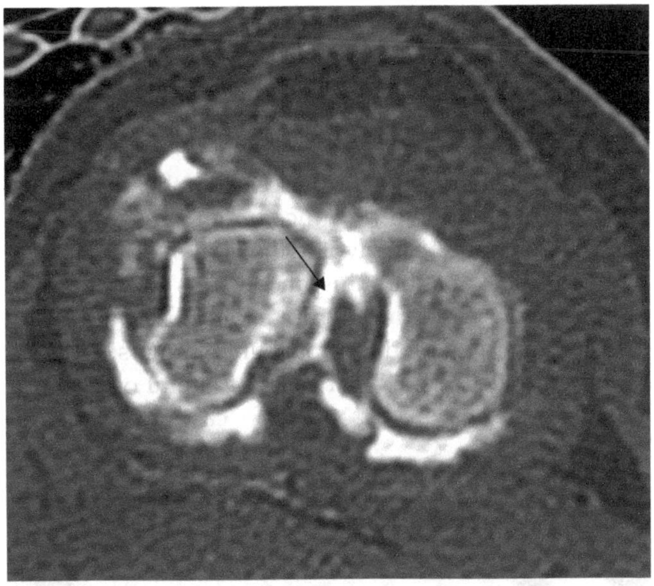

Figure 38.31 CT arthrogram of a mid-body, complete cranial cruciate tear (arrow) in a dog.

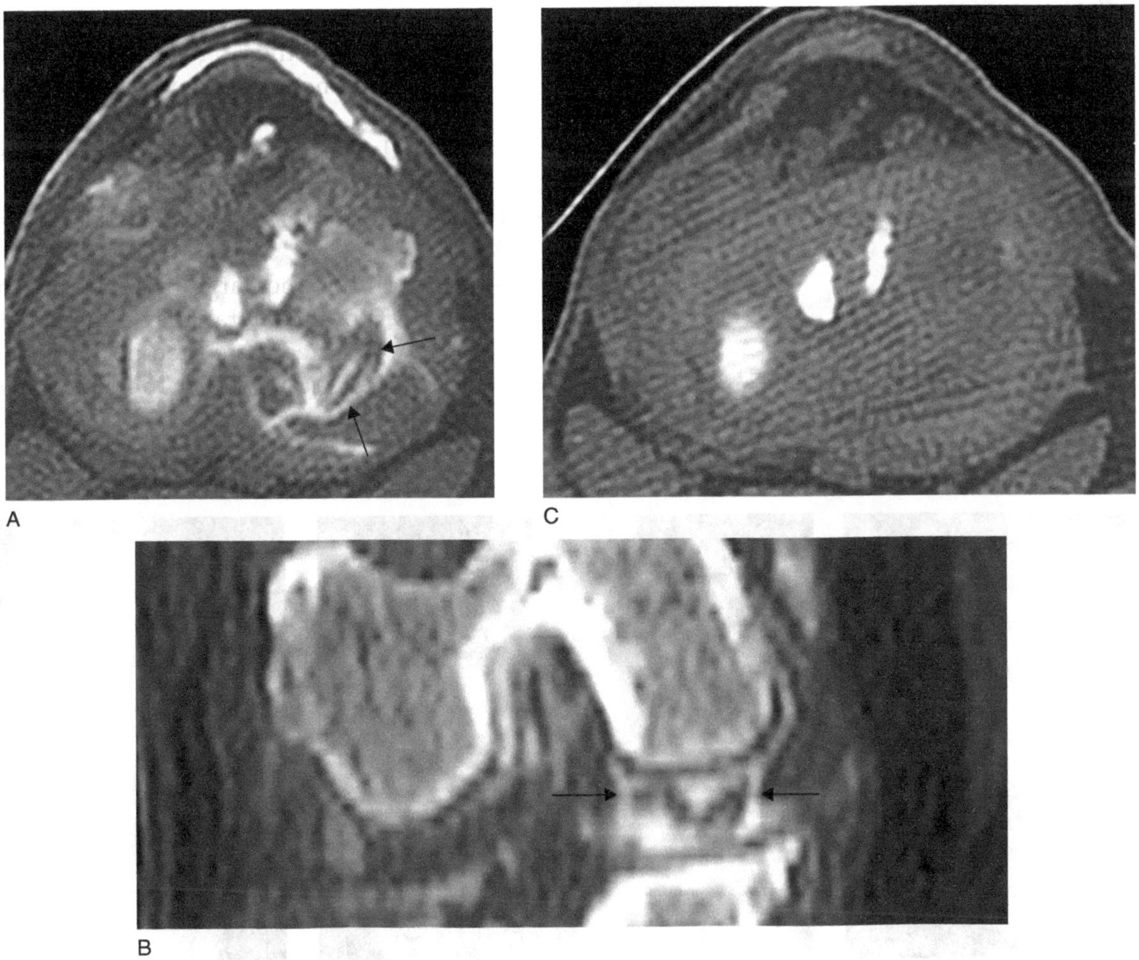

Figure 38.32 (A) Transverse CT arthrogram, (B) frontally reformatted arthrogram and (C) transverse CT image (same level as A) show a bucket handle medial meniscal tear in an adult dog (arrows).

The Tarsal Joint

Developmental

Osteochondritis dissecans

In the dog, osteochondritis dissecans of the tarsocrural joint is a well-known but uncommon cause of lameness. The disorder can involve the medial or the lateral trochlear ridge of the talus and results in instability, pain, lameness and degenerative joint disease.

Using an extended protocol including six radiographic projections, 27% of cases of lateral osteochondritis dissecans and 10% of cases of medial osteochondritis dissecans can be missed. The higher percentage of missed cases in lateral ridge can be explained by the supplementary superimposition of the calcaneus. These percentages increase to 72% using only two standard projections (mediolateral and dorsoplantar, both extended).

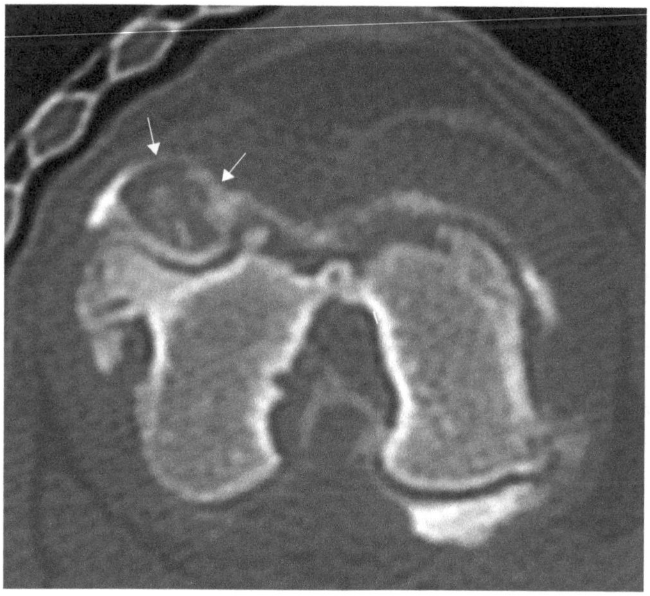

Figure 38.33 Adult dog with long digital extensor tendonitis in a dog. Transverse CT arthrogram shows an enlarged tendon that is increased in density (arrows).

Significant differences exist between lateral and medial tarsocrural lesions. The size of lateral tarsocrural lesions is significantly larger than those of medial lesions. With bilateral lesions, the lameness is present in the joint with the largest defects in 30% of cases. The non-clinical tarsocrural lesions are significantly smaller than the clinical ones. The prognosis after surgical or arthroscopic removal depends on the size of the defect.

CT features

- Osteochondritis dissecans medial talar ridge (Figure 38.34):
  - On the transverse images, radiolucent defects surrounded with sclerosis can be seen. Most of the time several fragments associated with these defects can be observed.
  - Most defects are located in the proximal and dorsal part of the ridge. The number and location of fragments is essential information for the surgeon.
  - Frontal and sagittal reconstructions allow inspection of the entire joint.
- Osteochondritis dissecans lateral talar ridge (Figure 38.35):
  - Most of the time, large fragments in the proximal part of the lateral talar ridge are observed.
  - Rarely fragments are seen in the distal part of the lateral ridge, which demands a different surgical approach.

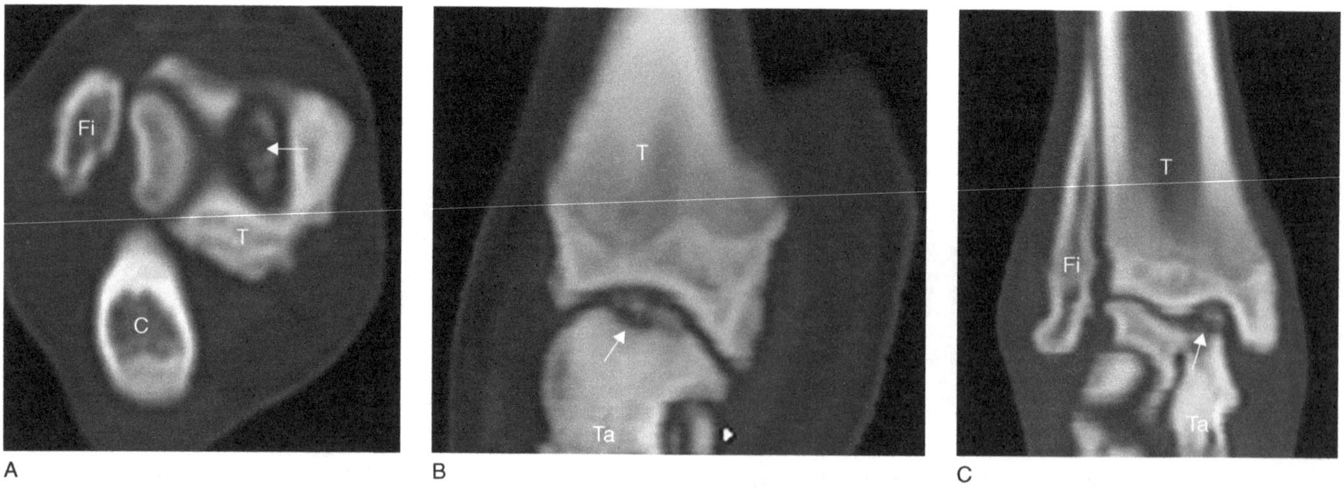

Figure 38.34 Young dog with medial osteochondritis dissecans. (A) Transverse, (B) sagittally reconstructed and (C) frontally reconstructed CT images show multiple detached fragments (white arrows). C = calcaneus; Fi = fibula; T = tibia; Ta = talus.

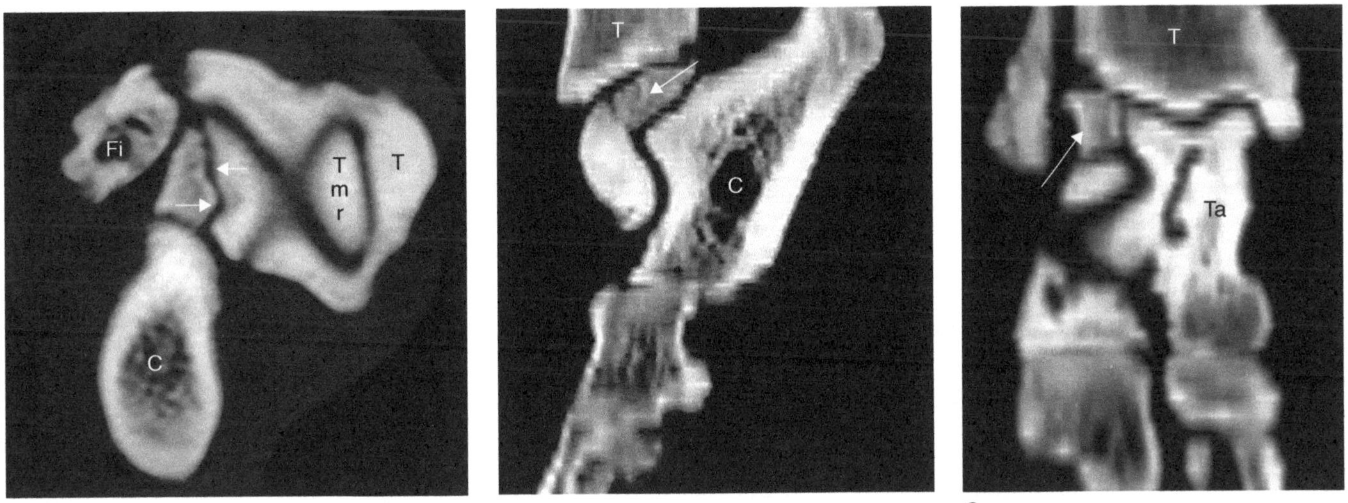

A B C

Figure 38.35 Young dog with lateral tarsocrural osteochondritis dissecans. (A) Transverse, (B) sagittally reconstructed and (C) frontally reconstructed CT images show a large detached fragment (white arrows). C = calcaneus; Fi = fibula; T = tibia; Ta = talus; Tmr = medial tarsal ridge.

Further reading

Cavanaugh RP, Carey K, Fischetti AJ and Samii VF (2007) What is your diagnosis? *J Am Vet Med Assoc* **230**: 1809–10.

Crawford JT, Manley PA and Adams WM (2003) Comparison of computed tomography, tangential view radiography and conventional radiography in evaluation of canine pelvic trauma. *Vet Radiol Ultrasound* **44**: 619–28.

De Rycke LM, Gielen IM, van Bree H *et al.* (2002) Computed tomography of the elbow joint in clinically normal dogs. *Am J Vet Res* **63**: 1400–7.

Dueland RT, Adams WM, Fialkowski JP, Patricelli AJ, Mathews KG and Nordheim EV (2001) Effects of pubic symphysiodesis in dysplastic puppies. *Vet Surg* **30**: 201–17.

Fitch RB, Wilson ER, Hathcock JT and Montgomery RD (1997) Radiographic, computed tomographic and magnetic resonance imaging evaluation of a chronic long digital extensor tendon avulsion in a dog. *Vet Radiol Ultrasound* **38**: 177–81.

Gemmill T (2004) Completing the picture: use of CT to investigate elbow dysplasia. *J Small Anim Pract* **45**: 429–30.

Gemmill TJ, Hammond G, Mellor D *et al.* (2006) Use of reconstructed computed tomography for the assessment of joint spaces in the canine elbow. *J Small Anim Pract* **47**: 66–74.

Gielen I, De Rycke L, van Bree H and Simoens P (2001) Computed tomography of the tarsal joint in clinically normal dogs. *Am J Vet Res* **62**: 1911–15.

Gielen I, van Bree H, Van Ryssen B, De Clercq T and de Rooster H (2002) Radiographic, computed tomographic and arthroscopic findings in 23 dogs with osteochondrosis of the tarsocrural joint. *Vet Rec* **150**: 442–7.

Gielen I, Van Ryssen B and van Bree H (2005) Computerized tomography compared with radiography in the diagnosis of lateral trochlear ridge talar osteochondritis dissecans in dogs. *Vet Comp Orthop Traumatol* **18**: 77–81.

Grundmann S and Montavon PM (2001) Stenosing tenosynovitis of the abductor pollicis longus muscle in dogs. *Vet Comp Orthop Traumatol* **14**: 95–100.

Holsworth IG, Wisner ER, Scherrer WE *et al.* (2005) Accuracy of computerized tomographic evaluation of canine radio-ulnar incongruence in vitro. *Vet Surg* **34**: 108–13.

Kramer A, Holsworth IG, Wisner ER *et al.* (2006) Computed tomographic evaluation of canine radioulnar incongruence in vivo. *Vet Surg* **35**: 24–9.

Mahoney PN and Lamb CR (1996) Articular, periarticular and juxtaarticular calcified bodies in the dog and cat: A radiologic review. *Vet Radiol Ultrasound* **37**: 3–15.

Reichle JK, Park RD and Bahr AM (2000) Computed tomographic findings of dogs with cubital joint lameness. *Vet Radiol Ultrasound* **41**: 125–30.

Samii VF and Dyce J (2004) Computed tomographic arthrography of the normal canine stifle. *Vet Radiol Ultrasound* **45**: 402–6.

Samii VF, Dyce J, Pozzi A *et al.* (2009) Computed tomographic arthrography of the stifle for detection of cranial and caudal cruciate and meniscal tears in dogs. *Vet Radiol Ultrasound* **50**: 144–50.

Smallwood JE and George TF (1993) Anatomic atlas for computed tomography in the mesaticephalic dog: caudal abdomen and pelvis. *Vet Radiol Ultrasound* **34**: 143–67.

Tivers MS, Mahoney P and Corr SA (2008) Canine stifle positive contrast computed tomography arthrography for assessment of caudal horn meniscal injury: a cadaver study. *Vet Surg* **37**: 269–77.

van Bree H, Gielen I, Van Ryssen B *et al.* (2002) Comparative joint imaging in small animals. *Eur J Comp Anim Pract* **12**: 25–36.

CHAPTER THIRTY-NINE

Particularities of Equine CT

Jimmy Saunders, Alastair Nelson and Katrien Vanderperren

Scanning Technique (Including Facilities and Equipment)

CT on the anesthetized horse

Recovery box and transport to the CT room

The sedation and anesthesia of the horse is ideally done in a recovery box located as close as possible to the CT machine and equipped with a hoist to allow the horse to be positioned on the CT table.

If such an infrastructure is unavailable, the induction can be done in a recovery box located elsewhere, and the horse can be transported to the CT machine by means of the CT table itself, a forklift or another moving table. If another table is used, then hoists should be available inside the CT room.

The CT room

The optimal size for the CT room is 8 m in length, 8 m in width and 5 m in height (including workstation and anesthetic material). These measurements allow easy positioning of the horse in dorsal (Figure 39.1A) as well as in lateral (Figure 39.1B) recumbency.

The CT machine

In adult horses, CT is limited to the head, neck and legs. How much of the body can be scanned depends on the gantry diameter, which ranges from 30 cm (portable system) to 90 cm (large-bore). Using a large-bore CT, the neck can be scanned up to C4 or C6 depending on the size of the horse, the forelimbs up to the elbow joint and the hindlimbs up to the stifle joint.

Specific CT equipment for horses (Figure 39.2)

Instead of the standard table designed for humans, a custom-built horse table has to be installed specifically allowing the imaging of subjects up to approximately 2000–2500 lb. The CT table should preferably be linked to the table drive, allowing helical scanning. Such a table can be made by the manufacturer or can be self-made. If the table proves unlinkable, it can be advanced manually by means of a hand crank, but this prevents the use of helical scanning. An alternative is the use of a stationary table and a CT gantry that advances on the table. Any table should be adjustable. Thick cushions, ropes and other containment and positioning materials, as well as a power injector for contrast studies, are mandatory for most studies of the brain and limbs.

CT on the standing horse

A system has been developed at the Rainbow Equine Clinic in North Yorkshire in the UK, to carry out CT scanning of the horse's head and cranial neck.

The main adaptation has been that the head/neck can be positioned within the scanner while the horse remains standing in a pit (Figure 39.3).

Another adaptation is that the CT gantry is reversed, so that the horse is being presented to that side of the gantry which is normally next to the patient table. The reason for this is that most scanners are designed with one side of the scanner having a shorter distance to the scan plane than the other.

The patient table is used to move the area to be scanned during helical scanning. When scanning the head and neck the table is linked to the platform the horse is standing on. This platform is mounted on air

Veterinary Computed Tomography, First Edition. Edited by Tobias Schwarz, Jimmy Saunders.

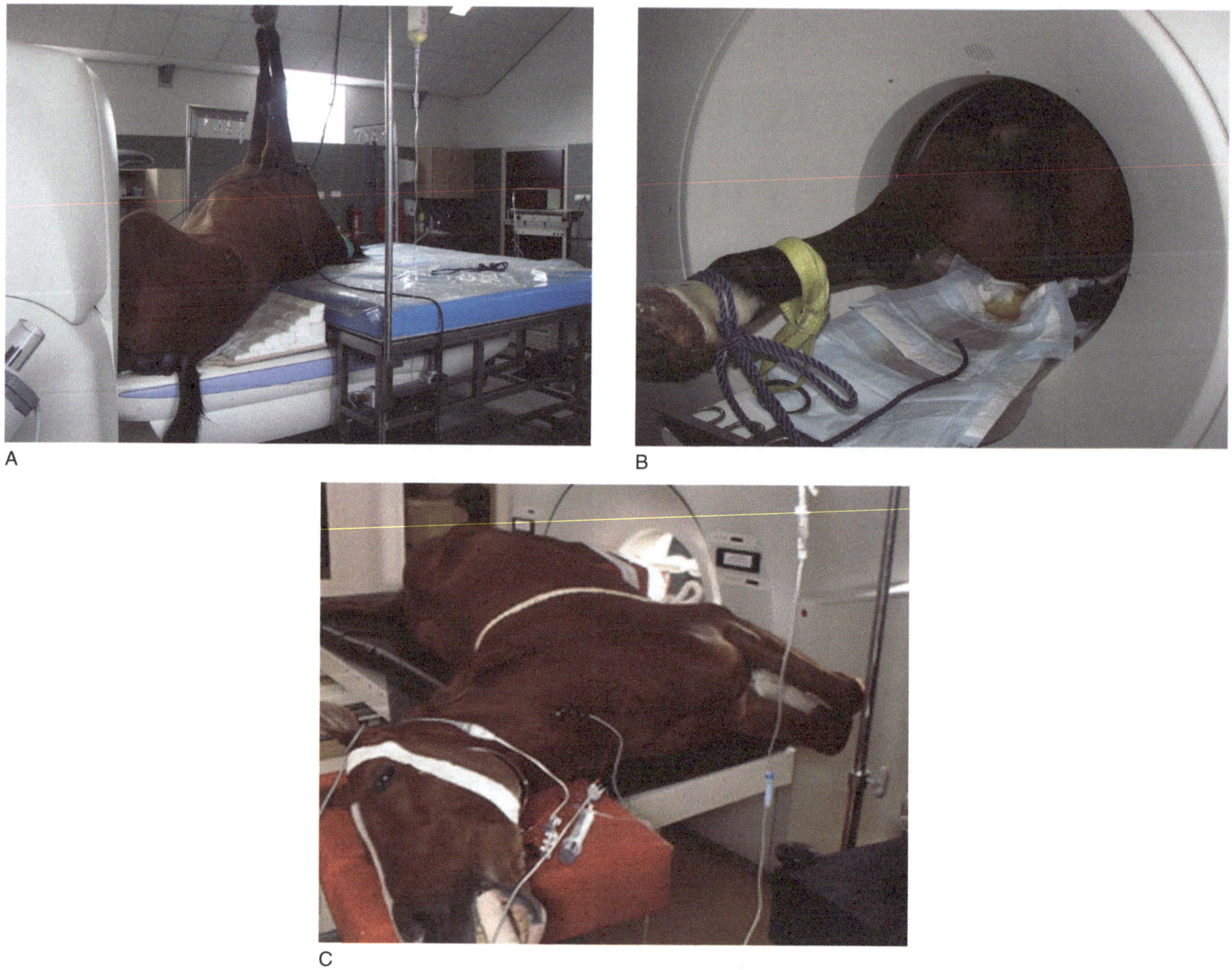

Figure 39.1 A CT room must be large enough to allow scanning of horses in (A,B) dorsal/dorsolateral decubitus (head and neck, stifle) as well as (C) in lateral decubitus (lower limbs) (images courtesy of H.E. Bergman, Lingehoeve, Netherlands).

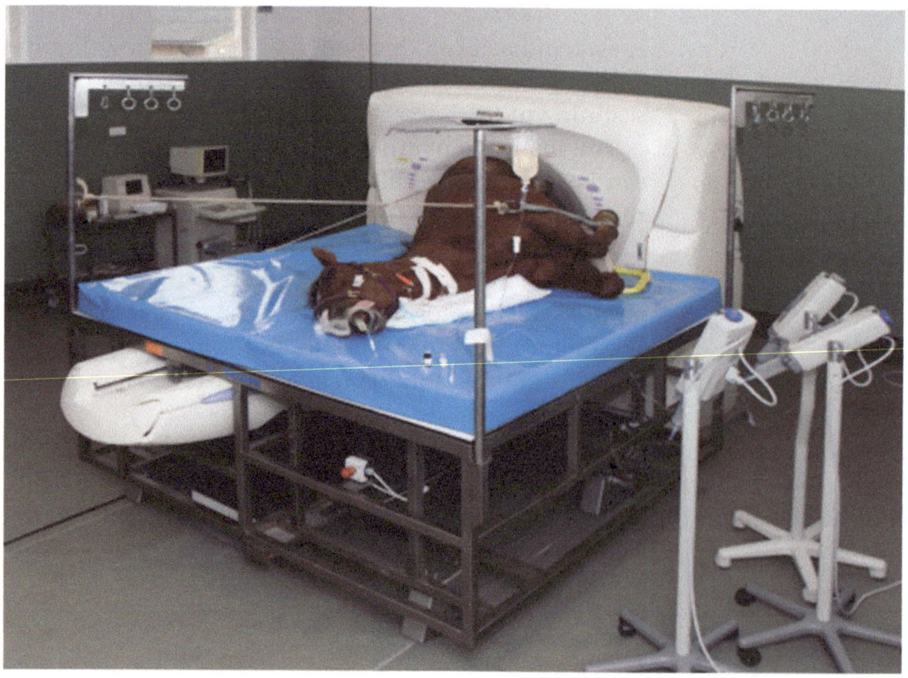

Figure 39.2 CT table specifically designed for horses (image courtesy of H.E. Bergman, Lingehoeve, Netherlands).

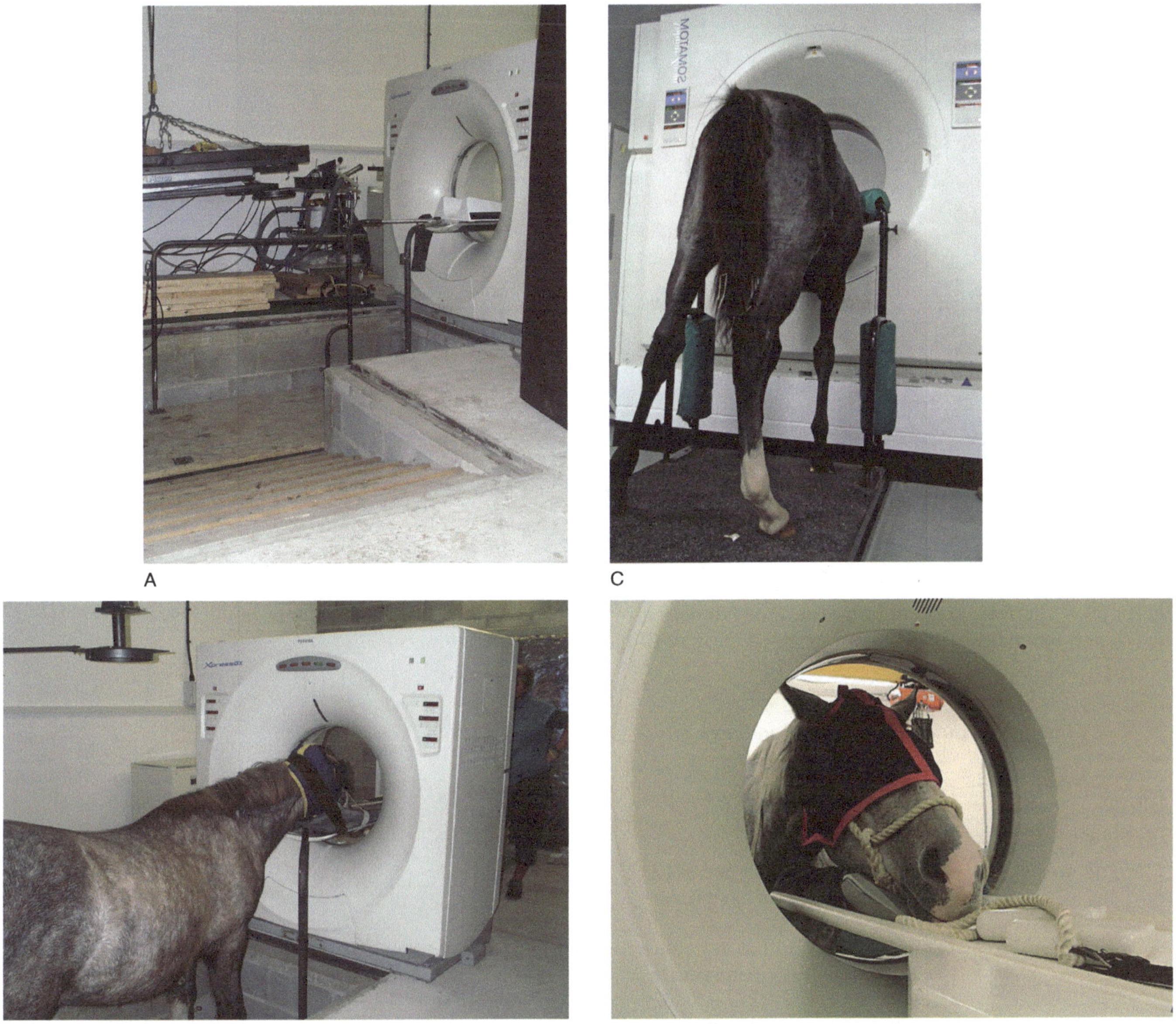

Figure 39.3 CT examination of the head and neck can be performed with a fixed CT on the standing horse. (A) A pit has been built right in front of the gantry CT scanner. (B) Horse standing in the pit during scanning. (C,D) Position of the head of the horse in the gantry during scanning (images courtesy of S.E. Powell, Rossdales Equines Diagnostic Centre, Suffolk, UK).

skates, which allow frictionless movement of the platform and horse. The disadvantages of the system include the following:

- Horses tolerate helical scanning of the head well, but the movement of the patient table during scout acquisition is too rapid and so the acquisition cannot be carried out.
- Movement blur may necessitate repeating a scan of the area affected by movement, mainly only a small section of the area. Movement blur may degrade the quality of MPR and 3-D reconstructions.
- A handler is present during scanning. The handler scanning behind a lead screen directly adjacent to the gantry, which acts as a radiation shield, reduces the radiation dose to a minimum.

A peripheral quantitative computed tomography (pQCT) scanner, was designed to image the limbs of the horse, both in standing or recumbent position in the Equine Clinic Desbrosses (Figure 39.4). These systems have a reduced image quality compared with conventional CT machines.

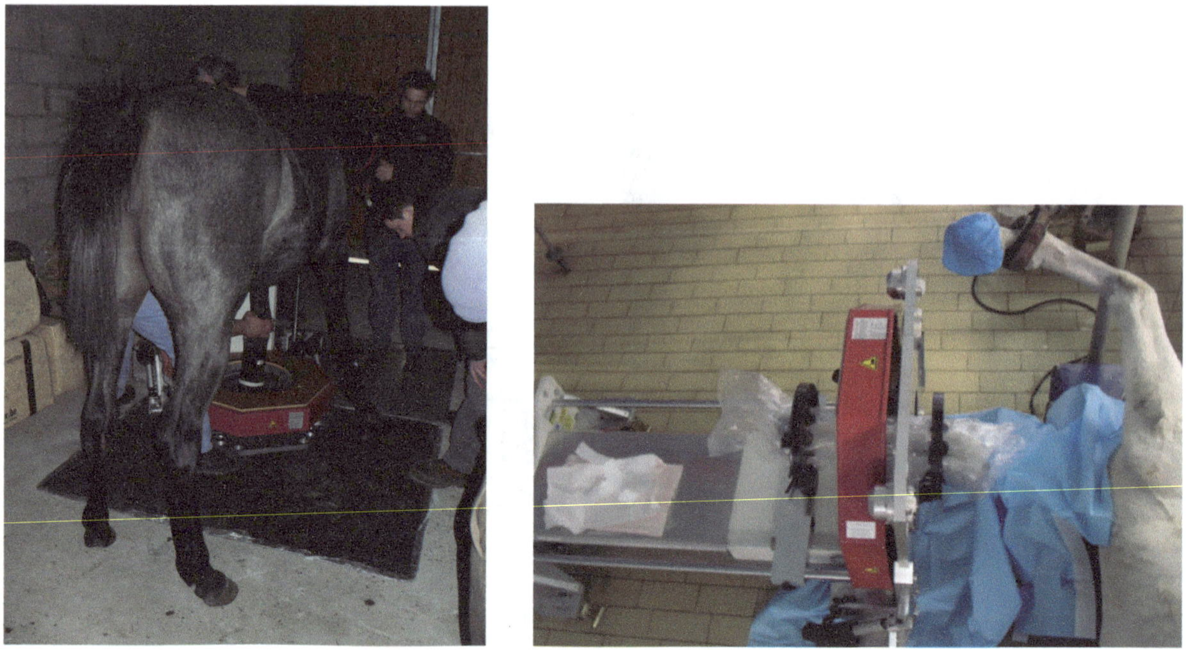

A B

Figure 39.4 Peripheral quantitative computed tomography scanner designed to image the limbs of the horse, both in standing (A) and recumbent (B) position (image courtesy of Clinique Desbrosses, France).

Table 39.1
CT imaging protocol for the head and neck.

Series	Pre- and post-contrast	Bone
Decubitus	Dorsal	
Scan margins	**Head/Brain:** Rostral orbit → C1 **Neck:** Occiput → as caudal as possible **Sinonasal and dental:** Foal: Nostrils ←→ caudal aspect of bony orbit Adult: Nostrils ←→ temporomandibular joint	
Voltage (kVp)	120	
Current (mAs)	280	
Tube rotation time (s)	1	
Slice width (mm)	5	2.5
Kernel frequency	Medium	High
Collimator pitch	1–1.5	1
Helical image reconstruction interval	2.5	1.25
Window level (HU)	+50 Dental: +2000 sinonasal	+400
Window width (HU)	150 Dental: 5000	2000

Imaging Protocols

Imaging protocols for vascular contrast CT are described in Chapter 5.

Axial skeleton (including brain)

Standard CT (Table 39.1)

Anesthetized horses are positioned in dorsal recumbency during examination of the head, which may result in an artifactual edema of the nasal turbinates.

CT myelography (Table 39.2)

Joints

Native joints (Table 39.3)

CT arthrography (Table 39.4)

Table 39.2
CT imaging protocol for myelographic studies.

Series	CT myelography
Access site	Cervical (cisternal): atlanto-occipal joint
Scan margin	Following conventional myelography include two vertebral bodies cranial and caudal to region of interest for improved multiplanar reconstructions. If possible (foals), complete spine up to T1
Contrast medium application	Preferably ultrasound-guided cervical injection
Contrast medium type	Non-ionic, monomeric, iodinated contrast medium only
Contrast medium dose	30 mg iodine/kg bw (0.1 ml/kg of 300 mg I/ml)
Contrast medium injection mode	Manual
Scan delay post start contrast injection	As soon as possible
Side effects	Post-myelogram seizures Iatrogenic brainstem injury
Undesired effect	Accidental epi- or subdural injection (reduced risk if ultrasound-guided)
Additional comment	CSF samples should be collected prior to contrast medium injection, as the contrast medium alters the differential cell count within 24 h and can affect the growth of bacteria in culture

Table 39.3
CT protocol for joint studies.

Series	Pre- and post-contrast	Bone
Decubitus	Lateral – limb of interest down	
Special positioning	**Distal extremity, carpus, tarsus:** limb of interest down with horse in lateral decubitus. Contralateral limb out of gantry whenever possible **Stifle:** limb of interest down in full extension with horse in lateral/dorsolateral decubitus. Contralateral limb flexed out of gantry (Figure 39.1A,B)	
Scan margins	**Stifle:** scan as proximal as possible (adult horse = complete femoro-tibial joints and distal part femoro-tibial joint (→ 5 cm distal to tibial crest)) **Tarsus:** distal tibia → proximal metacarpus (attachment suspensory ligament included) **Carpus:** distal radius → proximal metacarpus (attachment suspensory ligament included) **Fetlock:** distal extremity (metacarpus/metatarsus) – distal hoof wall **Foot:** fetlock joint → distal phalanx including laminae ROI* or proximal border DSB → distal end of ROI or distal insertion DDFT	
Voltage (kVp)	120	
Current (mAs)	120–350	
Tube rotation time (s)	0.85–1	
Slice width (mm)	2	1 or 2 (fetlock) Intra-articular 0.6 mm
Sequential slice interval (mm)	2	1
Collimator pitch	0.85–1	
Kernel frequency	Medium	High
Motion control	Breath hold – hyperventilate to produce transient apnea	
Window level (HU)	+40–80 (120)	+750 (700)
Window width (HU)	200–400	2000 (3200)

Table 39.4
CT imaging protocol for arthrographic studies.

Access site	Standard site for joint centesis
Route of administration	Intra-articular (surgical preparation mandatory)
Catheter size	22 ga (tarsus 18 ga)
Injection method	Blind (aspirate to confirm needle position and for synovial fluid sampling) or ultrasound-guided manual injection
Contrast agent	Iodinated
Contrast medium type	Non-ionic, dimeric
Generic name	Omnipaque
Contrast medium concentration	30–40 mg iodine/ml (1/10 dilution of Omnipaque 300 mg with saline)
Volume	Until distention is reached *Guidelines* – **Carpal region:** radiocarpal 15–25 ml; intercarpal with carpometacarpal 15–25 ml; carpal sheath: 50–80 ml – **Coffin joint:** 20–30 ml – **Fetlock joint:** 20 (front)–30 ml (hind) – **Stifle joint:** femoropatellar 80 ml, others 60 ml each – **Tarsal joint:** 60 ml (tarso-crural), 3 ml others – **Tendon sheath:** 50–80 ml
Rate of injection	0.5 ml/s
Scan delay	After several joint flexions and extensions
Side effects	Mild synovitis
Undesired effects	– Extra-articular injection of contrast medium (reduced risk with ultrasound-guided injection) – Iatrogenic joint infection secondary to failure to perform surgical preparation prior to joint centesis and arthrography

CHAPTER FORTY

Equine Sinonasal and Dental

Jimmy Saunders and Zoe Windley

Dental and Periodontal CT: Anatomy and Normal Variants

The horse has 24 deciduous teeth (2 × Di 3/3, Dc 0/0, Dpm 3/3) and 36 to 44 permanent teeth (2 × I 3/3, C 1/1 or 0/0, PM 3/3 or 4/4, M 3/3) that are mostly named using the Triadan system (Figure 40.1).

As in most mammals, the equine tooth is composed of enamel, cementum, dentine and dental pulp and is supported by the periodontium (periodontal ligament, alveolar bone and gum) (Figure 40.2). Each of these structures has a specific density on CT that is not age-related (Table 40.1).

However, equine teeth also have their specificities determined by evolution.

- All permanent teeth in horses are hypsodont, which means that tooth eruption continues throughout life (at a rate of 23 mm/year). This process compensates for wear at the tooth's occlusal surface due to the prolonged mastication (up to 20 h/day) of abrasive forage (Figure 40.3).
- Due to the permanent abrasion, the horse's teeth need to continuously lay down secondary dentine to prevent occlusal pulp exposure. The permanent eruption forces the periodontal ligament and the alveolar bone to be very flexible. For this reason, an area of spongy and porous bone is present between the lamina dura (thin layer of compact bone attached to the periodontal ligament) and the mandibular and maxillary trabeculae.
- The cheek teeth have between five and eight pulp horns (Figure 40.2B).
- The maxillary cheek teeth have two enamel invaginations, called infundibula, that penetrate the occlusal surface. These correspond to remnants of vascular channels and are filled by cementum, often incompletely (Figure 40.2A).
- Infundibular changes are observed with age. Some of these changes have no clinical relevance. However, the differentiation between normal variations and clinically relevant/pathological changes has still to be defined (Figure 40.4).
- Enamel and cementum in horses can be peripheral (primary) or infundibular (secondary). The dentine forming the skeleton of the tooth is called primary, while the dentine that is laid down at the occlusal surface is termed secondary.
- As a consequence of the continuous eruption, the detailed morphology of equine teeth continuously changes over time. An increase in age is associated with a decrease in pulp volume, in the number of communications between pulp horns, in the distance the pulp extend apically within individual roots and in the length of the reserve crown, and with an increase in the number of apical foramina per root.
- Vessels in the apical pulp afford nutrition to the developing tooth via wide apical foramina. In the maxillary teeth additional vessels descend from the coronal surface into the infundibula. This strong vascular supply gives an optimal protection against infection. In the adult tooth, the apical foramina progressively become smaller, as does the pulp cavity, and the vascular supply from the infundibula dramatically reduces or may disappear completely, thereby decreasing the regenerating capabilities of the adult tooth.

Veterinary Computed Tomography, First Edition. Edited by Tobias Schwarz, Jimmy Saunders.

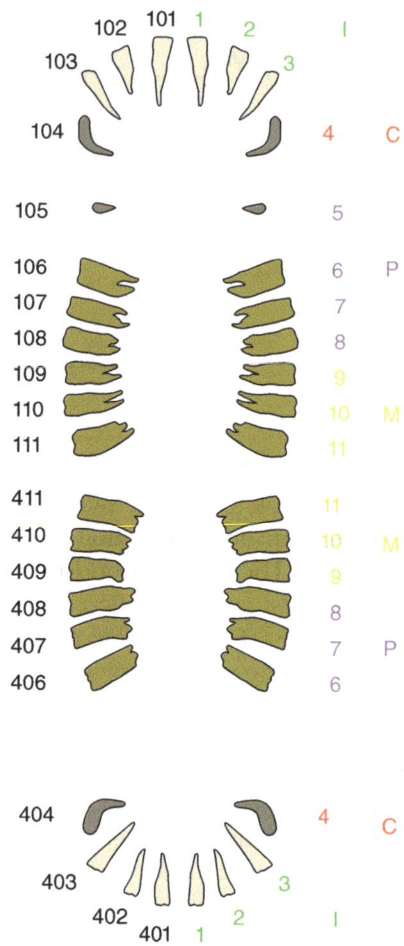

Figure 40.1 Triadan (left on the image) and traditional anatomic chart (right on the image) of the equine dental nomenclature of the permanent teeth.

Dental and Periodontal Disorders

Dental developmental disorders: cemental and enamel hypoplasia

Hypoplasia of the dental tissues is mostly benign. However, it may also be a predisposing factor for infectious dental and periodontal disease.

Infundibular cemental hypoplasia is present to some degree in all maxillary check teeth and affects more frequently the rostral infundibulum. This inadequate cementum deposition may be due to premature eruption, premature removal of protective deciduous teeth (caps) or compromised infundibular blood supply in the young horse. The latter may be due to an excessive deposition of infundibular cementum near the occlusal surface constricting the blood supply to cementocytes deeper within the infundibulum.

Peripheral cemental hypoplasia varies in severity. When large areas of the tooth are affected, the vascular supply of the cementum and even the stability of the tooth may be affected. Significant peripheral cemental hypoplasia may be associated with the presence of periodontal disease.

Enamel hypoplasia may induce both infundibular and peripheral cemental hypoplasia, as any defect in the enamel is directly transferred to the surrounding tissues (dentine and cementum).

CT features

- Infundibular cemental hypoplasia (Figure 40.5):
  - hypodense area within the infundibulum (rostral > caudal)
  - consequent deposit/presence of organic material within the infundibulum.
- Peripheral cemental hypoplasia
  - defect in the normal cemental outline (between the hyperdense peripheral enamel and the thin hypodense periodontal ligament).
- Enamel hypoplasia (Figure 40.6):
  - defect in the normal/hyperdense enamel outline, mostly multifocal. Three-dimensional reconstructions greatly facilitate a global evaluation.

Dental fracture

Horses can acquire fractures through external trauma (mandibular > maxillary) or iatrogenic trauma during dental treatment. However, in half the cases there is no evidence of trauma and the fracture is described as idiopathic. Most idiopathic cheek teeth fractures (±80%) are lateral slab fractures involving the pulp horns. Idiopathic lateral slab fractures are most common in the maxillary cheek teeth, with the Tridan 09 teeth being most commonly affected. Although it is commonly accepted that these fractures appear at locations of anatomical weakness ('thin' calcified tissue), which are subjected to enormous masticatory forces, the precise reason for weakness is not fully understood. The remaining idiopathic fractures (±20%) are midline sagittal infundibular fractures caused by the presence of infundibular cemental hypoplasia. This results in food entrapment, infundibular caries and finally a weakened tooth that is unable to support the force of mastication.

CT features (Figure 40.7)

- Presence of one or more hypodense (fracture) line(s) visible on at least two contiguous sections without continuation into adjacent tissue.

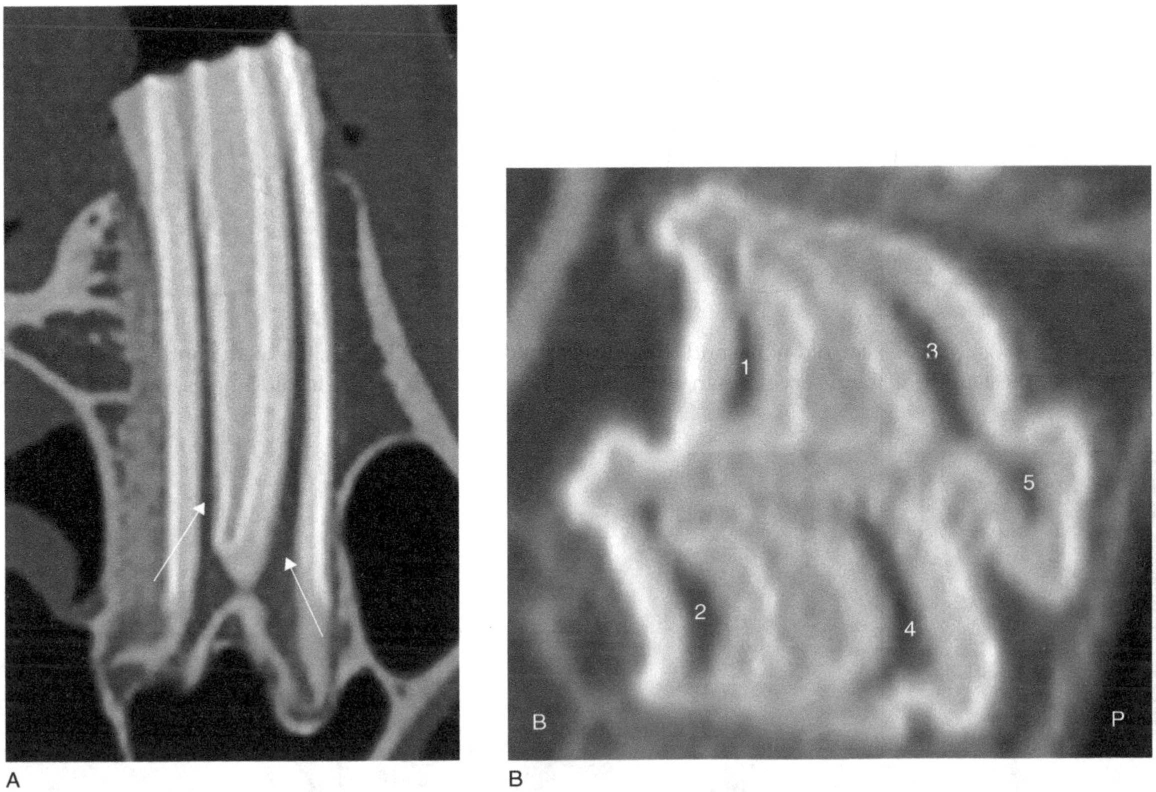

Figure 40.2 Normal Triadan (107) tooth with an eruption age of 2 years. (A) Transverse CT image shows the pulp (arrows). The infundibula are normal and no defects within the infundibular cementum are visible. (B) Dorsally reconstructed CT image shows the pulp horns (1–5). The palatal pulp horns (3,4) are of greater diameter than the buccal ones (1,2). The pulp horns have an elongated appearance in young and adult horses and become more rounded with increasing age. B = buccal; P = palatal.

Table 40.1
CT density of main dental structures.

Anatomical area	Hounsfield units
Enamel	+2000 to +3700
Cementum	+500 to +2400
- peripheral	+1780 to +2420
- infundibular	+1545 to +2376
Dentin	+950 to +3000
- primary	+1852 to +2686
- secondary	+1332 to +1977
Dental pulp	−1024 to +700

- Associated soft tissue lesions.
- Chronic dental fracture may be associated with dystrophic calcification(s) invading the nasal cavities.

Infection/Inflammation: infundibular caries

Infundibular caries is classified in five categories (with degree 0 = normal) using the modified Honma classification, which is based on the severity and the involvement of different dental structures at the occlusal surface. The process starts with defects in the cementum (degree 1) allowing debris, microorganisms and food to track down the central channel. This material is packed in anaerobic conditions at the apical aspect resulting in fermentation, acid production and decalcification of the infundibular cementum. Further progression of the process through the enamel (degree 2) then dentine (degree 3) may result in an apical abscessation or tooth fracture (degree 4).

CT features (Figures 40.8 and 40.9)

- Degree 1:
  - complete or incomplete, hypodense line along the infundibulum
  - large hypodense areas or expansion, forming a radiolucent bulbous shape at the apical extension of the infundibulum.
- Degree 2–4: cemental, enamel, dentin defects, apical abscessation, tooth fracture.

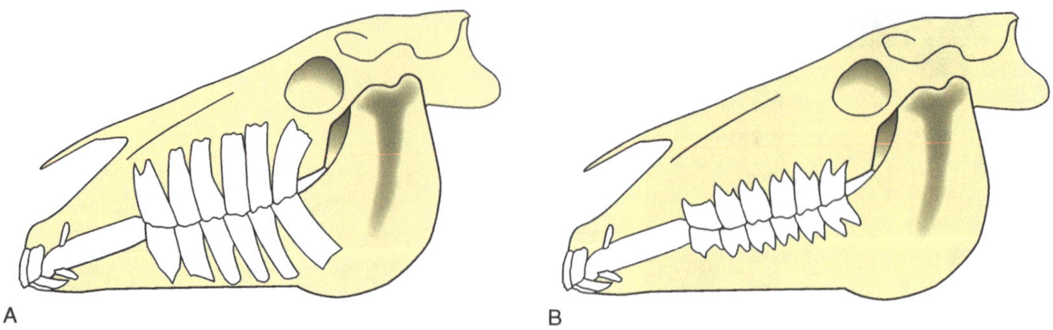

Figure 40.3 Dentition in (A) a 4-year-old horse and (B) a 20-year-old horse. In horses, the teeth continuously erupt throughout life. With time, the length of the reserve crown shortens and the roots develop. In old horses, only a small amount of tooth is left.

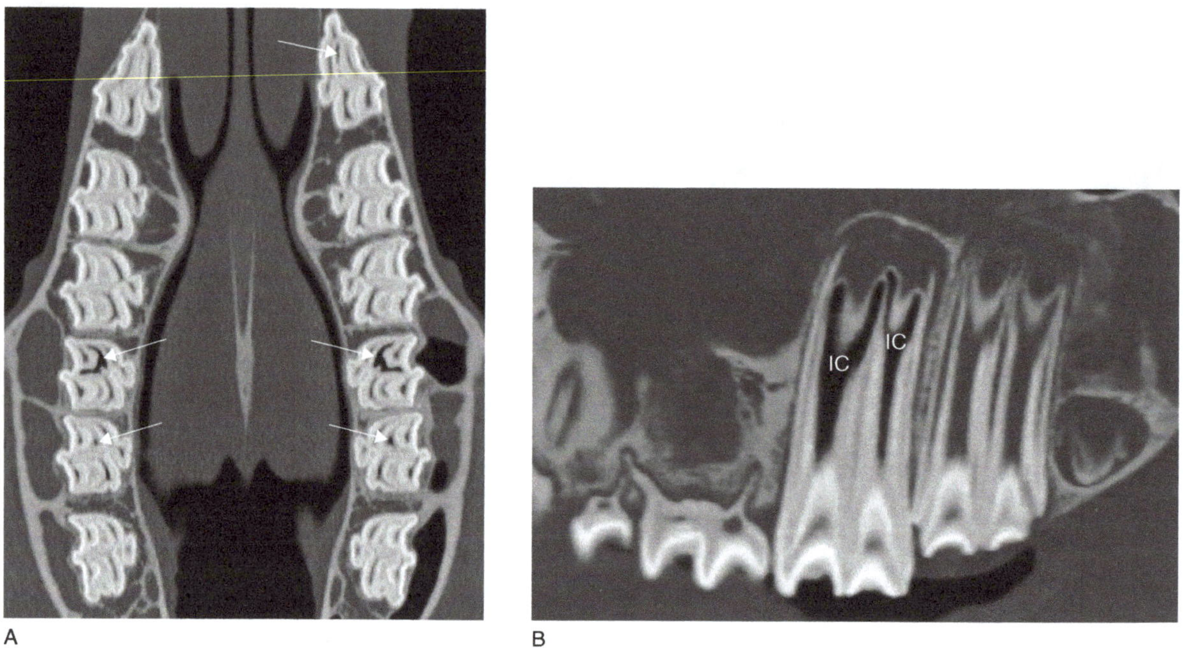

Figure 40.4 Infundibular changes found incidentally during CT examination of two patients. (A) Dorsally reconstructed CT image of the maxilla shows infundibular lesions (arrows) of the rostral infundibula of Triadan 109, 110, 206, 209 and 210. (B) Infundibular caries (IC) were seen in another horse, illustrated on this sagittally reconstructed CT image.

Degenerative/Acquired: pulpar exposure/pulpitis

Excessive attrition or reduction in secondary dentine deposition may cause pulpar exposure. Reduced secondary dentine deposition may be due to trauma or thermal damage during dental treatment (direct), or to a decrease or loss of vascular supply (indirect). Pulpitis secondary to infection after tooth fracture or cemental necrosis is mostly severe.

CT features (Figure 40.10)

- Heterogeneous density of the pulp due to the presence of areas of gas.
- Increased volume and irregular margin of the pulp horns.

Infectious/Inflammatory: apical abscess/alveolitis

There are numerous potential etiologies for equine apical abscesses. An apical abscess may be primary (unknown etiology) or secondary. This latter further classifies as developmental or acquired. Secondary developmental abscesses may arise from polydontia, dental displacement or rotation, dental dysplasia or the previously discussed hypoplasia. Acquired apical abscesses arise due to post-traumatic or idiopathic fractures (tooth, bone, both), caries, wear disorders, anachoretic pulpitis or periodontal disease. Apical infection caused by deep periodontal disease is uncommon in young teeth that may have a reserve crown in excess of 80 mm.

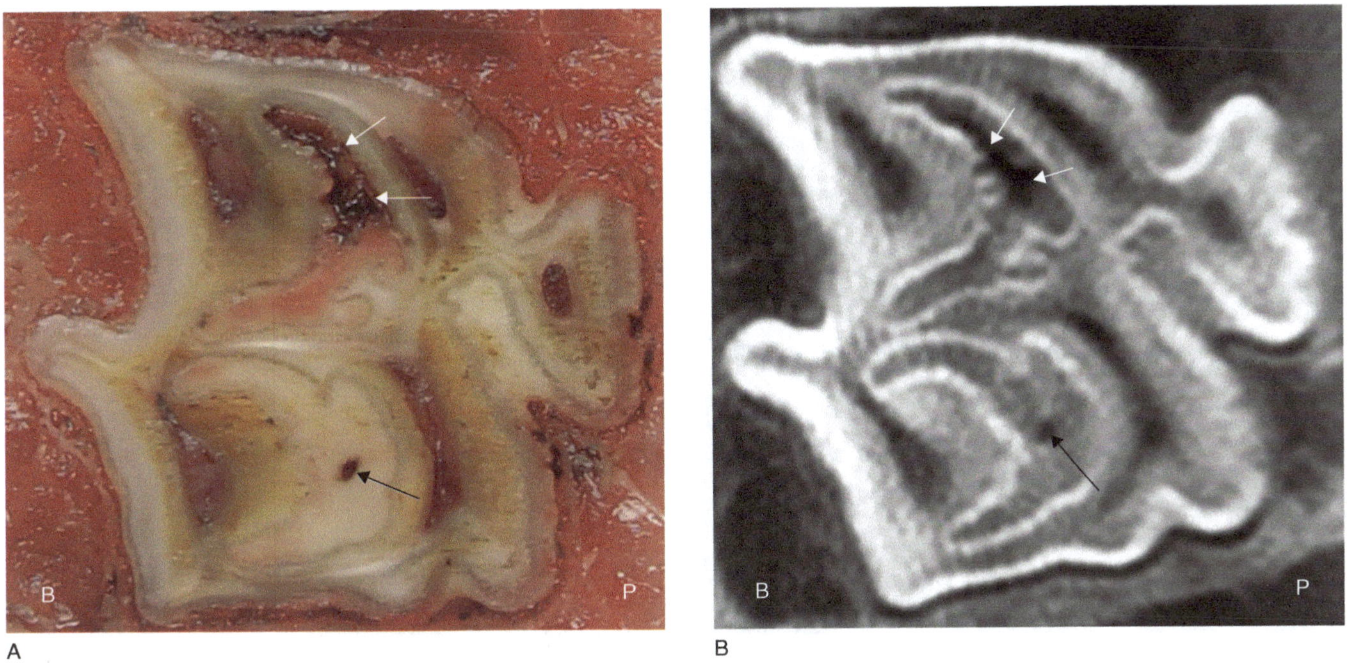

Figure 40.5 Five-year-old horse with infundibular cemental hypoplasia. (A) Dorsal anatomical section and (B) dorsal CT image. The rostral infundibulum is strongly enlarged (white arrows) and hypodense on CT. The caudal infundibulum (black arrow) shows an enlarged central lucent area indicative of infundibular cemental hypoplasia.

CT features (Figure 40.11)

- Destruction of the dentine between infundibula.
- Tooth roots damaged: destroyed, distorted, increased density, clubbed.
- Hypodense area around the apex.
- Fragmentation of tooth, masses of cement.
- Deposits of cement, fragments of unstructured mineralized tissue (cement pearls) adjacent to the infected tooth.
- Loss of lamina dura.
- Midline sagittal fractures (tooth fracture).
- Alveolar bone sclerosis, proliferations (osteitis).
- Sinusitis.

Periodontal disorders

Primary periodontal disease is uncommon in the horse. Secondary periodontal disorders are quite common and can be grouped in four categories: inflammation, dystrophy, neoplastic and other anomalies. Inflammation is the most frequently reported and can lead to a 'domino cycle' (Figure 40.12).

Periodontal disorders are quite frequent in the young horse due to the physiological process of tooth eruption and may resolve once normal occlusion is achieved. In older animals, apical infections usually cause infection of the supporting bones and depending on the tooth involved, cause facial swellings, fistulae or sinusitis.

CT features (Figure 40.13)

- Loss of alveolar bone.
- Dental loss, displacement, malocclusion.
- Diastemata presence, location, configuration.
- CT signs the primary disorder (mass, fracture).

Dental tumors

Odontogenic tumors are rare in general, although they seem to be more frequent in horses than in other species.

Ameloblastoma, cementoma, odontoma (complex or compound), ameloblastic odontoma and cysts/hamartoma should be differentiated from tumor-like processes such as aneurismal bone cysts, fibrous dysplasia, lymphosarcoma or bone tumors (osteoma, osteosarcoma).

CT features (Figure 40.14)

- Ameloblastoma (mandibula > maxilla): locally destructive roughly spherical or multilocular cystic and expansile process.
- Cementoma: hyperdense (sheets of cementum-like material) alteration crown structure, alveolar infection or proliferation.
- Odontoma: multiple small-lobulated foci of enamel within a well-defined cyst-like structure at the root of a maxillary tooth.

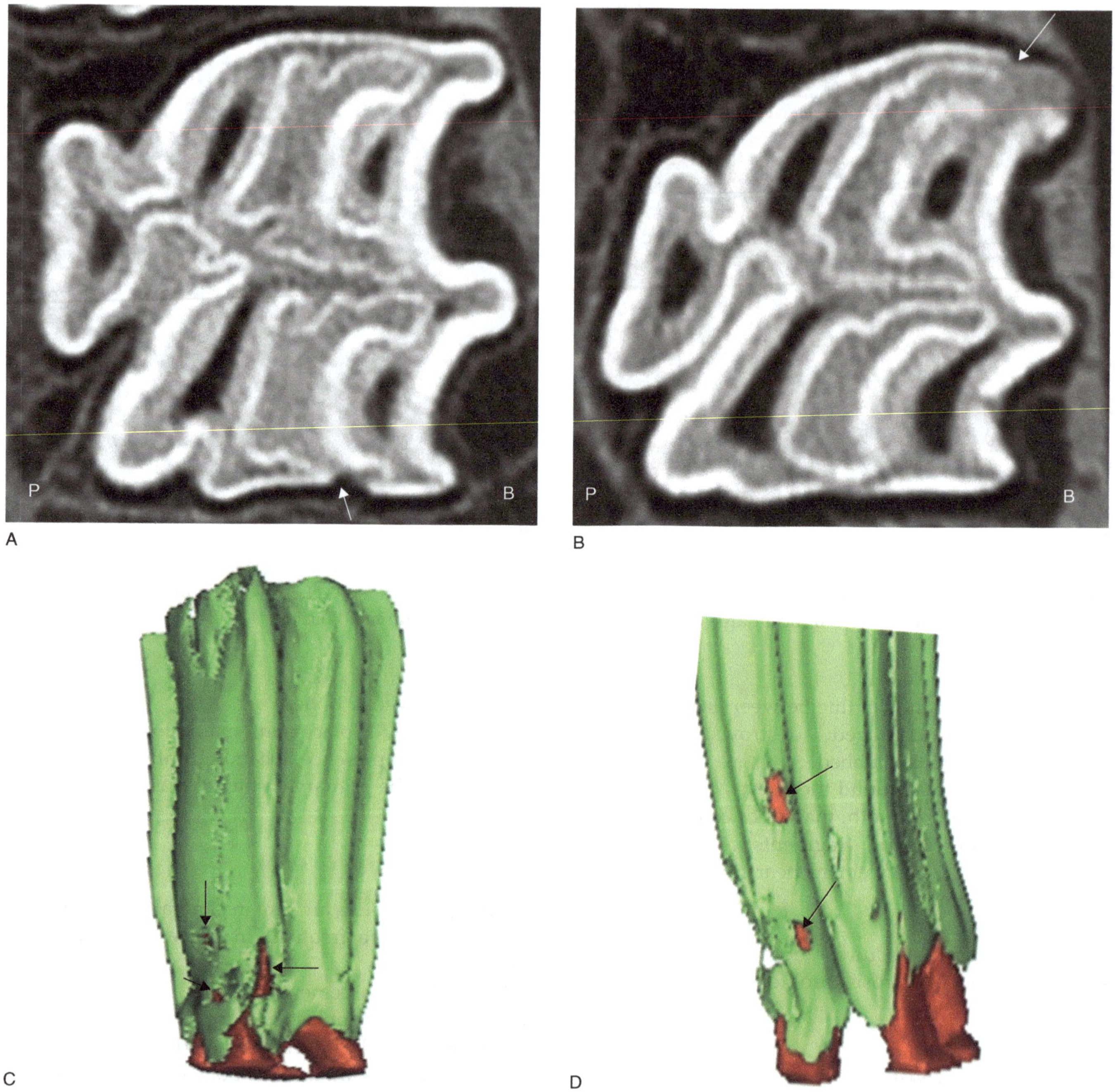

Figure 40.6 Adult horse with enamel hypoplasia of a Triadan 108 tooth (0.5 years post eruption). (A,B) Dorsal CT images and (C,D) 3-D reconstructed CT images show multifocal defects in the enamel outline (arrows). B = buccal; P = palatal.

Sinonasal: CT Anatomy and Normal Variants (Figure 40.15)

The nasal septum divides the nasal cavities into a left and right part. The rostral aspect of the equine nasal cavity is composed of strongly developed dorsal and ventral conchae that divide the nasal cavity longitudinally into a dorsal, a middle and a large ventral meatus. These conchae consist of single scrolls in a simple arrangement, leaving quite big spaces within them. In the caudal aspect of the nasal cavity, six endoturbinates (ethmoturbinates) and 25 delicate ectoturbinates with secondary lamellae form the ethmoid labyrinth that extends rostrally from the cribiform plate of the ethmoid.

The frontal and maxillary sinuses are air-filled spaces formed by the evagination of the frontal and maxillary

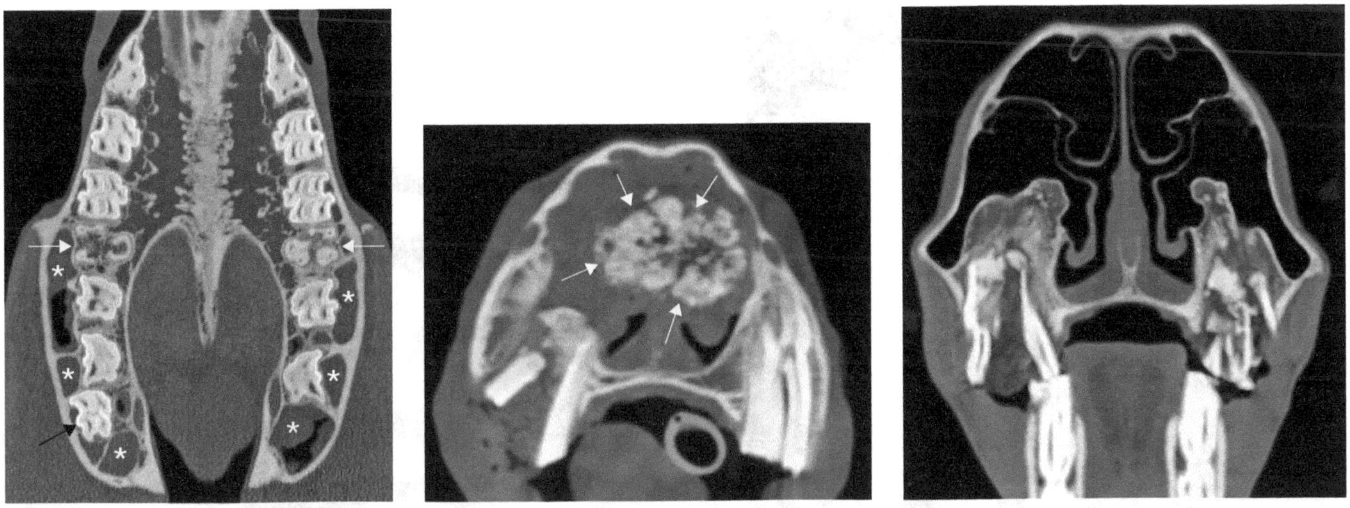

A B C

Figure 40.7 Dental fractures in three patients. (A) Dorsally reconstructed CT image shows fracture of Triadan 109 and 209 (white arrows). A supernumerary tooth is present in the right maxilla (black arrow) and soft tissue density is present bilaterally in the maxillary sinuses, indicating secondary sinusitis (asterisks). (B) Transverse CT image shows a fracture of Triadan 106 with two fragments and food trapped between them. Bone reaction is present at the dorsal aspect of the medial fragment and a calcified mass is present in the nasal cavities (arrows). These findings suggest a chronic fracture with secondary infection and dystrophic calicification. (C) Transverse CT image in a horse with bilateral dental fracture secondary to infundibular caries. Triadan 109 is fragmented in two pieces, with food trapped in between. Triadan 209 is broken into several fragments. Both pulpar cavities are enlarged, extend till the infraorbital canal and contain mineral densities.

bones. These sinuses communicate with each other via a large oval opening and directly with the nasal cavity. The maxillary sinuses are divided into a rostral and a caudal part by a thin bony septum and into a medial and a lateral compartment by the infraorbital canal. In young horses, reserve crowns largely obliterate the maxillary sinuses but when the teeth erupt, the air space within the sinuses gradually increases. The rostral maxillary sinus usually overlies the apices of Triadan 08 and 09 and the caudal maxillary sinus the apices of Triadan 10 and 11. The conchal sinuses are the spaces within the caudal aspect of the conchae that communicate with the frontal sinus and opens within the caudal maxillary sinus (dorsal conchae) or with the rostral maxillary sinus (ventral conchae). The relationship between the various air cavities can be easily visualized on transverse CT images.

Sinonasal Disorders

Malformation/Developmental: sinus cysts

Sinus cysts, also called maxillary follicular cysts, are expansile, non-neoplastic, simple or complex, epithelial-lined, fluid-filled cavities that develop in the maxillary sinus and can extend into the (concho)frontal sinus and in a few cases the nasal cavities. Sinus cysts are nearly always unilateral and can completely fill the involved sinus. Their exact etiology has not been elucitated.

CT features

- Simple or complex, fluid-filled cavity.
- Maxillary and frontal bones: mostly deformation and thinning (osseous pressure atrophy), less commonly thickening.
- Nasal septum deviation.
- Dental distortion, displacement.
- Submandibular lymphadenopathy.
- Orbital extension with exophthalmos is uncommon.

Infection/Inflammation

Primary sinusitis

The sinusal mucosa produces daily a large quantity of mucus that is evacuated into the nasal cavity via active ciliary movement. Primary infectious sinusitis occurs when this active evacuation mechanism is inhibited because of an extension of a viral or bacterial upper respiratory tract infection into the paranasal sinuses. Mucus then accumulates in the sinus, which favors infection by opportunistic bacteria (*Streptococcus equi* and *zoöepidemicus*). Without successful therapy, pus accumulates and induces sinus mucosal hyperplasia,

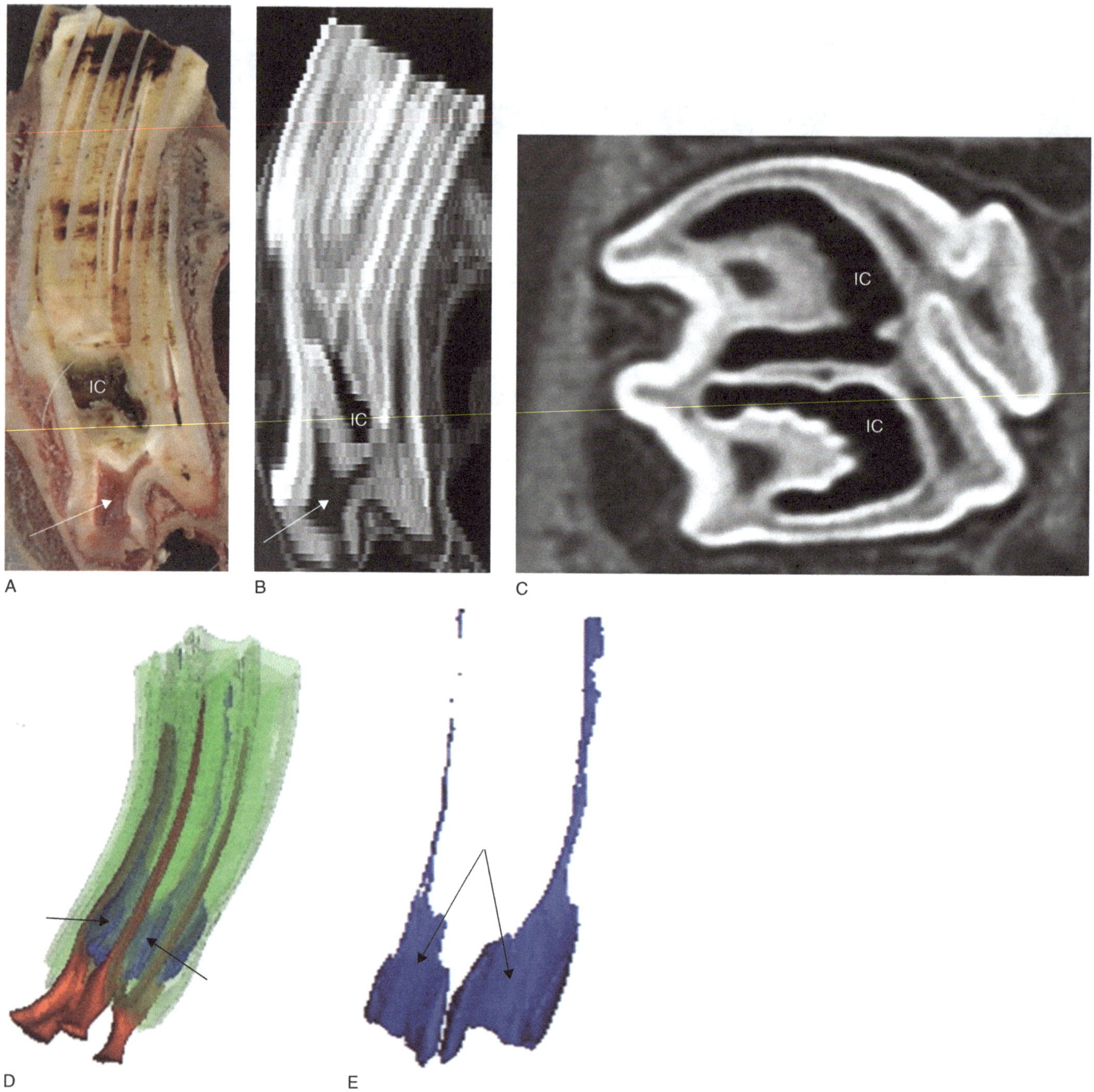

Figure 40.8 Adult horse with severe infundibular caries (IC) of a Triadan tooth 209 with an eruption age of 3 years. (A) Transverse anatomical section, (B) corresponding transverse reconstructed CT image, (C) dorsal CT image, (D) 3-D reconstructed CT image of the enamel, pulp (red) and infundibula (blue), (E) 3-D reconstructed CT image of the infundibula (blue). Both infundibula appear hypodense (A,B,C). They show bulbous enlargements (black arrows) at the apical extent of the infundibula (D,E). The pulp is illustrated with a white arrow in A and B.

necrosis and chronic empyema. The disorder is usually unilateral involving one or more sinuses.

CT features (Figure 40.16)

- Thickening of the sinusal mucosa.
- Fluid density filling the affected sinus.
- Chronic empyema may induce bone reactions.

Secondary sinusitis

Tooth disorders (M1>P4>P3 or a combination of these) are by far the main causes of secondary sinusitis. Other causes are open post-traumatic wounds in the region or destructive processes in the sinuses such as cysts, tumors and mycosis.

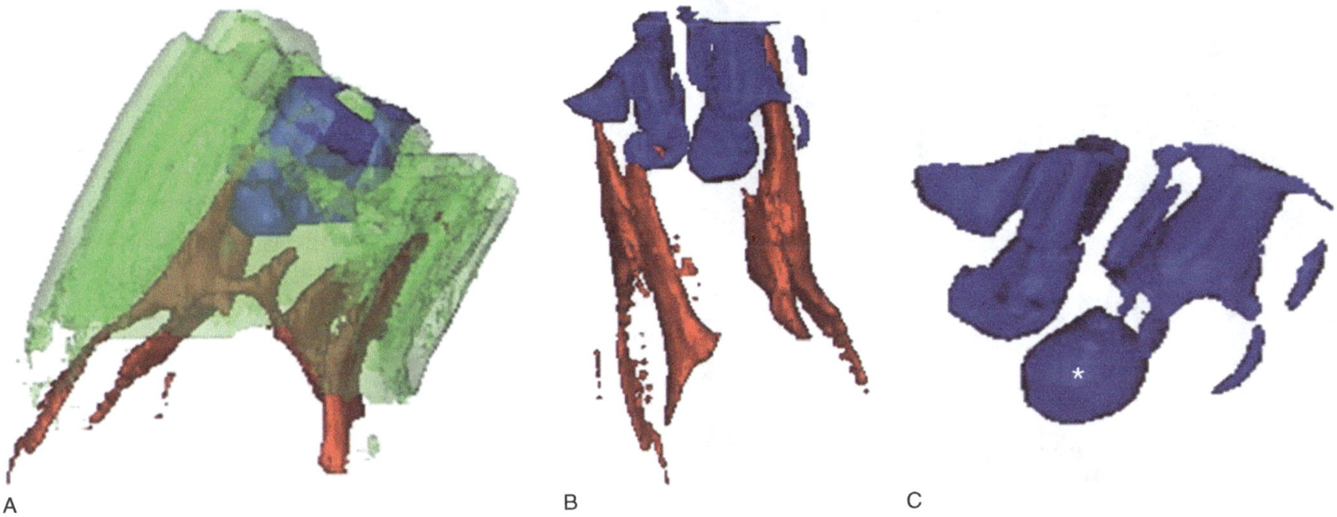

Figure 40.9 Adult horse with severe infundibular caries of a Triadan tooth 109 with an eruption age of 19 years. 3D-reconstructed CT images show (A) the enamel (green), pulp (red) and infundibula (blue) combined, (B) the pulp (red) and infundibula (blue), and (C) infundibular caries (blue) of a Triadan 109 tooth. The infundibula have a lucent appearance along their entire length and a spherical lesion (asterisk) of the caudal infundibulum is visible.

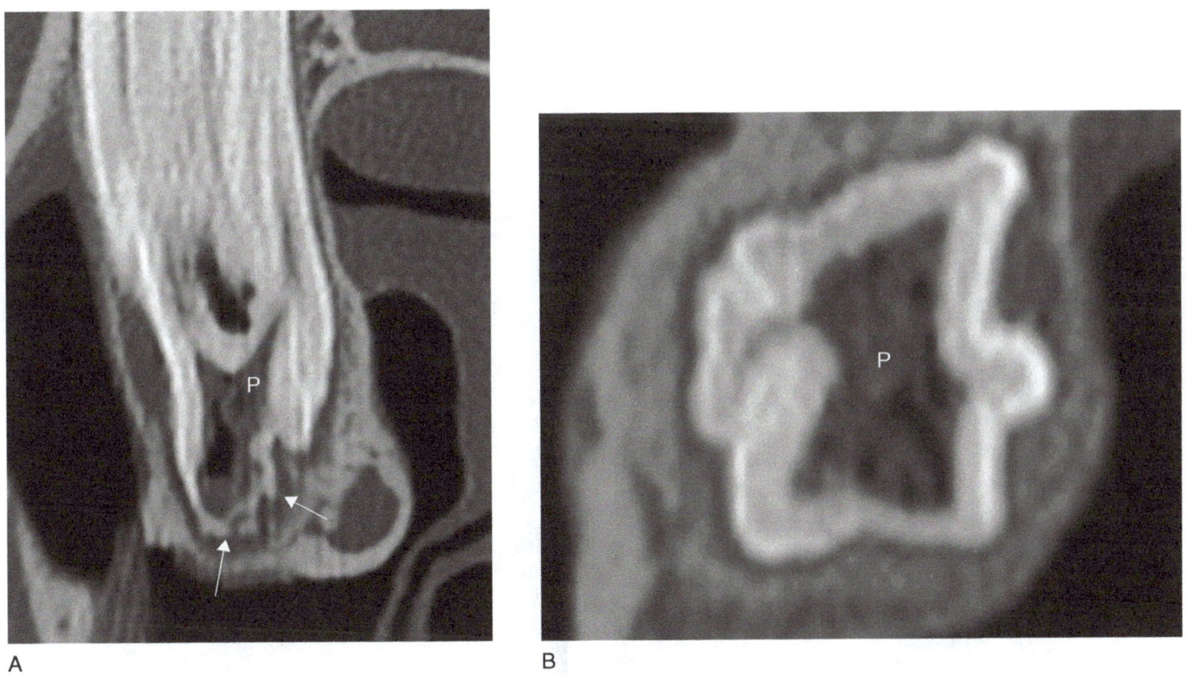

Figure 40.10 Adult horse with pulpitis. (A) Transverse and (B) dorsally reconstructed CT images show multiple hypodense areas in the pulpar cavity (P) with consequent heterogeneous density. The margins of the pulpar cavity appear irregular (arrows).

CT features (Figure 40.17)

- Affected sinus fluid filled, possible infiltration with gas.
- Signs of tooth disorder.
- Facial deformation (maxillary swelling, fistulae) is more frequent than with primary sinusitis but less frequent than with sinus cysts or neoplasia.
- Submandibular lymphadenopathy.

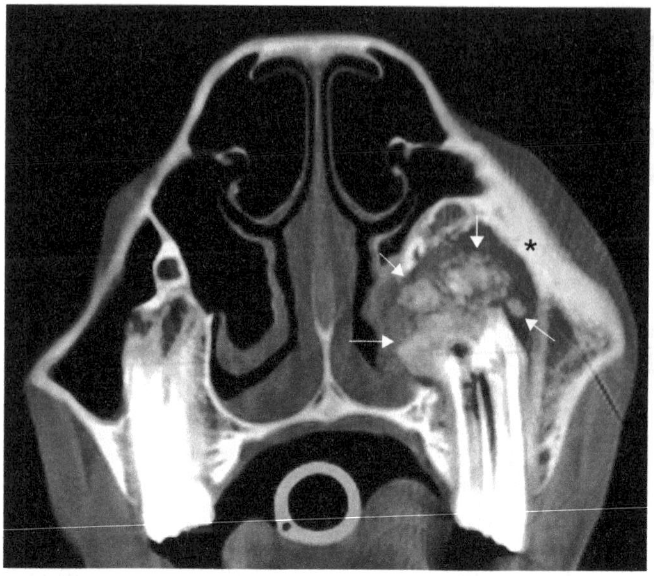

Figure 40.11 Adult horse with pyogranulomatous tooth inflammation and associated calcification. Transverse CT image shows soft tissue swelling, smoothly margined periosteal proliferation of the outer surface of the maxilla (asterisk). A calcified mass (arrows) is seen in contact and dorsal to the Triadan 208. The mass invades the ventral concha.

Sinonasal mycosis

Fungal infection caused by *Asp. fumigatus* is the most frequent sinonasal mycosis in Europe and is usually highly aggressive and destructive. It starts in the nasal cavities and can invade the sinuses (frontal > maxillary), the meninges or the brain. In warm humide climates, such as the Southern United States and Australia, other fungal organisms such as *Cryptococcus neoformans* or *Coccidiodes immitis* may cause mycotic granulomas.

CT features (Figure 40.18)

- Sinonasal aspergillosis:
  - turbinate (and conchae) destruction
  - bone reactions.

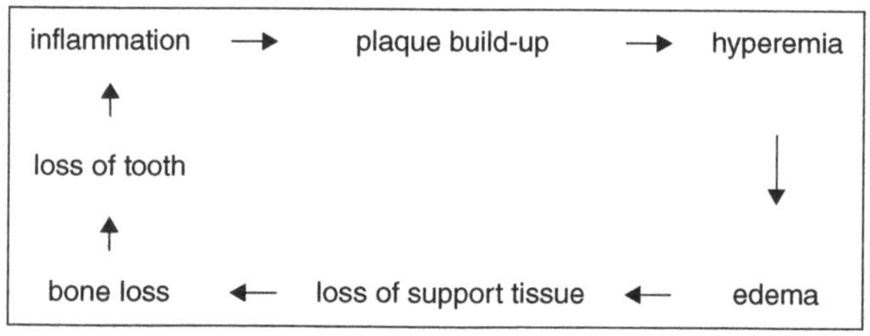

Figure 40.12 The 'domino cycle' in horses with secondary periodontal disease of inflammatory origin.

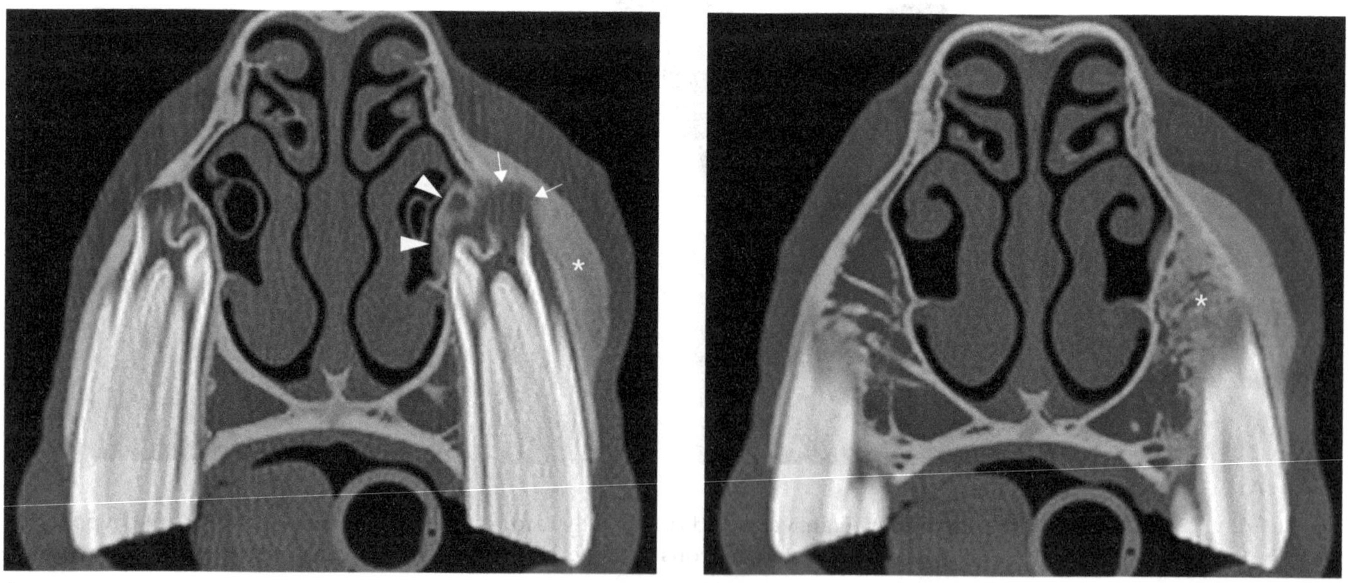

A B

Figure 40.13 Transverse CT images of a 5-year-old mare with pulpitis and alveolitis of Triadan 207 and associated maxillary osteomyelitis. (A) There is soft tissue swelling and smoothly margined periosteal proliferation of the outer surface of the maxilla (asterisk) overlying the left Triadan (207). The pulp chamber is increased in size and contains gas lucencies. A tract starts from the pulp and leads to a defect in the maxilla (arrows). Irregular bone margination is present at the buccal aspect of the tooth (arrowheads). (B) The density of the maxillary bone is increased (asterisk). The previously described soft tissue swelling and periosteal bone is visible.

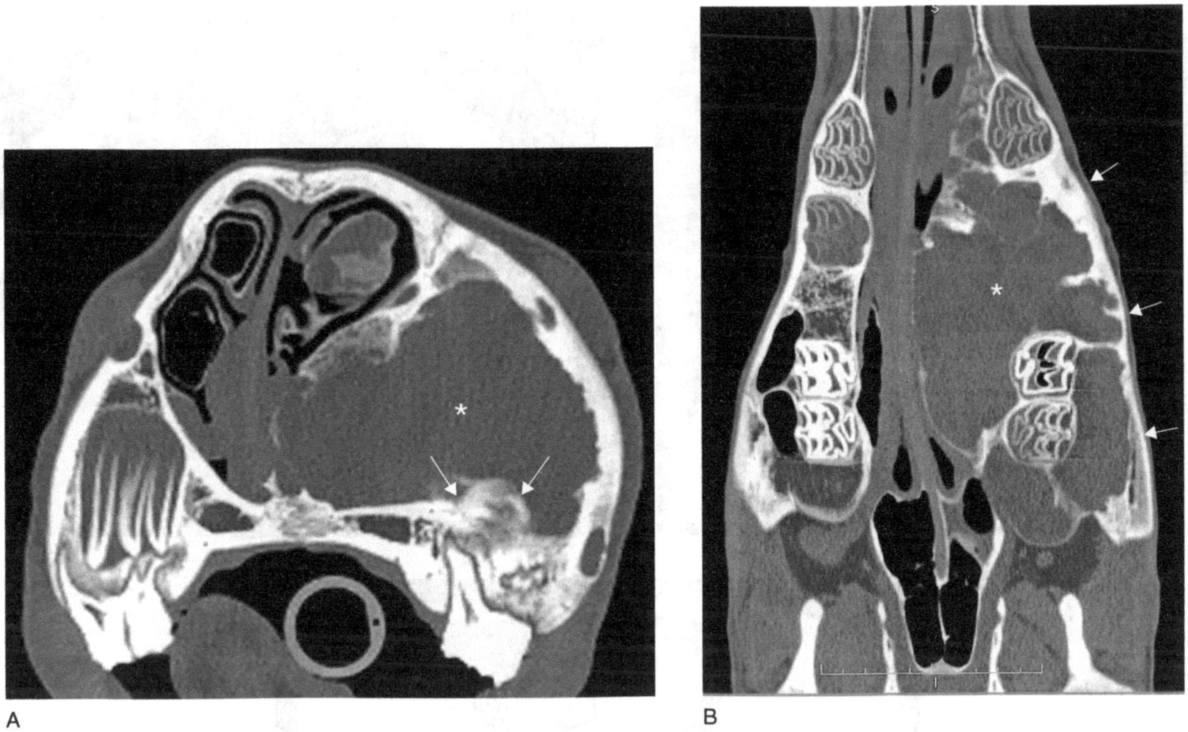

Figure 40.14 Two-year-old Welsh horse with dental ameloblastoma. (A) Transverse CT image shows an extensive, large, lobular, low-density (20 HU) soft tissue mass (asterisk) involving the left maxilla. The mass appears to arise from the germinal tissue of the Triadan 208 (arrows). The mass causes marked distortion of the inner surface of the maxilla and causes rightward deviation of the nasal septum to the right. (B) Dorsally reconstructed CT image shows the mass (asterisk) extending from Triadan 206 rostral to caudal to Triadan 211. The mass causes marked distortion of the inner surface of the maxilla (arrows) and causes rightwards deviation of the nasal septum. The medial aspect of the mass consists of a small/thin bone mineralized layer. There is gas present within the infundibula of Triadan 210.

- Tropical mycosis:
  - well-demarcated soft tissue density in the nasal passages and sinuses (mycotic granuloma).
- Submandibular lymphadenopathy.

Sinonasal neoplasia

Sinonasal tumors are rare in the horse. Most of them are malignant and have a bad prognosis. Squamous cell carcinoma is the most common tumor type. Clinical signs are similar to those of other sinonasal disorders but in a more aggressive way. Extensive tissue infiltration and destruction is frequent. Other tumor types to be considered are juvenile ossifying fibroma (young horse), sarcoid, melanoma, tumors of fibro-osseous origin, oral papilloma, epulis, salivary adenocarcinoma, myxoma/sarcoma and congenital tumors. Tumors of dental tissue origin may involve the nasal cavities and maxillary sinuses.

CT features (Figure 40.19)

- Mass of soft tissue density (homogeneous, compact) into the nasal conchae, sinuses with possible obliteration of one or both nasal cavities.
- Bone thinning or even bone lysis are common with consequent exposed infraorbital nerve, loose teeth, lesions to large arteries, extension to the soft palate, even the central nervous system giving rise to neurological symptoms and blindness.
- Metastases are uncommon. Secondary infection is mostly associated with aggressive tumors and increased tissue destruction.
- Post-contrast IV: marked enhancement.

Trauma

Sinonasal trauma is quite frequent in horses and affects mostly young stallions. Common reasons for trauma are a kick from another horse or collision with a fixed object, resulting in a closed or open wound and

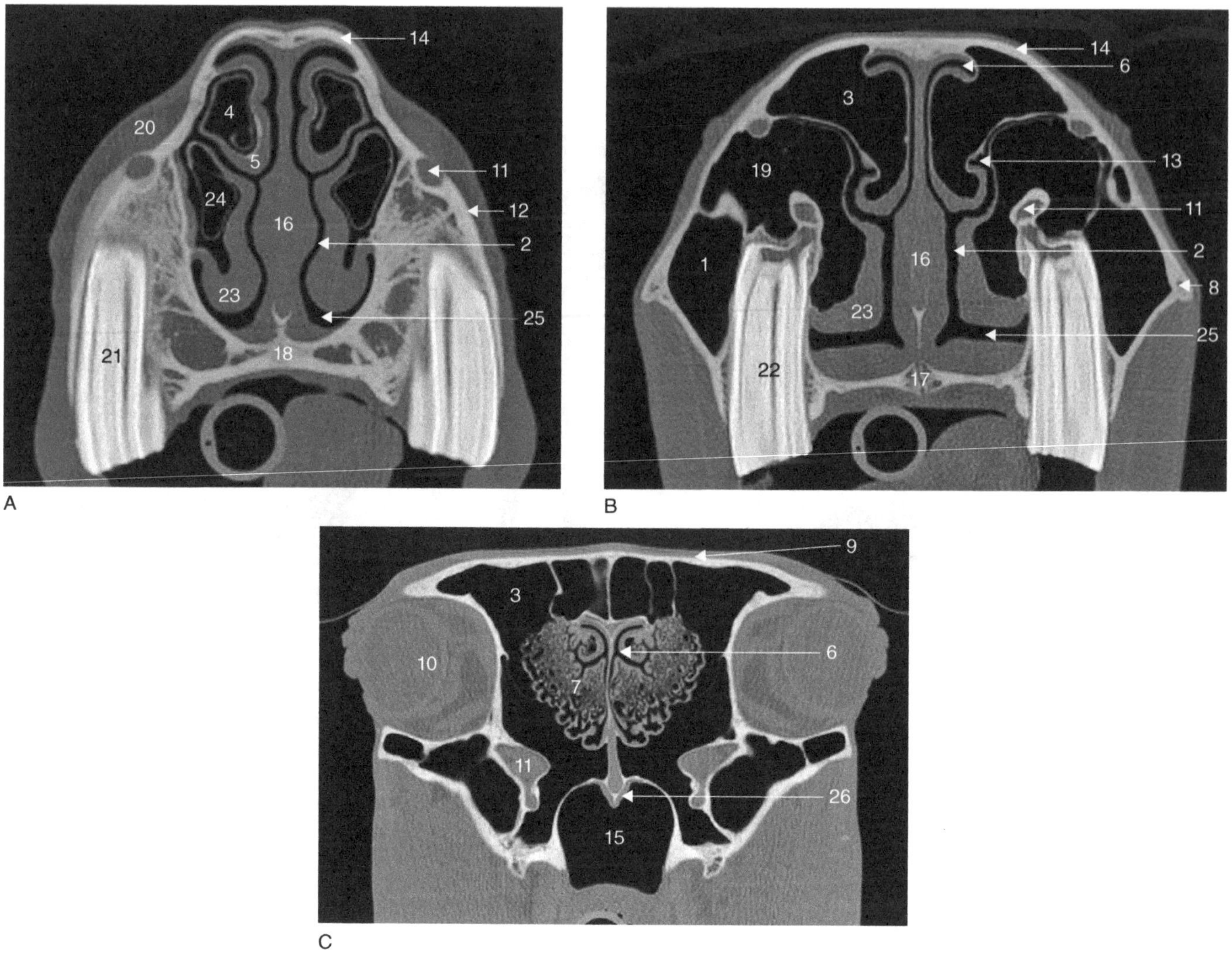

Figure 40.15 Transverse CT images of the nasal cavities and paranasal sinuses of a normal adult horse at the level of (A) Triadan 08, (B) Triadan 09 and (C) orbit. 1 = caudal maxillary sinus; 2 = common nasal meatus; 3 = conchofrontal sinus; 4 = dorsal nasal concha bulla; 5 = dorsal nasal concha; 6 = dorsal nasal meatus; 7 = ethmoid labyrinth; 8 = facial crest; 9 = frontal bone; 10 = globe; 11 = infraorbital canal; 12 = maxillary bone; 13 = middle nasal meatus; 14 = nasal bone; 15 = nasopharynx; 16 = nasal septum; 17 = palatine bone; 18 palatine process of maxillary bone; 19 = rostral maxillary sinus; 20 = superior labii elevator muscle; 21 = Triadan 208; 22 = Triadan 209; 23 = ventral nasal concha; 24 = ventral nasal concha bulla; 25 = ventral nasal meatus; 26 = vomer bone.

sometimes in facial deformation (with or without fracture), ocular lesions or even central nervous system disorders.

Impacted fractures, particularly in the region of the frontonasal suture, are a common fracture type, not always diagnosed by the owner. Sinusal bleeding can induce epistaxis and secondary sinusitis, particularly if a bone sequestrum (nasal fistulation) is present.

CT features (Figure 40.20)

- Discontinuity of bone margins.
- Displacement of bone fragments.
- Associated regions of hyperdensity due to hemorrhage.
- Fluid in involved sinus.
- Young horses:
  - periosteal proliferation/reaction in the region of the frontonasal suture
  - fluid in the maxillary sinus.

Ethmoid hematoma

Progressive ethmoid hematoma is a non-neoplastic, locally destructive process that develops because of repeated submucosal bleedings. Most hematomas

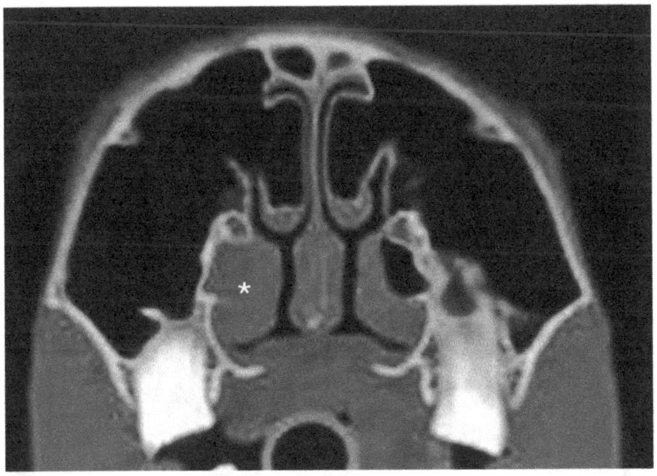

Figure 40.16 Twenty-year-old mare with primary sinusitis (inspissated pus was present within the ventral nasal concha on endoscopy). Transverse CT image shows obliteration of the right ventral nasal concha (asterisk) by soft tissue density (image courtesy of Justin Perkins, Royal Veterinary College, UK).

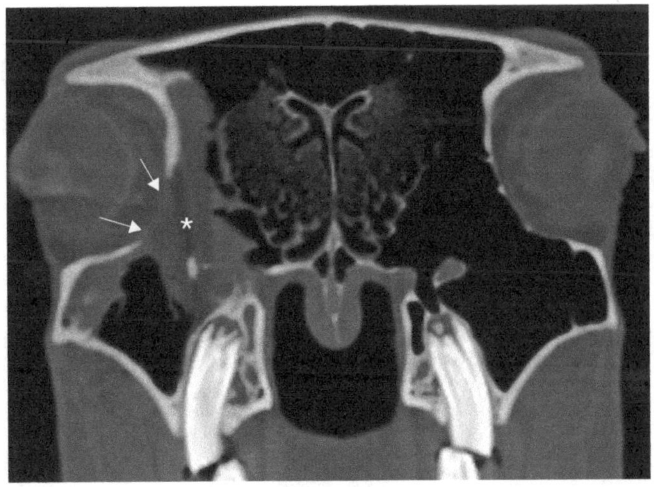

Figure 40.18 Adult horse with sinonasal mycosis. Transverse CT image shows soft tissue density (asterisk) in the conchofrontal sinus along the orbit extending to the ethmoid labyrinth and infraorbital canal. There is lysis of the frontal bone at the medial aspect of the orbit (arrows).

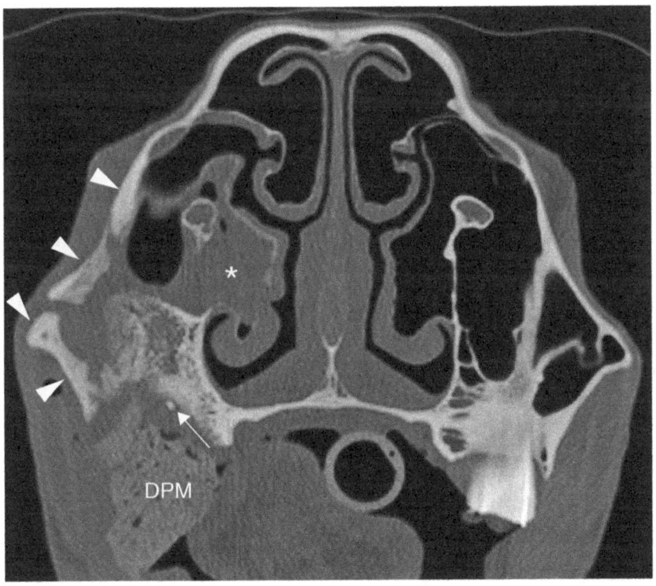

Figure 40.17 Transverse CT image in an adult horse with sinusitis secondary to dental disorders (postoperative CT study). There is bone remodeling (arrowheads) associated with the osteotomy lines in the right maxilla overlying the maxillary sinus (healing osteotomy). The mucosa of the caudal maxillary sinus is thickened. Porous-appearing dental packing material (DPM) is present within the socket of Triadan 110. A dental fragment (arrow) is seen on the buccal side of the dental packing material (may serve as a nidus for infection). Bone proliferation is present dorsal from this fragment. The ventral conchal sinus is full of soft tissue/fluid material (asterisk).

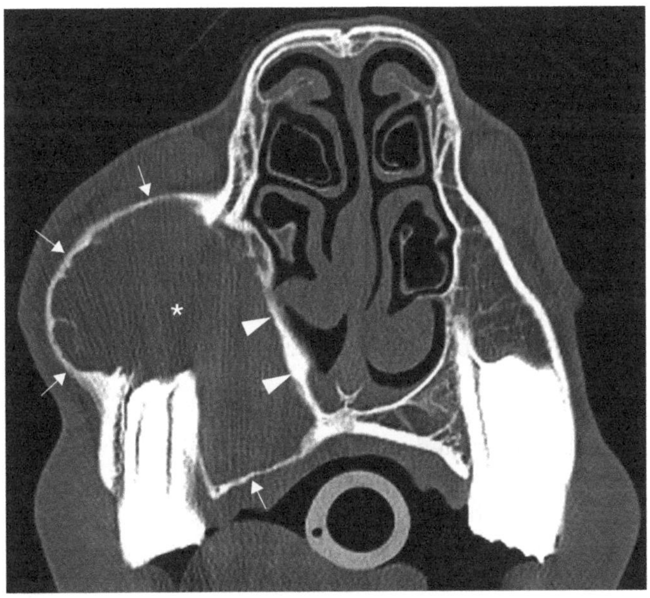

Figure 40.19 Transverse CT image (level Triadan 208) of a young horse with ossifying fibroma shows an expansile soft tissue mass density (asterisk) that displaces the surrounding bone structures. The ventral nasal concha is displaced and misshapen. The nasal septum is slightly deviated to the left. The outer wall and the palatine process of the maxilla are thinned (arrows), while the nasal aspect of the maxilla appears thickened (arrowheads).

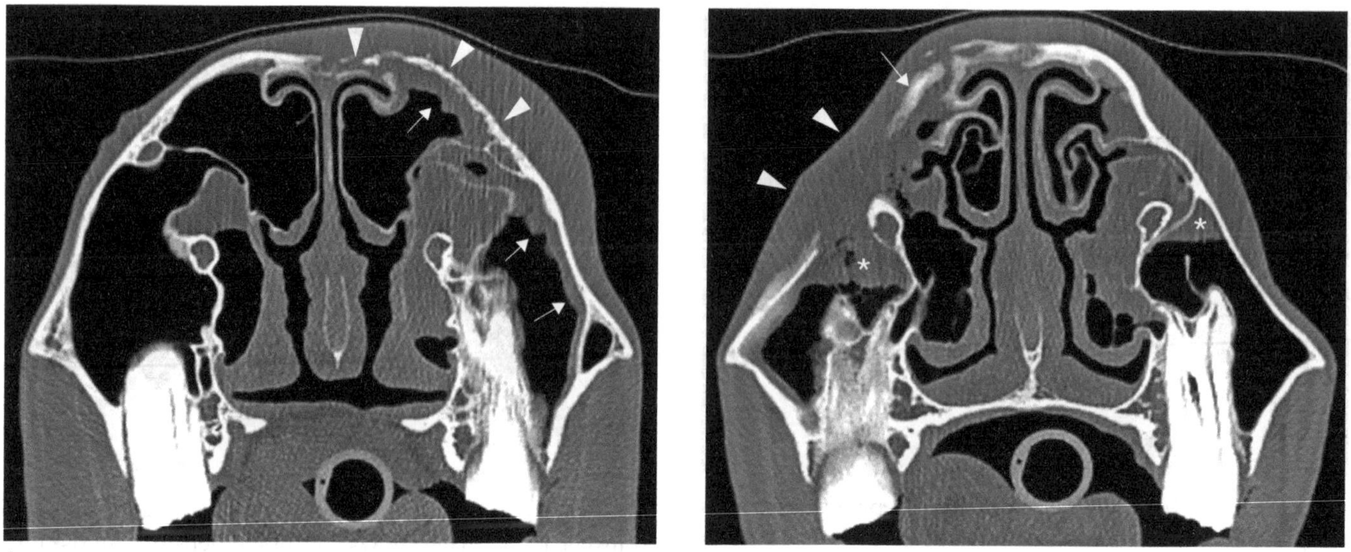

A B

Figure 40.20 Nine-year-old Warmblood mare with a head trauma and surgery for a fractured left maxilla 1 month ago. (A) Transverse CT image shows bone resorption associated with the most dorsal portion of the nasal bone (arrowheads) and mucosal thickening (arrows). Mucosal thickening in addition to soft tissue accumulation is present in the right rostral maxillary sinus. (B) Transverse CT image shows soft tissue swelling on the right side associated with bone resorption (arrowheads) and a probable sequestrum (arrow). The fracture margins are irregular with proliferation alternating with areas of resorption. Deep to this region there is soft tissue-dense material with internal gas. There is fluid accumulation (asterisk) or moderate mucosal thickening within both rostral maxillary sinuses.

appear in or around the ethmoid bone, while the less frequent small ones develop from the maxillary sinuses. They can cause destruction of the cribriform plate and involve the brain, which is a contraindication for intra-lesional formalin injection. The exact cause of ethmoid hematoma is still unknown.

CT features (Figure 40.21)

- Sinus-associated mass of mixed density (unilateral >> bilateral).
- Very large hematoma may occupy the entire maxillary sinus and the nasal cavities on one side.
- Facial deformation caused by necrotic pressure due to a large mass.
- Possible extension though cribriform plate.
- Post-contrast (IV):
  - hematoma: marked enhancement
  - brain: marked enhancement when involved.
- Dorsal and sagittal reconstructions help to define the origin and extension of the process and, the integrity the cribriform plate.
- Small ethmoid hematomas may be present on the contralateral side.

Nasal polyps

Nasal polyps are the result of mucosal hypertrophy or a proliferation of fibrous connective tissue secondary to a chronic inflammation originating from the nasal mucosa (septum >> conchae or tooth alveolus). Their exact etiology is unknown.

CT features (Figure 40.22)

- Smooth, well-delineated, single soft tissue density mass originating from a mucosal surface. Multiple masses are rare.
- Its size can vary greatly from a few centimeters to complete filling of the nasal cavity.
- Displacement and/or deformation of normal nasal structures is possible.
- Mostly unilateral, may be bilateral.

Idiopathic

Figure 40.23 illustrates an unusual sinonasal disorder.

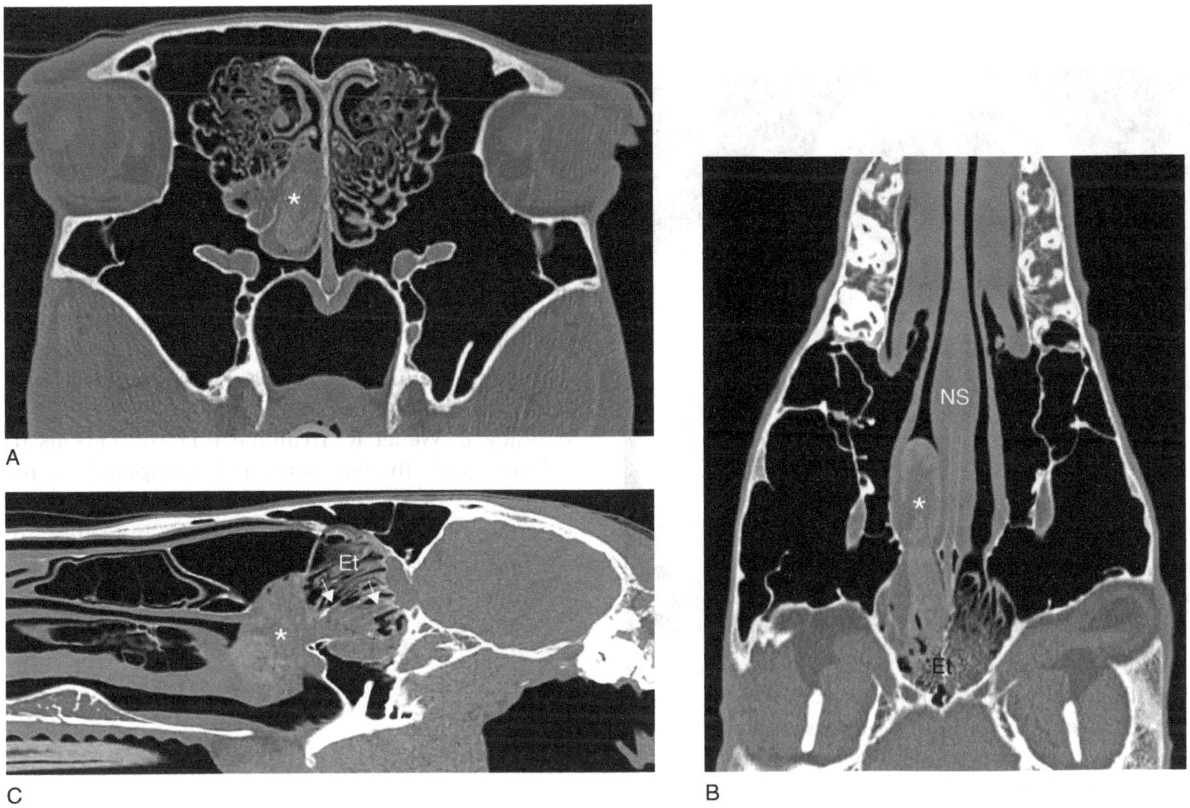

Figure 40.21 Adult horse with ethmoid hematoma. (A) Transverse CT image shows a slightly heterogeneous soft tissue density mass (asterisk) arising from the ventromedial aspect of the left ethmoturbinates. (B) Dorsally reconstructed CT image shows the mass extending rostrally in the caudal nasal passage (asterisk). (C) Sagittally reconstructed CT image shows the mass (asterisk) originating from the ethmoid turbinates (arrows). Et = ethmoid turbinates; NS = nasal septum.

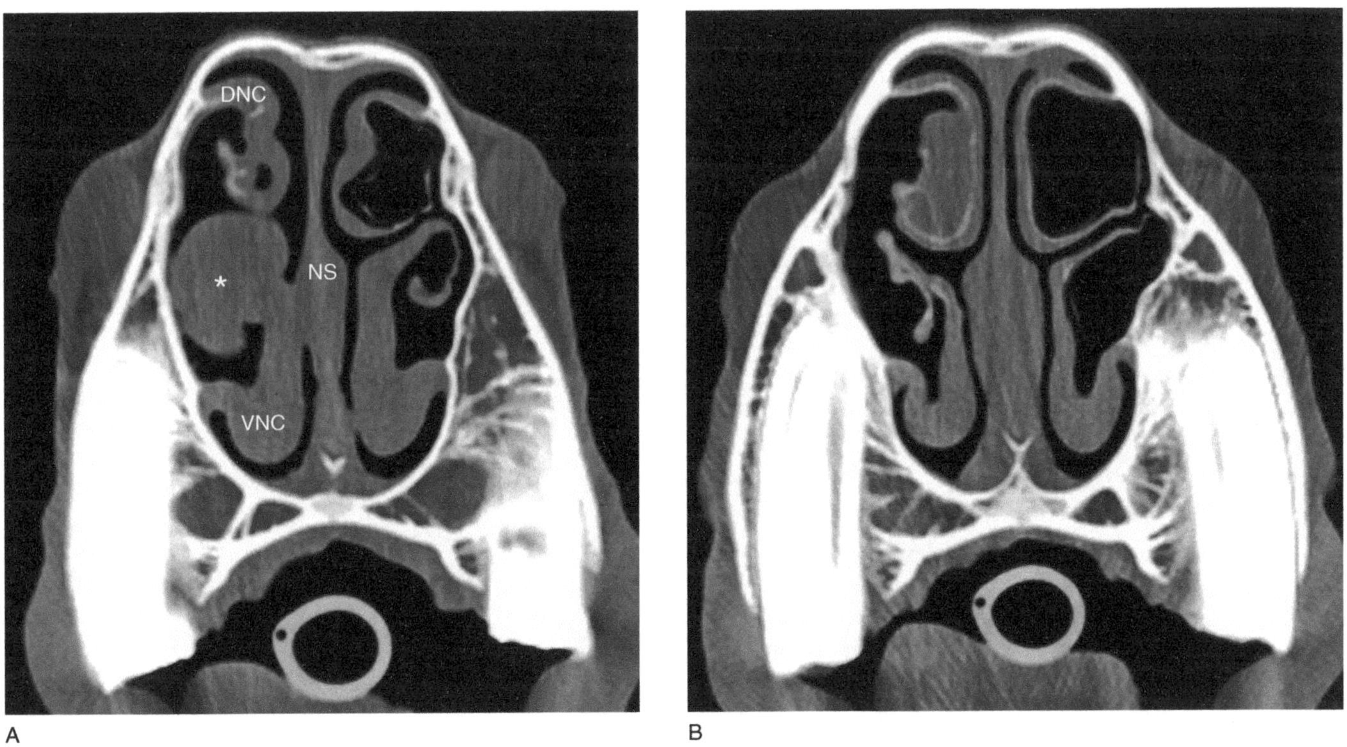

Figure 40.22 Adult horse with nasal polyp. Transverse CT images show (A) a sessile ovale mass (asterisk) originating from the ventral nasal concha (VNC) that contacts the nasal septum (NS). The dorsal nasal concha (DNC) is atrophied and (B) has a thickened mucosa.

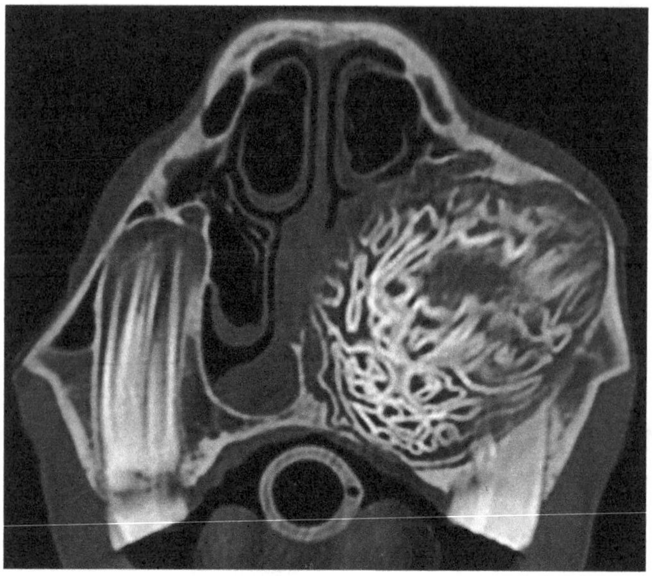

Figure 40.23 Transverse CT image of a 4-year-old mare with idiopathic tooth sinonasal disorder. There is a large 'dental' mass filling the ventral two-thirds of the left nasal cavity. The maxillary sinus is involved and the maxillary bone is displaced laterally.

Further reading

Morrow KL, Park RD, Spurgeon TL *et al.* (2000) Computed tomographic imaging of the equine head. *Vet Radiol Ultrasound* **41**: 491–7.

Windley Z, Weller R, Treamine WH and Perkins JD (2009) Two- and three-dimensional computed tomographic anatomy of the enamel, infundibulae and pulp of 126 equine cheek teeth. Part 1: Findings in teeth without macroscopic occlusal or computed tomographic lesions. *Eq Vet J* **41**: 433–40.

Windley Z, Weller R, Treamine WH and Perkins JD (2009) Two- and three-dimensional computed tomographic anatomy of the enamel, infundibulae and pulp of 126 equine cheek teeth. Part 2: Findings in teeth with macroscopic occlusal or computed tomographic lesions. *Eq Vet J* **41**: 441–7.

CHAPTER FORTY-ONE

Equine Calvarium, Brain and Pituitary Gland

Jennifer Kinns and Russ Tucker

Artifacts Associated with Imaging of the Equine Head (Figure 41.1)

The equine caudal fossa presents a specific problem in CT imaging. The beam hardening artifact from the surrounding dense bone results in hypodense bands across the brainstem, which confound interpretation. Thick-slice reformatting of sequential images acquired as thin slices can reduce this problem. Volume averaging can also be detrimental. The size of the equine calvarium necessitates thicker slice acquisition on many systems; this can result in multiple densities, such as those of bone and brain, averaged in one image voxel. Acquisition of thin slices in regions of concern can reduce the problem.

CT: Anatomy and Normal Variants

Calvarium (Figure 41.2)

Compared to other species, the calvarium, or roof of the skull, is relatively small. It is formed by the paired frontal, parietal and temporal bones, and the occipital bone. The occipital bone has a large paracondylar process rostral to the occipital condyle. There are large openings on each side of the occipital bone; the cranial opening (foramen lacerum) combines the oval and carotid foramina while the caudal opening represents the jugular foramen. Both the styloid and muscular processes of the temporal bone are prominent; the former forms the temporohyoid articulation with the large stylohyoid bone.

Temporomandibular joint (Figure 41.3)

The temporomandibular joint is a synovial condylar articulation. It is formed from the expanded, flat facet of the mandibular condyle and the articular surface of the temporal bone, which has a rostral condyle and caudal glenoid cavity. It has two non-communicating ventral and dorsal synovial pouches, an articular disk, joint capsule, and rostral and caudal ligaments. On CT images the joint extends further laterally at its rostral aspect where the mandibular condyle is wide and flat. Caudally the articulation is narrower and more axial in location. The thick intra-articular disk can be seen with difficulty on CT, but the associated fibrous lateral and elastic caudal ligaments cannot.

Brain (Figure 41.4)

Due to the large size and associated artifacts, particularly in the caudal fossa, CT of the equine brain provides a poor contrast image compared to that of small animals. Gray/white matter differentiation is not good, and subtle lesions can be missed. The forebrain and midbrain are more readily examinable than the cerebellum and brainstem, but caution should be exercised in the interpretation of subtle changes in density.

Disease Features

Malformation/Developmental

Dentigerous cyst

A dentigerous cyst is a congenital defect that arises due to incomplete closure of the first branchial cleft. It appears as a cyst surrounding the crown of a tooth, which is commonly fixed to the temporal bone. The

Veterinary Computed Tomography, First Edition. Edited by Tobias Schwarz, Jimmy Saunders.

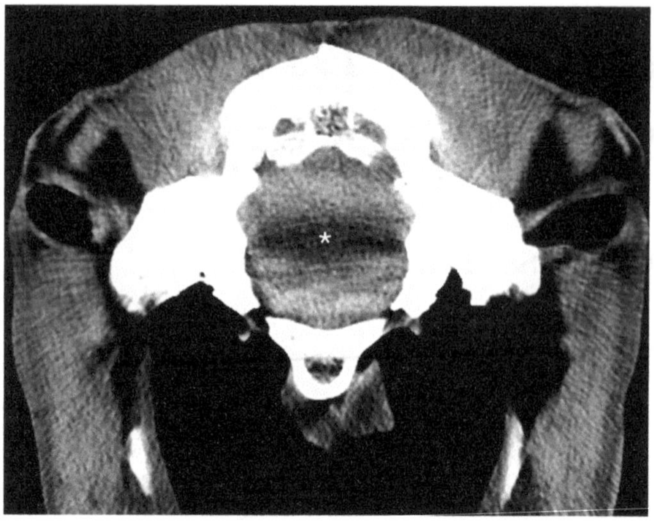

Figure 41.1 Transverse CT image (caudal fossa region) in a horse. The dark band (asterisk) extending across the region is a beam-hardening artifact.

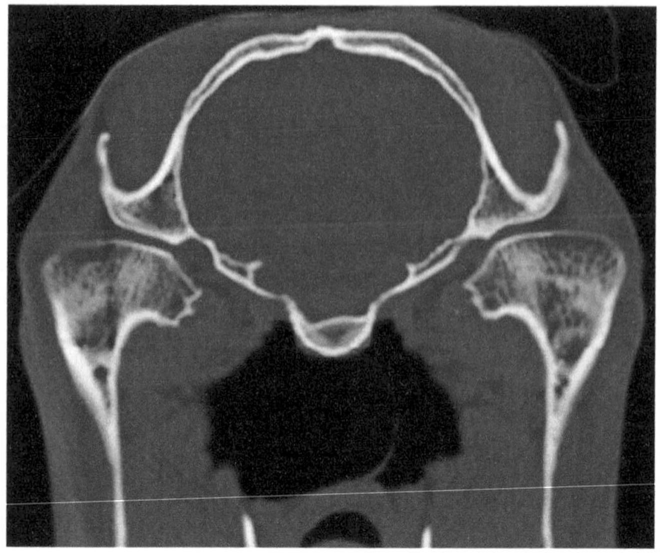

Figure 41.3 Transverse CT image (temporomandibular joint) of a normal horse.

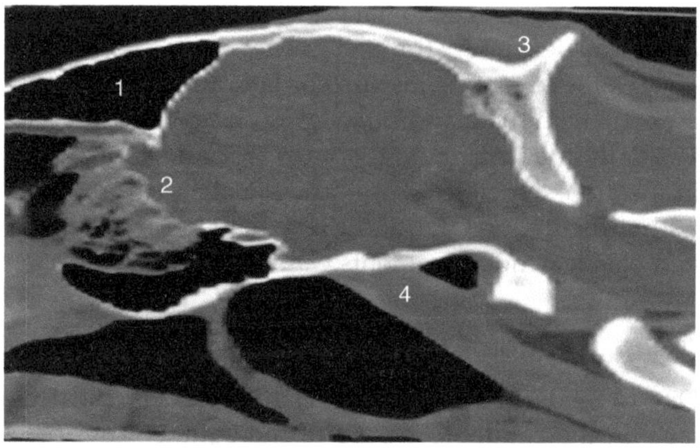

Figure 41.2 Sagittally reconstructed image of a CT study of the normal equine calvarium, viewed with a bone window. 1 = frontal bone; 2 = cribriform plate; 3 = external occipital protuberance; 4 = region of attachment of rectus capitis on the base of the skull.

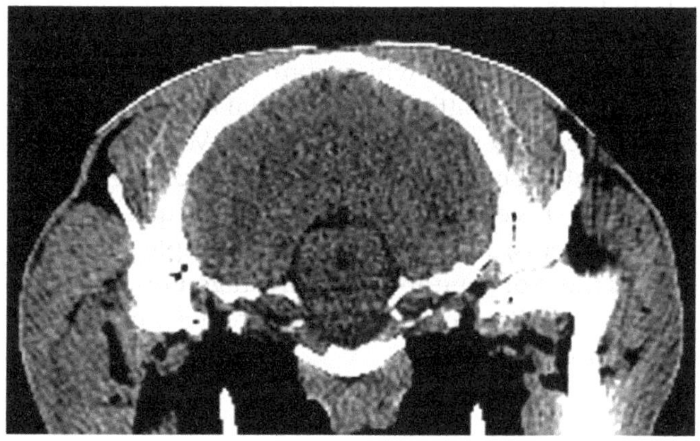

Figure 41.4 Transverse CT image (midbrain) of a normal horse. The mesencephalic aqueduct is clearly visible. Gray/white matter differentiation is poor.

clinical presentation is usually of a firm swelling and often intermittent seromucoid or seropurulent discharge from the region. Although the tooth structure is normally visible radiographically, it can be difficult to identify without multiple oblique projections, and CT improves delineation of the lesion.

CT features (Figure 41.5)

- Hyperdense tooth-like structure in an aberrant location, often adjacent to the calvarium.
- Tooth is most often single but can be multiple.
- Often surrounded by a hypodense rim.
- Rarely occur within the paranasal sinuses.

Cerebellar abiotrophy

Cerebellar abiotrophy is an inherited degenerative disease of the cerebellum that occurs in Arabians and part-Arabians. Most affected animals appear normal at birth with clinical signs typically appearing in the first year. Hypoplasia of the cerebellar vermis is a separate reported syndrome in horses that may occur in association with cystic dilation of the fourth ventricle (Dandy–Walker syndrome).

CT features

- Small cerebellum.

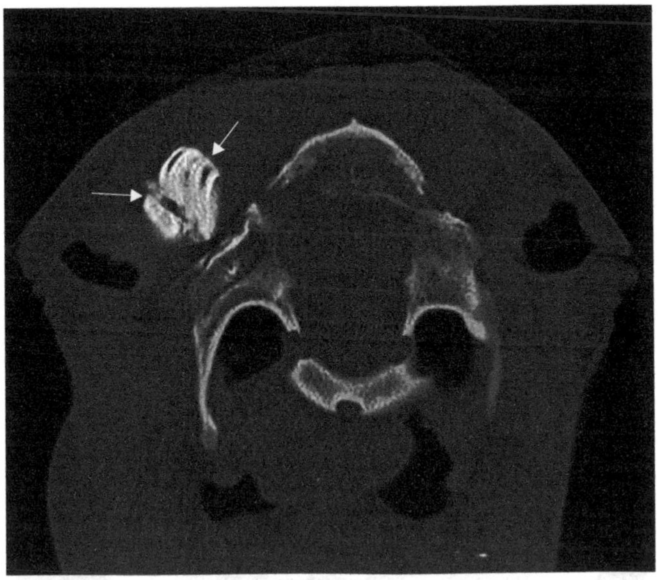

Figure 41.5 Transverse CT image (caudal occipital bone) of a dentigerous cyst (arrows) in a 4-year-old horse.

Hydrocephalus

Hydrocephalus is an uncommon condition of equine neonates. Horses born with congenital hydrocephalus have severe neurological deficits. Ventricular dilatation may be confined to the lateral ventricles or involve the whole ventricular system. The accumulation of cerebrospinal fluid (CSF) is most often due to obstruction of CSF drainage, though the cause of obstruction is not usually identified ante-mortem.

CT features

- Marked ventricular dilatation with fluid dense content.
- Thin rim of cortex.

Trauma

Imaging protocol for head trauma

Administration of contrast medium may not be necessary in acute trauma cases. Regions of hemorrhage will appear hyperdense on non-contrast images. Contrast medium may allow identification of active bleeding if the timing of the scan is appropriate to capture a vascular phase. Thin-slice acquisition through the basilar region can be helpful where basilar trauma is suspected, and reconstruction of this region in multiple planes is recommended.

Skull fracture

CT is the modality of choice for evaluating bone disruption in head trauma cases. While head radiographs can be difficult to interpret due to superimposition, CT permits accurate evaluation of the calvarium and basilar region. Sagittal and dorsal plane reconstructions are recommended. Fractures of the base of the skull (basisphenoid and basioccipital) may occur if the horse rears and falls over backwards; this is due to avulsion of the insertion of the rectus capitis ventralis muscle. This type of fracture is usually associated with guttural pouch hemorrhage. Fractures of the orbit are common and are associated with direct trauma, such as kick wounds; they may involve the frontal and lacrimal bones and the zygomatic process of the frontal and temporal bones.

CT features

- Discontinuity of bone margins.
- Displacement of bone fragments.
- Associated regions of hyperdensity due to hemorrhage.
- Intracranial free gas may occur secondary to open fractures or those that involve the sinuses or nasopharynx.
- Orbital fractures are often of a depression type.

Brain trauma

Brain contusion can occur with or without the presence of skull fractures. Clinical signs will depend on the site and extent of the injury.

CT features

- Initial appearance is of areas of low density (edema) mixed with high density (hemorrhage).
- Both edema and hemorrhage may increase over several days.
- Possible mass effect, especially if a large hematoma forms.

Epidural and subdural hematoma

Epidural hematoma usually results from vascular injury, and most often occurs in association with fracture. Clinically hematomas are often associated with deterioration of clinical signs after trauma. Subdural hematomas are not confined between the dura and bone, and are often associated with parenchymal contusion.

CT features (Figure 41.6)

- Epidural hematoma appears as localized regions of high density (around 70 HU, but depends on the age of the lesion) outside the brain with convex margins or a lentiform shape.

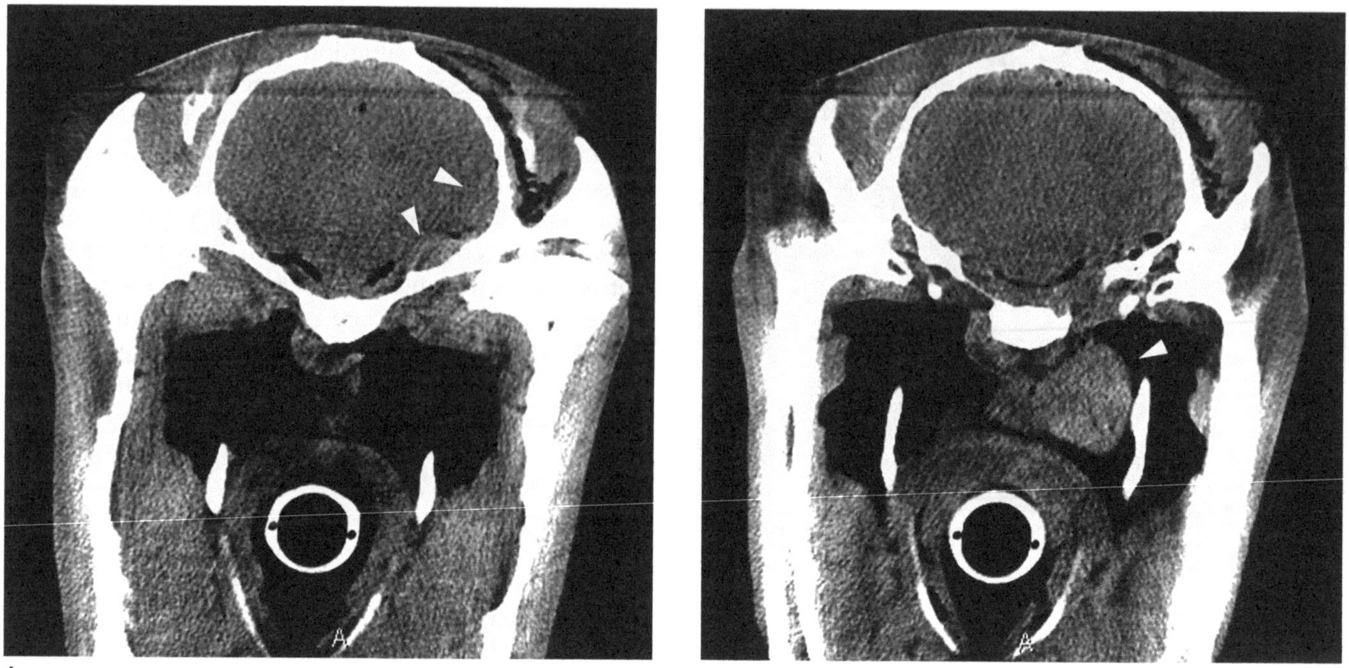

A B

Figure 41.6 Fifteen-year-old Morgan stallion that fell while lunging and had altered mentation. (A) Transverse CT image of the brain shows a hyperdense broad-based subdural hematoma (arrowheads) that was confirmed at post-mortem. Gas is also present within the brain parenchyma. (B) Further transverse CT image of the same horse (guttural pouch) shows a large hematoma (arrowhead) within the medial compartment (images courtesy of Nathan Nelson, The Ohio State University).

- Subdural hematomas appear wider and do not have a convex margin.

Infection/Inflammation

Abscess

There are several stages of abscess formation. Initially an acute cerebritis is present with surrounding edema. This progresses to confluent areas of necrosis with a capsule finally developing around the necrotic core. The early stages of abscess formation may not be apparent on CT.

CT features

- Mass effect.
- The center of the lesion is hypodense to the adjacent brain parenchyma and the rim may be hyperdense.
- An area of hypodense edema may surround the lesion.
- Post-contrast (IV): typically rim enhancement.

Encephalitis

Viral encephalitis in horses may be caused by Eastern, Western or Venezuelan equine enchaphalitis viruses, West Nile virus, rabies virus or herpes virus (EHV-1). The incidence of most is geographically dependent, though EHV-1 is ubiquitous. Equine protozoal myeloencephalitis (EPM) is the most common form of encephalitis in North America, and is caused by coccidian parasites. Verminous encephalitis is rare and may occur due to aberrant migration of nematodes.

CT features

- CT may be normal.
- The CT appearance of the different forms of encephalitis is non-specific.
- Areas of hypodensity (edema), hyperdensity (hemorrhage) or patchy enhancement may be present.
- Lesions are usually bilateral but asymmetric.
- Mass lesions with a hypodense center may be present with EPM cysts.

Fistulous tract

Sinus tracts most often develop in association with a foreign body. The purpose of CT is to determine the extent of the tract and the presence and location of any foreign material. Often the material is not directly visualized but the delineation of the tract facilitates appropriate surgical intervention. Fistulous tracts may also be associated with temporomandibular joint (TMJ) sepsis (see below).

CT protocol

Intravenous contrast medium application is most useful for delineating the extent of inflammation associated with the draining tract. A CT fistulogram can also be used to highlight the tract, and may demonstrate a foreign body as a filling defect. If a fistulogram is performed a Foley catheter will prevent backflow of contrast. The head should be positioned such that gravity assists flow of contrast in to the lesion and the CT scan should be commenced immediately after contrast has been injected to the point of back pressure.

CT features (Figure 41.7)

- Gas or hypodense fluid within a tract communicating with the skin surface.
- Contrast enhancement of the walls of the tract and adjacent tissue.
- Foreign body density depends on material (wood = hypodense).

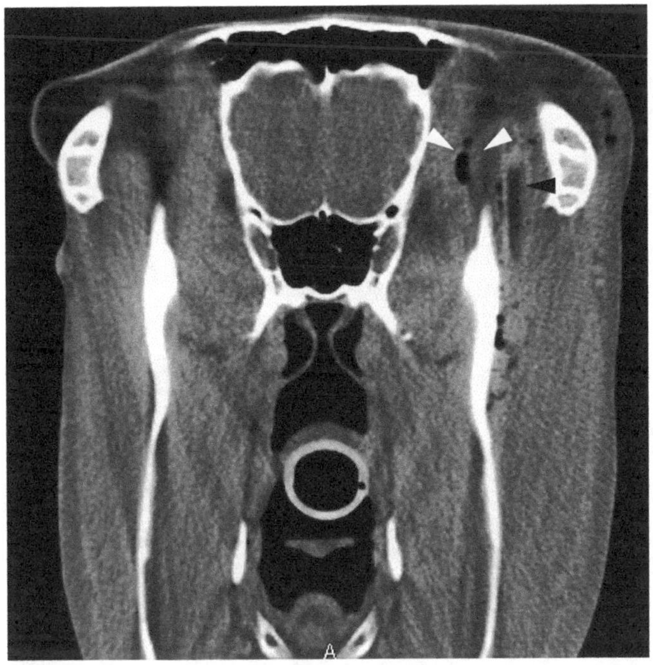

Figure 41.7 Adult Tennessee Walker gelding with a 48-hour history of a draining wound over the left eye. Transverse CT image shows a linear hypodense wood foreign body (black arrowhead) medial to the caudal orbit with adjacent pockets of gas (white arrowheads) (image courtesy of Nathan Nelson, The Ohio State University).

Osteitis

Infection and inflammation of the bones of the calvarium may occur secondary to penetrating trauma. Sequestration of bone fragments associated with calvarial trauma is also possible.

CT features

- Lysis and irregularity of bone margins.
- Periosteal proliferation is irregular, but is not always present.
- Sequestered bone fragments of increased density with a surrounding region of hypodensity (involucrum).

Temporomandibular joint sepsis

Temporomandibular joint sepsis is rare, and may be associated with a fistulous tract on presentation. The cause is often unknown.

CT features (Figure 41.8)

- Areas of lysis of the mandibular condyle, temporal tubercle or both.
- Gas may be present within the joint.
- Communication with fistulous tract, if present.

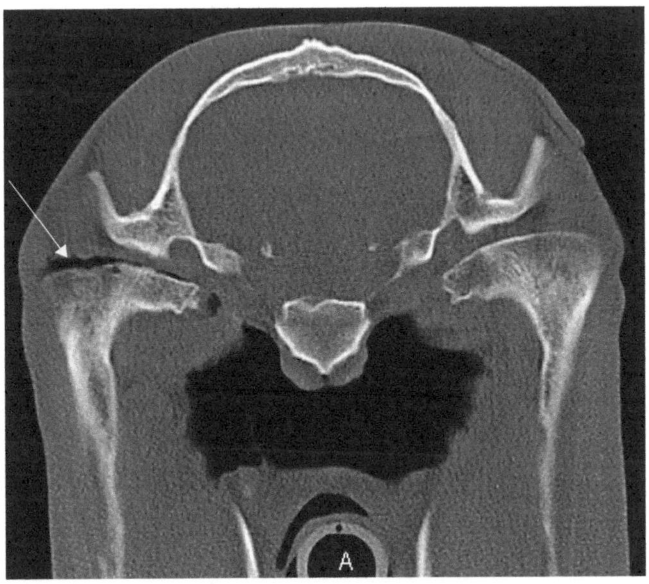

Figure 41.8 Adult Appaloosa gelding with septic temporomandibular joint. Transverse CT image shows gas within the joint (arrow) and an irregular margin to the mandibular condyle. Stylohyoid osteomyelitis was also present (not visible on this image) (image courtesy of Nathan Nelson, The Ohio State University).

Temporohyoid osteoarthropathy

Temporohyoid osteopathy is a specific condition in horses. The etiology is poorly understood but it may

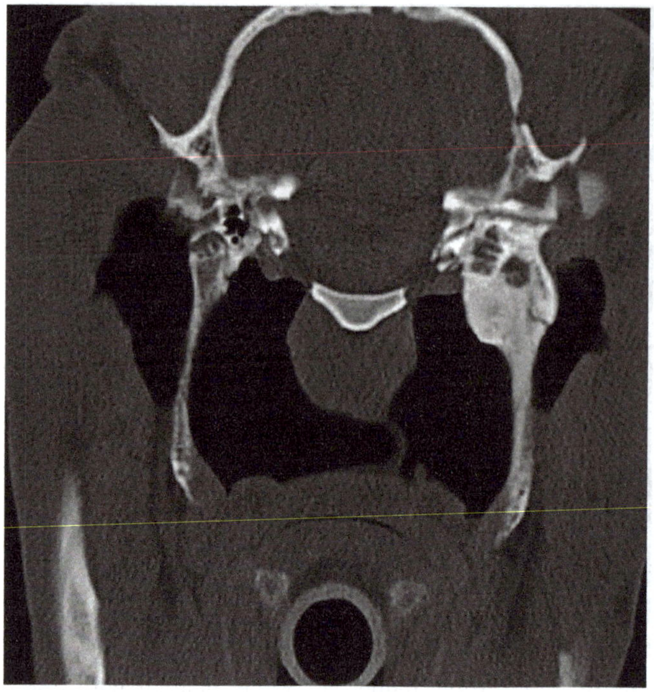

Figure 41.9 Adult Quarterhorse with left sided facial paralysis. Transverse CT image shows evidence of temporohyoid osteoarthropathy with a stylohyoid fracture and proliferation (image courtesy of Nathan Nelson, The Ohio State University).

occur as a sequela to otitis media, upper respiratory infection, or as a primary degenerative disease. It is typified by progressive osseous proliferation of the stylohyoid and can lead to fusion of the temporohyoid joint. The clinical presentation is typically that of vestibular signs and facial nerve dysfunction.

CT features (Figure 41.9)

- Bony proliferation of the stylohyoid bone and temporohyoid articulation.
- Thickening of the ceratohyoid bone and proliferation of the styloceratohyoid articulation may also be present.
- Bilateral changes common on CT in horses with unilateral clinical signs.
- Fluid within the tympanic bulla in some cases.

Neoplasia

Benign bone neoplasia

Primary bone neoplasia is rare in horses. Benign lesions, including osteomas and ossifying fibromas, can occur. The clinical presentation is typically one of progressive swelling.

CT features

- Smoothly marginated bone dense mass.
- May cause thinning of adjacent bone by pressure necrosis.

Malignant bone neoplasia

Osteosarcoma and metastatic carcinoma can both occur in the equine calvarium, though they are rare. The clinical presentation may be similar to that of benign and soft tissue neoplasia, and CT aids the differentiation of benign and aggressive lesions.

CT features

- Localized bone disruption and lysis.
- Variable irregular periosteal proliferation.
- Variable associated mass.
- Bone-dense material within the mass if osteosarcoma.

Intra-axial brain neoplasia

Neoplasms arising within the brain are rare in horses. Neurological signs prompt clinical investigation and are usually progressive.

CT features (Figure 41.10)

- Mass lesion that may cause a midline shift.
- Variable contrast enhancement.
- Variable surrounding hypodensity (edema).

Pituitary adenoma

Pituitary pars intermedia dysfunction is also known as equine Cushing's disease. It is caused by adenomatous hypertrophy of the intermediate lobe of the pituitary gland. Diagnosis is by the typical clinical picture (hirsutism predominantly and often chronic laminitis, bulging fat pads, polydipsia and polyuria) and endocrinological testing.

CT features (Figure 41.11)

- Enlarged pituitary width and height (normal is approximately $2 \times 2 \times 0.5$ cm length × width × height), though adenomatous glands may measure within normal limits.

Cholesterinic granulomas

Cholesterinic granulomas are benign growths of the choroid plexus. They are common, occurring in 15–20% of older horses. The lesions occur in the lateral and fourth ventricles and can cause neurological signs

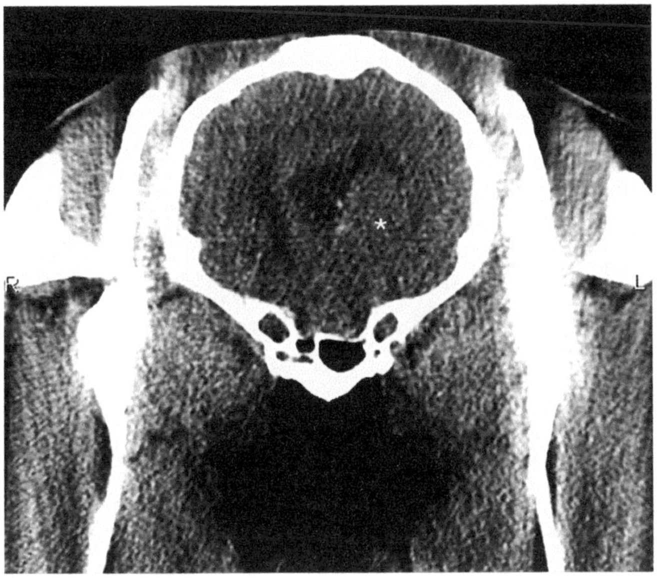

Figure 41.10 Four-year-old Quarterhorse mare with an oligodendroglioma arising from the olfactory lobe. Transverse CT image shows a mass (asterisk) growing into the left lateral ventricle causing dilation of the ventricle and a generalized mass effect. Focal hyperdensity on the axial margin represents dystrophic mineralization (image courtesy of Nathan Nelson, The Ohio State University).

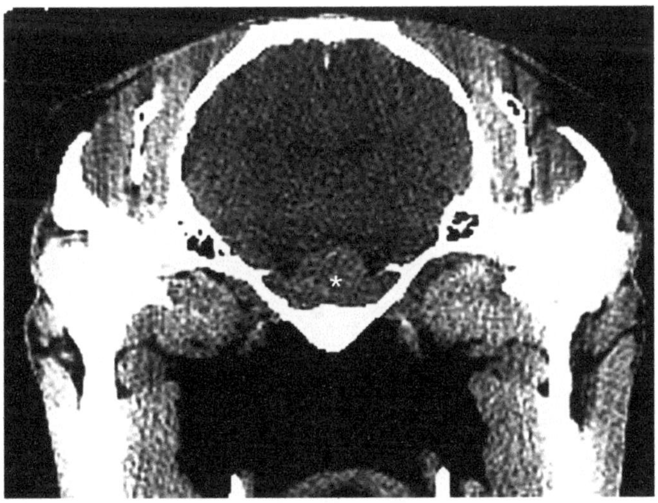

Figure 41.11 Adult Thoroughbred gelding with signs of Cushing's type disease. Transverse post-contrast CT image shows the enlarged and uniformly enhancing pituitary gland (asterisk).

due to an associated obstructive hydrocephalus or direct brain compression. CT-guided biopsy can allow differentiation from less common tumor types.

CT features (Figure 41.12)

- Often bilateral.
- Variable density.

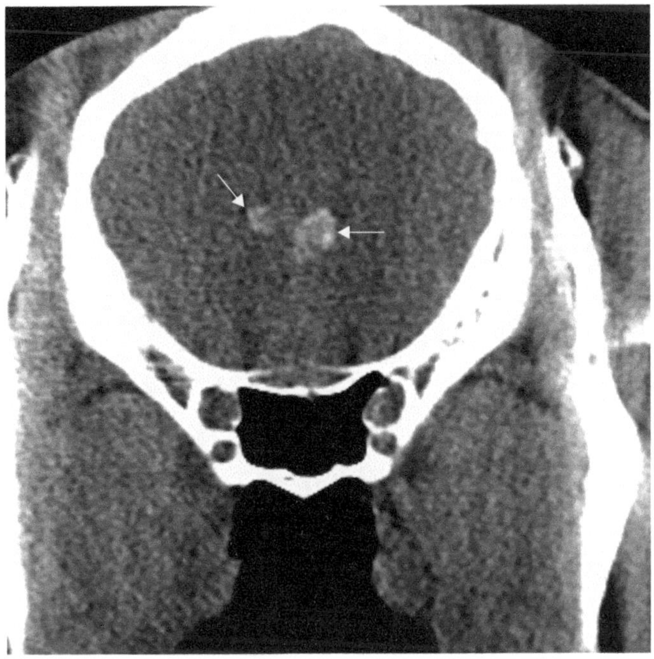

Figure 41.12 Transverse CT image of an adult Warmblood with bilateral cholesterinic granulomas in the lateral ventricles. The regions of hyperdensity (arrows) represent dystrophic mineralization (image courtesy of Nathan Nelson, The Ohio State University).

- Hyperdense foci may be present pre-contrast due to dystrophic mineralization.
- Contrast enhancement varies from mild patchy to marked diffuse.

Further Reading

Hilton H, Puchalski SM and Aleman M (2009) The computed tomographic appearance of equine temporohyoid osteoarthropathy. *Vet Radiol Ultrasound* **50**: 151–6.

McKlveen TL, Jones JC, Sponenberg DP, Scarratt K, Ward D and Aardema BS (2003) Assessment of the accuracy of computed tomography for measurement of normal equine pituitary glands. *Am J Vet Res* **64**: 1387–94.

Rodriguez MJ, Latorre R, López-Albors O *et al.* (2008) Computed tomographic anatomy of the temporomandibular joint in the young horse. *Eq Vet J* **40**: 566–71.

Porat-Mosenco Y, Schwarz T and Kass PH (2002) Thick-section reformatting of thinly collimated computed tomography for reduction of skull-base-related artifacts in dogs and horses. *Vet Radiol Ultrasound* **45**: 131–5.

Vink-Nooteboom M, Junker K, Van den Ingh TS and Dik KJ (1998) Computed tomography of cholesterinic granulomas in the choroid plexus of horses. *Vet Radiol Ultrasound* **39**: 512–16.

CHAPTER FORTY-TWO

EQUINE NECK AND SPINE

Jimmy Saunders and Hendrik-Jan Bergman

CT: ANATOMY AND NORMAL VARIANTS

The horse's neck comprises seven vertebrae. C3–C7 are connected with each other by paired joints on the left and right sides (the facet joints), by elastic fibrocartilages (the intervertebral disks) and by several ligaments. The spinal cord passes through each vertebra and nerve roots emerge between each vertebra.

The nuchal ligament is very developed in equines. Two parts, funiculus and laminae, insert at the external occipital protuberance of the occipital bone and run to the withers, supporting and holding the horse's head and neck in position (Figure 42.1A and B). The semispinalis capitis muscle originates on the cervical vertebrae and the first six to seven thoracic vertebrae and inserts with two symmetrical tendons on the occipital bone, on both sides of the nuchal ligament (Figure 42.1A and C). Incidental bone proliferation is frequently seen at the insertion of these two structures on the occipital bone (see below, Nuchal entheseopathy, Figure 42.4C).

DISEASE PROCESSES

Congenital/Developmental

Occipitoatlantoaxial malformation

Occipitoatlantoaxial malformation is an uncommon disorder described in Arabian and Friesian foals.

CT features

- Fusion of two or more vertebrae (occipito-atlanto-axial).
- Hypoplasia of atlas and/or the dens of the axis. An elongatation of the dens has rarely been described.
- Additional free axis.

Cervical vertebral malformation (cervical vertebral stenotic myelopathy)

Cervical vertebral malformation (Table 42.1) is one clinical entity in the group of equine developmental orthopedic diseases and also one of the most common causes of wobbler syndrome. It includes not only malformation but also malarticulation and degenerative changes of the joints, causing spinal cord compression.

The disorder is a main indication for CT myelography in horses suspected to have lateral compressive lesions. Minimum median diameter values can be measured on CT and correlate well with macroscopic necropsy measurements.

Table 42.1
Cervical vertebral malformation (CVM) types in horses.

Type I CVM	Type II CVM
Young (<2 years) rapidly growing horse	Older horse (young possible)
Male and Thoroughbreds at risk	Affects all horses
Midcervical vertebral column	Caudal neck (C5-C6, C6–C7)*
Dynamic stenotic compression when the neck is flexed	More static compression: osteoarthritis of the articular processes

*Not accessible with current CTs in living animals.

Veterinary Computed Tomography, First Edition. Edited by Tobias Schwarz, Jimmy Saunders.

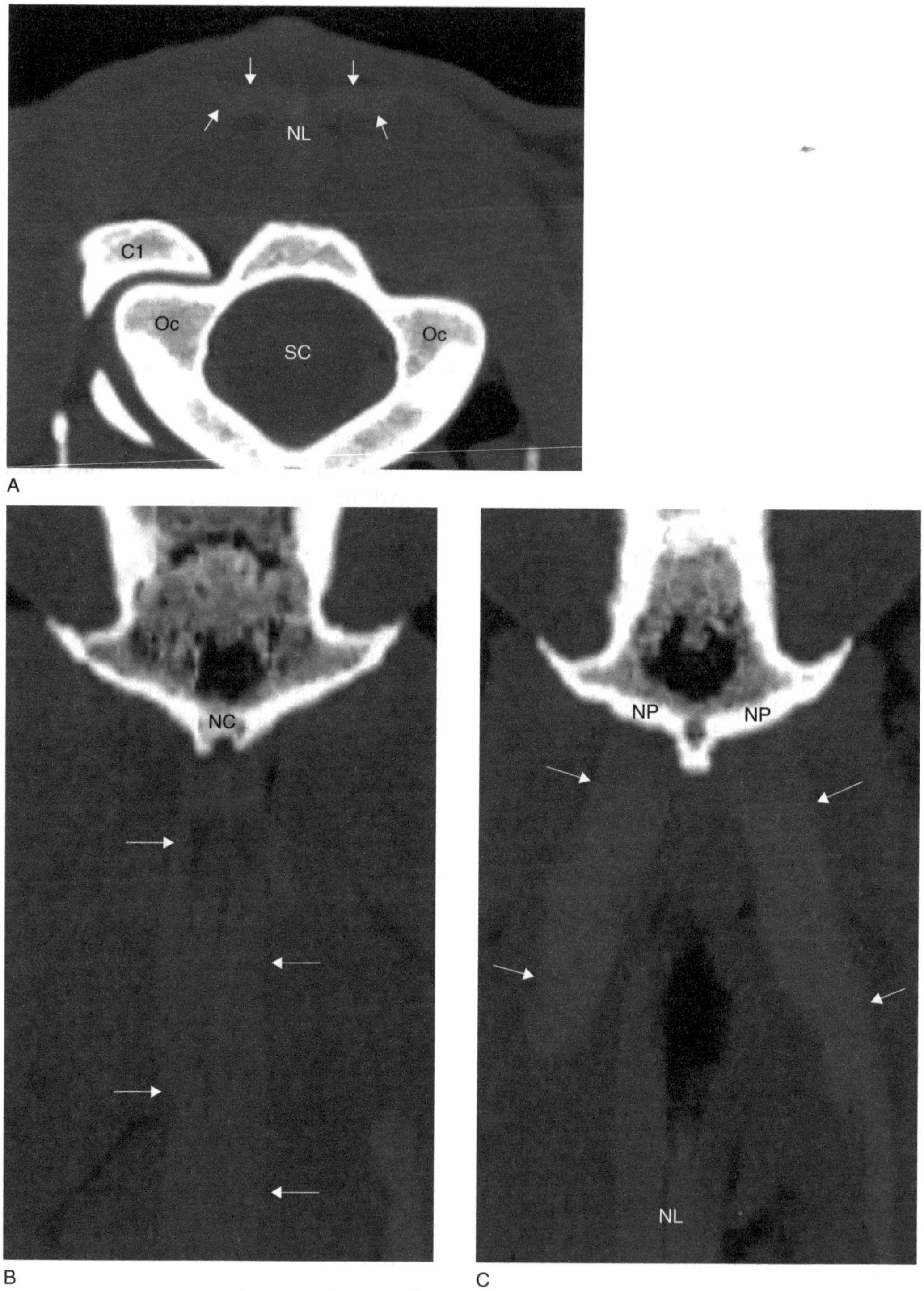

Figure 42.1 Normal aspect of the attachment of the nuchal ligament and semispinalis capitis tendons. (A) Transverse CT image shows the nuchal ligament (NL) and semispinalis tendons (arrows). (B) Dorsally reconstructed CT image shows the cranial attachment of the nuchal ligament (arrows) on the nuchal crest (NC) of the occipital bone. (C) Dorsally reconstructed CT image a few mm dorsal to (B) shows the attachment of the semispinalis tendons (arrows) on the nuchal plane (NP). C1 = atlas; Oc = occipital condyle; SC = spinal cord.

CT features (only Type I)

- Have not been reported.
- Anticipated CT features:
  - absolute or dynamic stenosis of the vertebral canal (vertebral malalignment)
  - malformation (including osteochondrosis) or osteoarthritis to the articular processes
  - angular deviations of the vertebrae, associated with physeal lesions (dorsal flare caudal epiphyses, enlargement)
  - soft tissue pathology associated with spinal cord compression: ligamentum flavum hypertrophy, joint capsule swelling and hypertrophy, synovial cysts
  - CT myelography: spinal cord compression as circumferential loss of contrast agent due to stenosis of the vertebral canal or lateral impingement of the dural sac by a malformed articular facet; proximal intervertebral foramen impingement: compression of the nerve root by a malformed articular facet.

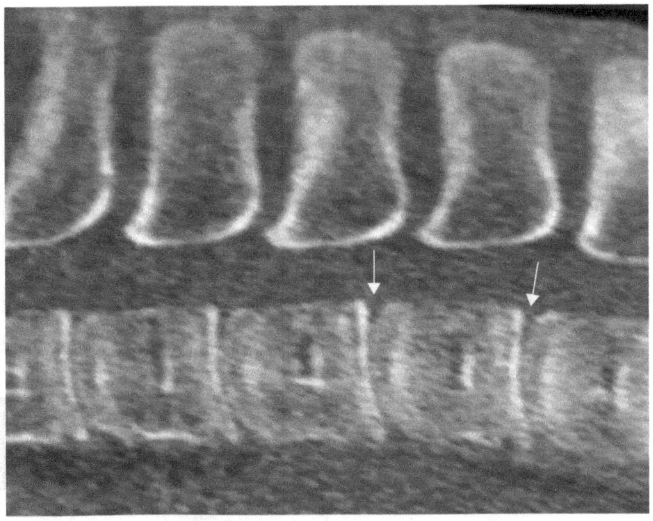

Figure 42.2 Six-month-old stallion with kyphosis of the thoracolumbar region secondary to trauma (two months earlier). Sagittally reconstructed CT image shows vertebral malalignment (arrows). The cranial vertebral physes are closed while the caudal physes are not suggesting discrepancy in their closure time.

Fractures, luxations

Cervical fractures are common in foals and often involve epiphyseal separation, particularly of the dens of the axis. In adult horses, fractures occur more commonly in high-speed paddock or race accidents and affect mostly the midcervical and caudal cervical vertebrae. Associated tearing of joint capsule and dislocation/fracture of the dorsal articular processes is not rare, allowing vertebral subluxation and spinal cord contusion. Subtle fractures or the complexity of comminuted fractures are better demonstrated using CT compared to radiography.

A specific type of fracture in the adult horse is the avulsion fracture at the insertion of the nuchal ligament and/or semispinalis capitis tendons, which has to be differentiated from a nuchal enthesopathy.

CT features

- Fracture/Luxation of the vertebral column (Figures 42.2 and 42.3):
  - multiple bone fragments
  - best visible on the dorsally reformatted images
  - spinal cord displacement.
- Avulsion fracture of the nuchal ligament/semispinalis capitis tendon (Figure 42.4):
  - bone fragment close to the external occipital protuberance of the occipital bone
  - a nidus in the ventral aspect of the nuchal crest is sometimes visible
  - nuchal ligament/semispinalis capitis tendon enlarged, asymmetric and/or heterogeneous with irregular margins
  - with chronicity, bone proliferation on the caudal occipital bone.

Degenerative

Nuchal enthesopathy

Bone proliferation is frequently present at the cranial attachment of the nuchal ligament or of the semispinalis tendon, especially in dressage and jumping horses. Most of these horses do not show pain or diminution of performance. However, in some, unwillingness, head shaking or stiffness may emerge.

CT features (Figure 42.5)

- Bone proliferation at the attachment on the nuchal crest or nuchal plane.
- Separate fragments may be present bone nodules, mineralization inside the ligament.
- Nuchal ligament/semispinalis capitis tendons ill-defined, thickened, irregularly marginated, heterogeneous or, for the muscle, asymmetric.

Neoplasia

Neoplasms affecting the vertebral canal are a rare occurrence in the horse. They are mostly metastases of

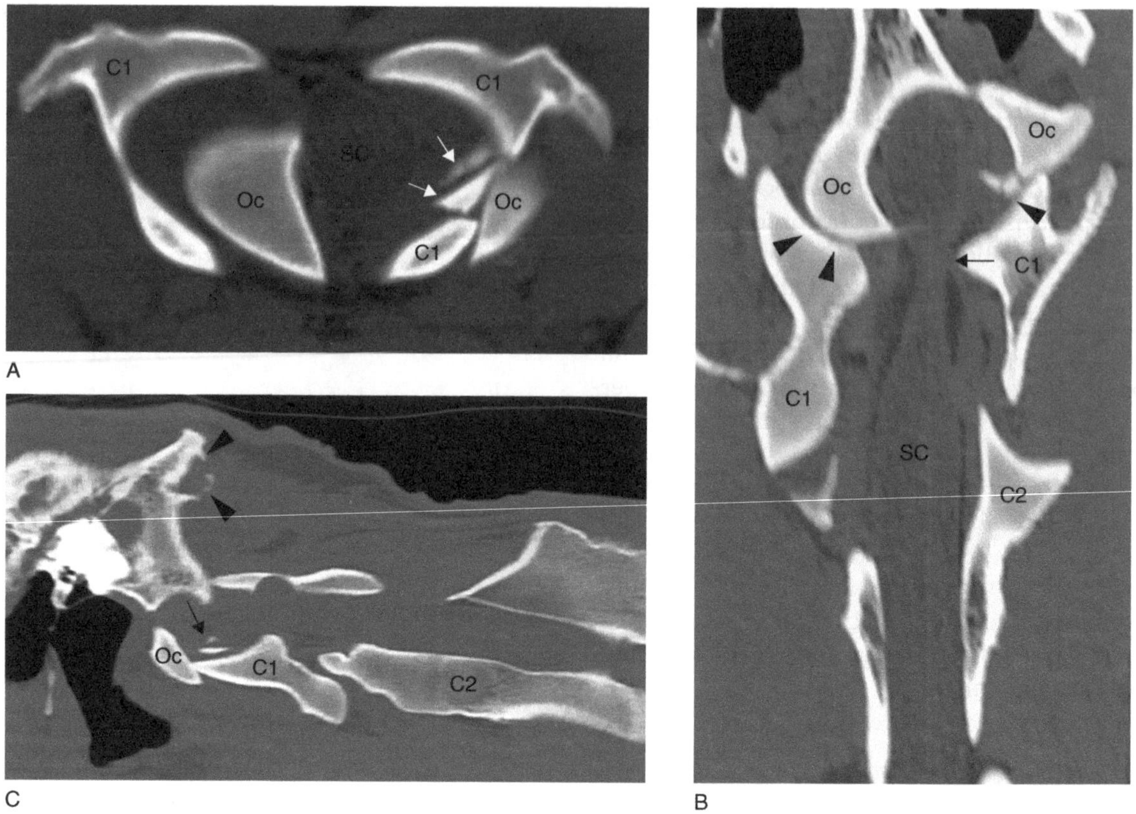

Figure 42.3 Adult horse with fracture of the atlas and subluxation of its atlanto-occipital joint. (A) Transverse CT image shows multiple, sharply margined, bone fragments (arrows) associated with the left pedicle of the atlas. The fragments are just axial to the left occipital condyle (Oc) within the spinal canal. (B) Dorsally reconstructed CT image shows a subluxation of the atlanto-occipital joint (arrowheads). The dura is clearly demarcated and a compression of the left subarachnoid space is visible (arrow). The spinal cord is visible and appears displaced to the left. (C) Sagittally reconstructed CT image shows the previously described fragments at the bottom of the vertebral canal (arrow). Bone reactions are visible on the caudal aspect of the occipital bone (arrowheads). C1 = atlas; C2 = axis; Oc = occipital condyle; SC = spinal cord.

non-neural origin causing extradural compression of the spinal cord with other primary foci in the body. Melanoma in the spinal canal in mature gray horses has been described. Other reported neoplasms include squamous cell carcinoma, hemangiosarcoma, osteosarcoma, intestinal adenocarcinoma, plasma cell myeloma, fibrosarcoma, pheochromocytoma and lymphoma. Guided biopsy is necessary for final diagnosis.

CT features (Figure 42.6)

- Lytic bone lesion.
- Extradural soft tissue mass causing spinal cord compression.
- Possible involvement of the paravertebral musculature.

Further Reading

Mayhew GJ (1999) The diseased spinal cord. *Proc Am Assoc Eq Pract* **45**: 67–84.

Moore BR, Holbrook TC, Stefanacci JD, Reed SM, Tate LP and Menard MC (1992) Contrast-enhanced computed tomography and myelography in six horses with cervical stenotic myelopathy. *Eq Vet J* **24**: 197–202.

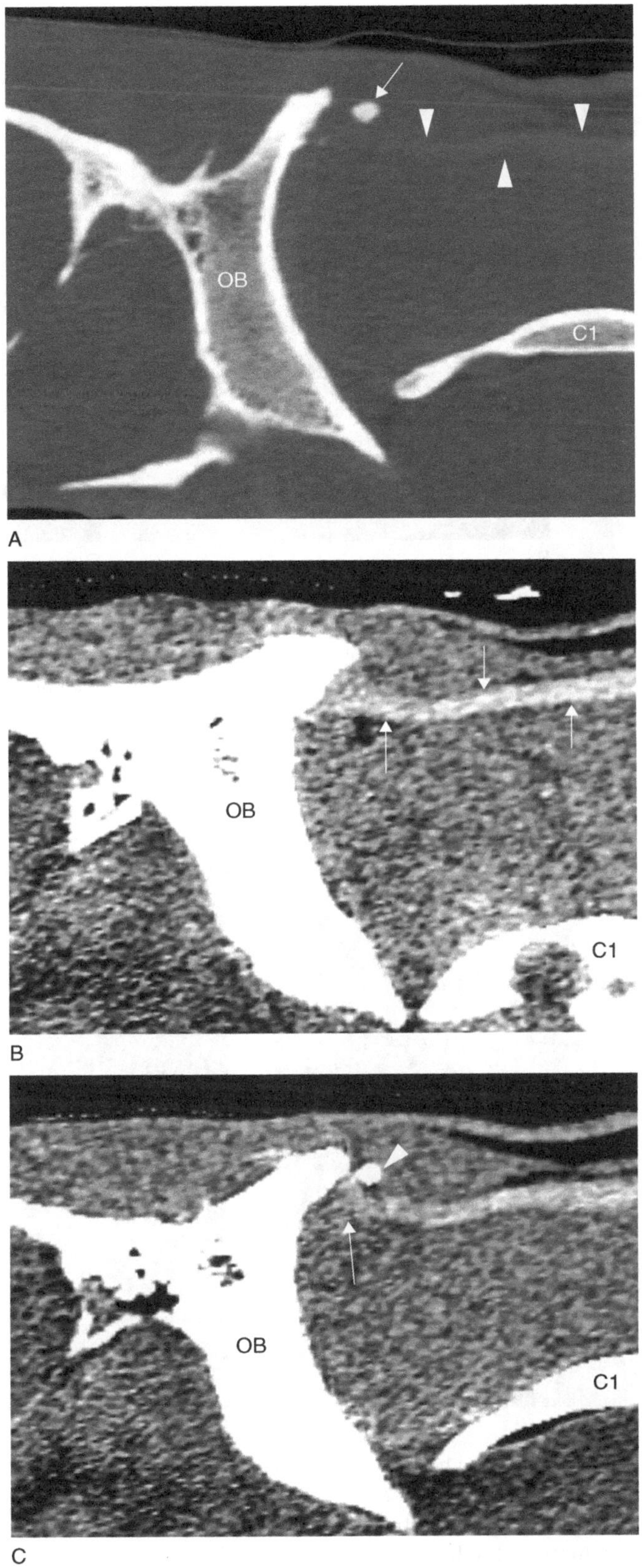

Figure 42.4 Four-year-old Anglo-Arab mare with long history of sudden resistance to riding in frame and a final diagnosis of chronic avulsion fracture at the insertion of the right side of the semispinalis capitis tendon. (A) Sagittally reconstructed CT image shows a rounded bone fragment (arrow) just ventral and caudal to the external occipital protuberance of the occipital bone. The semispinalis capitis tendon is visible (arrowheads). (B) Sagittally reconstructed CT image shows the normal left semispinalis capitis tendon entheses (arrows) and its attachment to the occipital bone. (C) Sagittally reconstructed CT image shows the right semispinalis capitis tendon entheses (arrow). The semispinalis tendon appears heterogeneous and irregularly delineated at its insertion. The previously described fragment is still visible (arrowhead). The tendon at the level of its entheses appears enlarged. C1 = atlas; OB = occipital bone.

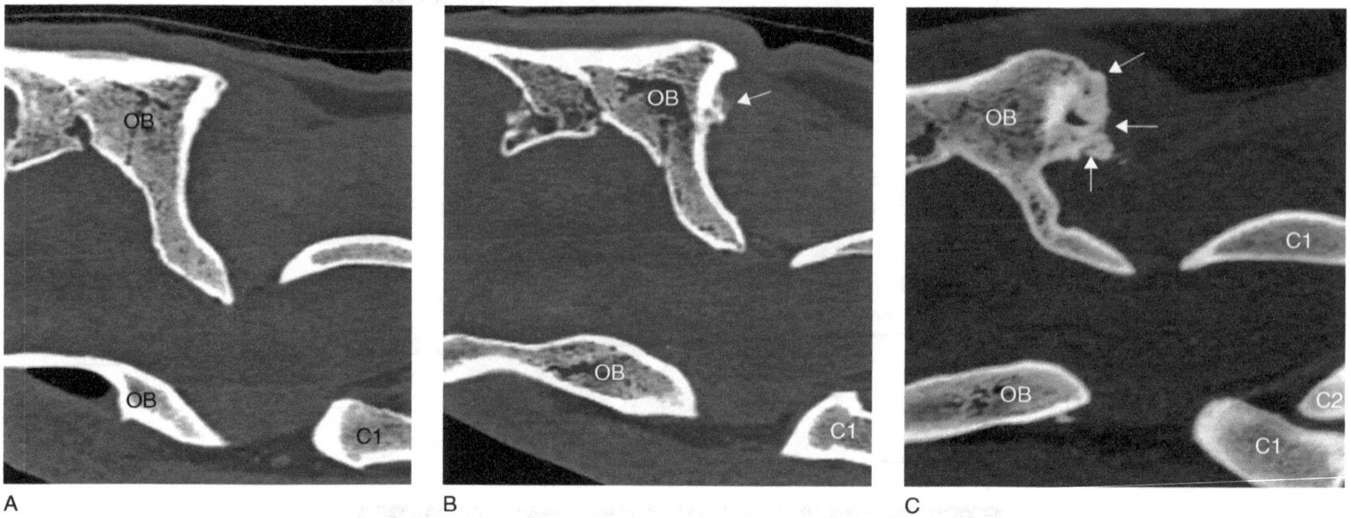

Figure 42.5 (A) Sagittal reference CT image of the occipital bone in a normal horse. (B) Seven-year-old horse with intermittent headshaking and a diagnosis of nuchal entheseopathy. On a sagittally reconstructed CT image, the ventral aspect of the attachment of the nuchal ligament is irregular with bone proliferation extending caudally from the occipital bone (arrow). (C) Nine-year-old horse without clinical signs. Sagittally reconstructed CT image shows severe chronic bone proliferation at the attachment site of the nuchal ligament (arrows). C1 = atlas; OB = occipital bone.

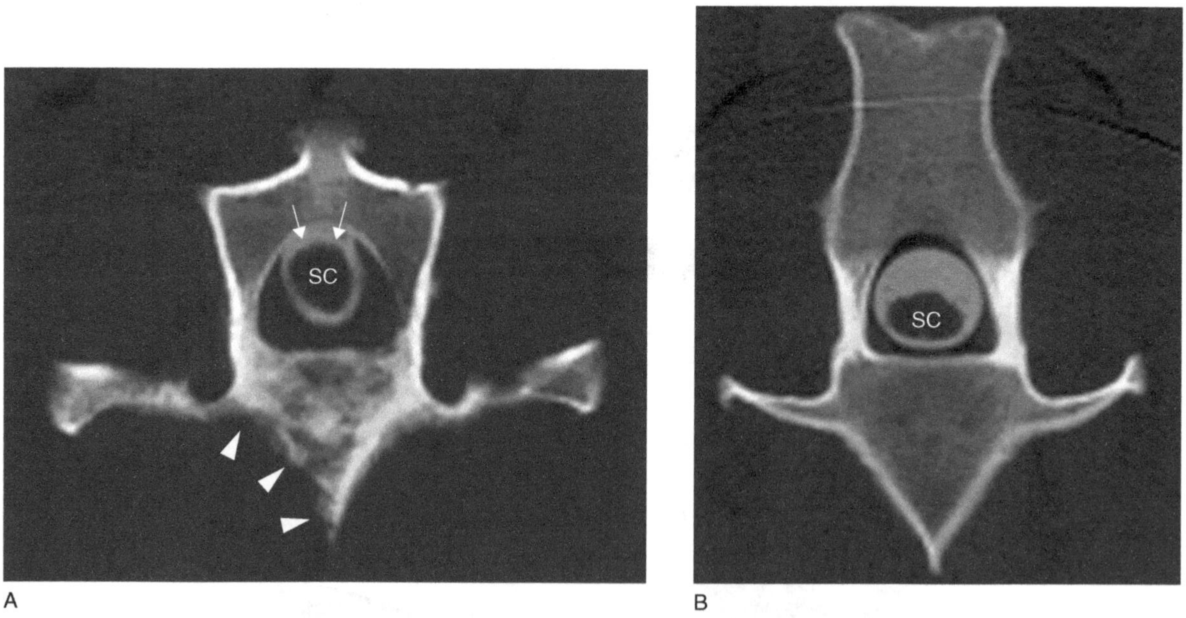

Figure 42.6 Eleven-year-old horse with vertebral hemangiosarcoma (metastases were found in the kidneys, liver and lungs). (A) Transverse CT myelogram at the level of C3 shows severe osteolysis of the vertebral body (arrowheads). The spinal cord is dorsally displaced and is misshapen. The dorsal contrast column is thinned dorsally (arrows). (B) Transverse reference CT myelogram of the normal contrast column at the level of C3. SC = spinal cord.

CHAPTER FORTY-THREE

EQUINE FRACTURES

Hendrik-Jan Bergman and Jimmy Saunders

INTRODUCTION

As CT provides an excellent bone detail, it can be of great value to demonstrate the precise nature of fractures when other imaging modalities remain inconclusive. CT is very useful for diagnosis of subtle bone lesions such as fissures, stress fractures or subchondral bone fractures, for diagnosis of fractures in complex joints (joints comprising many bones) or for better understanding of comminuted fractures.

CT angiography can be used to evaluate vascular integrity in horses with trauma to the distal extremities with regard to their prognosis.

FISSURES, STRESS FRACTURES AND SUBTLE SUBCHONDRAL BONE FRACTURES

Fissures and stress fractures are two types of incomplete fractures. Their diagnosis can be difficult but is critical to prevent progression to a catastrophic complete fracture. Even several weeks after the clinical and scintigraphic confirmation, the estimated frequency of continued negative radiography is 20–50%. In such cases, other advanced imaging modalities are required for diagnosis directly improving management and prognosis.

A fissure is a crack extending from a surface into, but not through, a bone. Fissures are quite common in horses and are mostly the result of a kick from another horse. Most fissures run longitudinally. Their most common locations are the proximal, typically the dorsal sagittal groove in the proximal articular surface, middle and distal phalanx. This condition is also commonly seen in the metacarpal/metatarsal condyles (lateral > medial).

Stress fractures are overuse injuries most commonly recognized in equine athletes undergoing continual high-load, repetitive activities. These fractures are usually seen in the third metacarpal/metatarsal bone, particularly the dorsolateral aspect, as a severe form of bucked shins. Stress fractures have also been describe in the upper limb (humerus, tibia and scapula) and in the axial skeleton (pelvis and vertebrae).

Subchondral bone fractures involve traumatic damage to the cartilage and subchondral bone caused by contusion, excessive shearing and/or rotational forces. They may be associated with the formation of loose intra-articular osteochondral fragments.

CT features

Fissure (Figures 43.1 and 43.2).

- Prior to contrast medium administration:
  - small lucent/hypodense line in bone, mostly regular
  - the fissure line may be surrounded by a lucent defect in the subchondral bone or subchondral bone sclerosis
  - optimal visualization may require the use of MPR reconstructions.
- After intra-articular contrast medium administration
  - contrast medium can be present in the fissure.

Stress fracture

- Lucent fracture line(s).
- Asymmetrical subchondral bone formation.
- Callus formation: (benign) periosteal reactions and cortical thickening.

Subchondral bone fracture (Figure 43.3)

- Disruption/irregularity in cortical bone.
- Partial or complete fragment separation.

Veterinary Computed Tomography, First Edition. Edited by Tobias Schwarz, Jimmy Saunders.

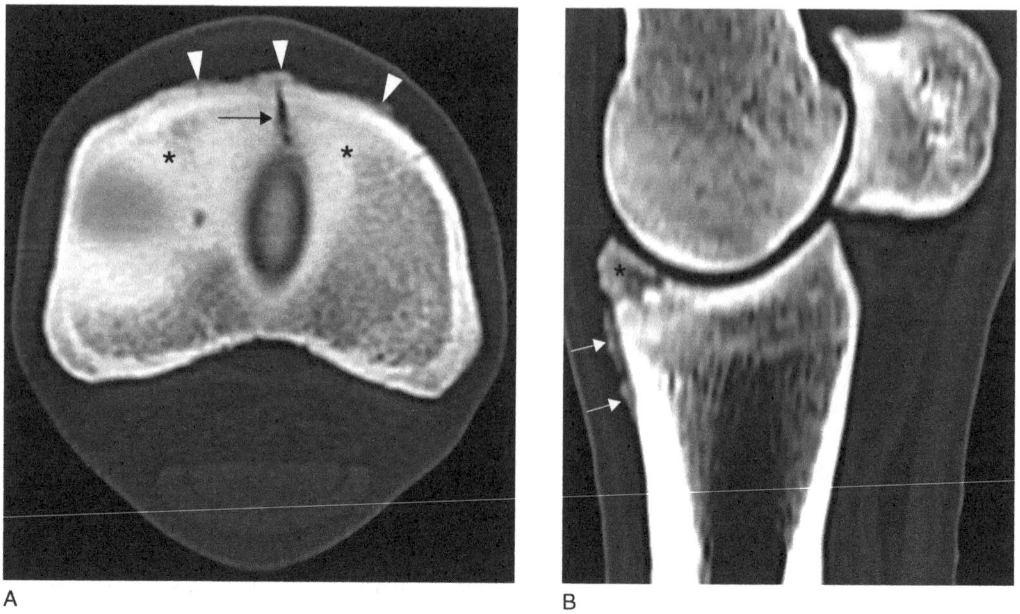

Figure 43.1 (A) Transverse CT image showing a fissure line (arrow) surrounded by sclerosis (asterisks) on the midline in the dorsal portion of the proximal phalanx of a left forelimb. There is irregularly margined periosteal proliferation over the dorsal surface of the proximal phalanx, more pronounced at the level of the fissure line (arrowheads). (B) Sagittally reconstructed CT image showing subchondral lucency (asterisk). There is irregularly margined periosteal proliferation over the dorsal surfaces of the proximal phalanx extending distally to the proximal diaphyseal region (arrows).

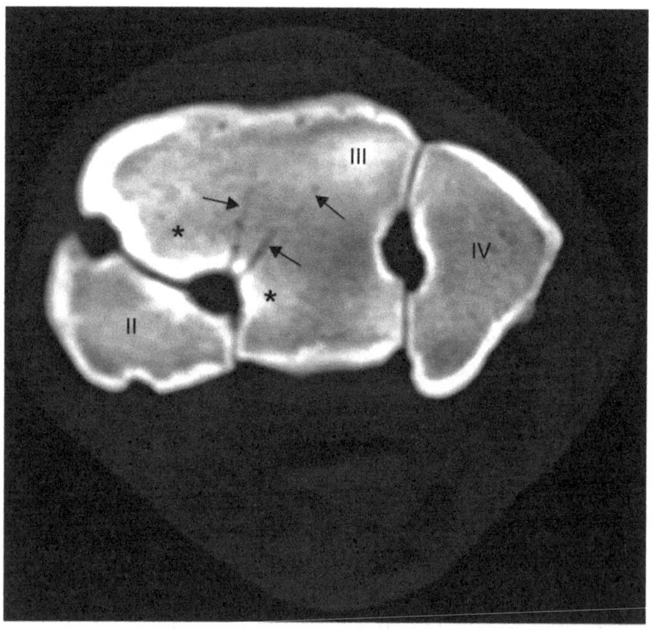

Figure 43.2 Transverse CT image of a left carpus showing the second (II), third (III) and fourth (IV) carpal bones. There is an incomplete palmar cortical fracture in the medial aspect of the third carpal bone (arrows) surrounded by regional sclerosis (asterisks).

- Fragment(s) may be non-displaced or displaced, and possibly become intra-articular, free floating.

Salter–Harris Fractures

The Salter–Harris classification of growth plate injuries (I–VI) can be applied to all domestic animals. Type II fractures are the most common type of physeal injury. CT can help to diagnose the fracture, define a possible intra-articular component and give additional information for surgical planning. The CT features depend of the type of fracture (Figure 43.4).

Comminuted Fractures

In case of a comminuted fracture, the bone is broken, splintered or crushed into three or more pieces. The radiological examination of the geometric pattern of multiple fractures can be challenging, considering the complex superimposition of the 3-D anatomy of a region onto a 2-D image. CT is highly superior to radiography for evaluating the spatial configuration and completeness of the fracture as well as the relationship between the fracture and adjacent lesions (such as osseous cyst-like lesion, secondary degenerative joint disease) or joints (Figure 43.5). CT is essential to select

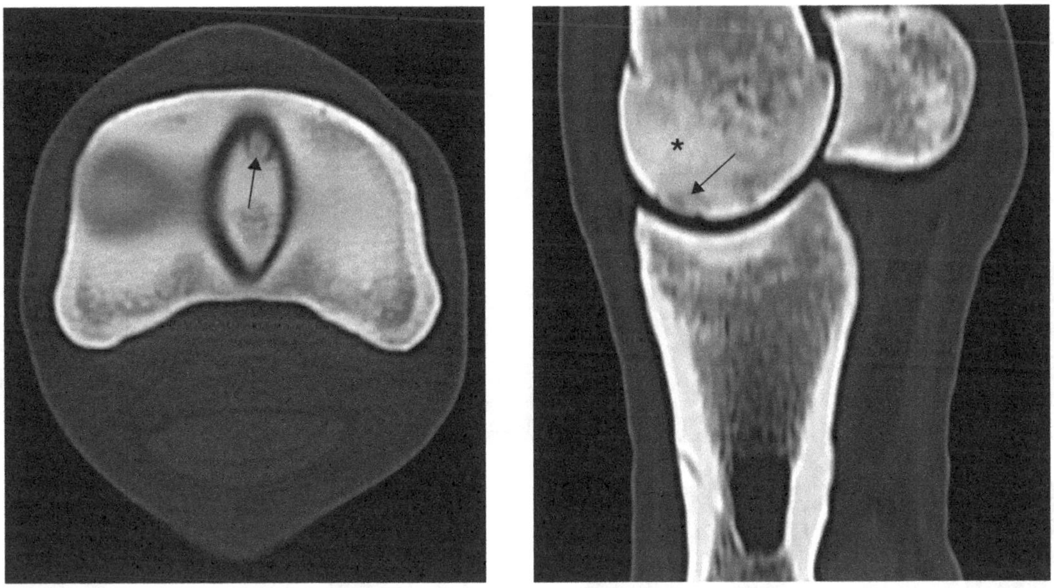

A B

Figure 43.3 (A) Transverse CT image of a left metacarpophalangeal joint showing an ovoid fracture at the distodorsal aspect of the sagittal ridge of the third metacarpal bone, which is associated with an incompletely separated osseous fragment (arrow). (B) Sagittally reconstructed CT image showing a radiolucent region (arrow) adjacent to this lesion. There is a large, ill-defined region of sclerosis (asterisk) involving the distodorsal aspect of the sagittal ridge.

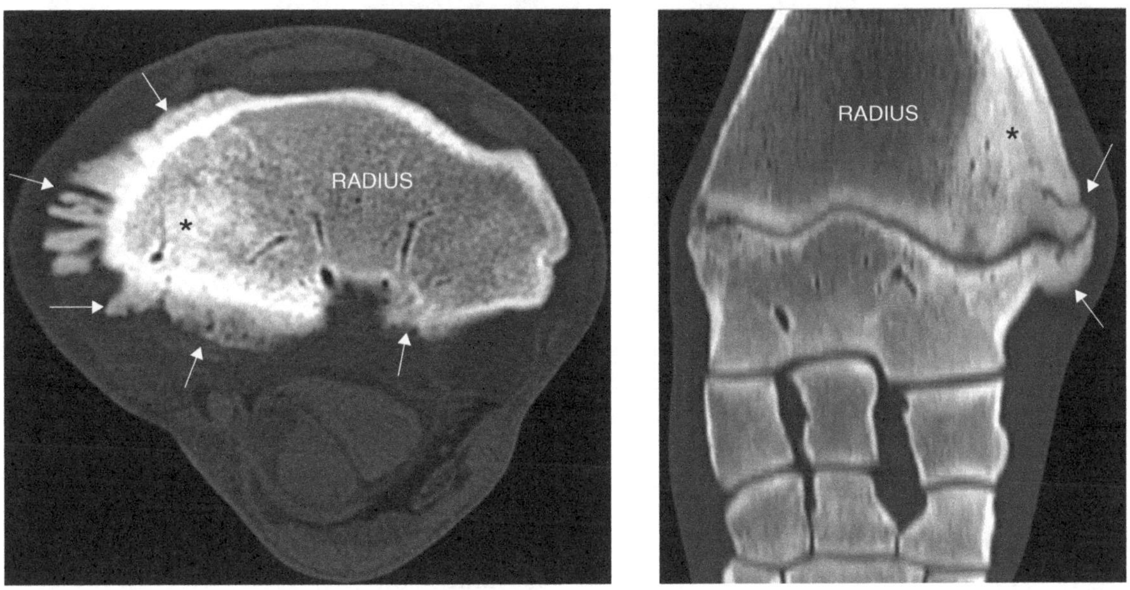

A B

Figure 43.4 (A) Transverse CT image showing extensive new bone formation (arrows) along the dorsomedial, medial and palmaromedial aspects of the distal physis of the radius. Severe bone sclerosis (asterisk) can be seen, indicating chronic disease. (B) Frontally reconstructed image showing the distal growth plate of the radius. The medial aspect of the distal physis is elongated (arrows) and an extensive sclerosis is present at the medial aspect of the metaphysis (asterisk). The medial aspect of the distal epiphysis of the radius is shorter than the lateral epiphysis. These changes were consecutive to a Salter–Harris fracture.

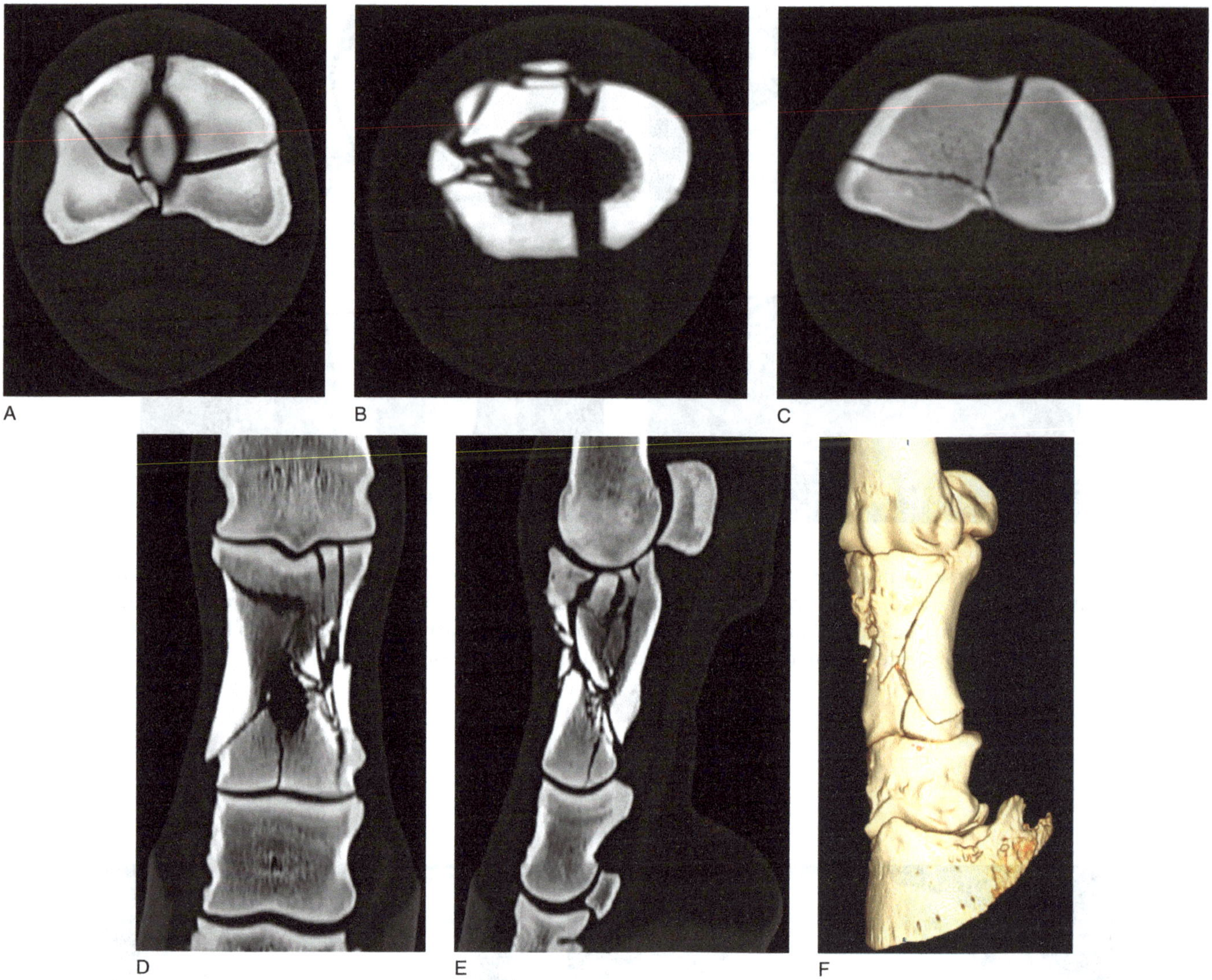

Figure 43.5 Transverse CT images of a comminuted fracture of the proximal phalanx at the level of (A) the distal metaphysis, (B) mid-diaphysis and (C) proximal metaphysis. (D) Frontal and (E) sagittal images, and (F) a 3-D reconstruction illustrating the intra-articular component and the complexity of the fracture.

the most appropriate treatment option (conservative versus surgical) and for optimal surgical planning. Most common comminuted fractures are fractures involving the proximal and middle phalanx, and the carpal bones.

Complex Joints (Carpus, Tarsus)

The detection of fractures in complex joints is sometimes difficult by radiography because of the superimposition of the different bone structures. In these cases CT can be used for fracture detection or for defining the exact fracture location and configuration. This important information gained from CT can give a more accurate diagnosis and can be used in selecting the most appropiate treatment and in determining the prognosis.

Specific fractures that are involved are chip and slab fractures of the carpal joint (Figure 43.6) and slab fractures of the tarsal bones (third tarsal bone > central tarsal bone > second and fourth tarsal bones) (Figures 43.7 and 43.8).

Further Reading

Collins JN, Galuppo LD, Thomas HL, Wisner ER and Hornof WJ (2004) Use of computed tomography angiography to evaluate the vacular anatomy of the distal portion of the forelimb of horses. *Am J Vet Res* **65**: 1409–20.

Martens P, Ihler CF and Rennesund J (1999) Detection of a radiographically occult fracture of the lateral palmar process of the distal phalanx in a horse using computed tomography. *Vet Radiol Ultrasound* **40**: 346–9.

Rose PL, Seeherman H and O'Callaghan M (1997) Computed tomographic evaluation of comminuted middle phalangeal fractures in the horse. *Vet Radiol Ultrasound* **38**: 424–9.

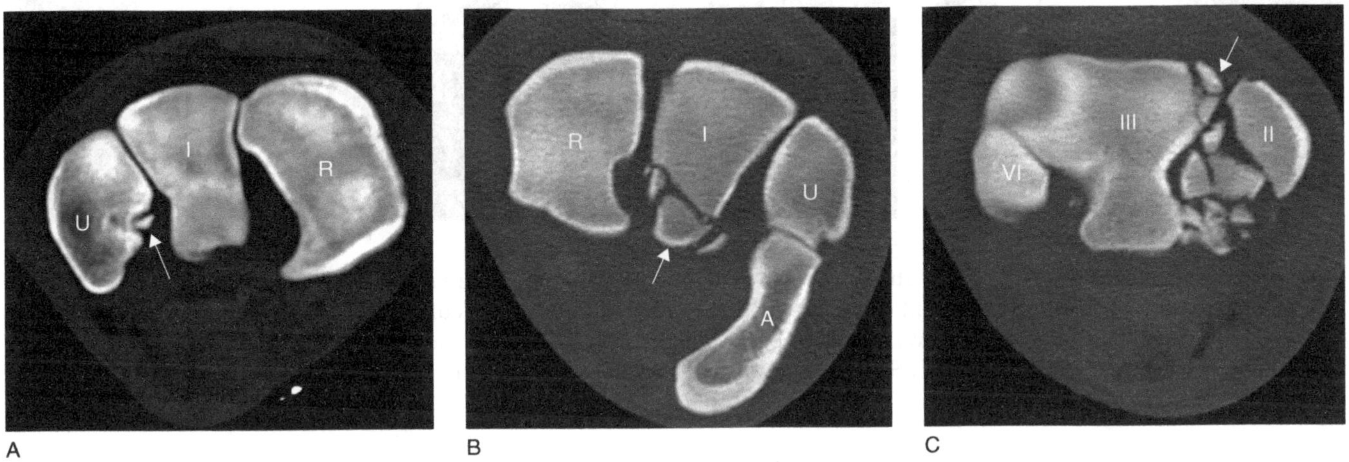

Figure 43.6 Transverse CT images illustrating fractures of a carpus in three different horses. (A) A small fracture fragment (arrow) is visible at the medial aspect of the right ulnar carpal bone (U). (B) Fracture of the palmar aspect of the intermediate carpal bone (I) of a left carpus (arrow). (C) Comminuted fracture of the second carpal bone (II) of a right carpus. Three small bone fragments (arrow) are visible at the dorsomedial aspect of the third carpal bone (III). IV = fourth carpal bone; A = accessory carpal bone; R = radial carpal bone.

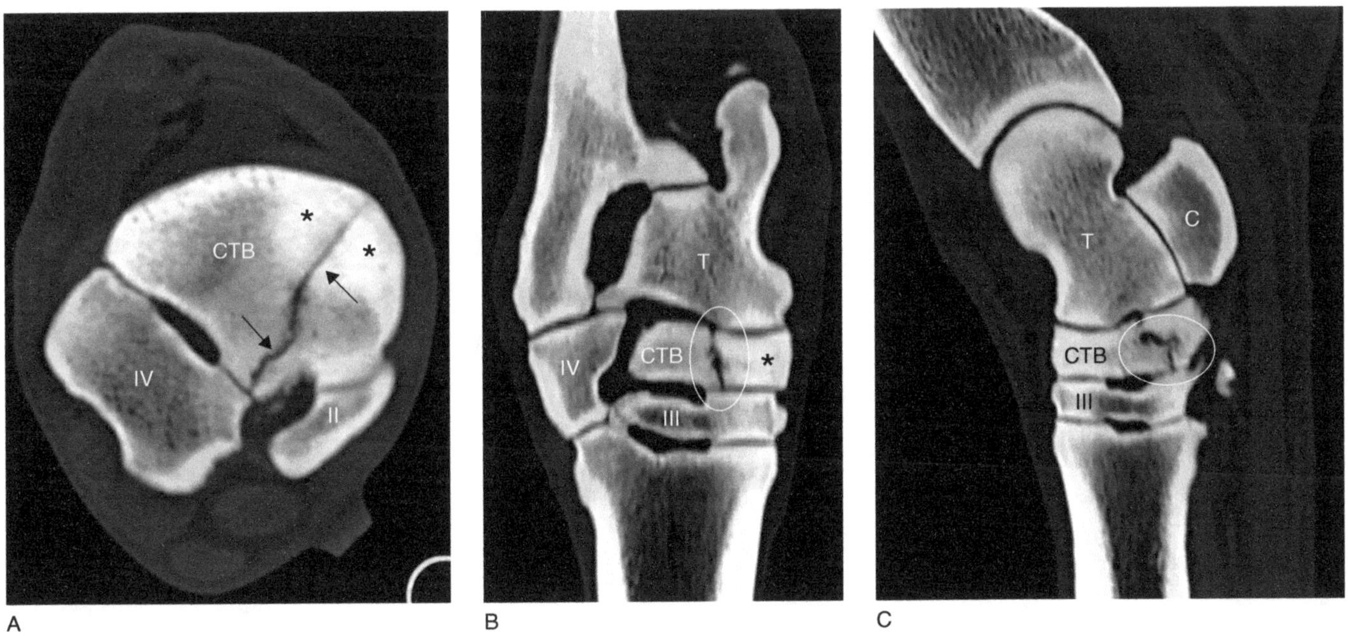

Figure 43.7 (A) Transverse CT image illustrating a complete fracture of central tarsal bone (CTB) (arrows) surrounded by sclerosis (asterisks). (B) Frontally reconstructed CT image showing a longitudinal fracture (circle) in the mid-portion of the central tarsal bone. Sclerosis is visible (asterisk). (C) On a sagittally reconstructed CT image, the previously described fracture (circle) is seen at the plantar aspect of the central tarsal bone. A marked sclerosis of the central tarsal bone is visible on the three images (asterisks). II = second tarsal bone; III = third tarsal bone; IV = fourth tarsal bone; C = calcaneus; T = talus.

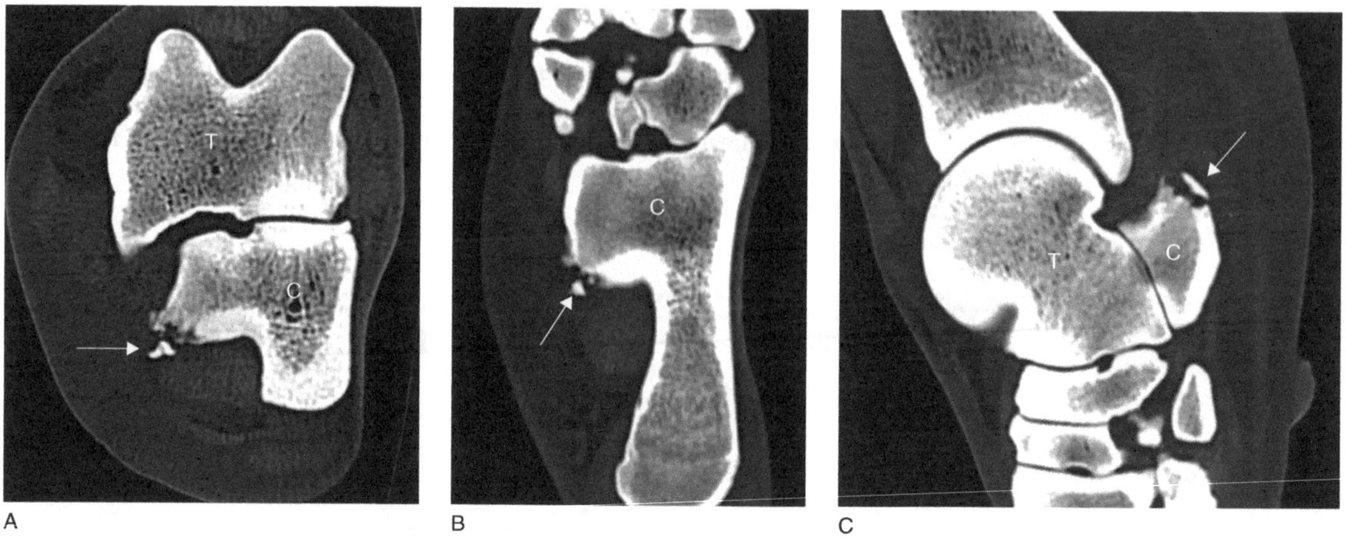

Figure 43.8 (A) Transverse CT image showing a bone fragment (arrow) at the plantomedial aspect of the sustentaculum tali. Smooth periosteal reaction is present along the medial border of the sustentaculum tali. (B) Frontally reconstructed CT image showing the same fragment (arrow) as well as periosteal reaction adjacent to the fragment. The bone cortex is thickened at the level of the sustentaculum tali. (C) Sagittally reconstructed image showing the avulsed fragment (arrow) adjacent to a bone defect. C = calcaneus; T = talus.

CHAPTER FORTY-FOUR

Equine Foot

Sarah Puchalski

CT: Anatomy and Normal Variants

The equine hoof capsule houses all components of the musculoskeletal system in addition to laminae, vasculature and neural tissue. Anatomic structures of clinical importance that lie within the hoof capsule include the middle and distal phalanges, comprising the distal interphalangeal (DIP) joint along with the collateral ligaments (CLs) of this joint.

The podotrochlear apparatus includes the deep digital flexor tendon (DDFT), the podotrochlear bursa (from now called navicular bursa), distal sesamoid bone (following called navicular bone), distal sesamoidean impar ligament and the collateral sesamoidean ligament (CSL) or suspensory ligament of the navicular bone. The distal portion of the digital sheath and distal digital annular ligament are also housed within the hoof capsule.

Deep digital flexor tendon

The distal portion of this DDFT is housed within the hoof. Distal to the fetlock joint, the DDFT has two symmetric lobes (Figure 44.1). In the pastern region, the tendon lobes are round but become ovoid to fusiform until the level of the proximal border of the navicular bone. At this level, the tendon maintains a slightly bilobed appearance but the lobes become flattened in a dorsal to palmar direction (Figure 44.2). Over the flexor cortex of the navicular bone, the tendon flattens and widens as it approaches its insertion onto the palmar flexoria fasciae of the distal phalanx. Distal to the navicular bone, the DDFT is thin and difficult to differentiate from the distal digital annular ligament (Figure 44.3). The fibers of the tendon run in a slightly diverging pattern to their insertion. On angiographic studies, a small blood vessel is consistently present on midline, running between the tendon lobes. One small vessel extends across the dorsal aspect of the DDFT connecting to the midline vessel at the level of the collateral sesamoidean ligament (CSL) (Figure 44.4). The DDFT is homogeneous and generally around 100 HU. In the distal pastern and heel bulb region, the digital sheath appears as a thin hypodense rim around the DDFT (Figure 44.2).

Distal interphalangeal collateral ligaments

The CLs of the DIP are paired, symmetric soft tissue structures that are housed almost completely below the coronary band. Proximally, the ligaments arise from the epicondylar fossae of the middle phalanx, abaxial and slightly dorsal. Near their proximal attachment their shape is ovoid to rectangular. These ligaments change in shape to become flatter in a medial to lateral direction and longer in a dorsal to palmar direction as they course distally. This change in shape appears as 'fanning' out on gross specimens. The CLs are homogeneous but their margins can be difficult to clearly delineate, particularly near their distal attachment to the distal phalanx. The CLs are slightly less dense than the DDFT at ± 80 HU.

Collateral sesamoidean ligament

The CSL is also known as the suspensory ligament of the navicular bone or, occasionally, the proximal ligament of the navicular bone. The ligamentous tissue is present as a tough band of soft tissue that crosses the entire proximal border of the navicular bone. At the proximal extremities of the bone, the ligament sends off the proximal attachments, medially and laterally. The proximal portions of both medial and lateral ligament extend proximally and dorsally to attach to the distal, dorsal aspect of the proximal phalanx.

Veterinary Computed Tomography, First Edition. Edited by Tobias Schwarz, Jimmy Saunders.

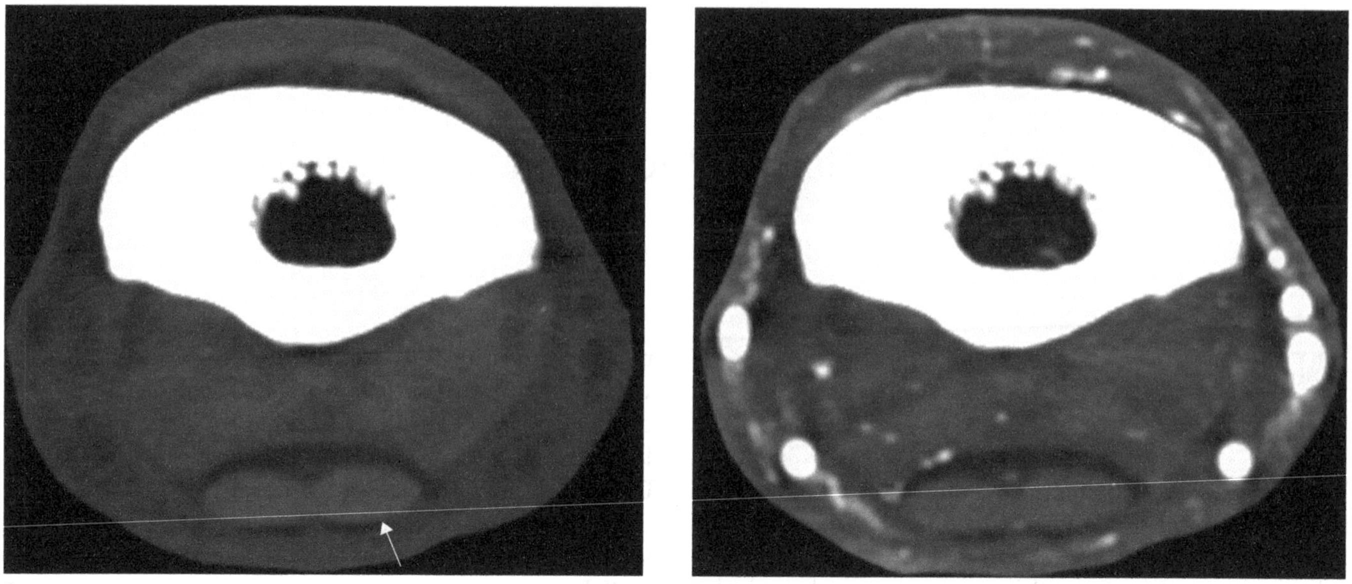

A B

Figure 44.1 Normal transverse CT images (A) without contrast and (B) with intra-arterial contrast made at the level of the distal aspect of the proximal phalanx. The DDFT has a bilobed, symmetric shape and is surrounded by the digital sheath (arrow).

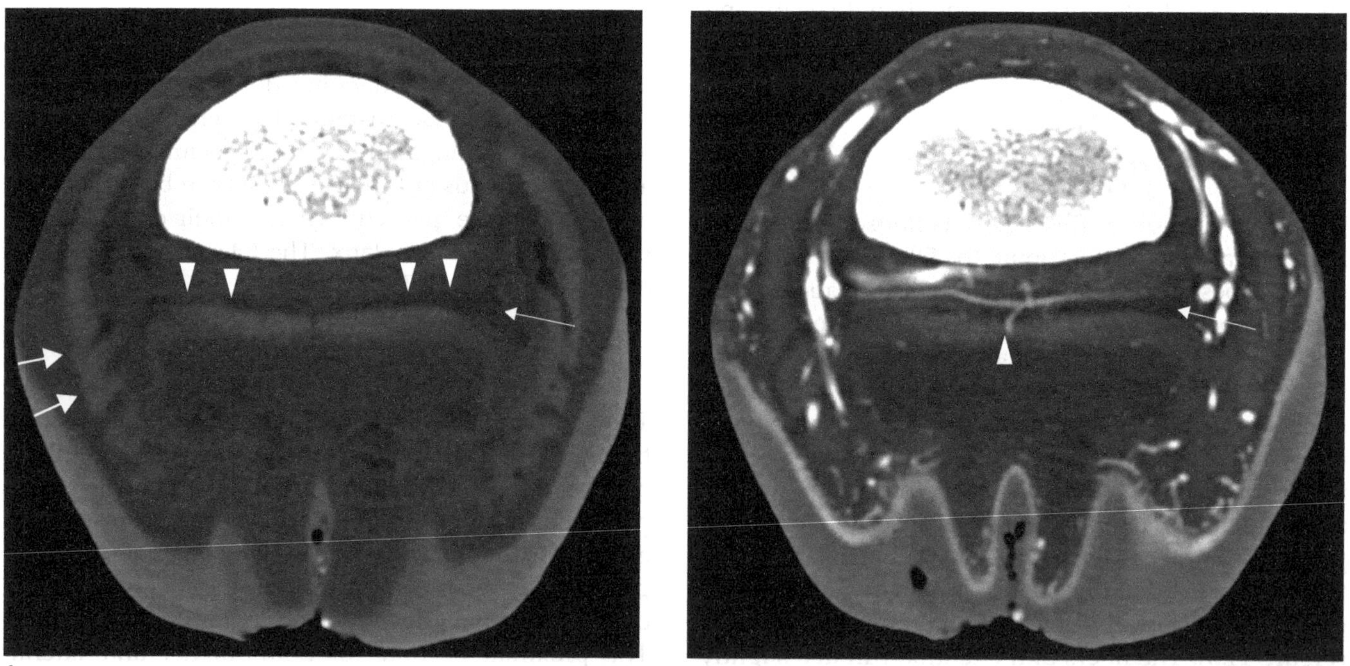

A B

Figure 44.2 Normal (A) pre- and (B) post-intra-arterial transverse CT images (level of the middle phalanx and navicular bursa). (A) The DDFT is flattened in a dorsal to palmar direction. There is a small amount of hypodense fluid within the navicular bursa (white arrow). The dorsal border of the navicular bursa is bound to the CSL (white arrowheads). The collateral or ungual cartilages are intermediate attenuation to hoof wall and soft tissues (large white arrows). (B) A small blood vessel crosses the entire dorsal aspect of the navicular bursa and a branch extends into the DDFT on mid-line (arrowhead).

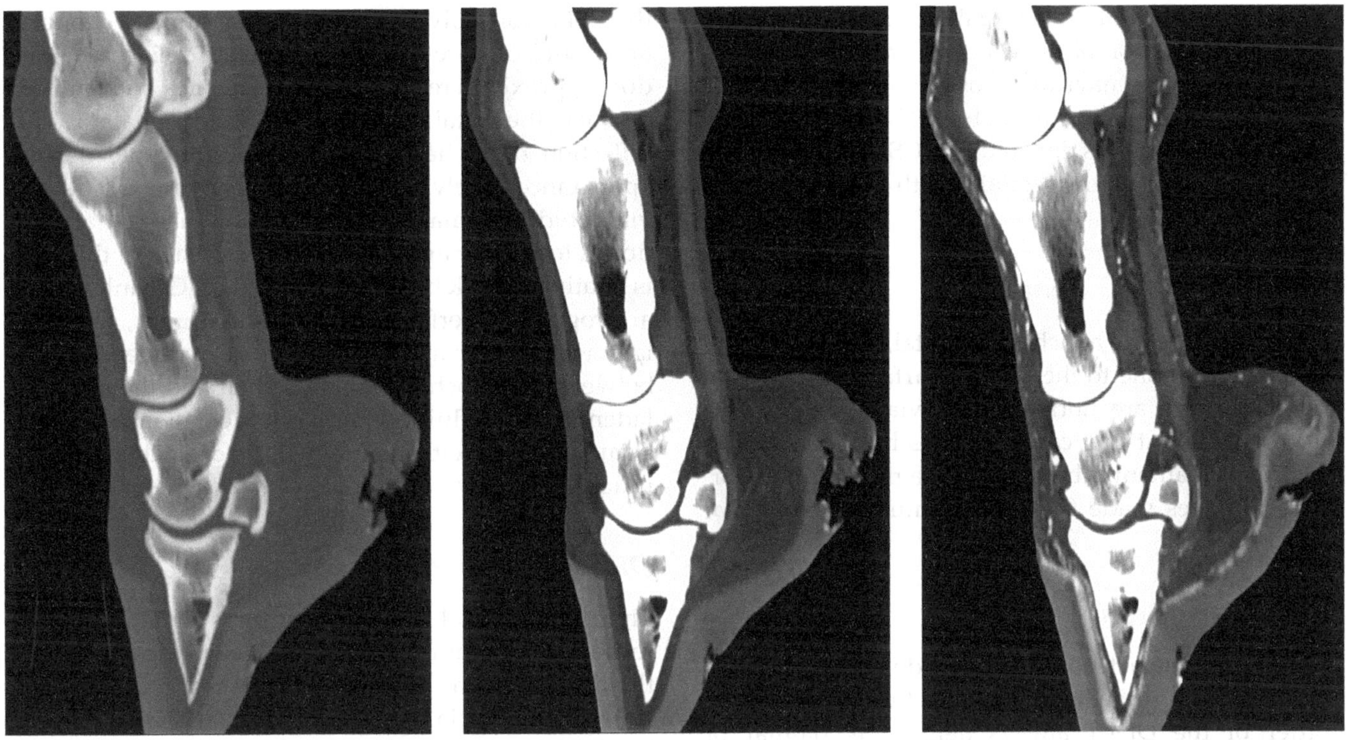

A B C

Figure 44.3 Normal sagittally reconstructed CT images in (A) a bone window, (B) a soft tissue window without contrast medium and (C) with intra-arterial contrast medium application.

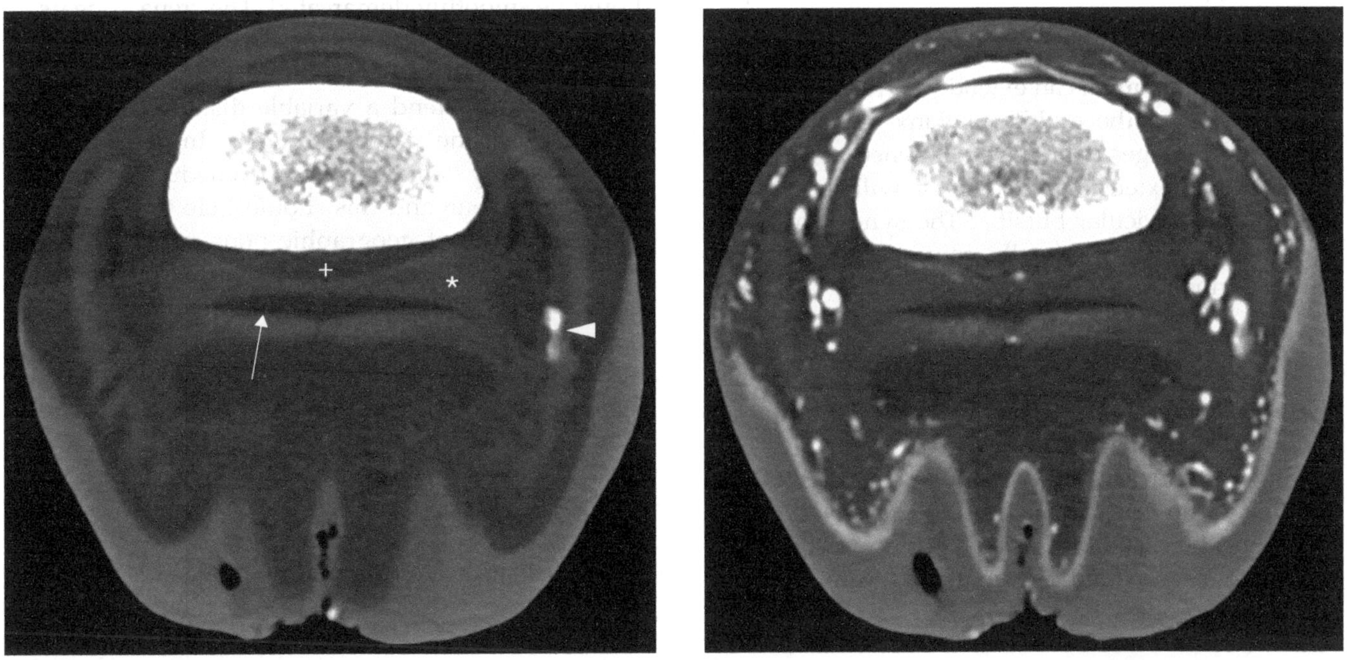

A B

Figure 44.4 Normal (A) pre- and (B) post-intra-arterial-contrast transverse CT images (level of the middle phalanx, navicular bursa and distal interphalangeal joint (+)) show a small amount of fluid in the navicular bursa (arrow). The collateral sesamoidean ligament is symmetric (asterisk). There is partial ossification of one collateral cartilage (arrowhead).

Proximally, the CSL is difficult to identify on CT images. The portion of the CSL that crosses the proximal border of the navicular bone separates the three synovial compartments of the foot. The palmar reflection of the DIP joint is dorsal to the CSL, the navicular bursa is palmar and the digital sheath is proximal and slightly palmar.

Navicular impar ligament

This small structure attaches the distal, flexor cortex of the navicular bone to the palmar surface of the distal phalanx. There are normally synovial invaginations into the ligament that can appear as hypodense mottling. This ligament is best seen on sagittal plane reformatted images made from thin (1 mm) transverse or helical images.

Navicular bursa

Locating the structures that provide its boundaries best identifies this synovial structure. The dorsal border of the DDFT always defines its palmar or plantar border. Distally, the palmar border of the impar ligament defines its dorsal border. The flexor cortex and fibrocartilage of the flexor cortex of the navicular bone define its dorsal border at this level. Proximal to the navicular bone, the proximal portion of the CSL defines its dorsal border. The synovial fluid of the bursa is hypodense and in the normal horse may protrude very slightly beyond the abaxial margins of the DDFT proximal to the navicular bone. The proximal reflection of the bursa can extend proximally to about the mid-level of the middle phalanx but on sagittal reformatted images maintains a flattened appearance. The proximal extension of the bursa will change dramatically in navicular bursitis. The synovium of the navicular bursa is minimally contrast enhancing on contrast-enhanced studies.

Collateral or ungual cartilage

These structures have density characteristics that are intermediate to the DDFT and the hoof capsule. These also have a robust system of vascular channels that are illuminated on contrast studies. They are well visualized from the distal and abaxial surface of the distal phalanx as they extend proximally to terminate proximal to the coronary band.

Distal interphalangeal joint

This joint is comprised of the middle and distal phalanges, the navicular bone, the impar ligament and the CSL. Normally, the peri-articular and subchondral bone surfaces are smooth and well delineated. The dorsal, proximal reflection of the joint can be identified dorsal to the distal condyle of the middle phalanx. This reflection often has a mottled, intermediate density appearance, likely representing synovium and synovial fluid. Normally, this reflection has a flattened dorsal to palmar appearance. The cartilage of this joint is relatively thick but not identified on CT unless a CT arthrogram is performed. On arthrography, the cartilage will appear as a thick layer of hypodense tissue between the subchondral bone shelf and the contrast-laden synovial fluid. It should appear symmetric and homogeneous with contrast limited to the synovial fluid.

Distal phalanx

There are several anatomic features of interest with respect to foot lameness. An exhaustive description of the distal phalanx anatomy will be reserved for other sources. The fascia flexoria of the distal phalanx should be smoothly margined with a clear line of demarcation between the dense bone of the soft tissue attachments and the trabecular bone of the marrow cavity. The distal attachments of the CL of the DIP joint are relatively shallow, narrow fossae that are located on the dorsolateral and dorsomedial aspects of the distal phalanx. The dorsal surface of the distal phalanx should be smoothly demarcated. The crena appears as a smoothly margined semi-circular indent in the dorsal border of the distal phalanx and is present in some horses. It will extend a variable distance proximally depending on the size of the crena. In general, there will be a clearly demarcated corticomedullary junction deep to the crena and this should help to distinguish it from an area of geographic bone lysis as seen in septic osteitis. The solar margin can appear irregularly margined with variably sized and orientated vascular canals. There is a vascular canal in the palmar processes that enters and exits at the periphery of the distal phalanx that can cause the false appearance of a solar margin fracture.

Middle phalanx

The dorsal surface of the middle phalanx is smoothly margined deep to the dorsal, proximal reflection of the DIP joint. The dorsal aspect of the epicondylar fossae at the proximal attachment of the CLs should be smooth and symmetric. The scutum of the palmar proximal aspect of the middle phalanx is the attachment of multiple soft tissues.

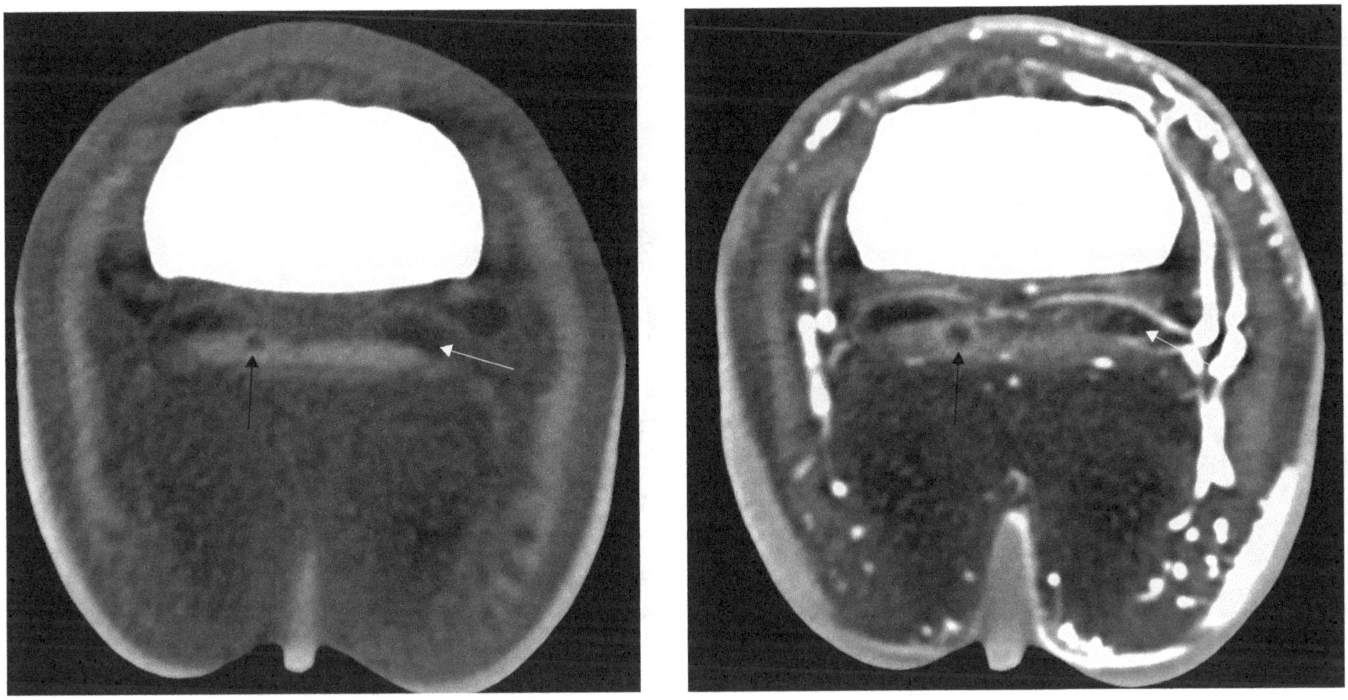

A B

Figure 44.5 (A) Pre- and (B) post-intra-arterial-contrast transverse (level of the middle phalanx) CT images of a horse with a peripherally enhancing DDFT lesion in one lobe (black arrow). Note the concurrent navicular bursa effusion (white arrow) with enhancement of the synovium.

Disease Features

Computed tomographic examination of the equine foot can be performed with or without contrast media. Evaluation of the bone column is adequately assessed in the absence of contrast medium; however, evaluation of the major soft tissue structures implicated in lameness arising from the foot is greatly improved by the addition of intra-arterial contrast media. Protocols allow for high quality, standardized image acquisition. When routine imaging protocols fail to yield a satisfactory answer for the clinical question at hand, the imaging clinician should consider other contrast-ameliorated procedures such as arthrography or bursography. This is of particular importance when we consider that most diagnostic anesthesia techniques are relatively non-specific.

Deep digital flexor tendinopathy

Deep digital flexor tendon injury can occur anywhere in the distal limb, and occasionally, multiple non-contiguous lesions will be identified. Lesions result in alterations in classic roentgenologic findings and often DDFT lesions will involve only one lobe thereby providing an internal control for comparison.

CT features (Figures 44.5 and 44.6)

- Prior to contrast administration:
  - enlarged injured tendon lobe resulting in shape change
  - poorly defined and irregular tendon margins
  - decreased tendon density, with the exception of chronic injury when soft tissue mineralization may occur
  - insertion site onto the distal phalanx: enthesopathy appearing as irregular marginations, proliferation or lysis.
- During regional intra-arterial infusion of contrast material:
  - the vast majority of DDFT injuries have a component of contrast enhancement through extravasation of contrast media or neovessel formation.

Distal interphalangeal collateral desmopathy

The anatomic location and orientation of the DIP collateral ligaments make them a difficult anatomic structure to evaluate with any imaging modality.

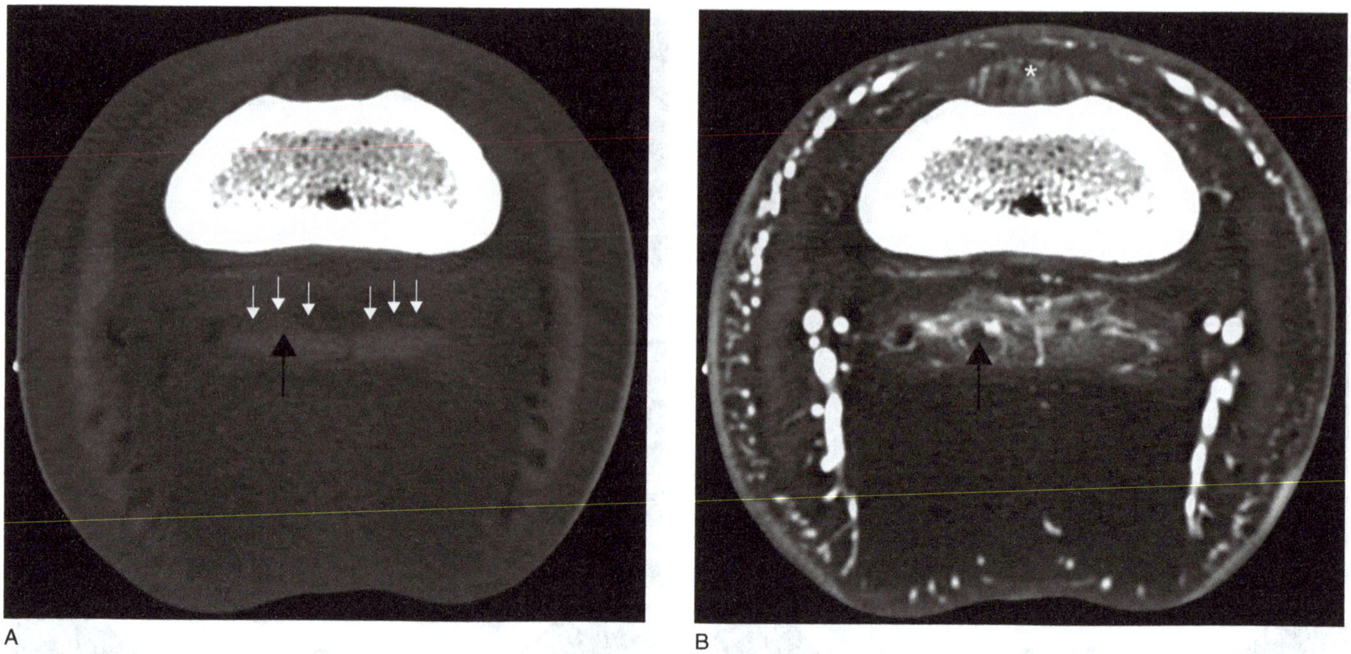

Figure 44.6 Adult horse with deep digital flexor tendinopathy. Transverse CT images made (level of the middle phalanx) (A) without contrast and (B) with intra-arterial contrast show bi-axial dorsal border erosions (white arrows) and a core to dorsal border lesion in one lobe (black arrow). Note that the entire dorsal border of the tendon is abnormally enhancing and new vessel formation is present in association with the core lesion. There is also synovial proliferation and enhancement in the dorsal reflection of the distal interphalangeal joint (asterisk).

CT features (Figure 44.7)

- Prior to contrast medium administration:
  - CLs regionally or focally hypodense
  - enlargement can be difficult to detect because of their confined anatomic location
  - the proximal and distal attachment sites should be carefully evaluated for bone proliferation or lysis.
- During regional intra-arterial infusion of contrast medium:
  - in general, the hypodense regions are expected to contrast enhance
  - infrequently, particularly with acute ligament injury, swelling within the hoof capsule will cause a regional perfusion deficit limited to the region of the CL.
- After intra-articular contrast medium administration:
  - contrast-laden synovial fluid will occasionally extend into defects in the CLs.

Collateral sesamoidean desmitis

Collateral sesamoidean desmitis commonly occurs with other podotrochlear apparatus pathology such as deep digital flexor tendonopathy, navicular bursitis and distal interphalangeal synovitis.

CT features

- Prior to contrast administration:
  - Enlargement and shape change of the ligament as it crosses the proximal border of the navicular bone. It is often best evaluated on reformatted sagittal plane images.
  - Frequently, this structure, when injured cannot be separated from the dorsal aspect of the deep digital flexor tendon.
  - The proximal portions of the ligament are difficult to identify on CT images.
- During regional intra-arterial infusion of contrast medium:
  - it is often heterogeneously moderately contrast enhancing.

Navicular impar desmitis

This diminutive ligament is difficult to evaluate on transverse images unless they are made perpendicular to its long axis. It is best evaluated on reformatted

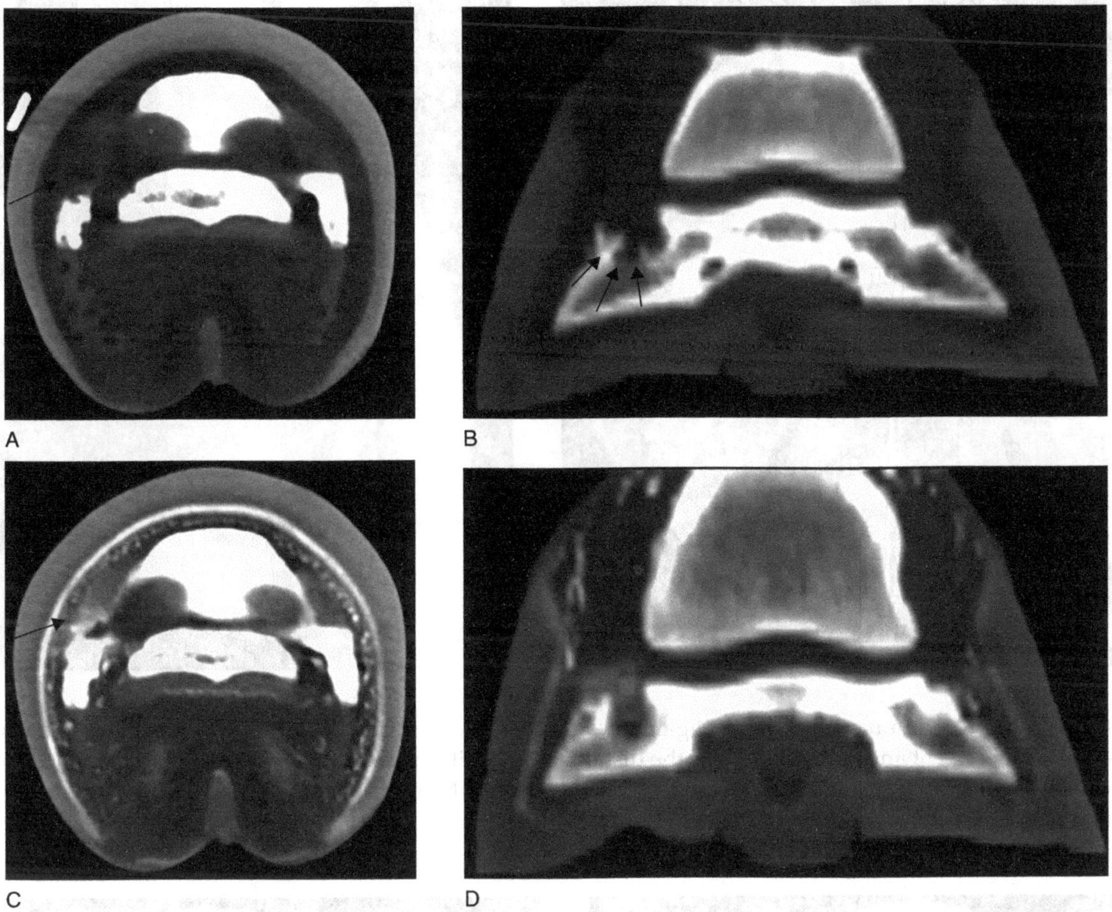

Figure 44.7 Adult horse with a severe desmopathy and enthesopathy of the lateral collateral ligament (LCL) of the distal interphalangeal joint. Pre-contrast (A) transverse and (B) frontally reconstructed CT images, and intra-arterial contrast (C) transverse and (D) frontally reconstructed CT images are shown. The LCL is enlarged and heterogeneous (large black arrow) when compared with the medial ligament. There is irregularly margined osseous resorption of the distal phalanx at the distal attachment site (small black arrows). There is amorphous contrast enhancement of the distal aspect of the LCL.

images made either in a sagittal plane or transverse to its long axis. Depending on the orientation of the distal limb during scanning, this can require reformatting from volume data.

CT features (Figure 44.8)

- Prior to contrast medium administration:
  - enlargement of the ligament, loss of the normally mottled architecture.
- During regional intra-arterial infusion of contrast medium:
  - contrast enhancement distal to the navicular bone.

Navicular bursitis

The hallmark feature of bursitis is synovial effusion. It is important to consider the underlying cause of bursitis, and the deep digital flexor tendon dorsal border and palmar navicular bone should be closely scrutinized for lesions.

CT features (Figure 44.9)

- Prior to contrast medium administration:
  - distention of the bursa with low-density fluid within the expected anatomic limits of the structure
  - the fluid accumulation can cause dorsal displacement of the soft tissues dividing the palmar aspect of the DIP joint and the dorsal aspect of the navicular bursa
  - subacute and chronic bursal distention will cause extension of the synovial space abaxially and proximally.
- During regional intra-arterial infusion of contrast medium:
  - the synovial lining is variably contrast enhancing but generally moderate to markedly enhancing with active synovitis.

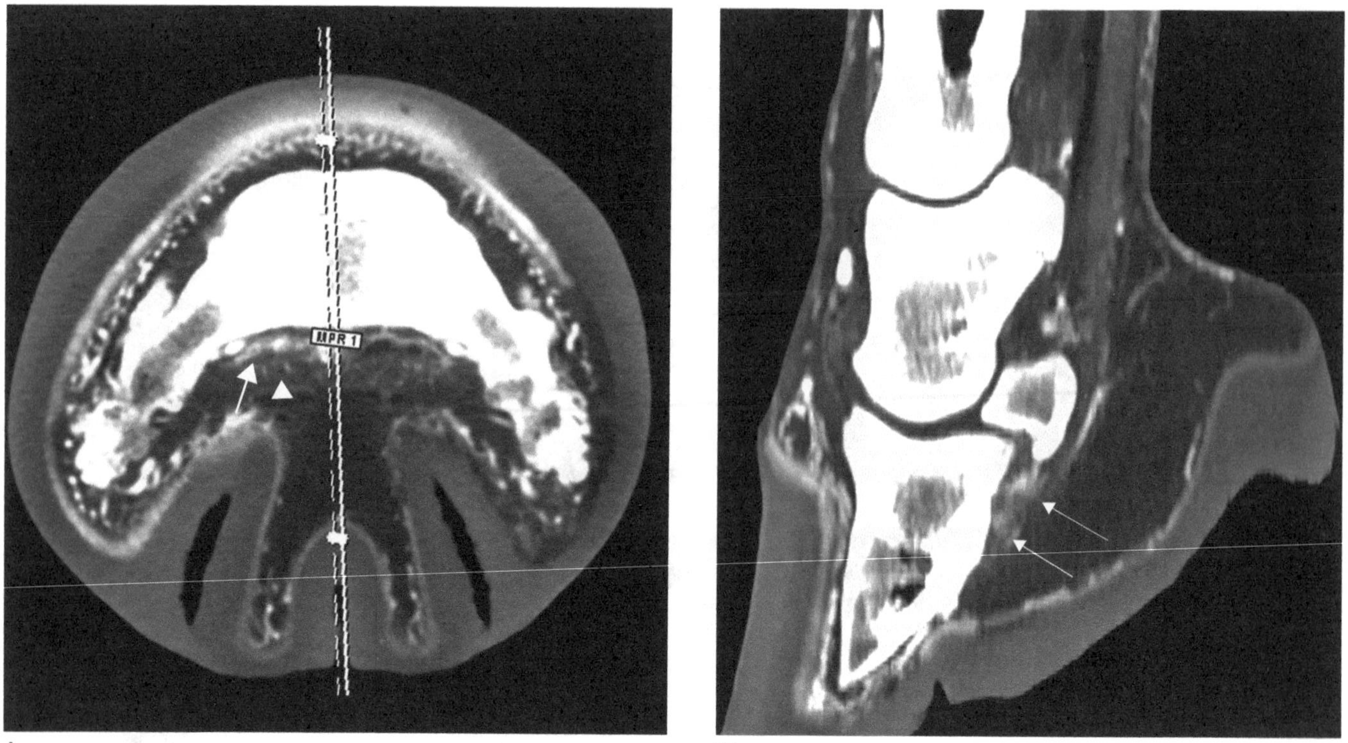

A B

Figure 44.8 Adult horse with navicular impar ligament desmitis. Intra-arterial (A) transverse (level of the distal phalanx) CT image shows enlargement and enhancement of the distal DDFT (white arrowhead) and the impar ligament (white arrow). (B) This shows well on the sagittally reconstructed CT image where the impar ligament and the DDFT can no longer be identified as separate structures (white arrows).

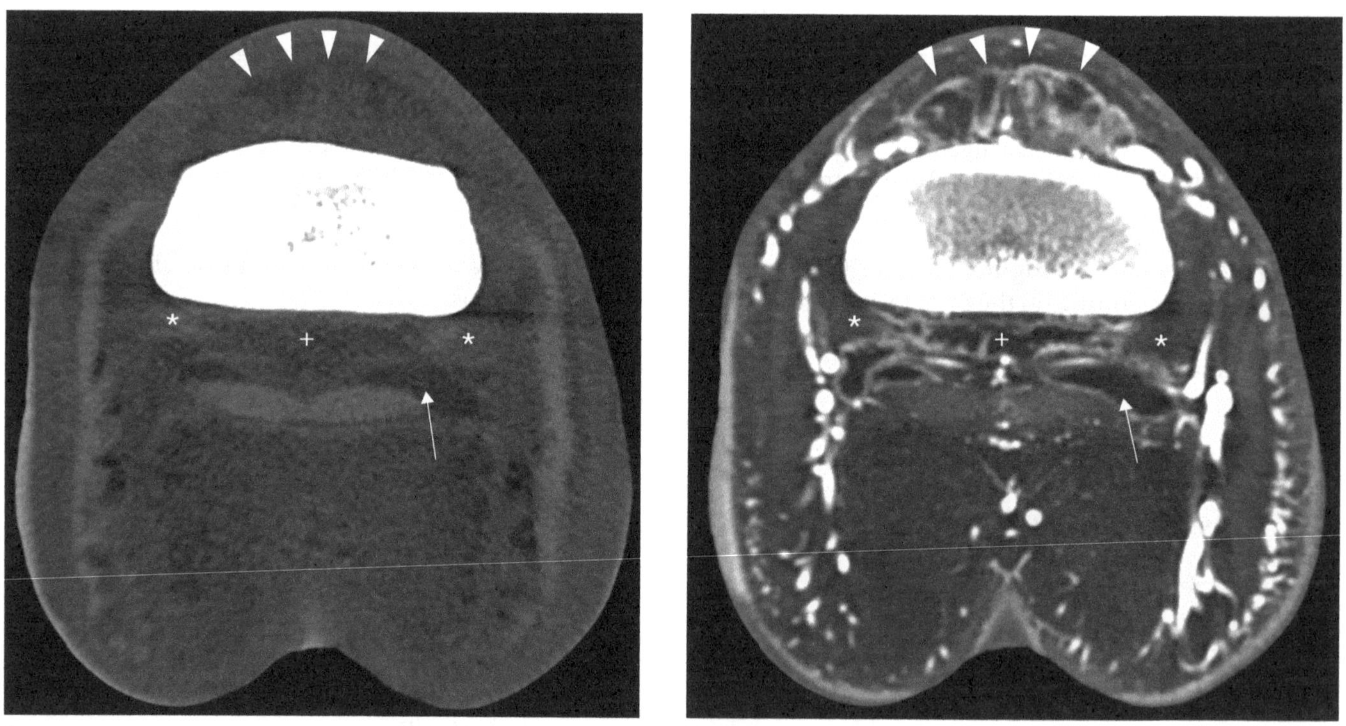

A B

Figure 44.9 Adult horse with synovitis of the distal interphalangeal (DIP) joint and navicular bursitis. Transverse CT images (A) without contrast and (B) with intra-arterial contrast (level of the middle phalanx, navicular bursa and DIP joint) show a severe effusion of the navicular bursa (white arrow) and DIP joint (+). The dorsal reflection of the DIP joint has synovial proliferation and marked synovial enhancement (white arrowheads). The collateral sesamoidean ligament is asymmetric (asterisk).

Ossification of the collateral cartilages

Mineralization of the collateral cartilages is readily identified on CT. Its significance must be evaluated in light of the clinical signs and presence of other pathology.

Contrast enhancement and tendon healing

The pattern of contrast enhancement in tendon injuries changes over time. Two common patterns are most frequently seen.

- Lesions that are seen to have a peripheral rim of contrast enhancement with a central avascular portion will fill in with vascularized tissue.
- Lesions that have amorphous enhancement will become more organized, frequently with a decrease in the overall quantity of enhancement. Vessel ingrowth will also occur with more clearly defined blood vessels margins.

Further Reading

Puchalski SM, Galuppo LD, Hornof WJ and Wisner ER (2007) Intraarterial contrast-enhanced computed tomography of the equine distal extremity. *Vet Radiol Ultrasound* **48**: 21–9.

Puchalski SM, Galuppo LD, Drew CP and Wisner ER (2009) Use of contrast-enhanced computed tomography to assess angiogenesis in deep digital flexor tendonopathy in a horse. *Vet Radiol Ultrasound* **44**: 292–7.

Puchalski SM, Snyder JR, Hornof WJ, Macdonald MH and Galuppo LD (2005) Contrast enhanced computed tomography of the equine distal extremity. In: 51 Annual Convention of the AAEP, ivis.org, Seattle, WA, USA.

CHAPTER FORTY-FIVE

EQUINE FETLOCK

Katrien Vanderperren and Hendrik-Jan Bergman

CT: ANATOMY AND NORMAL VARIANTS (FIGURES 45.1 AND 45.2)

The equine fetlock joint is a high motion joint composed of the third metacarpal/metatarsal bone, the proximal phalanx and two proximal sesamoid bones.

The bony components of the joint can be seen in great detail with CT. There is some shape variation between the proximal sesamoid bones with the medial proximal sesamoid bone being more cuboidal than the lateral one and with the proximal sesamoid bones of the forelimbs being more elongated and triangular than the ones of the hindlimb.

Anatomic variation in thickness and bone density of the subchondral bone exists between different regions of the distal condyles of the third metacarpal/metatarsal bones. This variation is dependent on training and is generally more marked in horses undergoing intense training. A zone of increased density runs obliquely from the palmar/plantar apical region of the third metacarpal/metatarsal bone to the dorsal proximal aspect of the distal epiphysis. The subchondral bone of the palmar/plantar distal aspect of the condyles is more dense compared to the bone deep to the sagittal ridge on the palmar/plantar aspects. The lateral condyle usually appears more dense than the medial.

Most soft tissue components of the fetlock region can be well identified by using the soft tissue settings. However, the distinction of structures with the same density remains difficult (i.e. superficial and deep parts of the collateral ligaments, distal sesamoidean ligaments (short and oblique; cruciate and straight), collateral sesamoidean ligaments with superficial part of the collateral ligaments). Regional intra-arterial contrast infusion can be used for the evaluation of these soft tissue structures. The main indication of CT in the fetlock region is desmitis of the distal sesamoidean ligaments. The straight, oblique, cruciate and short sesamoidean ligaments are a part of the suspensory apparatus, preventing hyperextension of the fetlock joint. All distal sesamoidean ligaments originate from the base of the proximal sesamoid bones and the palmar ligament. The straight sesamoidean ligament inserts on the proximal aspect of the middle phalanx, whereas the other distal sesamoidean ligaments insert on the proximal phalanx.

The articular cartilage in the fetlock joint is 1 mm thick at the proximal aspect of the joint and becomes thinner distally (0.4–0.5 mm); it can be identified after the administration of intra-articular contrast medium.

DISEASE FEATURES

Osteoarthrosis

The fetlock joint is frequently affected by osteoarthritic changes, which can be primary or secondary. Primary osteoarthrosis refers to an age-related disease of the joint, whereas secondary osteoarthrosis is associated with previous damage to the joint. Chronic mechanical overload leads to a common fetlock osteoarthrosis in the palmar/plantar aspect of the metacarpal/metatarsal condyles of racehorses, also called palmar/plantar osteochondral disease.

CT features (Figures 45.1 and 45.3–45.5)

- Prior to contrast medium administration:
  - joint distention due to effusion and swelling
  - resorptive subchondral bone lesions
  - changes in subchondral density
  - subchondral bone sclerosis
  - osteophytes at joint margins and/or enthesiophytes at sites of capsular/ligaments insertions
  - narrowing of joint space
  - palmar/plantar osteochondral disease: resorptive subchondral bone lesions in the palmar/plantar aspect of the metacarpal/metatarsal condyles.

Veterinary Computed Tomography, First Edition. Edited by Tobias Schwarz, Jimmy Saunders.

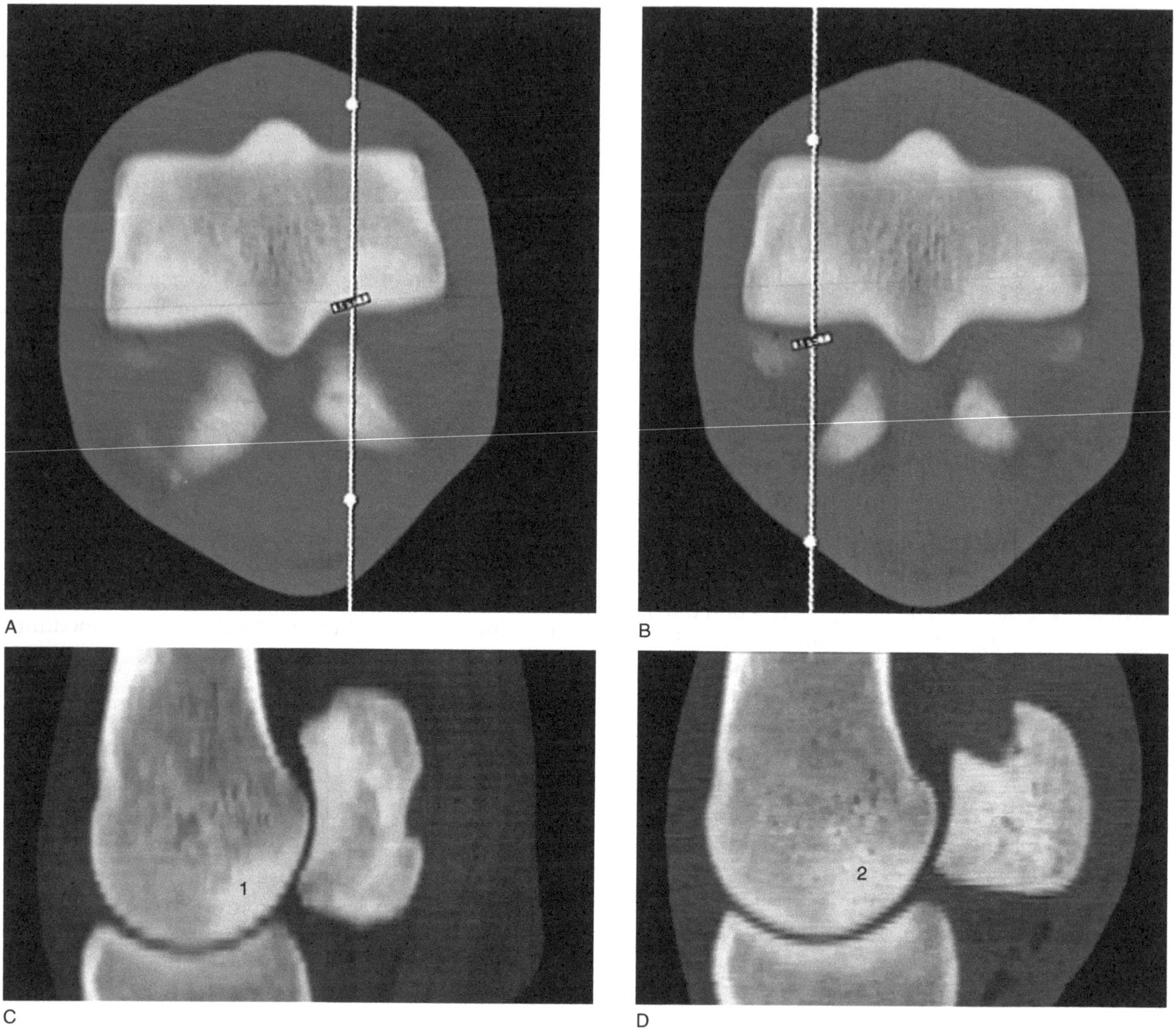

Figure 45.1 (A,B) Transverse and (C,D) sagittal reconstructed CT images of a right fetlock joint of thoroughbred race horse in training. (A) The lateral aspect of the condyle shows mild sclerosis and (B) the medial aspect shows moderate sclerosis of the palmar aspect of the metacarpal condyle. 1 = mild degree of sclerosis; 2 = moderate increase of subchondral bone sclerosis. White lines in (A) and (B) denote scan plane for (C) and (D) respectively (images courtesy of Sarah Puchalski, University of Davis, California).

- After intra-articular contrast medium administration:
  - cartilage defects: partial to full penetration of contrast medium in the articular cartilage
  - cartilage fragment can also be present
  - cartilage thickening/thinning: increased/decreased space between the subchondral bone and contrast medium
  - palmar/plantar osteochondral disease: minimal to severe disruption of articular cartilage, collapse of the articular surface in the palmar/plantar aspect of the metacarpal/metatarsal condyles.

Subchondral bone cysts

Subchondral bone cysts or 'osseous cyst like lesions' are usually seen in young horses. Trauma to the cartilage or subchondral bone, infiltration of synovial fluid through an articular defect, chronic osteoarthritis, fracture, ischemia and inflammation have been proposed as potential causes. Subchondral cystic lesions may

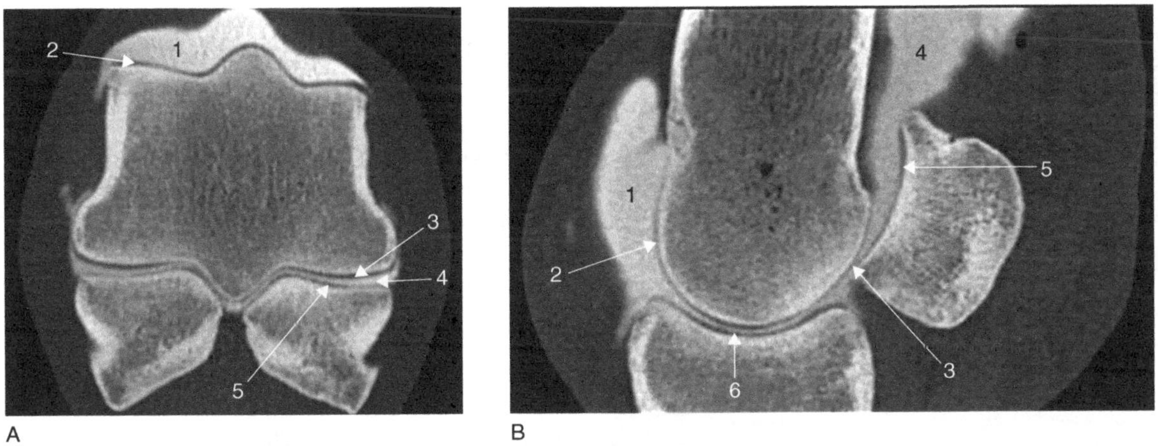

Figure 45.2 (A) Transverse and (B) sagittally reconstructed CT images obtained after intra-articular administration of contrast medium in a left fetlock joint of a normal horse demonstrating the cartilage. 1 = contrast medium in the dorsal synovial recess; 2 = cartilage of the dorsal aspect of the condyle of the third metacarpal bone; 3 = cartilage of the palmar aspect of the condyle of the third metacarpal bone; 4 = contrast medium in the palmar synovial recess; 5 = cartilage of the proximal sesamoid bone; 6 = cartilage of the proximal phalanx.

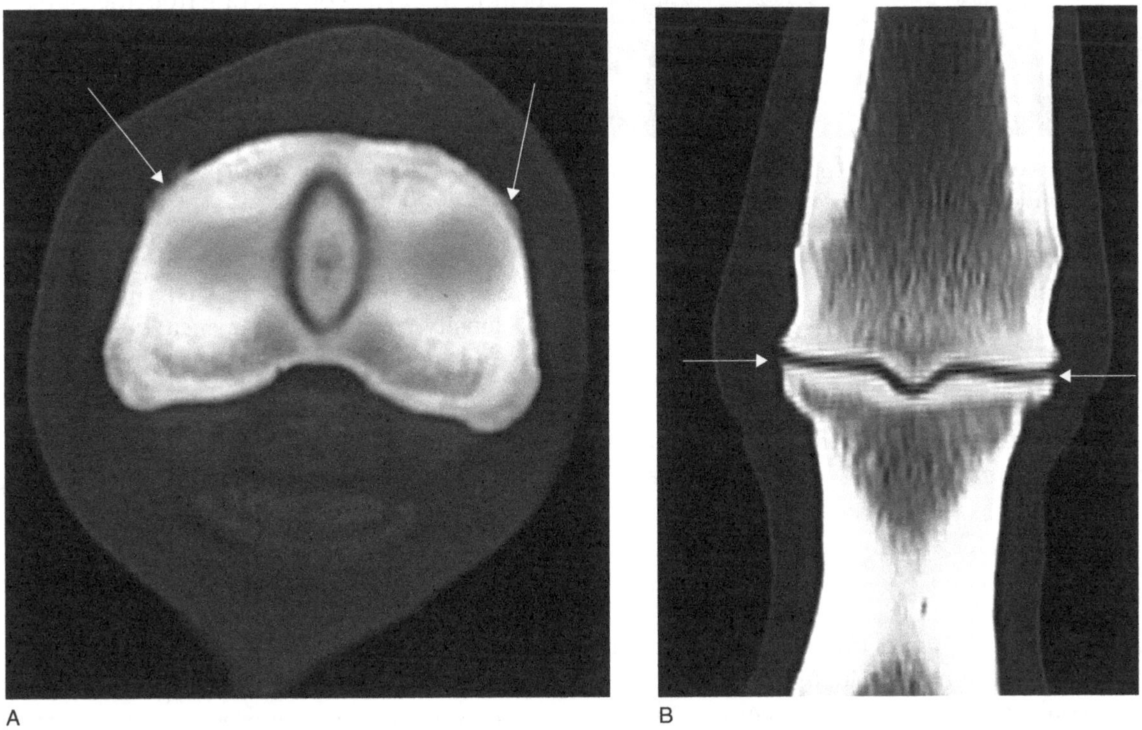

Figure 45.3 (A) Transverse and (B) frontally reconstructed CT images of a right fetlock joint with osteoarthrosis. 1 = rim of periarticular new bone formation on the dorsomedial and dorsolateral aspect of the proximal phalanx is present; 2 = new bone formation at the articular margins.

occur in the condyles (medial > lateral) of the distal third metacarpal, less frequently metatarsal bone, the proximal sesamoid bones and the proximal phalanx.

CT features (Figure 45.6)

- Prior to contrast medium administration:
  - hypodense focus (lucent defect), varying in size and shape, surrounded by a sclerotic border (rim)
  - communication with the adjacent joint is often identifiable. Most subchondral cystic lesions of the condyles open to the joint just dorsal to the transverse ridge.
- During regional intra-arterial infusion of contrast medium:
  - enhancement of the soft tissue within the defect.

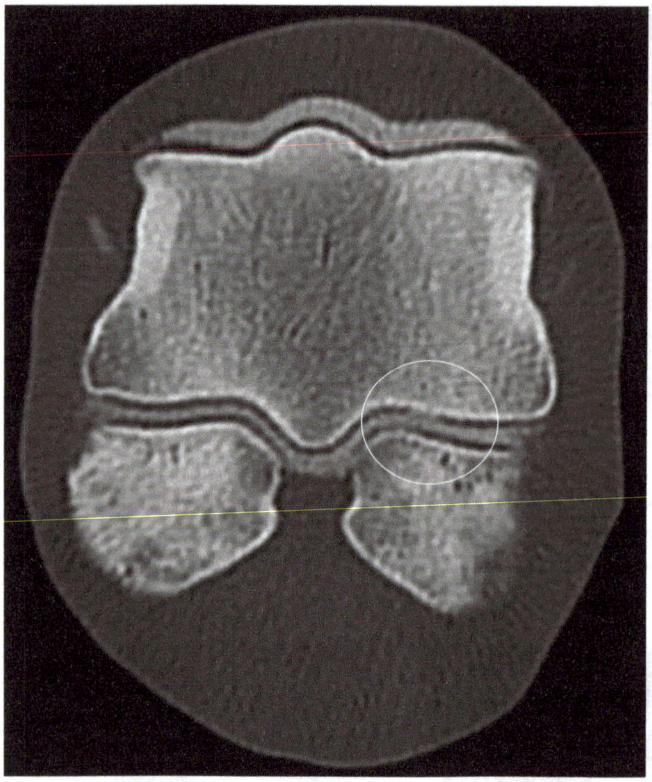

Figure 45.4 Transverse CT image obtained after intra-articular administration of contrast medium in a right fetlock joint with a small full-thickness cartilage lesion in the medial palmar condyle. A small defect in the cartilage is filled with contrast material (circle).

- After intra-articular contrast administration:
  - contrast medium can enter (fill) the defect confirming a communication with the joint space.

Osteomyelitis of the proximal sesamoid bones

The entire proximal sesamoid bone can be affected. However, an unusual sesamoidean infection involving most of the axial borders of the proximal sesamoids has been described, where either one or both proximal sesamoid bones can be affected. This disorder is typically associated with inflammation of the palmar (intersesamoidean) ligament.

CT features (Figures 45.7 and 45.8)

- Prior to contrast medium administration:
  - cavitary lesions within cancellous bone
  - axial border bone destruction (primarily at the mid-body and apical region of the axial borders, although the whole proximal sesamoid bone can be involved).
- During regional intra-arterial infusion of contrast medium:
  - disruption/reduction/thickening of the palmar ligament
  - contrast enhancing palmar ligament
  - new vessel formation.
- After intra-articular contrast medium administration:
  - detection of possible communication of the joint space with the lytic lesions.

Osteochondral fragments

Fragments in the fetlock joint occur at different sites. In the dorsal part of the joint, fragments can be seen at the sagittal ridge or the condyles of the third metacarpal/metatarsal bone, in the synovial pad and at the dorsoproximal end of the proximal phalanx. Fragments at the palmar (plantar) aspect of the fetlock joint include fragments originating from the palmar/plantar aspect of the proximal phalanx immediately medial or lateral to the sagittal groove, fragments arising from the palmar/plantar eminence of the proximal phalanx, fragments deriving from the base of the proximal sesamoid bone and fragments originating from the palmar/plantar condyles.

CT features (Figure 45.9)

- Separate osseous fragments with a low density or density similar to the cortical bone.
- Adjacent indentation (not always present).

Fractures

Fractures of the fetlock joint are discussed in Chapter 43.

Soft tissue injuries

Desmitis of the sesamoidean ligaments

Injuries of the oblique and straight sesamoidean ligaments are common. Injuries of the cruciate sesamoidean ligaments have been described, whereas desmitis of the short sesamoidean ligaments has not been reported.

CT features (Figures 45.10 and 45.11)

- Prior to contrast medium administration:
  - enlargement of the ligament
  - heterogeneous, hypodense appearance of the ligament
  - hypodense defects at the attachments of the ligaments
  - small bony fragments at the attachment sites.

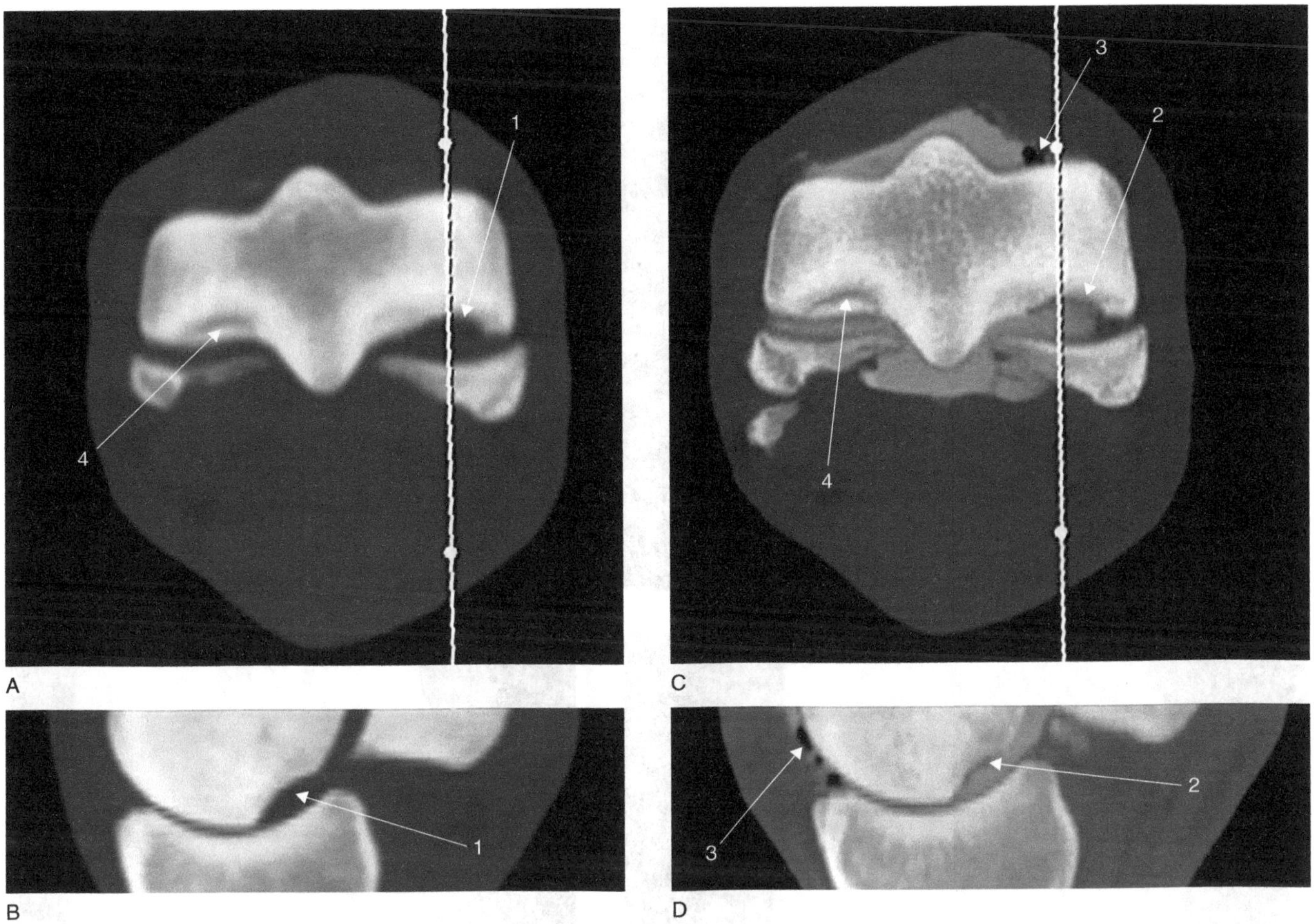

Figure 45.5 (A,C) Transverse and (B,D) sagittally reconstructed CT images of the left front fetlock joint before and after administration of intra-articular contrast medium in a horse with palmar osteochondral disease. 1 = bone defect in the palmarodistal aspect of the medial metacarpal condyle surrounded by sclerosis; 2 = loss of articular cartilage and subchondral bone; 3 = small air bubbles due to intra-articular injection of contrast medium; 4 = small osteochondral fragment at the palmar aspect of the lateral condyle. White lines in (A) and (C) denote scan plane for (B) and (D) respectively (images courtesy of Sarah Puchalski, University of Davis, California).

- During regional intra-arterial infusion of contrast medium:
  - mild to severe, focal to diffuse enhancement of the ligament
  - new vessel formation.

Further Reading

Firth EC, Rogers CW, Doube M and Jopson NB (2005) Musculoskeletal responses of 2-year old Thoroughbred horses to early training. 6. Bone parameters in the third metacarpal and third metatarsal bones. *NZ Vet J* **53**: 101–12.

Hanson JA, Seeherman HJ, Kirker-Head CA and O'Callaghan MW (1996) The role of computed tomography in evaluation of subchondral osseous lesions in seven horses with chronic synovitis. *Eq Vet J* **28**: 480–8.

Riggs CM, Whitehouse GH and Boyde A (1999) Structural variation of the distal condyles of the third metacarpal and third metatarsal bones in the horse. *Eq Vet J* **31**: 130–9.

Rijkenhuizen ABM, van den Top GB and van den Belt AJ (2005) The role of computer tomography in the surgical management of cystic lesions. *Pferdeheilkunde* **21**: 317–21.

Vanderperren K, Ghaye B, Snaps F and Saunders JH (2008) Evaluation of computed tomographic anatomy of the equine metacarpophalangeal joint. *Am J Vet Res* **69**: 631–8.

Young BD, Samii VF, Mattoon JS, Weisbrode SE and Bertone AL (2007) Subchondral bone density and cartilage degeneration patterns in osteoarthritic metacarpal condyles of horses. *Am J Vet Res* **68**: 841–9.

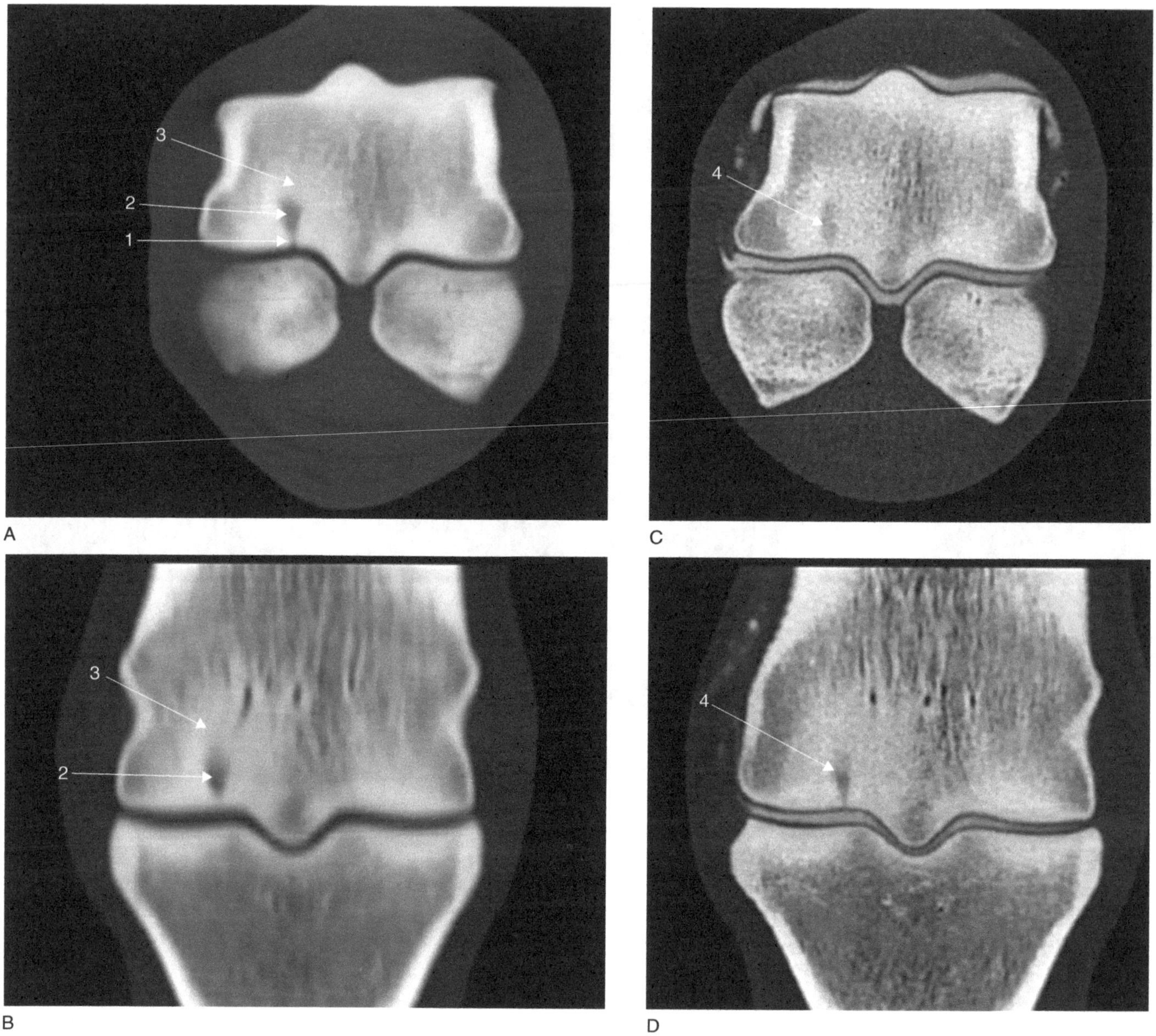

Figure 45.6 (A,C) Transverse and (B,D) frontally reconstructed CT images obtained before and after intra-articular administration of contrast medium of a horse with an incomplete fracture of the distal third metacarpal condyle with osseous cyst like lesion formation (right fetlock joint). There is a lucent fissure (1) extending from the palmar aspect of the distal third metacarpal condyle. As it extends dorsally, it enlarges into a cystic lucency (2) with a surrounding rim of sclerosis (3). After the arthrogram, contrast medium is suspected to be within the lucent lesion (4).

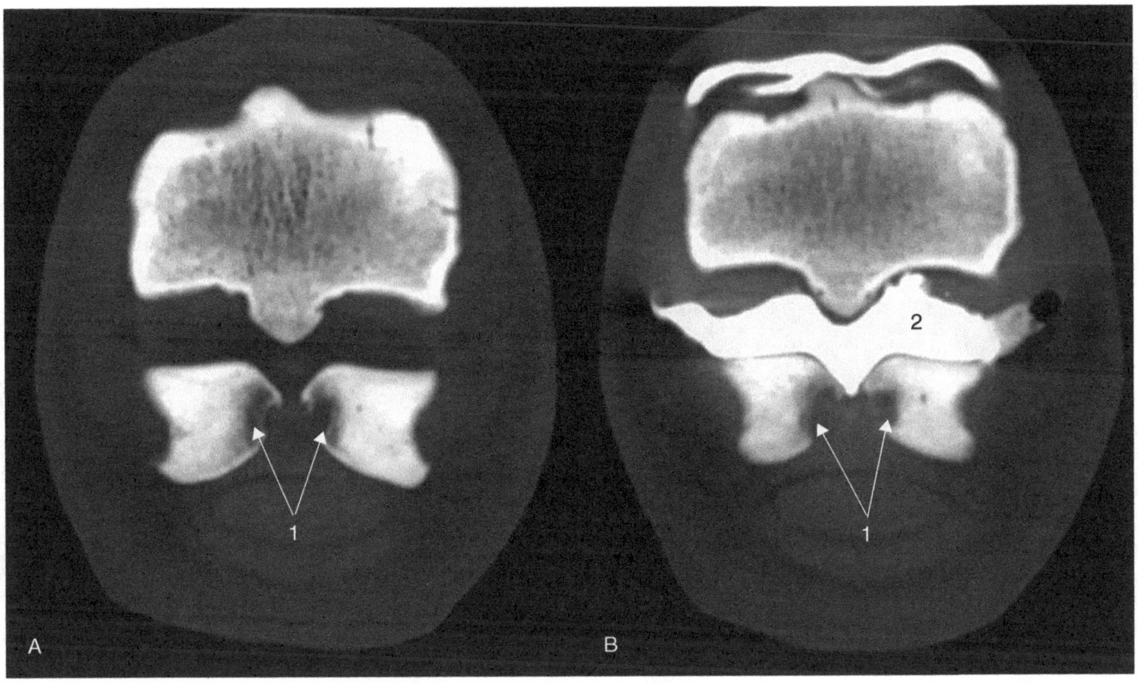

Figure 45.7 Transverse CT images of the right metatarsophalangeal joint prior to (A) and after (B) administration of intra-articular contrast medium. 1 = osteolysis of the axial aspects of both proximal sesamoid bones. After administration of contrast medium (2) into the metatarsophalangeal joint, the plantar aspect of the joint margin is maintained. No direct communication of the joint space and the lytic lesions is identified.

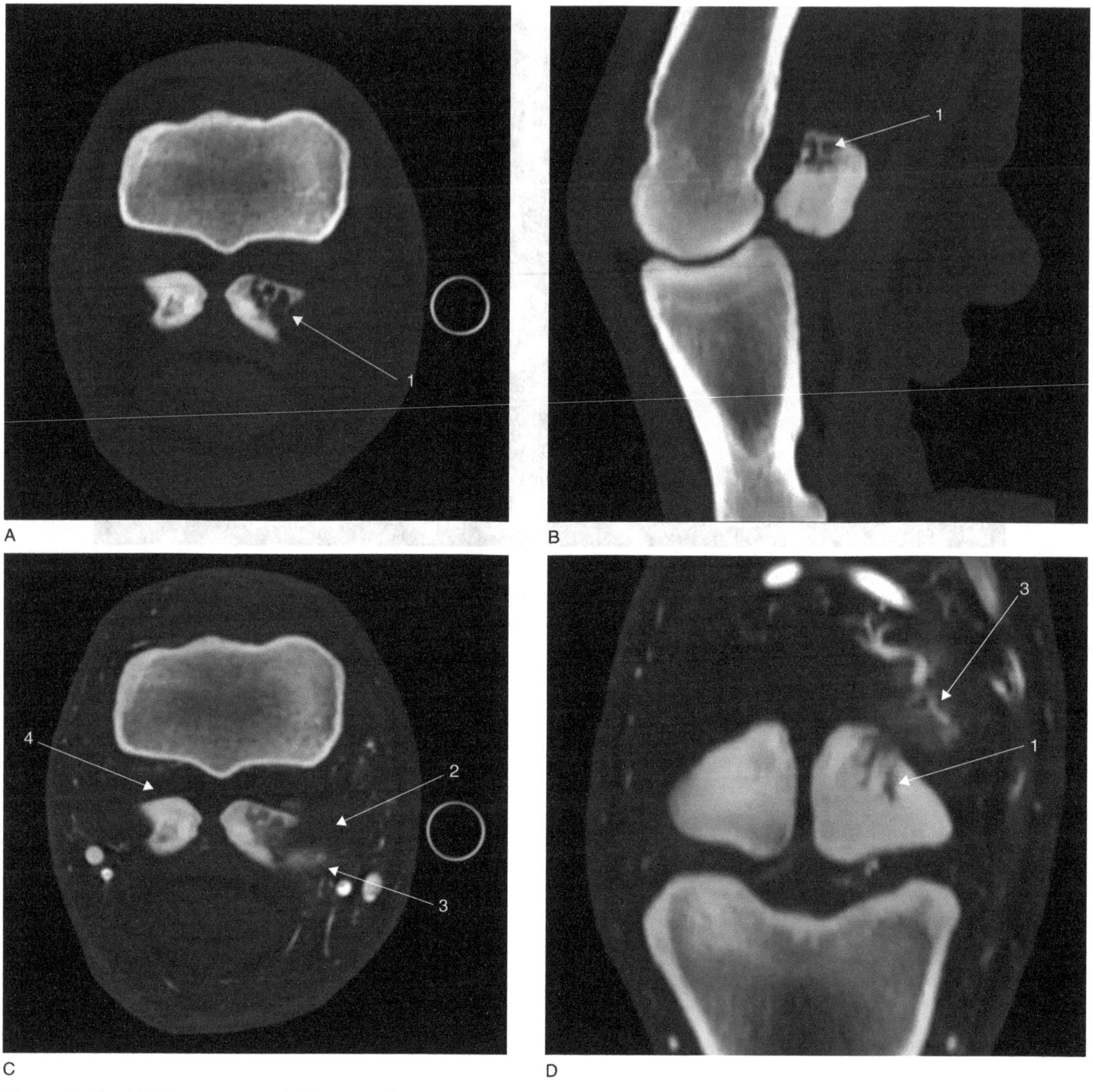

Figure 45.8 (A) Transverse and (B) sagittally reconstructed CT images prior to and (C) transverse and (D) frontally reconstructed CT images after regional intra-arterial administration of contrast medium of a hindlimb with osteomyelitis of the medial proximal sesamoid bone and severe desmopathy of the suspensory ligament at the proximal sesamoid bone on a right fetlock joint. 1 = marked, irregularly margined osteolysis of the entire medial proximal sesamoid bone, most pronounced at the abaxial border; 2 = enlarged, hypodense, irregularly margined medial branch of the suspensory ligament; 3 = the ligament is markedly contrast enhancing. Note also the marked soft tissue swelling surrounding the medial suspensory branch; 4 = moderate metatarsophalangeal joint effusion.

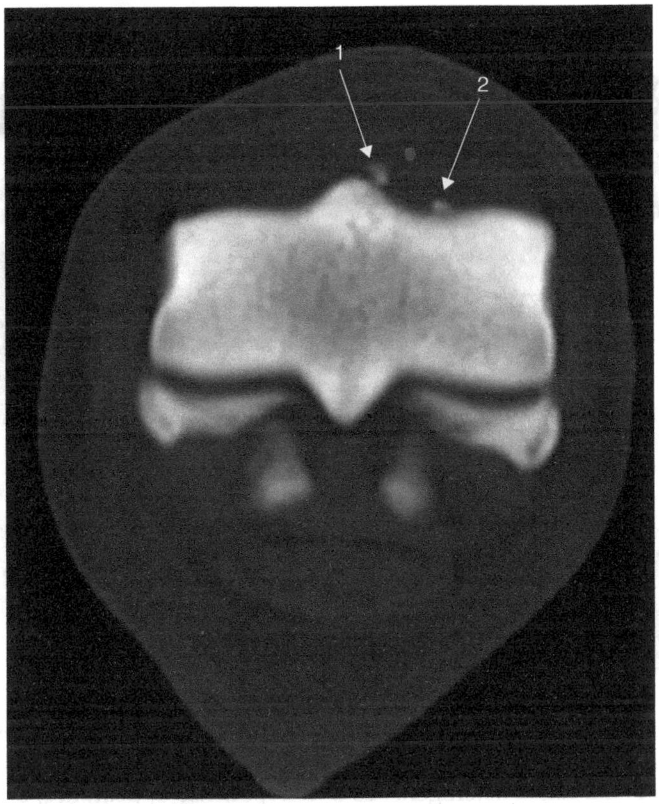

Figure 45.9 Transverse CT image of a horse with two osseous fragments in the dorsal compartment of the right fetlock joint. 1 = small low-density fragment dorsal to the sagittal ridge; 2 = smaller low-density fragment just dorsal to the medial condyle.

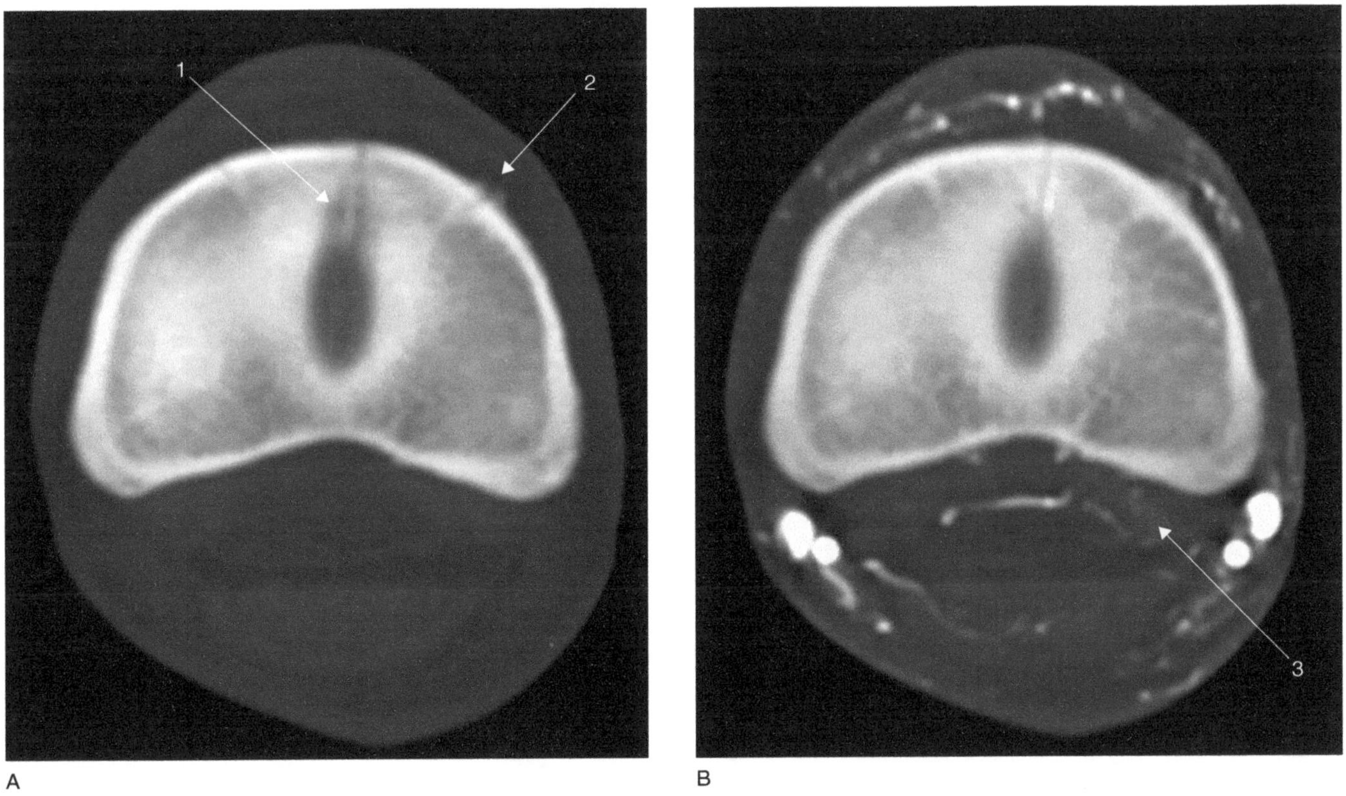

Figure 45.10 (A) Transverse pre-contrast and (B) post-contrast CT images of a horse with an incomplete fracture of the first phalanx and lateral oblique sesamoidean ligament injury (left fetlock). This horse was lame for 6 weeks and radiographs and ultrasound were negative. 1 = clearly demarcated cleft in the proximal subchondral bone plate of the proximal first phalanx; 2 = irregular periosteal proliferation at the dorsal margin of the proximal phalanx; 3 = lateral oblique sesamoidean ligament with marked contrast enhancement. These two conditions are sometimes seen together.

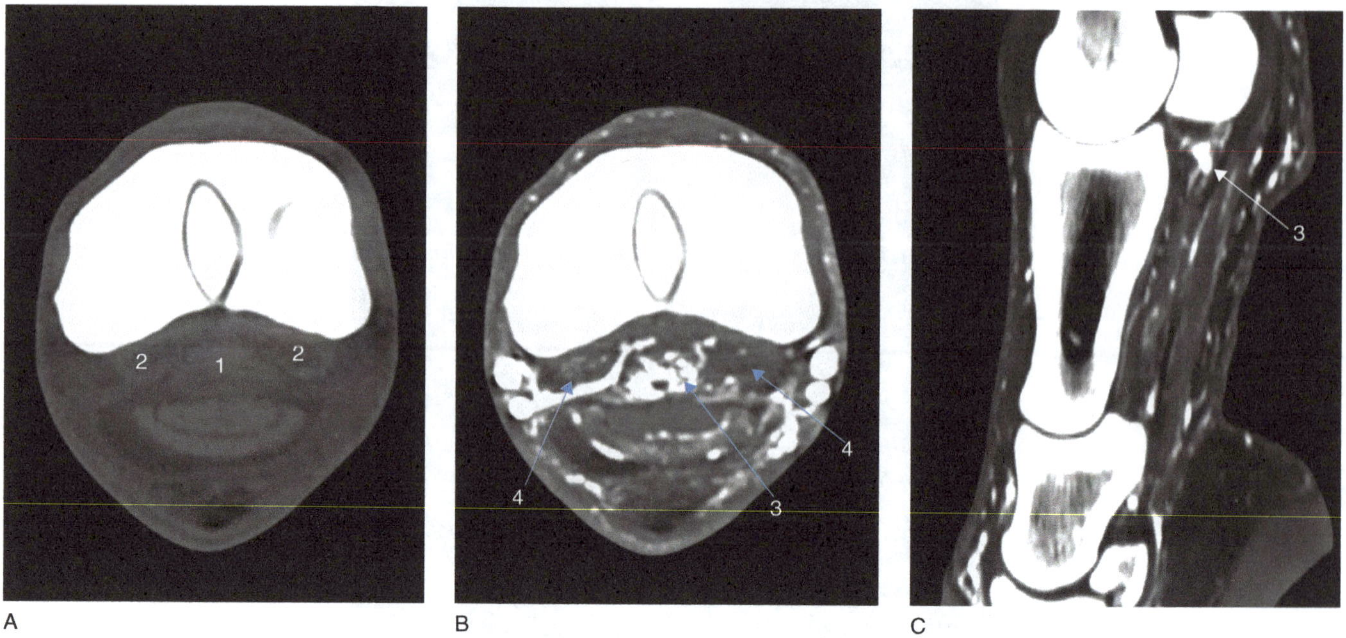

Figure 45.11 (A) Transverse pre-contrast, (B) transverse and (C) sagittal post-contrast CT images of a horse with a proximal straight sesamoidean ligament desmopathy and mild bi-axial oblique sesamoidean desmitis (left fetlock). 1 = the straight sesamoidean ligament is enlarged and has a heterogeneous and hypodense appearance; 2 = the oblique sesamoidean ligaments are mildly hypodense; 3 = diffuse contrast enhancement of the straight sesamoidean ligament; 4 = the oblique sesamoidean ligaments show mild contrast enhancement.

CHAPTER FORTY-SIX

Equine Upper Limbs (Carpus, Tarsus, Stifle)

Hendrik-Jan Bergman and Jimmy Saunders

The disorders discussed in this chapter will be restricted to those for which CT represents a clear diagnostic surplus value compared with other imaging modalities.

CT: Anatomy and Normal Variants (Table 46.1)

A detailed CT anatomy description of the carpal, tarsal and stifle joints already exists. The CT anatomy will focus on the features relevant for the clinical disorders that are discussed in this chapter.

The carpal region

CT is particularly useful for diagnosis of injuries affecting the carpal bones (sclerosis, fracture), the wall and contents of the carpal sheath (deep digital flexor tendon, superficial digital flexor tendon, accessory ligament of the superficial digital flexor tendon, flexor retinaculum, palmar carpal ligament), and the proximal attachment of the suspensory ligament. The use of regional intra-arterial contrast infusion is mandatory for evaluation of these soft tissue structures. CT arthrography is an interesting option for cartilage disorders of the radiocarpal, intercarpal or carpometacarpal joint, or disorders of the small interosseus/carpal ligaments. A separate evaluation of these short ligaments is not possible on native CT.

The carpus includes the distal radius, the radial, intermediate, ulnar and accessory bones in the proximal row, the second, third and fourth bones in the distal row, and the proximal metacarpi and the structures adjacent to these osseous components. Occasionally, a first and/or fifth carpal bone is present. It contains three carpal joints: radiocarpal, intercarpal and carpometacarpal. This latter joint is a plane joint with minimal movement. The carpal synovial sheath encloses the digital flexor tendons of the forelimb starting from a level of ±10 cm proximal to the radiocarpal joint to near the middle of the third metacarpus. The palmar carpal ligament is thick and dense, is closely attached to the carpal bones and forms the dorsal wall of the carpal canal. The accessory carpal bone and its corresponding ligaments form the lateral wall of this canal, whereas the mediopalmar wall is formed by the carpal flexor retinaculum. The interosseus medius muscle (suspensory ligament) arises at the level of the distal row of the carpal bones and the proximal part of the third metacarpal bone.

The tarsal joint

Native CT of the tarsus is sufficient for evaluation of the bone and soft tissue structures. CT arthrography of the tarsus may be useful for the detection of cartilage lesions, while intra-arterial contrast administration is indicated for evaluation of the proximal suspensory ligament.

The equine tarsus is an anatomically complex region with many joints, ligaments and tendons. This joint consists of two large (talus, calcaneus) and four small (central, fused first and second, third and fourth tarsal bones) bones, which are kept together by numerous ligaments. Only the ligaments relevant for this chapter will be discussed. The interosseus talocalcaneal ligament fills the tarsal sinus, connecting the talus and calcaneus. The tarsal foramina at the talocalcaneal-centroquartal, talocentrodistal and tarsometatarsal joints are filled with interosseus ligaments connecting

Veterinary Computed Tomography, First Edition. Edited by Tobias Schwarz, Jimmy Saunders.

Table 46.1
Procedures included in a routine CT examination of the upper joints.

	Carpus	Tarsus	Stifle
Native CT	yes	yes	yes
CT arthrogram	yes	yes	yes
Intra-arterial CT	yes	yes	no

the distal talus with the proximal central tarsal bone, the distal central tarsal bone with the proximal third tarsal bone and the distal third tarsal bone with the proximal canon bone. The distal plantar ligament attaches at the distal aspect of the sustentaculum tali. Having a fibrocartilagenous structure it contributes to the delineation of the dorsal wall of the tarsal sheath. The distal plantar ligament covers the suspensory ligament, continuing distally as the distal check ligament.

The stifle joint

CT is particularly useful to diagnose injuries affecting the femorotibial joints (mainly menisci and cranial meniscotibial ligaments) and the cruciate ligaments. Disorders affecting these structures are difficult, or even impossible to diagnose using other imaging modalities. The use of CT arthrography is mandatory for accurate visualization. CT arthrography requires the injection of contrast medium in the three compartments of the joint performed individually as the communication between them is far less frequent than reported. Ultrasound guidance facilitates the injection of contrast medium.

The stifle joint has three compartments: femoropatellar, femorotibial medial and lateral. Two menisci are present between the articular cartilage surfaces of the femur and tibia condyles of the latter joint. They are attached to the tibia by the cranial and caudal meniscotibial ligaments. Their semi-lunar (proximal concave, distal convex) shape compensates for the incongruence of the femorotibial articular surfaces. The femur and tibia are joined by two extra-articular cruciate ligaments, which support and stabilize the joint. The cranial cruciate ligament runs in a craniodistal direction, originating from the caudal lateral surface of the intercondylar region of the femur and inserting cranially and medially on the medial eminence of the tibia, whereas the caudal cruciate ligament is oriented in a caudodistal direction, starting at the cranial medial aspect of the intercondylar fossa of the femur and inserts on the popliteal notch of the tibia.

DISEASE FEATURES

General disorders

Fractures, luxations

Fractures of these complex joints, a main indication for CT, will be discussed in Chapter 43.

Subchondral bone cysts

Subchondral bone cysts or 'osseous cyst-like lesions' are usually seen in young horses. Trauma to the cartilage or subchondral bone, infiltration of synovial fluid through an articular defect, chronic osteoarthritis, fracture, ischemia and inflammation have been proposed as potential causes.

CT features (Figures 46.1–46.3)

- Prior to contrast medium administration:
  - solitary or multiple circumscribed hypodense focus (lucent defect), varying in size and shape, often surrounded by a sclerotic border (rim)
  - communication with the adjacent joint is often identifiable.
- During regional intra-arterial infusion of contrast medium:
  - enhancement of the soft tissue within the possible defect.
- After intra-articular contrast medium administration:
  - contrast medium can enter (fill) the defect confirming a communication with the joint space.

Cartilage lesions

Cartilage lesions may be associated with developmental (e.g. osteochondrosis) or acquired (e.g. trauma, osteoarthrosis) disorders. The cartilage may appear thicker, thinner or may show a fissure/fracture depending on the disease process. Cartilaginous abnormalities without other joint lesions are not always associated with clinical signs in horses.

CT features (Figures 46.4 and 46.5)

- After intra-articular contrast medium administration:
  - cartilage thickening: increased space between the subchondral bone and contrast medium
  - cartilage thinning: decreased space between the subchondral bone and contrast medium
  - cartilage defect partial or full:
    - direct contact between the contrast medium (layer) and the adjacent subchondral bone
    - partial to full penetration of contrast medium in the articular cartilage.

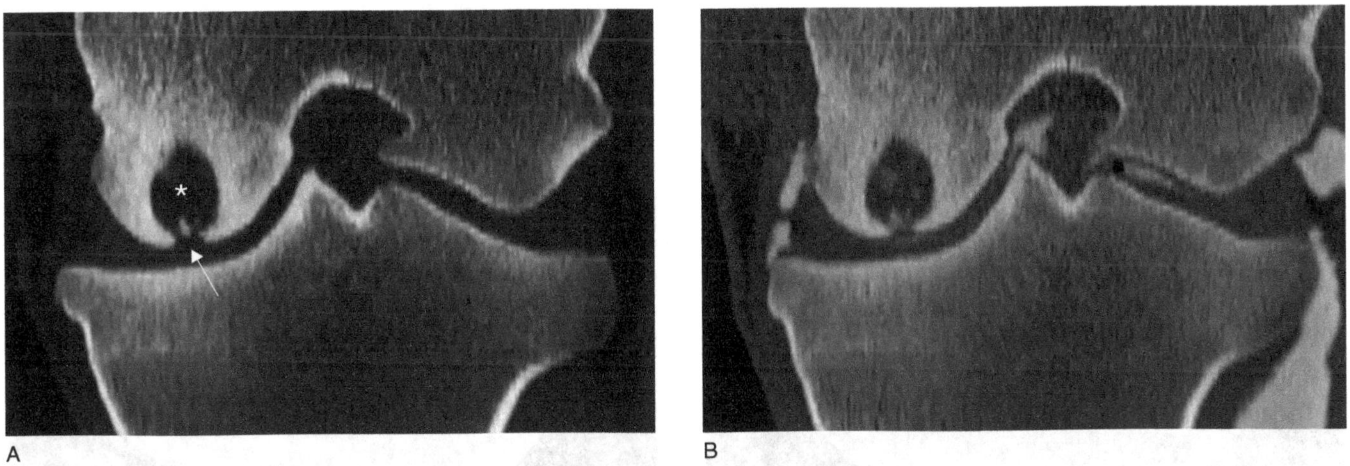

Figure 46.1 Nine-year-old Warmblood gelding with a subchondral bone cyst of the stifle joint. (A) Pre-contrast frontally reconstructed CT image shows a large rounded lucency in the distal portion of the medial femoral condyle (asterisk) with an apparent communication with the articular surface (arrow). (B) CT arthrogram (of the three joints) shows contrast medium extending into the cyst confirming communication with the joint.

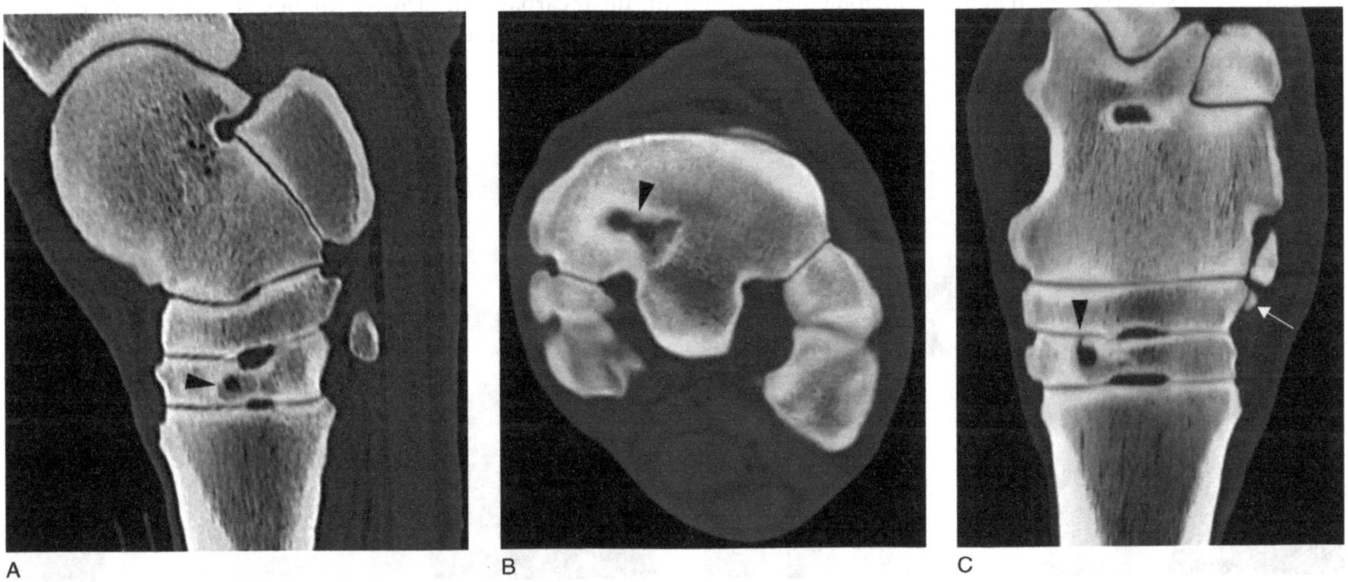

Figure 46.2 Ten-year-old Warmblood mare with diagnosis of subchondral cyst-like lesion of the third tarsal bone. (A) Sagittally reconstructed, (B) transverse and (C) frontally reconstructed CT images show an irregularly margined, lobular lucent lesion in the mid-portion of the third tarsal bone (arrowhead). There is also a small osseous fragment at the dorsal, proximal aspect of the central tarsal bone at the proximal intertarsal joint (arrow).

Specific disorders of the carpal, tarsal and stifle joint

The carpal joint

Sclerosis of the carpal bones

Sclerosis of the third carpal bone is common in racehorses. The third carpal bone shows a rapid response to relatively small amounts of high-speed exercise by increasing bone mineral density and altering bone architecture. This increased stiffness is detrimental to bone compliance and results in vulnerability to mechanical damage. The end stage of third carpal bone disease is thought to be slab fractures; the prognosis for return to athletic function is guarded. However, it is not known at what point increases in sclerosis indicate the onset of disease or increased risk of third carpal bone fracture. Subchondral lucency and cartilage lesions of the radial and intermediate facet of third carpal bone may involve the same

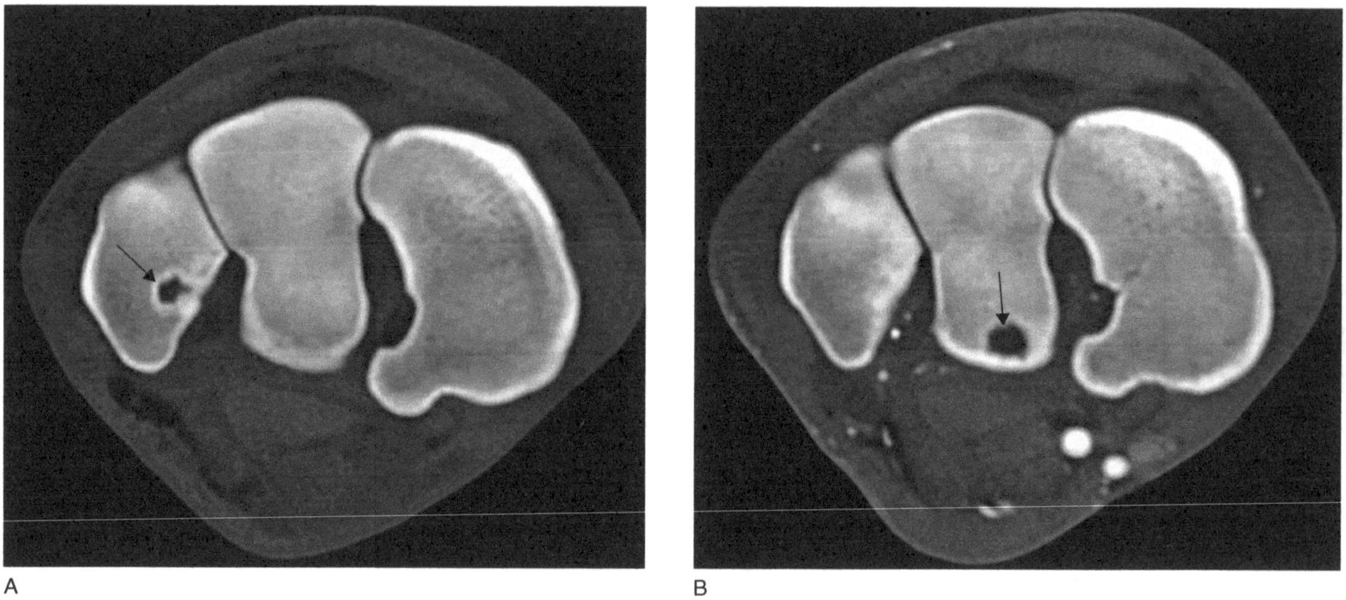

Figure 46.3 Subchondral bone cyst in the carpus of two different patients. (A) Fifteen-year-old Warmblood mare. Transverse CT image shows a lucent lesion in the palmaromedial aspect of the ulnar carpal bone (arrow). (B) Eleven-year-old Warmblood gelding. Transverse CT image obtained during intra-arterial infusion shows a round subchondral lucency at the palmar aspect of the intermediate carpal bone (arrow).

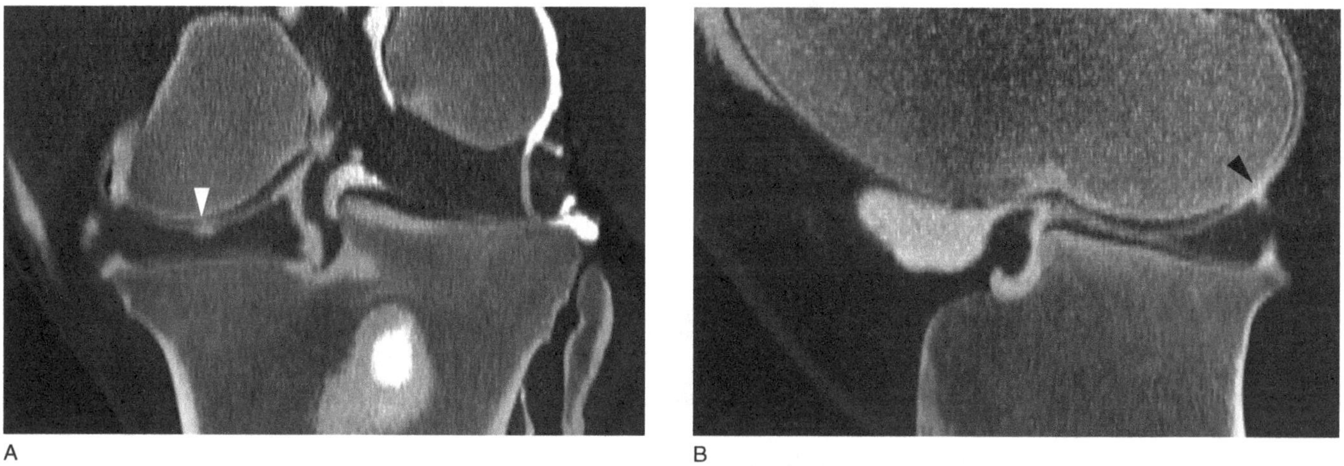

Figure 46.4 Adult horse with evidence of cartilage injury (multiple fragments were present in the joint). A CT study was performed with contrast material in the medial and lateral femorotibial joints. (A) Frontally and (B) sagittally reconstructed CT image of a full-thickness cartilage lesion shows contrast medium that abuts the subchondral bone of the femoral condyle (arrowhead).

pathophysiological process and perhaps precede slab fractures.

CT features (Figure 46.6)

- Increased density (sclerosis) of the third carpal bone (radial facet).
- Commonly in combination with subchondral lucency(ies).
- Degenerative bone damages with active sclerosis.

Tear/Desmitis/Avulsion of the intercarpal ligaments

Tearing of the intercarpal ligaments has been recognized as a cause of effusion and occasionally lameness in racehorses. The medial palmar intercarpal ligament is more commonly affected than lateral one. In contrast to racehorses, these lesions can be identified in nonracehorses without associated osteochondral abnor-

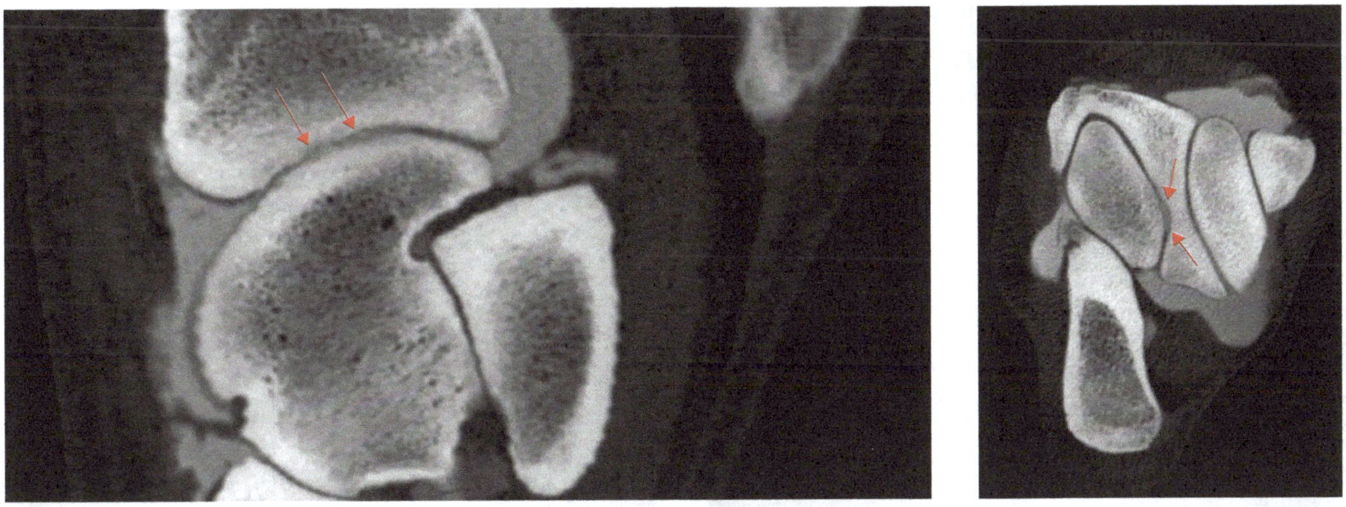

Figure 46.5 Adult horse with cartilage injury of the left tarsal joint. (A) Sagittally reconstructed and (B) transverse CT arthrogram show focal full-thickness cartilage defect (contrast medium in contact with subchondral bone) at the proximal part of the medial aspect of the lateral talar ridge (arrows).

malities. Injuries of other intercarpal ligaments, such as between the second and third carpal bones can also be observed.

CT features (Figure 46.7)

- Prior to contrast medium administration:
  - subchondral bone damage/osteochondral fragmentation
  - associated bone lesions with avulsion of the lateral palmar intercarpal ligament: lucent zones in the ulnar carpal bone, avulsion fragments originating from the medial palmar aspect of the ulnar carpal bone.
- During regional intra-arterial infusion of contrast medium:
  - contrast enhancement within the affected intercarpal ligaments
  - possible enlargement of the intercarpal ligament
  - new vessel formation.
- After intra-articular contrast medium administration:
  - possible cartilage erosion (partial or full thickness).

Carpal canal (tunnel) syndrome

Carpal canal syndrome (carpal sheath effusion) is recognized in horses mainly due to distal radial osteochondromas, injuries of carpal sheath contents (flexor tendons, accessory ligament of the superficial digital flexor tendon), injuries of carpal sheath wall (palmar carpal ligament), exostosis distal radius or carpal bone injuries. Most of these are due to hyperextension injury.

CT features (Figures 46.8 and 46.9)

- Prior to contrast medium administration:
  - enlargement of the involved structures resulting in shape change (tendon injury)
  - decrease in tendon density (hypodense)
  - carpal sheath distention with or without synovial proliferation
  - associated bone/carpal sheath wall (palmar carpal ligament) lesions.
- During regional intra-arterial infusion of contrast medium:
  - moderate to marked contrast enhancement of the involved structure
  - new vessel formation(s)
  - arterial displacement/compression.

Common palmar carpal ligament desmitis/enthesopathy

A particular disorder of the carpal sheath is palmar carpal ligament desmitis and enthesopathy.

CT features (Figures 46.10 and 46.11)

- Prior to contrast medium administration:
  - local thickening and heterogeneous density of the common palmar carpal ligament, affecting mostly the lateral part; diffuse thickening is less common

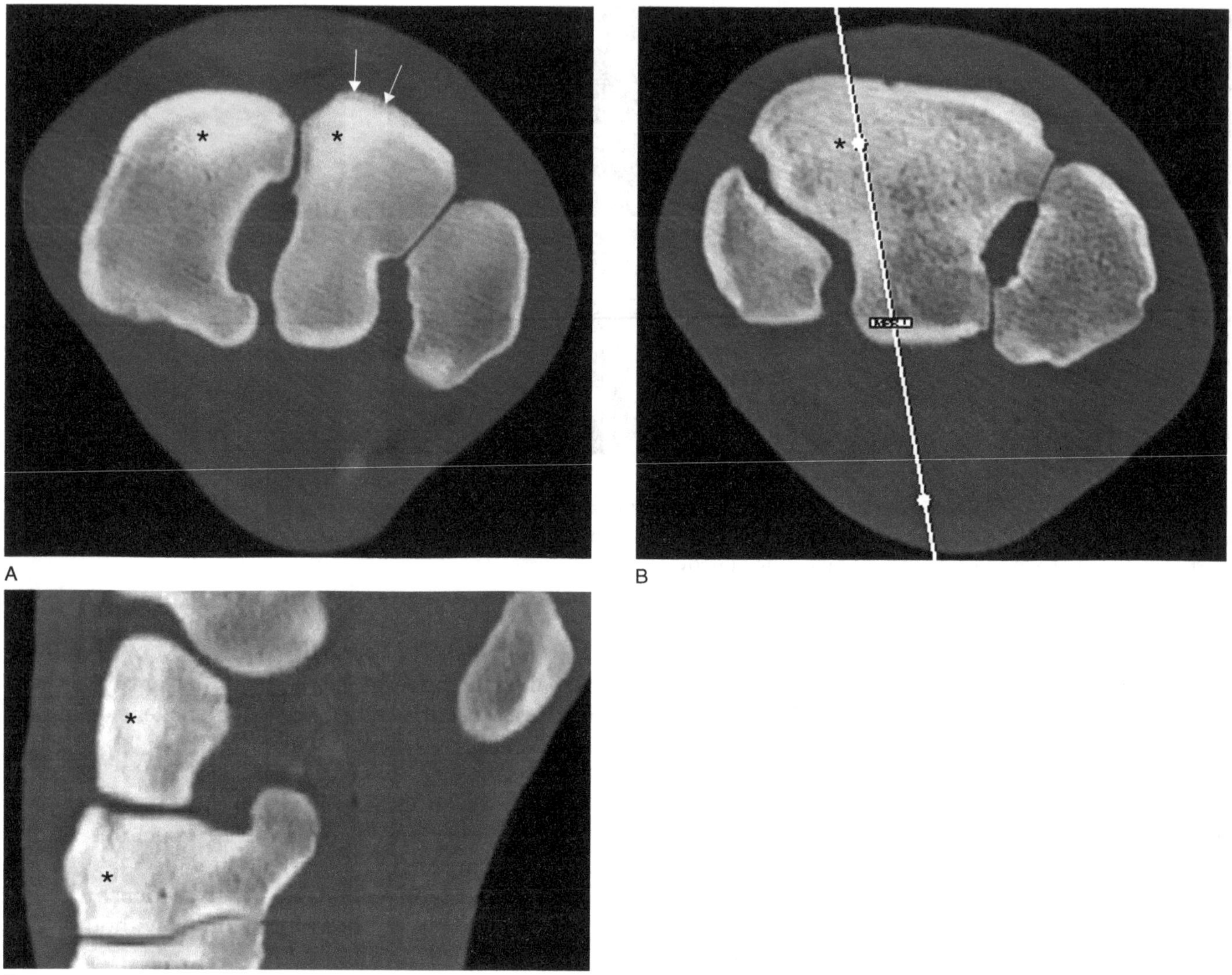

Figure 46.6 Adult horse with third carpal bone sclerosis on the right front leg. (A) Transverse CT image shows increased density at the dorsal aspect of the radial carpal bone (asterisk) and the dorsomedial aspect of the intermediate carpal bone (asterisk). Smooth periosteal reactions are visible at the dorsal aspect of the intermediate carpal bone (arrows). (B) Transverse CT image shows increased density at the dorsal aspect of the radial facet of the third carpal bone (asterisk). (C) Sagittally reconstructed CT image (as shown by white line in B) shows increased density at the dorsal aspect of the intermediate and third carpal bones (asterisks).

  - partial disruption of the proximal aspect of the ligament
  - carpal canal effusion often associated
  - palmar aspect of the distal radial physeal scar irregular at the proximal attachment of the common palmar carpal ligament.
- During regional intra-arterial infusion of contrast medium:
  - local or diffuse, irregularly marginated, heterogeneous contrast enhancement
  - new vessel formation due to inflammation.

Proximal suspensory desmitis (enthesopathy)

Proximal suspensory desmitis is a primary, multifactorial degenerative condition that may affect both fore- and hindlimbs, uni- or bilaterally. Conformational abnormalities and high-level performance training have been suggested as predisposing factors.

CT features (Figures 46.12 and 46.13)

- Prior to contrast medium administration:
  - Thickening of one (asymmetry of the heads) or both heads of the suspensory ligament with

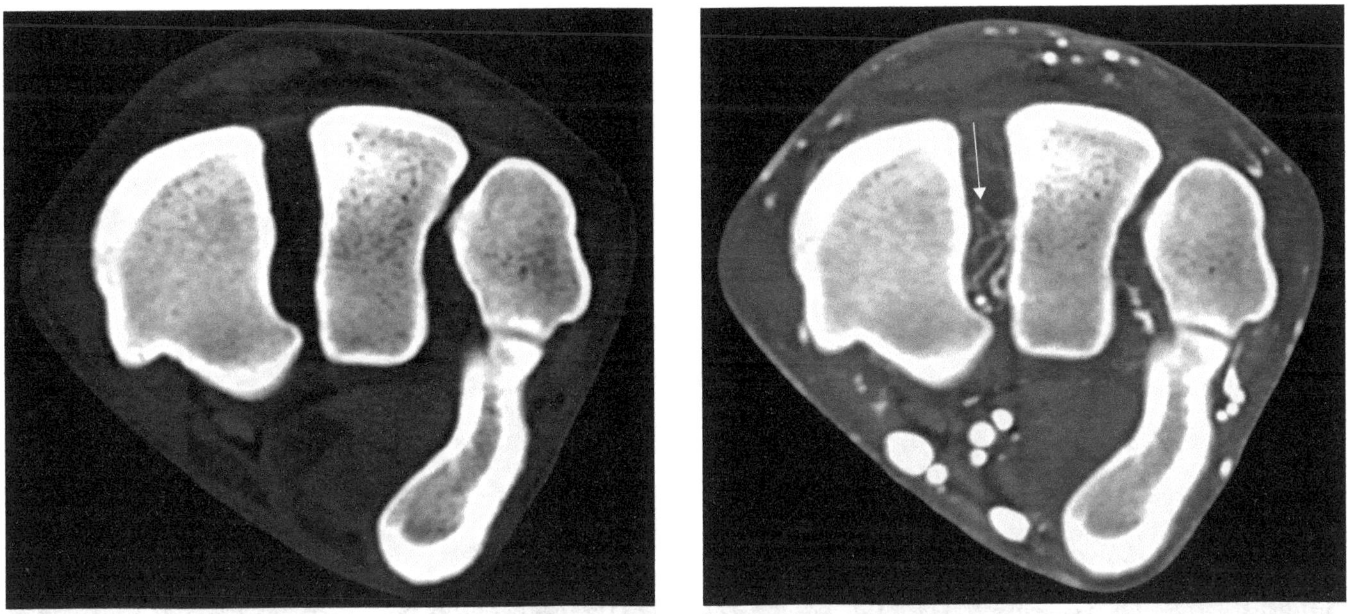

A B

Figure 46.7 Seven-year-old Warmblood mare with intercarpal ligament injury of the left carpus. (A) Pre-contrast transverse CT image appears normal. (B) Transverse CT image during regional intra-arterial infusion of contrast medium shows irregular enhancement and new vessel formation within the intercarpal ligament between the radial and intermediate carpal bones (arrow).

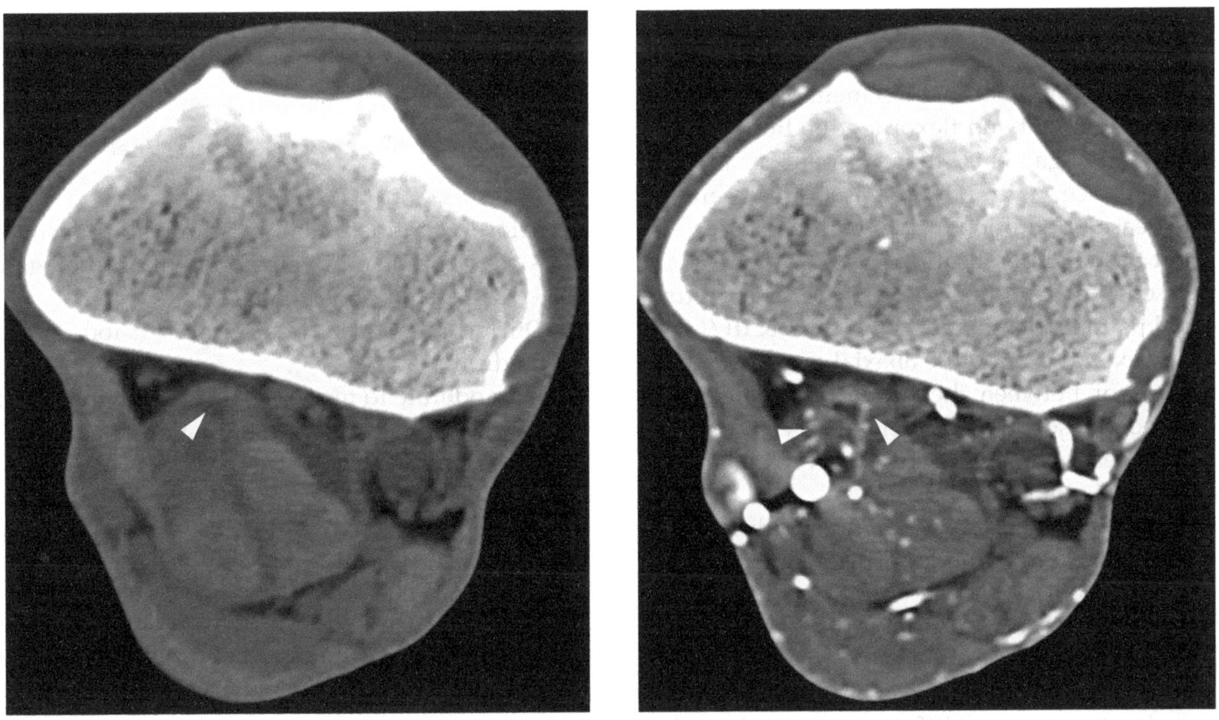

A B

Figure 46.8 Nine-year-old, Arab gelding with a tear in the distal part of the superior check ligament. (A) Pre-contrast transverse CT image shows a hypodense lesion (arrowhead) within the superior check ligament. (B) CT image obtained during regional intra-arterial infusion of contrast medium shows an irregularly shaped hypodense region in the distal portion of the superior check ligament with peripheral contrast enhancement (arrowheads).

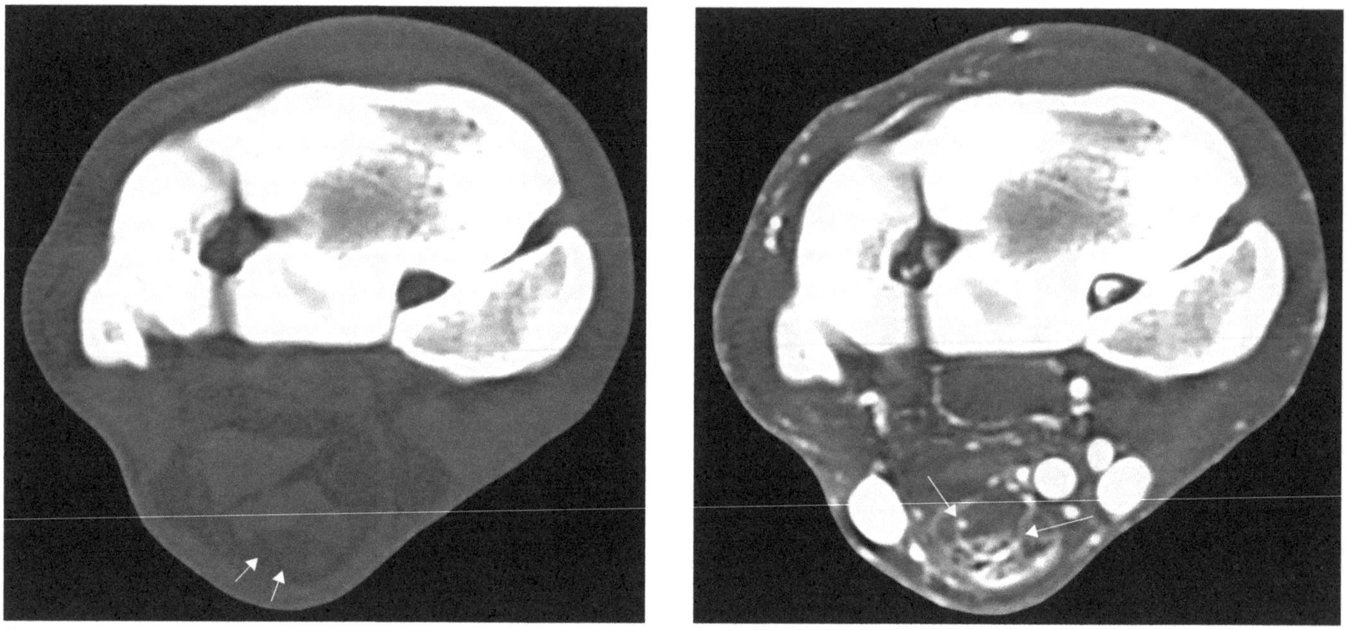

A B

Figure 46.9 Adult Warmblood gelding with superficial digital flexor tendinopathy with associated carpal canal synovitis on the left carpus. (A) Pre-contrast transverse CT image shows an enlarged superficial digital flexor tendon containing a hypodense area (arrows) just distal to its musculotendinous junction within the carpal canal. There is moderate carpal canal effusion. (B) Transverse CT image obtained during regional intra-arterial infusion of contrast medium (same level as A) shows marked contrast enhancement with marked neovascular formation of the previously mentioned superficial digital flexor tendon lesion (arrows).

consequent palmar displacement of the inferior check ligament and flexor tendon bundle.
  - Affected ligaments may present a mottled appearance with hypodense areas and a decreased definition of the margins.
  - Soft tissue mineralization.
  - Osseous proliferations (exostosis) at the proximal palmar/plantar aspect of the MCIII/MTIII may extend around the abaxial margins of both heads or between the heads of the ligament. Osseous resorption is rarely observed.
  - Endosteal sclerosis may be observed deep to the ligament attachment.
  - Syndesmopathies of the second and third metatarsal bones – third and fourth metacarpal bones (Figure 46.14).
- During regional intra-arterial infusion of contrast medium:
  - Contrast enhancement may be absent, minimal, moderate or severe, diffuse or local, bilateral or unilateral, heterogeneous or homogeneous.
  - Hypodense ligament with peripheral enhancement.
  - Contrast medium extravasation and new vessel formation.

The tarsal joint

Distal plantar ligament desmitis/desmopathy

CT features (Figure 46.15)

- Prior to contrast medium administration:
  - dystrophic mineralization within the ligament
  - associated bone changes.
- During regional intra-arterial infusion of contrast medium:
  - moderate to marked contrast enhancement due to extravasation (inflammation) and new vessel formation.

Desmitis interosseous tarsal ligaments

Lesions in the small interosseous ligaments are sometimes the only morphological abnormality observed in horses with tarsal pain.

CT features (Figure 46.15)

- Prior to contrast medium administration:
  - osseous proliferations at the attachment sites of the affected ligament.

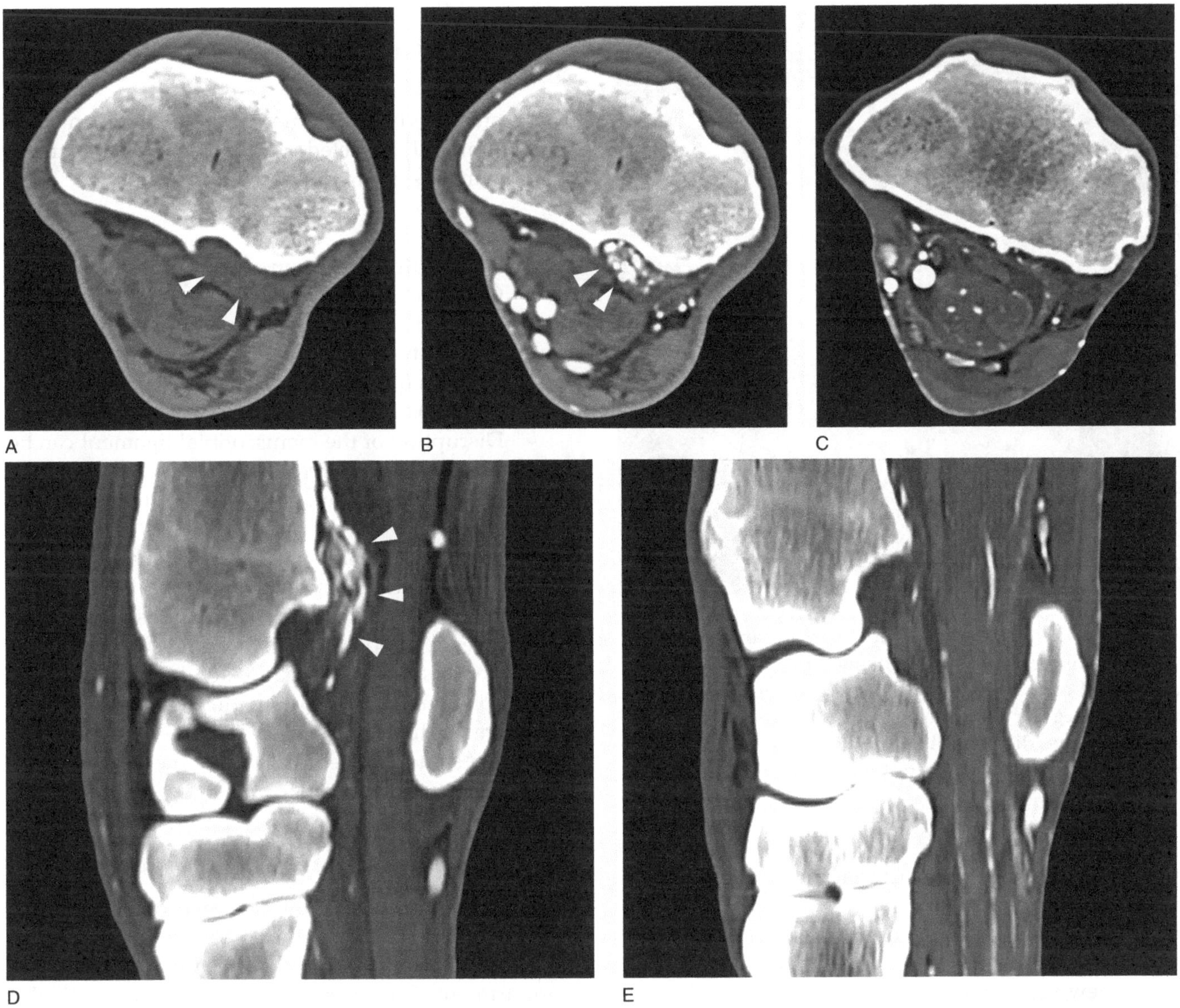

Figure 46.10 Friesian mare with regionally extensive palmar carpal ligament injury. (A) On a pre-contrast transverse CT image the palmar carpal ligament is thickened at the origin of the lateral aspect (arrowheads). The abnormality is accompanied by osseous remodeling along the caudal aspect of the distal radius. (B) Transverse CT image obtained during intra-arterial infusion of contrast medium (same level as A) shows marked contrast enhancement of the lesion described in (A) (arrowheads). (C) Reference transverse CT image of a different horse obtained during intra-arterial infusion of contrast medium at the same level as A and B. (D) Sagittally reconstructed CT image obtained during intra-arterial infusion of contrast medium shows marked palmar carpal ligament enhancement (arrowheads) extending distally up to the level of the accessory carpal bone. (E) Reference sagittally reconstructed CT image of a different horse obtained after intra-arterial contrast administration at the same level as D.

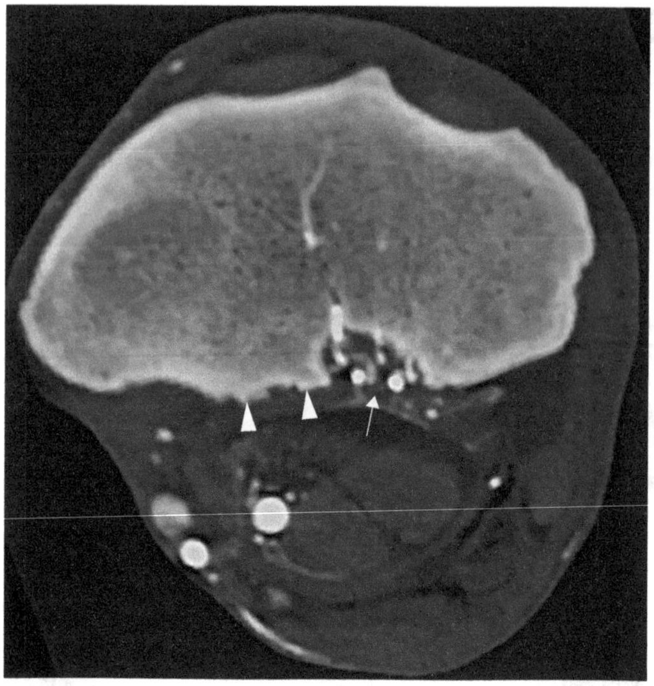

Figure 46.11 Adult horse with palmar carpal ligament injury. Transverse CT image obtained during intra-arterial infusion of contrast material shows moderate carpal sheath effusion, irregular bone proliferation along the caudo-lateral aspect of the distal radius (arrowheads) and moderate palmar carpal ligament contrast enhancement (arrow).

- During regional intra-arterial infusion of contrast medium:
  - irregular contrast enhancement within the affected ligament
  - new vessel formation.

Proximal suspensory desmitis (desmopathy)

See Carpus.

The stifle joint

The majority of disorders affecting the equine stifle joint are traumatic or degenerative in origin.

Meniscotibial ligament desmopathy/enthesopathy (Figures 46.16–46.19)

The cranial and caudal meniscotibial ligaments are most commonly affected (cranial > caudal). Tears in these ligaments are frequently seen.

CT features

- Prior to contrast medium administration:
  - Osseous changes at the attachment site on the tibia of the cranial medial meniscotibial ligament (cranial >>> caudal). Resorption is more frequent than proliferation (irregular >> smooth).
  - Disruption of the meniscotibial ligament can be observed in severe cases.
- After intra-articular contrast medium administration:
  - Contrast medium within the cranial medial or caudal medial meniscotibial ligament. The outline of contrast is mostly irregular and is more or less extended depending on the gravity of the lesion.
  - Contrast medium may extend in the adjacent bone (tibia) or between the ligament and the cranial horn of the meniscus.
  - The same changes rarely affect the cranial lateral meniscotibial ligament.

Meniscal injuries (Figures 46.18 and 46.19)

Meniscal tears are frequently seen in the cranial aspect of the femorotibial joint, although lesions are occasionally encountered caudally, especially in the medial compartment. Concurrent disorders, mainly articular cartilage disease but also cruciate ligament lesions, are frequently present in horses with meniscal injuries.

CT features

- Prior to contrast medium administration:
  - abnormal shape of the cranial horn of the medial meniscus
  - meniscal extrusion or protrusion can be seen on frontally reformatted images.

Figure 46.12 Seven-year-old Warmblood gelding with bilateral suspensory desmitis. (A) Pre-contrast transverse CT image of the left proximal metacarpus shows the proximal suspensory ligament (arrows) and thickening of the palmar cortex of the third metacarpus (asterisk). (B) On a transverse CT image obtained during regional intra-arterial administration of contrast medium (same level as A) the proximal suspensory ligament is heterogeneous with contrast enhancement within both the medial and lateral lobes. Within the lateral lobe, the enhancement is irregular and central (arrow). (C) Pre-contrast transverse CT image of the right proximal metacarpus shows the body of the suspensory ligament severely enlarged and heterogeneous (asterisk). (D) On a transverse CT image obtained during regional intra-arterial administration of contrast medium (same level as C), the body of the suspensory ligament is severely enlarged and markedly contrast enhancing. Within its body, several peripherally enhancing regions without central enhancement are identified.

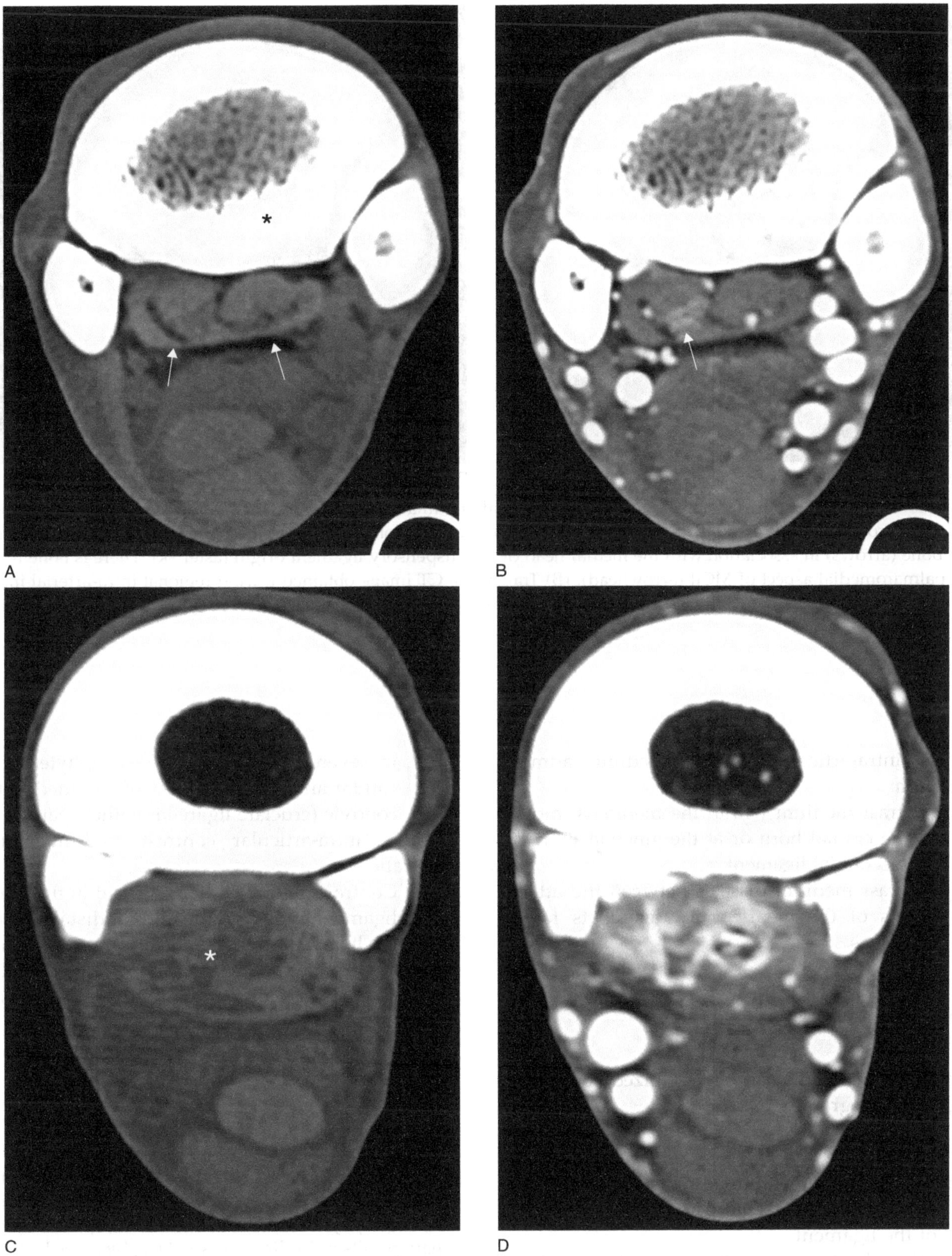
A
B
C
D

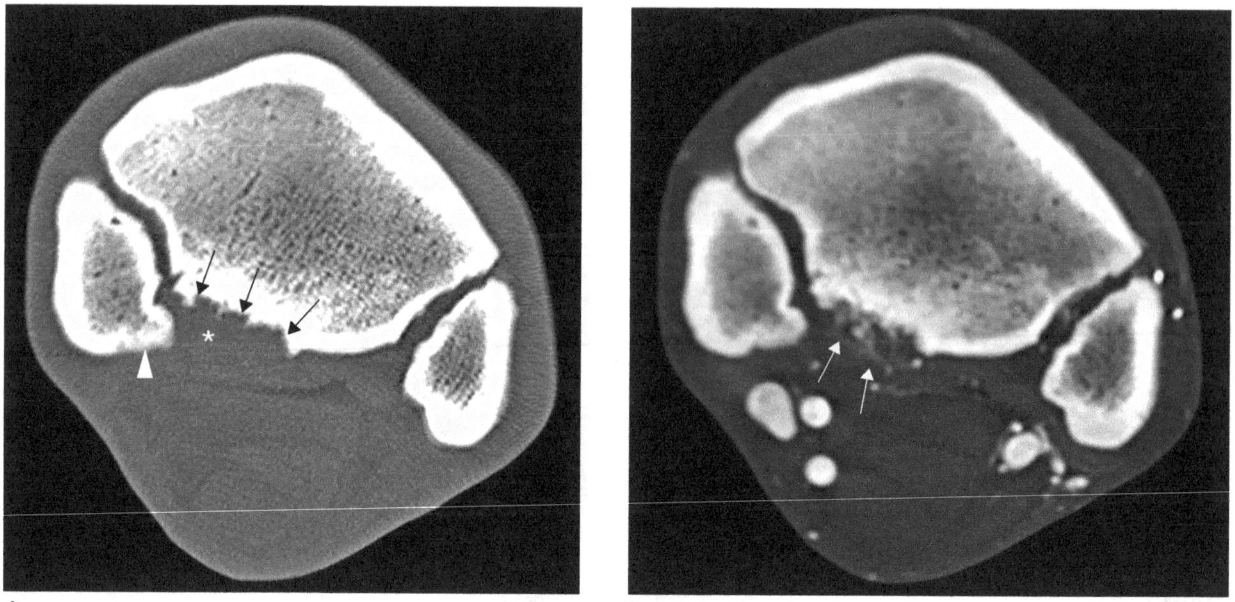

Figure 46.13 Four-year-old Warmblood gelding with medial proximal suspensory ligament injury and associated enthesopathy. (A) Pre-contrast transverse CT image shows regions of irregular bone reaction at the palmar aspect of the third metacarpal bone (arrows) in association with the medial head of the suspensory ligament origin (asterisk). There is bone reaction at the palmaromedial aspect of MCII (arrowhead). (B) Transverse CT image obtained during regional intra-arterial infusion of contrast shows marked neovascularization of the medial head of the proximal suspensory ligament (arrows).

- After intra-articular contrast medium administration:
  - contrast medium within the meniscus, mostly in the cranial horn or at the junction with the meniscotibial ligament
  - contrast medium dissects between the attachments of the meniscotibial ligaments to the meniscus.

Cruciate ligaments injuries (Figures 46.20 and 46.21)

The cruciate ligaments can be visualized completely using CT arthrography.

CT features

- Prior to contrast medium administration:
  - enlargement (thickening) and irregular margins of the ligament
  - mineralization (smooth, osseous fragments) is sometimes present in the cruciate ligament
  - evidence of bone resorption or bone proliferation at an attachment site of the cruciate ligament
  - in severe cases, a rim of osteophytes on the caudal and medial aspect of the medial tibial condyle (cruciate ligament enthesopathy).
- After intra-articular contrast medium administration:
  - Contrast medium extension within the cruciate ligament, mostly in the mid- or distal portion of the ligament. Both cranial and caudal ligaments are affected with the same frequency. These changes are compatible with a partial cruciate ligament tear.

Further Reading

Bergman EHJ, Puchalski SM, van der Veen H and Wiemer P (2007) Computed tomography and computed tomography arthrography of the equine stifle: technique and preliminary results in 16 clinical cases. *Proc Am Assoc Eq Pract* **53**: 46–55.

Kaser-Hotz B, Sartoretti-Schefer S and Weiss R (1994) Computed tomography and magnetic resonance imaging of the normal equine carpus. *Vet Radiol Ultrasound* **35**: 457–61.

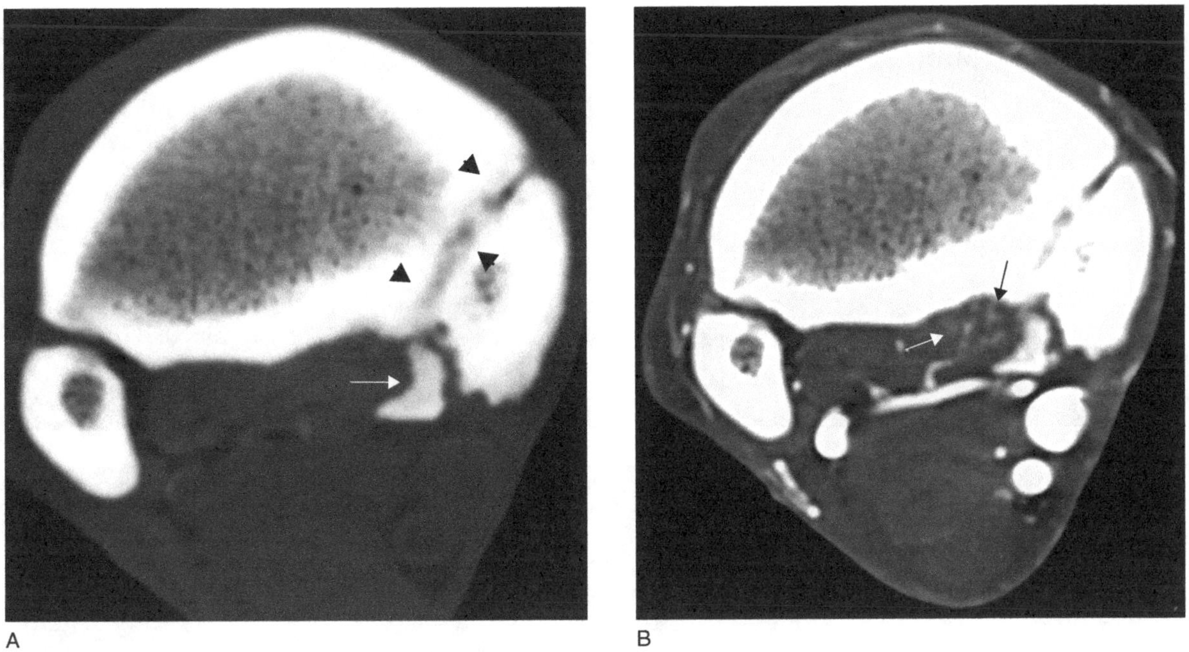

Figure 46.14 Adult horse with syndesmopathy and associated suspensory ligament desmitis. (A) Transverse CT image shows bone reactions between the second and third metacarpal bones (arrowheads) and a bone fragmentation/mineralization at the medial aspect of the second metacarpal bone (arrow). (B) Transverse CT image (same level as A) obtained during regional intra-arterial infusion of contrast medium shows marked moderate neovascularization of the medial branch of the suspensory ligament (arrows).

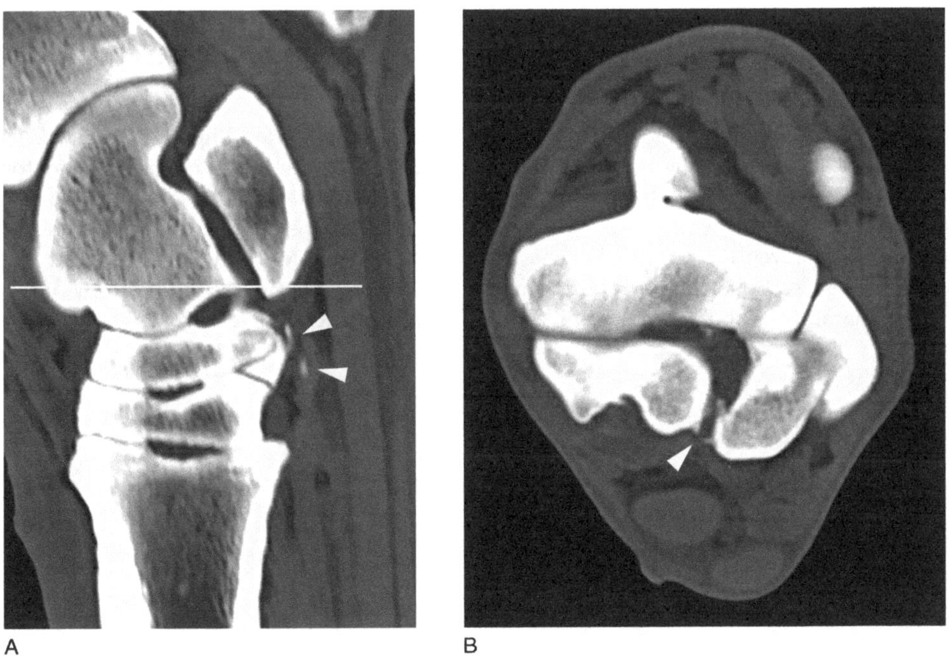

Figure 46.15 Adult horse with degenerative changes into the distal plantar ligament. (A) Sagittally reconstructed CT image shows dystrophic mineralizations in the proximal aspect of the distal plantar ligament (arrowheads). (B) Transverse CT image, obtained at the level as shown with the line in A, shows bone reactions (enthesiophytosis) at the insertion sites of the interosseus talocalcaneal ligament (arrowhead).

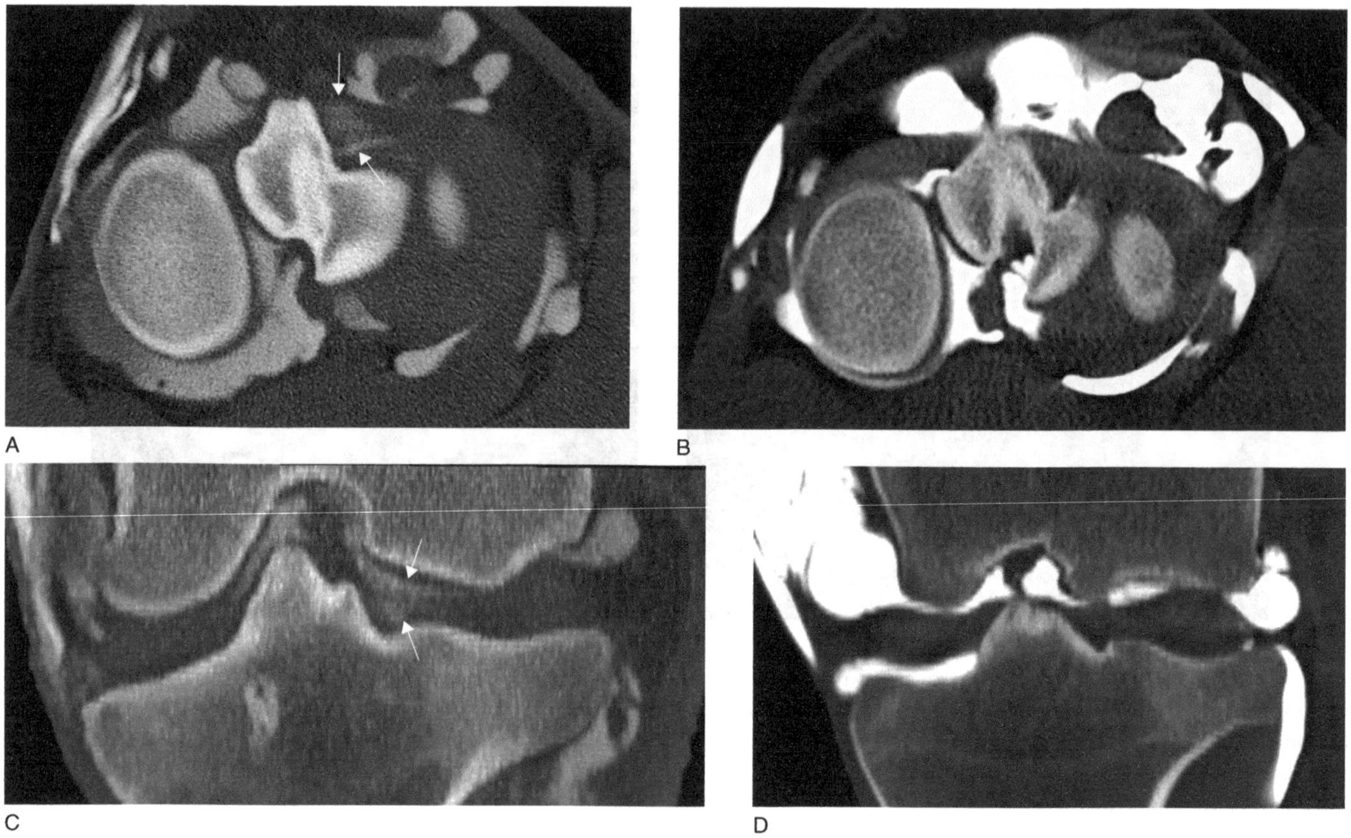

Figure 46.16 Fifteen-year-old Appaloosa gelding with hind lateral meniscotibial ligament tearing. (A) Transverse and (C) frontally reconstructed CT-arthrogram shows extensive, irregularly margined contrast uptake within the lateral meniscotibial ligament (arrows). (B,D) Reference images of a normal joint at the same level.

Mayrhofer W, Stanek C, Lutz H and Heidbrink U (2006) The value of clinical, radiological and computed tomographical examination in the diagnosis of carpal joint diseases in the horse. *Pferdeheilkunde* **22**: 773–84.

Raes E, Bergman EHJ, Vanderperren K, Van der Vekens E and Saunders JH (2011) Cross-sectional anatomy and comparative computed tomography of the equine tarsus. *Am J Vet Res* (in press).

Tomlinson, JE, Redding WR, Berry C and Smallwood JE (2003) Computed tomographic anatomy of the equine tarsus. *Vet Radiol Ultrasound* **44**: 174–8.

Van der Vekens E, Bergman EHJ, Vanderperren K, Raes EV, Puchalski SM, van Bree HJ and Saunders JH (2011) Computed tomographic anatomy of the equine stifle joint. *Am J Vet Res* **72**: 512–21.

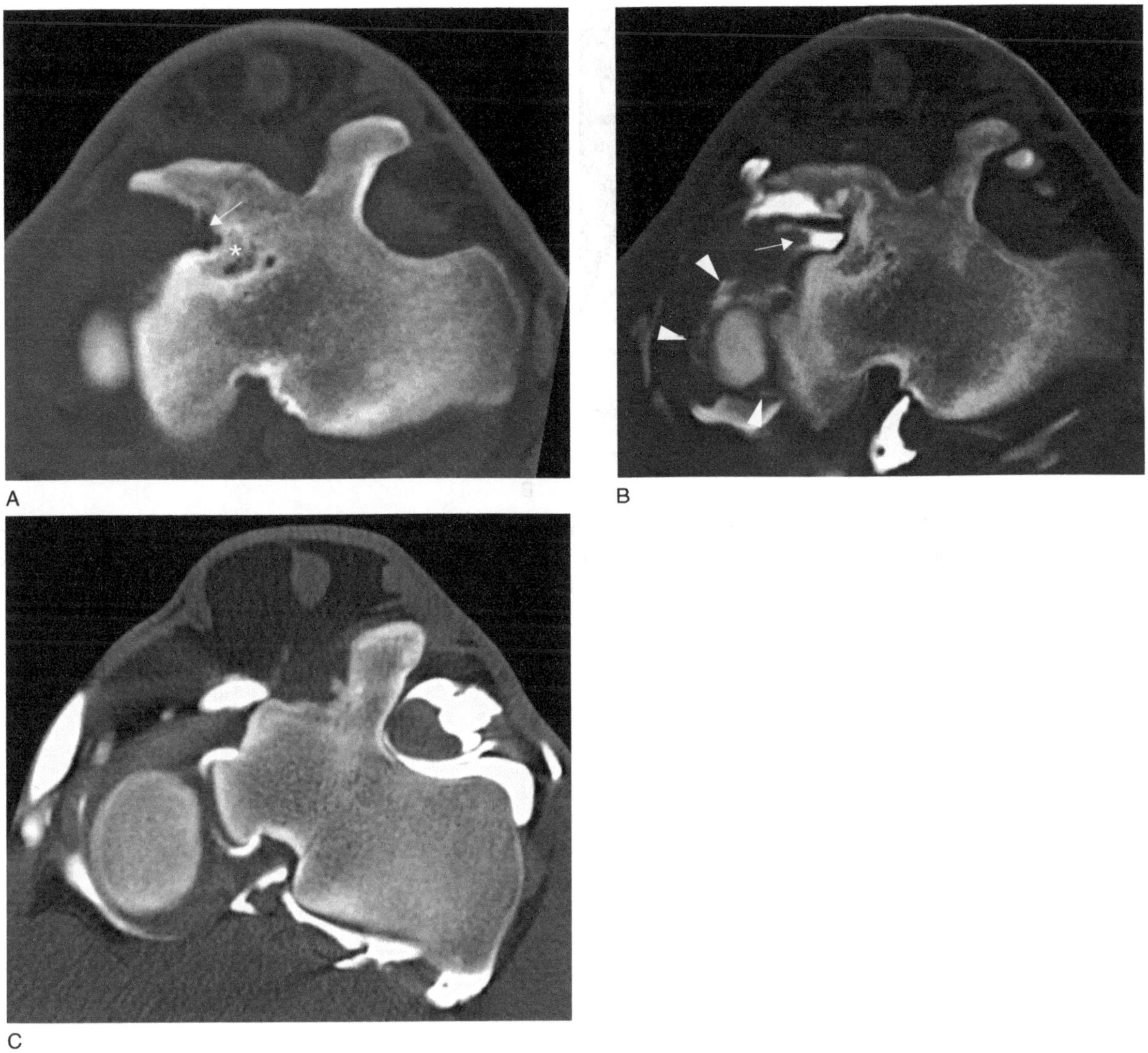

Figure 46.17 Nine-year-old Warmblood gelding jumper with hind medial meniscal and cranial meniscotibial ligament injuries. (A) Pre-contrast transverse CT image shows bone resorption and irregular proliferation at the insertion site of the cranial medial meniscotibial ligament (arrow) indicative of enthesopathy of this ligament. There is a large, irregularly shaped lucent lesion with a sclerotic rim in the subchondral bone of the proximal tibia near the insertion of the cranial medial meniscotibial ligament (asterisk). (B) Transverse CT arthrogram (same level as A) shows that the contrast material does not communicate with the previously described osseous lesion in the proximal tibia. Contrast medium is seen dissecting through the cranial medial meniscotibial ligament (arrow). Multiple radial tears are present in the medial meniscus (arrowheads). (C) Reference image of a normal stifle joint at the same level.

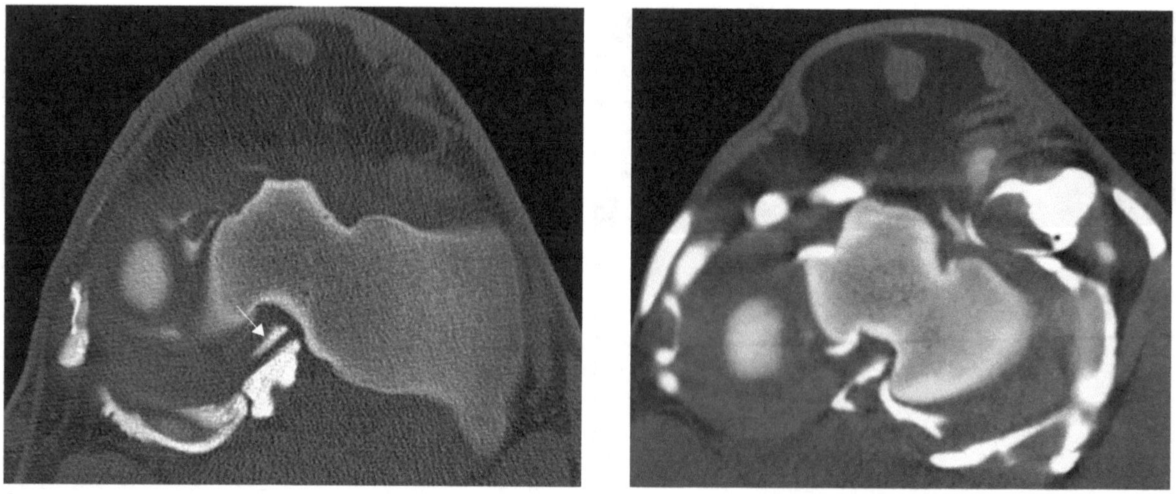

A B

Figure 46.18 Seven-year-old gelding with right medial meniscus and meniscotibial ligament tearing. (A) Transverse CT arthrogram (medial femorotibial joint) shows contrast medium that linearly dissects within the caudal medial meniscotibial ligament (arrow). Contrast medium surrounds the meniscus. (B) Reference image of a normal stifle joint at the same level.

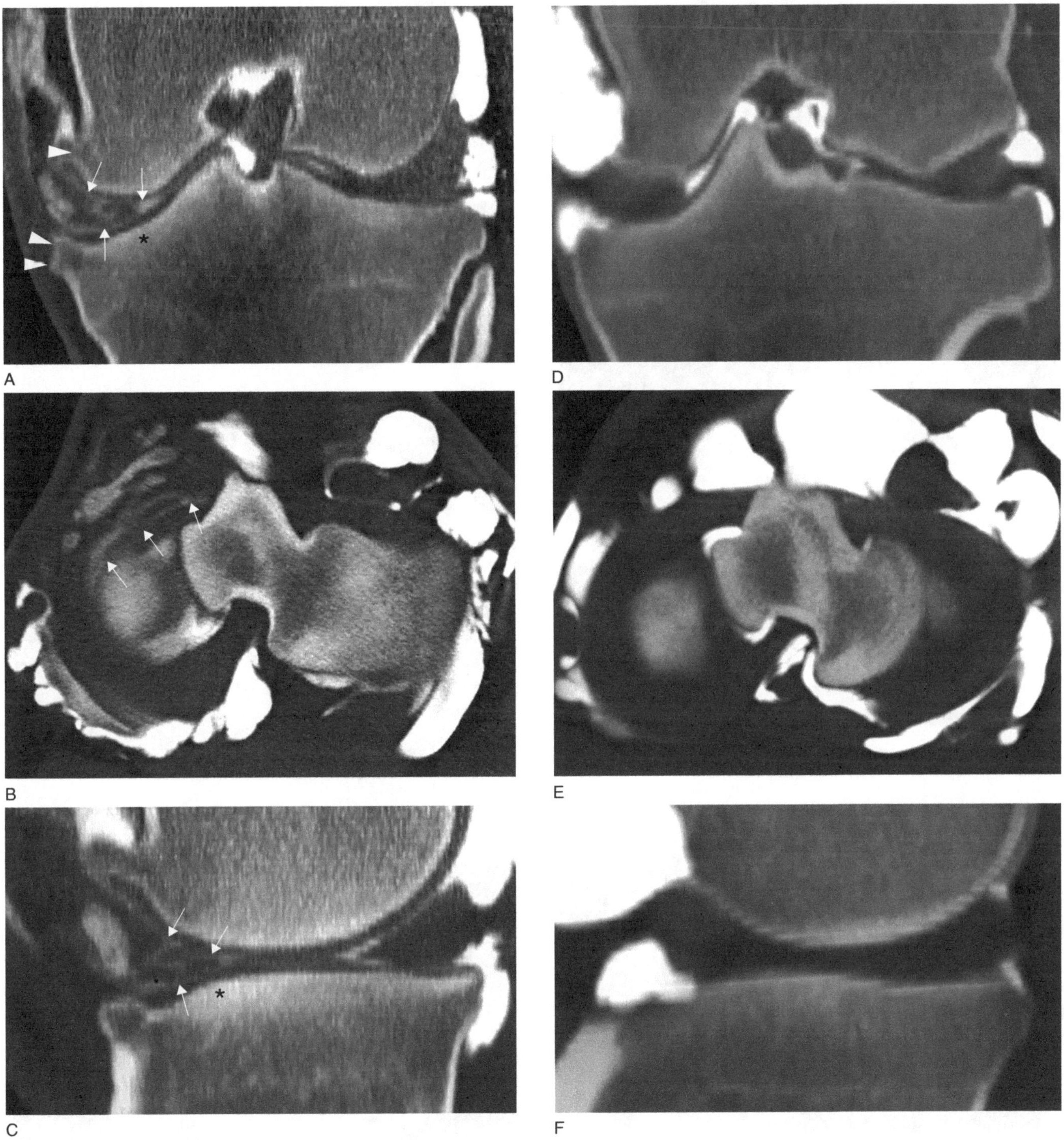

Figure 46.19 Ten-year-old Friesian mare with medial meniscal and medial meniscotibial ligament tearing and severe osteoarthrosis. (A) Frontally reconstructed, (B) transverse and (C) sagittally reconstructed CT arthrogram (medial and lateral femorotibial joints) show a complex pattern of contrast uptake into the cranial horn of the medial meniscus and in its cranial meniscotibial ligament (arrows). There is extensive new bone production along the medial aspect of the distal femur in the medial epicondylar and condylar region and on the medial aspect of the tibia in the periarticular region (arrowheads). There is subtle subchondral sclerosis of the medial plateau of the tibia and the medial condyle of the femur (asterisk). (D,E,F) Reference images of a normal stifle joint at the same level.

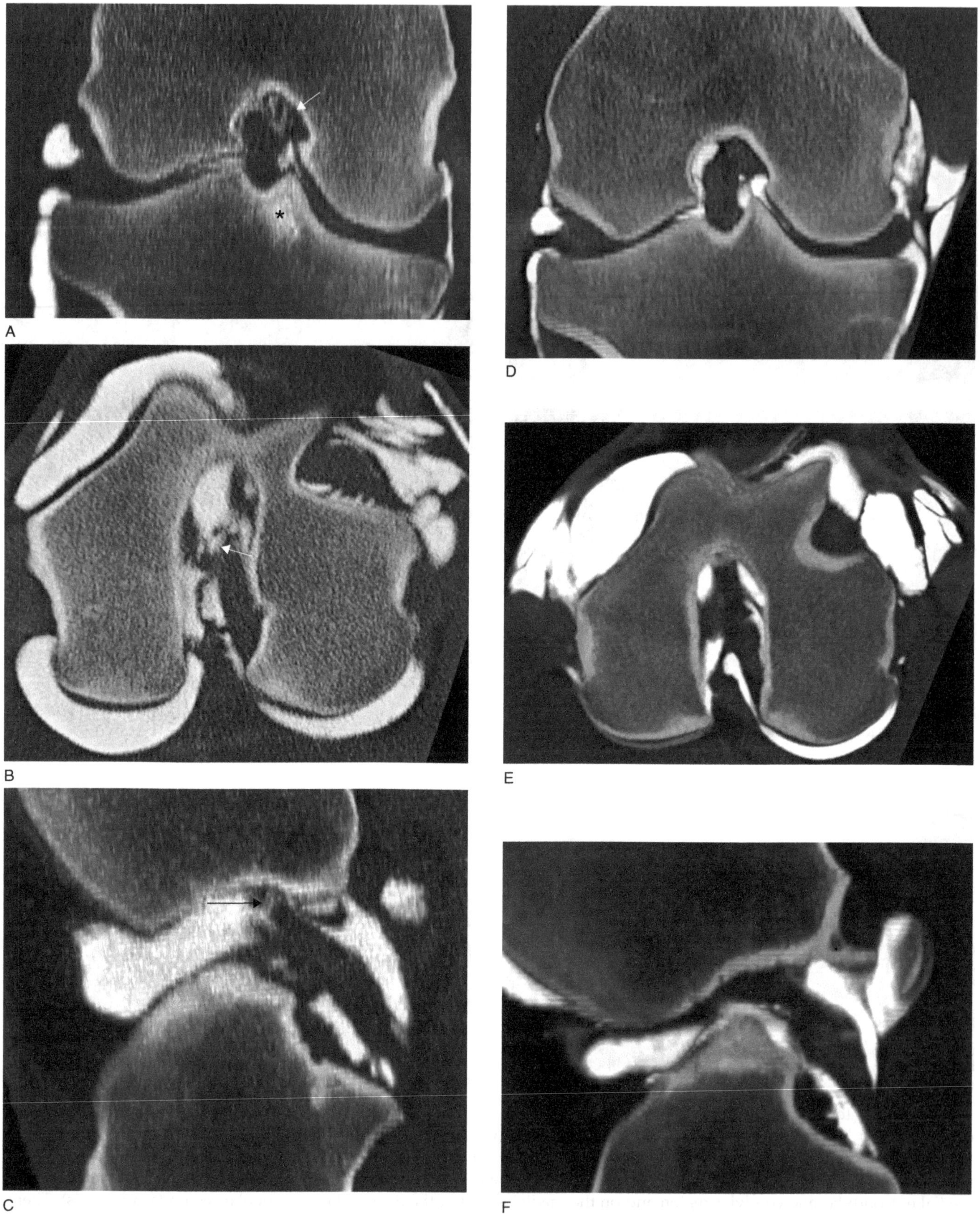

Figure 46.20 Adult Warmblood gelding with caudal cruciate ligament tear. (A) Frontally reconstructed, (B) transverse and (C) sagittally reconstructed CT arthrogram (medial and lateral femorotibial joints) show irregularly shaped contrast medium accumulation in the proximal portion of the caudal cruciate ligament near its proximal attachment (arrow). There is bone sclerosis in the proximal tibia medial eminentia (asterisk). (D,E,F) Reference images of a normal stifle joint at the same level.

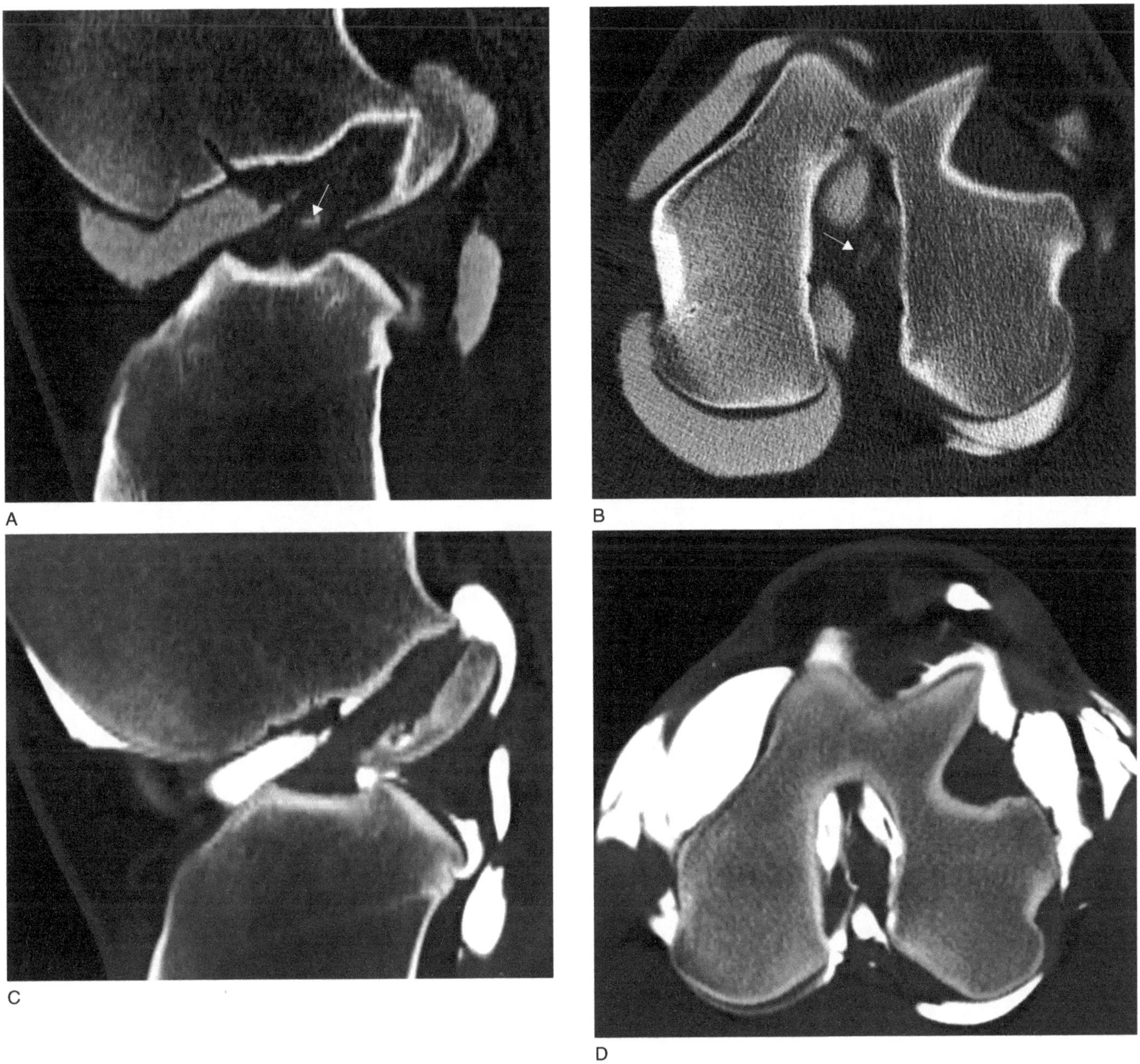

Figure 46.21 Eight-year-old Warmblood gelding with left cranial cruciate ligament tear. (A) Sagittally reconstructed and (B) transverse CT arthrogram (three joints) show contrast in several linear defects in the mid-portion of the cranial cruciate ligament (arrow). (C,D) Reference images of a normal stifle joint at the same level.

CHAPTER FORTY-SEVEN

Ruminant and Porcine

Fintan McEvoy and Stefanie Ohlerth

Ruminant CT

Imaging protocol

In general, CT is not commonly performed in ruminants because of the high cost and anesthesia. However, in very valuable animals, rare breeds, pet animals, exotic ruminants and camelides, or occasionally with livestock problems, CT may represent a highly useful tool for the work-up of skeletal, central nervous, upper digestive and airway tract as well as other thoracic diseases.

For CT studies in large and small ruminants, positioning and scan parameters may be chosen according to the scan protocols for horses or small animals. For the application of contrast media in slaughter animals, the withdrawal time has to be taken into account.

CT disease features

There is a whole variety of infectious/parasitic and metabolic diseases of the central nervous system in ruminants, which may be associated with meningitis, encephalitis, myelitis, encephalomalacia or cerebellar hypoplasia. Single or multiple abscesses in the brain and spinal cord may be seen in ruminants due to hematogeneous infection or direct spread from head trauma or nasopharyngeal injury. Brain abscesses may also represent a sequel to dehorning, placement of a nose ring, rhinitis or otitis media.

Fractures and infectious bone lesions such as osteomyelitis occur rather frequently in ruminants. In the spine, traumatic lesions and spondylitis may be found (Figure 47.1).

Congenital or neoplastic diseases of the central nervous system, other than leucosis, are rather uncommon as they are in general in ruminants.

CT may be very helpful to identify abscesses, neoplastic lesions (e.g. leucosis, adenocarcinoma or sarcomas), perforating trauma or foreign bodies associated with the upper digestive apparatus.

Upper airway diseases are excellent to work up with CT and the most common problems in ruminants include rhinitis, sinusitis, cysts in young animals (Figure 47.2) and trauma. Space-occupying lesions such as granulomas (e.g. with actinomycosis), abscesses or tumor-like adenocarcinoma are occasionally seen. Sinusitis may develop secondary to dehorning, trauma, cysts or parasites. In cows with poor healing of sinusitis, CT may be indicated for the detection of a sequestrum that has developed secondary to the sinusitis.

Dental diseases may be diagnosed in camelides, where a tooth root abscess, subsequent osteomyelitis and sequestrum formation may be seen (Figure 47.3). There is a high prevalence of lower airway diseases in ruminants due to viral, bacterial, parasitic or non-infectious causes. CT lung patterns in small ruminants or young animals are very similar to those described in dogs. However, CT is not the method of choice in ruminants for their diagnosis.

Porcine CT

Imaging protocol

Pigs up to approximately 300 kg can be scanned on CT tables designed for use with humans. For whole-body scanning ventral recumbency is best tolerated, the thoracic and pelvic limbs should be drawn cranially and caudally respectively. Sedation using Azaperone 1–2 mg/kg (Stresnil, Mallinckrodt, USA) provides adequate restraint. Fasting 12–16 h prior to scanning will reduce artifacts due to intestinal content. For whole-body scanning (shoulders to pelvis) a slice thickness of 0.5 cm, 110 kVp, 140 mAs will permit scan completion in approximately 80 s in pigs up to 100 kg using a single-slice helical scanner. Body composition studies

Veterinary Computed Tomography, First Edition. Edited by Tobias Schwarz, Jimmy Saunders.

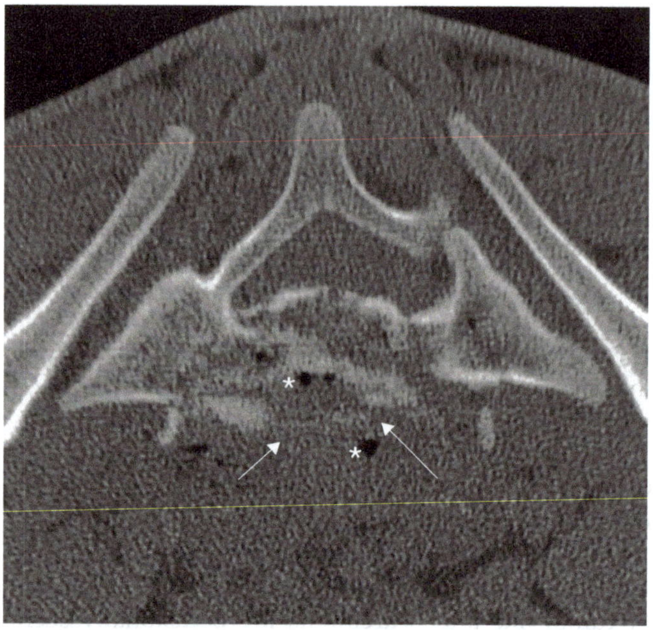

A

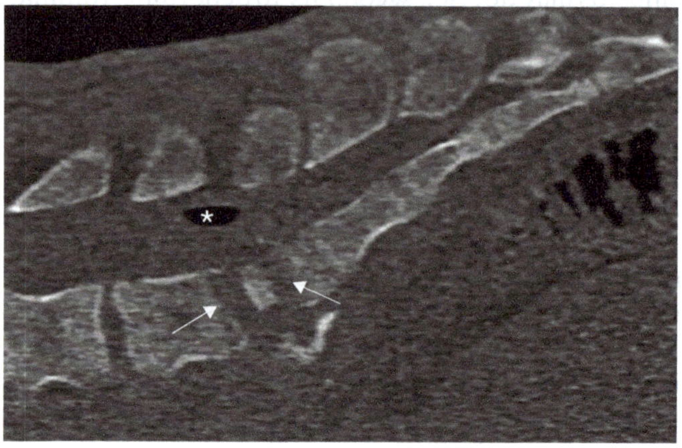

B

Figure 47.1 Two-month-old calf with infectious spondylitis /discospondylitis. (A) Transverse CT image shows a marked lysis of the sacrum (arrows) with free gas (asterisk) in the adjacent soft tissue. (B) Sagittally reconstructed CT image confirms lysis of the caudal endplate of L6 and of the sacrum (arrows) and shows free gas (asterisk) in the vertebral canal.

require a kernel optimized for soft tissue contrast, while skeletal studies should include images processed with a kernel optimized for spatial resolution. If densitometry is to be performed, the kernel should be standardized as it will influence the recorded tissue CT numbers.

CT anatomy and normal variants

Production pigs are an extremely uniform population. Slight variation exists in the number of lumbar vertebrae. The shape of the spinous process of the scapula is considered important for the predisposition to shoulder abscesses, a common problem in housed breeding sows. Intestinal volume is not as great as in small ruminants.

CT disease features

For economic reasons, CT is rarely performed as an aid to diagnosis in individual pigs. Accounts of its use in clinical veterinary medicine are few. Osteochondrosis and osteomyelitis are known problems in production pigs and these conditions lend themselves to CT diagnosis (Figure 47.4).

CT in porcine animal models

There is considerable use of pigs as animal models of human disease. CT has been used in models of experimentally induced pyelonephritis, cryoablation of liver tumors and ocular foreign bodies.

CT in production pigs

The principal application of CT in pigs relates to the examination of body composition. The proportion by weight or volume of adipose to lean tissue must be optimized for optimal feed conversion, reproductive performance and slaughter characterized to meet market demand. CT can be used as a non-invasive tool in the selection of breeding stock and in the validation of other methods, e.g. measurement using ultrasound of tissue thickness, that can be applied under farm conditions. Industrial CT is an advanced topic in itself and there is current research into the use and feasibility of CT to grade carcasses and guide automated cutting systems in abattoirs.

At its simplest, body composition estimates require that image slices are segmented into relevant groups, lean, fat and bone. Since the three tissues have very different HU, this is readily achieved (Figure 47.5A). Estimates can be based on data from whole-body or selected transverse scans by calculating the proportion of voxels in the HU range for the various tissue types. Three important issues have to be addressed in these studies. The first is a particular problem in live pigs as opposed to carcasses, where due to slice thickness artIfact a voxel at the junction, for example between intestinal gas and intestinal wall, may be mistakenly interpreted as a fat-containing voxel. There are various strategies, for example by examining neighboring voxels, to minimize the effect of these 'mixed voxels'. The second issue when segmenting tissue by HU is the

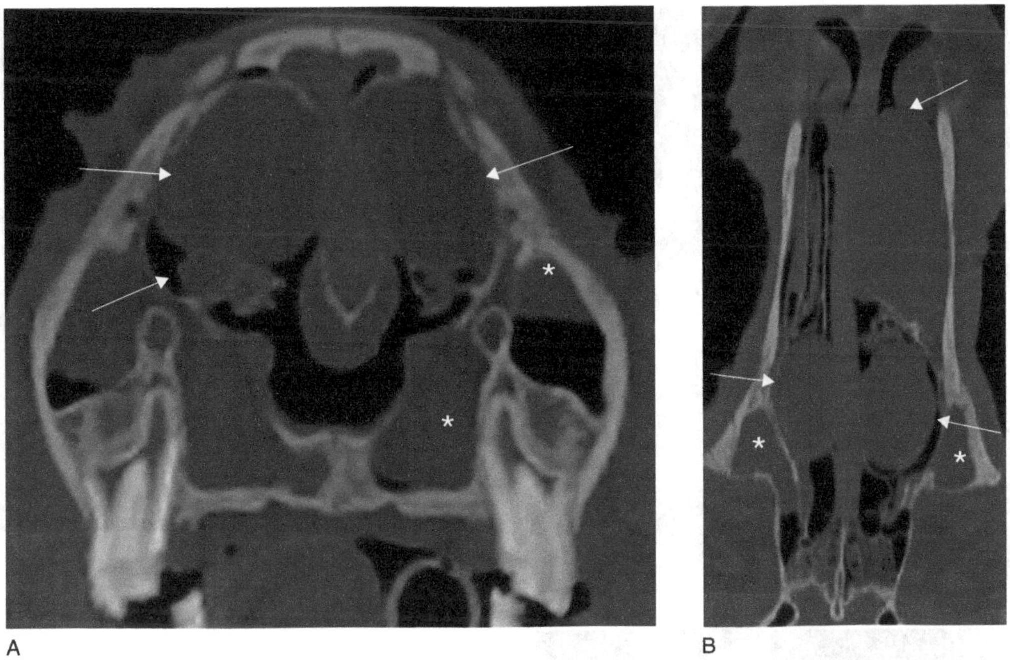

Figure 47.2 Young cow with nasal cysts and sinusitis. (A) Transverse CT image shows multiple cysts of different size in the nasal cavities (arrows) and maxillary sinusitis (asterisks) bilaterally. There is mild deformation of the skull. (B) Dorsally reconstructed CT image shows the cysts (arrows) and sinusitis (asterisks). There is moderate deviation of the nasal septum to the right. The CT study was performed in dorsal recumbency.

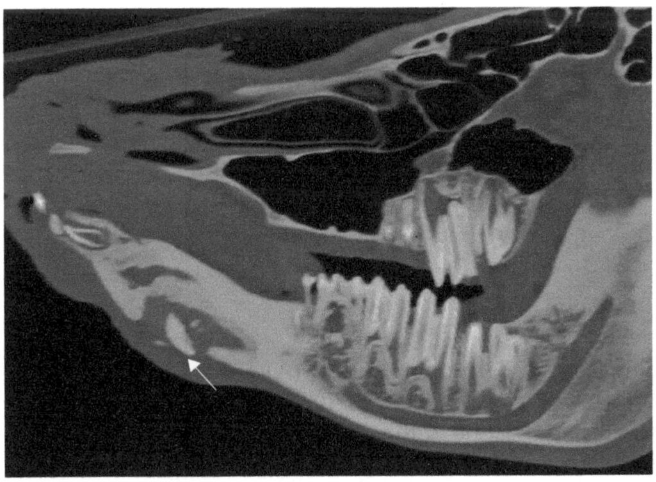

Figure 47.3 Adult cow with chronic fistulous tract formation along the mandibula (old partially healed fracture). Sagittally reconstructed CT image shows soft tissue swelling, marked smooth new bone formation, sclerosis within the right mandibula and a sequestrum (arrow). The CT study was performed in dorsal recumbency.

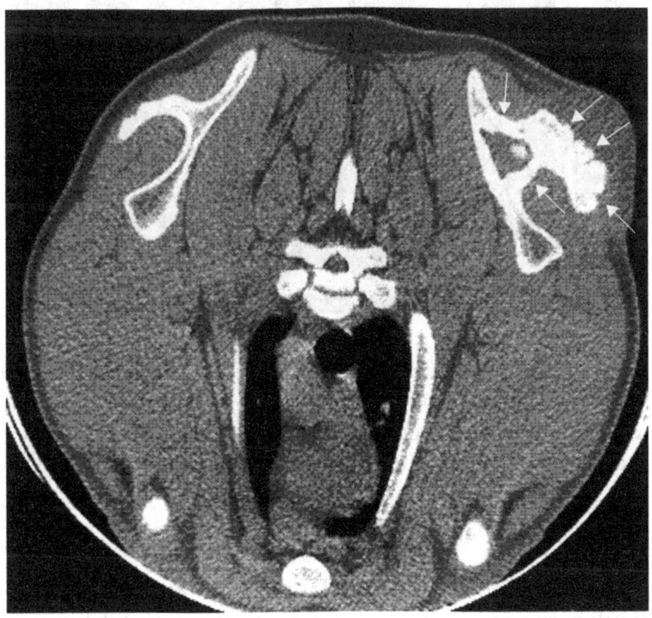

Figure 47.4 Adult pig with an osteomyelitis of the scapula associated with an abscess in the shoulder region. Transverse CT image shows thickening of the spine and body of the scapula and an irregular outline of the spine of the scapula (arrows). There is an overlying soft tissue swelling. Mathematical models are currently being explored to describe the shape of the scapula and test if certain shapes predispose to this problem. (Courtesy Jørgen Kongsro, Norsvin, Norway.)

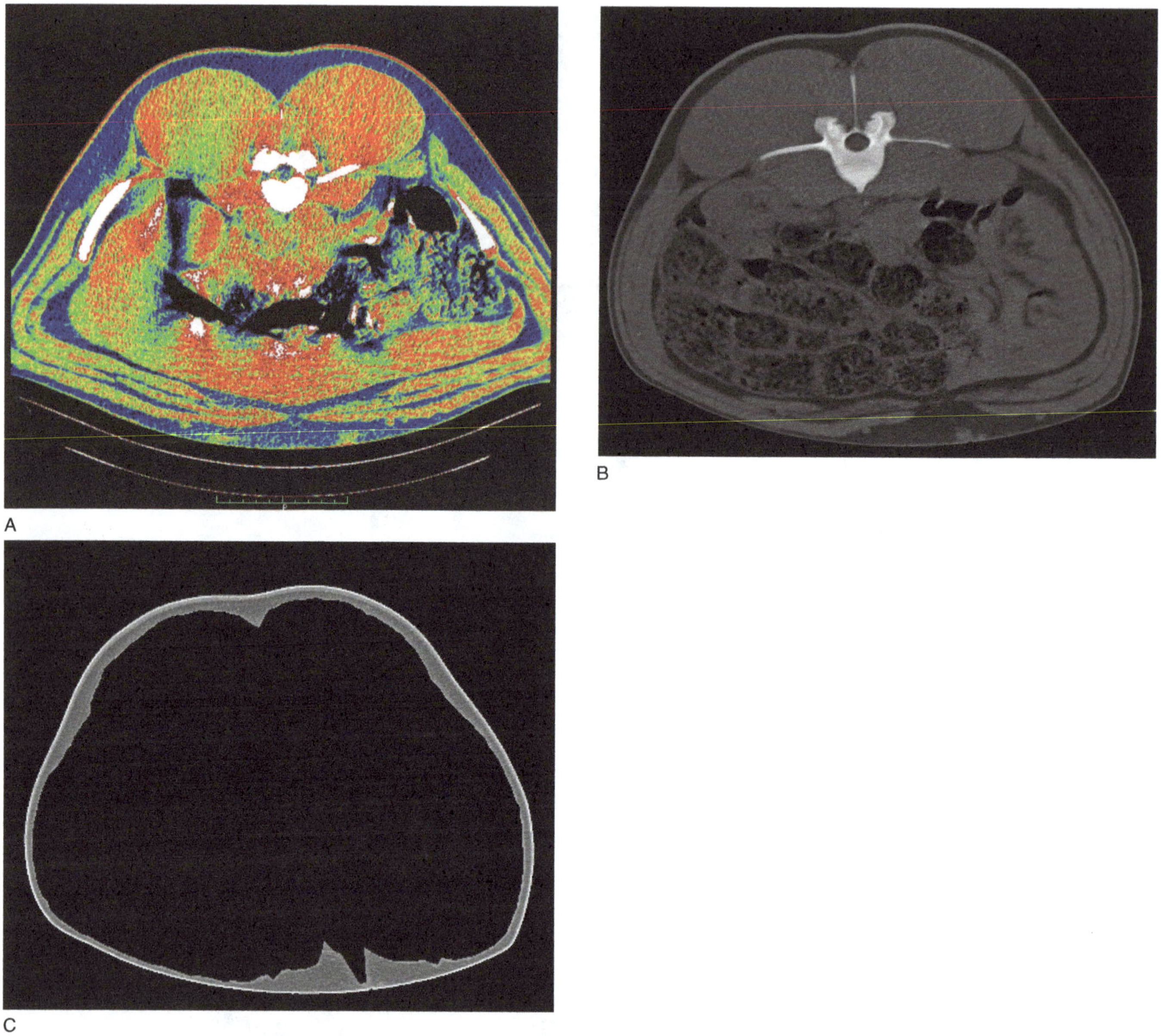

Figure 47.5 Transverse CT images (abdomen) of a pig undergoing tests for body composition. (A) The color look-up table separates adipose from other tissues (blue is assigned a –50 to –200 HU). (B) Grayscale image. (C) Automatic detection of the junction between subcutaneous adipose tissue and underlying muscle and deletion of the area inside this junction. This procedure allows separating descriptions of subcutaneous and visceral adipose tissue.

influence of the choice of HU range to apply to a particular tissue on final estimates. Various tables are available showing typical HU for different tissues. These can be taken as guides only as it has been shown in pigs that the HU for a particular tissue type varies from individual to individual and within individuals with age and location. Optimal accuracy may require that a CT range be determined for the particular individual at a particular time point. Finally, data sets can be very large given that a whole-body scan will contain 100 or more slices and the number of scans required can be high to achieve statistical power or if the method is used as a selection procedure for breeding stock. For this reason automated image analysis is essential.

Adipose tissue is metabolically active and differs in function and chemical composition from location to location throughout the body. Excessive visceral adipose deposits, for example, are associated with obesity-related diseases to a greater extent than subcutaneous. The subcutaneous adipose layer in the pig is itself composed of three layers (detectable by ultrasound but not CT) that differ in their rate of development, heritability and correlation with other body characteristics such as the size of intramuscular fat depots. Pigs have been used to investigate differences between these various adipose depots, an analysis that requires that image segmentation strategies are capable of separating one fat depot from another. This is a more challenging task than the simple segmenting adipose tissue from other tissues such as muscle or bone that have very different HU. Various image feature recognition techniques can be used to isolate these depots. Subcutaneous adipose tissue, for example, can be isolated because it is bounded by skin and muscle, both of which have HU greater than zero (Figures 47.5B and 47.5C). A software algorithm that can recognize this transition zone can be used to select this tissue from each image slice. Such software is available commercially or can be written on site. Volume or HU analysis can thus be performed in the isolated tissue. Work in this area has shown that the HU of adipose tissue in pigs varies with distance from the skin surface and with age possibly reflecting location dependent differences in chemical and physical adipose tissue composition.

The application of CT in production pigs is different to that seen in companion or sport animal species. The pig industry invests large sums of money into genetic improvement programs using CT. Some testing centers are performing in excess of 3000 CT examinations annually. This application of CT is relevant in its own right for the veterinarian and also as a source of data that can give insights into the general topic of obesity or other diseases where the pig can be used as a model.

Further Reading

Kolstad K, Brenøe UT and Vangen O (2002) Genetic differences in energy partitioning in growing pigs. *Acta Agriculturae Scandinavica, Section A – Animal Science* **52**: 213–20.

Vester-Christensena M, Erbou SGH, Hansen MF *et al.* (2009) Virtual dissection of pig carcasses. *Meat Science* **81**: 699–704.

CHAPTER FORTY-EIGHT

Rabbits and Rodents

Randi Drees

Imaging Protocol

See Table 48.1.

CT: Anatomy and Normal Variants

Head (Figure 48.1, Table 48.2)

Rabbits and rodents have aradicular hypsodont teeth that grow throughout life. In hamsters and rats only the incisors are aradicular hypsodont, the cheek teeth are anelodont brachydont. In guinea pigs the apex of the incisors extends lingual to the level of the second cheek tooth. Only in rabbits is deciduous dentition present at birth. The occlusal surface of the cheek teeth in guinea pigs is oriented in an oblique plane: the mandibular teeth are curved lingually and the maxillary cheek teeth are curved buccally. In chinchillas and rabbits the occlusal surface is almost horizontally oriented. CT allows accurate evaluation of the teeth, periodontium and alveolar bone as well as the oral soft tissues and bony structures of the skull.

In the normal guinea pig the ventral auricular cartilages are commonly mineralized. The tympanic bullae of chinchillas are large, thin-walled and septated; in other rodents and rabbits they are comparably small.

Thorax

The heart takes up a relatively large portion of the thoracic cavity in rabbits and rodents. Thymic remnants may be seen in the ventral cranial mediastinum of the adult rabbit and rodent. Otherwise thoracic structures are similar to those of mammals.

Abdomen

The stomach of rabbits and rodents is comparably small and hook-shaped and mostly located in the right cranial abdomen. The duodenum in rabbits has a slight enlargement at the level of the termination of the bile duct. The small intestines are commonly located in the right cranial abdomen in rabbits and rodents. The ileum has a thick-walled expansion (sacculus rotundus), most prominent in rabbits. The C-shaped large cecum is located in the mid and ventral portion of the peritoneal cavity and is normally filled with gas and ingesta in rabbits and rodents. The ascending colon in the rabbit is subdivided in four regions, of which the first are distinguishable by their teniae and haustra. The major portion of the liver is located in the right cranial abdomen. The spleen is usually small. In rabbits, the right lobe of the pancreas can be diffuse in the mesoduodenum. The kidneys and bladder are comparable in shape and location to those of other mammals; mineral-dense sediment in the urinary bladder of the rabbit can be seen as a normal variant. In guinea pigs the ischiopubic symphysis dilates to allow passage of the large fetal head. It fuses at 7–8 months if no breeding has occurred up to this point and then may contribute to dystocia in later pregnancies.

Musculoskeletal

Periarticular mineralized bodies and linear dystrophic mineralization of entheses and muscles is commonly seen in rabbits and rodents and is usually of minor clinical significance.

Metabolic

Normal serum calcium concentration in rabbits is 30–50% higher than in other mammals. Resorption of calcium via the intestinal tract is achieved by passive diffusion and active transport; excretion of calcium into the gastrointestinal tract is independent of serum calcium levels. Renal calcium excretion or conservation according to metabolic needs is control-

Veterinary Computed Tomography, First Edition. Edited by Tobias Schwarz, Jimmy Saunders.

Table 48.1
CT imaging protocol for rabbits and rodents.

Decubitus	• Head, thorax: ventral • Abdomen: dorsal or ventral* • Spine and myelo-CT: dorsal • Other: ventral, dorsal, lateral depending on area of interest

Special positioning	• Head:
	  • Transverse plane: hard palate perpendicular to gantry (head on foam pad or similar)
	  • Direct dorsal plane: hard palate parallel to gantry (animal on foam pad)
	• Myelo-CT: scan plane aligned with intervertebral disk space in region of interest
	  • Accurate straight positioning in trough

Scan margins	• Head: tip of the nose ←→ cranial neck • Thorax: thoracic inlet ←→ caudal margin of diaphragm • Abdomen: cranial end of diaphragmatic cupola ←→ anus • Spine and myelo-CT: cranial ←→ caudal margin of neurolocalized segment or region of interest • Others: cranial ←→ caudal margin of region of interest
Voltage (kVp)	120
Current (mAs)	100
Tube rotation time (s)	≤1
Slice width (mm)	• Head: 1 mm • Thorax, abdomen: 2–3 mm • Spine and myelo-CT: 1 mm • Other: 1–3 mm depending on region of interest
Sequential slice interval (mm)	• Head: 1 mm • Spine and myelo-CT: 1 mm • Other: 1–3 mm depending on region of interest
Helical image reconstruction interval	• Thorax, abdomen: 2–3 mm
Pitch	• Thorax, abdomen: 1.4
Kernel frequency	• Pre- and post-contrast: medium • Bone: high • Myelo-CT: medium and high frequency
Contrast medium application site	• Intra-venous: cephalic or saphenous catheter • Myelo-CT: subarachnoid puncture
Contrast medium type	• Intra-venous: ionic or non-ionic iodinated contrast medium • Myelo-CT: non-ionic iodinated contrast medium
Contrast medium dose	• Intra-venous: 700–800 mg I/kg • Myelo-CT: 0.33 ml/kg or until sufficient opacification verified under image guidance
Contrast medium injection mode	Manual
Scan delay post start contrast injection	Intra-venous: 1 min
Window level (HU)	• Pre- and post-contrast, myelo-CT: +250 • Bone: +500
Window width (HU)	• Pre- and post-contrast, myelo-CT: +50 • Bone: +3500

*Respiratory motion is less in dorsal recumbency, however ventral recumbency is often better tolerated by the patient.

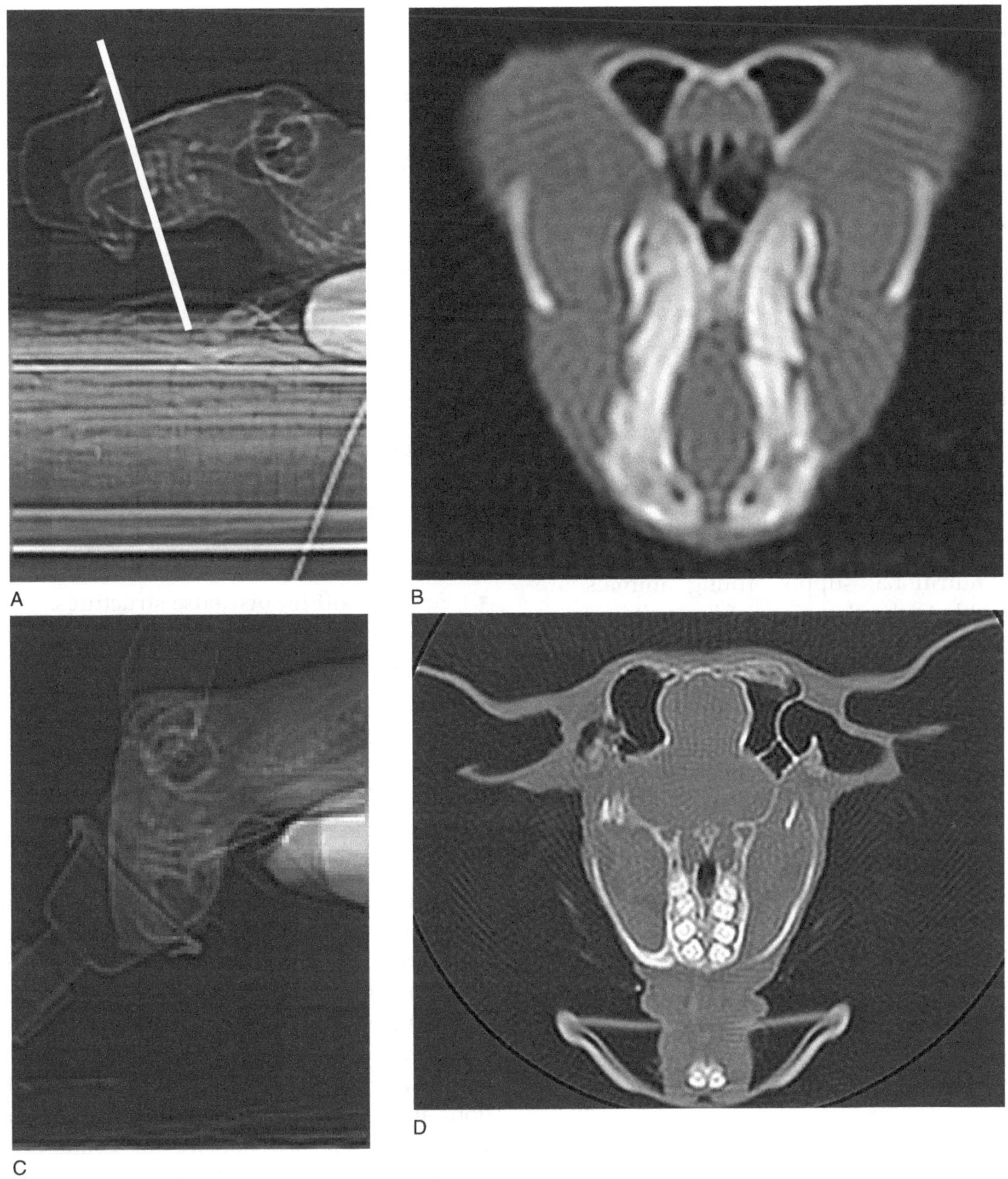

Figure 48.1 Positioning for head CT for rabbit and rodent patients. (A) Alignment of the gantry (white line) perpendicular to the hard palate for transverse plane (B) acquisition. (C) Parallel alignment of the gantry to the hard palate for direct dorsal plane (D) acquisition can be helpful for evaluation of dental and periodontal structures.

Table 48.2
Dental formula in rabbits and rodents.

Dental formula	Rabbit	Guinea pig, chinchilla	Hamster, rat
Deciduous	$\frac{2030}{1020}=16$	N/A	N/A
Permanent	$\frac{2033}{1023}=28$	$\frac{1013}{1013}=20$	$\frac{1003\,(2H)}{1003\,(2H)}=14\text{–}16$

led by pituitary-dependent hormone and vitamin D; however, vitamin D has less impact than in other mammals. Renal failure therefore sequentially leads to failure of serum calcium regulation.

Lameness and lethargy in adult guinea pigs are commonly attributed to vitamin C deficiency, as they depend on nutritional supply. Young animals are more susceptible to develop signs of hypovitaminosis C (scurvy), such as ceasing skeletal maturation, epiphyseal dysplasia and progressive osteopenia. Alternatively, osteodystrophy due to secondary nutritional or renal hyperparathyroidism should be considered as a cause of lameness or can be found incidentally. Specifically, osteodystrophia fibrosa has been described in guinea pigs, with an increased incidence in satin breed guinea pigs. Osteodystrophia fibrosa presents with decreased bone opacity (ostopenia, double cortical line), patchy osteosclerois, coarse bone trabeculation, arthropathies and pathologic fractures.

CT Disease Features

Trauma

Spinal trauma

Rabbits are prone to spinal fractures and (sub)luxations, commonly associated with restraint-induced self trauma. CT examination can additionally be performed after subarachnoid contrast injection (myelogram).

CT features

- Sharp-margined fracture lines or fragments in acute cases.
- Malalignment of vertebrae.
- Myelo-CT: deviation or obliteration of the contrast columns indicating compression of the spinal cord, contrast medium in the spinal cord (myelomalacia), leakage of contrast medium out of the subarachnoid space (dural laceration).

Fractures and soft tissue trauma

Fractures of the skull or other skeletal structures can be seen in rodents and rabbits, usually due to bite or step injuries.

CT features

- Severed soft tissue-dense structures.
- Sharp-margined fracture lines or fragments and malaligned skeletal structures.

Infection/Inflammation

Dental and periodontal disease

The progressive syndrome of acquired dental disease is commonly seen in rabbits and rodents, leading to deterioration of tooth quality, acquired malocclusion, elongation of tooth roots and periapical disease. Secondary osteomyelitis and abscesses in or adjacent to the maxilla, mandible or retrobulbar space are seen in advanced disease. Predisposing factors are weakened alveolar support of the tooth due to underlying metabolic bone disease, dietary texture and composition, and genetic predisposition. Direct dorsal plane CT acquisition is beneficial for evaluation of tooth alignment and periodontal disease.

CT features (Figures 48.2 and 48.3)

- Curvature and elongation of the teeth with hook formation in the oral cavity: usually oral curvature of the maxillary incisors and rostral curvature of the mandibular incisors, lingual hooks on mandibular cheek teeth, buccal hooks on maxillary cheek teeth. Elongation of tooth roots with possible periosteal penetration. Distortion of teeth alignment, loss of occlusal line.
- Dental decay: loss of vertical enamel lining, hypodense tooth center, tooth fragmentation.
- Widening of the periodontal space with periodontal disease.

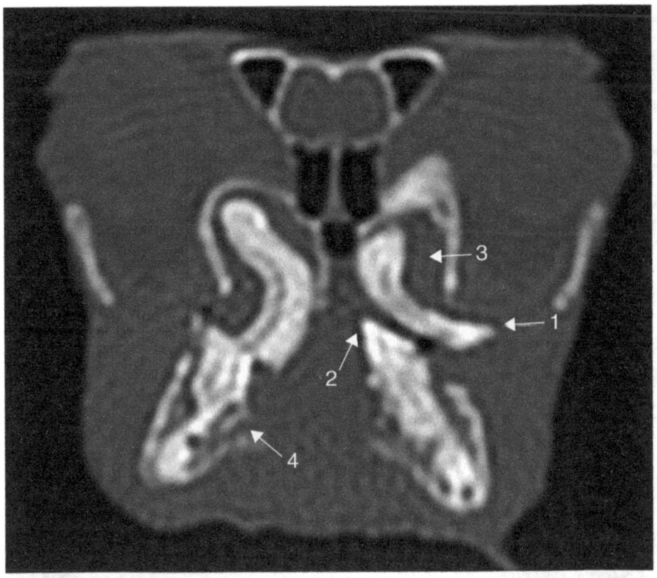

Figure 48.2 Adult chinchilla with dental and periodontal disease. Transverse CT image shows an overgrowth and curvature of mandibular and maxillary cheek teeth with buccal (1) and lingual (2) hook formation. There is also widening of the periodontal spaces (3) and irregular lysis of the alveolar bone (4).

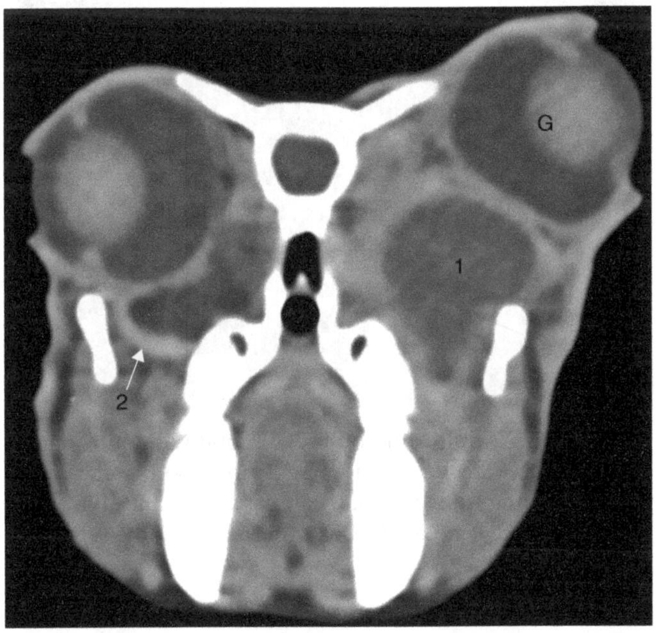

Figure 48.3 Adult Dutch rabbit with bilateral retrobulbar abscesses. Transverse post-contrast CT image shows abscesses with a fluid-dense, non-enhancing center (1) and a soft tissue-dense, contrast-enhancing rim (2). The left globe (G) is displaced dorsolaterally and deformed.

- Loss of normal root structure, definition of lamina dura and alveolar bone; in advanced cases tooth root abscesses with lysis of the surrounding alveolus and possibly extensive osteomyelitis of the adjacent bone.
- Dystrophic mineralization of the alveolus with chronic alveolitis.
- Thinned ventral mandibular and incisive cortex.
- All over loss of bone opacity in the skull.
- Lingual and/or buccal soft tissue swelling in regions of trauma due to dental hooks or overgrowth.
- Abscess: fluid or soft tissue-dense mass possibly containing gas; rim enhancement on post-contrast series.

Upper and lower airway disease

Upper and possible consequential lower airway infection with *Pasteurella* spp., *Bordetella* spp. and *Staphylococcus* spp. are common causes for sneezing, nasal discharge and possible pneumonitis or bronchopneumonia in rabbits and rodents. CT enables evaluation of the extent of upper airway disease and differentiation from nasal discharge related to tooth root abscess formation. A small amount of recumbency-dependent atelectasis is commonly seen as a normal variant and has to be differentiated from consolidation.

CT features (Figure 48.4)

- *Rhinitis:* soft tissue dense material in the nasal cavity, commonly bilaterally. Possible destruction of the turbinates and the bony nasal septum with chronic rhinitis.
- *Bronchitis:* bronchial thickening, peribronchial infiltrates, bronchial plugs.
- *Pneumonia:* diffuse interstitial pattern and/or consolidation.

Otitis

Lop-eared rabbits are prone to develop otitis externa. Otitis media in rabbits commonly occurs in conjunction with upper airway infections (*Pasteurella* spp.) and patients can present with severe head tilt. Ruling out otitis is important if *Encephalitozoon cuniculi* infection is suspected in rabbits. In guinea pigs otitis media is usually due to infection with *Streptococcus pneumoniae*; this infection has an increased likelihood with prolonged subclinical vitamin C deficiency.

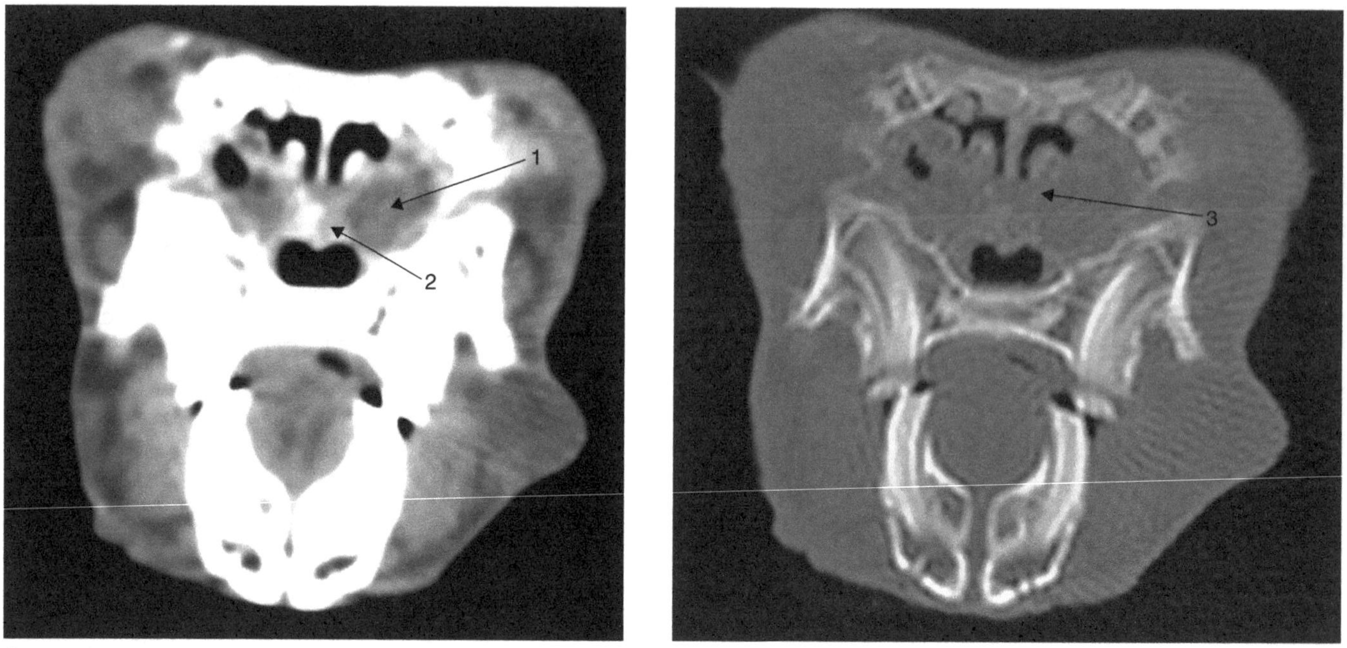

Figure 48.4 Transverse CT images of an adult Dutch rabbit with a rhinitis due to infection with *Pasteurella* spp. (A) The nasal cavities are partially obliterated with fluid- (1) and soft tissue-dense material (2). (B) The nasal turbinates are partially destroyed (3).

CT features (Figure 48.5)

- *Otitis externa:* increased enhancement and thickness of the ear canal lining. Overall subjective narrowing of the external ear canal. Increased amount of non-enhancing soft tissue-dense material in the external ear canal and possible mineralization of auricular cartilages (chronic).
- *Otitis media:* fluid or inspissated soft tissue to mineral-dense material within the tympanic cavity, possible contrast enhancement of the lining of the tympanic bulla, sclerosis and thickening of the tympanic bulla, and possible lysis of the bulla in severe and chronic cases.
- *Otitis interna:* none, or alteration of the small bony structures of the inner ear.

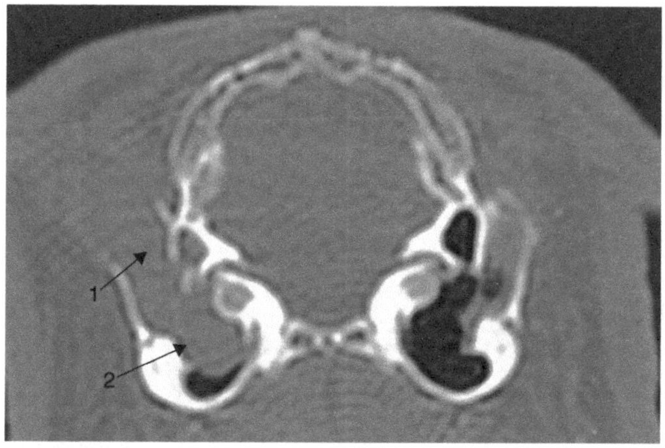

Figure 48.5 Adult Mini lop breed rabbit with otitis media and externa. Transverse CT image shows soft tissue-dense material filling the external ear canal (1) and tympanic bulla (2). There is no evidence of thickening of the tympanic bulla.

Gastrointestinal disease

Rabbits commonly have a moderate amount of hair in the stomach. Formation of trichobezoars usually results in and is not a cause of gastrointestinal dysfunction. Intestinal obstruction often occurs with ingestion of foreign material. The etiology of cecal impaction is incompletely understood but thought to be related to stress and sequential hypomotility. Mucoid enteropathy is mostly seen in adult pet rabbits, often after stressful incidents. Almost all gastrointestinal disorders lead to additional gas collection in the gastrointestinal system. Mildly increased gas accumulation in the gastrointestinal tract can be related to anesthetic procedures.

CT features

- Possible soft tissue-dense trichobezoar visible in the stomach.
- Gas-distended gastrointestinal tract.

- Enlarged mesenteric lymph nodes: reactive lymphadenopathy.
- Cecal impaction: cecal dilatation with gas and impacted ingesta.
- Mucoid enteropathy: large amount of fluid to soft tissue-dense mucus in the colon, often with cecal impaction. Stomach and small intestines can be distended with fluid and gas.

Urinary system

In rabbits, mineral urinary sediment is a normal variant. Renal, ureteral, cystic and urethral urolithiasis is caused by increased urine concentration of stone-forming ions and can lead to mechanical obstruction and irritation in rabbits and rodents. Cystitis is often present with cystic urolithiasis. Guinea pigs often present with urethral urolithiasis. Renal failure leads to alterations in calcium metabolism in rabbits. Granulomatous lesions of the kidney associated with *Encephalitozoon cuniculi* infection in rabbits are seen on necropsy or histologic samples. Abyssinian breed guinea pigs are prone to develop non-insulin-dependent diabetes mellitus. Secondary cystitis can lead to urinary bladder wall hypertrophy and voiding dysfunction.

CT features

- Gravity-dependent mineral sediment in the urinary bladder (normal variant in rabbits).
- Gravity-dependent mineral (less commonly soft tissue-dense) stones in the urinary system.
- Renal failure in rabbits: renomegaly, urolithiasis, increased bone opacity (osteosclerosis), metastatic soft tissue mineralization,
- Urinary bladder wall hypertrophy: distended urinary bladder and subjectively thickened wall.

Genital system

Pyometra or other inflammatory conditions of the uterus are seen in female rabbits and rodents. Mastitis and mammary neoplasia is usually identified on clinical examination; thoracic CT for metastasis check may be indicated.

CT features

- Enlarged uterus filled with fluid-dense material.

Osteomyelitis

Osteomyelitis is seen with similar etiology as in small animals but rarely occurs in rabbits and rodents.

CT features

- Osteolytic lesions in affected bones, possibly associated with severed soft tissues if related to wounds.

Neoplasia

Most commonly observed neoplasia in rabbits and rodents are lymphoma, thymoma, mammary neoplasia and uterine neoplasia. Pulmonary neoplasia is common in rodents >3 years. Other neoplasms seen in small animals can also affect the rabbit and rodent patient.

Lymphoma and thymoma

Intrathoracic lymph node enlargement or cranial mediastinal masses are commonly observed in rabbits and guinea pigs with lymphoma. However, all other forms of lymphoma can occur in the rabbit and rodent. Differentiating between thymoma and lymphoma may depend on cytologic analysis.

CT features (Figure 48.6)

- Lymphoma: cranial mediastinal, sternal and tracheobronchial lymph node enlargement; peripheral lymph node enlargement; hepatosplenomegaly; gastrointestinal masses. Less commonly pulmonary infiltrates.
- Thymoma: ventral cranial mediastinal mass, often cystic components and poor contrast enhancement.

Genital neoplasia and cystic disorders

Mammary neoplasia is seen in middle-aged to older rabbits and rodents and can be benign or malignant. Malignant mammary neoplasia can metastasize to the sternal lymph nodes and lung. Uterine, uterine stump or cervical neoplasia is commonly seen in guinea pigs and can be mineralized. Guinea pigs often present with cystic ovarian disease with or without associated hormonal imbalances; endometrial hyperplasia or leiomyoma occur sequentially.

CT features (Figure 48.7)

- Soft tissue-dense mammary masses with variable contrast enhancement and possible mineralization, sternal lymphadenopathy, lung nodules.
- Uterine or cervical masses with/without mineral content.
- Ovarian cysts: fluid-dense cystic structures arising from the ovaries, caudodorsal to the kidneys, commonly bilaterally.

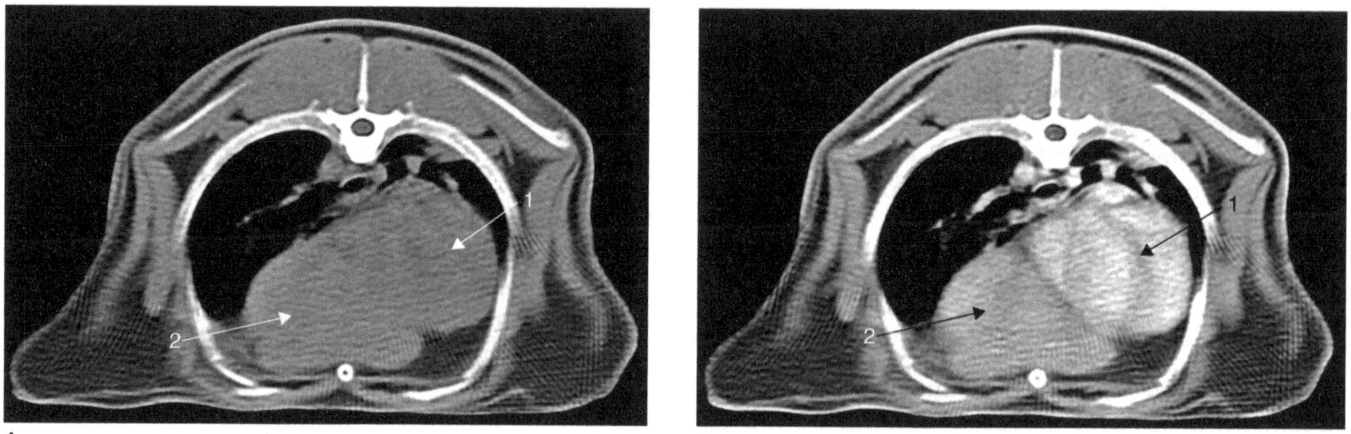

A B

Figure 48.6 Adult Dutch rabbit with a thymoma. (A) Transverse CT image shows the heart (1) displaced laterally by a large soft tissue-dense mediastinal mass (2). (B) On post-intravenous transverse contrast CT, the mass (2) moderately enhances.

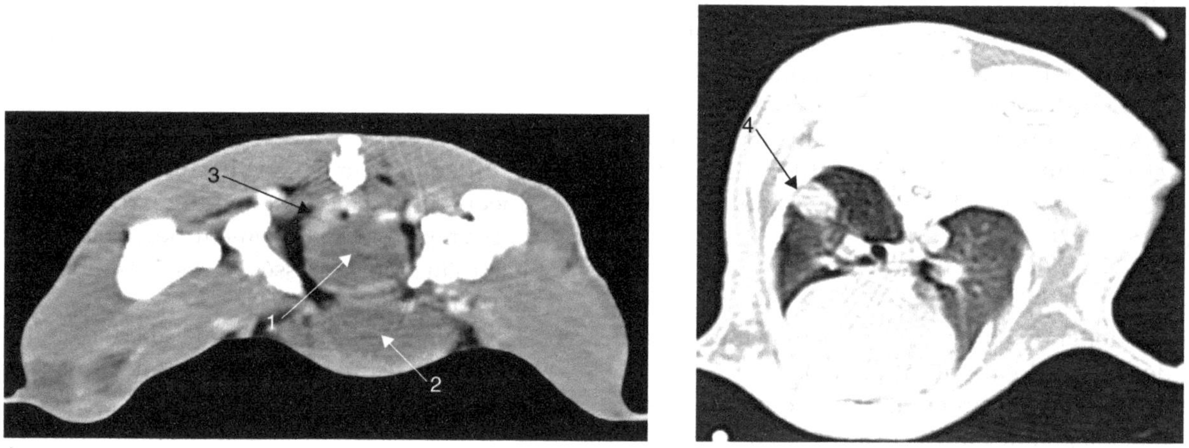

A B

Figure 48.7 Adult Angora rabbit with uterine stump adenocarcinoma. (A) Transverse CT image of the caudal abdomen at the level of the coxofemoral joints. The mixed soft tissue- and fluid-dense mass (1) is heterogeneously enhancing following intravenous contrast injection. It is located dorsally to the urinary bladder (2) and displaces the colon (3) dorsally and to the right. (B) Transverse CT image shows soft tissue nodules (4) in the lung parenchyma, consistent with metastatic disease.

Further Reading

Beregi A, Zorn S and Felkai F (1999) Ultrasonic diagnosis of ovarian cysts in ten guinea pigs. *Vet Radiol Ultrasound* **40**: 74–6.

Capello V and Cauduro A (2008) Clinical technique: application of computed tomography for diagnosis of dental disease in the rabbit, guinea pig, and chinchilla. *J Exotic Pet Med* **17**: 93–101.

Harcourt-Brown F (2007) Radiographic signs of renal disease in rabbits. *Vet Rec* **160**: 787–94.

Legendre LF (2002) Malocclusions in guinea pigs, chinchillas and rabbits. *Can Vet J* **43**: 385–90.

Reiter AM (2008) Pathophysiology of dental disease in the rabbit, guinea pig and chinchilla. *J Exotic Pet Med* **17**: 70–7.

CHAPTER FORTY-NINE

Avian

Michaela Gumpenberger

Imaging Protocol

See Tables 49.1 and 49.2.

Imaging Technique

Routine CT in birds is performed under general anesthesia, mostly with isoflurane and a head chamber. Exceptionally, some regions (coelomic cavity, lung) of larger, weak individuals may be scanned in conscious animals (Figure 49.1). They can be strapped to the table or may be positioned in a box. However, diagnoses in delicate regions such as the spine or head should always be done in anesthetized birds.

The positioning for head scans depends on the shape of the beak, head and neck. Birds with spherical heads, smaller beaks and shorter necks (e.g. birds of prey, most parrots) will be easier scanned in dorsal recumbency or sometimes even lateral recumbency. Avian species with elongated heads, beaks and necks (e.g. water fowl) are easier positioned in sternal recumbency. Therefore heads will be scanned in dorsal or transversal plane depending on the species. Paper tissues, foam wedges or cardboard boxes can be used as additional devices for correct positioning.

Smaller avian species can be positioned crosswise to the longitudinal axis of the patient table. The resulting sagittal scan is performed much quicker than the axial one. This may be of special interest in critical care patients or in slower, single-slice CT machines.

Slice thickness and distance may vary from 0.5 mm in tiny birds to 5 mm when scanning the coelomic cavity in larger species (e.g. swans). Diagnoses of the spine or head should always be done with small slices. Sagittal scans result in more artifacts than transverse scans caused by grit in the intestines and metallic footrings.

Intravenous contrast medium is administered manually into the jugular vein in small species (e.g. budgerigars). Prior to the removal of the patient from the table for contrast medium application it is recommended to sketch the bird's silhouette with a marker on paper towels. Repositioning after contrast medium application will then be possible with only minimal dislocation. Administration of contrast medium into the basilic vein can be managed in dorsal recumbency without major displacement of the bird.

Barium sulfate suspension (10–20 ml/kg body weight of 5–10%) can be administered with a crop tube 60–90 min prior to the CT examination. The barium will enable better differentiation of the gastrointestinal tract, especially if no intravenous contrast medium will be used.

Analysis of coelomic disorders may be easier in sagittal scans/reconstructions that resemble the more familiar lateral radiograph.

CT Anatomy and Normal Variants (Figure 49.2, Table 49.3)

Today more than 9700 different avian species are known. Although the basic anatomy is similar, each species has its own characteristics. Radiographs still offer a good overview to gain general knowledge of a patient. Rare species (e.g. dead individuals of a zoological garden or museum) should be radiographed and scanned whenever available to build up an archive of reference images.

Disease Features: General Remarks

Most skeletal disorders like fractures or hyperostosis as well as lead intoxication can usually be confirmed

Veterinary Computed Tomography, First Edition. Edited by Tobias Schwarz, Jimmy Saunders.

Table 49.1
CT Imaging protocol of the coelomic cavity of avians.

Series	Pre- and post-contrast bone	Additional remarks
Positioning, routine	Dorsal	Wings should be flexed and attached to the body while the legs should be extended caudally to minimize artifacts
Positioning of weak animal, critical care	Sternal	In emaciated patients the sharp-edged carina may compromise symmetric positioning
Scan margins	Shoulder ←→ Cloaca	
Voltage (kVp)	100 to 120	Depending on the size of bird
Current (mAs)	100 to 130	Depending on the size of bird
Tube rotation time (s)	1 or 2	
Slice width (mm)	1–3	Budgerigar to swan
Sequential slice interval (mm)	1–3	Budgerigar to swan
Kernel frequency	Pre-contrast: soft tissue/medium Bone: bone	
Window level (HU)	Pre-contrast: +40 Bone: +350	Modified soft tissue window: 50–160
Window width (HU)	Pre-contrast: 400 Bone: 3200	Modified soft tissue window: 500–640

Table 49.2
Intravenous contrast protocol.

Contrast medium application site	Jugular vein (small birds) or basilic vein
Contrast medium type	Iodinated
Contrast medium dose	150–300 mg I/kg bw
Contrast medium injection mode	Manual
Scan delay post start contrast injection	1 min, repetition after 3–5 min
Kernel frequency	Soft tissue/standard
Window level (HU)	+40
Window width (HU)	350

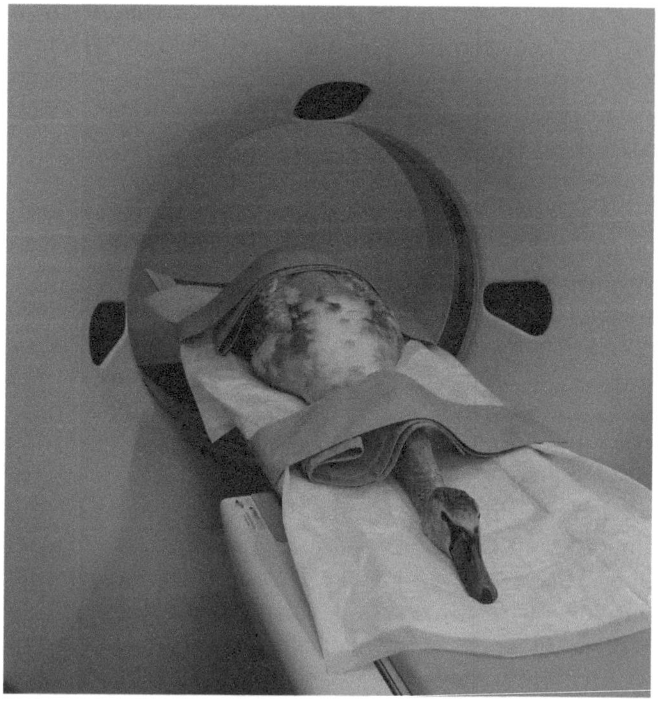

Figure 49.1 Conscious, but weak mute swan (*Cygnus olor*) positioned within the gantry.

Figure 49.2 (A) Scout for sagittal scans in figure 49.2B to demonstrate the normal anatomy of the coelomic organs of a domestic pigeon (*Columba livia f. domestica*). B = bowel loops; Lu = lung; H = heart; Li = liver; V = ventriculus. 1: right lateral scan; 2: right sagittal; 3: left sagittal; 4: left lateral scan. (B) Anatomy of a domestic pigeon, sagittal slices (frozen) and scans (soft tissue and lung window): (B) to (D) right lateral scan, (E) to (G) right paramedian, (H) to (J) left sagittal, (K) to (M) left lateral scan. B = bowel loops; Bm = breast muscle; H = heart; K = kidneys; L = lung; Li = liver; P = proventriculus; V = ventriculus.

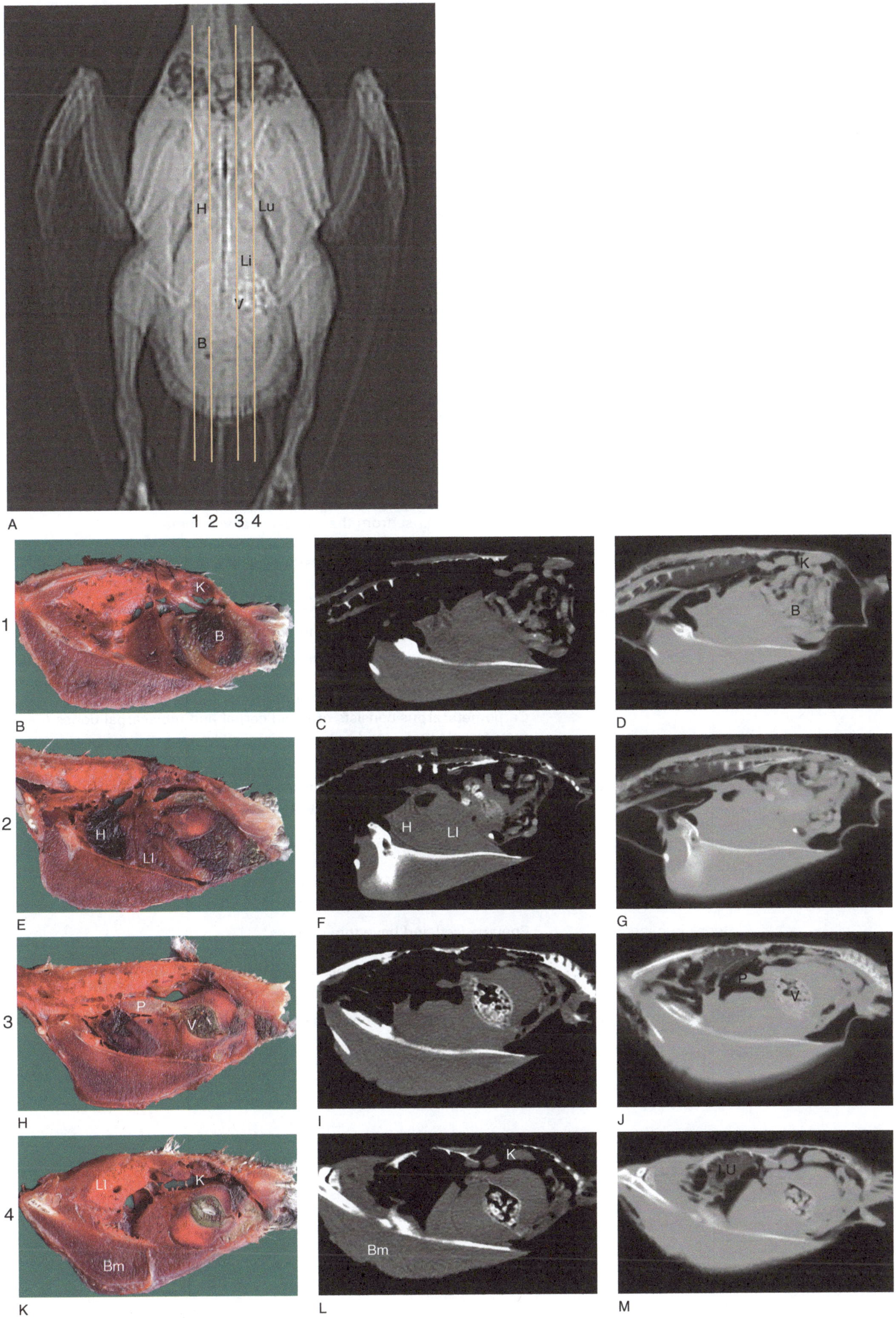

H
Lu
Li
V
B
A
1 2 3 4
1
K
B
B
C
K
B
D
2
H
LI
E
H
LI
F
G
3
P
V
H
I
P
V
J
4
LI
K
Bm
K
K
Bm
L
LU
M

Table 49.3
Anatomy – most important variations compared with mammals.

	Organ	Anatomical details
Head	Head	Infraorbital sinus (better: paranasal sinus with infraorbital, preorbital and postorbital part) connected to nasal cavity
	Eyes	Septum interorbitale between large bulbi Scleral bones support lens attachment Pecten oculi: cannot be differentiated within vitreous in plain CT
Skeleton	Cervical spine	Single condylus occipitalis articulates with atlas and allows rotation of head and neck 180° Number of cervicic vertebrae varies with species
	Thoracic spine	Most cranial thoracic vertebrae are fused and form the notarium (os dorsale) in galliformes and pigeons Single mobile thoracic vertebra connects notarium with synsacrum
	Lumbar spine	Last thoracic, all lumbar and sacral vertebrae as well as first caudal vertebrae are fused to form the synsacrum (os lumbosacrale)
	Caudal spine	Pygostyle – fusion of last caudal vertebrae
	Ribs	Floating ribs arise from the last cervical vertebrae 5–6 pairs connect sternum to thoracic spine Uncinate processes are directed caudally and are connected with the following rib
	Sternum	Not segmented Carina or keel supports attachment of massive flight muscles
	Forelimbs	Clavicles unite and form the furcula Ulna larger than radius Only two carpal bones (os carpi radiale and ulnare) Carpometacarpus consists of fused carpal and metacarpal bones (os metacarpale majus and minus) Digits II, III and IV
	Pelvis and hindlimbs	Pelvis firmly connected to synsacrum, but open ventrally Tibiotarsus: fusion of tibia and part of tarsus, longer than femur Fibula only rudimental Tarsometatarsus: fused distal tarsal bones and metatarsal bones (II to IV) Os metatarsale I: builds first toe Digit I-IV have two, three, four and five phalanges
	Bones in general	Pneumatized and have thin cortices Hyperostosis: especially long bones may show increased density with loss of medullary space under hormone influence (estrogen): egg development as well as ovarial cysts or neoplasias
	Musculoskeletal system	Tendons of limbs, sometimes of the TMJ and some dorsal muscles tend to ossify

Table 49.3
(Continued)

	Organ	Anatomical details
Coelomic organs	Diaphragm	Does not exist
	Heart	Very close to liver, cannot usually be differentiated in plain CT
	Liver	Right (larger, perforated by caudal vena cava) and left (dorsal and ventral) lobe, additional processus vary with species Homogeneous, mean density in domestic pigeons 55–65 HU, nearly impossible to differentiate form the heart in plain CT
	Gallbladder	At visceral surface of right liver lobe Not present in most pigeons and parrots
	Spleen	Right sagittally positioned, medial to proventriculus, in most cage birds small and round (budgerigar = 1 mm, Amazon parrot = 6 mm)
	Pancreas	Lies between the limbs of the duodenum, trilobated, usually not differentiable in CT
	Esophagus	First dorsal to trachea, then at the right side of the neck
	Crop	Extension of esophagus at the level of the thoracic inlet Expansile to ventral and laterocaudal, depending on filling degree
	Stomach	Consists of proventriculus and ventriculus (gizzard): especially in herbivore and granivore species Gizzard is thick walled, mean density in domestic pigeons 60–70 HU, mostly grit in lumen (responsible for artifacts) Single, very expansile stomach in seagulls and storks Small stomach in fruit eaters or nectar-feeding birds Usually does not contain gas
	Small intestines	Duodenum at the right, forms a tight U-shaped loop Duodenojejunal junction close to stomach Jejunum forms some loops, not differentiable from ileum Usually does not contain gas
	Large intestines	Paired ceca in hens, small ceca in pigeons, not present in parrots and carnivore species Short rectum continues to cloaca Usually contains gas
	Kidneys	Trilobated, positioned ventral to synsacrum Mean density in domestic pigeons 35–60 HU
	Ureters	Only visible with contrast media
	Urinary bladder	Does not exist
	Gonads	Males: two testicles cranioventral to cranial pole of kidneys, enlarge during mating season (do not misinterpret as renomegaly) Females: only left ovary developed; follicles appear as round structures of various sizes
	Lung	Not lobated Tertiary bronchia responsible for honeycombed lung pattern Does not expand during breathing Density reported in various parrots: –600 to –650 HU
	Air sac system	Unpaired: clavicular air sac Paired: cervical (unpaired in hens), cranial thoracic, caudal thoracic and abdominal air sacs

radiographically in a straightforward way. Hence the following tables will focus on selected disorders that are diagnosed more precisely with CT. Besides some case reports only very few papers of advanced CT studies in avian species exist. Therefore the given examples mostly reflect the experiences of the author.

Disease Features: Skeleton and Head (Table 49.4)

Disease Features: Coelomic Organs (Table 49.5)

Additionally, CT is used in chickens to predict values for the amount of abdominal fat or breast cut for commercial reasons.

Table 49.4
Disease features: skeleton and head.

Organ system	Pathological changes	Manifestation	CT characteristics	Figure
Head	Malformation, developmental	Meningo-encephalocele and cranial malformations in domestic ducks with feather crests	Variable bone formations and skull defects, protrusion of mostly fatty tissue	
	Trauma, dislocation	Mostly collisions with cars or windows, cause fractures and intracranial hemorrhage	Similar to mammals; eye: fractures of scleral bones; sub-/luxation of lens	49.3
	Infection, inflammation, degeneration	Sinusitis, sometimes otitis	Obstruction of usually aerated sinuidal system	
	Infection, inflammation, degeneration (eye)		Cataract or lyses of lens	49.3
	Neoplasia	Single case reports of pituitary adenomas, retrobulbar and intracranial masses	Space-occupying masses, similar to mammals	49.4 49.5
Vertebral column	Trauma, dislocation	Fractures, luxations	Hemorrhage, loss of pneumatized chambers within bony structures; sagittal reconstruction helpful	49.6
	Infection, inflammation, degeneration	Mostly systemic aspergillosis or bacterial infection	Increased density, loss of detail; very rarely involvement of intervertebral meniscus: thickening and hyperdensity, mild protrusion, sclerosis of neighboring vertebral endplates	49.7
Extremities	Trauma, dislocation	Delicate fractures and luxation of especially coxofemoral joint and furcula/shoulder	Additional to fracture/fissure lines increased densities within pneumatized bones (resembling hemorrhage), often peripheral emphysema and soft tissue swelling; frontal/sagittal reconstruction helpful	49.8 49.9
	Infection, inflammation, degeneration	Arthritis	Periosteal reactions (less than in mammals), soft tissue swelling; massive osteolytic reactions may indicate septic arthritis	

Table 49.5
Disease features: coelomic organs.

Organ system	Pathological changes	Pathogenesis	CT characteristics	Figure
Liver	Hepatomegaly	Infection, degenerative/metabolic (lipidosis; hemochromatosis – mostly in mynah birds), neoplasia	Liver extends caudal to the sternum, stomach displaced to dorsal (and caudal), loss of hourglass-shaped waist on dorsal reconstructions, compression of air sacs; in fatty liver disease density lower than 20–30 HU	49.10
Spleen	Splenomegaly	Chronic infection (chlamydia, mycobacteria), leucosis, neoplasia; sometimes metabolic (lipidosis); psittacosis often accompanied with inflammation of lung and air sacs	Enlarged round structure dorsal to stomach, ventral to cranial and medial division of kidneys; stomach may be displaced cranioventrally and to the left	49.11
Gastrointestinal tract	Dilatation of stomach	Proventricular dilatation due to neurogene proventricular dilatation disease, going-light-syndrome of budgerigars (megabacteria), parasites or mycoses, rarely ileus	Abnormal shape, often thin-walled, often gas-filled	49.12
	Dilatation of bowel loops	Severe inflammation, foreign bodies, parasites (similar to mammals)	Gas and fluid accumulation	
	Dilatation of cloaca	Spinal trauma or neoplasia involving sacral nerves (e.g. renal neoplasia); rare idiopathic dilatation	May protrude caudally, may displace small bowel loops cranially	
Kidney	Renomegaly	Mostly neplasias (adenocarcinoma, fibrosarcoma), also infection (chlamydia) /inflammation/ degeneration (gout, lipidosis, cystic degeneration)	Bowel loops displaced ventrally, sometimes caudoventrally (enlargement of cranial division or gonads), cranioventrally (enlargement of caudal division of gonads); compression of abdominal air sacs makes differentiation of severely enlarged kidneys on plain CT nearly impossible	49.13 49.14
	Increased density	Kidney gout with calcinosis, nephrosis, severe dehydration	More than 70 HU (in domestic pigeons and parrots), may be enlarged and heterogeneous	
Female genital tract	Dystocia, egg-related peritonitis	Usually incomplete or soft shell, impacted yolk or follicles	Loss of detail, compression of air sacs, ventral displacement of gastrointestinal tract	49.15
Male genital tract	Enlargement of testis	Mostly caused by neoplasia (often in budgerigars); moderate enlargement normal during breeding season	Compression of air sacs, displacement of gastrointestinal tract to (caudo-) ventral, stomach in severe enlargement displaced cranially; functional sertoli cell tumors may cause hyperostosis	49.16

(*Continued*)

Table 49.5
(Continued)

Organ system	Pathological changes	Pathogenesis	CT characteristics	Figure
Lung	Opacification	Aspergillosis, tuberculosis, broncho-/pneumonia (foreign body aspiration, bacterial, hypovitaminosis A), rarely fibrosis	Patches of increased density within the lung, peribronchial infiltrates, thickened walls of bronchi and the air sacs (aerosacculitis); granulomas (which tend to ossify) and abscesses possible; loss of definition of vessels and bronchi	49.17
	Bronchiectasis	Described in pneumonia and fibrosis	Increased diameter of bronchi	
Air sacs	Thickening/ opacification	Inflammation/infection, often accompanied by pneumonia	Thickening of walls, fluid or substrate in lumina	
	Dilatation	Mainly abdominal air sacs = 'air-trapping'	Caused by stenosis of upper respiratory tract and lung, often mycosis	
Coelomic cavity	Ascites	Mostly accompany heart failure and hepatic disease (such as hemochromatosis)	Loss of detail, compression or filling of air sacs	49.18

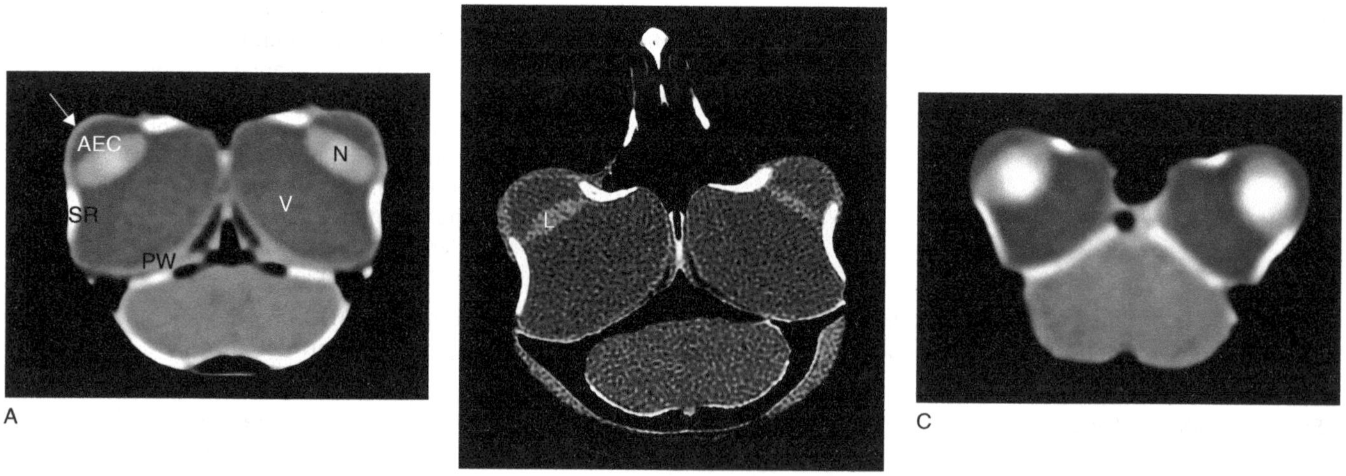

Figure 49.3 (A) Dorsal CT image (head) of a normal common buzzard *(Buteo buteo)*. Note the globular shape of the bulbus that is typical for diurnal birds. The huge bulbi are only separated by the interorbital septum. (B) Dorsal CT image (head) of an eagle owl (*Bubo bubo*). The lenses are flattened and mildly hypodense. No nuclei are present. The bird suffered from a bilateral severe cataract. Note the tubular shape of the bulbus of nocturnal birds. (C) Dorsal CT image (head) of a long eared owl (*Asio otus*). The left lens is subluxated to anterior medially. Cornea (arrow); AEC = anterior eye chamber; L = lens; N = nucleus lentis; PW = posterior wall; SR = bony scleral ring; V = vitreous.

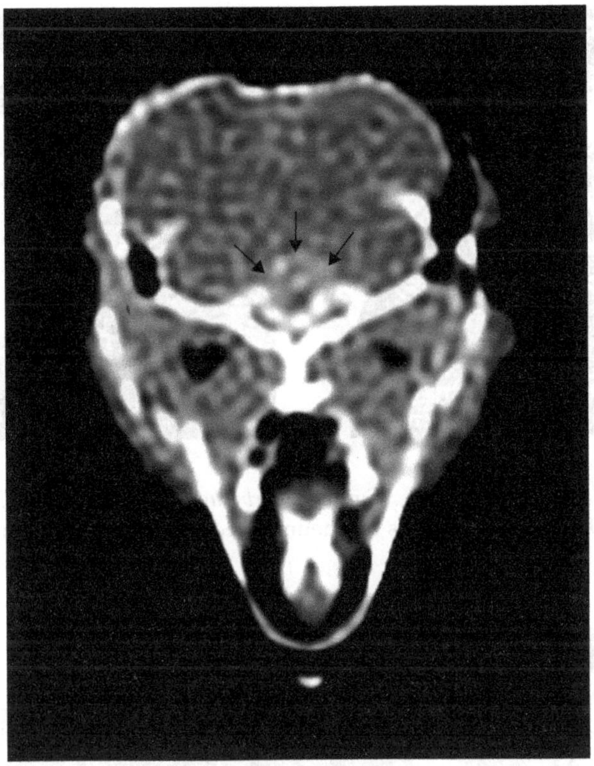

Figure 49.4 Dorsal CT image (head) of a cockatiel (*Nymphicus hollandicus*) with pituitary adenoma. A rounded mildly hyperdense structure (arrows) is visible.

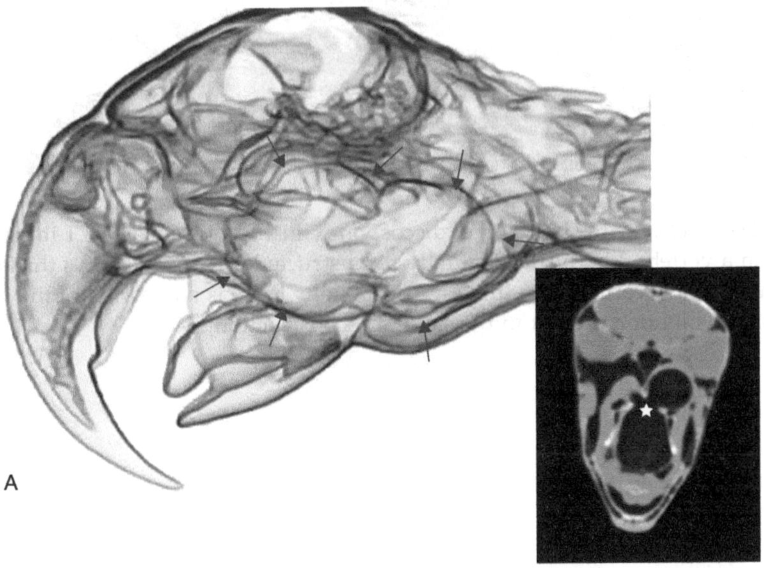

A

B

Figure 49.5 (A) 3D reconstruction (head) of a Scarlet macaw (*Ara Macao*). There is a bilobated bullous emphysema (arrows), originating from the choana. (B) Transverse CT image shows the origin (asterisk) of the bulla obstructing the upper respiratory tract.

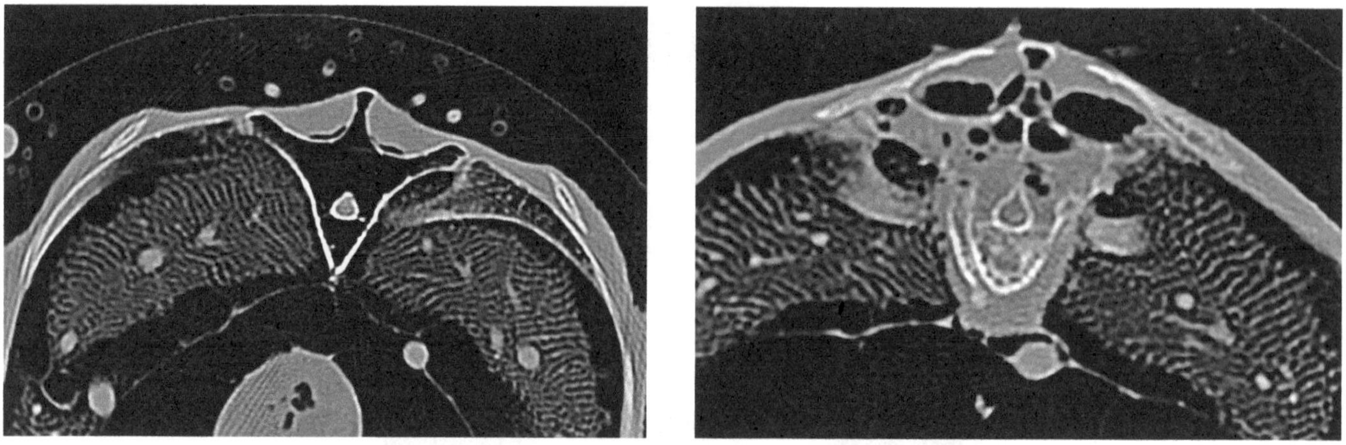

A B

Figure 49.6 Vertebral column of a bearded vulture (*Gypaetus barbatus*). (A) Transverse CT image of a normal vertebra. (B) Transverse CT image of a fractured vertebra with loss of pneumatized spaces due to hemorrhage.

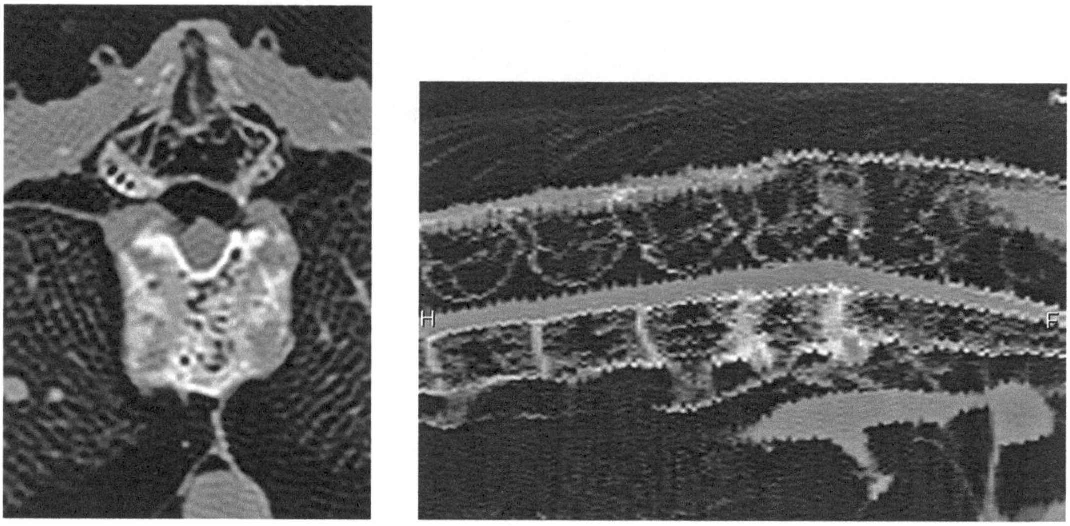

A B

Figure 49.7 Mute swan (*Cygnus olor*) with suspicion of discospondylitis. (A) Transverse CT image (vertebral column) shows areas of sclerosis and lysis in a vertebral body. (B) Sagittally reconstructed CT image shows thickening, sclerosis and hyperdensity of the intervertebral disk and vertebral endplates. Additionally there is narrowing of the intervertebral foramina due to moderate protrusion. Note the motion artifact in the sagittal reconstruction.

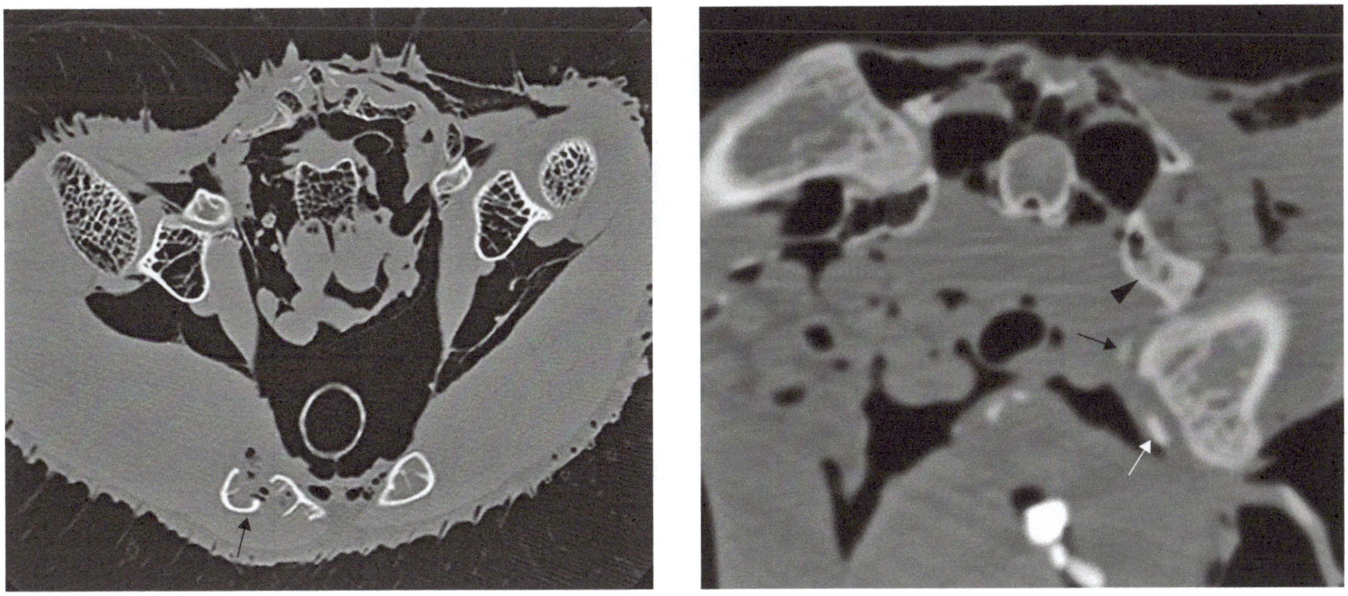

A B

Figure 49.8 Transverse CT images (shoulder girdle and pelvis) of mute swans (*Cygnus olor*) with fractures. (A) There is a fractured furcula (arrow) with subcutaneous emphysema. (B) There is a luxated left femoral head and some small avulsion fractures (arrow), typical hemorrhage (arrowhead) within pelvic bone and surrounding emphysema.

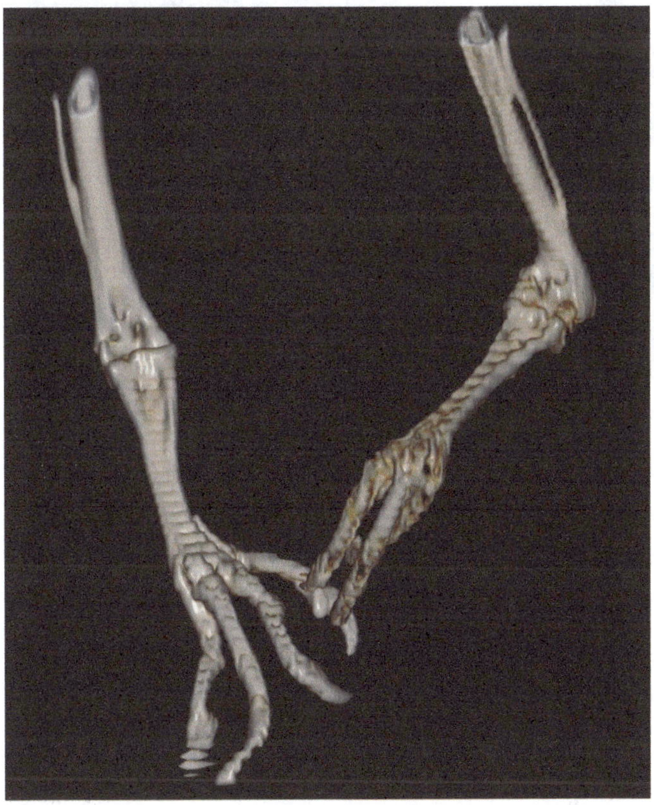

Figure 49.9 3D reconstruction of both legs of a saker falcon (*Falco cherrug*) with an old fracture of the left distal tibiotarsus. While the particular position of the condyle was not understood on transversal images, the 3D model helps to diagnose the angulation of the distal epiphyses.

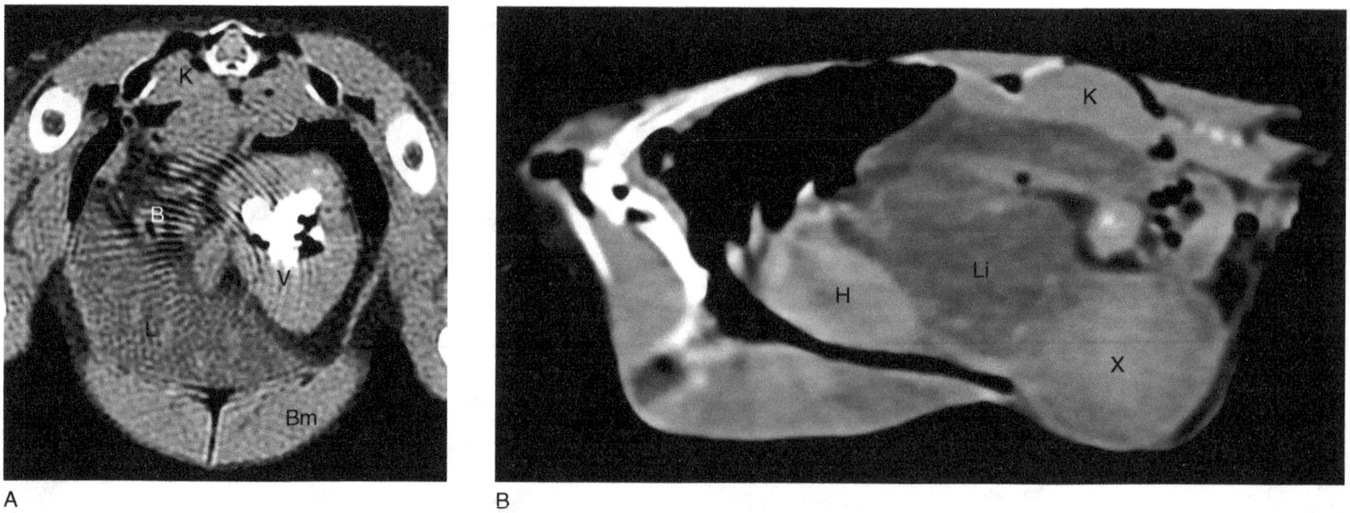

Figure 49.10 (A) Transverse CT image of a domestic pigeon with fatty liver disease. The liver (L) measured –10 HU and the coelomic fat –160 HU. Vessels can be differentiated within the liver parenchyma. Artifacts caused by grit in the ventriculus are visible. B = bowel loops; Bm = breast muscle; V = ventriculus. (B) Right sagittal CT image of a galah (*Eolophus roseicapillus*) with fatty liver (Li) disease (–5 HU) with protruding xanthoma (X) of the liver. The heart (H) measured mean 62 HU. K = kidneys.

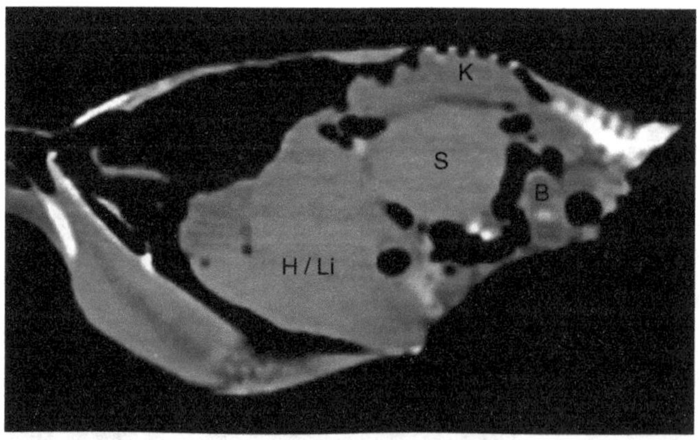

Figure 49.11 Mealy parrot (*Amazona farinosa*) with leucosis. Right sagittal CT image shows a markedly enlarged spleen (S). B = bowel loops; H/Li = heart and liver; K = kidney.

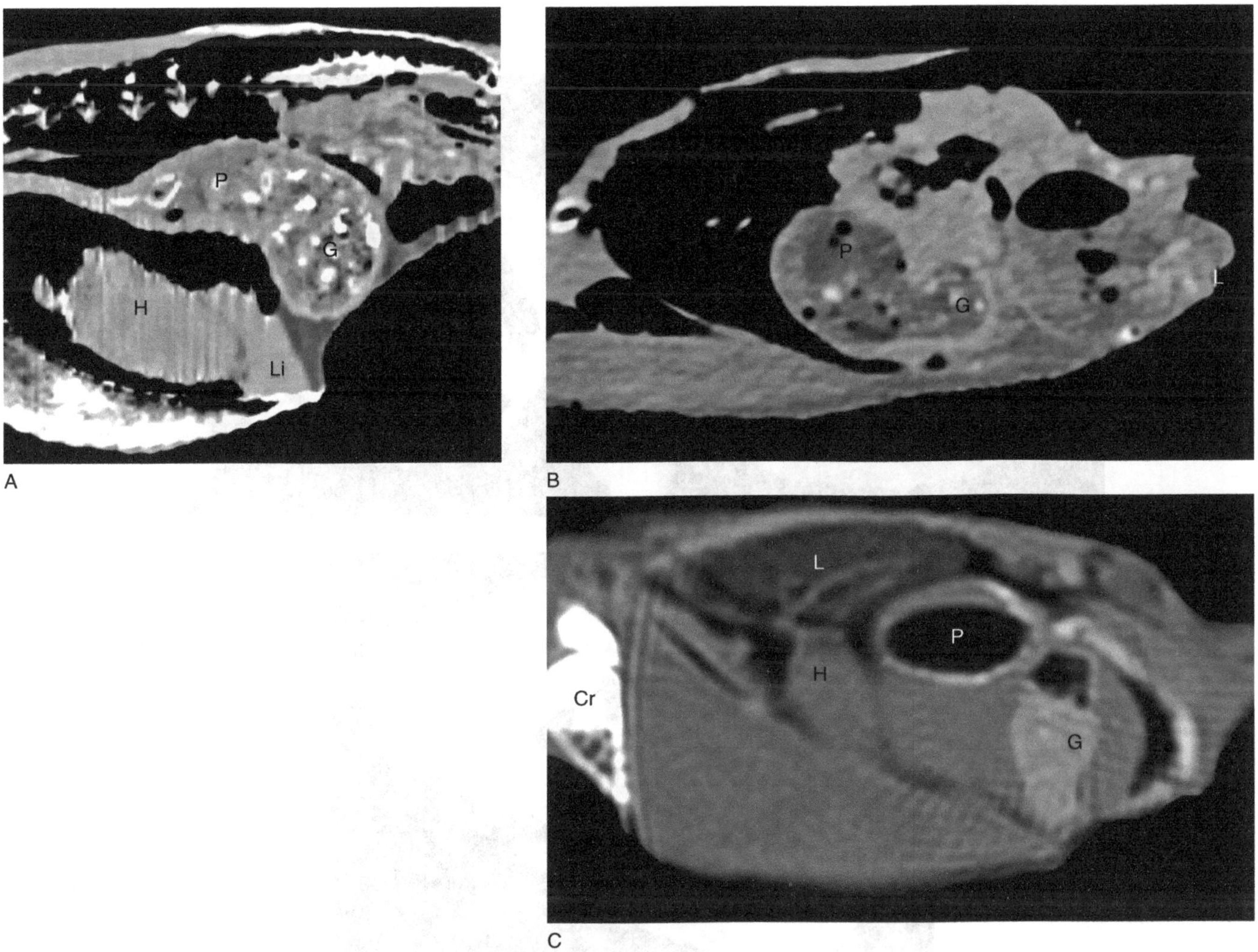

Figure 49.12 (A) Sagittally reconstructed CT image of a normal Egyptian vulture (*Neophron percnopterus*) showing the large proventriculus (P) and gizzard (G) after feeding. (B) Sagittal CT image of a yellow-fronted Amazon parrot (*Amazona ochrocephala*) with proventricular dilatation disease. The proventriculus is severely enlarged, has an abnormal shape and continues to an abnormally thin-walled gizzard. (C) Sagittal CT image of a budgerigar (*Melopsittacus undulatus*) with going-light-syndrome showing a gas distended proventriculus, normal wall and shape of gizzard. Cr = crop; H = heart; L = lung; Li = liver.

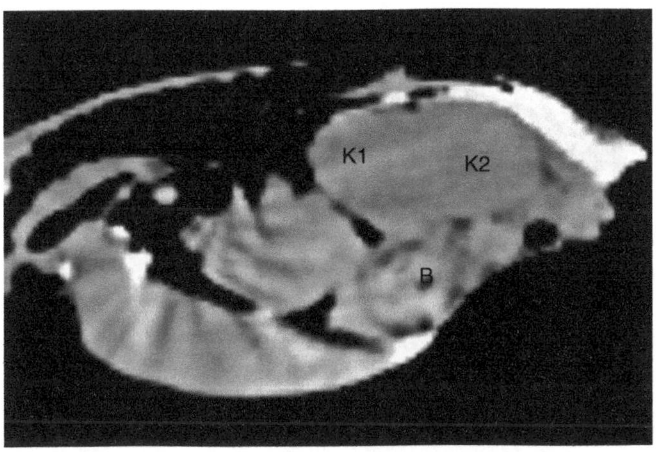

Figure 49.13 Blue-fronted Amazon (*Amazona aestiva*) with renal adenocarcinoma. Sagittal CT image shows a marked kidney enlargement with compression of abdominal air sacs. Nevertheless the origin of the mass is clearly visible from the cranial (K1) and middle division (K2) of the kidney (compare Figure 49.14). The small bowel loops (B) are displaced ventrally.

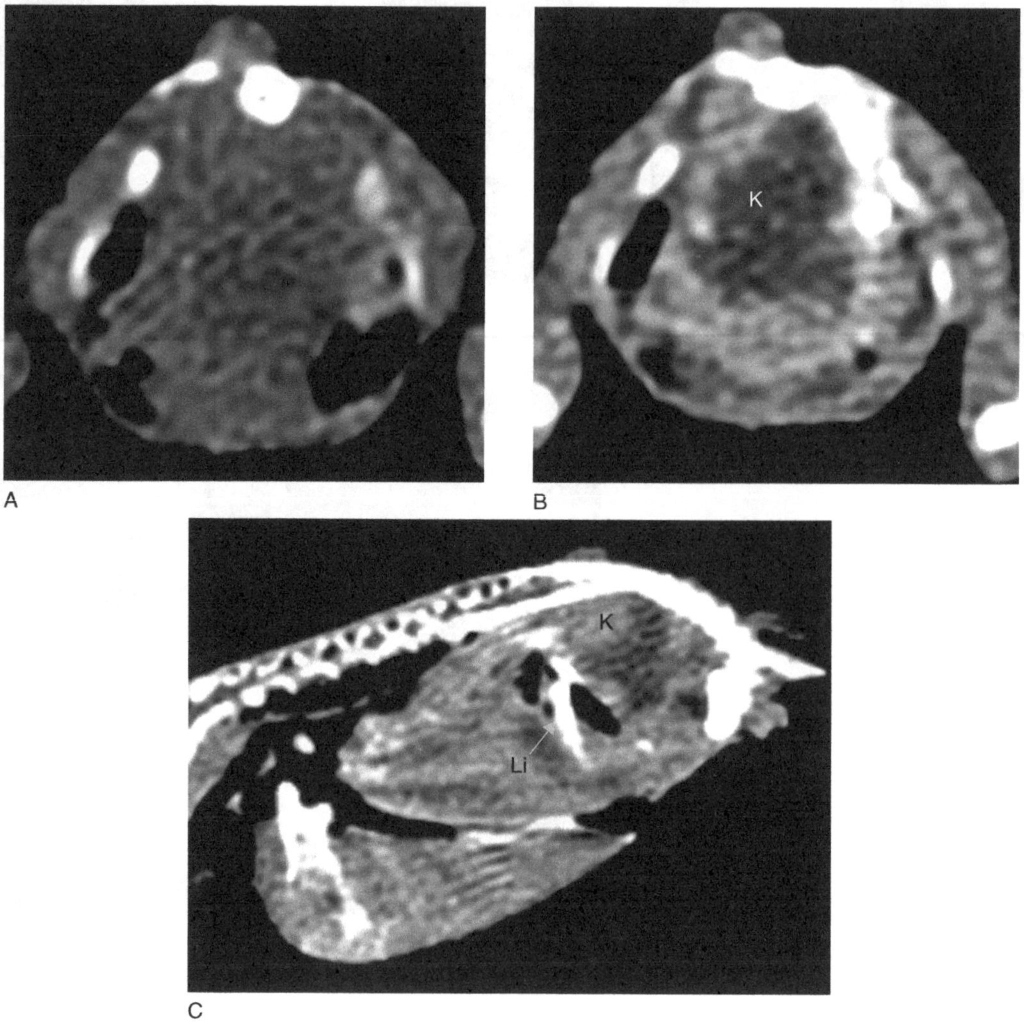

Figure 49.14 Budgerigar (*Melopsittacus undulatus*) with renal adenocarcinoma. (A) Transverse CT image shows a soft tissue mass originating from the kidney region. (B) Post-intravenous transverse contrast CT image and (C) Sagittally reconstructed CT image. The thickened ureter (arrow) is displaced ventrally, the kidneys (K) appear as a heterogeneous, partially non-enhancing and severely enlarged mass. Li = liver.

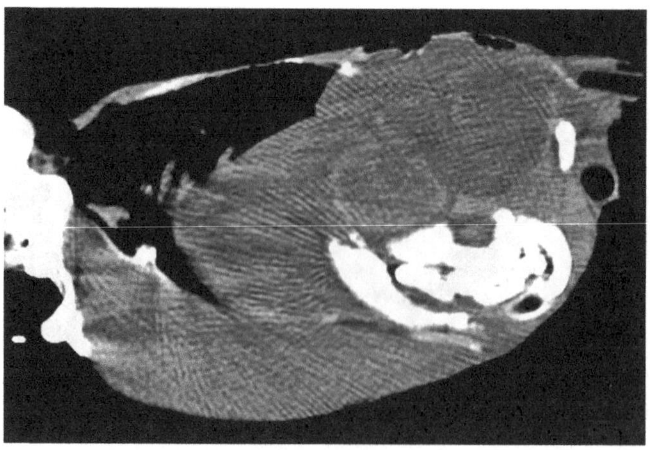

Figure 49.15 Domestic pigeon with multiple adhered follicles and peritonitis. Sagittal CT image shows poor coelomic detail. A soft tissue mass, consisting of multiple round, peripherally mildly hyperdense structures displaces the contrast medium filled gastrointestinal tract ventrally.

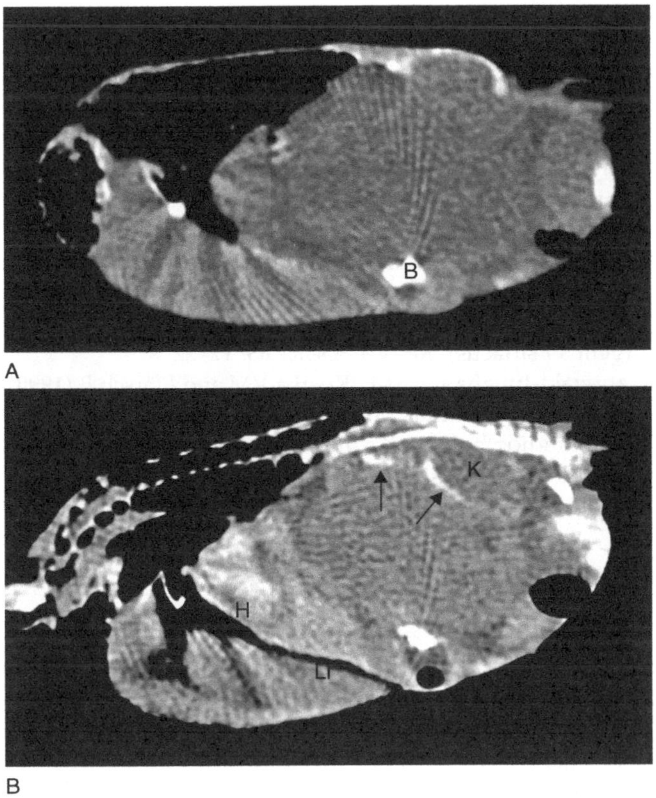

Figure 49.16 Cockatiel (*Nymphicus hollandicus*) with a gonadal tumor (seminoma). (A) Sagittal CT image shows the contrast filled bowel loops (B) displaced ventrally by a soft tissue mass originating from kidney region. (B) On the post-intravenous contrast sagittal CT image, the ureter (arrows) defines the ventral border of normal sized kidneys (K). H = heart; Li = liver.

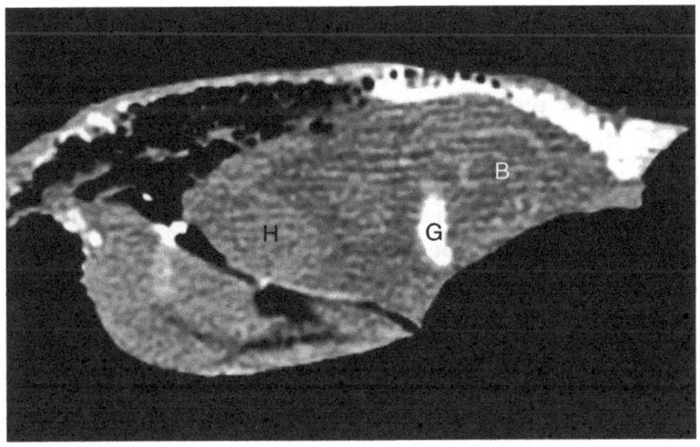

Figure 49.18 Cockatiel (*Nymphicus hollandicus*) with ascites caused by cardiac insufficiency. Sagittal CT image shows loss of coelomic differentiation. The heart (H) is visible due to the decreased density of the neighboring liver. Part of the gizzard (G) and some bowel loops (B) with remnants of contrast medium are in normal position.

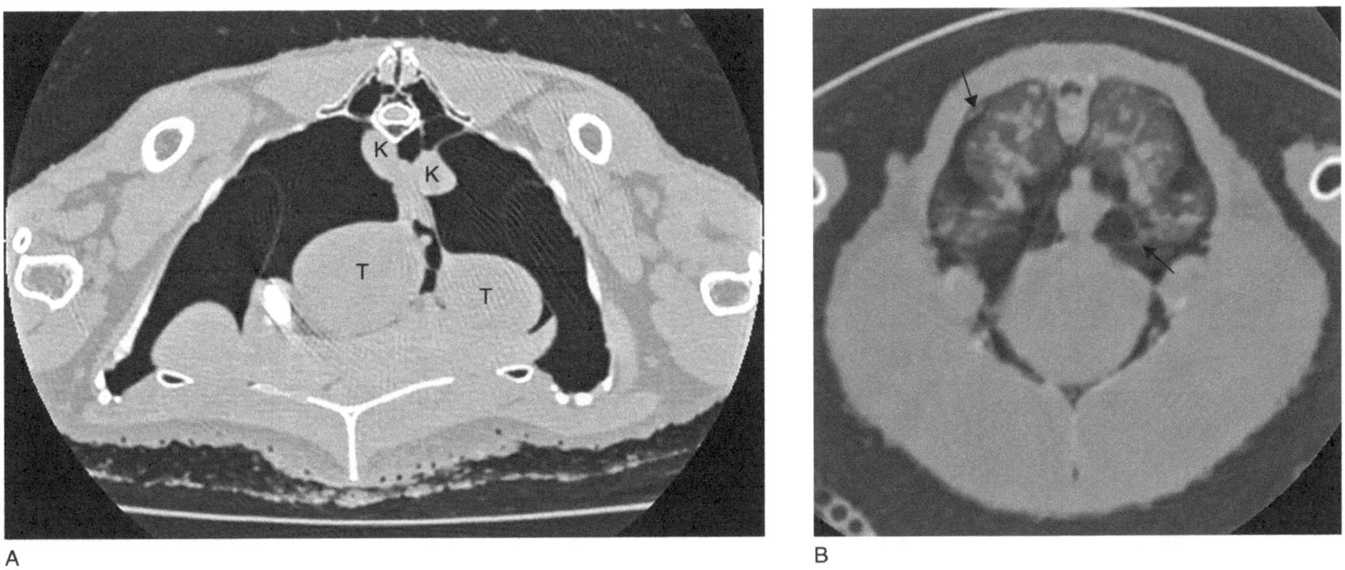

Figure 49.17 (A) Transverse CT image of a domestic duck showing thin-walled normal air sacs. (B) Transverse CT image of a blue-fronted amazon bird (*Amazona aestiva*) with aspergillosis. There are heterogeneous patchy lungs, peribronchial infiltration and mild focal thickening of air sac wall (arrows). K = kidneys; T = testicles.

Acknowledgement

The author would like to thank Dr Alexandra Scope, Clinic for Avian, Reptile and Fish Medicine and the Institute of Pathology and Forensic Veterinary Medicine, both University of Veterinary Medicine, Vienna, for the cooperation in avian patients.

Further Reading

Amann O, Kik MJL, Passon-Vastenburg MH, Westerhof I, Lumeij JT and Schoemaker NJ (2007) Chronic pulmonary interstitial fibrosis in a blue-fronted Amazon parrot (*Amazona aestiva aestiva*). *Avian Dis* **51**: 150–3.

Artmann A and Henninger W (2001) Psittacine paranasal sinus – a new definition of compartments. *J Zoo Wildl Med* **32**: 447–58.

Gumpenberger M and Henninger W (2001) The use of computed tomography in avian and reptile medicine. *Semin Avian Exotic Pet Med* **10**: 174–80.

Gumpenberger M and Kolm G (2006) Ultrasonographic and computed tomographic examinations of the avian eye: physiologic appearance, pathologic findings, and comparative biometric measurement. *Vet Radiol Ultrasound* **47**: 492–502.

Krautwald-Junghanns ME (1998) CT-assisted versus silicone rubber cast morphometry of the lower respiratory tract in healthy amazons (genus Amazona) and grey parrots (genus Psittacus). *Res Vet Science* **65**: 17–22.

Krautwald-Junghanns M-E, Kostka VM and Dörsch B (1998) Comparative studies on the diagnostic value of conventional radiography and computed tomography in evaluating the heads of psittacine and raptorial birds. *J Avian Med Surg* **12**: 149–57.

CHAPTER FIFTY

Chelonians

Michaela Gumpenberger

Chelonians are enclosed in their, usually, bony shell. Therefore physical examination differs and is limited in comparison with lizards or snakes. Diagnostic imaging is often essential to gain a diagnosis. This chapter focuses on chelonians as representatives of reptiles.

Imaging Protocol

See Tables 50.1 and 50.2.

Imaging Techniques

Routine CT of the coelomic cavity can be performed without anesthesia in most chelonians, except for head scans. The legs are taped into the shell in physiological position while the head and tail are able to move. The animals have to be placed on a cardboard box or block of styrofoam or plastic. Otherwise they may annul themselves out of proper position with the tail. Calm animals can sometimes rest in a box without further restraint. Larger species like African spurred tortoises (*Geochelone sulcata*) can be strapped on a first-aid stretcher or anesthetized. Soft-shelled turtles may rest in a smaller shaded box or be anesthetized, too.

Smaller individuals can be positioned crosswise to the longitudinal axis of the patient table. The resulting sagittal scan is performed much quicker than the axial one. Movement artifacts may arise from head movement but usually do not hinder diagnosis. Existing protocols for head scans for dogs and horses may be used and adapted for chelonians in general.

Intravenous contrast medium is administered manually into the jugular or coccygeal vein. The correct repositioning of the patient is guaranteed when using the various scales of the shell for orientation. The center of the scan should be the middle of the neural shields. Repositioning after contrast medium administration will then be possible with no or only minimal dislocation. Reptiles are poikilothermal animals. Therefore they need to be warmed up to an optimal body temperature (mostly 28–30°C) to ensure metabolization of the similarly warmed contrast media.

Analysis of coelomic disorders may be easier in sagittal scans or reconstructions, which resemble the more familiar lateral radiograph. Interpretation of the most common 'whole-body scans' should in general follow a strict hierarchy, for example: heart/liver, gastrointestinal tract, urogenital tract, respiratory tract, skeletal system, other structures. Dorsal reconstructions should be orientated parallel to the plastron.

CT: Anatomy and Normal Variants

The clade of tortoises and turtles is represented by hundreds of different subspecies with different anatomy. Therefore Table 50.3 focuses on the general anatomy of Mediterranean tortoises.

The general schematic anatomy of tortoises is demonstrated in Figure 50.1.

Disease Features: Skeleton and Head

Table 50.4 provides an overview of the most likely findings in chelonians. CT characteristics are described in more detail when they differ significantly from dogs

Veterinary Computed Tomography, First Edition. Edited by Tobias Schwarz, Jimmy Saunders.

Table 50.1
Imaging protocol of the coelomic cavity of chelonians.

Series	Pre- and post-contrast bone	Additional remarks
Positioning	Sternal	Legs taped into the shell in physiological position (see further remarks in text)
Scan margins	Axial scan: cranial rim of shell → caudal rim of shell Sagittal scan from right to left: right shell bridge → neural shields → left shell bridge	
Voltage (kVp)	100–130	Depending on the size
Current (mAs)	100–200	Depending on the size
Tube rotation time (s)	1–2	
Slice width (mm)	1–5	Small to giant species
Sequential slice interval (mm)	1–4	Small to giant species
Kernel frequency	Pre-contrast: soft tissue/medium Bone: bone	
Window level (HU)	Pre-contrast: +50 to +100 Bone: +350 to +500	Lungs: –200 to –400
Window width (HU)	Pre-contrast: 350–450 Bone: 2500	Lungs: 1600–2000

Table 50.2
Intravenous contrast protocol.

Contrast medium application site	Jugular vein or coccygeal vein
Contrast medium type	Iodine based, ionic or non-ionic – warmed
Contrast medium dose	600 mg I/kg body weight
Contrast injection mode	Manual
Scan delay post start contrast injection	1 min, repetition after 3–10 min
Kernel frequency	Soft tissue/medium
Window level (HU)	+100
Window width (HU)	350

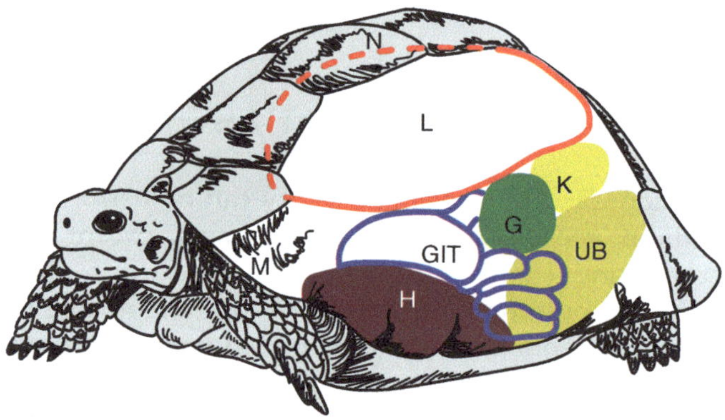

Figure 50.1 Schematic basic anatomy of the coelomic organs of a Mediterranean tortoise. G = gonads; GIT = gastrointestinal tract; H = liver; K = kidneys; L = lung; M = marginal shield; N = neural shield; UB = urinary bladder.

and cats. Otherwise the author would kindly refer the reader to the particular chapter of the present book.

Disease Features: Coelomic Organs

Table 50.5 provides an overview of the most likely findings in chelonians.

Further Reading

Gumpenberger M (2007) Diagnostic imaging of dyspnoic chelonians. In: Seybold J and Mutschmann F (eds) *Proceedings 7th International Symposium on Pathology and Medicine in Reptiles and Amphibians* (Berlin 2004). Chimaira, pp. 217–22.

Gumpenberger M and Filip Th (2007) Computed tomography and use of intravenous contrast media in imaging chelonian kidneys. *Proceedings 14th Annual Meeting of ARAV*, New Orleans, Louisiana, USA, p. 5.

Gumpenberger M and Henninger W (2001) The use of computed tomography in avian and reptile medicine. *Semin Avian Exotic Pet Med* **10**: 174–80.

Table 50.3
Anatomy – most important variations to mammals.

	Organ	Anatomical details	Figures
Head	Head	Differs in each species – check special literature	
	Eyes	Scleral ossicles support the globe	
Skeleton in chelonians	Shell	Consists of carapace (dorsal part), plastron (ventral part) and bridge. Each built by numerous bony plates that are derived from dermal ossification, ribs, vertebrae and clavicles Hinges present in some species Compacta = 1200–1400 HU, medullary space = 700–750 HU in Mediterranean tortoises	50.2
	Cervical spine	Eight vertebrae, movable	
	Thoracal and lumbar spine	Nine vertebrae, not movable, fused with carapace	
	Caudal spine	Movable, various number depending on length of tail	
	Shoulder and pelvic girdle	Enclosed in shell Extremities usually have five toes	
Coelomic organs	Diaphragm	Lacking	
	Heart and main vessels	Three-chambered, complete atrial septum Flanked by liver lobes Paired carotid arteries and jugular veins Paired ventral abdominal vein and renal portal system present	50.4 50.5
	Thyroid gland	Anterior to the heart, mean density in Herman's tortoises 40–50 HU, in juvenile animals maybe more (to 70 HU)	50.5 50.27
	Liver	Two major lobes; the right one larger than the left Homogeneous, mean density in Herman's tortoises 50–70 HU	50.3
	Gallbladder	Located at right liver lobe	
	Spleen	Oval, dorsomedial to stomach, right sagittal Mean density in Herman's tortoises 40–50 HU, may be denser in juvenile animals (to 75 HU)	50.3
	Pancreas	Close to stomach and duodenum, caudal to gall bladder	
	Esophagus	Dorsal to trachea Longitudinal folds for great distensibility	
	Stomach	Positioned in the left cranial half of the shell, across the caudal face of the liver, pylorus positioned right sagittal or central	
	Small intestines	Many loops	50.4
	Large intestines	Cecum in the right caudal quarter of the coelomen Prominent colon in herbivorous tortoises	50.3 50.5
	Kidneys	No pelvis, macroscopically no medulla or cortex Positioned at level of or dorsocranial to hip joints Normal density 25–40 HU (in Herman's tortoises)	
	Urinary bladder	Single sac or central structure with bilateral accessory bladders	
	Gonads	Cranioventral to cranial pole of kidneys Females: follicles appear as round structures of various sizes, may occupy nearly whole coelomic cavity in chelonians Medium-sized to large follicles in Herman's tortoises measure 60–75 HU	50.3 50.4 50.5
	Adrenals	Associated with kidneys	
	Trachea	Two main bronchi branch off in the first half of the neck	
	Lung	Paired; typical reticular or honeycomb pattern	50.2 50.4
	Lymph nodes	Lacking (except snapping turtle); but do have lymphatic system with perivascular lymph channels	

Table 50.4
Disease features: skeleton and head.

Organ system	Pathological changes	Manifestation	CT characteristics	Figures
Head	Infection, inflammation, degeneration	Otitis media	Protrusion of tympanic scale, obstruction of middle ear, variably affects bony structures (osteolyses)	
	Infection, inflammation, degeneration	Mandibular and maxillary osteomyelitis	Lytic process, hardly any periosteal new bone production	
Shell	Trauma, dislocation	Fractures, mostly caused by dog bites, dropping and car accidents	Check position of fractures (often impression fracture), lung hemorrhage/consolidation, spinal lesions	50.6
	Infection, inflammation, degeneration	(Mostly nutritional) secondary hyperparathyreoidism with demineralization (often accompanied by kidney disease)	Pyramidal shape of neural bone plates, flattening of carapace, heterogeneous, honeycomb or moth-eaten-like pattern of bony plates, loss of compacta (especially plastron, visceral surface), decreased density; in very severe cases most of the shell consists of fatty tissue, bone may not be visible in bony window	50.7 50.8 50.9
	Infection, inflammation, degeneration	Shell necrosis	Lytic areas within bony plates while the superficial horny shield may be healed, may be accompanied by intracoelomic abscessation	50.10
	Infection, inflammation, degeneration	Sequestration (after trauma or coeliotomy)	Isolated part of bony plates, hypodense halo, plastron more often affected	50.11
Vertebral spine and extremities	Trauma, dislocation	Fractures of proximal extremities rare due to protection of shell; may be assisted by abscesses	Similar to mammals; greenstick fracture: note thinned compacta; healing: fibrous fracture stabilization may be more prominent than osteous callus formation (complete healing may least 6–18 months)	
	Trauma, dislocation	Luxation of shoulder or hip joint, rare	Similar to mammals	50.9
	Infection, inflammation, degeneration	Arthrosis and pseudogout (calcium deposits)	Shell-like bony tissue around (shoulder, hip and knee) joints	50.12
	Infection, inflammation, degeneration	Arthritis	Soft tissue swelling and widened joint space, sometimes lytic bone, less periosteal reactions	
	Infection, inflammation, degeneration	Abscessation (may be caused by bites of, for example, mating partners or prey as well as by injections)	Mostly well defined (reptiles usually have caseous and often encapsulated pus), may calcify; sometimes necrotic process with bone involvement (progressively lytic process)	50.13
	Neoplasia	Primary as well as metastasis, rare	Seems to be more often lytic, may be followed by fractures	

Table 50.5
Disease features: coelomic organs.

Organ system	Pathological changes	Pathogenesis	CT characteristics	Figures
Cardiovascular system	Calcification	Excessive vitamin D3 and calcium, often accompanied by renal disease	Increased densities/mineralization of heart, more linear in vessels	50.14
	Pericardial effusion		Small amounts may be normal; large amounts cause displacement of coelomic organs, especially liver	50.14
Liver	Hepatomegaly	Mostly lipidosis	Liver extends to the inguinal window of the shell, in fatty liver disease density lower than 20 HU	50.16 50.17
Gastrointestinal tract	Dilatation of stomach	Stenosis	Enlarged stomach, displacing liver cranially, gravel signs may be present	50.15
	Dilatation of bowel loops	Stenosis, severe inflammation or parasitosis, sometimes foreign body (especially sea turtles) or abscessation	Gas and fluid accumulation; small bowel loop diameter one third or more of height of shell	
	Foreign bodies		Similar to mammals	
Kidney	Renomegaly	Degeneration: gout, nephrocalcinosis; also infection, inflammation, rarely neoplasia	Normal density does not notably increase with gout (uric acid deposits are not radiodense) but with calcinosis, shape more blunted and rounded, can cause lung compression	50.16 50.17
	Increased density	Kidney gout with calcinosis, nephrosis	Increased density, marble-like appearance; check for further mineralization at heart, large vessels and larger joints (knee)	50.14
Urinary bladder	Abnormal contents	Cystic calculi	Usually large (and singular), often layered	50.18
	Enlarged	Urinary retention	Severely enlarged urinary bladder; liver dislocated to cranial, bowel loops to dorsal, lung compression	50.19 50.20
Female genital tract	Preovulatory dystocia or follicular stasis		Atretic follicles, heterogeneous with hypodense areas, horizontal levelling of liquid contents – appearance does not improve on follow-up examinations	50.21
	Dystocia or egg binding		Enlarged, broken, incomplete or thickened shells; loss of ovoidal shape of yolk, builds horizontal fluid line, may have gas cap; displacement: ova may be found in urinary bladder (suspected on radiographs but proved with CT)	50.22 50.23
	Egg-related or egg-yolk coelomitis		Poor differentiation, loss of round shape of follicles, atretic follicles (see above)	50.24

(*Continued*)

Table 50.5
(Continued)

Organ system	Pathological changes	Pathogenesis	CT characteristics	Figures
Lung	Opacification of lumina	Mostly pneumonia	Loss of air chambers, mostly horizontal fluid line	50.25
	Thickening (and opacification) of septa	Pneumonia, hemorrhage, edema, contusion	Thickened septa, sometimes some fluid in air chambers or increased density of septa	50.26
	Abscessation	Pneumonia	Consolidation of lung, multiple roundish, mostly mild hyperdense structures replace normal lung tissue	50.27
	Emphysema	May accompany one-sided pneumonia	Loss of normal air chamber architecture, loss/rupture and thinning of septa	50.28
Coelomic cavity generally	Ascites	Rare event	Similar to mammals; liver elevated from plastron	
	Adiposity	Often accompanied by lipidosis	Fatty tissue at the inner surface of the shell and around shoulder and pelvic girdle	

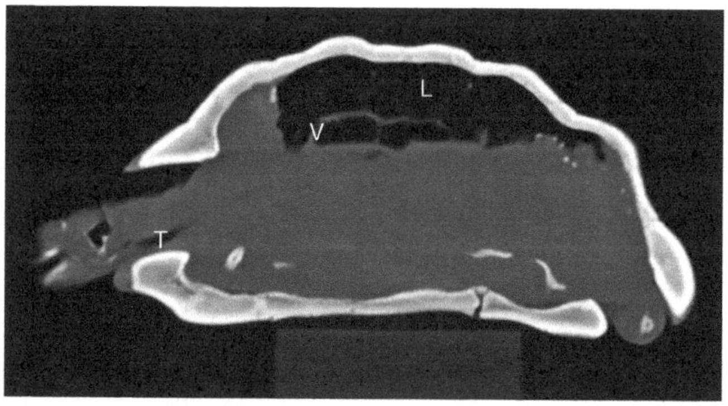

Figure 50.2 Left sagittal CT image of a normal spur-thighed tortoise shows perfect mineralization of the shell. The single bony plates are clearly differentiable, including compacta and spongiosa. Note the tortoise rests on a wooden block. L = lung; T = trachea; V = vessel in lung.

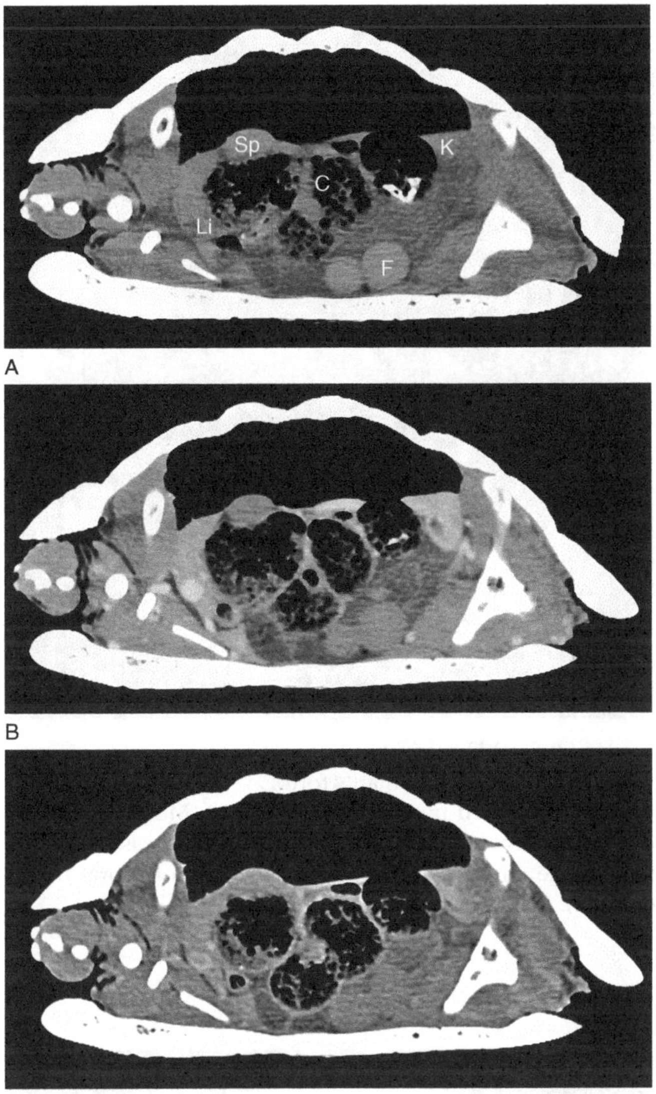

Figure 50.3 Right sagittal CT images (coelomic cavity) of a normal Herman's tortoise. (A) Pre-contrast CT image. The liver (Li) is small and homogeneous, some follicles (F) are present. The spleen (Sp) presents caudal to the liver and dorsomedial to the stomach. The kidneys (K) are poorly differentiable. Gas and feces are present in cecum/colon (C). (B) Early and (C) late post-contrast images. The large vessels within the liver parenchyma and the kidneys show early, strong enhancement. The ureter is visible as an undulating structure at the caudal end of the kidney on the early post-contrast image. The spleen (Sp) shows late contrast enhancement.

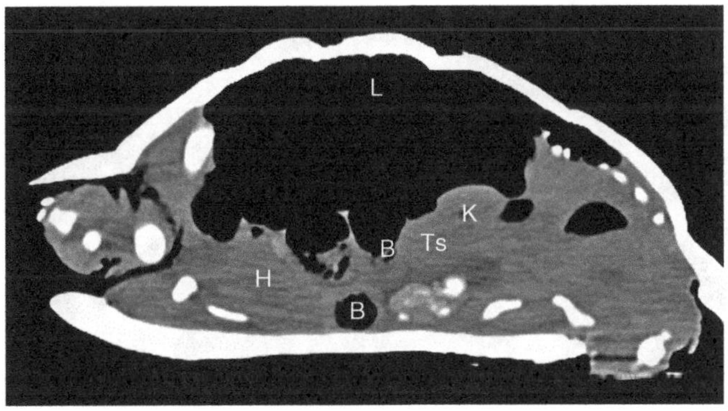

Figure 50.4 Sagittal CT image of a normal Herman's tortoise. The poor coelomic detail is normal in chelonians. The testes (Ts) are located immediately cranial to the kidneys (K). B = bowel loops; H = heart; L = lung.

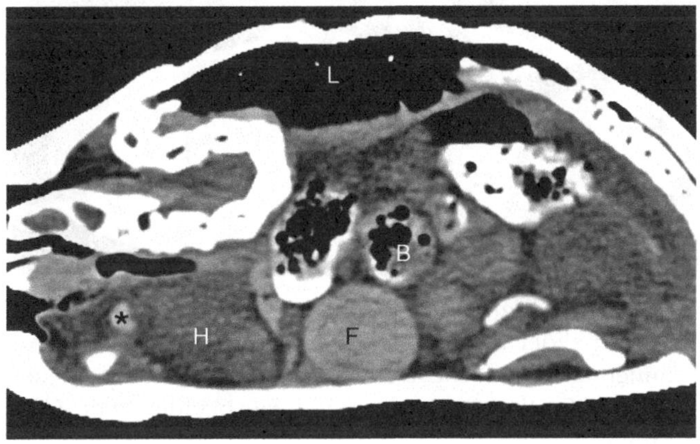

Figure 50.5 Sagittal CT image of a normal Herman's tortoise. The head is retracted. Consequently, the neck superimposes and compresses the lung (L). Asterisk = thyroid gland; B = bowel loops with feces; F = normal homogeneous hyperdense follicle; H = heart.

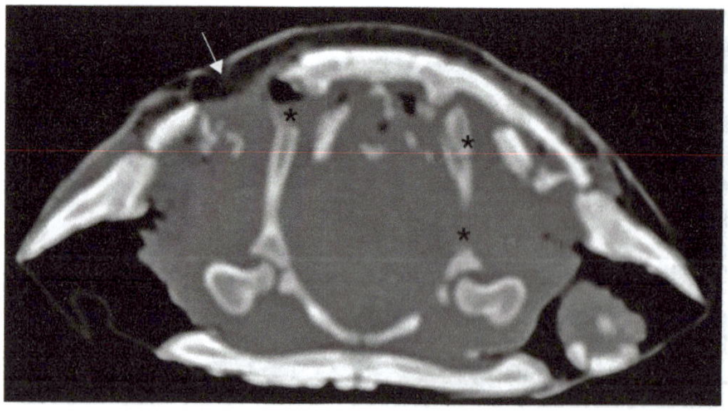

Figure 50.6 Herman's tortoise after dog bite. Transverse CT image at the level of the hip joints shows a fracture of the carapace (arrow), fracture of the pelvis (asterisks) and hemorrhage in the most caudal lung fields.

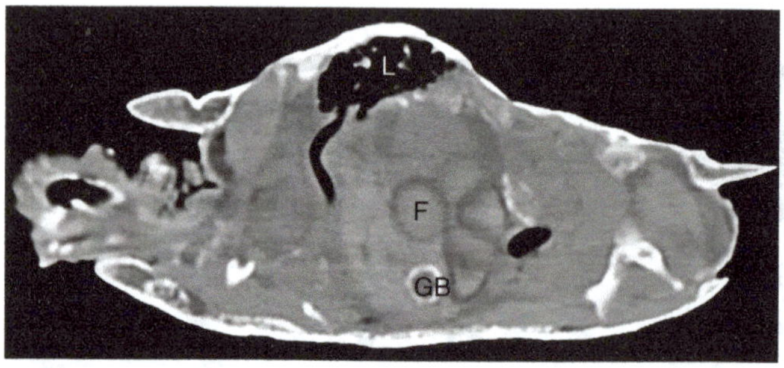

Figure 50.7 Right sagittal CT image (coelomic cavity) of a red-eared slider turtle. There is a severe malformation and demineralization of the shell causing lung (L) compression. Some calcification is visible in the gall bladder wall (GB). F = follicles.

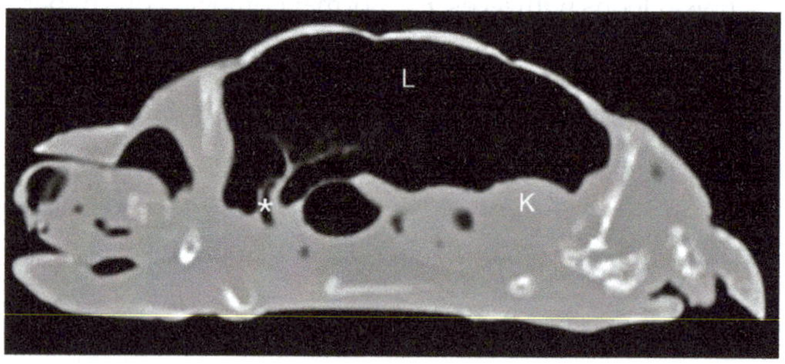

Figure 50.8 Spur-thighed tortoise with severe secondary hyperparathyroidism. Left sagittal scan shows a barely mineralized skeleton. The medullary space measures 20–27 HU (normal range: 700–750 HU). The soft tissues of the coelomic organs occupy one third of the height of the shell – lean tortoise. Asterisk = main bronchi with accompanying vessel; K = kidney; L = lung.

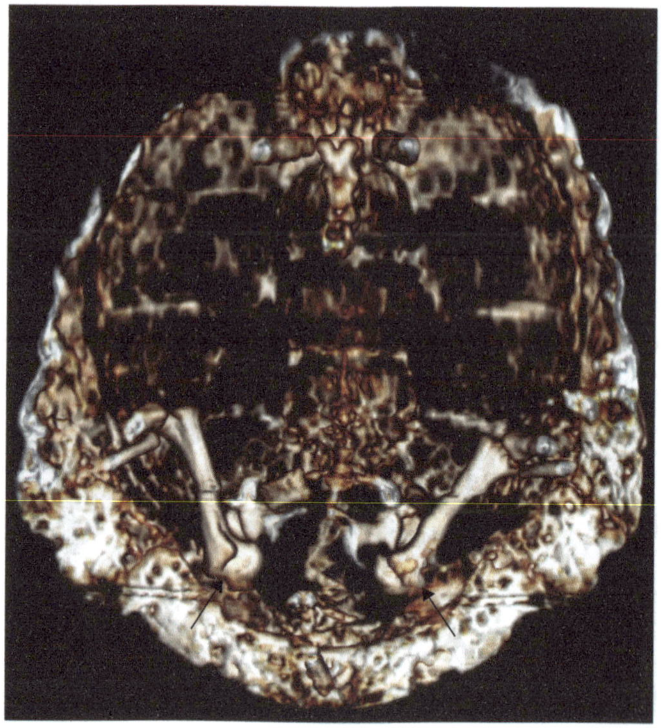

Figure 50.9 3-D reconstruction (dorsal view, carapace partially removed) of a Herman's tortoise with renal hyperparathyroidism caused by severe kidney gout. Most of the shell lacks sufficient mineralization, huge lytic areas represent fatty tissue. There is caudal luxation of both femoral heads (arrows).

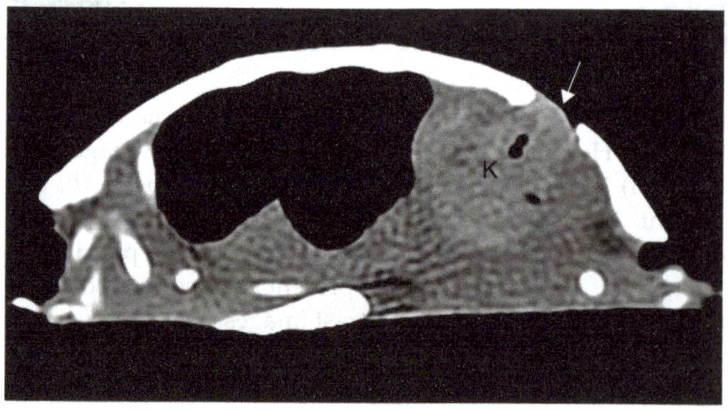

Figure 50.10 Sagittal CT image of a musk turtle. There is kidney abscessation (K) secondary to shell necrosis (arrow).

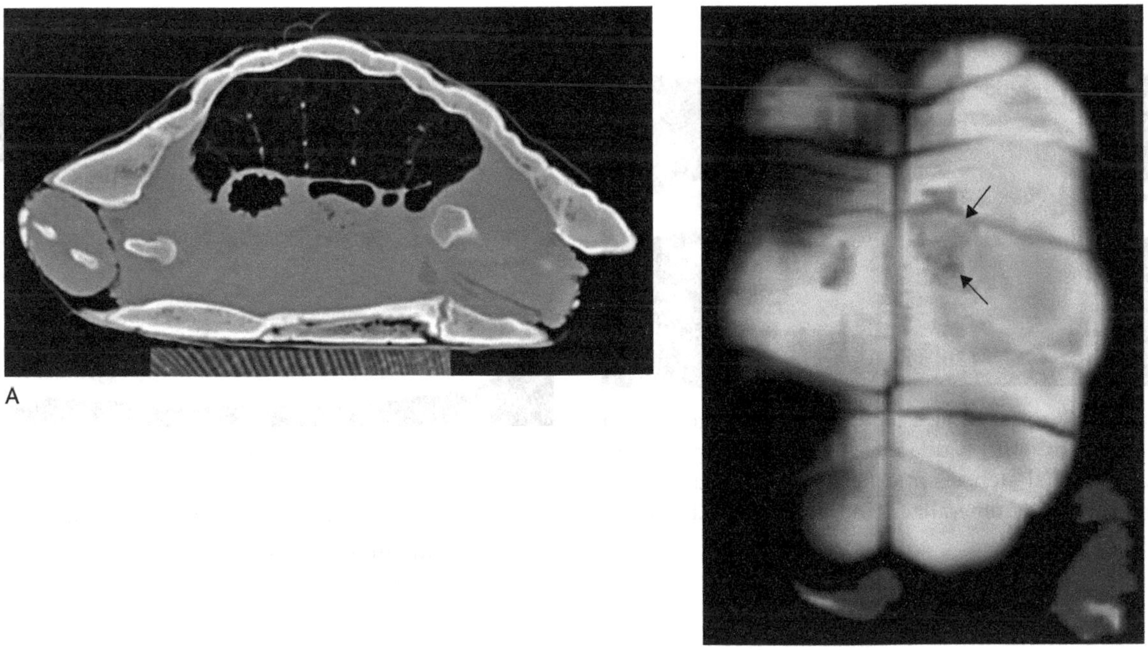

Figure 50.11 (A) Herman's tortoise that underwent a coeliotomy some months ago. Sagittal CT image shows a huge sequestrum in the abdominal bony plate. A new bony plate is growing while the surgically created flap is isolated. Some air invades the space between sequestrum and new bone. (B) Dorsally reconstructed CT image of the plastron of another Herman's tortoise. While it was hardly differentiable on single sagittal images, a huge sequestrum (arrows) is visible in the abdominal bony plate. Suspected origin was dropping on a stone floor.

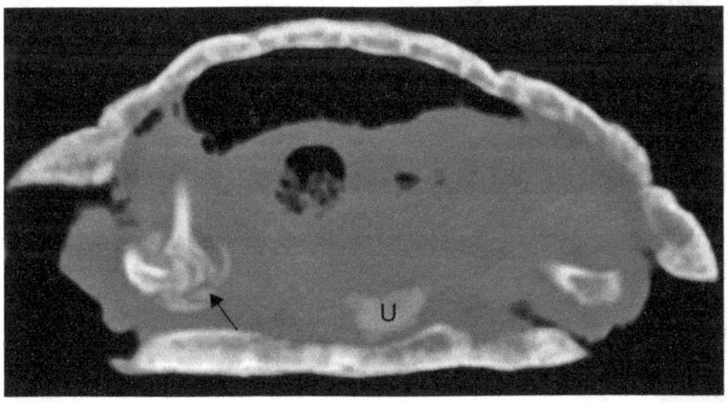

Figure 50.12 Herman's tortoise with pseudogout. Sagittal CT image shows moderate demineralization and ring like calcifications around the shoulder joint (arrow). Urate (U) accumulation is visible within the urinary bladder.

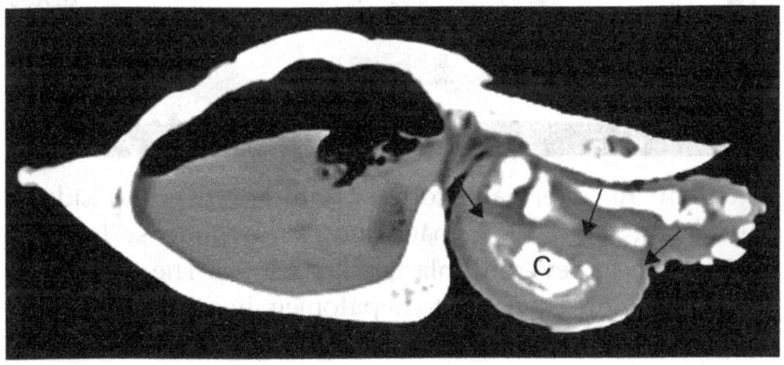

Figure 50.13 Left sagittal image of one hindlimb of a Herman's tortoise. A well-demarcated (arrows) abscess with central calcification (C) causes massive soft tissue swelling cranial to the left tibia and fibula. These bones are not involved.

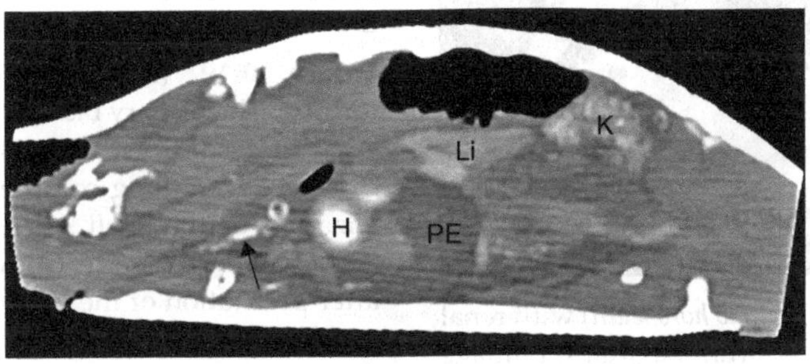

Figure 50.14 Long-necked turtle with nephritis and nephrocalcinosis accompanied by heart disease. Right sagittal scan shows severe calcification of the heart (H) and main vessels (arrow). Additionally, severe pericardial effusion (PE) is present. The liver (Li) is displaced caudodorsally by the enlarged heart. The kidneys (K) show similar calcifications and mild enlargement. The lung is compressed.

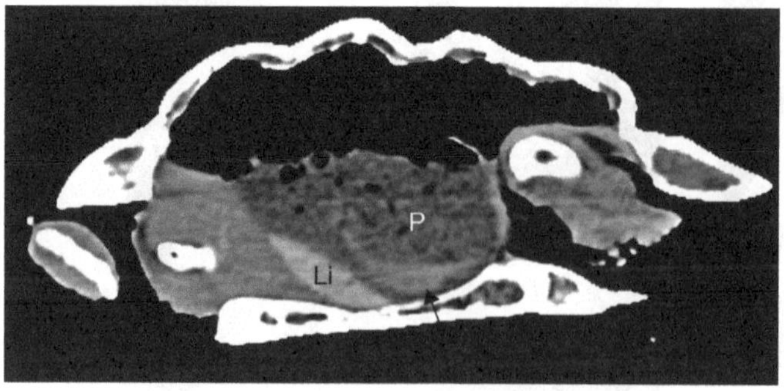

Figure 50.15 Right sagittal CT image of a Mediterranean tortoise. The pylorus (P) is dilated with gravel sign (arrow) ventrally, functional stenosis and hemorrhage of unknown origin. The shell is demineralized and deformed. Li = liver.

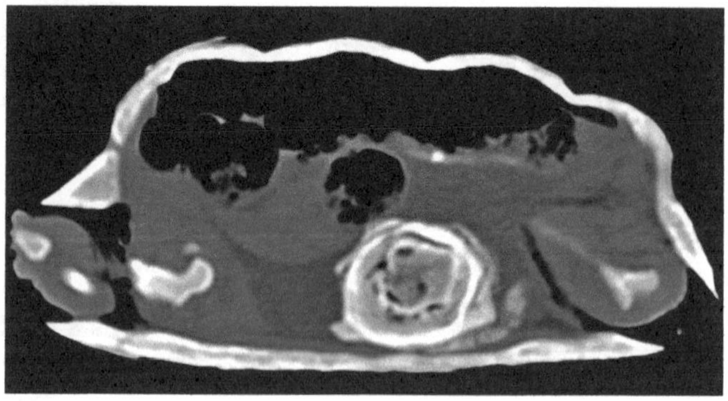

Figure 50.18 Right sagittal CT image of an African spurred tortoise (*Geochelone sulcata*). A huge onion shell-like urinary bladder stone is accompanied by lots of fragments. On conventional radiographs only the main stone was visible, mimicking dystocia.

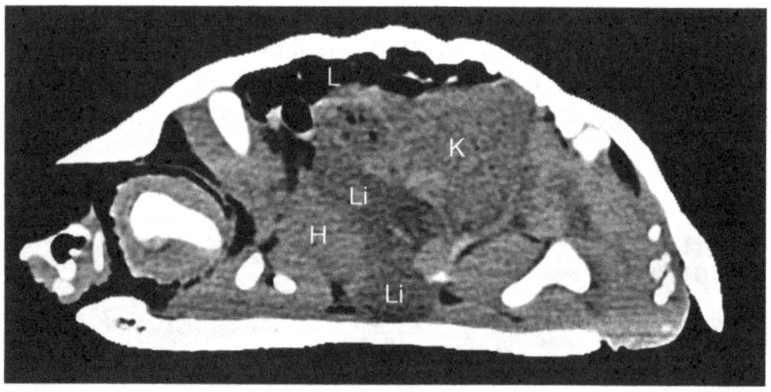

Figure 50.16 Herman's tortoise with lipidosis and kidney gout. Right sagittal CT image shows a hypodense (–2 HU) liver (Li) and a severely enlarged kidney (K). There is severe lung (L) compression due to hepatomegaly and renomegaly. H = heart.

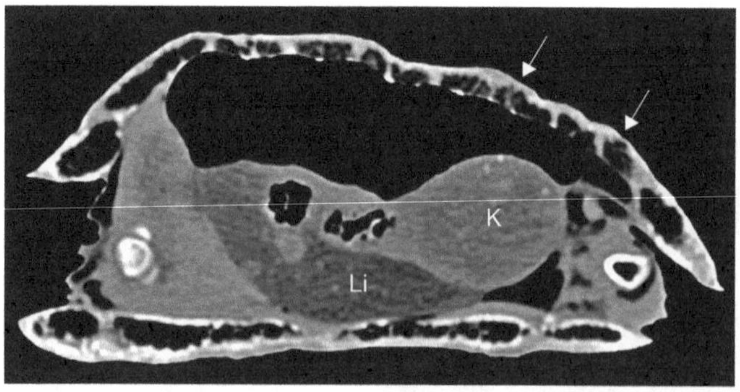

Figure 50.17 Russian tortoise (*Testudo horsfieldii*) with renal adenocarcinoma and liver lipidosis (Li). Sagittal CT image shows an enlarged, rounded kidney (K) that contains some bright spots. There is severe demineralization and flattening of the carapace (arrows).

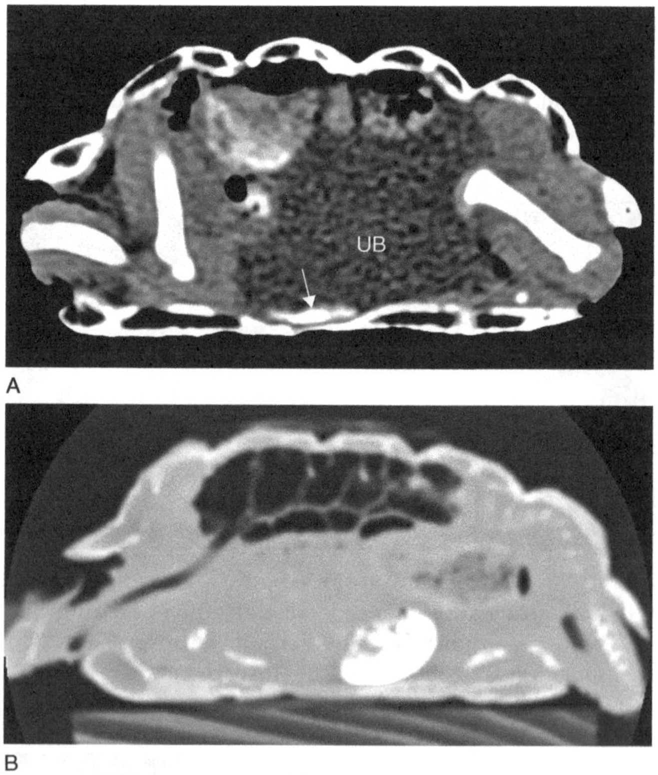

Figure 50.19 (A) Right sagittal CT image of a Herman's tortoise. The urinary bladder (UB) is severely distended with some urates (arrow) and displaces the bowel loops dorsally causing severe lung compression. There is severe demineralization of the shell giving a bumpy appearance to the surface of the carapace. (B) Aerated unfold aspect of the lung after punctation of the urinary bladder in the same animal.

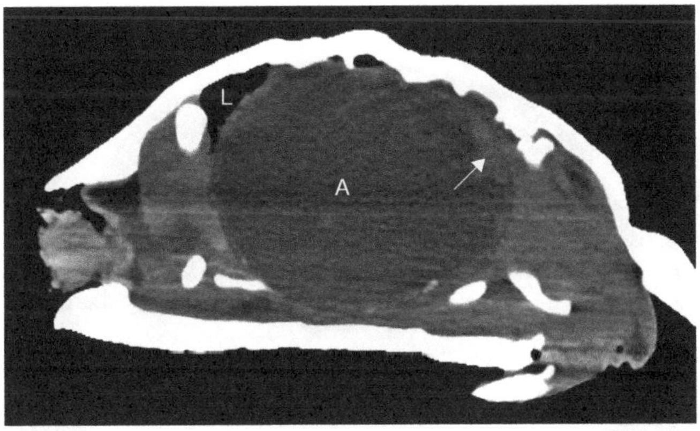

Figure 50.20 Herman's tortoise with a huge intra-coelomic abscess originating from a fissure in the carapace. Right sagittal CT image shows the abscess (A) with an irregular wall (arrow) causing severe lung (L) compression. Such an abscess should be differentiated from a dilated urinary bladder.

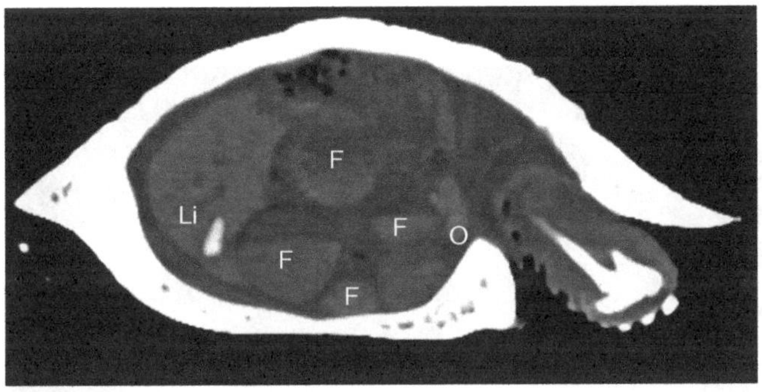

Figure 50.21 Right lateral sagittal CT image of a Herman's tortoise showing atretic follicles (F) with abnormal horizontal levelling of their contents and abnormal density. The oviduct (O) is typically hyperdense and curled. There is also focal mineralization of the liver (Li).

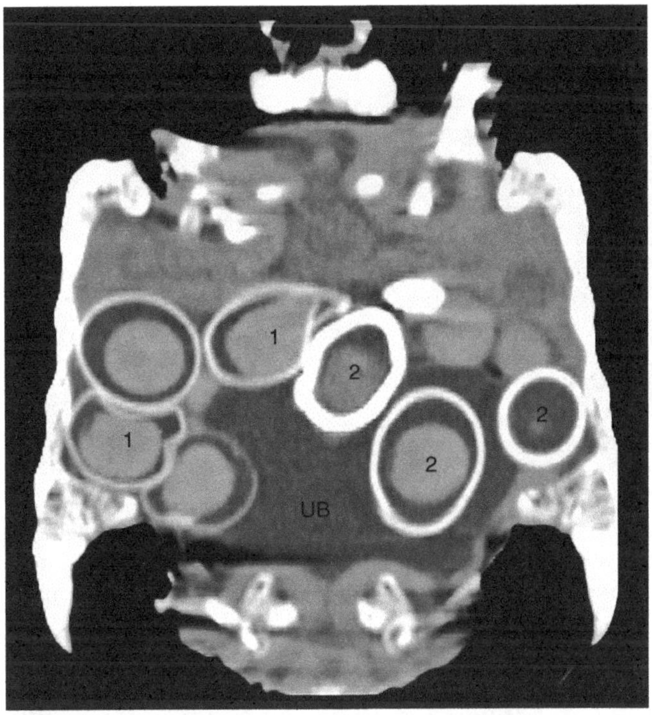

Figure 50.23 Herman's tortoise with chronic dystocia. Dorsally reconstructed CT image of the ventral half of the body (level shoulder and hip joints) shows some broken shells (1) within the oviduct and three thickened shells (2) within the urinary bladder (UB). Displacement of eggs into the urinary bladder may be caused by improper treatment or obstruction of the cloaca during deposition of a clutch.

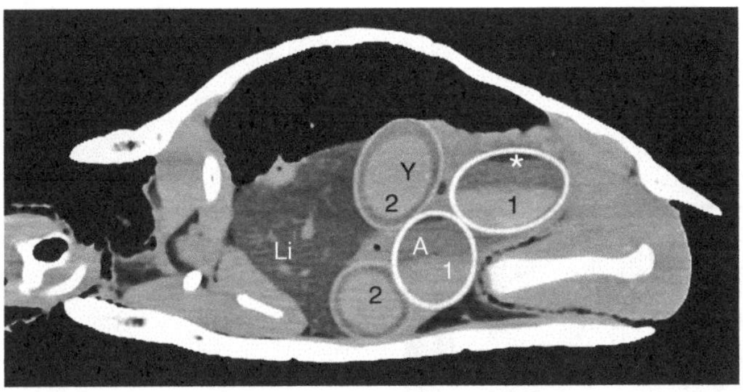

Figure 50.22 Red-eared slider turtle with dystocia. Right sagittal CT image shows two calcified egg shells (1) that contain an abnormal horizontally levelled yolk (Y) and albumen (A) in addition to a small gas bubble (asterisk). Two other poorly mineralized ova (2) have a normal centered oval-shaped yolk with a peripheral ring of albumen. The hepatic tissue (Li) is hypodense (lipidosis).

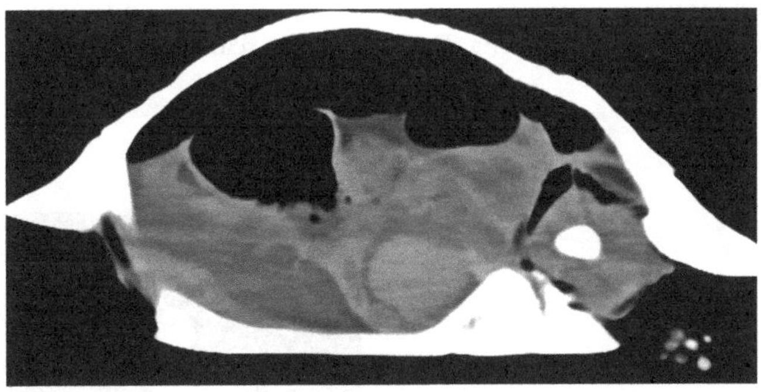

Figure 50.24 Herman's tortoise with peritonitis caused by yolk. Sagittal CT image shows very poor detail in the caudal half of the coelomic cavity. Some rounded structures seem to be visible.

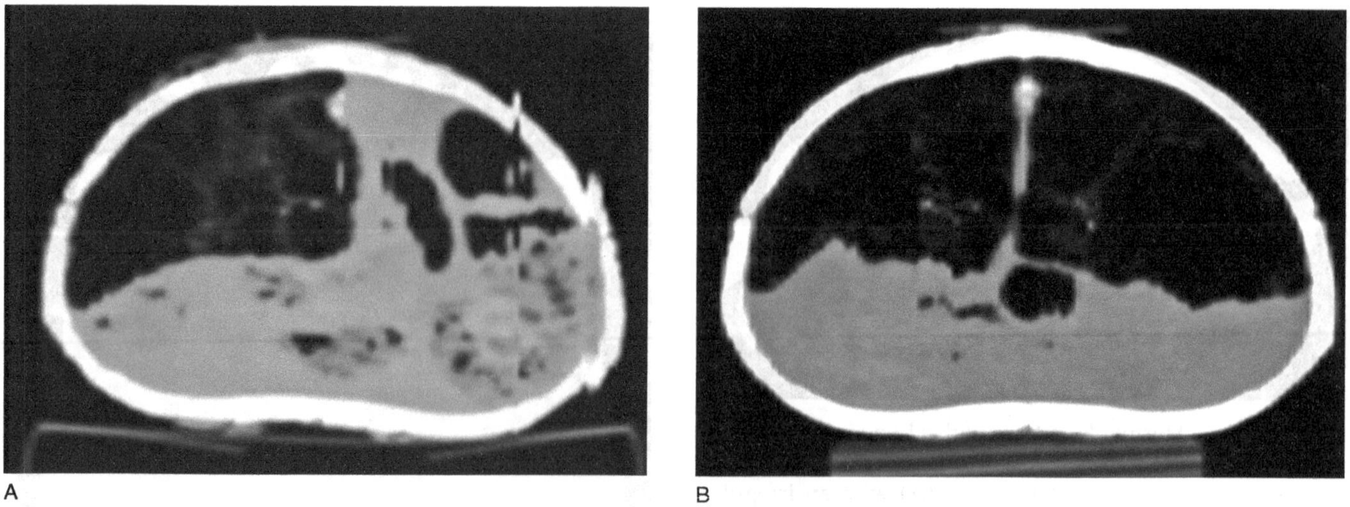

Figure 50.25 Spur-thighed tortoise with severe unilateral pneumonia. (A) Transverse CT image shows mild thickening of the reticular patterns in the right lung. The left lung is not differentiable and is fluid-filled. (B) Transverse CT image of the same animal after 20 days' therapy. Both lungs are normal.

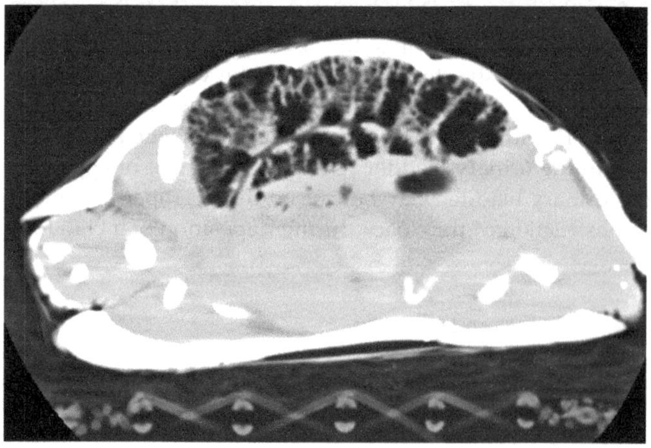

Figure 50.26 Spur-thighed tortoise with severe 'interstitial' pneumonia. Sagittal CT image shows thickened and hyperdense reticular patterns. The animal was scanned in a wicker basket.

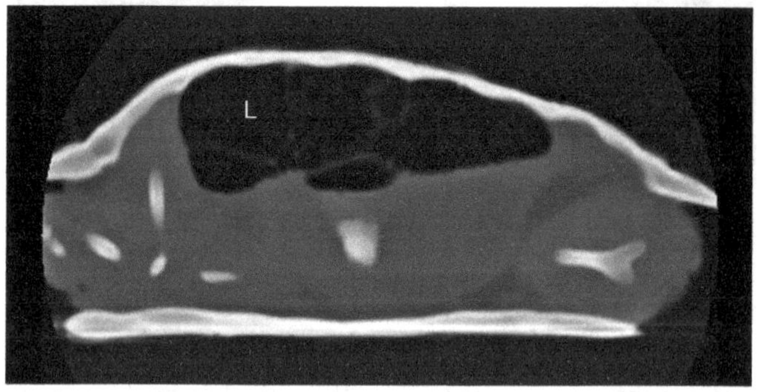

Figure 50.28 Red-eared slider turtle with severe lung emphysema. Right sagittal CT image shows loss of normal reticular lung (L) pattern and merged air chambers. Severe emphysema of one lung usually takes place in pneumonia or obstruction of the contralateral lung.

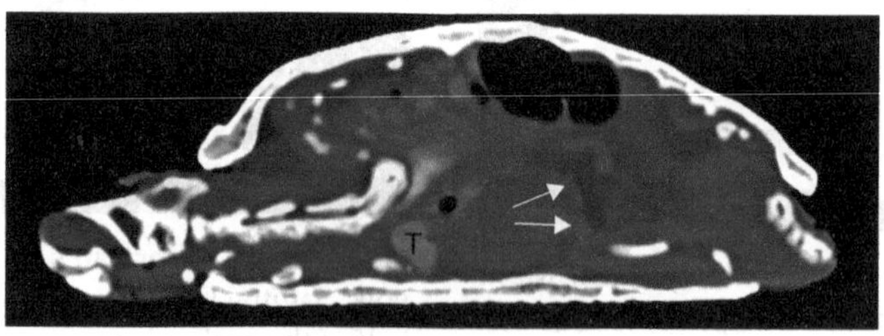

Figure 50.27 Red-eared slider turtle with lung abscessation. Median sagittal CT image shows that the cranial half of the lung contains multiple rounded abscesses. More abscesses (arrows) were found in the coelomic cavity. The thyroid gland (T) is enlarged. This animal was kept like a Herman's tortoise for several years.

INDEX

Page numbers in *italics* indicate figures; those in **bold** indicate tables.

Veterinary Computed Tomography, First Edition. Edited by Tobias Schwarz, Jimmy Saunders.

Printed in the USA/Agawam, MA
September 17, 2026

910661.046